THE NEW ANGIOTHERAPY

THE NEW ANGIOTHERAPY

Edited by

TAI-PING D. FAN, PhD

University of Cambridge, UK

and

ELISE C. KOHN, MD

National Institutes of Health, Bethesda, MD

Foreword by

JUDAH FOLKMAN, MD

Department of Surgery, Children's Hospital,
Harvard Medical School, Boston, MA

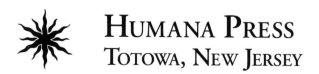

HUMANA PRESS
TOTOWA, NEW JERSEY

© 2002 Humana Press Inc.
999 Riverview Drive, Suite 208
Totowa, New Jersey 07512

humanapress.com

For additional copies, pricing for bulk purchases, and/or information about other Humana titles, contact Humana at the above address or at any of the following numbers: Tel: 973-256-1699; Fax: 973-256-8341; E-mail: humana@humanapr.com or visit our Website at http://humanapress.com

Due diligence has been taken by the publishers, editors, and authors of this book to assure the accuracy of the information published and to describe generally accepted practices. The contributors herein have carefully checked to ensure that the drug selections and dosages set forth in this text are accurate and in accord with the standards accepted at the time of publication. Notwithstanding, as new research, changes in government regulations, and knowledge from clinical experience relating to drug therapy and drug reactions constantly occurs, the reader is advised to check the product information provided by the manufacturer of each drug for any change in dosages or for additional warnings and contraindications. This is of utmost importance when the recommended drug herein is a new or infrequently used drug. It is the responsibility of the treating physician to determine dosages and treatment strategies for individual patients. Further it is the responsibility of the health care provider to ascertain the Food and Drug Administration status of each drug or device used in their clinical practice. The publisher, editors, and authors are not responsible for errors or omissions or for any consequences from the application of the information presented in this book and make no warranty, express or implied, with respect to the contents in this publication.

This publication is printed on acid-free paper. ∞

ANSI Z39.48-1984 (American National Standards Institute)
Permanence of Paper for Printed Library Materials.

Production Editor: Jason Runnion

Cover design by Patricia F. Cleary.

Cover illustration: Fig. 6 from Chapter 2, Angiogenesis - Regulating Cytokines, by M. S. Pepper, S. J. Mandriota, and R. Montesano.

Printed in the United States of America.   10 9 8 7 6 5 4 3 2 1

Library of Congress Cataloging-in-Publication Data

The new angiotherapy/edited by Tai-Ping Fan and Elise C. Kohn
    p.; cm.
  Includes bibliographical references and index.
  ISBN 0-89603-464-X (alk. paper)
  1. Neovascularization. 2. Neovascularization inhibitors. I. Fan, Tai-Ping D.   II. Kohn, Elise C.
  [DNLM: 1. Neovascularization, Pathologic.   2. Neovascularization, Physiologic.   WG 500 N5324 2001]
  QP106.6 .N49 2001
  612.1'3—dc21
                                                                        00-050029

DEDICATION

To Dorothy, our two children, Victoria and Patrick, as a token of my love and appreciation for their immense patience and many sacrifices in making my dreams come true. Also to my grandmother, parents, and brothers and sisters for their constant encouragement.-TPF

To my husband, Gary Claxton, for his loving support, to my mentor, Dr. Lance Liotta, for his valuable advice and encouragement, and to very dear friends without whom this book could not have been finished.-ECK

FOREWORD

In this very timely and informative book, Tai-Ping Fan and Elise Kohn have assembled, in *The New Angiotherapy*, chapters written by many of the leading scientists in the field of angiogenesis research. The molecular underpinnings of the angiogenic process in reproduction, development, repair, and disease are clearly developed. Broad coverage is given to preclinical and clinical applications of angiogenesis inhibitors, and the book is a valuable source of references to the many aspects of the angiogenic process. It is, however, far more than a reference book. It is organized so that the reader begins to recognize the emergence of unifying themes in the study of angiogenesis.

The growth of new microvessels from resting vessels is the outcome of a fine balance between molecules that are either positive or negative regulators of angiogenesis. Some of these regulators reside in the extracellular matrix, while others circulate. Several angiogenesis regulators are cleavage products of larger proteins that have different functions.

An analogy of the angiogenic process to the clotting process, in which approximately 40 proteins determine whether or not a clot will form, is not too farfetched. Negative regulators of angiogenesis—angiogenesis inhibitors—can be thought of as a new class of drugs. They are being tested in clinical trials for neoplastic and non-neoplastic diseases. Certain of these drugs are fairly specific angiogenesis inhibitors and block mainly the endothelial cells in the tumor bed. Other inhibitors block endothelial cell proliferation, but also have direct antitumor effects (2-methoxy-estradiol, for example). It is even possible to shift the effect of certain conventional cytotoxic agents toward an anti-angiogenic function by changes in dose and schedule. It may be prudent to distinguish between "indirect" angiogenesis inhibitors that block a tumor from producing an angiogenic factor (such as small molecules designed to target an oncogene product such as vascular endothelial growth factor) in contrast to "direct" inhibitors that block vascular endothelial cells from responding to a spectrum of angiogenic factors.

The need for surrogate markers that could measure efficacy of anti-angiogenic therapy or could indicate in some way the angiogenic activity of a tumor is thoroughly discussed in *The New Angiotherapy*. It is now recognized that angiogenesis inhibitors may be most effective if the dose is titrated against total angiogenic output of a patient's tumor, in much the same way that insulin is titrated against the pulse rate, and coumarin dose is adjusted according to prothombin level. In other words, as Sir James Black has emphasized for drugs like propranolol, clinical trials may be optimally designed with a goal of equal effect, rather than equal dose.

The importance of quantifying the effectiveness of anti-angiogenic therapy is just one of many new directions in angiogenesis research, both basic and clinical, that are highlighted by the authors. Future directions are also emphasized in the chapters on gene therapy, and therapeutic angiogenesis for ischemic disease of the heart and limbs, as well as in new thinking about preventive anti-angiogenesis therapy.

Judah Folkman, MD
Children's Hospital,
Harvard Medical School,
Boston, MA

PREFACE

Angiogenesis is the development of new blood vessels from an existing vascular bed. Normal vascular proliferation occurs only during embryonic development, the female reproductive cycle, and wound repair. Many pathological conditions are characterized by persistent, unregulated angiogenesis, such as cancer, atherosclerosis, rheumatoid arthritis, and diabetic neuropathy. Conversely, inadequate angiogenesis can often lead to chronic pressure ulcers, duodenal ulcers, and myocardial infarction. Control of vascular development will permit new therapeutic approaches to these disorders, whereas enhancement of angiogenesis by exogenous growth factors can prevent or limit the damage in chronic wounds and duodenal ulcers.

The New Angiotherapy covers the recent progress in basic and applied research in angiogenesis. Critical reviews contributed by an international team of experts discuss the fundamental concepts in the physiology and pathophysiology of angiogenesis and evaluate the potential of angiotherapy in the management of angiogenic disease, highlighting some of the angiogenics and antiangiogenics both in development and in clinical trials. The future prospects of receptor antagonists, enzyme inhibitors, and vascular targeted approaches, especially that of gene therapy in the development of angiotherapy, are also covered.

Over the past five years, angiogenesis research has been expanding rapidly. To keep abreast of the most recent developments in the principles and practice of angiotherapy, we recommend *Angiogenesis*—the only specialist journal in the field. Please visit the website at http://www.wkap.nl/journalhome.htm/0969-6970.

We would like to thank the following colleagues for their generous assistance in reviewing some of the manuscripts: Adriana Albini, Robert Auerbach, Lee Ellis, Arjan Griffieon, Pamela Jones, Pieter Koolwijk, Macro Presta, David Walsh, Johannes Waltenberger, and David West.

Tai-Ping D. Fan, PhD
Elise C. Kohn, MD

CONTENTS

VI Angiotherapy in the Clinic

CONTRIBUTORS

Takayuki Asahara • *Department of Cardiology and Biomedical Research, St. Elizabeth's Medical Center, Tufts University School of Medicine, Boston, MA*

Robert Auerbach • *Laboratory of Developmental Biology, University of Wisconsin, Madison, WI*

Wanda Auerbach • *Laboratory of Developmental Biology, University of Wisconsin, Madison, WI*

Jane E. Barker, *Bernard O'Brien Institute of Microsurgery, St. Vincent's Hospital, Fitzroy, Australia*

Roy Bicknell • *Molecular Angiogenesis Laboratory, Imperial Cancer Research Fund, Institute of Molecular Medicine, University of Oxford, John Radcliffe Hospital, Oxford, UK*

Amy D. Bradshaw, *Department of Biological Structure, University of Washington, Seattle, WA*

Peter C. Brooks • *Department of Biochemistry and Molecular Biology, Norris Cancer Center, USC School of Medicine, Los Angeles, CA*

Margaret D. Brown • *School of Sport and Exercise Sciences, University of Birmingham, Birmingham, UK*

Peter D. Brown • *Department of Clinical Research, British Biotech Pharmaceuticals, Oxford, UK*

Robert A. Brown • *University College London, Plastic and Reconstructive Surgery, Tissue Repair Unit, London, UK*

D. Stephen Charnock-Jones • *Reproductive Molecular Research Group, Department of Obstetrics and Gynaecology, University of Cambridge, The Rosie Hospital, Cambridge, UK*

Xiaoming Deng • *Departments of Pathology and Pharmacology, University of California, Irvine, CA; and Pathology and Laboratory Medicine Service, VA Medical Center, Long Beach, CA*

Tai-Ping D. Fan • *Angiogenesis Laboratory, Department of Pharmacology, University of Cambridge, Cambridge, UK*

M. Judah Folkman • *Department of Surgery, Children's Hospital, Harvard Medical School, Boston, MA*

T. Annie T. Fong • *Preclinical and Pharmaceutical Development, SUGEN, South San Francisco, CA*

Stephen B. Fox • *Department of Anatomical Pathology, Canterbury Health Laboratories, Christchurch School of Medicine, Christchurch Hospital, Christchurch, New Zealand*

Zoltan Gombos • *Departments of Pathology and Pharmacology, University of California, Irvine, CA; and Pathology and Laboratory Medicine Service, VA Medical Center, Long Beach, CA*

Derrick S. Grant • *Jefferson Medical College, Thomas Jefferson University, Philadelphia, PA*

Shawn J. Green • *EntreMed, Rockville, MD*

Adrian L. Harris • *Molecular Oncology Laboratory, Imperial Cancer Research Fund, University of Oxford Institute of Molecular Medicine, John Radcliffe Hospital, Oxford, UK*

Yulong He • Reproductive Molecular Research Group, Department of Obstetrics and Gynaecology, University of Cambridge, Cambridge, UK

Vinzenz Hombach • Department of Internal Medicine II, Ulm University Medical Center, Ulm, Germany

Olga Hudlická • Department of Physiology, University of Birmingham, Birmingham, UK

Jeffrey M. Isner • St. Elizabeth's Medical Center, Boston, MA

Pamela F. Jones • Molecular Medicine Unit, University of Leeds, Clinical Sciences Building, St. James's University Hospital, Leeds, UK

Tetayana Khomenko • Departments of Pathology and Pharmacology, University of California, Irvine, CA; and Pathology and Laboratory Medicine Service, VA Medical Center, Long Beach, CA

Hynda K. Kleinman • Cell Biology Section, National Institute of Dental Research, NIH, Bethesda, MD

Tamara Konopka • Department of Pharmacology, University of Melbourne, Parkville, Australia

Elise C. Kohn • Chief, Molecular Signaling Section, Laboratory of Pathology, National Cancer Institute, National Institutes of Health, Bethesda, MD

Shant Kumar • Department of Immunology, Roswell Park Cancer Institute, Buffalo, NY

Kelvin K. W. Lau • Molecular Angiogenesis Laboratory, Imperial Cancer Research Fund, Institute of Molecular Medicine, University of Oxford, Oxford, UK

Theresa M. LaVallee • EntreMed, Rockville, MD

William W. Li • The Angiogenesis Foundation, Cambridge, MA

Vincent W. Li • The Angiogenesis Foundation, Cambridge, MA

Kenneth E. Lipson • Preclinical and Pharmaceutical Development, SUGEN, South San Francisco, CA

Katherine M. Malinda • Cell Biology Section, National Institute of Dental Research, National Institutes of Health, Bethesda, MD

Stefano J. Mandriota • Department of Morphology, University of Geneva Medical Center, Geneva, Switzerland

Clive D. McFarland • CSIRO, Division of Biomolecular Engineering, Sydney Laboratory, North Ryde, New South Wales, Australia

Gerald McMahon • Preclinical and Pharmaceutical Development, SUGEN, South San Francisco, CA

Geraldine M. Mitchell, Bernard O'Brien Institute of Microsurgery, St. Vincent's Hospital, Fitzroy, Australia

Jadwiga M. Miotla, Kennedy Institute of Rheumatology, London, UK

Roberto Montesano, Department of Morphology, University of Geneva Medical Center, Geneva, Switzerland

Lucia Morbidelli • Institute of Pharmacological Sciences, University of Siena, Siena, Italy

Wayne A. Morrison • Bernard O'Brien Institute of Microsurgery, St. Vincent's Hospital, Fitzroy, Australia

Cliff Murray • University of Nottingham Lab of Molecular Oncology, CRC Department of Clinical Oncology, City Hospital, Nottingham, UK

Tsutomu Oikawa • Department of Cancer Therapeutics, The Tokyo Metropolitan Institute of Medical Science (Rinshoken), Tokyo, Japan

Ewa M. Paleolog • *Endothelial Cell Biology Group, Kennedy Institute of Rheumatology, London, UK*

Michael S. Pepper • *Department of Morphology, University of Geneva Medical Center, Geneva, Switzerland*

Marco Presta • *General Pathology and Immunology, University of Brescia School of Medicine, Brescia, Italy*

Victor S. Pribluda • *EntreMed, Rockville, MD*

Dorothy Rodriguez • *Department of Biochemistry and Molecular Biology, Norris Cancer Center, University of Southern California School of Medicine, Los Angeles, CA*

Marco Rusnati • *Unit of General Pathology and Immunology, Department of Biomedical Science and Biotechnology, University of Brescia School of Medicine, Brescia, Italy*

E. Helene Sage • *Department of Biological Structure, University of Washington, Seattle, WA*

Ben K. Seon • *Department of Immunology, Roswell Park Cancer Institute, Buffalo, NY*

Laura K. Shawver • *Preclinical and Pharmaceutical Development, SUGEN, South San Francisco, CA*

Yuen Shing • *Department of Surgery, Children's Hospital, Harvard Medical School, Boston, MA*

Stephen K. Smith • *Reproductive Molecular Research Group, Department of Obstetrics and Gynaecology, University of Cambridge, Cambridge, UK*

William G. Stetler-Stevenson • *The Extracellular Matrix Pathology Section, Laboratory of Pathology, National Cancer Institute, Bethesda, MD*

Alastair G. Stewart • *Department of Pharmacology, University of Melbourne, Parkville, Australia*

Laurie M. Strawn • *Preclinical and Pharmaceutical Development, SUGEN, South San Francisco, CA*

Sandor Szabo • *Pathology and Laboratory Medicine Service, VA Medical Center, Long Beach, CA; Departments of Pathology and Pharmacology, University of California, Irvine, CA*

Maarten Tas • *University of Nottingham Lab of Molecular Oncology, CRC Department of Clinical Oncology, City Hospital, Nottingham, UK*

Giorgio Terenghi • *Blond-McIndoe Research Center, Queen Victoria Hospital, East Grinstead, Sussex, UK*

Philip E. Thorpe • *Harold C. Simmons Comprehensive Cancer Center, Dallas, TX*

Dimitris Tsakayannis • *The Angiogenesis Foundation, Cambridge, MA*

Giovanni Tulipano • *Unit of General Pathology and Immunology, Department of Biomedical Science and Biotechnology, University of Brescia School of Medicine, Brescia, Italy*

Aron Vincze • *Departments of Pathology and Pharmacology, University of California, Irvine, CA; and Pathology and Laboratory Medicine Service, VA Medical Center, Long Beach, CA*

David Andrew Walsh • *Academic Rheumatology, University of Nottingham Clinical Sciences Building, City Hospital, Nottingham, UK*

Johannes Waltenberger • *Department of Internal Medicine II (Cardiology), Ulm University Medical Center, Ulm, Germany*

David C. West • Department of Immunology, Faculty of Medicine, The University of Liverpool, UK

J. Wilson • Department of Immunology, Faculty of Medicine, The University of Liverpool, Liverpool, UK

Masashi Yoshida • Departments of Pathology and Pharmacology, University of California, Irvine, CA; and Pathology and Laboratory Medicine Service, VA Medical Center, Long Beach, CA

Marina Ziche • Institute of Pharmacological Sciences, University of Siena, Siena, Italy

COLOR PLATES

Color plate for Chapter 15 appears as an insert following page 262. Color plates for Chapters 23 and 26 appear as an insert following page 490.

Plate 1 (Fig. 2. from Chapter 15, for full caption *see* page 255)
Plate 2 (Fig. 1. from Chapter 23, for full caption *see* page 457)
Plate 3 (Fig. 2. from Chapter 23, for full caption *see* page 461)
Plate 4 (Fig. 3. from Chapter 26, for full caption *see* page 506)
Plate 5 (Fig. 8. from Chapter 26, for full caption *see* page 512)

I CONCEPTS

1

Vasculogenesis and Angiogenesis

Robert Auerbach and Wanda Auerbach

INTRODUCTION

The principle that underlies the targeting of blood vessels, "Angiotherapy," is that the differentiation, maintenance, and homeostasis of blood vessels may be targets for intervention in a variety of normal and disease processes. Wound healing, placenta development, estrus-associated uterine changes, vascular events accompanying hair growth, and normal vessel maintenance are among the many normal processes that may benefit from angiotherapy. Tumor-associated angiogenesis, ocular neovascularization, inflammation-associated vascular manifestations, autoimmune disease-related neovascularization, vascular repair following myocardial damage, dermatological vascular pathologies associated with scleroderma and psoriasis — there is an almost unending list of "angiogenic diseases" where angiotherapy can be of critical importance.

In this context it is of paramount significance that the mechanisms underlying blood-vessel development are by no means fully understood. Where conflicting views have emerged from the many experimental studies of blood-vessel formation, they have led to efforts to define and compartmentalize these views, thereby generating a sense of confidence concerning our understanding of vascular development that tends to over-shadow our uncertainties.

The origin of blood vessels during embryogenesis has been a subject of debate at least since the middle of the 19th century when His proposed that all blood vessels originate from pre-existing blood vessels (1). This view was widely accepted until the 1920s when, in a series of experimental studies of avian and mammalian embryos, Sabin, Regan, Clarke, and others reported on *de novo in situ* development of blood vessels during the differentiation of various organ rudiments (2–4). For a detailed discussion of these historically important experiments, see reviews by Wagner (5) and Auerbach and Joseph (6).

From: *The New Angiotherapy*
Edited by: T.-P. D. Fan and E. C. Kohn © Humana Press Inc., Totowa, NJ

More recently, two types of experiments have been used to further our understanding of blood vessel development. In the first, organ rudiments from one type of embryo have been grafted into another embryo. For example, mouse metanephric rudiments were transplanted onto the chorio-allantoic membrane (CAM) of a chick embryo *(7)*. Simple histological preparations using staining of DNA as well as comparison of nuclear size could readily distinguish mouse from chick nuclei, because mouse nuclei were larger and contained about four times as much DNA as chicken nuclei. These experiments clearly showed that chicken blood vessels invaded the grafted mouse metanephric rudiment, thus supporting His's early concepts of vascular origins.

The second type of experiment was superficially similar, and involved the grafting of quail embryonic tissues into chicken embryos *(8)*. Again nuclear morphology and DNA staining (Feulgen) could be used to distinguish donor from host cells and tissues. However, by using more primitive sources of donor tissues, donor cells could be found in blood vessels throughout the embryo, even in regions distant from the original graft site. These results supported the view that blood vessel development occurred by differentiation of precursor cells found within a developing organ rudiment rather than by extension of existing blood vessels.

In an effort to resolve these differences, Poole and Coffin *(9)* and Werner Risau *(see* ref. *10*) proposed two definitions: "Vasculogenesis" was defined as the development of blood vessels from precursor cells (angioblasts). "Angiogenesis" was defined as the formation of new blood vessels by extension of existing blood vessels. Vasculogenesis was seen as a process restricted to early embryonic development, whereas angiogenesis was associated with new blood-vessel formation operative during subsequent organogenesis and continuing throughout the life span of the individual. These definitions have found general acceptance. By those definitions, angiotherapy may aim to induce angiogenesis, as, for example, in the eliciting of collateral blood vessels in the heart, or it may aim to inhibit angiogenesis, as in the control of tumor growth and metastasis. Vasculogenesis is seen to be of little or no significance in angiotherapy.

But we are in danger of oversimplifying in an effort to understand blood-vessel development and thereby missing important aspects of angiotherapy. Foremost is the idea that vasculogenesis and angiogenesis are mutually exclusive. This idea is simply wrong. As we have pointed out previously *(11)* blood-vessel development in the metanephros involves both angiogenesis and vasculogenesis.

Still, these are embryonic rudiments, and therefore do not answer the important question of whether vasculogenesis may still occur in adults. That this is in fact the case is argued best by combining two types of experimental results: tumor transplantation experiments, and recovery from vascular insult. In tumor transplantation experiments carried out with adult mice, Wang et al. *(12)* were able to show that individual primitive endothelial cells could participate in angiogenesis, i.e., embryonic endothelial cells or precursor cells, co-injected subcutaneously with tumor cells gave rise to new blood vessels associated with the growing tumor. Isner and his group *(13,14)* showed that there were circulating angioblasts in adults, and that these could assist in (or give rise to) endothelial cells during neovascularization or vascular repair. Moreover, it had long been reported and recently confirmed that there are angioblasts (endothelial-cell precursors) in the adult bone marrow, and that these can pass through the circulation to contribute cells to blood vessels arising during neovascularization.

ANGIOGENESIS AND VASCULOGENESIS COEXIST DURING EMBRYONIC DEVELOPMENT

Vascular development in the mouse metanephros serves well to illustrate the changing attitude that we must adopt in considering angiogenesis vs vasculogenesis, especially because of the early studies that so "clearly" demonstrated that blood vessels in the mouse metanephros are entirely of extrinsic origin. As mentioned earlier, the Ekblom et al. experiments involved grafting of the 12-d mouse kidney rudiment to the CAM of chick embryos, and this grafting resulted in all vessels originating from the chick embryo (7,15). When Robert et al. (16) cultured 12-d mouse rudiments in vitro, they were able to find only scattered flk-1+ cells, (flk-1 marking angioblasts) and no vessels developed in vitro, supporting the Ekblom findings. However, when they then grafted these rudiments into syngeneic adult hosts, numerous flk-1+ endothelial cells developed in the vessels and glomeruli of the graft, and all were of donor origin. Thus, it appears that the xenograft experiments may have led to misleading conclusions concerning the origin of at least some of the vasculature of the developing kidney.

The developing brain rudiment has always been considered the prime example for a vasculature that is exclusively derived by angiogenesis (10,17). In our own laboratory we have shown that yolk-sac endothelial cells co-cultured with brain rudiments develop brain-specific properties (18). However, although this in vitro model demonstrated that individual endothelial cells could acquire organ specificity when introduced into developing embryonic rudiments such as the brain, the model did not distinguish between the possibility that such organ-specific differentiation would occur if endothelial cells migrated as a sheet from pre-existing blood vessels and the alternative that they entered as individual cells through the circulation. Hatzopoulas et al. (19) recently injected cultured endothelial cells originating from isolates of early mouse embryonic mesoderm into the extra-embryonic chick-embryo circulation, and these cells were subsequently localized in several sites, including the brain vasculature. These studies suggest, although they do not give conclusive evidence, that vasculogenesis plays a role in brain blood-vessel development, and especially supports the idea that maintenance of a healthy vasculature may depend on a repopulating pool of endothelial cell precursors (see also the earlier studies of Stewart and Wiley, ref. 20).

The developing limb is yet another organ whose vascularization was always believed to be entirely through the process of angiogenesis, but has now also been shown to involve both angiogenesis and vasculogenesis (21). These investigators use the terms "angiotrophic" and "angioblastic" to describe blood-vessel formation, a terminology that, although not adopted generally, is clearer, because vessel formation (literally, vasculogenesis) involves both formation of blood vessels by extension of existing vessels and by de novo formation from angioblasts.

Even the early embryonic neural tube, long thought to be comprised entirely of neurogenic cells, has been shown to become vascularized both by sprouting of pre-existing endothelial cells and by angioblasts that have entered the neural tube prior to establishment of patent blood vessels (22).

ANGIOGENESIS AND VASCULOGENESIS IN THE ADULT

The fact that hematopoietic and endothelial stem cells can both develop from a single precursor cell, the hemangioblast, and that endothelial cells and hematopoietic cells originate in close apposition during development of the embryonic yolk sac and the fetal liver suggested that a similar close relationship between endothelial and hematopoietic precursor cells could exist in adult life as well (23). That this was so was clearly reported by Shi et al. (13). In vitro experiments demonstrated that human CD34+ hematopoietic precursor cells generated adherent endothelial cells with high proliferation potential when cultured in the presence of vascular endothelial growth factor (VEGF). Moreover, using molecular markers to distinguish host from donor cells in a canine model of bone marrow transplantation, these investigators demonstrated that 12 wk after placing a Dacron graft in dog recipients, bone marrow-derived donor cells were the only source of the CD34+ endothelial cells in the newly vascularized graft. The authors conclude that "vasculogenesis is not only restricted to early embryogenesis, but may play a physiological role as demonstrated in this study, or may contribute to the pathology of vascular diseases in adults" (13).

The results were not, in fact, unexpected. In the 1960s, Stump et al. (24) and Gonzales et al. (25) had shown that endothelial cells, apparently derived from the circulation, could seed Dacron grafts in vivo. There was, however, no direct evidence that these cells were originally of bone marrow origin. On the other hand, the in vitro and in vivo results of Shi et al. (13) extend the earlier finding that bone marrow CFU-A (in vitro) and CFU-F (in vivo) colonies obtained from adult bone marrow can exhibit endothelial-cell phenotypes (26).

The results of Asahara et al., demonstrating that circulating CD34+ cells contribute to new blood vessel formation in adults are most readily interpreted as the result of release of bone marrow-derived progenitor cells. In this connection it is interesting that these investigators have also reported unpublished observations that indicate angioblast contributions to VEGF-induced corneal neovascularization (27). This finding is particularly important, because the corneal model has universally been accepted as a model for angiogenesis and not for vasculogenesis. It is particularly intriguing that endothelial-cell progenitors may express tie-2, the receptor for angiopoietin 1 and 2 (28), growth factors whose action previously were considered only as affecting angiogenesis and not vasculogenesis.

If one accepts the concept that angioblasts in the circulation can give rise to new blood vessels, then vasculogenesis as well as angiogenesis should become a target for angiotherapy. Targetting vasculogenesis may require different strategies than those used when targetting angiogenesis: for example, angioblasts express many cell-surface receptors shared with hematopoietic stem cells, receptors that to a large extent are no longer expressed on mature endothelial cells. Critical among these are homing (adhesion) molecules, for in order to participate in local blood-vessel formation they must recognize a target-site receptor, attach, and extravasate from the circulation. Differentiated endothelial cells resident within blood vessels need no such homing devices, but, on the other hand, must be able to traverse the basement membranes/extracellular matrix that stabilize mature blood vessels.

Targeting only angiogenesis or only vasculogenesis, moreover, may not be sufficient to prevent neovascularization. One may draw an analogy from hematopoietic repair following irradiation. There are short-term and long-term aspects to hematopoiesis, and distinctions are best seen when comparing low-dose and high-dose irradiation. Short-term restitution may be achieved by transplanting bone marrow cells, most of which disappear within a few weeks after transplantation. Long-term restitution is also achieved with bone marrow transplantation, but here the source of cells is a minority CD34+ stem-cell population whose differentiation, with time, leads to complete restitution.

CONCLUDING COMMENTS

This review has focused on the potential cooperation between two processes, angiogenesis and vasculogenesis. This does not mean that each of these cannot occur independently of the other. There is, for example, no compelling evidence that vasculogenesis, i.e., the differentiation of angioblasts during blood-vessel formation, is an obligatory component of tumor-induced angiogenesis. However, because circulating precursor cells can enter new blood vessels, and because these cells have been clearly demonstrated to exist, it would seem reasonable to assume that they do, in fact, participate in neovascularization. Similarly, although there is no doubt that vasculogenesis is the mode of origin of the initial vascular plexus of the yolk sac, three-dimensional structures that form even before the circulation is established may well provide a platform from which sprouting, i.e., angiogenesis, can become a major element during even the primitive blood-vessel development of the early embryo.

At present, most, if not all, angiotherapeutic protocols target blood vessels forming during the process of angiogenesis. As we learn more about the intricate interplay between angioblasts and the expanding sprouting vasculature, we may be able to improve long-term efficacy of treatment by including the angioblast and the process of vasculogenesis in angiotherapeutic protocols.

REFERENCES

1. His, W. (1868) Untersuchungen über die erste Anlage des Wirbelthierleibes. Leipzig, F. C. W. Vogel, Germany.
2. Sabin, F. R. (1917) Origin and development of the primitive vessels of the chick and of the pig. *Contrib. Embryo. Carnegie Inst. Publ. (Washington)* **6,** 61–124.
3. Reagan, P. R. (1917) Experimental studies on the origin of vascular endothelium and of erythrocytes. *Amer. J. Anat.* **21,** 39–176.
4. Clark, E. R. and Clark, E. L. (1935) Observations on changes in blood vascular endothelium in the living animal. *Am. J. Anat.* **57,** 385–438.
5. Wagner, R. C. (1980) Endothelial cell embryology and growth. *Adv. Microcirc.* 9, 45–75.
6. Auerbach, R. and Joseph, J. (1984) Cell surface markers on endothelial cells: a developmental perspective, in *Biology of Endothelial Cells* (Jaffe, E. A., ed.), Martinus Nijhoff, Boston, pp. 393–400.
7. Ekblom, P., Sariola, H., Karkinen, M., and Saxen L. The origin of the glomerular endothelium. *Cell Diff.* **11,** 35–39.
8. Noden, D. M. (1991) Development of craniofacial blood vessels, in *The Development of the Vascular System [Issues in Biomedicine 14]* (Feinberg, R., Shearer, G., and Auerbach, R., eds.), Karger, pp. 1–24.
9. Poole, T. J. and Coffin, J. D. (1989) Vasculogenesis and angiogenesis: Two distinct morphogenetic mechanisms establish embryonic vascular pattern. *J. Exp. Zool.* **251,** 224–231.
10. Risau, W. (1997) Mechanisms of angiogenesis. *Nature* **386,** 671–674.
11. Auerbach, R. and Auerbach, W. (1997) Profound effects on vascular development caused by perturbations during organogenesis. *Am. J. Pathol.* **151,** 1183–1186.
12. Wang, S. J., Greer, P., and Auerbach, R. (1996) Isolation and propagation of yolk sac-derived endothelial cells from a hypervascular transgenic mouse expressing a gain-of-function *fps/fes* proto-oncogene. *In Vitro Cell. Dev. Biol.* **32,** 292–299.
13. Shi, Q., Raffi, S., Wu, M. H-D., Wijelath, E. S., Yu, C., Ishida, A., et al. (1998) Evidence for circulating bone marrow-derived endothelial cells. *Blood* **92,** 362–367.
14. Van Belle, E., Bauter, C., Asahara, T., and Isner, J. M. (1998) Endothelial regrowth after arterial injury: from vascular repair to therapeutics. *Cardiovasc. Res.* **38,** 54–68.
15. Sariola, H., Ekblom, P., Lehtonen, E., and Saxen, L. (1983) *Dev. Biol.* **96,** 427–435.
16. Robert, R., St. John, P. L., Hyink, D. P., and Abrahamson, D. R. (1996) Evidence that embryonic kidney cells expressing flk-1 are intrinsic, vasculogenic angioblasts. *Am. J. Physiol.* **271,** F744–F753.
17. Risau, W. and Flamme, I. (1995) Vasculogenesis. *Annu. Rev. Cell Dev. Biol.* **11,** 73–91.

18. Yu, D. and Auerbach, R. (1999) Brain-specific differentiation of mouse yolk sac endothelial cells. *Brain Res. Dev. Brain Res.* **117(2),** 159–169. [cf. Yu, D. (1999) Mouse yolk sac endothelial cells and their organ specific differentiation. PhD dissertation, University of Wisconsin.]

19. Hatzopoulos A. K., Folkman, J., Evasile, E., Eiselen, G. K., and Rosenberg, R. D. (1998) Isolation and characterization of endothelial progenitor cells from mouse embryos. *Development* **125,** 1457–1468.

20. Stewart, P. A. and Wiley M. J. (1981) Developing nervous tissue induces formation of blood-brain characteristics in invading endothelial cells: a study using quail-chick transplantation chimaeras. *Dev. Biol.* **84,** 183–192.

21. Brand-Saberi, B., Seifert, R., Grim, M., Wilting, J., Kuehlewein, M., and Christ, B. (1994) Blood vessel formation in the avian limb bud involves angioblastic and angiotrophic growth. *Dev. Dynam.* **202,** 181–194.

22. Kurz. H., Gartner, T., Eggli, P. S., and Christ, B. (1996) First blood vessels in the avian neural tube are formed by a combination of dorsal angioblast immigration and ventral sprouting of endothelial cells. *Dev. Biol.* **173,** 133–147.

23. Choi, K., Kennedy, M., Kazarovc, A., Papadimitriou, J. C., and Keller, G. (1998) A common precursor for hematopoietic and endothelial cells. *Development* **125,** 725–732.

24. Stump, M. M., Jordan, G. L., Jr., DeBakey, M. E., and Halpert, E. (1963) Endothelium grown from circulating blood on isolated intravascular Dacron hub. *Am. J. Pathol.* **43,** 361–367.

25. Gonzalez, I. E., Ehrenfeld, W. K., and Vermuelen, F. (1969) Relationship between circulating blood and pathogenesis of atherosclerosis. *Israeli J. Med. Sci.* **5,** 648–651.

26. Eckmann, L., Freshney, M., Wright, E. G., Sprout, A., Wilkie, N., and Pragnell, I. B. (1988) A novel in vitro assay for murine haematopoietic stem cells. *Br. J. Cancer Suppl.* **9,** 36–40.

27. Asahara, T., Chen, D., Takahashi, T., Fujikawa, K., Kearney, M., Magner, M., et al. (1998) Tie2 receptor ligands, angiopoietin-1 and angiopoietin-2, modulate VEGF-induced postnatal neovascularization. *Circ. Res.* **83,** 233–240.

28. Asahara T., Murohara T., Sullivan A., Silver, M., van der Zee, R., Li, T., et al. (1997) Isolation of putative progenitor endothelial cells for angiogenesis. *Science* **275,** 965–967.

2
Angiogenesis-Regulating Cytokines

Michael S. Pepper, Stefano J. Mandriota, and Roberto Montesano

CONTENTS

INTRODUCTION

The establishment and maintenance of a vascular supply is an absolute requirement for the growth of normal and neoplastic tissues, and as might be predicted, the cardiovascular system is the first organ system to develop and to become functional during embryogenesis. Both during development and in postnatal life, all new blood vessels begin as simple endothelial-lined tubes. Some become capillaries after developing an intimate association with pericytes, whereas others develop into vessels of larger diameter (arteries and veins) and acquire a variable number of concentrically disposed smooth-muscle cell layers. Traditionally, the formation of new blood vessels has been ascribed to two interrelated but separable processes, vasculogenesis, and angiogenesis (Fig. 1).

Definitions

Vasculogenesis is a series of differentiation and morphogenetic events which result in the formation of a primary capillary plexus, and is comprised of at least three stages: 1) the *in situ* differentiation of mesodermal cells into angioblasts or hemangioblasts; 2) the differentiation of angioblasts and hemangioblasts into endothelial cells (and hematopoietic cells in the case of the hemangioblast); and 3) the organization of newly formed endothelial cells into a primary capillary plexus. The existence of the angioblast, which differentiates exclusively into endothelial cells, has been well-established. However, definitive proof for the existence of the hemangioblast, which is purported to have the dual capacity to differentiate into either endothelial or hematopoietic cells, is still lacking (reviewed in refs. *1–4*).

From: *The New Angiotherapy*
Edited by: T.-P. D. Fan and E. C. Kohn © Humana Press Inc., Totowa, NJ

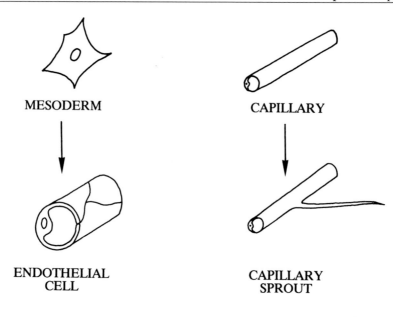

MESODERM   CAPILLARY

ENDOTHELIAL   CAPILLARY
CELL   SPROUT

VASCULOGENESIS   **ANGIOGENESIS**

Fig. 1. Vasculogenesis and angiogenesis. Blood vessels are formed by two processes: vasculogenesis, the *in situ* differentiation of mesodermal precursors into endothelial cells, which subsequently organize into tube-like capillaries to form a primary capillary plexus, and angiogenesis, in which new capillaries are formed by a process of sprouting from pre-existing capillaries or post capillary venules. Adapted from ref. *21*, with copyright permission from Springer-Verlag GmbH & Co. KG.

The term angiogenesis, derived from the Greek words "angeion" and "genesis," meaning vessel and production respectively, was coined by Hertig in 1935 *(5)* to describe the formation of new blood vessels in the placenta. As will become apparent however, angiogenesis is not limited to this setting, and a more contemporary definition would be "the formation of new capillary blood vessels by a process of sprouting from pre-existing vessels in a variety of developmental, physiological, and pathological settings." A similar although far less well-studied process also occurs in the lymphatic system, and is sometimes referred to as lymphangiogenesis.

Evidence has recently been provided for the existence, in the peripheral circulation, of an endothelial-cell precursor that contributes to the formation of new blood vessels in postnatal life *(6)*. These findings are likely to have a major impact on the current definition of angiogenesis. Recall that although the formation of capillary-like tubes is implicit in the definitions of both vasculogenesis and angiogenesis, primary differentiation of mesoderm into angioblasts is a process that is limited exclusively to vasculogenesis. Because mesoderm does not persist into postnatal life, the definition of vasculogenesis is unlikely to be affected by this new finding. However, the existence of a circulating endothelial precursor does mean that the source of new endothelium during angiogenesis can no longer be ascribed exclusively to sprouting from pre-existing vessels. Thus the definition of angiogenesis will have to be extended to include the incorporation of endothelial progenitors and/or their progeny into newly forming vessels. Important questions concerning the origin of circulating precursors (possibly from the bone marrow) as well as their precise relationship to angioblasts (and hemangioblasts) remain to be answered.

As indicated earlier, the immature endothelial-lined tubes that arise during vasculogenesis and angiogenesis subsequently differentiate into capillaries (after association with pericytes) or into larger vessels such as arteries and veins (after forming a media composed essentially of smooth-muscle cells). Furthermore, capillaries in many organs undergo further differentiation and develop organ-specific functions. Examples include formation of the blood-brain barrier (BBB) in the central nervous system (CNS), formation of fenestrated endothelium in endocrine and other organs, formation of sinusoids in the liver and spleen, and formation of high endothelial venules in lymph nodes. These processes, which occur in primitive vessels resulting either from vasculogenesis or angiogenesis, should be referred to as secondary differentiation, in order to distinguish them clearly from primary angioblast and endothelial cell differentiation.

The multiple cell functions that occur during angiogenesis belong either to a phase of activation or to a phase of resolution. The activation phase encompasses initiation and progression, and includes: 1) increased vascular permeability and extravascular fibrin deposition; 2) basement-membrane degradation; 3) cell migration and extracellular matrix invasion; 4) endothelial-cell proliferation; and 5) capillary lumen formation. The phase of resolution encompasses termination and vessel maturation, and includes: 1) inhibition of endothelial cell proliferation; 2) cessation of cell migration; 3) basement-membrane reconstitution; and 4) junctional complex maturation. As indicated earlier, the definition of vasculogenesis includes both primary endothelial-cell differentiation, as well as the organization of these endothelial cells into capillary-like tubes. With respect to the phases of activation and resolution, many components are equally as applicable to vasculogenesis as they are to angiogenesis. Although a great deal is known about those factors that induce the activation phase, very little is known about the factors involved in the phase of resolution, in which the dominant activity of negative regulators is called into play. Furthermore, it is at present unclear as to whether the resolution phase is an active phase, or whether it is the consequence of exhaustion of positive regulators that predominated during the phase of activation. If the latter hypothesis is correct, this assumes that endothelial cells have the inherent capacity to synthesize their own basement membrane and to organize into capillary-like tubes, and that this is mediated in part by the autocrine activity of endogenous regulators.

Angiogenesis in Pre- and Postnatal Life

Although, by definition, vasculogenesis must precede angiogenesis, the two processes continue in parallel during early development. However, unlike vasculogenesis, which appears to be restricted to early development, angiogenesis is also required for the maintenance of functional and structural integrity of the organism in postnatal life. Thus it occurs during wound healing, in inflammation, in situations of ischemia, and in female reproductive organs (in the ovary during ovulation and corpus luteum formation; in the placenta and mammary gland during pregnancy). Angiogenesis in these situations is tightly regulated, and is limited by the metabolic demands of the tissues concerned. Angiogenesis also occurs in pathological situations such as proliferative retinopathy, rheumatoid arthritis (RA) and juvenile hemangioma (reviewed in refs. 7–9).

Much of our interest in angiogenesis comes from the notion that for tumors to grow beyond a critical size, they must recruit endothelial cells from the surrounding stroma to form their own endogenous microcirculation (reviewed in ref. *10*). Thus during tumor progression, two phases can be recognized: a prevascular phase and a vascular phase. The transition from the prevascular to the vascular phase is referred to as the "angiogenic switch." The prevascular phase is characterized by an initial increase in tumor growth followed by a plateau in which the rate of tumor-cell proliferation is balanced by an equivalent rate of cell death (apoptosis). This phase may persist for many years, and can be recognized clinically as carcinoma *in situ*, which is characterized by few or no metastases. During the vascular phase, which is characterized by exponential growth, tissue invasion, and the hematogenous spread of tumor cells, the rapid increase in tumor growth is largely because of a decrease in the rate of tumor-cell apoptosis *(11,12)*. An inverse relationship thus exists between tumor dormancy/tumor-cell apoptosis and tumor angiogenesis. In a sense, tumor angiogenesis might almost be considered as "appropriate," in that newly formed vessels serve to meet the metabolic demands of the rapidly growing tumor. Although this may be beneficial to the tumor itself, it is clearly detrimental to the organism, because it is permissive for tumor growth, for the dissemination of tumor cells, and for the formation of metastasis.

Regulation of Angiogenesis: Balance and Context

It is usually stated that with the exception of angiogenesis that occurs in response to tissue injury or in female reproductive organs, endothelial-cell turnover in the healthy adult organism is very low. The maintenance of endothelial quiescence is thought to be caused by the presence of endogenous negative regulators, because positive regulators are frequently detected in adult tissues in which there is apparently no angiogenesis. The converse is also true, namely that positive and negative regulators often co-exist in tissues in which endothelial-cell turnover is increased. This has led to the notion of the "angiogenic switch," in which endothelial activation status is determined by a balance between positive and negative regulators: in activated (angiogenic) endothelium, positive regulators predominate, whereas endothelial quiescence is achieved and maintained by the dominance of negative regulators (Fig. 2) (reviewed in ref. *13*). Used initially in the context of tumor progression to describe the passage from the prevascular to the vascular phase, the notion of the "switch" can also be applied in the context of developmental, physiological, and pathological angiogenesis. Although it still remains to be definitively demonstrated in vivo, the current working hypothesis is that the "switch" involves either the induction of a positive regulator and/or the loss of a negative regulator. With respect to activated endothelium, an important distinction needs to be made between physiological and pathological settings: although many of the same positive and negative regulators are operative in both, endothelial-cell proliferation in the former is tightly controlled, whereas in the latter, uncontrolled angiogenesis implies the continuous dominance of positive regulators, which results in unchecked endothelial-cell growth.

Among the factors that affect endothelial-cell activation status, either positively or negatively, are cytokines and chemokines (chemotactic cytokines) produced by normal and tumor cells. Cytokines are polypeptide regulatory factors involved in the control of cellular proliferation and differentiation. Released by living cells or from extracellular matrix, cytokines act at picomolar to nanomolar concentrations to affect cellular function. Based on the observation that a given tissue can profoundly influence the way in which its cellular components respond to a given cytokine, it has been suggested that cytokines

POTENTIAL ENDOGENOUS REGULATORS OF ANGIOGENESIS

POSITIVE	NEGATIVE
Adipocyte lipids	Angiostatin
Angiogenin	C-X-C chemokines:
Angiopoietins	- Platelet factor 4
EGF/TGF-α	- IP-10, gro-β
FGFs	Endostatin
G-CSF	Hyaluronan
HGF	IL-12
Hyaluronan oligosaccharides	Interferons
Hypoxia	MMP & PA inhibitors
IL-8	16Kd prolactin fragment
PDGF-BB	Proliferin-related protein
PlGF	Retinoids
Proliferin	Ribonuclease inhibitor
Prostaglandins	Steroids/metabolites:
TGF-β	- glucocorticoids
Thymidine phosphorylase/PD-ECGF	- 2-methoxyestradiol
Tissue factor	TGF-β
TNF-α	Thrombospondin
VEGFs/VPF	TNF-α

Fig. 2. Potential endogenous positive and negative regulators of angiogenesis. A large number of factors, listed here alphabetically, have been shown to regulate angiogenesis in the experimental setting. For many of these factors, definitive studies are still required to demonstrate their role in the endogenous regulation of angiogenesis. It is nonetheless generally assumed that the switch to the angiogenic state may involve either the loss of a negative regulator or the induction of a positive regulator, or both, although definitive proof for this notion is also still awaited. Adapted from ref. 8, with copyright permission from Arnold Publishers.

should be seen as "specialized symbols in a language of intercellular communication, whose meaning is controlled by context" *(14)*. Context is determined by (at least) three parameters: first, by the presence and concentration of other cytokines in the pericellular environment of the responding cell; second, by interactions between cells, cytokines, and the extracellular matrix; and third, by the geometric configuration of the cells (and thus their cytoskeleton).

With respect to angiogenesis, the molecular mechanisms underlying the notions of both the "angiogenic switch" as well as "context," are likely to be central to the regulation of this process. With respect to vasculogenesis, although the notions of the "switch" and "context" are not at present widely used, both are also likely to be important.

IN VIVO AND IN VITRO MODELS FOR THE STUDY OF ANGIOGENESIS

The two most widely used in vivo angiogenesis assays are the chick-embryo chorioallantoic membrane (CAM) and the rabbit corneal micropocket. Direct subcutaneous injection or infusion of substances of interest has also been used to assess their pro- or anti-angiogenic effects. Quantitative in vivo assays involve subcutaneous implantation of various three-dimensional substrates to which putative angiogenesis-regulating factors can be added. These include polyester sponges, expanded polyfluorotetraethylene (ePTFE) tubes filled with collagen, polyvinyl-alcohol foam discs covered on both sides by millipore filters (the disc angiogenesis system), and Matrigel, a basement membrane-rich extracellular matrix. These assays are essential to establish whether a given molecule stimulates blood-vessel formation in the intact organism; however, their interpretation is frequently complicated by the fact that the experimental conditions may inadvertently favor inflammation, and that under these conditions the angiogenic response is elicited indirectly, at least in part, through the activation of inflammatory or other nonendothelial cells. Although this may be relevant to some settings in which angiogenesis occurs in vivo, it does not allow one to study the consequences of the direct interaction of angiogenesis regulators with endothelial cells. To circumvent this drawback, in vitro assays using populations of cultured endothelial cells have been developed for several of the cellular components of the angiogenic process, and based on the geometry of the assay, these can be classified as either two-dimensional or three-dimensional. Conventional two-dimensional assays include measurement of endothelial cell proliferation, migration, and production of proteolytic enzymes such as matrix metalloproteinases (MMPs) and plasminogen activators (PAs). Three-dimensional assays have as their end-point the formation of capillary-like cords or tubes by endothelial-cells cultured either on the surface of (planar models) or within simplified extracellular matrices. These assays include: 1) long-term culture of endothelial cells in dishes coated with a thin layer of matrix proteins; 2) short-term culture of endothelial cells on a thick gel of basement membrane-like matrix; 3) suspension of endothelial cells within three-dimensional gels composed of collagen or fibrin; 4) radial growth of branching tubules from rings of rat aorta or from fragments of either rat adipose-tissue microvessels or human placental blood vessels embedded in collagen or fibrin gels; 5) radial growth of tubular sprouts from endothelial cells grown on microcarrier beads embedded in a fibrin gel (reviewed in ref. *15*).

In our own studies, we have employed an in vitro model of angiogenesis that assays both for the invasive capacity of stimulated endothelial cells as well as their capacity for histotypic morphogenesis, i.e., the formation of capillary-like tubes. The model consists of cultivating endothelial cells on the surface of three-dimensional collagen *(16)* or fibrin *(17)* gels; under these conditions, the cells form a monolayer on the surface of the gel and do not invade the underlying matrix (Fig. 3A). When the monolayer is treated with an angiogenic factor such as basic fibroblast growth factor (bFGF) *(18)* or vascular endothelial growth factor (VEGF) *(19)*, the cells are induced to invade the underlying gel, and by adjusting the plane of focus beneath the surface monolayer, branching and anastomosing cell cords can be seen within the gel (Fig. 3B). In cross-section, the presence of tube-like structures resembling capillaries can be observed beneath the surface monolayer (Fig. 3C). Invasion can be quantitated by measuring the total additive length of all cells that have penetrated into the underlying gel to form cell cords *(19)*. Unlike planar models of in vitro angiogenesis, the model we have developed has the advantage of accurately recapitulating the invasive nature of the angiogenic process, and by virtue of its three-dimensional nature, is also permissive for histotypic morphogenesis, i.e., for the formation of patent capillary-like tubes whose abluminal surfaces are in direct contact with the extracellular matrix.

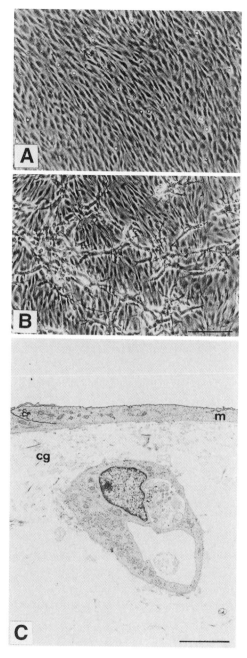

Fig. 3. Collagen gel invasion model for the study of angiogenesis in vitro. **(A)** When viewed from above by phase-contrast microscopy, endothelial cells grown on the surface of a three-dimensional collagen gel form a confluent monolayer without invading the underlying matrix. **(B)** Addition of angiogenic cytokines such as bFGF or VEGF induces the cells to invade the underlying gel and to form a network of branching cords, which can be viewed by focussing beneath the surface monolayer. **(C)** When the invading cell cords are viewed in cross-section by electron microscopy, their tubular nature, morphologically similar to capillaries seen in vivo, can be appreciated ("cg" = collagen gel, and "m" = surface monolayer.) Bar in **(A,B)** = 150 μm and in **(C)** = 10 μm. **(A,B)** adapted from ref. *18*; **(C)** adapted from ref. *21*, with copyright permission from Springer-Verlag GmbH & Co. KG.

ANGIOGENESIS-REGULATING CYTOKINES

The ultimate target for both positive and negative regulators of angiogenesis is the endothelial cell. This has led to the notion that angiogenesis regulators may either act directly on endothelial cells, or indirectly by inducing the production of direct-acting regulators by inflammatory and other nonendothelial cells. The most extensively studied cytokines involved in the positive regulation of angiogenesis are VEGF and acidic and basic FGFs (aFGF, bFGF). However, although a regulatory role for VEGF in developmental, physiological, and pathological angiogenesis has been well defined, much controversy still exists as to whether the FGFs are relevant to the endogenous control of angiogenesis in vivo. The finding that in vitro, VEGF and FGF positively regulate many endothelial-cell functions including proliferation, migration, and extracellular proteolytic activity, has led to the notion that these factors are direct-acting positive regulators. In contrast, transforming growth factor-β1 (TGF-β1) and tumor necrosis factor-α (TNF-α1) inhibit endothelial-cell growth in vitro, and have therefore been considered as direct-acting negative regulators. However, both TGF-β1 and TNF-α are angiogenic in vivo, and it has been demonstrated that these cytokines induce angiogenesis indirectly by stimulating the production of direct-acting positive regulators from stromal and chemoattracted inflammatory cells. In this context then, TGF-β1 and TNF-α are considered to be indirect positive regulators. In view of TGF-β's capacity to directly inhibit endothelial-cell proliferation and migration, to reduce extracellular proteolysis, and to promote matrix deposition in vitro, as well as to promote the organization of single endothelial cells embedded in three-dimensional collagen gels into tube-like structures, TGF-β has also been proposed to be a potential mediator of the phase of resolution (reviewed in refs. 20–22).

Other cytokines which have been reported to regulate angiogenesis in vivo include hepatocyte growth factor (HGF), epidermal growth factor/transforming growth factor-α (EGF/TGF-α), platelet-derived growth factor-BB (PDGF-BB), interleukins (IL-1, IL-6, and IL-12), interferons, granulocyte colony stimulating factor (G-CSF), placental growth factor (PlGF), proliferin and proliferin-related protein. Chemokines that regulate angiogenesis in vivo have to date only been identified in the -C-X-C- family, and include IL-8, platelet factor 4, and gro-β. Angiogenesis can also be regulated by a variety of noncytokine factors including enzymes (angiogenin, platelet-derived endothelial-cell growth factor/thymidine phosphorylase [PD-ECGF/TP], inhibitors of matrix-degrading proteolytic enzymes (tissue inhibitors of metalloproteinases [TIMPs] and plasminogen-activator inhibitors [PAIs]), extracellular matrix components/coagulation factors or fragments thereof (thrombospondin, angiostatin, hyaluronan and its oligosaccharides, endostatin), soluble cytokine receptors, prostaglandins, adipocyte lipids, and copper ions (Fig. 2) (reviewed in refs. 7,20,21,23).

It is crucial to bear in mind that although a large number of factors have been shown to be active in the experimental setting, it does not necessarily follow that these factors are relevant to the endogenous regulation of new blood-vessel formation, i.e., that they are relevant to the control of vasculogenesis or angiogenesis in the intact organism. In the case of molecules that are active during the phase of activation, only one, namely VEGF, meets most of the criteria required for the definition of a vasculogenic or angiogenic factor (21,24).

Vascular Endothelial Growth Factor

Vascular endothelial growth factor (VEGF) is a highly conserved multifunctional glycoprotein that exerts several possibly independent functions on vascular endothelium.

VEGF was initially described as a tumor-secreted protein that increases the permeability of microvessels, hence its alternate (and possibly more appropriate) name, vascular permeability factor. This extremely potent function of VPF/VEGF is 50,000 times greater than that of histamine. In vivo, VEGF is also a potent positive regulator of angiogenesis, and in vitro, VEGF induces endothelial-cell migration and proliferation and alters endothelial cell gene expression (including the production of matrix-degrading proteolytic enzymes). Although the mitogenic properties of VEGF appear to be endothelial cell-specific, in vitro this effect is relatively weak when compared to other positive regulating cytokines such as bFGF. VEGF contains a signal peptide and is therefore secreted from producer cells. At least three VEGF isoforms, which vary in their relative proportions in different tissues, are generated through alternative splicing of a single mRNA that arises from a gene containing 8 coding exons. The most abundant and most extensively studied 165 amino acid isoform (VEGF$_{165}$; 164 amino acids in rodents), arising from exons 1–5, 7, and 8, has been detected in both soluble and cell/matrix-bound forms. (This isoform will be referred to simply as VEGF throughout this chapter.) A 121 amino acid form (VEGF$_{121}$; 120 amino acids in rodents), arising from exons 1-5 and 8, has been detected only in soluble form, whereas a 189 amino acid isoform (VEGF$_{189}$; 188 amino acids in rodents), arising from exons 1-8 appears to be localized exclusively to the cell surface and extracellular matrix. A polymerase chain reaction (PCR) product inferring the presence of a fourth isoform, VEGF$_{206}$, has also been described in humans, although its biological significance remains to be determined. Although VEGF was initially purified on the basis of its affinity for heparin, this is substantially lower than that of other heparin-binding growth factors such as bFGF. VEGF$_{121}$ does not bind to heparin. VEGF isoforms exist as disulfide-bonded homodimers, and have a significant degree of similarity to placenta growth factor (PlGF, approx 50% identity) and platelet-derived growth factor (PDGF, approx 20% identity). The PlGF gene contains 7 coding exons from which two alternatively spliced forms can be generated. PlGF can form biologically active heterodimers with VEGF. VEGF expression is regulated by hypoxia, glucose deprivation, prostaglandins and estrogens, as well as by a number of cytokines (reviewed in refs. *25–28*).

The importance of VEGF in experimental primary and metastatic tumor growth in vivo has been clearly demonstrated using a variety of approaches including anti-VEGF antibodies, soluble VEGF receptors (VEGFRs), antisense VEGF, a VEGF-toxin conjugate, as well as a dominant negative approach using a truncated form of VEGFR-2. The inhibitory effect of soluble VEGFR chimeric proteins and antisense VEGF oligonucleotides in a murine model of proliferative retinopathy has also been described (reviewed in ref. *9*). However, the most dramatic demonstration of the requirement for VEGF in the development of the vascular tree comes from genetic studies involving targeted gene disruption in mice. In a manner that is unprecedented for a gene that does not undergo imprinting, heterozygosity for VEGF inactivation was embryonic lethal *(29,30)*. The observation that the phenotype of VEGF –/– mice was more severe than that of VEGF+/– mice, demonstrates the existence of a dose-dependent requirement for VEGF during embryogenesis, and implies that minimal amounts of VEGF are required in a tightly regulated manner for normal vascular development. Essentially, although endothelial-cell development was delayed in VEGF-deficient mice, resulting in the formation of abnormal vascular structures and massive tissue necrosis, it was not entirely aborted. This is in contrast to VEGF receptor-2 (Flk-1)-deficient mice, in which endothelial-cell development was completely absent (*see* below). These findings point to the existence of VEGFR-2 ligands other than VEGF. Because of embryonic lethality, the homozygous phenotype was inaccessible by standard (germ-line) breeding; this required the use of embryonic stem (ES) cell aggregates combined with tetraploid mouse embryos. Under these conditions, the resulting fetuses contain a mutant ES-derived embryonic compartment (in which VEGF is inactivated) and wild-type, tetraploid-derived extraembryonic membranes. This approach allows for rapid examination of mutant phenotypes derived from genetically altered ES cells without the need for germ-line transmission *(31)*. With the exception of conditional VEGF knockouts, which are likely to add significantly to our understanding of the role of this cytokine, the ES-tetraploid system is currently the only method available to assess the effect of homozygous deficiency of a gene that is embryonic lethal in the heterozygous state. Finally, when a nude mouse model was used to determine the role of VEGF in ES-cell tumorigenesis (i.e., formation of teratomas), VEGF–/– ES cell-induced tumor and associated blood-vessel growth were strikingly reduced when compared to wild-type ES cells *(30)*.

Two proteins with structural homology to VEGF have recently been described. The first has been called VEGF-B *(32)* or, alternatively, VEGF-related factor (VRF) *(33,34)*. VEGF-B transcripts are alternatively spliced, and the overall genomic organization of VEGF-B is conserved between other members of the VEGF gene family (VEGF, PlGF, PDGF). VEGF-B is primarily cell-associated, and is capable of forming heterodimers with VEGF. VEGF-B increases [^{3}H]thymidine incorporation in human and bovine endothelial cells. Whether VEGF-B/VRF binds to the same receptors as other members of the VEGF family (*see* below) remains to be elucidated. VEGF-B is co-expressed with VEGF in some tissues, and is particularly abundant in embryonic and adult striated (cardiac and skeletal) muscle; however, unlike VEGF, elevated levels of VEGF-B mRNA were not found in glioblastomas, breast, or renal carcinomas *(32,33,35)*.

The second protein with structural homology to VEGF has been called VEGF-C *(36)*, or alternatively, VEGF-related protein (VRP) *(37)*. VEGF-C was isolated during a search for a ligand for VEGFR-3 (Flt-4). VEGF-C displays a high degree of similarity with VEGF, including conservation of the eight cysteine residues involved in intra- and intermolecular disulfide bonding. It appears that the VEGF-C mRNA is first translated into a precursor from which the mature ligand is derived by cell-associated proteolytic processing. The cysteine-rich C-terminal half, which increases the length of the VEGF-C polypeptide relative to other ligands of this family, shows a pattern of spacing of cysteine residues reminiscent of the Balbiani ring 3 protein repeat. Like VEGF and VEGF-B, VEGF-C/VRP transcripts are alternatively spliced to give a number of major isoforms. VEGF-C binds to the extracellular domain of VEGFR-3 and induces VEGFR-3 tyrosine phosphorylation. In addition to VEGFR-3, VEGF-C appears to bind to and induce phosphorylation of VEGFR-2 (Flk-1/KDR). VEGF-C/VRP transcripts are detectable in many adult and fetal human tissues and in a number of cell lines. Patterns of VEGF-C expression during development suggest that this cytokine plays an important role in lymphangiogenesis *(38)*.

Alterations in endothelial-cell function induced by members of the VEGF family are mediated via transmembrane tyrosine kinase receptors that at present include VEGFR-1 (Flt-1), VEGFR-2, and VEGFR-3. Ligands for VEGFR-1 include VEGF and PlGF; ligands for VEGFR-2 include VEGF and VEGF-C; whereas the only ligand reported so far for VEGFR-3 is VEGF-C *(27,39*; for references on VEGF-B/VRF and VEGF-C/VRP, *see* above). Whether VEGF-B binds to the same receptors as other members of the

VEGF family remains to be described. VEGFRs are expressed in many adult tissues, despite the apparent lack of constitutive angiogenesis. VEGFRs are however clearly upregulated in endothelial cells during development and in certain angiogenesis-associated/dependent pathological situations including tumor growth (reviewed in refs. 25,28). The phenotypes of both VEGFR-1- and VEGFR-2-deficient mice have been described. VEGFR-1-deficient mice die in utero at mid-somite stages, and although homozygous deficient mice are capable of forming endothelial cells in both intra- and extra-embryonic regions, assembly of these cells into vessels is perturbed, resulting in the formation of abnormal vascular channels. The authors conclude that VEGFR-1 signaling pathways may regulate normal endothelial cell-cell or cell-matrix interactions during vascular development (40). VEGFR-2-deficient mice also die in utero between 8.5 and 9.5 d postcoitum, although in contrast to VEGFR-1, this appears to be owing to abortive development of endothelial-cell precursors. Yolk-sac blood islands and organized embryonic blood vessels were not detectable at any stage of development. The development of hematopoietic precursors was also severely reduced (41). By using a dominant-negative approach, the requirement for VEGFR-2 has also been clearly demonstrated in tumor angiogenesis (42,43). Gene targeting and dominant negative approaches have therefore clearly defined an essential role for VEGFRs in developmental and tumor angiogenesis.

Because VEGFR-expressing endothelial cells are located adjacent to regions of tumor ischemia and necrosis, it is possible that the increase in VEGFR expression is mediated by hypoxia (44; reviewed in ref. 45). In this context, it has been demonstrated in some in vitro studies that hypoxia increases high-affinity VEGF binding to endothelial cells and induces an increase in VEGFR-2 number (without alterations in receptor affinity), and that this is associated with increased VEGF-induced mitogenicity and VEGFR-2 tyrosine phosphorylation in endothelial cells (46,47). It has also been reported that hypoxia increases expression of VEGFR -1 and -2 mRNA in endothelial cells both in vivo and ex vivo in rat lungs (48). Of particular interest is the observation that conditioned medium from hypoxic skeletal myoblasts or smooth muscle cells contains a factor that markedly increases VEGFR-2 number (without alterations in receptor affinity) in endothelial cells in vitro (49). On the basis of neutralizing antibody studies, it was concluded that this factor is neither VEGF, bFGF, TNF-α, or TGF-β1. Taken together, these findings suggest that hypoxia can increase the effect of VEGF via the paracrine induction of VEGFRs in metabolically deprived tissues. With the exception of hypoxia, other factors that increase VEGFR expression have not been published. However, we have observed that high and low glucose concentrations increase VEGFR-2 mRNA levels in bovine microvascular but not large vessel-derived endothelial cells in vitro (S.J. Mandriota and M.S. Pepper, unpublished observations). We have also studied the effect of bFGF on VEGFR-2 expression in bovine endothelial cells, and have found that although bFGF increases levels of VEGFR-2 mRNA and total protein, cell surface protein is diminished. This may be owing to the fact that bFGF concomitantly increases expression of VEGF and VEGF-C, which upon secretion may interact with and promote internalization of VEGFR-2 (S. J. Mandriota and M. S. Pepper, unpublished observations). Downregulation of VEGFR expression in endothelial cells *in* vitro has been seen with nitric oxide (NO) or an NO-related metabolite in rat lungs ex vivo (48), with TGF-β (50), and with TNF-α (51).

Basic Fibroblast Growth Factor

Basic fibroblast growth factor (bFGF), also known as FGF-2 (or heparin-binding growth factor-2), is a member of the FGF superfamily that comprises more than 14 distinct gene products. bFGF is a cationic polypeptide (pI 9.6) with potent angiogenesis-inducing properties in vivo (reviewed in refs. 52–56).

Application of neutralizing antibodies to bFGF to the chick embryo CAM has been reported to inhibit vascularization *(57)*. Although these findings suggest that endogenous bFGF is rate-limiting in CAM vascularization, they do not allow one to determine whether the target for bFGF in this process is the endothelium. In contrast to the clear inhibitory effect on tumor growth observed in studies with neutralizing antibodies to VEGF, use of neutralizing antibodies to bFGF has been reported to inhibit tumor growth in some studies *(58–60)* but not in others *(61,62)*. One study reported a significantly lower degree of neovascularization in animals that received anti-bFGF antibody *(60)*, suggesting that in this tumor model, angiogenesis is bFGF-dependent. It is difficult however to conclude whether the reduction in tumor growth in the other studies was mediated through inhibition of angiogenesis, because bFGF mitogenicity is not endothelial cell-specific. With respect to genetic studies in transgenic mice, unlike FGFs -3, -4, and -5 (reviewed in refs. *54,63*), the effects of a homozygous null mutation in bFGF have not been reported. The phenotype of transgenic mice in which full length human bFGF was overexpressed in all tissues and through all stages of development under the control of a phosphoglycerate kinase promoter has recently been described *(64)*. These mice develop severe abnormalities in the skeletal system with no obvious features related to aberrant vascular morphogenesis or growth. In particular, there were no signs of hemangioma or microangiopathy, and overexpression of bFGF did not increase the overall susceptibility to tumor formation.

Basic FGF-induced endothelial responses are mediated via transmembrane tyrosine kinase receptors (FGFRs). To date, high-affinity FGFRs 1–4 have been described, and the existence of a large number of FGFR variants (generated by alternative mRNA splicing and differential polyadenylation) further increases FGFR diversity. This diversity results in a complex pattern of overlapping binding specificities for the various FGFs. It has been demonstrated that bFGF binds with high affinity to all four FGF receptors (or alternatively spliced variants) (reviewed in refs. *56,65–67*). The importance of FGFR-1 has recently been demonstrated by targeted gene disruption in mice. Post-implantation growth and mesodermal patterning were affected, resulting in recessive embryonic lethality during gastrulation *(68,69)*. Although mesoderm was formed, specification of cell fate and regional patterning were severely disrupted. With respect to the cardiovascular system, in a few embryos that had progressed to the appropriate stage, the heart and blood islands were present, and VEGFR-2-positive cells (endothelial precursors) were found in appropriate locations in the lateral plate and yolk-sac mesoderm. This suggests that FGFR-1 is not required for differentiation of endothelial-cell precursors. In humans, genetic alterations in the FGFRs 1–3 have recently been linked to craniofacial and limb developmental defects and achondroplasia (reviewed in refs. *54,63*).

The controversy that has arisen over the role of bFGF as an endogenous regulator of angiogenesis stems from the following observations. First, as indicated earlier, there is a lack of consensus regarding inhibitory studies, and bFGF gain of function and FGFR gene-inactivation approaches have failed to clearly delineate a requirement for bFGF in endothelial function during development and in postnatal life. Second, the stimulatory effects of bFGF on proliferation and migration are not restricted to endothelial cells. Third, in contrast to VEGF, bFGF lacks a signal peptide and therefore fails to enter the classical secretory pathway. Its mode of cellular export is at present unknown. bFGF is synthesized as both an 18 kDa and higher molecular weight *(22–25 kDa)* isoforms, resulting from the use of alternate start codons, in which translation is initiated at CUG rather than AUG. The 18 kDa form is stored in the cytoplasm of its producer cells, whereas the higher molecular weight forms contain an amino-terminal nuclear localization/retention sequence that appears to mediate intranuclear accumulation. Although bFGF does not enter the classical secretory pathway, the 18 kDa form can be detected outside the cell. 18 kDa bFGF export may involve cell injury/death and possibly an active and regulatable nonclassical secretory mechanism. As a consequence of its extracellular localization, it appears that access to the transmembrane FGFRs is limited only to 18 kDa bFGF and not to its high molecular-weight isoforms (reviewed in refs. *52,70,71*).

Although endothelial cells express FGFRs 1, 2 and 4 in vitro, which may be a consequence of culture conditions and/or serial passaging, the fourth and perhaps most significant issue concerning the endogenous angiogenic activity of bFGF is whether or not endothelial cells of the microvasculature express FGFRs in vivo. This is important because new capillary blood vessels arise from pre-existing capillaries or postcapillary venules. A limited number of studies have reported the presence of immunoreactive FGFR-1 in endothelial cells of the microvasculature (predominantly postcapillary venules) of a wide range of normal and neoplastic adult tissues, as well as in newly formed vessels of atherosclerotic plaques and underlying adventitial vessels. However, FGFRs have been undetectable in microvascular endothelial cells in virtually all settings in which there is active angiogenesis, and in which expression of high-affinity VEGFRs has been clearly demonstrated (reviewed in refs. *21,44,56*).

bFGF immunoreactivity has been demonstrated in the vascular intima (endothelial cells and underlying basement membrane) in a wide variety of settings in vivo. These include embryonic and normal adult tissues, chronic inflammatory tissues, juvenile hemangiomas, the endothelium of newly formed vessels in atherosclerotic plaques in human vessels, angiogenesis associated with thyroid hyperplasia, and a variety of tumors including glioblastomas. However, the presence of bFGF immunoreactivity gives no information as to the origin of the molecule nor the molecular nature of the structures to which it is bound. Extracellular matrix-bound bFGF is extremely stable, and because bFGF immunoreactivity but not mRNA is detectable in quiescent endothelial cells in vivo, it is possible that endothelium-associated bFGF may have a nonendothelial origin (circulation or medial smooth muscle cells), or that it may have been deposited in the matrix during development and postnatal growth. In contrast, bFGF mRNA has been detected by *in situ* hybridization in endothelial cells of brain tumors including glioblastomas, and bFGF mRNA is induced during endothelial regeneration in the rat aorta, which demonstrates that activated endothelium has the capacity to synthesize bFGF. bFGF-like activity, protein, and mRNA are present in cultured endothelial cells, all of which can be increased by serial passaging, and bFGF expression by cultured endothelial cells is density-dependent: levels are greater in sparse (low-density) cultures, in which cells migrate and proliferate, than in confluent (high-density) cultures in which cell migration and proliferation are virtually absent. The aforementioned observations suggest that cultured endothelial cells are phenotypically closer to activated/angiogenic endothelium than to the resting endothelium from which they were derived (reviewed in ref. *21*).

If one accepts that the FGFs are indeed endogenous regulators of angiogenesis despite the fact that microvascular endothelial cells cannot be convincingly shown to express FGFRs in vivo, a number of alternative hypotheses can be envisaged. The first two follow on from the observation that bFGF immunoreactivity can be detected in endothelium in vivo. First, bFGF-dependent, FGFR-independent signaling may occur in endothelial cells through other cell surface molecules such as heparan sulfate proteoglycans (HSPGs)

(72). Second, the observation that bFGF lacks a signal peptide and that its high molecular-weight forms have nuclear localization/retention signals, raises the possibility of an autocrine/intracrine role for bFGF in vivo. A third scenario might be that bFGF is an indirect angiogenic factor that acts by stimulating the production of direct acting cytokines by adjacent nonendothelial cells. However, it is important to note that none of these alternate hypotheses that have been proposed to explain bFGF-dependent, FGFR-independent endothelial-cell activation have yet been clearly substantiated in vivo.

As a general observation, it appears that providing justification for the role of bFGF in the regulation of endogenous angiogenesis requires extensive and elaborate argument when compared to VEGF, although it is possible that the role of bFGF may be more subtle than that of VEGF.

Transforming Growth Factor-β

TGF-β is a member of a large superfamily of cytokines including activins, inhibins, bone morphogenetic proteins, and others. Three TGF-βs (1, 2, and 3) have been described in mammals. TGF-βs are secreted from cells or purified from platelets as a high molecular-weight latent complex in which the C-terminal mature homodimer is noncovalently associated with a dimer of its N-terminal pro-region (also known as latency-associated peptide or LAP). Cleavage of the dimerized TGF-β precursor to form the TGF-β/LAP complex occurs in the secretory pathway and is mediated by a furin peptidase. LAP in turn may be disulfide bonded to structurally and genetically unrelated TGF-β binding proteins. Following secretion, the latent TGF-β/LAP complex, which is unable to bind TGF-β receptors, is activated in the extracellular milieu. Although the latent complex can be activated in vitro by plasmin, cathepsin D, and low pH, the physiological mechanisms that activate TGF-β in vivo are unknown. LAP, when independently expressed, associates noncovalently with mature TGF-β, thereby inactivating its biological activity (reviewed in refs. *73–75*).

TGF-βs achieve their biological effects through binding to cell-surface receptors (TGF-βRs) designated types I, II, and III. TGF-β binds directly to TGF-βR II, which exists on the cell surface as a homo-oligomer. Binding is followed by recruitment of TGF-βR I and the formation of a stable ternary complex. The cytoplasmic domain of TGF-βR II is autophosphorylated and constitutively active. Following recruitment, TGF-βR I, which is not phosphorylated in the absence of TGF-β, is phosphorylated on serine/threonine by TGF-βR II. This is followed by TGF-βR I-mediated activation of intracellular signal transduction. Therefore, the kinase activities of TGF-βRs I and II are both required for transducing TGF-β's signals. Furthermore, the components of the heterotrimeric complex are interdependent, as TGF-βR I requires TGF-βR II to bind TGF-β, whereas TGF-βR II requires TGF-βR I to signal. TGF-βR III is betaglycan, a transmembrane proteoglycan with a short cytoplasmic domain, containing both heparan sulfate and chondroitin sulfate glycosaminoglycans. TGF-βR III does not appear to be required for signal transduction, but may serve to present or deliver TGF-β to the signaling receptors. Endothelial cells also express endoglin, a protein with structural homology to the TGF-βR III. TGF-β also binds to the decorin core protein, which neutralizes its activity, as well as to thrombospondin, a large multifunctional glycoprotein that mediates the adhesion of both endothelial and nonendothelial cells to the extracellular matrix (reviewed in refs. *76–79*).

TGF-β1 has featured prominently among cytokines studied for their capacity to regulate new blood vessel formation. However, it is still unclear as to precisely how TGF-β is involved in the endogenous regulation of this process. Thus, a number of in vivo studies have demonstrated that exogenous application of TGF-β1 induces angiogenesis in the experimental setting. However, the lack of extensive angiogenesis in the face of other major tissue alterations in transgenic mice that overexpress TGF-β1 in a tissue-specific manner, suggests that when angiogenesis does occur in vivo, this is dependent on local inflammation, which may either be initiated or exacerbated by TGF-β. If one accepts that TGF-β is important for angiogenesis outside of the experimental setting, then an indirect inflammatory cell-mediated mode of activity may be applicable to physiological or pathological angiogenesis associated with acute and chronic inflammation, wound healing, and tumor growth. With respect to in vitro studies, it is likely that different models recapitulate different phases of the angiogenic process, and therefore when interacting directly with endothelial cells, TGF-β has different functions on vessel formation at different stages of the process. Thus TGF-β regulates the phase of activation by potentiating or inhibiting the activity of positive regulators like bFGF and VEGF in a concentration-dependent manner (see below). On the other hand, once a new vessel has formed, TGF-β1 promotes the phase of resolution by maintaining endothelial cell quiescence and inducing vessel maturation. Thus, with respect to its direct effect on endothelial cells, in vitro studies suggest that the response depends on whether TGF-β1 is present during the activation or resolution phases of angiogenesis, as well as on the local concentration of active cytokine. However, very few of the effects of TGF-β1 on endothelial cells in vitro have been confirmed in vivo. These include inhibition of proliferation and migration, the maintenance of endothelial quiescence, alterations in gene expression affecting matrix synthesis and extracellular proteolysis, and the induction of apoptosis. With respect to TGF-βRs, in vitro findings point to the importance of TGF-βRs I, II and III in TGF-β-mediated signaling in endothelial cells. However, the consistent inability to detect TGF-βRs in endothelial cells in vivo and the observation that the type II and III receptors are downregulated in three-dimensional cultures in vitro, suggests that expression of TGF-β receptors in two-dimensional cultures in vitro is consequence of endothelial cell activation (reviewed in refs. *22,80–83*).

Although there has been much controversy concerning the interpretation of studies with TGF-β on experimental angiogenesis both in vivo and in vitro, genetic studies in humans and mouse have recently revealed a role for this cytokine in embryonic vascular assembly and in the maintenance of vessel wall integrity. TGF-β1 is expressed in many tissues during embryogenesis (including endothelial and hematopoietic precursors) *(84)*, and targeted disruption of the TGF-β1 gene results in mortality at three distinct times: prior to organogenesis, during midgestation, or at 3 wk postpartum *(85–88)*. With respect to the group that dies during mid-gestation, this is owing to defects in the extraembryonic tissues, namely the yolk-sac vasculature and the hematopoietic system. TGF-β1–/– embryos per se, unlike their yolk sacs, had no specific abnormalities, although generalized developmental retardation, ischemia, and necrosis did occur, which may have been secondary to the extraembryonic lesions. In particular, intraembryonic endothelial cells expressing high levels of VEGFR-2 appeared to have developed normally. With respect to the yolk sac, initial differentiation of mesodermal precursors into endothelial cells appeared to have occurred, although there was a reduction in the number of VEGFR-2-expressing cells. Differentiation into capillary-like tubes was also defective, resulting in vessels with increased wall fragility: contacts between endothelial cells had either not formed or had been disrupted, resulting in leakage of blood cells into the yolk-sac cavity.

As indicated earlier, the definition of vasculogenesis includes both the primary differentiation of mesodermal precursors into endothelial cells as well as the organization of these endothelial cells into capillary-like tubes. It is not possible at present to say whether the reduction in the number of VEGFR-2-expressing endothelial cells in the yolk sac was owing to reduced angioblast differentiation, or to inefficient network formation by newly differentiated endothelial cells. (With respect to the latter, TGF-β1 has been shown to potentiate VEGF and bFGF-dependent capillary sprout formation in vitro; *see* below.) However, what is clear is that TGF-β1 is an important positive regulator of extraembryonic endothelial-cell differentiation, the establishment of vessel-wall integrity, and yolk-sac hematopoiesis. The earlier findings also suggest that intraembryonic and extraembryoinc vasculogenesis and hematopoiesis are regulated differently.

Of great significance is a recent report that has revealed that the three categories of lethality that occur in the absence of TGF-β1, namely early pre-organogenesis loss, mid-gestation yolk-sac failure, and postnatal death, are determined by genetic background. A major co-dominant modifier gene, which is responsible in part for the distribution of the three lethal phenotypes, has been mapped to proximal mouse chromosome 5 *(88)*.

The phenotype of TGF-βR II deficient mice has also recently been reported *(89)*. These mice are highly reminiscent of TGF-β1 null mice described earlier. Thus, homozygous deficiency was lethal at about 10.5 d gestation, and this resulted from defects in yolk-sac hematopoiesis and vasculogenesis. As with TGF-β1-deficient mice, TGF-βR II null mice were capable of forming blood vessels, but these were dilated and incompletely attached to the adjacent mesothelial and endodermal cell layers. Generalized embryonic growth retardation also occurred, although this was thought to result from the extraembryonic defects. It is striking that the expression patterns of TGF-β1 and TGF-βR II are highly coincidental during embryogenesis *(90)*.

The phenotype of vessel-wall fragility in homozygous TGF-β1- and TGF-βR II-deficient embryos is strikingly reminiscent of the vascular lesions that occur in patients with hereditary hemorrhagic telangiectasia (HHT). HHT is an autosomal, dominant, single-gene disorder characterized by multisystemic vascular dysplasia and recurrent hemorrhage. The earliest detectable change in the telangiectatic lesions is dilatation of postcapillary venules in the upper dermis; the endothelial cells themselves, including intercellular junctions, appear to be normal (reviewed in ref. *91*). The genes for HHT have recently been identified, and their identification has led to the definition of two HHT subtypes. The gene for HHT type I is endoglin *(92)*, which displays regions of structural homology to betaglycan, the type III TGF-βR. The gene for HHT type 2 is ALK-1 *(93)*, a TGF-β-binding type I receptor that is expressed at high levels in endothelial cells in vitro *(94)*.

The pathogenesis of the vascular lesions seen in TGF-β1- and TGF-βR II-deficient mice as well as in individuals with HHT is not known. Nonetheless, because TGF-β induces the synthesis and assembly the endothelial-cell extracellular matrix (*see* above), one of the consequences of defective TGF-βR signaling may be the formation of structurally incompetent basement membranes. It is striking that with respect to the vasculature, the phenotype of mice lacking either fibronectin or the α_5 integrin subunit *(95,96)* closely mimicks the phenotype of TGF-β- and TGF-βR-deficient mice, particularly because TGF-β1 has been shown to increase expression of fibronectin and its specific integrin, $\alpha_5\beta_1$ (reviewed in ref. *22*). It is also noteworthy that vascular lesions in HHT are well-localized, and that vascular integrity is maintained outside of the lesions; this suggests that some local event, possibly trauma, initiates vascular repair, which in the case of HHT patients is defective. An additional and intriguing possibility comes from the observation that a similar phenotype of vessel dilatation and increased vessel-wall fragility occurs in mice deficient in PDGF-B *(97)*, in PDGF receptor-β (PDGFR-β) *(98)* as well as in mouse embryos exposed to anti-PDGF-A neutralizing antibodies *in utero (99)*. It has been demonstrated that TGF-β1 induces PDGF-A and -B chain synthesis in endothelial cells *(100–102)*. In addition, TGF-β1 increases PDGFR-β expression in fibroblasts and smooth-muscle cells *(103,104)*. Because it is possible that endothelial-cell derived PDGF may mediate the differentiation of vascular wall cells (pericytes and smooth-muscle cells) from the surrounding mesenchyme, and promote their recruitment to newly formed capillaries, the absence of TGF-β signaling in endothelial cells may result in defective assembly of other cellular components of the vessel wall, which under normal circumstances would be expected to contribute to vascular stability. It should also be recalled that TGF-βs themselves affect many smooth-muscle cell functions including migration and proliferation, and that some of these effects may in turn be mediated through the autocrine regulation of PDGFs and their receptors (reviewed in refs. *82,83,105,106*). Vessels that form in the absence of the ligand or its receptors are ectatic both in vivo and in vitro. This is likely to be owing to incomplete vessel-wall maturation, which following an increase in hemodynamic pressure during development results in vessel-wall rupture and hemorrhage. It is noteworthy that during development in the mouse this occurs in extraembryonic but not in intraembryonic tissues, and that in humans, the phenotype of vessel-wall fragility generally becomes apparent during the second or third decades, although lesions can appear at any time from infancy to old age. However, ectatic vessels which form in the absence of exogenous TGF-β in vitro (*see* below) do so in the absence of circulating blood; this suggests that although intravascular hemodynamic pressure is likely to be responsible for vessel rupture and hemorrhage, the formation of dilated vessels can occur in its absence.

In summary, the role of TGF-β and its receptors in the maintenance of vascular integrity has been clearly established from genetic studies in humans and mouse. They appear to be required for capillary sprout maturation, as well as for promoting interactions with other vascular-wall cells including recruitment and differentiation of smooth-muscle cells. The observation that the phenotype of TGF-β null mice depends on genetic background points to the importance of modifier proteins in determining the penetrance and severity of the phenotype. This in itself may turn out to be an excellent example of "context." With respect to angiogenesis, the notion of the "angiogenic switch" is at present not as clearly applicable to TGF-β as it is to other cytokines such as VEGF; correlative in vivo and in vitro data nonetheless suggest that in addition to its indirect angiogenic effect, TGF-β1 can either promote or inhibit angiogenesis when interacting directly with endothelial cells, depending on whether it is present during the activation or resolution phases of this process. In this respect, the response of endothelial cells to TGF-β1 during angiogenesis further highlights the notion of "context," a notion to which TGF-β appears to be particularly well-suited.

CONTEXTUAL ACTIVITY OF ANGIOGENESIS-REGULATING CYTOKINES

Despite the unambiguous demonstration of VEGF's relevance in the endogenous regulation of angiogenesis, a number of important questions remain. The first arises from the observation that both VEGF and its receptors are expressed at high levels in a variety of adult tissues in which there is apparently no angiogenesis. This might mean that VEGF has additional functions not directly related to angiogenesis: 1) VEGF is clearly involved in the regulation of vascular permeability *(25)*; 2) VEGF may be important for endothelial survival (trophic effect); 3) VEGF may be required for the maintenance of organ-specific endothelial characteristics such as fenestrae *(107,108)*. Despite the dogma that endothelial cell turnover in the adult organism is very low, the presence of VEGF may indicate the requirement for a constant low-grade angiogenesis that is necessary to regenerate capillaries in organs with high rates of blood flow (lung and kidney). The absence of extensive angiogenesis in the face of high levels of VEGF (and its receptors) might also indicate the dominance of negative regulators, which serve to prevent uncontrolled angiogenesis in these organs.

The second question arises from the observation that levels of VEGF and its receptors appear to be unchanged in certain organs and tumors in which there is extensive angiogenesis. These include, although are unlikely to be limited to, the mammary gland during pregnancy *(108a)* and some experimental tumors, in which the levels of VEGF are similar in the prevascular and vascular phases of tumor progression *(109)*. One explanation might be that in these tissues, angiogenesis is in fact VEGF-dependent, but that the angiogenic switch involves the loss of a negative regulator. Alternatively, it may imply that some other positive regulator might be acting in these settings. A third hypothesis, namely that of context, implies that VEGF-induced angiogenesis depends on interactions with other regulatory molecules. Based on results from our own laboratory, we will describe three examples of context.

Synergism Between VEGF and bFGF

Because it is likely that endothelial cells are rarely if ever exposed to a single cytokine, and based on the observation that VEGF and bFGF are often co-expressed in settings in which angiogenesis occurs in vivo, we assessed the effect of simultaneous addition of VEGF and bFGF on the in vitro angiogenic response. We found that when added separately at equimolar concentrations, bFGF was about twice as potent as VEGF. However, when added simultaneously, VEGF and bFGF induced a synergistic invasive response (Figs. 4 and 5A), which occurred with greater rapidity than the response to either cytokine alone *(19)*. The synergistic interaction between VEGF and bFGF was subsequently confirmed in an independent study using a related three-dimensional in vitro assay *(110)*, and synergism has been observed in vivo in a rabbit model of hind-limb ischemia *(111)* as well as in the rat sponge implant model *(112)*. These results demonstrate that, when acting in concert, VEGF and bFGF have a potent synergistic effect on the induction of angiogenesis both in vivo and in vitro.

What are the mechanisms responsible for this synergistic effect? Although co-addition of VEGF and bFGF in conventional two-dimensional in vitro assays of endothelial-cell proliferation, migration, and PA-mediated extracellular proteolysis has failed to reveal synergism *(113–115)*, synergism is detected at the level of endothelial proliferation when cells are grown in a three-dimensional collagen matrix *(110,110a)*. An additional approach has been to determine whether bFGF and VEGF modulate expression of FGFRs and VEGFRs in monolayer culture. None of the endothelial-cell lines we have used express VEGFR-1 *(50)*. However, although neither cytokine, either alone or in combination, is capable of significantly modulating expression of FGFR-1, bFGF increases expression of VEGFR-2 at the level of mRNA and total protein. bFGF also induces the

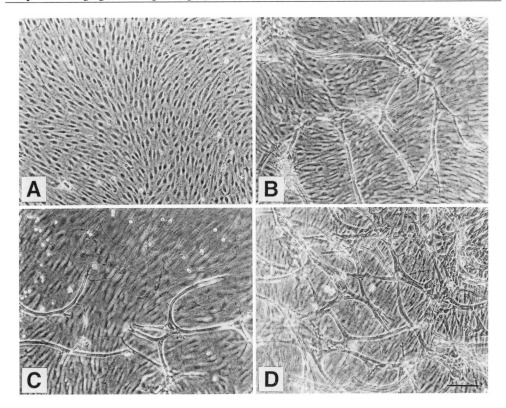

Fig. 4. Synergistic effect of co-added bFGF and VEGF on angiogenesis in vitro. (**A**) Endothelial cells are grown on the surface of a three-dimensional collagen gel as described in Fig. 3. Under these conditions, the cells do not invade the underlying matrix. When treated with bFGF (10 ng/mL) (**B**) or VEGF (30 ng/mL) (**C**) for 4 d, the cells invade the underlying matrix and form branching cell cords within the gel. When co-added (**D**), bFGF and VEGF induce an invasive response that is greater than additive. Bar = 100 μm. Adapted from ref. *15*, with copyright permission from Marcel Dekker, Inc.

ligands for this receptor, namely VEGF and VEGF-C, which may explain why in contrast to total protein, bFGF decreases cell surface VEGFR-2, possibly by promoting internalization of the VEGF/VEGFR-2 complex (S.J. Mandriota and M.S. Pepper, unpublished observation). The observation that bFGF increases both VEGF and VEGFR-2, raises the possibility that bFGF-induced in vitro angiogenesis is mediated by an autocrine VEGF/VEGFR-2 loop. Indeed, we have observed that bFGF-induced in vitro angiogenesis can be inhibited by at least 50% by co-administration of VEGF antagonists (J.-C. Tille et al., manuscript submitted). At least in vitro therefore, VEGF-induced invasion might require the presence of a second cytokine such as bFGF, which increases VEGFR-2-mediated signal transduction above a critical threshold required for mitosis, migration, and increased proteolytic activity, all of which are necessary for the formation of new capillary sprouts. It is important to bear in mind that if we wish to extrapolate the results from our in vitro studies to the in vivo setting, we must assume that in vivo, endothelial cells are able to respond to exogenous bFGF through its interaction with the cell surface (e.g., FGFRs or HSPGs). Findings obtained thus far in vivo do not allow us to comment on this possibility. Nor do they allow us to rule out the possibility that in vivo, bFGF is acting

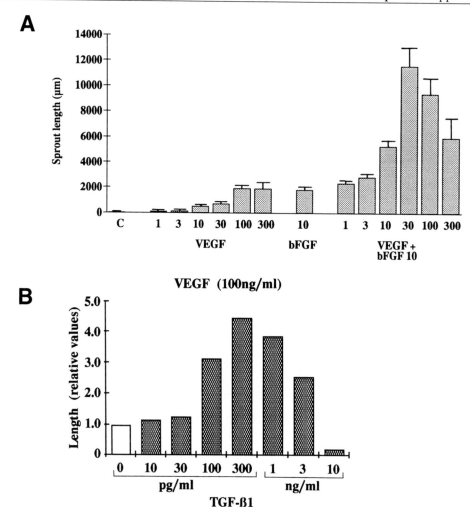

Fig. 5. Interactions between angiogenesis-regulating cytokines. Randomly selected fields of bovine microvascular endothelial cell monolayers treated with VEGF, bFGF, and/or TGF-β1 for 4 d were photographed at a single level beneath the surface monolayer. Endothelial-cell invasion was quantitated by measuring the total additive length of all cell cords, and values are expressed as mean ± SEM from at least three experiments per condition. **(A)** Synergistic effect of bFGF and VEGF on in vitro angiogenesis. VEGF-induced invasion is dose-dependent. Co-addition of bFGF at a single concentration induces an invasive response that was greater that additive. **(B)** Biphasic effect of TGF-β1 on VEGF-induced in vitro angiogenesis. VEGF (100 ng/mL)-induced invasion is potentiated by TGF-β1 at 100 pg/l–3ng/mL and inhibited by TGF-β1 at 10 ng/mL. (A) is adapted from ref. *19* and (B) is adapted from ref. *117*, with copyright permission from Academic Press.

indirectly by inducing the production of a positive regulator by nonendothelial cells, which in turn contributes to the synergistic effect. Recent observations using inhibitory anti-bFGF antibodies indicate that VEGF-induced in vitro angiogenesis as well as the VEGF-induced increase in urokinase-type PA and tissue-type PA activity are dependent on endogenous bFGF *(115a)*. These findings raise the possibility that VEGF-induced endothelial responses are dependent on endogenous bFGF. Taken together, these findings demonstrate that VEGF- and bFGF-mediated in vitro angiogenic responses are themselves a form of synergism, in that they are dependent on the presence of both cytokines concomitantly.

What is the significance of these findings? First, the levels of VEGF and its receptors appear to be unchanged in certain organs and tumors in which there is extensive angiogenesis (see above). Although, as mentioned earlier, some controversy still exists concerning its role as an endogenous regulator of angiogenesis, it has recently been demonstrated that bFGF is expressed in the mammary gland during early pregnancy, i.e., during the phase of active angiogenesis, and declines during late pregnancy and lactation (116), at which time angiogenesis is markedly reduced. In addition, induction of the vascular phase in certain experimental tumors in which VEGF levels are unchanged appears to coincide with the export of bFGF from tumor cells (117). These findings suggest that VEGF-dependent angiogenesis in certain settings may require the presence of a second positive regulator. Although this hypothesis is based on findings obtained from our in vitro invasion assay, in which bFGF is clearly angiogenic, endogenous regulators of synergism might include cytokines other than bFGF as well as hypoxia. Second, our observations might provide a partial explanation for the observation that VEGF and its receptors are expressed, sometimes at relatively high levels, in adult tissues in which angiogenesis is apparently not occurring. The lack of angiogenesis in these tissues might indicate the absence of a synergistic co-factor required for VEGF-dependent angiogenesis (and/or the presence of a dominant, negative regulator). Third, modulation of new capillary blood-vessel formation may serve as an alternative/adjunct to current therapeutic modalities in several angiogenesis-associated diseases. At first sight, the redundancy of angiogenesis-regulating cytokines might suggest that therapeutic strategies based on neutralization of single angiogenic factors might be unrealistic. If however the synergism which we have observed in vitro is relevant to the endogenous regulation of angiogenesis in vivo, angiogenesis would be more prominent in tumors or other pathologic settings in which more than one angiogenic factor is produced. This may justify anti-angiogenesis strategies based on the neutralization of a single angiogenic factor, because this would reduce the synergistic effect. On the other hand, recent work has demonstrated that administration of angiogenic factors can enhance the growth of collateral vessels in animal models of coronary, peripheral and cerebral arterial occlusion (reviewed in ref. 9). In this context, we predicted that the therapeutic effect of co-addition of two cytokines whose interaction is synergistic would be greater than that derived from addition of one of these cytokines alone (19). Support for this hypothesis has been provided by an in vivo study in which co-administered VEGF and bFGF synergized in the induction of collateral blood-vessel formation in a rabbit model of hind-limb ischemia (111). In summary, our findings on the synergism between VEGF and bFGF may have relevance both to understanding the mechanisms of angiogenesis as well as to positive and negative therapeutic modulation of this process. Furthermore, our observations highlight the importance of a three-dimensional environment for the study of angiogenesis in vitro: had we relied exclusively on traditional two-dimensional assays of proliferation, migration, or proteolysis, synergism between VEGF and bFGF would not have been detected.

Biphasic Effect of TGFβ-1

TGFβ-1 is an angiogenesis-modulating cytokine that has been described as being proor anti-angiogenic depending on the nature of the assay (see previous Subheading). These findings have led to the proposal that this cytokine has different functions on vessel formation at different stages of the angiogenic process. Thus when acting directly on endothelial cells, TGF-β-1 may inhibit invasion and vessel formation, and once sprout formation has occurred, it may be necessary for the inhibition of further endothelial-cell replication and migration, and may induce vessel organization and functional maturation. An additional possibility is that TGF-β-mediated angiogenesis is contextual, in that this requires the presence of other positive regulators, whose activity is potentiated in the presence of TGF-β. Furthermore, because TGF-β has been described as a bifunctional regulator in a variety of biological processes, it is likely that the direct effect of this cytokine on endothelial-cell function is concentration-dependent *(14)*. To address these issues, the effect of a wide range of concentrations of TGF-β1 on the response of microvascular endothelial cells to VEGF or bFGF was assessed in our in vitro model of angiogenesis, which assays both for endothelial cell invasion and capillary morphogenesis. Unlike VEGF and bFGF, when tested on its own over a wide range of concentrations TGF-β1 had no effect. However, VEGF- or bFGF-induced invasion of collagen or fibrin gels was markedly increased when TGF-β1 was co-added at 200–500 pg/mL, and decreased when TGF-β1 was added at 5–10 ng/mL (Fig. 5B and 6) *(118)*. Similar findings have been reported with large-vessel (aortic) endothelial cells *(119)*, and a biphasic effect has been noted when endothelial cells are grown in suspension in collagen gels: TGF-βs -1 and -3 at 500 pg/mL promoted angiogenesis in a manner similar to that seen with bFGF, whereas TGF-β1 at 5 ng/mL was slightly inhibitory *(120,121)*. This biphasic effect is in accord with the observations that endothelial-cell wound-induced migration *(122,123)* and invasion of three-dimensional collagen gels *(123)* or the explanted amnion *(124)* are inhibited at relatively high concentrations (1–10 ng/mL) of TGF-β1, whereas 500 pg/mL TGF-β1 potentiated two-dimensional, wound-induced migration (118; M.S. Pepper, unpublished observation). With respect to proliferation, although one study has demonstrated a similar biphasic effect of TGF-β1 in subconfluent endothelial-cell cultures *(125)*, the vast majority of studies have demonstrated that this cytokine is inhibitory over a wide range of concen-trations (reviewed in ref. *22*). Finally, not only was invasion affected by TGF-β1 in a concentration-dependent manner, but lumen formation in the resulting tube-like structures was progressively reduced with increasing concentrations of cytokine. Thus, in the absence of TGF-β1, bFGF-induced cell cords within fibrin gels contain widely patent lumina. Co-addition of TGF-β1 at 500 pg/mL reduced lumen diameter to a more physiological size (Fig. 6) *(118)*. Addition of TGF-β1 at a 10-fold higher concentration, namely 5 ng/mL, completely inhibited lumen formation in the invading cell cords *(126)*. It is interesting to note that the presence of ectatic or cavernous lumina in the absence of TGF-β1, which are reduced in size in the presence of this cytokine in vitro, are strikingly reminiscent of the vascular phenotype seen in TGF-β1-deficient mice (*see* above).

The mechanisms responsible for the in vitro biphasic effect are not known. One hypothesis is based on alterations in the net balance of extracellular proteolysis *(127,128)*. Thus at the dose of TGF-β1 that potentiates bFGF- or VEGF-induced invasion, an optimal balance between proteases and protease inhibitors might be achieved, which allows for focal pericel-lular matrix degradation, while at the same time protecting the matrix against inappropriate degradation. This hypothesis may also apply to the regulation of lumen formation, in as much as the linear dose-dependent increase in PAI-1 can be correlated with a progressive reduction in lumen size. The observation that PAI-1 competes with the urokinase-type PA receptor and integrin $\alpha_v\beta_3$ for binding to vitronectin *(129,130)*, also raises the possibility that higher concentrations of TGF-β1-induced PAI-1 might inhibit migration by interfering with cell

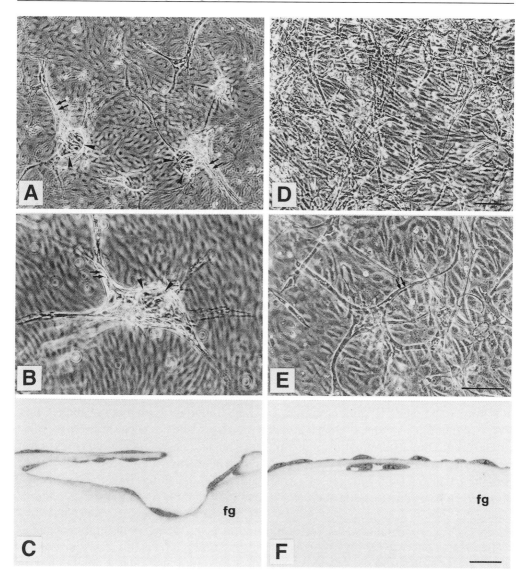

Fig. 6. TGF-β1 modulates lumen size during in vitro angiogenesis. bFGF (30 ng/mL) was added without (**A,B,C**) or with 500 pg/mL TGF-β1 (**D,E,F**) to confluent monolayers of microvascular endothelial cells grown on fibrin gels in the presence of Trasylol. The resulting capillary-like tubular structures were viewed by phase-contrast microscopy (**A,B,D** and **E**) and semi-thin sections (**C** and **F**). bFGF induced endothelial cells to invade from a circular opening in the surface monolayer (arrow-heads in **A** and **B**), to form well organized cell cords with a clearly visible refringent lumen (arrows in **A** and **B**), which tapered down progressively in the distal part of the cords. Semi-thin sectioning revealed that the proximal part of the cords was often cavernous (**C**). When 500 pg/mL TGF-β1 was co-added with bFGF, the total additive length of the invading cell cords was increased (compare **A** and **D**, and *see* Fig. 5B for quantitation), and clearly distinguishable lumina were present beneath the surface monolayer (white refringent line indicated by the arrows in **E**). Semi-thin sectioning revealed that the lumen was reduced to a more physiological size when compared to cultures treated with bFGF alone (compare **C** and **F**). Bars in (**A**), (**D**) = 100 µm, in (**B**), (**E**) = 50 µm, and in (**C**), (**F**) = 20 µm. Adapted from ref. *117*, with copyright permission from Academic Press.

adhesion. A second explanation may come from the observation that TGF-β1 decreases VEGFR-2 expression at concentrations that inhibit in vitro angiogenesis (50,118). A third possibility might be related to alterations in integrin expression and ligand-binding affinity (131,132). Because TGF-β alters endothelial-cell integrin expression (reviewed in ref. 22; 133a), it is likely that maximal invasion occurs in the presence of an optimal degree of cellular adhesion, and that submaximal invasion occurs when adhesion is either greater or less than that achieved with the potentiating dose of TGF-β1. The notion that 500 pg/mL TGF-β1 stimulates adhesion to an extent that is optimal for migration is consistent with the observation that 500 pg/mL TGF-β1 potentiates, whereas 5 ng/mL inhibits bFGF-induced, wound-induced, two-dimensional migration (119; M.S. Pepper, unpublished data). Differential regulation of integrin expression may also contribute to the alterations in lumen size that are seen with different concentrations of TGF-β1 in fibrin gels. Finally, the complete absence of lumen formation at 5 ng/mL may imply that at this concentration, TGF-β1 inhibits the cellular machinery responsible for maintaining endothelial-cell polarity, which in the case of angiogenesis is likely to be a major factor in driving histotypic morphogenesis, namely the formation of tube-like structures.

Synergism Between Hyaluronan Oligosaccharides and VEGF

In addition to diffusible cytokines, extracellular matrix components including collagens, fibronectin, laminin, and other glycoproteins have been shown to be important in angiogenesis. Hyaluronan (hyaluronic acid, HA), a glycosaminoglycan composed of repeating disaccharide units of D-glucuronate and N-acetylglucosamine, is one of the most abundant extracellular matrix constituents. Although initially considered primarily as a structural moiety, HA has now emerged as an important signaling molecule. Thus, HA is involved in a number of developmental processes, and has been shown to promote cell proliferation, differentiation, and motility. The diverse biological activities of HA are believed to be mediated, at least in part, through interaction with specific cell-surface receptors such as CD44, which results in activation of intracellular signaling events. HA obtained from different tissue sources exhibits considerable variation in size, and its biological activity has been shown to be critically dependent on molecular mass in a number of experimental systems, including angiogenesis. Thus, native high molecular-weight HA is anti-angiogenic, whereas HA degradation products of specific size (3–10 disaccharide units) stimulate endothelial-cell proliferation and migration, and induce angiogenesis in the chick chorioallantoic membrane (CAM) assay, in rat skin, and in a cryoinjured skin-graft model (reviewed in ref. 15).

We have used our collagen gel assay to determine whether HA and/or its degradation products influence endothelial-cell invasion. We found that like bFGF and VEGF (*see* above), oligosaccharides of HA (OHA) induce endothelial cells to invade the underlying gel within which they form capillary-like tubes, with an optimal effect at approx 0.5–2.0 µg/mL OHA. Co-addition of OHA (0.5–2.0 µg/mL) and VEGF (30 ng/mL), but not of OHA and bFGF (10 ng/mL), induced a striking in vitro angiogenic response that was greater than the sum of the effects elicited by either agent separately. In contrast to OHA, native high molecular-weight HA (nHA) was consistently inactive, either when added alone or when added in combination with VEGF or bFGF (Fig. 7) (133).

The mechanisms by which OHA stimulate endothelial-cell invasion of collagen gels are not known. However, in bovine endothelial cells, OHA have recently been found to induce phosphorylation and activation of MAP kinase (M. A. Slevin et al., manuscript

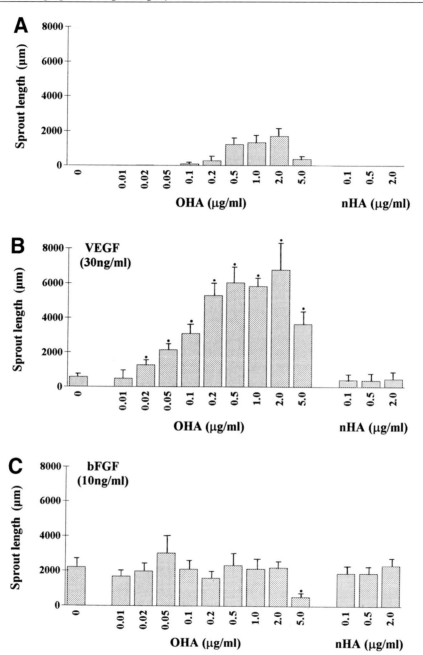

Fig. 7. Synergistic effect of OHA and VEGF on angiogenesis in vitro. Confluent monolayers of endothelial cells on collagen gels were treated with OHA or nHA at the indicated concentrations (**A**), cotreated with OHA or nHA and VEGF (**B**), or cotreated with OHA or nHA and bFGF (**C**). Invasion was quantified after 4 d and results are expressed as mean total additive length (in m)± s.e.m. of all sprouts that had penetrated beneath the surface monolayer in three randomly selected photographic fields from each of at least 3 separate experiments per experimental condition.*$p < 0.001$. OHA stimulate angiogenesis in vitro in a dose-dependent manner (**A**) and synergize with VEGF (**B**) but not with bFGF (**C**). nHA has no significant effect on invasion, either when added alone (**A**) or in combination with VEGF or bFGF (**B,C**). Adapted from ref. *132*, with copyright permission from Williams and Wilkins.

submitted), as well as upregulation of early response genes such as c-*fos*, c-*jun*, and *jun*-B *(134)*, which are known to control the expression of a number of other genes including those of matrix-degrading proteases. Because HA receptors, including a CD44-like transmembrane protein, have been identified in bovine endothelial cells *(135–138)*, it is conceivable that OHA promotes endothelial-cell invasion and tube formation by activating intracellular signaling pathways that ultimately result in modulation of pericellular proteolysis. The molecular mechanisms responsible for the specific synergistic interaction between OHA and VEGF in the induction of angiogenesis in vitro are also unknown. OHA and VEGF might activate independent but converging intracellular signaling pathways, resulting in a synergistic effect, or OHA might upregulate expression of high-affinity VEGF receptors such as Flk-1. Alternatively, as has been shown for heparin-like glycosaminoglycans, OHA may complex with VEGF molecules, thereby increasing ligand half-life or facilitating multivalent VEGF binding and receptor oligomerization.

Although exogenously-added OHA promotes angiogenesis in in vitro and in vivo assays, it has not yet been clearly established whether endogenous OHA can act as a physiological regulator of angiogenesis. Several observations nonetheless suggest the potential involvement of OHA in angiogenesis associated with reparative and pathological processes (reviewed in refs. *15,139*). In a number of clinical settings, including wound healing, rheumatoid arthritis (RA), vasoproliferative retinopathy, and cancer, angiogenesis occurs in close proximity to HA-rich tissues or fluids. HA catabolism has been shown to be very rapid: in skin for instance, up to 25% of injected HA is degraded locally in 24 h. Although most vertebrate hyaluronidases so far characterized are lysosomal, HA-degrading activities with near neutral pH optima have recently been shown to be expressed by tumor cells and to induce angiogenesis in vivo *(140,141)*. It is therefore conceivable that breakdown of high molecular-weight HA occurs in the extracellular space during pathological processes. This would result in the production of HA oligosaccharides, which in addition to being angiogenic on their own, could synergize with VEGF, which has been shown to be expressed in all the clinical settings mentioned earlier. Based on our in vitro studies, we propose that the potential therapeutic effect of co-administration of VEGF and OHA deserves to be investigated in situations that would benefit from stimulation of angiogenesis, particularly in animal models of coronary or peripheral arterial insufficiency.

FUTURE PERSPECTIVES

Although an enormous amount of progress has been made in identifying cytokines that regulate blood-vessel formation either positively or negatively, many important fundamental questions remain. A number of issues which merit further investigation are discussed below.

First, although it is currently assumed that vasculogenesis is limited to early development, the observation that circulating endothelial-cell precursors contribute to new blood-vessel formation in postnatal life is likely to significantly enhance our understanding of angiogenesis. Two important questions raised by this seminal observation include the origin of circulating precursors as well as their precise relationship to angioblasts (and hemangioblasts). From a therapeutic point of view, the existence of circulating precursors may have important implications both for stimulation and inhibition of angiogenesis.

Second, both vasculogenesis and angiogenesis result in the formation of simple endothelial-lined capillary-like tubes, and a significant body of information is now available concerning the mechanisms of these processes. However, the mechanisms of vessel-wall maturation, which include differentiation of contractile cells (pericytes and smooth-muscle cells) from adjacent mesenchyme as well as their organization into a functional vessel, remain for the present poorly understood. Nonetheless, in addition to TGF-β and PDGF as well as their respective cell-surface receptors (*see* above), evidence is at present emerging that implicates a third cytokine family, namely the angiopoietins, in the process of vessel-wall maturation. Angiopoietin-1 has recently been identified as the ligand for the TIE-2 tyrosine kinase receptor *(142)*, and gene-deletion studies have revealed an important role for this ligand-receptor pair in vessel-wall maturation *(143–145)*. It appears that angiopoietin-1 is expressed by stromal cells and TIE-2 by endothelial cells, and that in the absence of either the ligand or its receptor, smooth-muscle cell differentiation and recruitment are significantly reduced, resulting in the formation of dilated endothelial-lined vascular channels that fail to mature into arteries and veins. It will now be important to know which genes (including possibly TGF-β and PDGF) are regulated by angiopoietin-1 in TIE-2 expressing endothelial cells.

Third, we are clearly entering an era in which a genetic approach to understanding the pathogenesis of vascular disorders (reviewed in ref. *146*) will require identification of mutations in endothelial-cell receptor tyrosine kinases (VEGFRs-1, -2 and -3; TIE-1 and TIE-2) and other molecules involved in new blood-vessel formation. Mutations in these receptors would be expected to be important in the pathogenesis of vascular malformations, and may play a role in the development of hemangiomas as well as in chronic vasoproliferative disorders (cancer, arthritis, retinopathy), which are likely to be multigenic in origin. It will also be important to determine whether increased susceptibility/predisposition to some of these chronic disorders is linked to a genetically-based pro-angiogenic state that may result from increased activity of positive regulators (angiogenic factors and receptors) or decreased activity of inhibitors. With respect to vascular malformations, an activating mutation in Tie-2 has recently been shown to segregate with an autosomal dominant form of venous malformation in two independent families *(147)*, and candidate loci for the Klippel-Trenauny-Weber syndrome *(148)* and cerebral cavernous malformations *(149–151)* have been identified.

Finally, novel pharmacological and gene-therapy approaches need to be developed for the stimulation and inhibition of angiogenesis. In addition, extensive clinical evaluation of current therapeutic strategies will almost certainly require testing in multicenter trials. It will also be important to develop animal models that are relevant to angiogenesis-associated diseases, and that could be exploited in the search for novel therapeutic strategies. For example, the establishment of transgenic mice by site-directed overexpression of positive regulators (e.g., VEGF in the skin as a model for hemangiomas) could be combined with assessment of the therapeutic potential of novel angiogenesis inhibitors.

ACKNOWLEDGMENTS

We would like to thank Dr. J.-D. Vassalli for his important contributions to our work, and Dr. L. Orci for continued support, advice, and constructive criticism. We are also grateful to C. Di Sanza, M. Quayzin, and J. Rial-Robert for excellent ongoing technical assistance. Work performed in the authors' laboratory has been supported by the Swiss National Science Foundation, the Juvenile Diabetes Foundation International, and the Sir Jules Thorn Charitable Overseas Trust.

REFERENCES

1. Wagner, R. C. (1980) Endothelial cell embryology and growth. *Adv. Microcirc.* **9,** 45–75.
2. Dieterlen-Lièvre, F. (1993) La genèse du système sanguin chez l'embryon. *La Recherche* **254,** 528–534.
3. Risau, W. and Flamme, I. (1995) Vasculogenesis. *Ann. Rev. Cell Dev. Biol.* **11,** 73–91.

4. Wilting, J., Brand-Saberi, B., Kurz, H., and Christ B. (1995) Development of the embryonic vascular system. *Cell Mol. Biol. Res.* **41,** 219–232.

5. Hertig, A. T. (1935) Angiogenesis in the early human chorion and in the primary placenta of the macaque monkey. *Carnegie Contrib. Embryol.* **25,** 37–81.

6. Asahara, T., Murohara, T., Sullivan, A., Silver, M., van der Zee, R., Li, T., et al. (1997) Isolation of putative progenitor endothelial cells for angiogenesis. *Science* **275,** 964–967.

7. Folkman, J. (1995) Clinical applications of research on angiogenesis. *N. Engl. J. Med.* **333,** 1757–1763.

8. Pepper, M. S. (1996) Positive and negative regulation of angiogenesis: from cell biology to the clinic. *Vasc. Med.* **1,** 259–266.

9. Pepper, M. S. (1997) Manipulating angiogenesis: from basic science to the bedside. *Arterioscler. Thromb. Vasc. Biol.*, 17,605–17,619.

10. Folkman, J. (1974) Tumor angiogenesis. *Adv. Cancer Res.* **19,** 331–358.

11. Holmgren, L., O'Reilly, M. S., and Folkman, J. (1995) Dormancy of micrometastases: balanced proliferation and apoptosis in the presence of angiogenesis suppression. *Nature Med.* **1,** 149–153.

12. O'Reilly, M. S., Holmgren, L., Chen, C., and Folkman J. (1992) Angiostatin induces and sustains dormancy of human primary tumors in mice. *Nature Med.* **2,** 689–692.

13. Hanahan, D. and Folkman, J. (1996) Patterns and emerging mechanisms of the angiogenic switch during tumorigenesis. *Cell* **86,** 353–364.

14. Nathan, C. and Sporn, M. (1991) Cytokines in context. *J. Cell Biol.* **113,** 981–986.

15. Montesano, R. and Pepper, M. S. (2000) Capillary morphogenesis in vitro: cytokine interactions and balanced proteolysis, in *Tumor Angiogenesis and Microcirculation* (Voest, E. E. and D'Amore, P. A., eds.), Marcel Dekker, New York .

16. Montesano, R. and Orci, L. (1985) Tumor-promoting phorbol esters induce angiogenesis in vitro. *Cell* **42,** 469–477.

17. Montesano, R., Pepper, M. S., Vassalli, J.-D., and Orci, L. (1987) Phorbol ester induces cultured endothelial cells to invade a fibrin matrix in the presence of fibrinolytic inhibitors. *J. Cell Physiol.* **132,** 509–516.

18. Montesano, R., Vassalli, J.-D., Baird, A., Guillemin, R., and Orci, L. (1986) Basic fibroblast growth factor induces angiogenesis in vitro. *Proc. Natl. Acad. Sci. USA* **83,** 7297–7301.

19. Pepper, M. S., Ferrara, N., Orci, L., and Montesano, R. (1992) Potent synergism between vascular endothelial growth factor and basic fibroblast growth factor in the induction of angiogenesis in vitro. *Biochem. Biophys. Res. Commun.* **189,** 824–831.

20. Klagsbrun, M. and D'Amore, P. A. (1991) Regulators of angiogenesis. *Ann. Rev. Physiol.* **53,** 217–239.

21. Pepper, M. S., Mandriota, S., Vassalli, J.-D., Orci, L., and Montesano, R. (1996) Angiogenesis regulating cytokines: activities and interactions. *Curr. Top. Microbiol. Immunol.* **213/II,** 31–67.

22. Pepper, M. S. (1997) Transforming growth factor-beta: vasculogenesis, angiogenesis and vessel wall integrity. *Cytokine Growth Factor Res.* **8,** 21–43.

23. Leek, R. D., Harris, A. L., and Lewis, C. E. (1994) Cytokine networks in solid human tumors: regulation of angiogenesis. *J. Leukocyte Biol.* **56,** 423–435.

24. Risau, W. (1996) What, if anything, is an angiogenic factor ? *Cancer Metastasis Rev.* **15,** 149–151.

25. Dvorak, H. F., Brown, L. F., Detmar, M., and Dvorak, A. M. (1995) Vascular Permeability Factor/ Vascular Endothelial Growth Factor, microvascular hyperpermeability, and angiogenesis. *Am. J. Pathol.* **146,** 1029–1039.

26. Breier, G. and Risau, W. (1996) The role of vascular endothelial growth factor in blood vessel formation. *Trends Cell. Biol.* **6,** 454–456.

27. Thomas, K.A. (1996) Vascular endothelial growth factor, a potent and selective angiogenic agent. *J. Biol. Chem.* **271,** 603–606.

28. Ferrara, N. and Davis-Smyth, T. (1997) The biology of vascular endothelial growth factor. *Endocrine Rev.* **18,** 4–25.

29. Carmeliet, P., Ferreira, V., Breier, G., Pollefeyt, S., Kieckens, L., Gertsenstein, M., et al. (1996) Abnormal blood vessel development and lethality in embryos lacking a single VEGF allele. *Nature* **380,** 435–439.

30. Ferrara, N., Carver-Moore, K., Chen, H., Dowd, M., Lu, L., O'Shea, K. S., et al. (1996) Heterozygous embryonic lethality induced by targeted inactivation of the VEGF gene. *Nature* **380,** 439–442.

31. Nagy, A. and Rossant, J. (1996) Targeted mutagenesis: analysis of phenotype without germ line transmission. *J. Clin. Invest.* **97,** 1360–1365.

32. Olofsson, B., Pajusola, K., Kaipainen, A., von Euler, G., Joukov, V., Saksela, O., et al. (1996) Vascular endothelial growth factor B, a novel growth factor for endothelial cells. *Proc. Natl. Acad. Sci. USA* **93,** 2576–2581.

33. Grimmond, S., Lagercrantz, J., Drinkwater, C., Silins, G., Townson, S., Pollock, P., et al. (1996) Cloning and characterization of a novel human gene related to vascular endothelial growth factor. *Genome Res.* **6,** 124–131.

34. Townson, S., Lagercrantz, J., Grimmond, S., Silins, G., Nordenskjöld, M., Weber, G., and Hayward, N. (1996) Characterization of the murine VEGF-related factor gene. *Biochem. Biophys. Res. Commun.* **220,** 922–928.

35. Lagercrantz, J., Larsson, C., Grimmond, S., Fredriksson, M., Weber, G., and Piehl, F. (1996) Expression of the VEGF-related gene in pre- and postnatal mouse. Biochem Biophys *Res. Commun.* **220,** 147–152.

36. Joukov, V., Pajusola, K., Kaipainen, A., Chilov, D., Lahtinen, I., Kukk, E., et al. (1996) A novel vascular endothelial growth factor, VEGF-C, is a ligand for the Flt4 (VEGFR-3) and KDR (VEGFR-2) receptor tyrosine kinases. *EMBO J.* **15,** 290–298.

37. Lee, J., Gray, A., Yuan, J., Luoh, S.-M., Avraham, H., and Wood, W. I. (1996) Vascular endothelial growth factor-related protein: a ligand and specific activator of the tyrosine kinase receptor FLT4. *Proc. Natl. Acad. Sci. USA* **93,** 1988–1992.

38. Kukk, E., Lymboussaki, A., Taira, S., Kaipainen, A., Jeltsch M., Joukov, V., and Alitalo, K. (1996) VEGF-C receptor binding and pattern of expression with VEGFR-3 suggests a role in lymphatic vascular development. *Development* **122,** 3829–3827.

39. Mustonen, T. and Alitalo, K. (1995) Endothelial receptor tyrosine kinases involved in angiogenesis. *J. Cell Biol.* **129,** 895–898.

40. Fong, G.-H., Rossant, J., Gertsenstein, M., and Breitman, M.L. (1995) Role of the Flt-1 receptor tyrosine kinase in regulating the assembly of vascular endothelium. *Nature* **376,** 66–70.

41. Shalaby, F., Rossant, J., Yamaguchi, T. P., Gertsenstein, M., Wu, X.-F., Breitman, M. L., and Schuh, A. C. (1995) Failure of blood-island formation and vasculogenesis in Flk-1-deficient mice. *Nature* **376,** 62–66.

42. Millauer, B., Shawver, L. K., Plate, K. H., Risau, W., and Ullrich, A. (1994) Glioblastoma growth inhibited in vivo by a dominant negative Flk-1 mutant. *Nature* **367,** 576–579.

43. Millauer, B., Longhi, M. P., Plate, K. H., Shawver, L. K., Risau, W., Ullrich, A., and Strawn, L. M. (1996) Dominant negative inhibition of Flk-1 suppresses the growth of many tumor types in vivo. *Cancer Res.* **56,** 1615–1620.

44. Plate, K. H., Breier, G., Weich, H. A., and Risau, W. (1992) Vascular endothelial growth factor is a potent tumor angiogenesis factor in human gliomas in vivo. *Nature* **359,** 845–848.

45. Plate, K. H., Breier, G., and Risau, W. (1994) Molecular mechanisms of developmental and tumor angiogenesis. *Brain Pathol.* **4,** 207–218.

46. Thieme, H., Aiello, L. P., Takagi, H., Ferrara, N., and King, G. L. (1995) Comparative analysis of vascular endothelial growth factor receptors on retinal and aortic vascular endothelial cells. *Diabetes* **44,** 98–103.

47. Waltenberger, J., Mayr, U., Pentz, S., and Hombach, V. (1995) Vascular endothelial growth factor (VEGF) represents a survival factor for hypoxic endothelium. Potential role of the VEGF-receptor KDR for therapeutic angiogenesis. *Circulation* **92,** I–749.

48. Tuder, R. M., Flook, B. E., and Voelkel, N. F. (1995) Increased gene expression for VEGF and the VEGF receptors KDR/flk and flt in lungs exposed to acute or chronic hypoxia. *J. Clin. Invest.* **95,** 1798–1807.

49. Brogi, E., Schatteman, G., Wu, T., Kim, E. A., Vartikovski, L., Keyt, B., and Isner, J. M. (1996) Hypoxia-induced paracrine regulation of vascular endothelial growth factor receptor expression. *J. Clin. Invest.* **97,** 469–476.

50. Mandriota, S. J., Menoud, P.-A., and Pepper, M. S. (1996) Transforming growth factor-1 downregulates vascular endothelial growth factor receptor-2/flk-1 expression in vascular endothelial cells. *J. Biol. Chem.* **271,** 11,500–11,505.

51. Patterson, C., Perrella, M. A., Endege, W. O., Yoshizumi M., Lee, M.-E., and Haber, E. (1996) Downregulation of vascular endothelial growth fcator receptors by tumor necrosis factor-a in cultured human vascular endothelial cells. *J. Clin. Invest.* **98,** 490–496.

52. Basilico, C. and Moscatelli, D. (1992) The FGF family of growth factors and oncogenes. *Adv. Cancer Res.* **59,** 115–165.

53. Fernig, D. G. and Gallagher, J. T. (1994) Fibroblast growth factors and their receptors: an information network controlling tissue growth, morphogenesis and repair. *Prog. Growth Factor Res.* **5,** 353–377.

54. Wilkie, A. O. M., Morriss-Kay, G. M., Jones, E. Y., and Heath, J. K. (1995) Functions of fibroblast growth factors and their receptors. *Curr. Biol.* **5,** 500–507.

55. Birmbaum, D., Lovec, H., Coulier, F., Goldfarb, M., and Lopez-Ferber, M. (1997) Les FGF: une famille en croissance. *Médecine Sciences* **13,** 392–396.

56. Christofori, G. (1997) The role of fibroblast growth factors in tumour progression and angiogenesis in *Tumour Angiogenesis* (Bicknell, R., Lewis, C. E., and Ferrara, N., eds.), Oxford University Press, NY, 201–237.

57. Ribatti, D., Urbinati, C., Nico, B., Rusnati, M., Roncali, L., and Presta, M. (1995) Endogenous basic fibroblast growth factor is implicated in the vascularization of the chick embryo chorioallantoic membrane. *Dev. Biol.* **170,** 39–49.

58. Reilly, T. M., Taylor, D. S., Herblin, W. F., Thoolen, M. J., Chiu, A. T., Watson, D. W., and Timmermans, P. B. (1989) Monoclonal antibodies directed against basic fibroblast growth factor which inhibit its biological activity in vitro and in vivo. *Biochem. Biophys. Res. Commun.* **164,** 736–743.

59. Hori, A., Sasada, R., Matsutani, E., Naito, K., Sakura, Y., Fujita, T., and Kozai, Y. (1991) Suppression of solid tumor growth by immunoneutralizing monoclonal antibody against human basic fibroblast growth factor. *Cancer Res.* **51,** 6180–6184.

60. Stan, A. C., Nemati, M. N., Pietsch, T., Walter, G. F., and Dietz, H. (1995) In vivo inhibition of angiogenesis and growth of the human U-87 malignant glial tumor by treatment with an antibody against basic fibroblast growth factor. *J. Neurosurg.* **82,** 1044–1052.

61. Matsuzaki, K., Yoshitake, Y., Matuo, Y., Sasaki, H., and Nishikawa, K. (1989) Monoclonal antibodies against heparin-binding growth factor II/basic fibroblast growth factor that block its biological activity: invalidity of the antibodies for tumor angiogenesis. *Proc. Natl. Acad. Sci. USA* **86,** 9911–9915.

62. Dennis, P. A. and Rifkin, D. B. (1990) Studies on the role of basic fibroblast growth factor in vivo: inability of neutralizing antibodies to block tumor growth. *J. Cell. Physiol.* **144,** 84–98.

63. Yamaguchi, T. P. and Rossant, J. (1995) Fibroblast growth factors in mammalian development. *Curr. Opin. Genet. Dev.* **5,** 485–491.

64. Coffin, J. D., Florkiewicz, R. Z., Neumann, J., Mort-Hopkins, T., Dorn, G. W., Lightfoot, P., et al. (1995) Abnormal bone growth and selective translational regulation in basic fibroblast growth factor (FGF-2) transgenic mice. *Mol. Biol. Cell* **6,** 1861–1873.

65. Jaye, M., Schlessinger, J., and Dionne, C. A. (1992) Fibroblast growth factor receptor tyrosine kinases: molecular analysis and signal transduction. *Biochim. Biophys. Acta* **1135,** 185–199.

66. Givol, D. and Yayon, A. (1992) Complexity of FGF receptors: genetic basis for structural diversity and functional specificity. *FASEB J.* **6,** 3362–3369.

67. Johnson, D. E. and Williams, L. T. (1993) Structural and functional diversity in the FGF receptor multigene family. *Adv. Cancer Res.* **60,** 1–41.

68. Deng, C.-X., Wynshaw-Boris, A., Shen, M. M., Daugherty, C., Ornitz, D. M., and Leder, P. (1994) Murine FGFR-1 is required for early postimplantation growth and axial organization. *Genes Dev.* **8,** 3045–3057.

69. Yamaguchi, T. P., Harpal, K., Hankemeyer, M., and Rossant, J. (1994) FGFr-1 is required for embryonic growth and mesodermal patterning during mouse gastrulation. *Genes Dev.* **8,** 3032–3044.

70. Mignatti, P. and Rifkin, D. B. (1991) Release of basic fibroblast growth factor, an angiogenic factor devoid of secretory signal sequence; a trivial phenomenon or a novel secretion mechanism? *J. Cell Biochem.* **47,** 201–207.

71. Bikfalvi, A., Klein, S., Pintucci, G., and Rifkin, D. (1997) Biological roles of fibroblast growth factor-2. *Endocr. Rev.* **18,** 26–45.

72. Quarto, N. and Amalric, F. (1994) Heparan sulfate proteoglycans as transducers of FGF-2 signalling. *J. Cell Sci.* **107,** 3201–3212.

73. Miyazono, K., Ichijo, H., and Heldin, C.-H. (1993) Transforming growth factor-b: latent forms, binding proteins and receptors. *Growth Factors* **8,** 11–22.

74. Massagué, J., Attisano, L., and Wrana, J. L. (1994) The TGF-β family and its composite receptors. *Trends Cell Biol.* **4,** 172–178.

75. Kingsley, D. M. (1994) The TGF-β superfamily: new members, new receptors, and new genetic tests of function in different organisms. *Genes Dev.* **8,** 133–146.

76. Attisano, L., Wrana, J. L., López-Casillas, F., and Massagué, J. (1994) TGF-β receptors and actions. *Biochim. Biophys. Acta* **1222,** 71–80.

77. Derynck, R. (1994) TGF-β-receptor mediated signalling. *Trends Biochem. Sci.* **19,** 548–553.

78. Wrana, J. L., Attisano, L., Wieser, R., Ventura, F., and Massagué J. (1994) Mechanism of activation of the TGF-β receptor. *Nature* **370,** 341–347.

79. Yingling, J. M., Wang, X.-F., and Bassing, C.H. (1995) Signaling by the transforming growth factor-β receptors. *Biochim. Biophys. Acta* **1242,** 115–136.

80. Roberts, A. B. and Sporn, M. B. (1989) Regulation of endothelial cell growth, architecture, and matrix synthesis by TGF-β. *Amer. Rev. Resp. Dis.* **140,** 1126–1128.

81. RayChaudhury, A. and D'Amore, P. A. (1991) Endothelial cell regulation by transforming growth factor-beta. *J. Cell Biochem.* **47,** 224–229.

82. Madri, J. A., Kocher, O., Merwin, J. R., Bell, L., Tucker, A., and Basson, C. T. (1990) Interactions of vascular cells with transforming growth factors β. *Ann. NY Acad. Sci.* **593,** 243–258.

83. Madri, J. A., Bell, L., and Merwin J. R. (1992) Modulation of vascular cell behavior by transforming growth factors β. *Mol. Reprod. Dev.* **32,** 121–126.

84. Akhurst, R. J., Lehnert, S. A., Faissner, A. J., and Duffie, E. (1990) TGF beta in murine morphogenetic processes: the early embryo and cardiogenesis. *Development* **108,** 645–656.

85. Shull, M. M., Ormsby, I., Kier, A. B., Pawlowski, S., Diebold, R. J., Yin, M., et al. (1992) Targeted disruption of the mouse transforming growth factor-β1 gene results in multifocal inflammatory disease. *Nature* **359,** 693–699.

86. Kulkarni, A. B., Huh, C.-G., Becker, D., Geiser, A., Lyght, M., Flanders, K. C., et al. (1993) Transforming growth factor β1 null mutation in mice causes excessive inflammatory response and early death. *Proc. Natl. Acad. Sci. USA* **90,** 770–774

87. Dickson, M. C., Martin, J. S., Cousins, F. M., Kulkarni, A. B., Karlsson, S., and Akhurst, R. J. (1995) Defective haematopoiesis and vasculogenesis in transforming growth factor-β1 knock out mice. *Development* **121,** 1845–1854.

88. Bonyadi, M., Rusholme, S. A. B., Cousins, F. M., Su, H. C., Biron, C. A., Farrall, M., and Akhurst, R.J. (1997) Mapping of a major genetic modifier of embryonic lethality in TGFβ1 knockout mice. *Nature Genet.* **15,** 207–211.

89. Oshima, M., Oshima, H., and Taketo, M. M. (1996) TGF-β receptor type II deficiency results in defects of yolk sac hematopoiesis and vasculogenesis. *Dev. Biol.* **179,** 297–302.

90. Lawler, S., Candia, A. F., Ebner, R., Shum, L., Lopez, A. R., Moses, H. L., et al. (1994) The murine type II TGF-β receptor has a coincident embryonic expression and binding preference for TGF-β1. *Development* **120,** 165–175.

91. Guttmacher, A. E., Marchuk, D. A., and White, R. I. (1995) Hereditary hemorrhagic telangectasia. *N. Engl. J. Med.* **333,** 918–924.

92. McAllister, K. A., Grogg, K. M., Johnson, D. W., Gallione, C. J., Baldwin, M. A., Jackson, C. E., et al. (1994) Endoglin, a TGF-β binding protein of endothelial cells, is the gene for hereditary haemorrhagic telangiectasia type 1. *Nature Genet.* **8,** 345–351.

93. Johnson, D. W., Berg, J. N., Baldwin, M. A., Gallione, C. J., Marondel, I., Yoon, S.-J., et al. (1996) Mutations in the activin receptor-like kinase 1 gene in hereditary haemorrhagic telangectasia type 2. *Nature Genet.* **13,** 189–195.

94. Attisano, L., Carcamo, J., Ventura, F., Weis F. M. B., Massagué, J., and Wrana, J. L. (1993) Identification of human activin and TGFβ type I receptors that form heteromeric kinase complexes with type II receptors. *Cell* **75,** 671–680.

95. Yang, J. T., Rayburn, H., and Hynes, R. O. (1993) Embryonic mesodermal defects in α_5 integrin-deficient mice. *Development* **119,** 1093–1105.

96. George, E. L., Georges-Labouesse, E. N., Patel-King, R. S., Rayburn, H., and Hynes, R. O. (1993) Defects in mesoderm, neural tube and vascular development in mouse embryos lacking fibronectin. *Development* **119,** 1079β1091.

97. Levéen, P., Pekny, M., Gebre-Medhin, S., Swolin, B., Larsson, E., and Betsholtz, C. (1994) Mice deficient for PDGF B show renal, cardiovascular, and hematological abnormalities. *Genes Dev.* **8,** 1875–1887.

98. Soriano, P. (1994) Abnormal kidney development and hematological disorders in PDGF β-receptor mutant mice. *Genes Dev.* **8,** 1888–1896.

99. Schatteman, G. C., Loushin, C., Li, T., and Hart, C. E. (1996) PDGF-A is required for normal murine cardiovascular development. *Dev. Biol.* **176,** 133–142.

100. Daniel, T. O., Gibbs, V. C., Milfay, D. F., and Williams, L. T. (1987) Agents that increase cAMP accumulation block endothelial c-*sis* induction by thrombin and transforming growth factor-β. *J. Biol. Chem.* **262,** 11,893–11,896.

101. Starksen, N. F., Harsh, G. R., Gibbs, V. C., and Williams L. T. (1987) Regulated expression of the platelet-derived growth factor A chain gene in microvascular endothelial cells. *J. Biol. Chem.* **262,** 14,381–14,384.

102. Kavanaugh, W. M., Harsh, G. R., Starksen, N. F., Rocco, C. M., and Williams, L. T. (1988) Transcriptional regulation of the A and B chains of platelet-derived growth factor in microvascular endothelial cells. *J. Biol. Chem.* **263,** 8470–8472.

103. Gronwald, R. G. K., Seifert, R. A., and Bowen-Pope, D. F. (1989) Differential regulation of expression of two platelet-derived growth factor receptor subunits by transforming growth factor-β. *J. Biol. Chem.* **264,** 8120–8125.

104. Battegay, E. J., Raines, E. W., Seifert, R. A., Bowen-Pope, D. F., and Ross, R. (1990) TGF-β induces bimodal proliferation of connective tissue cells via complex control of an autocrine PDGF loop. *Cell* **63,** 515–524.

105. Casscells, W. (1992) Smooth muscle cell growth factors. *Prog. Growth Factor Res.* **3,** 177–206.
106. Schwartz, S. M., deBlois, D., and O'Brien, E. R. M. (1995) The intima. Soil for atherosclerosis and restenosis. *Circ. Res.* **77,** 445–465.
107. Roberts, W. G. and Palade, G. E. (1995) Increased microvascular permeability and endothelial fenestration induced by vascular endothelial growth factor. *J. Cell Sci.* **108,** 2369–2379.
108. Roberts, W. G. and Palade, G. E. (1997) Neovasculature induced by vascular endothelial growth factor is fenestrated. *Cancer Res.* **57,** 765–772.
108a. Pepper, M. S., Baetens, D., Mandriota, S. J., Sanza, C., Oikemus, S., Lane, T. F., Soriano, J. V., Montesano, R., and Iruela-Arispe, M. L. (2000) Regulation of VEGF and VEGF receptor expression in the rodent mammary gland during pregnancy, lacatation, and involution. *Dev. Dyn.* **218,** 507–524.
109. Christofori, G., Naik, P., and Hanahan, D. (1995) Vascular endothelial growth factor and its receptors, flt-1 and flk-1, are expressed in normal pancreatic islets and throughout islet cell tumorigenesis. *Endocrinology* **9,** 1760–1770.
110. Goto, F., Goto, K., Weindel, K., and Folkman, J. (1993) Synergistic effects of vascular endothelial growth factor and basic fibroblast growth factor on the proliferation and cord formation of bovine capillary endothelial cells within collagen gels. *Lab. Invest.* **69,** 508–517.
110a. Pepper, M. S. and Mandriota, S. J. (1998) Regulation of vascular endothelial growth factor receptor-2 (Flk-1) expression in vascular endothelial cells. *Exp. Cell Res.* **241,** 414–425.
111. Asahara, T., Bauters, C., Zheng, L. P., Takeshita, S., Bunting, S., Ferrara, N., et al. (1995) Synergistic effect of vascular endothelial growth factor and basic fibroblast growth factor on angiogenesis in vivo. *Circulation* **92(Suppl. II),** II–365–II371.
112. Hu, D. E. and Fan, T.-P.D. (1995) Suppression of VEGF-induced angiogenesis by the protein tyrosine kinase inhibitor, lavendustin. A. *Br. J. Pharmacol.* **114,** 262–268.
113. Pepper, M. S., Vassalli, J.-D., Orci, L., and Montesano, R. (1994) Angiogenesis in vitro: cytokine interactions and balanced extracellular proteolysis in *Angiogenesis. Molecular Biology, Clinical Aspects. NATO ASI Series A: Life Sciences,* vol. 263. (Maragoudakis, M. E., Gullino, P. M., and Lelkes, P. I., eds.), Plenum, New York, pp. 149–170.
114. Mandriota, S. J., Seghezzi, G., Vassalli, J.-D., Ferrara, N., Wasi, S., Mazzieri, R., et al. (1995) Vascular endothelial growth factor increases urokinase receptor expression in vascular endothelial cells. *J. Biol. Chem.* **270,** 9709–9716.
115. Yoshida, A., Anand-Apte, B., and Zetter, B. R. (1996) Differential endothelial migration and proliferation to basic fibroblast growth factor and vascular endothelial growth factor. *Growth Factors* **13,** 57–64.
115a. Mandriota, S. J. and Pepper, M. S. (1997) Vascular endothelial growth factor-induced in vitro angiogenesis and plasminogen activator expression are dependent on endogenous basic fibroblast growth factor. *J. Cell Sci.* **110,** 2293–2302.
116. Krnacik-Coleman, S. and Rosen, J. M. (1994) Differential temporal and spatial gene expression of fibroblast growth factor family members during mouse mammary gland development. *Mol. Endocrinol.* **8,** 218–229.
117. Christofori, G. and Hanahan, D. (1994) Molecular dissection of multi-stage tumorigenesis in transgenic mice. *Semin. Cancer Biol.* **5,** 3–12.
118. Pepper, M. S., Vassalli, J.-D., Orci, L., and Montesano, R. (1993) Biphasic effect of transforming growth factor-beta 1 on in vitro angiogenesis. *Exp. Cell Res.* **204,** 356–363.
119. Gajdusek, C. M., Luo, Z., and Mayberg, M. R. (1993) Basic fibroblast growth factor and transforming growth factor beta-1: synergistic mediators of angiogenesis in vitro. *J. Cell Physiol.* **157,** 133–144.
120. Merwin, J.R., Newman, W., Beall, L. D., Tucker, A., and Madri, J. (1991a) Vascular cells respond differentially to transforming growth factors beta1 and beta2 in vitro. *Am. J. Pathol.* **138,** 37–51.
121. Merwin, J. R., Roberts, A., Kondaiah, P., Tucker, A., and Madri, J. (1991b) Vascular cell responses to TGF-β3 mimick those of TGF-β1 in vitro. *Growth Factors* **5,** 149–158.
122. Heimark, R. L., Twardzik, D. R., and Schwartz, S. M. (1986) Inhibition of endothelial regeneration by type-beta transforming growth factor from platelets. *Science* **233,** 1078–1080.
123. Müller, G., Behrens, J., Nussbaumer, U., Böhlen, P., and Birchmeier, W. (1987) Inhibitory action of transforming growth factor-β on endothelial cells. *Proc. Natl. Acad. Sci. USA* **84,** 5600–5604.
124. Mignatti, P., Tsuboi, R., Robbins, E., and Rifkin, D. B. (1989) In vitro angiogenesis on the human amniotic membrane: requirements for basic fibroblast growth factor-induced proteases. *J. Cell Biol.* **108,** 671–682.
125. Myoken, Y., Kan, M., Sato, G. H., McKeehan, W. L., and Sato, D. (1990) Bifunctional effects of transforming growth factor-β (TGF-β) on endothelial cell growth correlate with phenotypes of TGF-β binding sites. *Exp. Cell Res.* **191,** 299–304.

126. Pepper, M. S., Belin, D., Montesano, R., Orci, L., and Vassalli, J.-D. (1990) Transforming growth factor beta-1 modulates basic fibroblast growth factor-induced proteolytic and angiogenic properties of endothelial cells in vitro. *J. Cell Biol.* **111,** 743–755.

127. Pepper, M. S. and Montesano, R. (1990) Proteolytic balance and capillary morphogenesis. *Cell Differ. Dev.* **32,** 319–328.

128. Pepper, M. S., Montesano, R., Mandriota, S., Orci, L., and Vassalli, J.-D. (1996b) Angiogenesis: a paradigm for balanced extracellular proteolysis during cell migration and morphogenesis. *Enzyme Protein* **49,** 138–162.

129. Deng, G., Curriden, S. A., Wang, S., Rosenberg, S., and Loskutoff, D. J. (1996) Is plasminogen activator inhibitor-1 the molecular switch that governs urokinase receptor-mediated cell adhesion and release ? *J. Cell. Biol.* **134,** 1563–1571.

130. Stefansson S. and Lawrence, D. A. (1996) The serpin PAI-1 inhibits cell migration by blocking integrin $\alpha_v\beta_3$ binding to vitronectin. *Nature* **383,** 441–443.

131. Giancotti, F. G. and Ruoslahti, E. (1990) Elevated levels of the $\alpha_5\beta_1$ fibronectin receptor suppress the transformed phenotype of Chinese hamster ovary cells. *Cell* **60,** 849–859.

132. Huttenlocher, A., Ginsberg, M. H., and Horwitz, A. F. (1996) Modulation of cell migration by integrin-mediated cytoskeletal linkages and ligand-binding affinity. *J. Cell Biol.* **134,** 1551–1562.

133. Montesano, R., Kumar, S., Orci, L., and Pepper, M. S. (1996) Synergistic effect of hyaluronan oligosaccharides and vascular endothelial growth factor on angiogenesis in vitro. *Lab. Invest.* **75,** 249–262.

133a. Collo, G. and Pepper, M. S. (1999) Endothelial cell integrin $\alpha5\beta1$ expression is modulated by cytokines and during migration in vitro. *J. Cell Sci.* **112,** 569–578.

133b. Slevin, M., Krupinski, J., Kumas, S., and Gaffney, J. (1998) Angiogenic oligosaccharides of hyaluronan induce protein tyrosine kinase activity in andothelial cells and activate a cytoplasmic signal transduction pathway resulting in proliferation. *Lab. Invest.* **78,** 987–1003.

134. Rooney, P., Kumar, S., Ponting, J., and Wang, M. (1995) The role of hyaluronan in tumor neovascularization. *Int. J. Cancer* **60,** 632–636.

135. Sattar, A., Kumar, S., and West, D. C. (1992) Does hyaluronan have a role in endothelial cell proliferation of the synovium? *Semin. Arthr. Rheum.* **22,** 37–43.

136. Bourguignon, L. Y. W., Lokeshwar, V. B., He, J., Chen, X., and Bourguignon, G. J. (1992) A CD44-like endothelial cell transmembrane glycoprotein (GP 116) interacts with extracellular matrix and ankyrin. *Mol. Cell. Biol.* **12,** 4464–4471.

137. Banerjee, S. D. and Toole, B. P. (1992) Hyaluronan-binding protein in endothelial cell morphogenesis. *J. Cell Biol.* **119,** 643–652.

138. Lokeshwar, V. B., Iida, N., and Bourguinon, L. Y. W. (1996) The cell adhesion molecule, GP 116, is a new CD44 variant (ex14/v10) involved in hyaluronic acid binding and endothelial proliferation. *J. Biol. Chem.* **271,** 23,853–23,864.

139. Laurent, T. C. and Fraser, J. R. E. (1992) Hyaluronan. *FASEB J.* **6,** 2397–2404.

140. Lokeshwar, V. B., Lokeshwar, B. L., Pham, H. T., and Block, N. L. (1996) Association of elevated levels of hyaluronidase, a matrix-degrading enzyme, with prostate cancer progression. *Cancer Res.* **56,** 651–657.

141. Liu, D., Pearlman, E., Diaconu, E., Guo, K., Mori, H., Haqqi, T., et al. (1996) Expression of hyaluronidase by tumor cells induces angiogenesis in vivo. *Proc. Natl. Acad. Sci. USA* **93,** 7832–7837.

142. Davis, S., Aldrich, T. H., Jones, P. F., Acheson, A., Compton, D. L., Jain, V., et al. (1996) Isolation of angiopoietin-1, a ligand for the TIE2 receptor, by secretion-trap expression cloning. *Cell* **87,** 1161–1169.

143. Dumont D. J., Gradwohl, G., Fong, G.-H., Puri, M., Gertsenstein, M., Auerbach, A., and Breitmen, M. (1994) Dominant-negative and targeted null mutations in the endothelial receptor tyrosine kinase, *tek,* reveal a critical role in vasculogenesis of the embryo. *Genes Dev.* **8,** 1897–1909.

144. Sato, T. N., Tozawa, Y., Deutsch, U., Wolburg-Buchholz, K., Fujiwara, Y., Gendron-Maguire, M., et al. (1995) Distinct roles of the receptor tyrosine kinases Tie-1 and Tie-2 in blood vessel formation. *Nature* **367,** 70–74.

145. Suri, C., Jones, P. F., Patan, S., Bartunkova, S., Maisonpierre, P. C., Davis, S., et al. (1996) Requisite role of angiopoietin-1, a ligand for the TIE2 receptor, during embryonic angiogenesis. *Cell* **87,** 1171–1180.

146. Shovlin, C. L. and Scott, J. (1996) Inhertied diseases of the vasculature. *Annu. Rev. Physiol.* **58,** 483–507.

147. Vikkula, M., Boon, L. M., Carraway, K. L., Calvert, J. T., Diamonti, A. J., Goumnerov, B., et al. (1996) Vascular dysmorphogenesis caused by an activating mutation in the receptor tyrosine kinase TIE2. *Cell* **87,** 1181–1190.

148. Whelan, A. J., Watson, M. S., Porter, F. D., and Steiner, R. D. (1995) Klippel-Trenaunay-Weber syndrome associated with a 5:11 balanced translocation. *Am. J. Med. Genet.* **59,** 492–494.

149. Dubovsky, J., Zabramski, J. M., Kurth, J., Spetzler, R. F., Rich, S. S., Orr, H. T., and Weber J. L. (1995) A gene responsible for cavernous malformations of the brain maps to chromosome 7q. *Hum. Mol. Genet.* **4,** 453–458.

150. Günel, M., Awad, I. A., Anson, J., and Lifton, R. P. (1995) Mapping a gene causing cerebral cavernous malformation to 7q11.2-q21. *Proc. Natl. Acad. Sci. USA* **92,** 6620–6624.

151. Marchuk, D. A., Gallione, C. J., Morrison, L. A., Clericuzio, C. L., Hart, B. L., Kosofsky, B. E., et al. (1995) A locus for cerebral cavernous malformations maps to chromosome 7q in two families. *Genomics* **28,** 311–314.

3

The Angiopoietins

Pamela F. Jones

CONTENTS

INTRODUCTION

Signaling mechanisms responsible for the formation and maintenance of a healthy, mature vasculature are not clearly understood. Vascularization occurs by two distinct processes: vasculogenesis, occurring only during embryogenesis, and angiogenesis, which comprises remodeling of the primitive embryonic network into the complex system of large and small vessels (reviewed in ref. *1*). Angiogenesis persists throughout adulthood, although there is relatively little remodeling of blood vessels, other than in the ovary and uterus throughout the menstrual cycle, placenta formation, and wound healing. There are undoubtedly numerous interactions between the balance of angiogenic inducers and inhibitors, working in concert to maintain the mature vasculature (reviewed in ref. *2*). Vessel sprouting, branching, and regression are all normal functions within vascular remodeling, requiring different combinations of positive and negative regulators. Orchestration of such a mixture of signals and responses must itself be a very complex process. Vascular dysfunctions potentially give rise to several pathological situations, including solid tumor growth, atherosclerosis, and diabetic retinopathy.

IDENTIFICATION OF THE ANGIOPOIETINS

Because receptor tyrosine kinase (RTK) signaling systems are fundamental in the proliferation of many cell types, attention focussed on endothelial cell-specific RTKs and their ligands as mediators of the endothelial-cell proliferation and differentiation necessary for angiogenesis (reviewed in ref. *3*). The vascular endothelial growth factor (VEGF) family and their associated receptors remain by far the best-characterized endothelial cell-specific receptor tyrosine kinase signaling systems, and are extensively described in

From: *The New Angiotherapy*
Edited by: T.-P. D. Fan and E. C. Kohn © Humana Press Inc., Totowa, NJ

the preceding chapter by Pepper et al. Mice defective for VEGF receptors show impaired vasculogenesis and angiogenesis (4,5). Mice containing a null mutation in the VEGF gene undergo some differentiation resulting in abnormal vasculature (6).

The Tie receptors, originally identified by polymerase chain reaction (PCR) between conserved regions of the tyrosine kinase domains, represent the only other known family of endothelial cell-specific receptors (7–15). This family comprises Tie1 (tyrosine kinase with immunoglobulin and epidermal growth factor homology domains) and Tie2, also known as tek (tunica interna endothelial cell kinase). Both Tie1 and Tie2 have been shown to be critically involved in vascularization. These RTKs show differences in their expression patterns; Tie2 expression is limited to the endothelium, whereas Tie1 is expressed in both endothelial cells and early hematopoietic cells (16–22). Both Tie1 and Tie2 are essential for normal development, as disruption of either gene is lethal. Disruption of Tie1 gene expression leads to edema and hemorrhaging, owing to disruption in the integrity of blood vessels (23,24). Mice deficient for Tie-2 die during development, at around E10.5, with defects in the remodeling of the primary vascular network, most prominent in the development of the endocardium of the heart (24,25).

Though Tie2 was first discovered in 1992, its ligand was only recently identified through the development of secretion-trap expression cloning (26). A source of Tie2 ligand was identified through the use of a probe molecule constructed from the ectodomain of human Tie2 fused to the Fc region of a human immunoglobulin. The recombinant fusion protein was coupled to the surface of a biosenor chip and used to screen media conditioned by a variety of cell lines. RNAs purified from two cell lines that gave specific binding to the probe molecule were used to construct cDNA libraries in the expression vector pJFE14. It had previously been demonstrated (27) that surface-bound molecules could be detected in COS cells using receptor-Fc fusion proteins, and hence that such molecules could be cloned. Because the ligand for Tie2 was known to be a secreted protein (as it had been detected in conditioned media), the cloning method had to be altered slightly in order to trap the ligand en route to the cell surface. Plasmid DNA was purified from each clone identified in the primary screen and amplified to produce an enriched pool. Subsequent rounds of COS cell transfection and staining identified positive pools, and these cycles continued until individual clones were isolated.

The ligand for Tie2, termed Angiopoietin-1, was cloned from both mouse and human, and shown to specifically recognize and bind to the Tie2 receptor (26). Angiopoietin-1 was shown by tyrosine phosphorylation assays to cause ligand-dependent activation of Tie2. However, Angiopoietin-1 has no apparent mitogenic effect on endothelial cells in culture. Similarly, Angiopoietin-1 had no effect on other angiogenic assays such as migration of endothelial cells, or their formation into tubules. Because other angiogenic factors, such as VEGF, induce dramatic cell proliferation, migration, and tubule-forming responses, it appears that Angiopoietin-1 must have a mode of action distinct from that of VEGF.

Following the identification and initial characterization of Angiopoietin-1, a second member of this protein family, Angiopoietin-2, was identified in both human and mouse by low-stringency homology cloning (28). Surprisingly, although Angiopoietin-2 shows ~60% identity to Angiopoietin-1 and binds to Tie2 with the same affinity, it does not elicit a phosphorylation response in the Tie2 receptor in endothelial cells (28). Moreover, in the context of an endothelial cell, Angiopoietin-2 acts as a functional antagonist of Angiopoietin-1, by inhibition of the Angiopoietin-1-dependent phosphorylation of the Tie2 receptor. However, fibroblasts stably expressing transfected Tie2 show receptor phosphorylation in response to

Angiopoietin-2. This suggests that endothelial cells can somehow discriminate between the two angiopoietins. This discriminatory ability of an endothelial cell has also been observed in studies where Angiopoietin-1 has been shown to act as a specific chemoattractant for endothelium in culture. Angiopoietin-2 acts as an antagonist, inhibiting the Angiopoietin-1-induced migration. However, fibroblasts stably transfected with Tie2 are chemotactic towards Angiopoietin-1, as well as Angiopoietin-2 *(29)*.

Further members of the angiopoietin family, which also recognize and specifically bind the Tie2 receptor, have recently been identified through low-stringency library-screening techniques *(30)*. Human Angiopoietin-1 and Angiopoietin-2 cDNA probes were used at low stringency to probe mouse genomic BAC library arrays leading to the identification of a novel sequence, subsequently termed Angiopoietin-3. A short genomic fragment was then used to obtain the full-length cDNA. Angiopoietin-4 was identified in a similar manner in a human genomic BAC library array and was subsequently cloned from human ovary cDNA. All four angiopoietins identified to date share a similar domain structure with an *N*-terminal region, an α-helical coiled-coil region, and a *C*-terminal fibrinogen-like domain.

Mouse Angiopoietin-3 and human Angiopoietin-4 are thought to represent orthologs of each other despite being more divergent than the other members of the family. Angiopoietin-1 and Angiopoietin-2 show 99 and 87% identity, respectively, between the human and mouse orthologs, whereas Angiopoietin-3 and Angiopoietin-4 are 54% identical. Human Angiopoietin-1 and Angiopoietin-2 map to distinct chrosomomal locations, 8q22.3-23 and 8p23 respectively *(31)*. Human Angiopoietin-4 has been mapped to chrosomosome 20p13.1 *(32)* and Angiopoietin-3 maps to a syntenic position of mouse chromsome 2 *(30)*. Continued efforts to identify orthologs of Angiopoietin-3 and Angiopoietin-4 have as yet not revealed any further angiopoietins, and hence the current hypothesis is that Angiopoietin-3 is the murine counterpart of Angiopoietin-4. Interestingly, Angiopoietin-3 and Angiopoietin-4, while showing more divergence in their amino acid sequence, are also divergent in their function. Expression studies show their tissue distributions are different, with Angiopoietin-3 more widely expressed, whereas in human, Angiopoietin-4 expression is high only in lung. In addition, endothelial Tie2 phosphorylation assays suggest that Angiopoietin-4 acts as an agonist, and Angiopoietin-3 as an antagonist, of the Tie2 receptor.

Angiopoietins have been identified in a variety of species in addition to the human and mouse proteins described earlier. Partial coding sequences have been identifed for bovine and rat Angiopoietin-1 and Angiopoietin-2 using a polymerase chain reaction (PCR)-based approach with degenerate oligos synthesized to regions conserved between human and mouse *(33)*. Chicken Angiopoietin-1 and a partial clone of chicken Angiopoietin-2 have been identified on the basis of low-stringency hybridizations using human Angiopoietin-1 and Angiopoietin-2 cDNA probes *(34)*. The high degree of conservation seen between human and mouse Angiopoietins-1 and -2 is also seen in the chicken orthologs. Human and chicken Angiopoietin-1 show 91% amino acid identity (human and mouse show 99%); chicken and human Angiopoietin-2 show 87% amino acid identity (human and mouse show 87%). Chicken Angiopoietin-1 and angiopoietin- 2 are 62% identical. The high degree of homology seen between the human and chicken orthologs, together with the degree of homology between Angiopoietin-1 and Angiopoietin-2 within species, again questions whether Angiopoietin-3 is the true ortholog of Angiopoietin-4. The identification of the chicken orthologs of Angiopoietin-3 and/or Angiopoietin-4, or the identification of angiopoietins in lower species, might help elucidate this enigma.

The protein sequence of the angiopoietins suggests that these proteins might function as multimers. α-helical coiled-coil domains have a tendency to multimerize *(35)*, and hence any angiopoietin has the potential to form multimers. It is also possible that the angiopoietins are capable of forming heterodimers in regions where multiple family members are expressed. For instance, Angiopoietin-1 and Angiopoietin-2 are both expressed at high levels in the placenta, and hence could potentially form hetero-multimers. Indeed, it has been shown that in the context of a hematopoietic cell stably expressing Tie2, a combination of Angiopoietin-1 and Angiopoietin-2 binds to the receptor better than either ligand alone *(36)*. The identification of Angiopoietin-3 and Angiopoietin-4 increase the potential number of heterodimers and multimers that may form, and increase the time- and tissue-specific repertoire that may be available.

It is possible that Tie1 and Tie2 can themselves form heterodimers in areas, such as endothelial cells, where both receptors are expressed. No ligands have as yet been identifed for Tie1, despite much effort expended on their isolation. Structural similarities between the extracellular domains of Tie1 and Tie2 suggest that their ligands may be very similar. It is plausible that the angiopoietins in some form are capable of binding to Tie1. It is known that these ligands cannot bind directly to Tie1 itself, but there may be some other component expressed in endothelial cells, that enables this interaction. Such a component may also be the discriminatory factor causing Angiopoietin-1 to act as an agonist, and Angiopoietin-2 to act as an antagonist. It is also possible that Tie2 presents bound ligand in a form that Tie1 can recognize and bind, and that it is a combination of receptors that permits signaling from Tie1 receptor. Given the apparent co-expression of Tie1 and Tie2 on endothelial cells, and the suggestion of multiple splice forms of both Tie1 and Tie2, it is conceivable that there is a set of receptor combinations whose composition may also be time- and tissue-dependent. The ability of an endothelial cell to respond to the binding of any of the angiopoietins, or multimers thereof, may alter as the combination of available receptors is altered.

BIOLOGICAL ROLES OF THE ANGIOPOIETINS

Although the direct biological activities of the angiopoietins remain unclear, there is mounting evidence to suggest that they are involved in the recruitment and stabilization of nonendothelial cells into the vessel wall. This evidence is accumulating from a variety of studies, including expression studies, in particular *in situ* hybridization analyses of ovary and more recently of a glioma tumor model, and detailed analyses of the expression patterns of the angiopoetins in both normal and genetically manipulated mice. Direct functional data, which are limited owing to the recent identification of this family of angiogenic factors, are accumulating from vascularization studies such as the mouse corneal pocket assay of neovascularization and the rabbit ischaemic limb assay of revascularization.

Northern analyses have shown that Angiopoietin-1 is quite widely expressed; mRNA can be detected in a variety of adult tissues including brain, small intestine, prostate, ovary, uterus, and placenta. Expression of Angiopoietin-2 appears to be very limited and is detected only in tissues that undergo vascular remodeling, such as ovary, uterus, and placenta *(28)*. Angiopoetin-3 is expressed in a wide range of tissues including heart, kidney, testis, lung, and liver; the highest level of Angiopoietin-4 is seen in the lung, with weaker expression detectable in a wider range of tissues *(30)*.

Normal functioning of the ovary is dependent on cyclic angiogenesis, causing hypervascularization of the corpus luteum, followed by vessel regression as the corpus luteum ages. *In situ* data show that the expression of Angiopoietin-1 is closely associated with the formation of mature blood vessels *(28)*. Angiopoietin-2 is expressed at sites of vessel invasion, at the leading edge of invading endothelial cells, where high levels of VEGF are also detected. VEGF is expressed through most of the ovarian cycle, except during regression of neovasculature of the corpus luteum *(37)*. During this stage, levels of Angiopoietin-2 are at their highest. These expression data suggest a role for the angiopoietins in the stabilization and destabilization of vasculature.

In situ hybridizations of E9-E11 mouse embryos show the prominent expression of Angiopoietin-1 in heart myocardium surrounding the endocardium *(38)*. Genetically engineered mice defective for Angiopoietin-1 expression die at embryonic day 12.5, showing defects in their vasculature reminiscent to those seen in mice lacking the Tie2 receptor, which die at embryonic day 10.5. This is most obvious in the development of the heart, which shows a much less intricately folded endocardium. The poor association between endothelial cells and the underlying matrix and failure to recruit and associate with periendothelial supporting cells, seen in both Angiopoietin-1$^{-/-}$ and Tie-2$^{-/-}$ mice, suggest this signaling serves at least in part to regulate endothelial-matrix interactions. A similar phenotype is seen in mice where overexpression of Angiopoietin-2 is driven by the endothelial-specific Tie-2 promoter. This overexpression causes the mice to die during development, with vascular defects observable by E9.5 *(38)*. These vascular defects, and in particular the apparent collapse and detachment of the endocardium from the myocardial layer in the heart, are very similar to those seen in Angiopoietin-1$^{-/-}$ and Tie-2$^{-/-}$ embryos. These observations support a role for Angiopoietin-1 in mediating interaction between endothelial cells and the underlying matrix, and support the hypothesis that Angiopoietin-2 is a functional antagonist of Angiopoietin-1, and thus destabilizes these interactions.

Further information about the role of Angiopoietin-1 has been obtained from genetically manipulated mice where overexpression of Angiopoietin-1 has been placed under the control of the keratin 14 gene promoter *(39)*. Transgenic mice overexpresing Angiopoietin in the skin are viable, but show a dramatic increase in the number, size, and branching pattern of blood vessels. Furthermore, Angiopoietin-1 has been shown to act as an chemoattractant for cultured endothelial cells *(29)*. Mice deficient for Tie2 show defective capillary sprouting in the neural tube; consistent with this is the finding that Angiopoietin-1 has the ability to induce capillary sprouting in vitro *(40)*. These observations suggest that although Angiopoietin-1, unlike VEGF, does not stimulate the proliferation of endothelial cells, it is capable of exerting a pro-angiogenic effect on the endothelium.

The mouse cornea micropocket assay of neovascularization has been used to show that neither Angiopoietin-1 nor Angiopoietin-2 alone affects the angiogenic response. However, when co-administered with VEGF, both angiopoietins were capable of enhancing the formation of blood vessels *(41)*. Treatment with VEGF and Angiopoietin-1 together caused an overall increase in the number of blood vessels, whereas Angiopoietin-2 plus VEGF affected the overall length of the vessels, and the number of endothelial cells at the leading edge of migration. Both these observations are consistent with the hypothesis that Angiopoietin-1 acts to stabilize mature vasculature, whereas Angiopoietin-2 acts to destabilize vasculature, leaving the endothelial cells open to respond to other pro-angiogenic factors such as VEGF.

Injection of naked DNA encoding VEGF directly into ischaemic muscle has previously been shown to augment revascularization into the area *(42)*. Similar treatment with Angiopoietin-1 has also shown increased vascularization into ischaemic areas *(43)*, whereas

Angiopoietin-2 has no apparent effect, consistent with its lack of chemoattractant activity *(29)*. It is interesting that both VEGF and Angiopoietin-1 show a similar effect on the ischaemic limb, although classic angiogenic assays show they must have a very different modes of action. Typically, angiogenic factors have been defined as those with mitogenic activity on endothelial cells: VEGF elicits a robust proliferation response on endothelium in culture, whereas none of the angiopoietins have a detectable effect. It is plausible that angiopoietin exerts its revascularization effects through its chemoattractant activity. However, it is also possible that Angiopoietin-1 acts in synergy with the elevated levels of VEGF that are induced by the hypoxic conditions caused by ischaemia *(44,45)*.

It is interesting that Angiopoietin-2 has no apparent inhibitory effect on the revascularization of the ischaemic limb. It has previously been postulated that the role of Angiopoietin-2 is in the disruption of stabilized vasculature to allow vessel sprouting or regression *(46)*. However, the inhibitory effect of Angiopoietin-2, as observed by receptor phosphorylation assays occurs when there is approx 10-fold more Angiopoietin-2 than Angiopoietin-1 *(28)*. Similarly, in the context of a hematopoietic cell stably expressing Tie2 receptors, a mixture of Angiopoietin-1 and a 10-fold molar excess of Angiopoietin-2 has been shown to bind 5–6 times more efficiently than the individual angiopoietins alone *(36)*. Hence the apparent lack of effect of Angiopoietin-2 on revascularization of the ischaemic limb may be owing to the Angiopoietin-2:Angiopoietin-1 ratio not being sufficiently high to be inhibitory. Conversely, in the light of the apparent synergy between Angiopoietin-2 and VEGF seen in the cornea micropocket assay *(41)*, it might be expected that the raised VEGF levels caused by hypoxia within the ischaemic limb would act in concert with Angiopoietin-2 to cause elongation of the revascularizing vessels.

That blood-vessel growth is required for tumor growth and metastasis is well documented *(47)*. Without an adequate blood supply, tumor cells become necrotic and potential tumors either die or remain dormant as a stable cell population, with dying cells replaced by new ones. It has generally been accepted that vascularization of a tumor occurs when angiogenic factors are expressed within the tumor, and these factors cause the proliferation and migration of normal endothelial cells towards that tumor *(48)*. However, there is increasing evidence that some tumors do not initially grow avascularly, but instead employ existing vessels for their blood supply *(49,50)*.

A recent study of the role of the angiopoietins in tumor angiogenesis, using the rat C6 glioma model, has shown that existing blood vessels are used to support the initial growth of the tumor. However, it appears that these co-opted vessels do not continue to support tumor growth, but rather undergo vessel regression concomitant with high levels of Angiopoietin-2 expression *(51)*. This leads to cell death of a large proportion of cells in the center of the tumor, which may be a natural defense against tumor growth. Angiogenesis then occurs at the periphery of the tumor, leading to vascularization amd continued growth of the tumor. These findings were also seen with an unrelated tumor model, the rat RBA mammary carcinoma, where increased Angiopoietin-2 expression reflected vessel regression. While Angiopoietin-2 and VEGF expression levels were both elevated, the level of Angiopoietin-1 mRNA appeared to be variable, and dependent on the tumor type. Low levels of Angiopoietin-1 would be expected in areas where regression of the vasculature occurs continually, because stablized, mature vessels would not be forming.

Tie2 expression has been shown to be upregulated in the endothelium of human gliomas, the most common and highly vascularized human brain tumor, which are known to overexpress VEGF. Angiopoietin mRNA levels are also increased, but in a cell type-specific manner *(52)*.

Angiopoietin-1 mRNA is expressed in the tumor cells, whereas Angiopoietin-2 mRNA is detected in the endothelial cells of a subset of glioblastoma blood vessels. The highest level of Angiopoietin-2 mRNA is seen in the small, actively growing capillaries. These studies suggest that Angiopoietin-2 may be an early marker of tumor angiogenesis, and hence may play a diagnostic role in the early identification of tumors and metastases. Given the elevated levels of VEGF also detected in these tumors, it appears likely that Angiopoietin-2 and VEGF act in synergy, leading to a rapid rate of capillary growth.

It is becoming increasingly apparent that the angiopoietins and VEGF act in a co-ordinated manner in the formation of vasculature. Owing to their opposing actions on the same receptor tyrosine kinase, it is proposed that Angiopoietin-1 affects the stability of the newly formed vessels, thus facilitating their formation, whereas Angiopoietin-2 destabilizes the existing vessels. The expression patterns show that Angiopoietin-2 is upregulated first, rendering the endothelium responsive to the later upregulation of VEGF. Angiopoietin-1 is expressed at a later point, causing stabilization of the newly formed vasculature. In the corneal micropocket model, Angiopoietin-1 and Angiopoietin-2 both individually failed to evoke an angiogenic response, whereas co-administration of either with VEGF resulted in augmented formation of new blood vessels. Hence Angiopoietin-1 and Angiopoietin-2 can both act in synergy with VEGF, albeit through different mechanisms. In the rat ischaemic limb model, Angiopoietin-1 has been shown to augment revascularization, whereas Angiopoietin-2 has no apparent effect. Because the hypoxic conditions present in the ischaemic limb cause elevation of VEGF, it might be expected that treatment with Angiopoietin-2 would also stimulate revascularization, in a similar manner to that seen in the corneal model. However, the two models are very different: the endothelial cells in the cornea and the hindlimb may express a different repertoire of factors involved in angiogeneisis, and hence may respond differently to VEGF, Angiopoietin-1, and Angiopoietin-2, either alone, or in combination. Also, the corneal micropocket assay does not induce an inflammatory response, such as is seen in other vascularisation models *(53)*. The presence (or absence) of a large infiltrate of neutrophils and macrophages, which themselves produce a wide range of factors, would undoubtedly influence the response to various exogenous angiogenic factors.

Do the angiopoietins represent a means of specifically targeting anti-angiogenic therapy? In the light of Angiopoietin-2 being an early marker of tumor angiogenesis, it would seem a reasonable candidate. However, if a tumor co-opts existing blood vessels, which then undergo regression, a considerable number of tumor cells are already destined to die. Blocking the action of Angiopoietin-2 would reduce this and hence appear to be less beneficial than enhancing its action. Furthermore, because Angiopoietin-1 and Angiopoietin-2 apparently have opposing actions in many situations, blocking the action of Angiopoietin-2 might allow greater pro-angiogenic activity by Angiopoietin-1. It is possible to target both Angiopoietin-1 and Angiopoietin-2 simultaneously, through the action of their shared receptor. If Tie2 action was blocked, one would predict, at least in the glioma model described earlier, that vascular regression, rapid growth of new vasculature, and stabilization of the new vasculature would be inhibited. Anti-tumor activity has been demonstrated using targeted expression of the extracellular domain of the Tie2 receptor. Using an adenoviral vector for systemic delivery of a soluble form of Tie2 (termed AdExTek), partial inhibition of the growth of tumors was demonstrated, as well as reduction in the number, size, and vascularization of metastases *(54)*. It has previously been shown that a similar soluble extracellular construct for VEGF R2 acts as a dominant-negative inhibitor, forming nonfunctional heterodimers with the endogenous cell-surface receptor *(55)*. A similar situation appears to be the case with AdExTeK, where the soluble form has been shown to co-immunoprecipitate with the normal form of the receptor *(54)*. Owing to accumulating evidence that the angiopoietins can act in synergy with VEGF, more complete inhibition of tumor growth might be achieved if both the VEGF receptor as well as the Tie2 receptor were targeted simultaneously.

SUMMARY

The angiopoietins represent a novel family of angiogenic factors critical for the formation and maintenance of the mature vascular system. That structurally related proteins that recognize and bind to the same cell-surface tyrosine kinase receptor is unprecedented in vertebrates and questions the need of Tie2 and its signaling pathway(s) for such precise signaling mechanism. The precise regulation of Angiopoietin-2 expression, both spatially and temporally, suggests a precise requirement of Tie2 for a signaling "off" switch. It is becoming clear that the angiopoietins and VEGF act in concert in some systems, highlighting the need for co-ordinated actions between vascular signaling molecules. This in turn implies that to disrupt vascularization effectively, multiple pathways need to be targeted simultaneously.

ACKNOWLEDGMENTS

I am grateful to Dr. Adam Craig for constructive criticisms and discussions. Research in the author's laboratory is supported by Yorkshire Cancer Research, British Heart Foundation, Medical Research Council, and the Royal Society.

REFERENCES

1. Risau, W. (1997) Mechanisms of angiogenesis. *Nature* **386,** 671–674.
2. Folkman, J. and D'Amore, P. A. (1996) Blood vessel formation: what is its molecular basis? *Cell* **87,** 1153–1155.
3. Mustonen, T. and Alitalo, K. (1995) Endothelial receptor tyrosine kinases involved in angiogenesis. *J. Cell Biol.* **129,** 895–896.
4. Shalaby, F., Rossant, J., Yamaguchi, T. P., Gertsernstein, M., Wu, X-F., Breitman, M., and Schuh, A. C. (1995) Failure of blood island formation and vasculogenesis in Flk-1-deficient mice. *Nature* **376,** 62–66.
5. Fong, G-H., Rossant, J., Gertsenstein, M., and Breitman, M. L. (1995) Role of the flt-1 receptor tyrosine kinase in regulating the assembly of vascular endothelium. *Nature* **376,** 66–70.
6. Carmeliet, P., Ferreira, V., Breier, G., Pollefeyt, S., Kieckens, L., Gertsenstein, M., et al. (1996) Abnormal blood vessel development and lethality in embryos lacking a single VEGF allele. *Nature* **380,** 435–439.
7. Dumont, D. J., Yamaguchi, T. P., Conlon, R. A., Rossant, J., and Breitman, M. L. (1992) Tek, a novel tyrosine kinase gene located on mouse chromosome 4, is expressed in endothelial cells and their presumptive precursors. *Oncogene* **7,** 1471–1480.
8. Dumont, D. J., Gradwohl, G., Fong, G.-H., Auerbach, A., and Breitman, M. L. (1993) The endothelial - specific receptor tyrosine kinase, tek, is a member of a new subfamily of receptors. *Oncogene* **8,** 1293–1301.
9. Iwama, A., Hamaguchi, I., Hashiyama, M., Murayama, Y., Yasunaga, K., and Suda, T. (1993) Molecular cloning and characterisation of mouse TIE and TEK receptor tyrosine kinase genes and their expression in hematopoietic stem cells. *BBRC* **195,** 301–309.
10. Maisonpierre, P. C., Goldfarb, M., Yancopoulos, G. D., and Gao, G. (1993) Distinct rat genes with related profiles of expression define a TIE receptor tyrosine kinase family. *Oncogene* **8,** 1631–1637.
11. Partanen, J., Armstrong, E., Makela, T. P., Korhonen, J., Sandberg, M., Renkonen, R., et al. (1992) A novel endothelial cell surface receptor tyrosine kinase with extracellular epidermal growth factor homology domains. *Mol. Cell. Biol.* **12,** 1698–1707.
12. Runting, A. S., Stacker, S. A., and Wilks, A. F. (1993) Tie2, a putative protein tyrosine kinase from a new class of cell surface receptor. *Growth Factors* **9,** 99–105.

13. Sato, T. N., Qin, Y., Kozak, C. A., and Audus, K. L. (1993) Tie-1 and tie-2 define another class of putative receptor tyrosine kinase genes expressed in early embryonic vascular system. *Proc. Natl. Acad. Sci. USA* **90,** 9355–9358.

14. Schnurch, H. and Risau, W. (1993) Expression of tie-2, a member of a novel family of receptor tyrosine kinases, in the endothelial cell lineage. *Development* **119,** 957–968.

15. Ziegler, S. F., Bird, T. A., Schneringer, J. A., Schooley, K. A., and Baum, P. R. (1993) Molecular cloning and characterization of a novel receptor protein tyrosine kinase from human placenta. *Oncogene* **8,** 663–670.

16. Armstrong, E., Korhonen, J., Silvennoinen, O., Cleveland, J. L., Lieberman, M. A., and Alitalo, R. (1993) Expression of tie receptor tyrosine kinase in leukaemia cell lines. *Leukemia* **7,** 1585–1591.

17. Batard, P., Sansilvestri, P., Scheinecker, C., Knapp, W., Debili, N., Vainchenker, W., et al. (1996) The tie receptor tyrosine kinase is expressed by human hematopoietic progenitor cells and by a subset of megakaryocytic cells. *Blood* **87,** 2212–2220.

18. Dumont D. J., Fong, G.-H., Puri, M. C., Gradwohl, G., Alitalo, K., and Breitman, M. L. (1995) Vascularisation of the mouse embryo: a study of flk-1, tek, tie and vascular endothelial growth factor expression during development. *Dev. Dyn.* **203,** 80–92.

19. Korhonen, J., Partanen, J., Armstrong, E., Vaahtokari, A., Elenius, K., Jalkanen, M., and Alitalo, K. (1992) Enhanced expression of the tie receptor tyrosine kinase in endothelial cells during neovascularisation. *Blood* **80,** 2548–2555.

20. Korhonen, J., Polvi, A., Partanen, J., and Alitalo, K. (1994) The mouse tie receptor tyrosine kinase gene: expression during embryonic angiogenesis. *Oncogene* **9,** 395–403.

21. Larsson-Blomberg, L. and Dzierzak, E. (1994) Isolation of tyrosine kinase related genes expressed in the early hematopoietic system. *FEBS Lett.* **348,** 119–125.

22. Rodewald, H. R. and Sato, T. N. (1996) Tie1, a receptor tyrosine kinase essential for vascular endothelial cell integrity, is not critical for the development of haematopoietic cells. *Oncogene* **12,** 397–404.

23. Puri, M. C., Rossant, J., Alitalo, K., Bernstein, A., and Partanen, J. (1995) The receptor tyrosine kinase TIE is required for integrity and survival of vascular endothelial cells. *EMBO J.* **14,** 5884–5891.

24. Sato, T. N., Tozawa, Y., Deutsch, U., Wolburg-Buchholz, K., Fujiwara, Y., Gendron-Maguire, M., et al. (1995) Distinct roles of the receptor tyrosine kinases Tie-1 and Tie-2 in blood vessel formation. *Nature* **376,** 70–74.

25. Dumont, D. J., Gradwohl, G., Fong, G.-H., Puri, M. C., Gertsenstein, M., Auerbach, A., and Breitman, M. L. (1994) Dominant-negative and targeted null mutations in the endothelial receptor tyrosine kinase, tek, reveal a critical role in vasculogenesis of the embryo. *Genes Dev.* **8,** 1897–1909.

26. Davis, S., Aldrich, T. H., Jones, P. F., Acheson, A., Compton, D. L., Jain, V., et al. (1996) Isolation of angiopoietin-1, a ligand for the TIE2 receptor, by secretion-trap expression cloning. *Cell* **87,** 1161–1169.

27. Davis, S., Gale, N. W., Aldrich, T. H., Maisonpierre, P. C., Lhotak, V., Pawson, T., et al. (1994) Ligands for the EPH-related receptor tyrosine kinases that require membrane attachment or clustering for activity. *Science* **266,** 816–819.

28. Maisonpierre, P. C., Suri, C., Jones, P. F., Bartunkova, S., Wiegand, S. J., Radziejeskwi, C., et al. (1997) Angiopoietin-2, a natural antagonist for Tie2 that disrupts in vivo angiogenesis. *Science* **277,** 55–60.

29. Witzenbichler, B., Maisonpierre, P. C., Jones, P. F., Yancopoulos, G. D., and Isner, J. M. (1998) Chemotactic properties of angiopoietin-1 and -2, ligands for the endothelial-specific receptor tyrosine kinase Tie2. *J. Biol. Chem.* **273,** 18,514–18,521.

30. Valenzuela, D. M., Griffiths, J., Rojas, J., Aldrich, T. H., Jones, P. F., Zhou, H., et al. (1999) Angiopoietin 3 and 4: Diverging gene counterparts in mouse and man. *Proc. Natl. Acad. Sci. USA* **96,** 1904–1909.

31. Cheung, A. H., Stewart, R. J., and Marsden, P. A. (1998) Endothelial Tie2/Tek ligands angiopoietin-1 (ANGPT1) and angiopoietin-2 (ANGPT-2): regional localisation of the human genes to 8q22.3-q23 and 8p23. *Genomics* **48,** 389–391.

32. Grosios, K., Leek, J. P., Markham, A. F., Yancopoulos, G. D., and Jones, P. F. (1999) Chromosomal localisation of the gene for angiopoietin-4, a further ligand for the Tie2 receptor tyrosine kinase. *Cytogenetics and Cell Genetics* **84,** 118–120.

33. Mandriota S. J. and Pepper, M. S. (1998) Regulation of angiopoietin-2 mRNA levels in bovine microvascular endothelial cells by cytokines and hypoxia. *Circ. Res.* **83,** 852–859.

34. Jones, P. F., McClain, J., Robinson, D. M., Sato, T. N., and Yancopoulos, G. D. (1999) Identification and characterisation of the chicken cDNAs encoding the endothelial cell-specific receptor tyrosine kinase Tie2 and its ligands, the angiopoietins. *Angiogenesis* **2,** 357–364.

35. Beck, K. and Brodsky, B. (1998) Supercoiled protein motifs: the collagen triple-helix and the alpha-helical coiled coil. *J. Struct. Biol.* **122,** 17–29.

36. Sato, A., Iwama, A., Takatura, N., Nishio, H., Yancopoulos, G. D., and Suda, T. (1998) Characterization of TEK receptor tyrosine kinase and its ligands, angiopoietins, in human hematopoietic progenitor cells. *Int. Immunol.* **10,** 1217–1227.

37. Goede, V., Schmidt, T., Kimmina, S., Kozian, D., and Augustin, H. G. (1998) Analysis of blood vessel maturation processes during cyclic ovarian angiogenesis. *Lab. Invest.* **78,** 1385–1394.

38. Suri, C., Jones. P. F., Patan, S., Bartunkova, S., Masonpierre, P. C., Davis, S., et al. (1996) Requisite role of angiopoietin-1, a ligand for the TIE2 receptor, during embryonic angiogenesis. *Cell* **87,** 1170–1180.

39. Suri, C., McClain, J., Thurston, G., McDonald, D. M., Zhou, H., Oldmixon, E. H., et al. (1998) Increased vascularization in mice overexpressing angiopoietin-1. *Science* **282,** 468–471.

40. Koblizek, T. I., Weiss, C., Yancopoulos, G., Deutsch, U., and Risau, W. (1998) Angiopoietin-1 induces sprouting angiogenesis in vitro. *Curr. Biol.* **8,** 529–532.

41. Asahara, T., Chen, D., Takahashi, T., Fujikawa, K., Kearney, M., Magner, M., et al. (1998) Tie2 receptor ligands, angiopoietin-1 and angiopoietin-2, modulate VEGF induced postnatal neovascularisation. *Circ. Res.* **83,** 233–240.

42. Tsurumi, Y., Takeshita, S., Chen, D., Kearney, M., Rossow, S. T., Passeri, J., et al. (1996) Direct intramuscular gene transfer of naked DNA encoding vascular endothelial growth factor augments collatoral development and tissue perfusion. *Circulation* **94,** 3281–3290.

43. Shyu, G., Manor, O., Magner, M., Yancopoulos, G. D., and Isner, J. M. (1998) Direct intramuscular injection of plasmid DNA encoding angiopoioetin-1 but not angiopoioetin-2 augments revascularisation on the rabbit ischaemic hindlimb. *Circulation* **98,** 2081–2087.

44. Namiki, A., Brogi, E., Kearney, M, Wu. T., Couffinhal, T., Varticovski, L., and Isner, J. M. (1995) Hypoxia induces vascular endothelial growth factor in cultured human endothelial cells. *J. Biol. Chem.* **270,** 31,189–31,195.

45. Enholm, B., Paavonen, K., Ristimake, A., Kumar, V., Gunji, Y., Klefstrom, J., et al. (1997) Comparison of VEGF, VEGF-B, VEGF-C and Ang-1 mRNA regulation by serum, growth factors, oncoproteins and hypoxia. *Oncogene* **14,** 2475–2483.

46. Hanahan, D. (1997) Signaling vascular morphogenesis and maintenance. *Science* **277,** 48–50.

47. Folkman, J. (1995) Angiogenesis in cancer, vascular, rheumatoid and other diseases. *Nature Med.* **1,** 27–31.

48. Hanahan, D. and Folkman, J. (1996) Patterns and emerging mechanisms of the angiogenic switch during tumorigenesis. *Cell* **86,** 353–364.

49. Nagano, N., Sasaki, H., Aoyagi, M., and Horakawa, K. (1993) Invasion of experimental rat brain tumor: early morphological changes following microinjection of C6 glioma cells. *Acta Neuropathol.* **86,** 117–125.

50. Pezzella, F., Fastorino, U., Taglizbue, E., Andreola, S., Sozzi, G., et al. (1997) Non-small-cell lung carcinoma tumor growth without morphological eveidence of neo-angiogenesis. *Am. J. Pathol.* **151,** 1417–1423.

51. Holash, J., Maisonpierre, P. C., Compton, D., Boland, P., Alexander, C. R., et al. (1999) A new model of tumor angiogenesis: dynamic balance between vascular growth and regression mediated by angiopoietin and VEGF. *Science* **284,** 1994–1998.

52. Stratmann, A., Risau, R., and Plate, K. H. (1998) Cell type-specific expression of angiopoietin-1 and angiopoietin-2 suggests a role in glioblastoma angiogenesis. *Am. J. Pathol.* **153,** 1459–1466.

53. Kenyon, B. M., Voest, E. E., Chen, C. C., Flynn, E., Folkman, J., and D'Amato, R. J. (1996) A model of angiogenesis in the mouse cornea. *Invest. Ophthalmol. Vis. Sci.* **37,** 1625–1632.

54. Lin, P., Buxton, J. A., Acheson, A., Radziejewski, C., Maisonpierre, P. C., Yancopoulos, G. D., et al. (1998) Antiangiogenic gene therapy targeting the endothelium-specific receptor tyrosine kinase Tie2. *Proc. Natl. Acad. Sci. USA* **95,** 8829–8834.

55. Lin, P. N., Sankar, S., Shan, S.-Q., Dewhirst, M. W., Polverini, P. J., Quinn, T. Q., and Peters, K. G. (1997) Inhibition of tumor growth by targeting tumor endothelium using a soluble vascular endothelial growth factor receptor. *Cell Growth Differ.* **9,** 49–58.

4

Regulation of Vascular Morphogenesis by Extracellular Matrix Proteins

Amy D. Bradshaw and E. Helene Sage

CONTENTS

INTRODUCTION

Two modes of vascularization have been defined that contribute to the development of the circulatory system. Vasculogenesis is the formation of blood vessels from endothelial cells in the absence of extant vessels, whereas angiogenesis is the formation of nascent vessels via sprouting of endothelial cells associated with established vasculature (1,2). Angiogenesis can be both beneficial to an organism, e.g., during development and wound healing, as well as detrimental, as in the vascularization of solid tumors. Deciphering the mechanisms governing endothelial-cell branching, migration, and vessel formation will contribute to the understanding of many processes including vascular development, wound healing, and cancer progression.

Both vasculogenesis and angiogenesis probably share many features that lead to the assembly of vessels. In angiogenesis, endothelial cells detach from the parent vessel; subsequently, degradation of the surrounding matrix occurs to allow for migration of the endothelial cells into the surrounding tissue. Finally, proliferation and alignment of the endothelial cells lead to the formation of a new vessel with a patent lumen (3). In vasculogenesis, newly differentiated endothelial cells are not required to detach from established vessels, but other processes such as endothelial-cell migration, proliferation, alignment, and adhesion, are common to both types of vascular morphogenesis (4). The extracellular matrix (ECM) is critical to many if not all of the activities associated with

From: *The New Angiotherapy*
Edited by: T.-P. D. Fan and E. C. Kohn © Humana Press Inc., Totowa, NJ

endothelial cells in developmental vascular morphogenesis, and in normal and pathological angiogenesis (5). A better understanding of molecular mechanisms by which
matrix and matrix-associated components influence cell behavior will lead to new and
improved methods for the control of pathological vascularization. In this chapter we
review a number of proteins that have been shown as essential for vascular development or ancillary to neovascularization (Table 1). These matrix components could be
future targets of angiotherapy.

COLLAGEN I

The collagen family of proteins makes up a significant percentage of the total protein
in all vertebrates. The collagens were originally considered as primarily structural
glycoproteins that provided mechanical support for an organism. Today, the collagens
are appreciated as crucial structural components as well as important regulatory proteins
that govern cell function through a variety of signal-transduction pathways.

Collagen I mRNA is detected first in embryonic day 8.5 (E8.5) embryos in the head
mesenchyme and persists through E12 (6). Similarly, collagen I protein is detected first
in E8 mice (3–4 somites), in which staining of the head mesenchyme and the basal lamina
between head mesenchyme and ectoderm is observed (7). Collagen I expression is also
detected in the capillaries generated by the fetus in the uteri of pregnant rats (8). Mov 13
mice provide an excellent model for the analysis of collagen I function in development,
as these mice have an insertion in the Col IA1 gene and consequently do not express
collagen I in the majority of cell types (odontoblasts and osteoblasts of long bones are the
exceptions; 9,10). Homozygous embryos are viable until approx E13, when death appears
to result from weak vasculature and consequent vessel rupture (11). In fact, preliminary
studies of mov 13 homozygous brain tissue indicate a reduction in vessel number relative
to that of age-matched, wild-type brains (A. Bradshaw, L. Iruela-Arispe, and E.H. Sage,
unpublished observations). Consequently, collagen I might be an important component
of angiogenesis as well. Models of angiogenesis with cultured endothelial cells also
support the significance of collagen I in this process. An increase in expression of collagen
I is associated with bovine aortic endothelial (BAE) cells undergoing cord/tube formation,
a process considered to reflect similar morphogenic events associated with angiogenesis
in vivo (12). BAE cells that do not express collagen I do not characteristically form cords
or tubes (13). Closer examination of cord-forming BAE cells reveals the polarization of
cells as they align along collagen fibers, a prerequisite to anastomosis and the final formation of capillary-like structures. Collagen I fibers might provide a scaffold upon which
endothelial cells assemble and initiate tube formation (3). In this model, establishment of
a functional lumen for the vessel would be facilitated by the breakdown of the collagen I
and its subsequent clearing from the channel. Evidence for the importance of collagenases
in angiogenesis is supported by studies in vitro and in vivo, in which emphasis has been
placed on the degradation of matrix to promote migration of endothelial cells (14,15).
Possibly, collagenases serve both to facilitate migration and orchestrate morphological
changes of endothelial cells. Recently, Fisher et al. (16) found that inhibition of the activity
of interstitial collagenases reduced the migration of human umbilical-vein endothelial cells
into collagen gels as well as tubule formation by these angiogenic cultures.

That Mov 13 homozygous embryos might be impaired in angiogenesis could reflect
a dependence of endothelial cells on 1) collagen I itself, or 2) another component of the
extracellular milieu that requires collagen I for its matrix association. In fact, localization

Table 1

Extracellular Matrix Proteins Associated with Vascular Morphogenesis

	Essential for vascular development	Expression in vivo coincident with angiogenesis	Functional role in angiogenesis in vivo	Expression in vitro coincident with angiogenesis	Functional role in angiogenesis in vitro
Collagen I	+[a]	+	+	+	+
Fibronectin	+	+	?[b]	+	+[c]
Vitronectin	–[d]	+	?	?	?
Thrombospondin 1	–	+	+	+	+
Tenascin-C	–	+	?	?	?
Osteopontin	–	+	?	?	?
SPARC	–	+	+[e]	+	+[e]

[a](+), Data are consistent with the expression of the protein, or with a functional role for the protein, during vascular events.
[b](?), Data are inconclusive or incomplete at this time. Refer to text for appropriate references.
[c]Adapted with permission from ref. (102).
[d](–), There are no data consistent with an essential functional role for the protein in vascular morphogenesis.
[e]Peptides derived from SPARC promote angiogenesis in vivo.

of secreted protein acidic and rich in cysteine (SPARC) in the ECM was observed to be compromised in homozygous *mov* 13 mice, although fibroblasts isolated from these embryos synthesized and secreted SPARC in vitro *(17)*. Apparently, when collagen I is unavailable as an ECM binding partner, secreted SPARC is not stable in the extracellular environment of these mice. Collagen I also associates with other components of the extracellular space, such as vitronectin and fibronectin *(18,19)*. Collagen I expression might therefore be of critical importance in the retention of these proteins in the ECM of tissues undergoing angiogenesis.

FIBRONECTIN

Fibronectin is a well-characterized glycoprotein present in both serum and most ECMs that supports the adhesion and spreading of many different cell types, including endothelial cells *(20)*. Fibronectin not only provides an adhesive surface for endothelial cells but also a structural framework for cell migration, cell-cell interaction, and deposition of other ECM proteins. In fact, fibronectin, in addition to collagen I, was one of the first matrix or matrix-associated proteins shown to be essential for vascular development.

Fibronectin is expressed widely in embryos during the onset of vasculogenesis and angiogenesis, predominantly by mesodermally derived tissues that include both extraembryonic and embryonic vascular structures *(21)*. In the early stages of brain vascularization, fibronectin is localized to capillary sprouts invading the neuroectoderm *(22)*. Likewise, fibronectin is associated with endothelial cells in the regions of vasculogenesis in neonatal rat retina *(23)*. A definitive role for fibronectin in vascular morphogenesis was established in mice in which the fibronectin gene was ablated by genetic recombination. Heart development was abnormal in these mice, but the degree of severity of the phenotype was variable. Likewise, the dorsal aorta was completely absent in some fibronectin-null mice, whereas others exhibited an abnormal and distended aorta with very few blood cells, relative to age-matched, wild-type animals *(21)*.

The high concentrations of fibronectin in circulating plasma could facilitate fibronectin deposition in the provisional matrix that is established during wound healing and provides a substratum that allows for cell migration and reorganization. Endothelial cells themselves produce fibronectin, and increased expression of fibronectin is associated with endothelial-cell proliferation and capillary ingrowth during the wound healing process *(24)*.

Fibronectin is recognized primarily by the $\alpha_5\beta_1$ integrin receptor expressed on both large- and small-vessel endothelium, although other integrins have also been shown to bind fibronectin *(25,26)*. Interestingly, the α_5 null mutation also exhibits vascular defects. Mice that do not express the integrin α_5 subunit develop a heart and a primitive circulatory system; however, the vessels are leaky and distended. The defects in the vascular system of these mice are thought to bring about embryonic lethality by E10-E11 *(27)*. The fact that the α_5-null mutant appears to be less severe in comparison to the fibronectin-null mouse could indicate that another fibronectin receptor exists that compensates somewhat for the absence of α_5. For example, the $\alpha_v\beta_3$ integrin has also been shown to function as a fibronectin receptor under some circumstances.

Alternatively, the severity of the fibronectin mutation might be owing to the lack of fibronectin in the ECM which, in itself, disrupts vascular morphogenesis because of a compromise in structure, i.e., other matrix components fail to localize to the appropriate extracellular space. Fibronectin has been shown to interact with proteins that are potentially important in vascular development, such as collagen I, tenascin, and osteopontin *(28–30)*.

The absence of fibronectin in the ECM might perturb the organization of the matrix and consequently affect endothelial-cell behavior, e.g., certain integrin receptors might not engage the appropriate ligand to activate a requisite signal-transduction pathway.

VITRONECTIN

Vitronectin is an abundant, multi-functional serum protein that is synthesized primarily by the liver but is found associated with the ECM in many tissues throughout the organism (31). A significant portion of the activity associated with serum to support cell adhesion and spreading is attributable to vitronectin. Vitronectin is thought to function in blood coagulation and fibrinolysis, as it binds to several of the proteins that participate in these processes: heparin, thrombin-antithrombin complex, plasminogen, plasminogen activator inhibitor (PAI-1), and urokinase plasminogen activator receptor (uPAR) (32,33). Because the binding of vitronectin to PAI-1 and to uPAR has also been shown to play a role in cell adhesion and migration in vitro, this interaction might be of importance in activities other than proteolysis (see below). Vitronectin is a potential mediator of angiogenesis and vasculogenesis, as it promotes endothelial cell attachment and migration and is associated coincidentally with vascular morphogenesis.

Whereas vitronectin expression in the adult is associated primarily with the liver, a wider distribution of expression is seen during development. In addition to the liver, other developing tissues also express vitronectin mRNA, e.g., capillaries of the meninges and brain as early as murine E10. Vessel walls, as well as endothelium, produced vitronectin mRNA, although vessels from other regions of the embryo appeared negative by in situ hybridization (34). In the avian embryo, vitronectin protein was detected in the lumen of the dorsal aorta concomitantly with vasculogenesis. The staining was associated with the basal surface of primordial endothelial cells, whereas the lumen of the vessel was negative for vitronectin protein. Whether the vitronectin is synthesized by the avian endothelial cells or another cell type is unknown (35). The spatial and temporal pattern of early vitronectin expression is suggestive of a possible role for this protein in vascular development. Since vitronectin-null mice exhibited no phenotypic abnormalities in blood-vessel structure or function, vitronectin is most likely not required for normal vascular morphogenesis but might influence endothelial-cell behavior during development (36).

Recently, a great deal of attention has been paid to the integrin $\alpha_v\beta_3$ in the regulation of angiogenesis. $\alpha_v\beta_3$ was characterized originally as a vitronectin receptor, although other ligands for this receptor have subsequently been identified: osteopontin, fibrinogen, von Willebrand factor (vWF), fibronectin, tenascin-C, thrombospondin-1, and denatured collagen I (25,37). Of the other integrins that have been implicated as receptors for vitronectin in vitro, $\alpha_v\beta_1$ and $\alpha_v\beta_5$ are expressed on some endothelial cells (26). Importantly, antagonists of $\alpha_v\beta_3$ and $\alpha_v\beta_5$ have been shown to inhibit angiogenesis in vitro and in vivo. In the chick chorioallantoic membrane (CAM) assay, the exposed position of the CAM permits the application of various factors, and the response can be measured by quantification of blood-vessel formation in this planar, transparent tissue. Function-blocking antibodies against $\alpha_v\beta_3$ and $\alpha_v\beta_5$ inhibited capillary formation in this assay (38). Furthermore, $\alpha_v\beta_3$ expression has been observed to be associated with endothelial cells undergoing angiogenesis in wound granulation tissue, ocular tissue, and human breast tumor-associated blood vessels (39–41). Antagonists of $\alpha_v\beta_3$ have been used to abrogate angiogenesis in mouse models of both ocular neovascularization and tumor-associated blood vessel growth (42,41). Apoptosis has been proposed as one mechanism by which $\alpha_v\beta_3$ inhibits angiogenesis. Cheresh and co-workers showed that factors interfering with the binding of $\alpha_v\beta_3$ receptors to their ligands initiated an apoptotic pathway within endothelial cells *(43)*. $\alpha_v\beta_3$-neutralizing reagents appear to have no effect on established vasculature in the studies carried out thus far. Consequently, factors that abolish $\alpha_v\beta_3$ activity are promising candidates for therapeutic agents to control pathological angiogenesis associated with many diseases including cancer, diabetic retinopathy, and macular degeneration *(44)*.

uPAR is another endothelial-cell surface protein that interacts with vitronectin and promotes cell adhesion in the absence of $\alpha_v\beta_3$ *(45)*. Vitronectin promotes cell motility via uPAR, although this process might be dependent upon the $\alpha_v\beta_5$ integrin signal-transduction pathway *(46)*. In fact, uPAR has been shown to form stable complexes with β_1 integrins and, consequently, to inhibit integrin function *(47)*. Hence, the vitronectin-uPAR pathway probably utilizes at least some shared components with the integrin signal-transduction pathway to manifest its activity. uPA enhances the interaction of vitronectin with uPAR, whereas PAI-1 inhibits this interaction *(48)*. The binding of PAI-1 to vitronectin is also known to stabilize PAI-1 in an active conformation and thus affect protease activity in the immediate environment of the cell surface. Interestingly, PAI-1 has also been shown to inhibit smooth-muscle cell migration on vitronectin through competition for $\alpha_v\beta_3$ integrin. $\alpha_v\beta_3$ itself has been implicated in the regulation of extracellular protease activity, as matrix metalloproteinase 2 (MMP-2) in its proteolytically active form binds $\alpha_v\beta_3$ on angiogenic endothelial cells as well as on invasive melanoma cells *(49)*. This interaction could allow endothelial cells to modify their extracellular milieu to facilitate cell movement. For example, MMP-2 cleaves native collagen I to expose a cryptic RGD sequence that subsequently binds to $\alpha_v\beta_3$. Consequently, numerous cell-surface interactions are in place to facilitate cell migration on vitronectin-containing matrices that could influence cell movement during angiogenesis.

THROMBOSPONDIN 1

Thrombospondin was characterized initially as a large glycoprotein released by platelets in response to stimulation by thrombin and other physiological activators. Today thrombospondin is known to be expressed by a number of different cell types, including endothelial cells, and to be one of a gene family made up of five known members (Tsp 1-5; *50*). Thrombospondin 1 has been characterized as a prototypic "matricellular protein," defined as an ECM-associated protein that interacts with a number of extracellular macromolecules including matrix proteins, cytokines, proteases, and cell-surface receptors. Although associated with the ECM, matricellular proteins are not structural and are therefore distinct from the more traditional ECM proteins such as collagen and fibronectin *(51)*. Matricellular proteins are also identified by their modular structure, in which certain domains of the protein can be assigned individual functions (Fig. 1). Activities assigned to thrombospondin 1 include cell adhesion/counteradhesion, proliferation, and migration *(51)*. Superficially, some of these functions appear contradictory. However, the variety of activities elicited by thrombospondin 1 might in part depend on cell-type expression of specific receptors as well as other extraneous factors that influence thrombospondin 1 activity.

Thrombospondin 1 probably does not play a vital role in early developmental vascular morphogenesis. *In situ* hybridization of thrombospondin 1 mRNA shows that the mRNA is expressed as early as E10, when a strong signal is detected in the head mesenchyme that declines by E14. Early expression of thrombospondin 1 is associated with hematopoietic

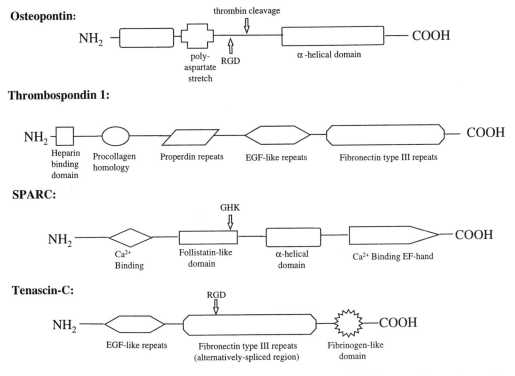

Fig. 1. A diagram representing the modular nature of the matricellular proteins osteopontin, thrombospondin 1, SPARC, and tenascin-C. Specific regions of the proteins mentioned in the text are indicated (refer to text for appropriate references). *RGD* and *GHK* refer to the locations of these tripeptides in the respective proteins. The recently-described extracellular Ca^{2+}-binding (EC) module of SPARC is comprised of both the α-helical and EF-hand domains *(101)*. Proteins/ domains are not drawn to scale.

cells in the lumen of blood vessels and probably derives from megakaryocytes, given the high levels of thrombospondin 1 expressed by platelets (3% of total platelet protein). Significant levels of thrombospondin 1 transcripts were not present in most developing vessels, although some mRNA was present in the cardiac endothelium coincidentally with septation *(52)*. Thus, the timing and expression pattern of thrombospondin 1 imply that it does not play a vital role in the early development of most blood vessels. Interestingly, thrombospondin 2 might be more significant in this regard, because it is expressed by endothelial cells during the early stages of vessel formation *(52)*. A nonessential role for thrombospondin 1 in development is also implied by the apparently normal embryogenesis of mice deficient in this protein *(53)*.

Although thrombospondin 1 does not appear to perform an essential function in developmental angiogenesis, this protein might prove subsequently to be important in later events that involve tissue repair or tumor survival. For example, thrombospondin 1 is not produced in normal skin; however, mRNA encoding thrombospondin 1 is detected early in wounds *(54)*. Furthermore, anti-sense thrombospondin 1 oligomers applied to wounds inhibited the level of thrombospondin 1 protein by 55–66% in the wound area and significantly delayed the re-epithelialization and dermal reorganization at the wound site *(55)*. A role for thrombospondin 1 in tumor progression was suggested by experiments using the metastatic MDA-MB-435 breast carcinoma cell line transfected with a thrombospondin 1 expression plasmid. These cells, injected into the fat pad of nude mice, were associated with inhibition of primary tumor growth and a decrease in metastasis. Tumors resulting from the transfected carcinoma cells exhibited a lower vessel count in comparison to nontransfected controls *(56)*. These data indicate that thrombospondin 1 might be a naturally occurring angiogenic inhibitor.

That thrombospondin 1 could be an important mediator of angiogenic events in vivo is supported by several experiments performed on endothelial cells in culture. Thrombospondin 1 has been shown to support adhesion and spreading of murine lung-capillary cells and BAE cells *(57)*. However, another study showed that thrombospondin 1 promoted attachment but not spreading of some BAE cells and identified the amino-terminal, heparin-binding domain of thrombospondin 1 (hep-1) as responsible for the dissociation of focal adhesions *(58)*. Consequently, BAE cells plated on fibronectin lost focal adhesions upon addition of thrombospondin 1 or a peptide representing the hep-1 domain (Fig. 1). A protein that destabilizes focal adhesions might be expected to promote migration as well. In accordance with this prediction, thrombospondin 1 was shown to be chemotactic for BAE cells *(57)*. Thrombospondin 1 also inhibited the mitogenic effects of serum and bFGF on endothelial cells *(57)*. Therefore, thrombospondin 1 presented to endothelial cells appeared to induce an inhibition of proliferation and a switch to a migratory phenotype.

Thrombospondin 1 has also been shown to elicit interesting activities in assays of angiogenesis in vitro. The addition of anti-thrombospondin 1 antibodies to BAE cells undergoing spontaneous angiogenesis in vitro was associated with an increase in the number of cords formed by these cells *(59)*. BAE cells transfected with antisense thrombospondin 1 mRNA exhibited a 10-fold increase over mock-transfected cells in migration toward bFGF and a twofold increase in the formation of capillary-like structures in a gelled basement membrane matrix (matrigel) *(60)*. Both of these studies are consistent with the function of thrombospondin 1 as an anti-angiogenic factor. Thrombospondin 1 has also been shown to stimulate angiogenesis in vitro, although this process was dependent on a factor secreted by myofibroblasts *(61)*.

Several receptors have been implicated in thrombospondin-mediated cell activities, such as both β_1 and β_3-containing integrins (especially $\alpha_v\beta_3$) *(37)*. Interestingly, thrombospondin 1 has also been shown to bind integrin-associated protein (IAP) and enhance the $\alpha_v\beta_3$-mediated signal transduction pathway in human melanoma cells plated on vitronectin *(62)*. The number of thrombospondin 1 receptors reflects the multitude of activities suggested for this protein. Many of the seemingly contradictory functions mediated by thrombospondin 1 might be owing in part to cell-type specific expression of different thrombospondin 1 receptors that mediate distinct signal-trandsduction pathways.

TENASCIN

Tenascin (myotendinous antigen, glioma-mesenchymal ECM antigen, cytotactin, J1) is an ECM-associated glycoprotein with a characteristic hexabranchion structure. Of the three tenascin family members currently identified, tenascin-C is the best characterized *(63)*. The role of tenascin in the vasculature is a relatively new area of research, but recent findings seem to indicate a functional significance for this protein in areas of neovascularization.

Tenascin is expressed widely during development in a variety of tissues including the mammary gland, kidney, gut, cartilage, bone, and the central and peripheral nervous systems (CNS/PNS). In contrast, a more limited expression pattern is seen in postnatal and adult tissue

(29). Interestingly, tenascin staining is seen in vessels and large veins of many different organs, e.g., skin, breast, lung, and liver *(64)*. Tenascin does not appear to be essential for developmental vascularization, as no defects in the circulatory system are observed in the tenascin-C-null mouse *(65)*. More subtle defects might be difficult to detect, however, as some neurological perturbations were found in this mutant only after careful scrutiny *(66)*.

Significantly higher levels of tenascin are also found associated with healing wounds and in tissues undergoing reparative or hyperplastic processes *(67,64)*. Expression of tenascin *de novo* has also been found in association with malignant tumors, particularly with capillary basement membranes. In fact, tumors that show a stronger expression of tenascin relative to fibronectin exhibited a higher degree of vascularization. Tenascin might therefore promote angiogenesis of these tumors to a greater degree than that observed for fibronectin *(68)*. Because high levels of tenascin expression were correlated with vascular hyperplasia in astrocytomas, tenascin might promote angiogenesis in this system as well *(69)*.

Tenascin has an adhesive activity as well as a counteradhesive activity on cultured cells. This apparent paradox could be owing to the conformation of tenascin on the plastic surface. For example, tenascin coated onto nitrocellulose promoted stronger adhesion of endothelial cells than was seen with tenascin coated on plastic. The length of time that tenascin was allowed to coat the dish prior to cell addition also appeared to influence its adhesive properties *(70)*. Whether the action of tenascin in vivo is to promote adhesion or counteradhesion probably depends upon the repertoire of cell-surface receptors as well as the conformation of tenascin in the matrix. In mouse-brain endothelial cultures, tenascin is expressed in vitro and promotes cell elongation with interconnecting processes, a morphology that might mimic angiogenesis in vivo *(71)*.

Endothelial cells express two known integrin receptors for tenascin: $\alpha_v\beta_3$ binds the RGD-containing repeat of tenascin (TNfn-3), and $\alpha_2\beta_1$ binds an unidentified region that could be the fibrinogen globular domain (Tnfbg, Fig. 1) *(71)*. Annexin II can also bind the alternatively-spliced repeat (Fn A-D) of tenascin that has been shown to disperse focal adhesions on endothelial cells, attenuate growth factor-induced mitosis, and promote cellular migration. Thus, annexin II appears to be the receptor on endothelial cells that is responsible for the activities elicited by these repeats of tenascin-C *(72)*. The counteradhesive activity of tenascin was observed when cells plated on fibronectin were found to round up upon the addition of tenascin *(73,74)*. Although fibronectin does interact with tenascin, the mechanism of counteradhesion does not appear to be mediated by this association. Possibly, the binding of annexin II to tenascin initiates a signal-transduction pathway that leads to cell rounding, as the counteradhesive properties of tenascin have been mapped to the domain which binds annexin II. Further experiments are necessary to determine whether all cell types sensitive to the counteradhesive activity of tenascin express annexin II and whether the activity is blocked by anti-annexin II antibodies.

OSTEOPONTIN

Although first characterized as a major extracellular component of bone matrices that participated in both mineralization and resorption of bone, osteopontin is now appreciated as a multi-functional protein expressed in a variety of different tissues *(75)*. Recently, osteopontin has also been implicated in vascular morphogenesis *(76)*. Osteopontin mRNA was found to be increased significantly in vascular smooth-muscle cells during neointima formation in rat carotid arteries *(77,78)*. Moreover, osteopontin protein promoted adhesion and migration of smooth-muscle cells and endothelial cells in vitro *(79)*. Like the matricellular protein SPARC *(see* below), osteopontin is often associated with cells in remodeling tissues. Weintraub et al. *(80)* showed that rat aortic smooth-muscle cells transfected with antisense osteopontin expression vectors exhibited decreased adhesion and invasion of collagen gels; moreover, activity could be restored to the cultures by the addition of exogenous osteopontin. Thus, osteopontin mediates cellular interactions with matrix components and promotes an invasive phenotype in smooth-muscle cells in vitro.

Like many of the matricellular proteins discussed in this chapter, osteopontin is probably not essential for vascular development, as osteopontin-null mice develop without overt phenotypic abnormalities *(53)*. Nomura et al. *(81)* used *in situ* hybridization to follow the pattern of osteopontin mRNA expression during development. Although osteopontin mRNA was detected in association with developing bone, transcripts were also found in a number of epithelial tissues including the embryonic kidney and the sensory epithelium of the ear. Although osteopontin mRNA was not detectable in developing vasculature, the isolation of an osteopontin cDNA from a rat pup aortic smooth-muscle cell library indicates that osteopontin is expressed, probably by smooth-muscle cells, in growing vessels *(77)*.

Three different α_v-containing integrins function as receptors for osteopontin: $\alpha_v\beta_1$, $\alpha_v\beta_5$, and $\alpha_v\beta_3$. Although all three receptors mediate adhesion to osteopontin, apparently only ligation of $\alpha_v\beta_3$ promotes migration of smooth-muscle cells *(82)*. Interestingly, osteopontin has a conserved thrombin cleavage site in close proximity to the RGD-binding domain. Endothelial cells showed an enhanced migratory response to an osteopontin that had been proteolyzed by thrombin *(83)*. In addition, Smith et al. *(84)* have also shown that a recombinant fusion protein mimicking the N-terminal fragment generated by thrombin cleavage contains a cryptic binding site for the integrin $\alpha_9\beta_1$, in addition to the $\alpha_v\beta_3$ (RGD) site. Thus, activation of thrombin could result in the generation of osteopontin polypeptides that exhibit properties separate from those of the native, intact protein. In fact, the proteolytic digestion of ECM-associated proteins to produce cleavage products with activities distinct from the parent protein might be a highly conserved means of controlling several different vascular pathways *(85)*.

SPARC

SPARC is a matricellular protein expressed by many cell types in diverse tissues. SPARC is also a component of serum. Different functions mediated by SPARC have been mapped to four separate regions of the protein, a characteristic common to the modular matricellular proteins (Fig. 1) *(86,51)*. SPARC is also sensitive to cleavage by a variety of proteinases, and in certain instances particular sequences of SPARC are released with activities distinct from those of the native protein *(85)*.

SPARC has an interesting expression pattern during development. Most tissues of the E10 chicken embryo express SPARC mRNA, notably the heart, aorta, and brain *(87)*. Similar to osteopontin, SPARC is expressed more broadly in embryonic tissues and becomes restricted in the adult to tissues associated with high levels of remodeling and proliferation, e.g., bone and gut *(86)*. SPARC is also expressed in *Xenopus* embryos, again in association with tissues undergoing rapid morphological development, such as the intersomitic clefts at the time of trunk myotome contraction *(88)*. In fact, *Xenopus* embryos injected with anti-SPARC antibodies exhibited a bending and shortening of the embryonic axis and consequently, highly disorganized myotome patterns *(89)*. A similar result has been shown in the invertebrate *Caenorhabditis elegans (90)*. A functional role for SPARC in vascular development might depend on specific proteolytic processing of extracellular SPARC. Iruela-Arispe and coworkers *(91)* showed that full-length SPARC had no angiogenic effect in the CAM assay; however, synthetic SPARC peptides from a domain of the protein containing a plasmin-sensitive region stimulated angiogenesis in a concentration-dependent manner. Plasmin activity was present at this time in the CAM and could serve as a regulator of SPARC function. SPARC has also been shown to be a source of copper-binding peptides containing the sequence KGHK *(92)*. Previously, GHK (also known as liver growth factor) had been described as a copper-binding peptide in serum that stimulated angiogenesis and wound healing *(93,94)*. Thus, SPARC is likely to have a number of functions, one of which is the regulation of angiogenesis upon proteolytic digestion.

In vitro, SPARC has been shown to act as a counteradhesive protein and potential regulator of angiogenesis. In the presence of SPARC protein, endothelial cells plated on a variety of substrates fail to spread and exhibit inhibition of the cell cycle *(95,96)*. Endothelial cells in cord-forming cultures also have increased levels of SPARC mRNA and protein *(12)*. Similar to thrombospondin 1, addition of SPARC diminished focal adhesions in BAE cells. Whereas the distribution of vinculin in SPARC-treated cells was disrupted, the integrin α_v remained localized to points of focal contacts *(97)*. SPARC is therefore not likely to inhibit integrin interaction with the ECM but might instead initiate a change in cell shape, perhaps through receptor-mediated signal transduction. Although a cell-surface receptor for SPARC has not yet been characterized, identification of a SPARC receptor will provide valuable insight into the mechanism of SPARC action and function.

SPARC has been shown to interact with a variety of ECM components including collagens, vitronectin, laminin, and thrombospondin 1. SPARC is not a structural component of the ECM and is difficult to detect in matrices associated with most quiescent cell types. However, SPARC is expressed abundantly in areas of rapid matrix turnover such as wound healing and sites of tumor expansion and metastasis. Of interest is a recent report that suppression of SPARC by an antisense expression vector transfected into melanoma cells reduced significantly the adhesive and invasive properties of these cells in vitro and completely abrogated their tumorigencity in vivo *(98)*. SPARC could serve as a dynamic regulator of the ECM through its specific interaction with matrix proteins. As mentioned earlier, *mov* 13 mice deficient in collagen I expression do not incorporate SPARC into the ECM. Possibly, some of the vascular defects manifested by these embryos could be attributable to a lack of SPARC activity, in combination with a lack of collagen I.

SUMMARY

The ECM and its associated matricellular proteins are important regulators of vascular morphogenesis. Cell-matrix interactions are thus reasonable targets of therapeutic agents to control angiogenesis under pathological conditions. Thrombospondin 1 has been characterized as an antiangiogenic tumor repressor, and the integrin $\alpha_v\beta_3$ also appears to be a promising target for diminution of undesirable vessel growth in vivo. In retrospect, this prediction is not surprising, as six of the seven ECM-associated proteins discussed in this chapter (all of which influence angiogenesis at some level) are claimed to be ligands for this integrin. It is interesting that no abnormalities in vascular development are observed in patients with Glanzmann's thrombocytopenia, a disease in which the β_3 integrin subunit is lacking. Because these patients do experience difficulties in wound healing, their ability to develop a normal vasculature may be owing in part to some redundancy conferred by the $\alpha_v\beta_5$ integrin. Moreover, mice lacking the α_v integrin subunit often die before birth and show abnormal development of brain vessels, although vascular development of other tissues appears to be normal *(53)*. Brain vascularization is entirely dependent on angiogenesis, in contrast to that of most other tissues in which vessel development also occurs through vasculogenesis *(99)*. α_v-deficient mice might contain endothelial cells that lack the capacity to participate in angiogenesis. It will therefore be interesting to see how endothelial cells isolated from these mice behave in assays of angiogenesis in vitro. For example, experiments could be designed to test specific aspects of angiogenesis in vitro to elucidate critical steps in the sequence.

It appears that the β_1 family of integrins is critical in the early stages of vasculogenesis, as antibodies specific for its various subunits perturb this process significantly *(100)*. Because the β_1 family comprises the majority of matrix-binding members, inhibition of β_1 abrogates interaction of cells with laminin, fibronectin, and native collagens, in addition to other ECM components. Clearly, the ability of endothelial cells to interact with ECM is a key event in both vasculogenesis and angiogenesis. An increased understanding of these processes will lead to improved methods of controlling pathological angiogenesis and a better understanding of vascular morphogenesis, a fascinating and complex phenomenon critical for multicellular life.

ACKNOWLEDGMENTS

We thank L. Iruela-Arispe for sharing unpublished results. A.D.B. was supported by National Institutes of Health fellowship F32 GM18705. Experiments cited in this review from the authors' laboratory were supported by National Institutes of Health grants GM40711, HL18645, and HL 03174.

REFERENCES

1. Noden, D. W. (1989) Embryonic origins and assembly of blood vessels. *Am. Rev. Respir. Dis.* **140**, 1097–1103.
2. Folkman J. and Klagsbrun, M. (1987) Angiogenic factors. *Science* **235**, 442–447.
3. Vernon R. B. and Sage E. H. (1995) Between molecules and morphology: Extracellular matrix and creation of vascular form. *Am. J. Pathol.* **14**, 873–883.
4. Risau W. and Flamme, I. (1995) Vasculogenesis. *Ann. Rev. Cell Dev. Biol.* **11**, 73–91.
5. Sage, E. H. and Vernon, R. B. (1994) Regulation of angiogenesis by extracellular matrix: the growth and the glue. *J. Hypertens.* **12**, S145–S152.
6. Niederreither, K., D'Souza, R., Metsaranta, M., Eberspaecher, H., Toman, P. D., Vuorio, E., and de Crombrugghe, B. (1994) Coordinate patterns of expression of type I and III collagens during mouse development. *Matrix Biol.* **14**, 705–713.
7. Leivo, I., Vaheri, A., Timpl, R., and Wartiovaara, J. (1980) Appearance and distribution of collagens and laminin in the early mouse embryo. *Dev. Biol.* **76**, 100–114.
8. Kitaoka, M., Iyama, K.-I., Yoshioka, H., Monda, M., and Usuku, G. (1994) Immunohistochemical localization of procollagen types I and III during placentation in pregnant rats by type-specific procollagen antibodies. *J. Histochem. Cytochem.* **42**, 1453–1461.
9. Harbers, K., Kuehn, M., Delius, H., and Jaenisch, R. (1984) Insertion of retrovirus into the first intron of the α1(I) collagen gene leads to embryonic lethal mutation in mice. *Proc. Natl. Acad. Sci. USA* **81**, 1504–1508.
10. Kratochwil, K., von der Mark, K., Kollar, E. J., Jaenisch, R., Mooslehner, K., Schwarz, M., et al. (1989) Retrovirus-induced insertional mutation in mov 13 mice affects collagen I expression in a tissue-specific manner. *Cell* **57**, 807–816.
11. Löhler, J., Timpl, R., and Jaenisch, R. (1984) Embryonic lethal mutation in the mouse collagen I gene causes rupture of blood vessels and is associated with erythropoietic and mesenchymal cell death. *Cell* **38**, 597–607.
12. Iruela-Arispe, L. M., Diglio, C. A., and Sage, E. H. (1991) Modulation of extracellular matrix proteins by endothelial cells undergoing angiogenesis in vitro. *Arterioscler. Thromb.* **11**, 805–815.

13. Vernon, R. B., Lara, S. L., Drake, C. J., Iruela-Arispe, M. L., Angello, J. C., Little, C. D., et al. (1995) Organized type I collagen influences endothelial patterns during "spontaneous angiogenesis in vitro" : Planar cultures as models of vascular development. *In Vitro Cell Dev. Biol.* **31,** 120–131.

14. Vernon, R. B. and Sage, E. H. (1996) Contraction of fibrillar type I collagen by endothelial cells: a study in vitro. *J. Cell Biochem.* **60,** 185–197.

15. Moses, M. A., Sudhalter, J., and Langer, R. (1990) Identification of an inhibitor of neovascularization from cartilage. *Science* **248,** 1408–1410.

16. Fisher, C., Gilbertson-Beading, S., Powers, E. A., Petzold, G., Poorman, R., and Mitchell, M. A. (1994) Interstitial collagenase is required for angiogenesis in vitro. *Dev. Biol.* **162,** 499–510.

17. Iruela-Arispe, L. M., Vernon, R. B., Wu, H., Jaenisch, R., and Sage, E. H. (1996) Type I collagen is required for the association of SPARC with the extracellular matrix in Mov 13 mice: implications for fibroblast function. *Dev. Dynam.* **207,** 171–183.

18. Gebb, C., Hayman, E. G., Engvall, E., and Ruoslahti, E. (1986) Interaction of vitronectin with collagen. *J. Biol. Chem.* **261,** 16,698–16,703.

19. Ingham, K. C., Brew, S. A., and Isaacs, B. S. (1988) Interaction of fibronectin and its gelatin-binding domains with fluorescent-labeled chains of type I collagen. *J. Biol. Chem.* **263,** 4624–4628.

20. Hynes, R. O. (1990) *Fibronectins*. Springer-Verlag, New York.

21. George, E. L., Georges-Labouesse, E. N., Patel-King, R. S., Rayburn, H., and Hynes R. O. (1993) Defects in mesoderm, neural tube, and vascular development in mouse embryos lacking fibronectin. *Development* **119,** 1079–1091.

22. Risau, W. and Lemmon, V. (1988) Changes in the vascular extracellular matrix during embryonic vasculogenesis and angiogenesis. *Dev. Biol.* **125,** 441–450.

23. Jiang, B., Liou, G. I., Behzdian, M. A., and Caldwell, R. B. (1994) Astrocytes modulate retinal vasculogenesis: effects on fibronectin expression. *J. Cell Sci.* **107,** 2499–2508.

24. Clark, R. A. F., Quinn, J. H., Winn, H. J., Lanigan, J. M., Dellepella, P., and Colvin, R. B. (1982) Fibronectin is produced by blood vessels in response to injury. *J. Exp. Med.* **156,** 646–651.

25. Hynes, R. O. (1992) Integrins: versatility, modulation, and signaling in cell adhesion. *Cell* **69,** 11–25.

26. Luscinska, F. W. and Lawler, J. (1994) Integrins as dynamic regulators of vascular function. *FASEB J.* **8,** 929–938.

27. Yang, J. T., Rayburn, H., and Hynes, R. O. (1993) Embryonic mesodermal defects in α5 integrin-deficient mice. *Development* **119,** 1093–1105.

28. Dzamba, B. J., Jaenisch, R., and Peters, D. M. (1993) Fibronectin binding site in type I collagen regulates fibronectin fibril formation. *J. Cell Biol.* **121,** 1165–1172.

29. Crossin, K. L. (1996) Tenascin: a multifunctional extracellular matrix protein with a restricted distribution in development and disease. *J. Cell. Biochem.* **61,** 592–598.

30. Mukherjee, B. B., Nemir, M., Beninati, S., Cordella-Miele, E., Singh, K., Chackalaparampil, I., et al. (1995) Interaction of osteopontin with fibronectin and other extracellular matrix molecules. *Ann. NY Acad. Sci.* **760,** 201–212.

31. Seiffert D., Keeton, M., Eguchi, Y., Sawdey, M., and Loskutoff, D. J. (1991) Detection of vitronectin mRNA in tissues and cells of the mouse. *Proc. Natl. Acad. Sci. USA* **88,** 9402–9406.

32. Felding-Habermann, B. and Cheresh, D. A. (1993). Vitronectin and its receptors. *Curr. Opin. Cell Biol.* **5,** 864–868.

33. Wei, Y., Waltz, D. A., Rao, N., Drummond, R. J., Rosenberg, S., and Chapman, H. A. (1994) Identification of the urokinase receptor as an adhesion receptor for vitronectin. *J. Biol. Chem.* **269,** 32,380–32,388.

34. Seiffert, D., Iruela-Arsipe, M. L., Sage, E. H., and Loskutoff, D. J. (1996) Distribution of vitronectin mRNA during murine development. *Dev. Dynam.* **203,** 71–79.

35. Drake, C. J., Cheresh, D. A., and Little, C. D. (1995) An antagonist of integrin $\alpha_v\beta_3$ prevents maturation of blood vessels during embryonic neovascularization. *J. Cell Sci.* **108,** 2655–2661.

36. Zheng, X., Saunders, T. L., Camper, S., Samuelson, L. C., and Ginsburg, D. (1995) Vitronectin is not essential for normal mammalian development. *Proc. Natl. Acad. Sci. USA* **92,** 12,426–12,430.

37. Haas, T. A. and Plow, E. F. (1994) Integrin-ligand interactions: a year in review. *Curr. Opin. Cell Biol.* **6,** 656–662.

38. Friedlander, M., Brooks, P. C., Shaffer, R. W., Kincaid, C. M., Varner, J. A., and Cheresh, D. A. (1995) Definition of two angiogenic pathways by distinct α_v integrins. *Science* **270,** 1500–1502.

39. Clark, R. A. F., Tonnesen, M. G., Gailit, J., and Cheresh, D. A. (1996) Transient functional expression of $\alpha_v\beta_3$ on vascular cells during wound repair. *Am. J. Pathol.* **148,** 1407–1421.

40. Friedlander, M., Theesfeld, C. L., Sugita, M., Fruttiger, M., Thomas, M. A., Chang, S., and Cheresh, D. A. (1996) Involvement of integrins $\alpha_v\beta_3$ and $\alpha_v\beta_5$ in ocular neovascular diseases. *Proc. Natl. Acad. Sci. USA* **93,** 9764–9769.

41. Brooks, P. C., Strombald, S., Klemke, R., Visscher, D., Sarkar, F. H., and Cheresh, D. A. (1995) Anti-integrin $\alpha_v\beta_3$ blocks human breast cancer growth and angiogenesis in human skin. *J. Clin. Invest.* **96,** 1696–1707.

42. Luna, J., Tobe, T., Mousa, S. A., Reilly, T. M., and Campochiaro, P. A. (1996) Antagonists of integrin $\alpha_v\beta_3$ inhibit retinal neovascularization in a murine model. *Lab. Invest.* **75,** 563–573.

43. Brooks, P. C., Montgomery, A. M. P., Rosenfeld, M., Reisfeld, R. A., Hu, T., Klier, G., and Cheresh, D. A. (1994) Integrin $\alpha_v\beta_3$ antagonists promote tumor regression by inducing apoptosis of angiogenic blood vessels. *Cell* **79,** 1157–1164.

44. Stromblad, S. and Cheresh, D. A. (1996) Cell adhesion and angiogenesis. *Trends Cell Biol.* **6,** 462–468.

45. Wei, Y., Waltz, D. A., Rao, N., Drummond, R. J., Rosenberg, S., and Chapman, H. A. (1994) Identification of the urokinase receptor as an adhesion receptor for vitronectin. *J. Biol. Chem.* **269,** 32,380–32,388.

46. Yebra, M., Parry, G. C. N., Stromblad, S., Mackman, N., Rosenberg, S., Mueller, B. M., and Cheresh, D. A. (1996) Requirement of receptor-bound urokinase-type plasminogen activator for integrin $\alpha_v\beta_5$-directed cell migration. *J. Biol. Chem.* **271,** 29,393–29,399.

47. Wei, Y., Lukashev, M., Simon, D. I., Bodary, S. C., Rosenberg, S., Doyle, M. V., and Chapman, H. A. (1996) Regulation of integrin function by the urokinase receptor. *Science* **273,** 1551–1555.

48. Deng, G., Curriden, S. A., Wang, S., Rosenberg, S., and Loskutoff, D. J. (1996) Is plasminogen activator inhibitor-1 the molecular switch that governs urokinase receptor-mediated cell adhesion and release? *J. Cell Biol.* **134,** 1563–1571.

49. Brooks, P. C., Stromblad, S., Sanders, L. C., von Schalscha, T. L., Aimes, R. T., Stetler-Stevenson, W. G., et al. (1996) Localization of matrix metalloproteinase MMP-2 to the surface of invasive cells by interaction with integrin $\alpha_v\beta_3$. *Cell* **85,** 683–693.

50. Lawler, J. (1996) Thrombospondins, In: *Tenascin and Counteradhesive Molecules of the Extracellular Matrix* (Crossin, K. L., ed.), Hardwood Acad., Amsterdam, Netherlands, pp. 109–125.

51. Bornstein, P. (1995) Diversity of function is inherent in matricelllular proteins: an appraisal of thrombospondin 1. *J. Cell Biol.* **130,** 503–506.

52. Iruela-Arispe, M. L., Liska, D. J., Sage, E. H., and Bornstein P. (1993) Differential expression of thrombospondin 1, 2, and 3, during murine development. *Dev. Dynam.* **197,** 40–56.

53. Hynes, R. O. (1996) Targeted mutations in cell adhesion genes: what have we learned from them? *Dev. Biol.* **180,** 402–412.

54. Reed, M. J., Puolakkainen, P., Lane, T. F., Dickerson, D., Bornstein, P., and Sage, E. H. (1993) Differential expression of SPARC and thrombospondin 1 in wound repair: immunolocalization and in situ hybridization. *J. Histochem. Cytochem.* **41,** 1467–1477.

55. DiPietro, L. A., Nissen, N. N., Gamelli, R. L., Koch, A. E., Pyle, J. M., and Polverini, P. J. (1996) Thrombospondin 1 synthesis and function in wound repair. *Am. J. Pathol.* **148,** 1851–1860.

56. Weinstat-Saslow, D. L., Zabrenetzky, V. S., VanHoutte, K., Frazier, W. A., Roberts, D. D., and Steeg, P. S. (1994) Transfection of thrombospondin 1 complementary DNA into a human breast carcinoma cell line reduces primary tumor growth, metastatic potential, and angiogenesis. *Cancer Res.* **54,** 6504–6511.

57. Taraboletti, G., Roberts, D., Liotta, L. A., and Giavazzi, R. (1990) Platelet thrombospondin modulates endothelial cell adhesion, motility, and growth: a potential angiogenesis regulatory factor. *J. Cell Biol.* **111,** 765–772.

58. Murphy-Ullrich J. E. and Höök, M. (1989) Thrombospondin modulates focal adhesions in endothelial cells. *J. Cell Biol.* **109,** 1309–1319.

59. Iruela-Arispe, M. L., Bornstein, P., and Sage, E. H. (1991) Thrombospondin exerts an antiangiogenic effect on cord formation by endothelial cells in vitro. *Proc. Natl. Acad. Sci. USA* **88,** 5026–5030.

60. DiPietro, L. A., Negben, D. R., and Polverini, P. J. (1994) Downregulation of endothelial cell thrombospondin 1 enhances in vitro angiogenesis. *J. Vasc. Res.* **31,** 178–185.

61. Nicosia, R. F. and Tuszynski, G. P. (1994) Matrix-bound thrombospondin promotes angiogenesis in vitro. *J. Cell Biol.* **124,** 183–193.

62. Gao, A-G, Lindberg, F. P., Dimitry, J. M., Brown, E. J., and Frazier, W. A. (1996) Thrombospondin modulates alpha v beta 3 function through integrin-associated protein. *J. Cell Biol.* **135,** 533–544.

63. Jones, F. S. and Copertino, D. W. (1996) The molecular biology of tenascin: structure, splice variants and regulation of gene expression, in *Tenascin and Counteradhesive Proteins of the Extracellular Matrix* (Crossin, K. L., ed.), Harwood Acad., Amsterdam, Netherlands, pp. 1–22.

64. Koukoulis, G. K., Gould, V. E., Bhattacharyya, A., Gould, J. E., Howeedy, A. A., and Virtanen, I. (1991) Tenascin in normal, reactive, hyperplastic, and neoplastic tissues: biological and pathologic implications. *Human Pathol.* **22,** 636–643.

65. Saga Y., Yagi, T., Ikawa, Y., Sakakura, T., and Aizawa, S. (1992) Mice develop normally without tenascin. *Genes Dev.* **6**, 1821–1831.
66. Steindler, D. A., Settles, D., Erickson, H. P., Laywell, E. D., Yoshiki, A., Faissner, A., and Kusakabe, M. (1995) Tenascin knockout mice: barrels, boundary molecules and glial scars. *J. Neurosci.* **15**, 1971–1983.
67. Mackie, E. J., Halfter, W., and Liverani, D. (1988) Induction of tenascin in healing wounds. *J. Cell Biol.* **107**, 2757–2767.
68. Higuchi, M., Ohnishi, T., Arita, N., Hiraga, S., and Hayakawa, T. (1993) Expression of tenascin in human gliomas: its relation to histological maligancy, tumor dedifferentiation and angiogenesis. *Acta Neuropathol.* **85**, 481–487.
69. Zagzag, D., Friedlander, D. R., Miller, D. C., Dosik, J., Cangiarella, J., Kostianovsky, M., et al. (1995) Tenascin expression in astrocytomas correlates with angiogenesis. *Cancer Res.* **55**, 907–914.
70. Joshi, P., Chung, C.-Y., Aukhil, I., and Erickson, H. P. (1993) Endothelial cells adhere to the RGD domain and the fibrinogen-like terminal knob of tenascin. *J. Cell Sci.* **106**, 389–400.
71. Sriramarao, P., Mendler, M., and Bourdon, M. A. (1993) Endothelial cell attachment and spreading on human tenascin is mediated by $\alpha_2\beta_1$ and $\alpha_v\beta_3$ integrins. *J. Cell Sci.* **105**, 1001–1012.
72. Chung, C. Y., Murphy-Ullrich, J. E., and Erickson, H. P. (1996) Mitogenesis, cell migration, and loss of focal adhesions induced by tenascin-C interacting with its cell surface receptor, annexin II. *Mol. Biol. Cell* **7**, 883–892.
73. Chiquet, M., Vrucinic-Filipi, N., Schenk, S., Beck, K., and Chiquet-Ehrismann, R. (1991) Isolation of chick tenascin variants and fragments. A C-terminal heparin-binding fragment produced by cleavage of the extra-domain from the largest subunit splicing variant. *Eur. J. Biochem.* **199**, 379–388.
74. Prieto, A. L., Andersson-Fisone, C., and Crossin, K. L. (1992) Characterisation of multi-adhesive and counter adhesive domains in the extracellular matrix protein cytotactin. *J. Cell Biol.* **119**, 663–678.
75. Denhardt, D. T. and Guo, X. (1993) Osteopontin: a protein with diverse functions. *FASEB J.* **7**, 1475–1482.
76. Giachelli, C. M., Liaw, L., Murry, C. E., Schwartz, S. M., and Almeida, M. (1995) Osteopontin expression in cardiovascular diseases. *Ann. NY Acad. Sci.* **760**, 109–126.
77. Giachelli, C. M., Bae, N., Lombardi, D., Majesky, M., and Schwartz, S. (1991) Molecular cloning and characterization of 2B7, a rat mRNA which distinguishes smooth muscle cell phenotypes in vitro and is identical to osteopontin (secreted phosphoprotein 1:2AR). *Biochem. Biophys. Res. Comm.* **177**, 867–873.
78. Giachelli, C. M., Bae, N., Almeida, M., Denhardt, D. T., Alpers, C. E., and Schwartz, S. M. (1993) Osteopontin is elevated during neointima formation in rat arteries and is a novel component of human atherosclerotic plaques. *J. Clin. Invest.* **92**, 1686–1696.
79. Liaw, L., Almeida, M., Hart, C. E., Schwartz, S. M., and Giachelli, C. M. (1994) Osteopontin promotes vascular cell adhesion and spreading and is chemotactic for smooth muscle cells in vitro. *Circ. Res.* **74**, 214–224.
80. Weintraub, A. S., Giachelli, C. M., Krauss, R. S., Almeida, M., and Taubman, M. B. (1996) Autocrine secretion of osteopontin by vascular smooth muscle cells regulates their adhesion to collagen gels. *Am. J. Pathol.* **149**, 259–272.
81. Nomura, S., Wills, A. J., Edwards, D. R., Heath, J. K., and Hogan, B. L. M. (1988) Developmental expression of 2ar (osteopontin) and SPARC (osteonectin) RNA as revealed by in situ hybridization. *J. Cell Biol.* **106**, 441–450.
82. Liaw, L., Skinner, M. P., Raines, E. W., Ross, R., Cheresh, D. A., and Schwartz, S. M. (1995) The adhesive and migratory effects of osteopontin are mediated via distinct cell surface integrins. *J. Clin. Invest.* **95**, 713–724.
83. Senger, D. R., Ledbetter, S. R., Claffey, K. P., Papdopoulos-Serfgiou, A., Perruzzi, C. A., and Detmar, M. (1996) Stimulation of endothelial cell migration by vascular permeability factor/vascular endothelial growth factor through the cooperative mechanisms involving the $\alpha_v\beta_3$ integrin, osteopontin and thrombin. *Am. J. Pathol.* **149**, 293–305.
84. Smith, L. L., Cheung, H.-K., Ling, L. E., Chen, J., Sheppard, D., Pytela, R., and Giachelli, C. M. (1996) Osteopontin N-terminal domain contains a cryptic adhesive sequence recognized by $\alpha_9\beta_1$ integrin. *J. Biol. Chem.* **45**, 28,485–28,491.
85. Sage, E. H. (1997) Pieces of eight: bioactive fragments of extracellular proteins as regulators of angiogenesis. *Trends Cell Biol.* **7**, 182–186.
86. Lane, T. E. and Sage, E. H. (1994) The biology of SPARC, a protein that modulates cell-matrix interactions. *FASEB J.* **8**, 163–173.
87. Bassuk, J. A., Iruela-Arispe, M. L., Lane, T. F., Benson, J. M., Berg, R. A., and Sage, E. H. (1993) Molecular analysis of chicken embryo SPARC (osteonectin). *Eur. J. Biochem.* **218**, 117–127.

88. Damjanovski, S., Malaval, L., and Ringuette, M. J. (1994) Transient expression of SPARC in the dorsal axis of early Xenopus embryos: correlation with calcium-dependent adhesion and electrical coupling. *Int. J. Dev. Biol.* **38**, 439–446.

89. Purcell, L., Gruia-Gray, J., Scanga, S., and Ringuette, M. (1993) Developmental anomalies of Xenopus embryos following microinjection of SPARC antibodies. *J. Exp. Zool.* **265**, 153–164.

90. Schwarzbauer, J. E. and Spencer, C. S. (1993) The Caenorhabditis elegans homologue of the extracellular calcium binding protein SPARC/osteonectin affects nematode body morphology and mobility. *Mol. Biol. Cell* **4**, 941–952.

91. Iruela-Arispe, M. L., Lane, T. L., Redmond, D., Reilly, M., Bolender, R. P., Kavanagh, T. J., and Sage, E. H. (1995) Expression of SPARC during development of the chicken chorioallantoic membrane: evidence for regulated proteolysis in vivo. *Mol. Biol. Cell* **6**, 327–343.

92. Lane, T. F., Iruela-Arispe, M. L., Johnson, R. S., and Sage, E. H. (1994) SPARC is a source of copper-binding peptides that stimulate angiogenesis. *J. Cell Biol.* **125**, 929–943.

93. Raju, K. S., Alessandri, G., Ziche, M., and Gullino, P. N., (1982) Ceruloplasmin, copper ions and angiogenesis. *J. Natl. Cancer Inst.* **69**, 81–88.

94. Pickart, L. (1983) The biological effects and mechanism of action of the plasma tripeptide glycyl-L-histidyl-L- lysine. *Lymphokines* **8**, 425–446.

95. Sage, H., Vernon, R. B., Funk, S. E., Everitt, E. A., and Angello, J. (1989) SPARC, a secreted protein associated with cellular proliferation, inhibits cell spreading in vitro and exhibits Ca^{2+}-dependent binding to the extracellular matrix. *J. Cell Biol.* **109**, 341–356.

96. Funk, S. E. and Sage, E. H. (1991) The Ca^{2+}-binding glycoprotein SPARC modulates cell cycle progression in bovine aortic endothelial cells. *Proc. Natl. Acad. Sci. USA* **88**, 2648–2652.

97. Murphy-Ullrich, J. E., Lane, T. F., Pallero, M. A., and Sage E. H. (1995) SPARC mediates focal adhesion disassembly in endothelial cells through a follistatin-like region and Ca^{2+} -binding EF-hand. *J. Cell. Biochem.* **57**, 341–350.

98. Ledda, M. F., Adris, S., Bravo, A. I., Kairiyama, C., Bover, L., Chernajovsky, Y., et al. (1997) Suppression of SPARC expression by antisense RNA abrogates the tumorgenicity of human melanoma cells. *Nature Med.* **3**, 171–176.

99. Bär, Th. (1980) The vascular system of the cerebral cortex. *Adv. Anat. Embryol. Cell Biol.* **59**, 1–62.

100. Drake, C. J., Davis, L. A., and Little, C. D. (1992) Antibodies to β1-integrins cause alterations of aortic vasculogenesis, in vivo. *Dev. Dynam.* **193**, 83–91.

101. Hohenester, E., Maurer, P., Hohenadl, C., Timpl, R., Jansonius, J. N., and Engel, J. (1996) Structure of a novel extracellular Ca^{2+} -binding module in BM-40. *Nature Struct. Biol.* **3**, 67–73.

102. Ingber, D. E. and Folkman, J. (1989) Mechanochemical switching between growth and differentiation during fibroblast growth factor-stimulated angiogenesis in vitro: role of extracellular matrix. *J. Cell Biol.* **109**, 317–330.

II ANGIOGENESIS IN HEALTH AND DISEASE

5

Integrin Receptors and the Regulation of Angiogenesis

Dorothy Rodriguez and Peter C. Brooks

INTRODUCTION

General Principles of New Blood-Vessel Development

Over the past several years a renewed interest has emerged in the biochemical and molecular mechanisms controlling vascular development and its implications in human disease. This renewed enthusiasm has lead many investigators towards the isolation and identification of molecules that regulate the formation of new blood vessels in hopes that targeting these molecules may provide novel strategies for the treatment of human vascular disorders. In general, the formation of new blood vessels can occur by either of two similar but distinct physiological processes termed "vasculogenesis" and "angiogenesis" *(1–4)*. Vasculogenesis is associated with the development of new blood vessels from precursor cells called angioblasts *(3,4)* and will not be discussed further in this chapter; instead, we will focus on angiogenesis. Angiogenesis is the process by which a network of new blood vessels form from a pre-existing vascular bed *(5,6)*. This complex process can be characterized by at least three general stages including: initiation by growth factors or cytokines; proteolytic remodeling of the extracellular matrix (ECM) and endothelial-cell migration; and finally, capillary differentiation and maturation *(7)*. These cellular events are tightly regulated and can occur during normal physiological processes such as trophoblast implantation, embryonic development, and wound healing *(1–7)*. However, during certain pathological conditions such as rheumatoid arthritis (RA), diabetic retinopathy, and tumor growth and metastasis, the tightly regulated control mechanisms are disrupted, leading to accelerated vascular growth *(1–7)*. Therefore, the identification and isolation of molecules that regulate angiogenesis will likely facilitate the development of novel approaches for the treatment of human neovascular diseases.

From: *The New Angiotherapy*
Edited by: T.-P. D. Fan and E. C. Kohn © Humana Press Inc., Totowa, NJ

Molecular Regulators of Angiogenesis

A number of distinct families of molecules have been identified that play a functional role in the angiogenic process including growth factors and their receptors, proteolytic enzymes, cell-adhesion receptors, and extracellular matrix components *(8–12)*. One of the most widely studied of these groups include the cytokine or growth-factor family. Some of these angiogenic factors include basic fibroblast growth factor (bFGF), vascular endothelial growth factor (VEGF), platelet-derived endothelial cell growth factor (PDECGF), and tumor necrosis factor-α (TNF-α) *(8)* . Although this is only a partial list of the growth factors and cytokines known to play a role in angiogenesis, other pro-angiogenic mediators have also been identified, including the recently described role for the circulating hormone leptin *(13)*. Moreover, recent studies have shown that angiopoietin-1 may also play a significant role in new blood-vessel formation *(14,15)*. Angiopoietin-1 has been identified as an important ligand for the endothelial cell-associated tyrosine kinase receptor Tie-2 *(14,15)*. Although angiopoietin-1 does not induce a strong angiogenic response in vitro, it has been shown to promote vessel remodeling and branching, suggesting that it may play a role in latter events during the angiogenic cascade *(14,15)*. In fact, recent studies by Suri and others showed that transgenic mice over expressing angiopoietin-1 had larger and more branched blood vessels providing addition support for its role in vascular development *(15)*. Importantly, many of the molecules mentioned above have been shown to be produced by a variety of cells including endothelial cells, tumor cells, macrophages, mast cells, and lymphocytes, all of which may be present within the vascular microenvironment *(16–18)*. A number of these soluble mediators are thought to activate endothelial cells by binding to specific tyrosine kinase receptors expressed on the cell surface *(19–23)*. These receptor-ligand interactions can result in a unique set of characteristics such as increased proliferation, elevated expression of cell-adhesion molecules, increased secretion of proteolytic enzymes, and increased cellular migration and invasion *(19–23)*.

In addition to cytokines and growth factors, the extracellular matrix (ECM) also plays an important role in angiogenesis. Vascular endothelial cells are capable of producing and subsequently interacting with a wide array of matrix molecules including fibronectin, laminin, heparan sulfate proteoglycans, and several types of collagen *(24–27)*. Interestingly, recent evidence suggests that proteolytic remodeling of ECM proteins plays an important role in the regulation of angiogenesis *(9,28–30)*. This proteolytic remodeling has been suggested to be mediated by a number of matrix degrading enzymes including members of the serine protease and matrix metalloproteinase (MMP) families *(9,28)*. Thus, vascular cells must have the capacity to interact with, and in turn respond to, the newly remodeled microenvironment. To this end, vascular cells express cell-adhesion receptors capable of interacting with ECM proteins and other vascular cells *(10,31–35)*. These adhesion receptors can be classified into at least four different families, including the selectins, the immunoglobulin supergene family, the cadherins, and the integrins *(10,35)*. Selectins are transmembrane molecules that play a role in mediating cell-cell interactions *(36)*. Neguyen and colleagues *(37)* and Koch and colleagues *(38)* have provided evidence that E-selectin may function as a critical component of capillary tube formation in vitro, thereby implicating it in angiogenesis. The immunoglobulin super-gene family (IgSF) has also been shown to mediate cell-cell adhesion *(31,38)*. Soluble VCAM-1, an important member of this group, was shown to induce chemotaxis in human endothelial cell in vitro and induce angiogenesis in vivo *(38)*. The cadherin family of receptors are known to mediate calcium-dependent homophillic cell-cell interactions and may be important in maintaining the integrity of both developing and mature blood vessels *(39)*. In fact, VE-cadherin is expressed predominately on endothelial cells and may play an important role in neovascularization *(40)*. Finally, the integrin family predominately mediates cell-ECM interactions, and will be the primary focus of this chapter.

THE INTEGRIN FAMILY OF CELL-ADHESION RECEPTORS

Integrins are a family of cell-surface, heterodimeric glycoproteins that are expressed by virtually all tissues in the human body, and play important roles in signal transduction and the regulation of cellular behavior *(41–42)*. These cell-adhesion receptors are composed of α and β subunits that are associated through noncovalent bonds. To date at least 15 α and 8 β subunits have been identified *(34,43,44)*. These subunits can form a variety of combinations and each heterodimer can have distinct cellular and adhesive specificities. This specificity allows the cell to recognize selectively a wide array of specific ECM ligands and may also help convey positional information to the cell *(41–44)*. Integrins expressed on vascular cells include members of the β_1, and α_v subfamilies (Table 1). These integrins are capable of binding a variety of adhesive proteins such as fibronectin, fibrinogen, vitronectin, thrombospondin, von Willebrand factor (vWF), and various types of collagen *(34,41–44)*. Interestingly, some integrin receptors such as those belonging to the β_1 and α_v subfamilies may have overlapping binding specificites. These overlapping binding abilities my represent examples of biological redundancy within the cell *(41–44)*. Alternatively, distinct signaling pathways may be activated by different integrins binding to a particular matrix component or the same integrin binding to distinct matrix components *(45,46)*. For example, $\alpha_2\beta_1$ on endothelial cells functions as a receptor for collagen and laminin, whereas integrin $\alpha_v\beta_3$ can bind to a number of ECM components including vitronectin, denatured collagen, fibrinogen, and fibronectin to name just a few *(34,41–46)*. Thus, the diversity of functions mediated by the integrins likely provides endothelial cells with the capacity to interact and in turn respond to their dynamic microenvironment.

A variety of important studies have demonstrated the ability of integrin receptors to regulate a diverse set of cellular responses including cellular adhesion, migration/invasion, gene expression, and cell survival *(47,48)*. Integrins provide an important link for the transmission of information between the ECM and the cells interior. These integrin-mediated signaling cascades are facilitated in part by the ability of integrins to interact with specific cytoskelatal components *(45–48)*. In fact, interactions between cytoskeletal molecules such as α-actinin and talin with β_1 integrins have been suggested to facilitate cellular responses such as adhesion and migration *(47–49)*. These protein-protein interactions have also been shown to contribute to transmembrane signaling events such as fluxes in intracellular calcium, changes in intracellular pH, protein phosphorylation, and regulation of gene expression *(45–49)*. In addition to interacting with cytoskeletal and ECM components, integrins can bind to a number of other important regulatory molecules including matrix-degrading proteases and their receptors as well as other cell-adhesion molecules *(50–56)*. In fact, recent studies have indicated that integrin $\alpha_v\beta_3$ can interact with the cell-cell adhesion molecules PECAM/CD31 and L1 CAM *(54,55)*. Moreover, some members of the β_2 integrin subfamily can help mediate homophillic and heterophillic cell-cell interactions with other integrin members *(57)*. The capacity of integrins to interact with other cell-adhesion molecules on adjacent cells may help facilitate angiogenesis by coordinating cell–cell interactions and contribute to the stable associations of endothelial cells and assessory cells *(54–56)*. Moreover, these cellular interactions may

Table 1
Vascular Cell Integrins

β_1 Integrin Family	α_v Integrin Family
$\alpha_1\beta_1$	$\alpha_v\beta_1$
$\alpha_2\beta_1$	$\alpha_v\beta_3$
$\alpha_3\beta_1$	$\alpha_v\beta_5$
$\alpha_4\beta_1$	
$\alpha_5\beta_1$	
$\alpha_6\beta_1$	

Integrin receptors known to be expressed in vascular endothelial cells.

also facilitate the coordinated induction of signal-transduction pathways mediated by cell-cell contact *(58,59)*. Interestingly, recent evidence has been accumulating that these multi-functional integrin receptors can also specifically interact with proteolytic enzymes. For example, integrin $\alpha_{2v}\beta_3$ can help localize the matrix-degrading enzyme MMP-2 in a proteolytically active form to the surface of invasive cells such as angiogenic endothelial cells *(50,59)*. This unique interaction appears to be mediated in part by the ability of $\alpha_v\beta_3$ to bind to the C-terminal hemopexin-like domain of MMP-2 *(59,60)*. Recent findings have revealed other important examples of protease and /or protease receptor-integrin interactions such as the ability of thrombin to bind to $\alpha_v\beta_3$ and the capacity of both β_1 and β_3 integrins to associate with the uPA receptor *(51–53)*. Therefore, integrins may help facilitate angiogenesis by regulating proteolytic cascades as well as localizing proteolytic activity to close cell-matrix contacts. Taken together, these findings suggest that integrins have the capacity to coordinate and regulate cellular behavior by a variety of mechanisms (Fig. 1). However a major question still remains: which specific integrin heterodimers actively contribute to the regulation of angiogenesis?

β_1 *Integrins in Angiogenesis*

The β_1 family of integrins plays an important role in mediating cellular interactions with the ECM. The $\beta1$ integrin subunit itself can noncovalently associate with a number of α subunits including a chains 1 through 9 and α_v *(41–43)*. Interestingly, many of the functions that have been ascribed to integrins have been suggested to be necessary for angiogenesis. Thus, β_1 integrins may represent an important family of regulatory molecules involved in neovascularization. Vascular endothelial cells express many β_1 integrins, including $\alpha_1\beta_1$, $\alpha_2\beta_1$, $\alpha_3\beta_1$, $\alpha_4\beta_1$, $\alpha_5\beta_1$, and $\alpha_6\beta_1$ *(34)*. However, simple expression of integrin receptors on the surface of endothelial cells dose not necessarily indicate that they play an active role in vascular development. Therefore, many investigators are currently designing experiments to determine which integrin receptors may be playing a role in angiogenesis.

Angiogenesis can be initiated by a number of distinct growth factors and cytokines *(16,17)*. Recent findings have indicated that specific growth factors can stimulate increased expression of β_1 and β_3 integrins on the surface of endothelial cells *(61–63)*. This regulated expression of β_1 and β_3 provides hints as to a possible role for these receptors during angiogenesis. Early studies by Grant and colleagues add to these findings in a functional manner by providing evidence that antibodies directed to the β_1 laminin receptor disrupted endothelial cell capillary-like tube formation in vitro *(64)*.

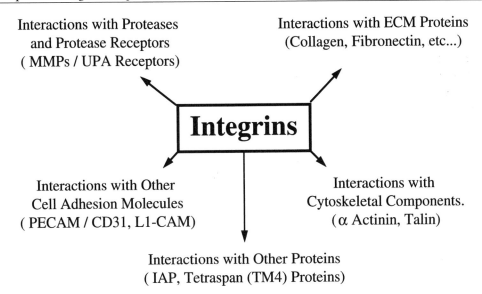

Interactions with Proteases
and Protease Receptors
(MMPs / UPA Receptors)

Interactions with ECM Proteins
(Collagen, Fibronectin, etc...)

Integrins

Interactions with Other
Cell Adhesion Molecules
(PECAM / CD31, L1-CAM)

Interactions with
Cytoskeletal Components.
(α Actinin, Talin)

Interactions with Other Proteins
(IAP, Tetraspan (TM4) Proteins)

Fig. 1. Protein-protein interactions with integrin receptors. The integrin family of cell-adhesion receptors are a group of heterodimeric transmembrane proteins known to mediate adhesive cellular functions. These multi-functional receptors have the capacity to interact with a number of distinct families of molecules including, proteases and protease receptors, extracellular matrix (ECM) proteins, cytoskeletal proteins, cell adhesion receptors, and other miscellaneous molecules. thus, integrins can serve to integrate information from the extracellular environment and intracellular compartments in order to regulate cellular behavior.

Although it is often difficult to extrapolate experimental results from tube-forming assays to true angiogenesis in vivo, these findings suggest that β_1 integrins participate in new blood-vessel development *(64)*.

Identification of Specific β_1 Integrins in Angiogenesis

While the experimental findings of Grant and colleagues demonstrated that an anti-β_1 antagonist could inhibit endothelial-tube formation, little evidence was available as to which specific β_1 integrins may be involved. Bauer and others documented that antibodies to either α_6 or β_1 integrin subunits could inhibit tube formation in vitro *(65)*. These results confirmed previous findings and helped establish a role for $\alpha_6\beta_1$ in vascular development.

Additional studies have now focused on other members of the β_1 integrin family such as $\alpha_2\beta_1$ *(66–69)*. Integrin $\alpha_2\beta_1$ is a collagen receptor for many cell types including endothelial cells, but has also been suggested to bind laminin *(70)*. In studies by Sanger and associates, Northern-blot analysis revealed that VEGF, a known angiogenesis-inducing growth factor, stimulated a better than fivefold induction of α_1 and α_2 mRNAs in endothelial cells *(68)*. Importantly, VEGF stimulation caused little if any change in expression of integrin $\alpha_3\beta_1$ in similar experiments. *(68)*. In other studies, Gamble and colleagues utilized anti-α_2 integrin antibodies to study endothelial cell tube formation in vitro *(66)*. These anti-α_2 antibodies caused an increase in tube formation rather than an inhibition. In contrast, Davis and others showed antibodies directed to α_2 and β_1 could block endothelial tube lumen formation *(67–69)*. Although these results may seem to be at odds, it should be noted that these studies utilized different antibodies that may have been directed to distinct domains within the integrin. In any event, these findings still suggest that integrin $\alpha_2\beta_1$ plays a functional role in the cellular processes associated with angiogenesis. These results were later confirmed in an in vivo microenvironment by Sanger and colleagues that utilized a mouse matrigel-plug assay *(68)*. Matrigel plugs containing tumor cells over expressing VEGF were implanted in nude mice. The mice were then treated subcutaneously with blocking antibodies directed to α_1 and α_2. Angiogenesis was inhibited by over 80% by antagonists directed to both α_1 and α_2, thus providing further evidence that $\alpha_1\beta_1$ and $\alpha_2\beta_1$ integrins actively participate in angiogenesis in vivo.

Additional evidence suggesting a role for β_1 integrins in angiogenesis was demonstrated Drake and others *(71)*. In this study, specific function-blocking antibodies directed to β_1 integrins were injected into quails during early embryonic development. Anti-β_1 monoclonal antibodies (MAbs) significantly disrupted vascular development, providing clear evidence that β_1 plays an important role in blood-vessel formation *(71)*. Finally, studies by Yang and colleagues provided evidence for a specific role for $\alpha_5\beta_1$ in vascular development *(72)*. Using gene-targeting techniques, α_5-deficient mice were generated. These studies showed that homozygous α_5 null mice had a number of mesodermal defects including defects in blood vessel formation. In fact, by day 9.5 of gestation, the mutant embryos showed evidence of disrupted and malformed blood vessels that appeared to be leaking blood cells *(72)*. Taken together, these in vivo and in vitro findings strongly suggest that a number of β_1 integrins including $\alpha_1\beta_1$, $\alpha_2\beta_1$, $\alpha_5\beta_1$, and $\alpha_6\beta_1$ all contribute to angiogenesis. With the growing interest in angiogenesis, combined with new molecular techniques and modern research tools, it will likely be only a matter of time before additional members of the integrin family are identified as critical components of the angiogenic cascade.

Potential Mechanisms by which β_1 Integrins Contribute to Angiogenesis

As mentioned previously, β_1 integrins can regulate a number of cell biological processes including cell adhesion, migration, proliferation, and cell survival *(41–48)*. Interestingly, recent studies by Meredith and others demonstrate that ligation of β_1 integrins can regulate endothelial-cell survival and that these signals may be associated with protein kinase- and/or phosphatase-signaling pathways *(43)*. Thus, β_1 integrins may contribute to angiogenesis by regulating signaling pathways associated with endothelial-cell survival. In other studies, specific β_1 integrins have been shown to regulate endothelial-cell adhesion and migration, processes that could also facilitate angiogenesis *(41,42)*. Finally, ligation of specific extracellular matrix components by β_1 integrins may regulate expression of matrix-degrading enzymes, which could facilitate matrix remodeling *(41–48)*. Although all these mechanisms could contribute to angiogenesis, which actually do contribute to vascular development is not clear and therefore awaits further investigation.

THE α_v INTEGRINS IN ANGIOGENESIS

The α_v chain can associate with a variety of integrin subunits including β_1, β_3, β_5, β_6, and β_8 *(41,42)*. Importantly, a number of these α_v integrins have been reported to be expressed on the surface of endothelial cells including $\alpha_v\beta_1$, $\alpha_v\beta_3$, and $\alpha_v\beta_5$ *(34)*. Little direct evidence is available to support a role for $\alpha_v\beta_5$ in angiogenesis and further research into the function of this integrin awaits new heterodimer-specific antibodies to assist in answering this question. However, over the past few years a wealth of information has been accumulating on the role of the vitronectin receptor $\alpha_v\beta_3$.

Integrin $\alpha_v\beta_3$ in Angiogenesis

Integrin $\alpha_v\beta_3$ is one of the more promiscuous members of the integrin family because it has the capacity to bind a wide variety of adhesive ligands including vitronectin, fibronectin, fibrinogen, thrombospondin, osteopontin, tenascin, vWF, and denatured collagens, to name just a few *(73–74)*. Many of these extracellular-matrix components contain the tripeptide sequence Arginine, Glycine, and Aspartic Acid (RGD), an amino acid sequence known to be recognized by a number of integrin receptors, including members of the α_v and β_1 subfamilies *(42,43)*. However this RGD dependency is not as strict as was once thought. In fact, evidence has been accumulating that proteins containing R/K(X)D, were X is any amino acid can be recognized by β_3 integrins *(75)*. Interestingly, $\alpha_v\beta_3$ has been suggested to be able to bind to molecules that do not contain an RGD tripeptide such as MMP-2 and CD31 *(50,51,54)*.

Control of $\alpha_v\beta_3$ Integrin Expression

A variety of studies have shown that $\alpha_v\beta_3$ is differentially expressed on vascular cells during angiogenesis *(62,76–79)*. In fact, $\alpha_v\beta_3$ was shown to be highly expressed on tumor vasculature in many animal models and within human-tumor biopsies, whereas little if any $\alpha_v\beta_3$ was expressed on normal quiescent blood vessels *(62,76–79)*. Further studies have demonstrated that a number of angiogenic cytokines and growth factors including bFGF can specifically up regulate the expression of $\alpha_v\beta_3$ both in vitro and in vivo *(62)*. However, to date, little is known concerning the molecular mechanisms regulating the expression of $\alpha_v\beta_3$. Recent studies by Boudreau and others have shed some new light on the molecular mechanisms regulating $\alpha_v\beta_3$ expression *(63)*. These studies indicated that expression of the transcriptional activator HOX D3 significantly induced β_3 integrin mRNA and subsequent surface expression of $\alpha_v\beta_3$ within endothelial cells *(63)*. Moreover, HOX D3 appeared to facilitate bFGF induced expression of $\alpha_v\beta_3$ *(63)*. Sustained expression of the HOX D3 in vivo caused abnormal vascular development *(63)*. These studies taken together with the differential expression of $\alpha_v\beta_3$ on vascular cells during angiogenesis implicate integrin $\alpha_v\beta_3$ in this process.

Experimental Evidence for a Functional Role of $\alpha_v\beta_3$ in Angiogenesis

In early studies by Davis and others, it was demonstrated that antibodies directed to $\alpha_v\beta_3$ could disrupt endothelial-cord formation in vitro *(80)*. Moreover, Nicosia and colleagues utilized RGD containing peptides to disrupt microvessel outgrowth from rings of rat aorta embedded in collagen gels *(81)*. These early in vitro studies suggested that $\alpha_v\beta_3$ may play a role in vascular development. However, without direct in vivo studies or heterodimer specific antagonists of $\alpha_v\beta_3$, it remained difficult to establish a functional role for $\alpha_v\beta_3$ in neovascularization. Recently, a number of in vivo studies have provided compelling evidence to support a direct role for $\alpha_v\beta_3$ in angiogenesis. Utilizing specific MAbs and peptides it was demonstrated that systemic administration of these antagonists inhibited cytokine and tumor-induced angiogenesis in vivo including the avian, and human/mouse chimeric models *(62,82,83)*. In addition, Friedlander and others demonstrated that antagonists of $\alpha_v\beta_3$ could disrupt retinal and corneal angiogenesis in both murine and rabbit models *(84,85)*. Importantly, recent findings by Ruegg and others demonstrated a role for $\alpha_v\beta_3$ in the inhibition of angiogenesis associated with TNF-α and interferon-γ (IFN-γ) treatments *(86)*. Finally, in elegant studies by Drake and colleagues, it was shown that $\alpha_v\beta_3$ antagonists could dramatically disrupt lumen formation and vascular patterning within quail embryos *(87)*. Taken together these in vivo studies clearly establish an important role for $\alpha_v\beta_3$ in vascular development.

Potential Mechanisms by which $\alpha_v\beta_3$ Contributes to Angiogenesis

Although little information is available concerning the mechanisms by which β_1 integrins facilitate angiogenesis, studies have provided many clues as to how $\alpha_v\beta_3$ may contribute to this process. In previous studies it was shown that antagonists of $\alpha_v\beta_3$ could inhibit angiogenesis by inducing apoptosis or programmed cell death within proliferating blood vessels (82). These data suggested one potential mechanism by which $\alpha_v\beta_3$ could regulate angiogenesis was by regulating endothelial-cell survival. Further support for this possibility was provided by studies from Stromblad and others where they showed that antagonists of $\alpha_v\beta_3$ could specifically activate DNA binding ability of p53 and increase the expression of the p53 inducable cell-cycle inhibitor p21 [WAF1/ CIP1] (88). Moreover, it was shown that ligation of $\alpha_v\beta_3$ could specifically upregulate expression of Bcl-2 and downregulate expression of Bax, two proteins known to regulate cell survival (88). In addition, studies by IsIk and colleagues showed that ligation of vitronectin by either $\alpha_v\beta_3$ or $\alpha_v\beta_5$ caused a decrease in endothelial-cell apoptosis in vitro (89). Taken together, these findings indicate that ligation of $\alpha_v\beta_3$ expressed in angiogenic endothelial cells may function in part by transmitting specific survival signals necessary for angiogenesis.

Previous results have demonstrated that ligation of $\alpha_v\beta_3$ integrin can regulate fluxes in cellular calcium concentrations (90). Importantly, Kohn and others demonstrated a role for calcium-dependent signaling for endothelial-cell proliferation (91). These studies also showed that the calcium-influx inhibitor CAI could significantly inhibit endothelial-cell proliferation and endothelial-cell cord formation in vitro. CAI was also shown to inhibit angiogenesis in the chick CAM model (91). These findings implicate calcium signaling in the regulation of vascular development. Therefore, a second mechanism by which $\alpha_v\beta_3$ may regulate angiogenesis is by regulating calcium-mediated signal transduction.

Because tyrosine kinase signaling has been shown to regulate a number of cell-biological functions and because integrin ligation has been shown to initiate kinase-signaling pathways, it is likely that tyrosine-kinase signaling is involved in angiogenesis. To this end, Eliceiri and others demonstrated that $\alpha_v\beta_3$ expressed in angiogenic blood vessels is required for sustained MAP kinase activity during angiogenesis and furthermore, that inhibition of MAP kinase activity by the MEK inhibitor disrupted $\alpha_v\beta_3$-dependent angiogenesis in vivo (92). Interestingly, antagonists of $\alpha_v\beta_3$ could disrupt sustained ERK activity in vessels occurring 4–20 h after bFGF stimulation, while having little if any effect on the initial wave of ERK activity occurring between 5–120 min poststimulation (92). Finally, it was shown that the inhibition of MAP kinase activity could also block growth factor induced endothelial-cell migration, suggesting $\alpha_v\beta_3$ may contribute to angiogenesis by regulating endothelial-cell migration and tyrosine kinase activity.

In recent studies, an additional mechanism by which $\alpha_v\beta_3$ may regulate angiogenesis was identified. This report indicated that $\alpha_v\beta_3$ could bind the matrix metalloproteinase MMP-2 to the surface of invasive cells such as angiogenic endothelial cells (50,60,93). This unique interaction may help facilitate ECM remodeling by localizing proteolytic activity to cell-ECM contact points thereby creating a microenvironment capable of supporting new vessel growth. Thus, numerous studies have provided evidence for multiple mechanisms by which $\alpha_v\beta_3$ may function during angiogenesis. These mechanisms may contribute individually at specific times during the angiogenic cascade or perhaps they may work cooperatively to facilitate $\alpha_v\beta_3$-dependent neovascularization.

Integrin $\alpha_v\beta_5$ *in Angiogenesis*

Integrin $\alpha_v\beta_5$ is an example of an alternative vitronectin receptor belonging to the α_v subfamily *(94,95)*. It was been shown to be distributed in a variety of tissues and cell types including endothelial cells *(94)*. Interestingly, $\alpha_v\beta_5$ was shown to be highly expressed on human vascular cells from patients with proliferative diabetic retinopathy (PDR) suggesting that $\alpha_v\beta_5$ may play an active role in retinal neovascularization *(85)*. To this end, Friedlander and colleagues demonstrated an important role for $\alpha_v\beta_5$ during angiogenesis *(84,85)*. Results from these studies indicated that MAb antagonists of $\alpha_v\beta_5$ could inhibit VEGF-induced angiogenesis in vivo, but had little effect on bFGF-induced angiogenesis *(84)*. These intriguing results helped define two potentially distinct pathways involved in angiogenesis. Furthermore, these results suggest that individual α_v containing integrins may have distinct roles depending on which growth factors are involved in initiating the angiogenic cascade. Although $\alpha_v\beta_5$ is similar to the related vitronectin receptor $\alpha_v\beta_3$, distinct differences also exist *(95,96)*. In fact, studies indicate that $\alpha_v\beta_3$ can mediate both cell adhesion and migration without a requirement for tyrosine kinase-dependent receptor activation *(96,97)*. However, while $\alpha_v\beta_5$ can mediate cell adhesion without receptor activation, a tyrosine kinase signaling cascade is necessary for $\alpha_v\beta_5$-dependent cell motility *(96,97)*. These distinct signaling requirements for avb5 dependent cellular migration may provide insight into its role in VEGF-dependent angiogenesis. Because many cytokines known to stimulate angiogenesis such as insulin, IGF-1 and EGF can activate $\alpha_v\beta_5$ dependent cellular motility, it is possible that $\alpha_v\beta_5$ may facilitate angiogenesis by regulating cellular migration. However, to date little direct evidence is available concerning the molecular mechanisms by which $\alpha_v\beta_5$ facilitates this process.

CONCLUSIONS

Over the past 10 years, our cumulative understanding of cell-adhesion and integrin biology has provided new insight into the role cell adhesion molecules play in numerous physiological processes. In particular, this wealth of information has lead to the speculation that integrin receptors may play an important role in angiogenesis. Over the past several years angiogenesis has emerged as an exciting and important field of biological research. In fact, the exciting new experimental findings discussed in this chapter provide compelling evidence that a number of specific integrin receptors actively participate in new blood-vessel development. Given the critical impact angiogenesis has on a variety of human disorders, understanding the molecular regulators of neovascularization is of paramount importance. Because angiogenesis encompasses a complicated cascade of interconnected cellular, biochemical, and molecular events, it has drawn interest from investigators in fields such as cell and developmental biology, biochemistry, molecular biology, organic chemistry, and physiology. The combined expertise from these diverse disciplines has paved the way to a new understanding of the complex mechanisms underlying the function of integrins during angiogenesis. This new understanding has prompted many investigators from both industry and academic institutions to assess the potential of integrin antagonists as anti-angiogenic reagents. In fact, integrin receptors such as $\alpha_v\beta_3$ are rapidly being considered as critical new therapeutic targets for the treatment of neovascular diseases. Thus, with the renewed excitement concerning modulating angiogenesis for therapeutic purposes, combined with the efforts of researcher from diverse scientific disciplines, our understanding of integrins in vascular development is rapidly coming into focus.

REFERENCES

1. Folkman, J. and Shing, Y. (1992) *Angiogenesis* **267,** 10,931–10,934.
2. Blood, C. H. and Zetter, B. R. (1990) Tumor interactions with the vasculature: angiogenesis and tumor metastasis. *Biochem. Biophys. Acta.* **1032,** 89–118.
3. Risau, W. and Flamme, I. (1995) Vasculogenesis. *Ann. Rev. Cell. Dev. Biol.* **11,** 73–91.
4. Flamme, I., Frolich, T., and Risau, W. (1997) Molecular mechanisms of vasculogenesis and embryonic angiogenesis. *J. Cell. Physiol.* **173,** 206–210.
5. Paku, S. and Paweletz, N. (1991) First steps of tumor–related angiogenesis. *Lab. Invest.* **65,** 334–345.
6. D'Amore, P. A. and Thompson, R. W. (1987) Mechanisms of Angiogenesis. *Ann. Rev. Physiol.* **49,** 453–464.
7. Varner, J. A., Brooks, P. C., and Cheresh, D. A. (1995) The integrin $\alpha_v\beta_3$: angiogenesis and apoptosis. *Cell. Adhes. Commun.* **3,** 367–374.
8. Leek, R. D., Harris, A. L., and Lewis, C. E. (1994) *J. Leuk. Biol. 56,* 423–433.
9. Pepper, M. S., Montesano, R., Mandriota, S. J., Orci, L., and Vassalli, J. (1996) Angiogenesis: a paradigm for balanced extracellular proteolysis during cell migration and morphogenesis. *Enzm. Prot.* **49,** 138–162.
10. Brooks, P. C. (1996) Cell adhesion molecules in angiogenesis. *Cancer. Met. Rev.* **15,** 187–194.
11. Polverini, P. J. (1996) Cell adhesion molecules: newly identified mediators of angiogenesis. *Am. J. Pathol.* **148,** 1023–1029.
12. Carey, D. J. (1991) Control of growth and differentiation of vascular cells by extracellular matrix proteins. *Ann. Rev. Physiol.* **53,** 161–177.
13. Sierra-Honigmann, M. R., Nath, A. K., Murakami, C., Garcia-Cardena, G., Papapetropoulos, A., Sessa, W. C., et al. (1998) Biological action of leptin as an angiogenic factor. *Science* **281,** 1683–1686.
14. Suri, C., Jones, P. F., Patan, S., Bartunkova, S., Maisonpierre, P. C., Davis, S., et al. (1996) Requisite role of angiopoietin-1, a ligand for the TIE-2 receptor, during embryonic angiogenesis. *Cell* **87,** 1171–1180.
15. Suri, C., McClain, J., Thurston, G., McDonald, D. M., Zhou, H., Oldmixon, E. H., et al. (1998) Increased vascularization in mice over expressing angiopoietin-1. *Science* **282,** 468–471.
16. Singh, R. K. and Fidler, I. J. (1996) Regulation of tumor angiogenesis by organ-specific cytokines. *Ann. Rev. Cell. Biol.* **18,** 1–11.
17. Pepper, M. S., Mandriota, S. J., Vassalli, J.-D., Orci, L., and Monitesano, R. (1996) Angiogenesis-regulating cytokines: activities and interactions. *Ann. Rev. Cell. Biol.* **18,** 31–67.
18. D'Amore, P. A. (1992) Capillary growth a two cell system. *Semin. Cancer. Biol.* **3,** 49–56.
19. Mustonen, T. and Alitalo, K. (1995) Endothelial receptor tyrosine kinases involved in angiogenesis. *J. Cell. Biol.* **129,** 895–898.
20. Heller, R. A. and Kronke, M. (1994) Tumor necrosis factor receptor-mediated signaling pathways. *J. Cell. Biol.* **126,** 5–9.
21. Waltenberger, J., Claesson, L., Siegbahn, A., Shibuya, M., and Heldin, C.-H. (1994) Different signal transduction properties of KDR and Flt1, two receptors for vascular endothelial growth factor. *J. Biol. Chem.* **269,** 26,988–26,995.
22. Marx, M., Perlmutter, R. A., and Madri, J. A. (1994) Regulation of platelet-derived growth factor receptor expression in microvascular endothelial cells during in vitro angiogenesis. *J. Clin. Invest.* **93,** 131–139.
23. Sato, T. N., Qin, Y., Kozak, C. A., and Audus, K. L. (1993) Tie-1 and tie-2 define another class of putative receptor tyrosine kinase genes expressed in early embryonic vascular system. *Proc. Natl. Acad. Sci. USA* **90,** 9355–9358.
24. Ingber, D. E. and Folkman, J. (1989) How does extracellular matrix control capillary morphogenesis. *Cell* **58,** 803–805.
25. Sephel, G. C., Kennedy, R., and Kudravi, S. (1996) Expression of capillary basement membrane components during sequential phases of wound angiogenesis. *Matrix. Biol.* **15,** 263–279.
26. Sage, H. E. (1997) Pieces of eight: bioactive fragments of extracellular proteins as regulators of angiogenesis. *Trends. Cell. Biol.* **7,** 182–186.
27. Risau, W. and Lemmon, V. (1988) Changes in the vascular extracellular matrix during embryonic vasculogenesis and angiogenesis. *Dev. Bol.* **125,** 441–450.
28. Yasunaga, C., Nakashima, Y., and Sueishi, K. (1989) A role of fibrinolytic activity in angiogenesis. *Lab. Invest.* **61,** 698–704.
29. Liotta, L. A., Steeg, P. S., and Stetler-Stevenson, W. G. (1991) Cancer metastasis and angiogenesis: an imbalance of positive and negative regulation. *Cell* **64,** 327–336.
30. Moses, M. A., Sudhalter, J., and Langer, R. (1990) Identification of an inhibitor of neovascularization from cartilage. *Science* **248,** 1408–1410.

31. Stad, R. K. and Burman, W. A. (1994) Current views on structure and function of endothelial adhesion molecules. *Cell Adhes. Comm.* **2,** 261–268.

32. Trochon, V., Mabilat, C., Bertrand, P., Legrand, Y., Smadja-Joffe, F., Soria, C., et al. (1996) Evidence of involvement of CD44 in endothelial cell proliferation, migration and angiogenesis in vitro. *Int. J. Cancer* **66,** 664–668.

33. Delisser, H. M., Christofidou-Solmidou, M., Strieter, R. M., Burdick, M. D., Robinson, C. S., Wexlewr, R. S., et al. (1997) Involvement of endothelial PECAM–1/CD31 in angiogenesis. *Am. J Pathol.* **151,** 671–677.

34. Luscinskas, F. W. and Lawer, J. (1994) Integrins as dynamic regulators of vascular function. *FASEB J.* **8,** 929–937.

35. Bischoff. J. (1995) Approaches to studying cell adhesion molecules in angiogenesis. *Trends. Cell. Biol.* **5,** 69–73.

36. Beviacaua, M. P. and Nelson, R. M. (1993) Selectins. *J. Clin. Invest.* **91,** 374–387.

37. Nguyen, M., Strubel, N. A., and Bischoff, J. (1993) A role for sialyl lewis–X/A glycoconjugates in capillary morphogenesis. *Nature* **365,** 267–269.

38. Koch, A. E., Halloran, M. M., Haskell, C. J., Shah, M. R., and Polverini, P. J. (1995) Angiogenesis mediated by soluble forms of E-selectin and vascular cell adhesion molecule-1. *Nature* **376,** 517–519.

39. Gumbiner, B. (1996) Cadherins: a family of ca+ dependent adhesion molecules. *Trends. Biochem. Sci.* **13,** 75–76.

40. Breier, G., Breviario, F., Caveda, L., Berthier, R., Schnurch, H., Gotsch, U., et al. (1996) Molecular cloning and expression of murine vascular endothelial-cadherin in early stage development of cardiovascular system. *Blood* **87,** 630–641.

41. Hynes, R. O. (1992) Integrins: versatility, modulation, and signaling in cell adhesion. *Cell* **69,** 11–25.

42. Ruoslahti, E. (1991) Integrins. *J. Clin. Invest.* **87,** 1–5.

43. Meredith, J. E., Fazeli, B., and Schwartz, M. A. (1993) The extracellular matrix as a survival factor. *Mol. Biol. Cell.* **4,** 953–961.

44. Humphries, M. J., Mould, P. A., and Tuckwell, S. (1993) Dynamic aspects of adhesion receptor function, integrins both twist and shout. *BioEssays* **15,** 391–397.

45. Lafrenie, R. M. and Yamada, K. M. (1996) Integrin dependent signal transduction. *J. Cell Biochem.* **61,** 543–553.

46. Schwartz, M. A. and Ingber, D. E. (1994) Integrating with integrins. *Mol. Biol. Cell.* **5,** 389–393.

47. Defilippi, P., Bozzo, C., Volpe, G., Romano, G., Venturino, M., Silengo, L., and Tarone, G. (1994) Integrin mediated signal transduction in human endothelial cells: analysis of tyrosine phosphorylation events. *Cell. Adhes. Comm.* **2,** 75–86.

48. Kolanus, W. and Seed, B. (1997) Integrins and inside–out signal transduction: converging signals from PKC and PIP3. *Curr. Opin. Cell. Biol.* **9,** 725–731.

49. Wary, K. K., Mainiero, F., Isakoff, S. J., Marcantonio, E. E., and Giancotti, F. G. (1996) The adapter protein Shc couples a class of integrins to the control of cell cycle progression. *Cell* **87,** 733–743.

50. Brooks, P. C., Stromblad, S., Sanders, L. C., von Schalscha, T. L., Aims, R. T., Stetler–Stevenson, W. G., et al. (1996) Localization of matrix metalloproteinase MMP-2 to the surface of invasive cells by interaction with integrin $\alpha_v\beta_3$. *Cell* **85,** 683–693.

51. Xue, W., Mizukami, I., Todd, R. F., and Petty, H. R. (1997) Urokinase-type plasminogen activator receptors associate with β_1 and β_3 integrins of fibrosarcoma cells: dependence on extracellular matrix components. *Cancer. Res.* **57,** 1682–1689.

52. Bar-Shavit, R., Sabbah, V., Lampugnani, M. G., Marchisio, P. C., Fenton, J. W., Vlodavsky, I., and Dejana, E. (1991) An Arg-Gly-Asp sequence within thrombin promotes endothelial cell adhesion. *J. Cell. Biol.* **112,** 335–344.

53. Buckley, C. D., Doyonnas, R., Newton, J. P., Blystone, S. D., Brown, E. J., Watt, S. M., and Simmons, D. L. (1996) Identification of $\alpha_v\beta_3$ as a heterotypic ligand for CD31/PECAM-1. *J. Cell. Sci.* **109,** 437–445.

54. Felding-Habermann, B., Silletti, S., Mei, F., Siu, C–H., Yip, P. M., Brooks, P. C., et al. (1997) A single immunogloglulin-like domain of human neural cell adhesion molecule L1 supports adhesion by multiple vascular and platelet integrins. *J. Cell. Biol.* **139,** 1567–1581.

55. Lobb, R. R., Antognetti, G., Pepinsky, R. B., Burkly, L. C., Leone, D. R., and Whitty, A. (1995) A direct binding assay for the vascular cell adhesion molecule-1 (VCAM1) interaction with α4 integrins. *Cell. Adhes. Comm.* **3,** 385–397.

56. Lampugnani, M. G. and Dejana, E. (1997) Interendothelial junctions: structure, signaling and functional roles. *Curr. Opin. Cell. Biol.* **9,** 674–682.

57. Ruoslahti, E. and Obrink, B. (1996) Common principles in cell adhesion. *Exp. Cell Res.* **227,** 1–11.

58. Brooks, P. C., Silletti, S., von Schalscha, T. L., Friendlander, M., and Cheresh, D. A. (1998) Disruption of angiogenesis by PEX, a noncatalytic metalloproteinase fragment with integrin binding activity. *Cell* **92**, 391–400.

59. Deryugina, E. I., Bourdon, M. A., Luo, G. X., Reisfeld, R. A., and Strongin, A. (1997) Matrix metalloproteinase-2 activation modulates glioma cell migration. *J. Cell. Sci.* **110**, 2473–2482.

60. Swerlick, R. A., Brown, E. J., Xu, Y., Lee, K. H., Manos, S., and Lawley, T. (1992) Expression and modulation of the vitronectin receptor on human dermal microvascular endothelial cells. *J. Invest. Dermatol.* **99**, 715–722.

61. Brooks, P. C., Clark, R. A. F., and Cheresh, D. A. (1994) Requirement of vascular integrin $\alpha_v\beta_3$ for angiogenesis. *Science* **264**, 569–571.

62. Boudreau, N., Andrews, C., Srebow, A., Ravanpay, A., and Cheresh, D. A. (1997) Induction of the angiogenic phenotype by HOX D3. *J. Cell. Biol.* **139**, 257–264.

63. Grant, D. S., Tashiro, K–I., Segui–Real, B., Yamada, Y., Martin, G. R., and Kleinman, H. K. (1989) Two different laminin domains mediate the differentiation of human endothelial cells into capillary-like structures in vitro. *Cell* **58**, 933–943.

64. Bauer, J., Margolis, M., Schreiner, C., Edgell, C–J., Azizkhan, J., Lazarowski, E., and Juliano, R. L. (1992) In vitro model of angiogenesis using a human endothelium-derived permanent cell line: contributions of induced gene expression, G-proteins, and integrins. *J. Cell. Physiol.* **153**, 437–449.

65. Gamble, J. R., Matthias, L. J., Meyer, G., Kaur, P., Russ, G., Faull, R., et al. (1993) Regulation of in vitro capillary tube formation by anti-integrin antibodies. *J. Cell. Biol.* **121**, 931–943.

66. Davis, G. E. and Camarillo, C. W. (1996) An $\alpha_2\beta_1$ integrin-dependent pinocytic mechanisms involving intracellular vacuole formation and coalescence regulates capillary lumen and tube formation in three-dimensional collagen matrix. *Exp. Cell. Res.* **224**, 39–51.

67. Senger, D. R., Claffey, K. P., Benes, J. E., Perruzzi, C. A., Sergiou, A. P., and Detmar, M. (1997) Angiogenesis promoted by vascular endothelial growth factor: regulation through $\alpha_1\beta_1$ and $\alpha_2\beta_1$ integrins. *Proc. Natl. Acad. Sci. USA* **94**, 13,612–13,617.

68. Meyer, G., Matthias, L. J., Noack, L., Vadas, M. A., and Gamble, J. R. (1997) Lumen formation during angiogenesis in vitro involves phagocytic activity, formation and secretion of vacuoles, cell death, and capillary tube remodeling by different populations of endothelial cells. *Anat. Rec.* **249**, 327–340.

69. Drake, C. J., Davis, L., and Little, C. (1992) Antibodies to β_1-integrins cause alterations of aortic vasculogenesis in vivo. *Dev. Dyn.* **193**, 83–91.

70. Yang, J. T., Rayburn, H., and Hynes, R. O. (1993) Embryonic mesodermal defects in α_5 integrin deficient mice. *Development* 119, 1093–1105.

71. Brooks, P. C. (1997) Integrin $\alpha_v\beta_3$: a therapeutic target. *DN&P* **10**, 456–461.

72. Horton, M. (1990) Current status review vitronectin receptor: tissue specific expression or adaptation to culture. *Int. J. Exp. Pathol.* **71**, 741–759.

73. Smith, J. W., Hu, D., Satterthwait, A., Pinz–Sweeney, S., and Barbas, C. F. (1994) Building synthetic antibodies as adhesive ligands for integrins. *J. Biol. Chem.* **269**, 32,788–32,795.

74. Enenstein, J. and Kramer, R. H. (1994) Confocal microscopic analysis of integrin expression on the microvasculature and its sprouts in the neonatal foreskin. *J. Invest. Dermatol.* **103**, 381–386.

75. Gladson, C. L. (1996) Expression of integrin $\alpha_v\beta_3$ in small blood vessels of glioblastoma tumors. *J. Neuropath. Exp. Neur.* **55**, 1143–1149.

76. Okada, Y., Copeland, B. R., Hamann, G. F., Koziol, J. A., Cheresh, D. A., and del Zoppo, G. J. (1996) Integrin $\alpha_v\beta_3$ is expressed in selected microvessels after focal cerebral ischemia. *Am. J. Pathol.* **149**, 37–44.

77. Max, R., Gerritsen, R. R., Nooijen, P., Goodman, S. L., Sutter, A., Keilholz, U., et al. (1997) Immuno-histochemical analysis of integrin $\alpha_v\beta_3$ expression on tumor–associated vessels of human carcinomas. *Int. J. Cancer* **71**, 320–324.

78. Davis, C. M., Danehower, S. C., Laurenza, A., and Molony, J. L. (1993) Identification of a role of the vitronectin receptor and protein kinase C in the induction of endothelial cell vascular formation. *J. Cell Biochem.* **51**, 206–218.

79. Nicosia, R. F. and Bonanno, E. (1991) Inhibition of angiogenesis in vitro by Arg-Gly-Asp-containing synthetic peptide. *Am. J. Pathol.* **138**, 829–833.

80. Brooks, P. C., Montgomery, A. M/P., Rosenfeld, M., Reisfeld, R. A., Hu, T., Klier, G., and Cheresh, D. A. (1994) Integrin $\alpha_v\beta_3$ antagonists promote tumor regression by inducing apoptosis of angiogenic blood vessels. *Cell* **79**, 1157–1164.

81. Brooks, P. C., Stromblad, S., Klemke, R., Visscher, D., Sarkar, F. H., and Cheresh, D. A. (1995) Antiintegrin $\alpha_v\beta_3$ blocks human breast cancer growth and angiogenesis in human skin. *J. Clin. Invest.* **96**, 1815–1822.

82. Friedlander, M., Brooks, P. C., Shaffer, R. W., Kincaid, C. M., Varner, J. A., and Cheresh, D. A. (1995) Definition of two angiogenic pathways by distinct α_v integrins. *Science* **270,** 1500–1502.

83. Friedlander, M., Thesefeld, C. L., Sugita, M., Fruitiger, M., Thomas, M. A., Chang, S., and Cheresh, D. A. (1996) Involvement of integrin $\alpha_v\beta_3$ and $\alpha_v\beta_5$ in ocular neovascular diseases. *Proc. Natl. Acad. Sci. USA* **93,** 9764–9769.

84. Ruegg, C., Yilmaz, A., Bierler, G., Bamat, J., Chaubert, P., and Lejeune, F. J. (1998) Evidence for the involvement of endothelial cell integrin $\alpha_v\beta_3$ in the disruption of the tumor vasculature induced by TNF and IFN-γ. *Nature Med.* **4,** 408–413.

85. Drake, C. J., Cheresh, D. A., and Little, C. D. (1995) An antagonists of integrin $\alpha_v\beta_3$ prevents maturation of blood vessels during embryonic neovascularization. *J. Cell. Sci.* **108,** 2655–2661.

86. Stromblad, S., Becker, J. C., Yebra, M., Brooks, P. C., and Cheresh, D. A. (1996) Suppression of p53 activity and p21[WAF1/CIP1] expression by vascular cell integrin $\alpha_v\beta_3$ during angiogenesis. *J. Clin. Invest.* **98,** 426–433.

87. Isik, F. F., Gibran, N. S., Jang, Y.-C., Sandell, L., and Schwartz, S. M. (1998) Vitronectin decreases microvascular endothelial cell apoptosis. *J. Cell. Physiol.* **175,** 149–155.

88. Schwartz, M. A. and Denninghoff, K. (1994) α_v Integrins mediate the rise in intracellular calcium in endothelial cells on fibronectin even though they play a minor role in adhesion. *J. Biol. Chem.* **269,** 11,133–11,137.

89. Kohn, E. C., Alessandro, R., Spoonster, J., Wersto, R. P., and Liotta, L. A. (1995) Angiogenesis: role of calcium-mediated signal transduction. *Proc. Natl. Acad. Sci. USA* **92,** 1307–1311.

90. Eliceiri, B. P., Klemke, R. Stromblad, S., and Cheresh, D. A. (1998) Integrin $\alpha_v\beta_3$ requirement for sustained mitogen-activated protein kinase activity during angiogenesis. *J. Cell Biol.* **140,** 1255–1263.

91. Pasqualini, R., Bodorova, J., Ye, S., and Hemler, M. E. (1993) A study of the structure, function and distribution of β5 integrins using novel anti-β5 monoclonal antibody. *J Cell. Sci.* **105,** 101–111.

92. Wayner, E. A., Orlando, R. A., and Cheresh, D. A. (1991) Integrins $\alpha_v\beta_3$ and $\alpha_v\beta_5$ contribute to cell attachment to vitronectin but differentially distribute on the cell surface. *J. Cell. Biol.* **113,** 919–929.

93. Klemke, R. L., Yebra, M., Bayna, E. M., and Cheresh, D. A. (1994) Receptor tyrosine kinase signaling required for integrin $\alpha_v\beta_3$-directed cell motility but not adhesion on vitronectin. *J. Cell. Biol.* **127,** 859–866.

94. Brooks, P. C., Klemke, R. L., Schon, S., Lewis, J. M., Schwartz, M. A., and Cheresh, D. A. (1997) Insulin-like growth factor receptor cooperates with integrin $\alpha_v\beta_5$ to promote tumor cell dissemination in vivo. *J. Clin. Invest.* 99, 1390–1398.

6

Vasoactive Peptides in Angiogenesis

David Andrew Walsh and Tai-Ping D. Fan

CONTENTS

INTRODUCTION

Angiogenesis, the formation of new from old vessels, occurs physiologically during the female reproductive cycle, and pathologically during tumor growth, diabetic retinopathy, and chronic inflammation. It may be either beneficial, for example in wound repair, or detrimental, for example in tumors. Neovascularization is a complex process rather than a single event, requiring endothelial cell migration and proliferation, capillary-tube formation, and anastomosis, recruitment of mural cells, and reorganization and maturation of the vascular bed. Each stage is regulated by a variety of factors and it is essential to complete all stages in order to establish a normal vasculature. Much research has focused on factors that are upregulated during angiogenesis, such as vascular endothelial growth factor (VEGF) and its receptors, and integrin $\alpha_v\beta_3$. Upregulation of angiogenic factors and endothelial cell-survival factors is essential to sustain angiogenesis and prevent regression of the neovasculature. In this chapter, we discuss a group of regulatory peptides, many of which are constitutively expressed in the mature vasculature, and even may be downregulated in neovasculature (Table 1, Fig. 1). None the less, these stimulate angiogenesis both in vitro and in vivo. We suggest that regulatory peptides may play important roles in the initiation of angiogenesis, before other growth factors have been upregulated. Peptides may, in addition, facilitate vascular survival (33). Constitutively produced vasoactive peptides may particularly be important for the survival of mature, appropriate blood vessels, following the downregulation of other vascular survival factors. Bradykinin and substance P are generated and released during the earliest stages of tissue injury, and it is appropriate that peptides that mediate acute inflammatory responses may simultaneously initiate processes such as angiogenesis that are essential for tissue repair. However, inappropriate initiation of angiogenesis by regulatory peptides may be a key process in several human diseases.

From: *The New Angiotherapy*
Edited by: T.-P. D. Fan and E. C. Kohn © Humana Press Inc., Totowa, NJ

Table 1
Angiogenic Actions of Vasoactive Peptides

Angiogenesis Model	Substance P	CGRP	Angiotensin II	Endothelins	Bradykinin
EC proliferation	(1–3)	(3,4)	(5,6)	(7,8)	(9,10)
EC migration	(2,11)		(12)	(7,13,14)	No effect (10)
EC wound repair				(15)	
Capillary-tube formation	(16)		(6)		
Capillary sprouting				(17)	
Chick CAM			(18,19)	No effect (20)	(21)
Rabbit cornea	(1,22)		(22)		
Rat sponge	(23)	(24)	(25,26)	No effect (25)	(27)
Heart					(28)
Carotid artery			(29)		
Renal collateral			(30)		
Cremaster muscle			(31,32)		

CAM, chorioallantoic membrane; CGRP, calcitonin gene-related peptide; EC, endothelial cell. Numbers in parentheses refer to cited references.

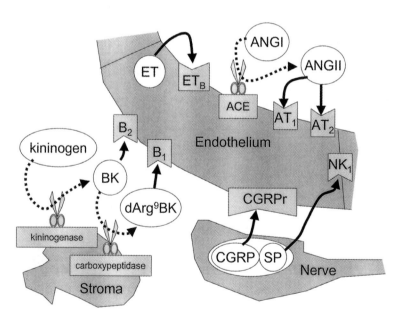

Fig. 1. Sources of vasoactive peptides. Broken arrows indicate enzymatic cleavage of precursors to generate active vasoactive peptide. Solid arrows indicate interaction of peptides with receptors on the endothelial-cell surface. The precise localization of receptors and enzymes requires further investigation, although current evidence supports the view that ACE is primarily localized to the luminal endothelial surface, whereas NK_1 receptors are localized to interendothelial junctions. Abbreviations: ACE, angiotensin-converting enzyme; ANGI, angiotensin I; ANGII; angiotensin II; AT_1, angiotensin receptor subtype AT_1; AT_2, angiotensin receptor subtype AT_2; BK, bradykinin; B_1, bradykinin receptor subtype B_1; B_2, bradykinin receptor subtype B_2; dArg⁹BK, des-Arg⁹-bradykinin; CGRP, calcitonin gene-related peptide; CGRPr, calcitonin gene-related peptide receptor; ET_b, endothelin receptor subtype ET_b; NK_1, neurokinin receptor subtype NK_1; SP, substance P.

NERVES AND ANGIOGENESIS

The mature microvasculature is associated with fine, unmyelinated nerve fibers containing neuropeptides. Sensory nerves contain substance P, neurokinin A (NKA), and calcitonin gene-related peptide (CGRP), and autonomic nerves contain neuropeptide Y (NPY) or vasoactive intestinal peptide (VIP). Substance P, the most intensively studied of these neuropeptides, is a member of the tachykinin family of peptides, which also includes neurokinin A (NKA) and neurokinin B (NKB) *(34)*. Substance P is translated from preprotachykinin A mRNA in the dorsal-root ganglia of the spinal cord and axonally transported to nerve terminals in peripheral tissues. Released substance P interacts with cell-surface, G protein-coupled receptors of the neurokinin (NK) family, with highest affinity for NK_1 receptors. NK_2 and NK_3 receptor subtypes are relatively selective for NKA and NKB, although both can also be activated by substance P. High (micromolar) doses of substance P can stimulate mast-cell degranulation independently of NK_1 receptor activation, through the direct activation of heterotrimeric G proteins *(35,36)*.

Neuropeptides are released from the peripheral-nerve terminal in response to electrical or chemical stimulation *(37,38)*. Release of sensory neuropeptides has also been demonstrated during acute inflammation *(39,40)*. Specific cell-surface, G protein-coupled receptors for many neuropeptides are localized to the vasculature and mediate actions on vascular tone, permeability, gene expression, and cell proliferation *(41–44)*. These neurovascular regulatory systems are compartmentalized with respect to arteries, capillaries, and venules, and functionally separated from surrounding stromal cells by membrane peptidases *(45)*. For example, substance P is degraded by neutral endopeptidase and angiotensin-converting enzyme, which are localized to perivascular fibroblasts and to the luminal surface of the vascular endothelium *(46,47)*.

Angiogenesis and nerves both are necessary for successful tissue repair. Smith and Wolpert *(48)* ascribed the requirement for nerves in amphibian limb regeneration to a permissive role in the vascularization of the blastema. In a series of elegant studies, they demonstrated that denervation before the limb became vascularized prevented subsequent vascularization, and that denervation after vascularization had begun resulted in abnormalities in vascular structure and organization. Denervation also impairs tissue healing in mammals, an effect that has been attributed to loss of sensory-efferent function *(49–51)*. Specific sensory denervation using the neurotoxin capsaicin, and selective antagonists of NK_1 receptors impair healing of skin wounds and gastric ulcers *(51–53)*. Conversely, stimulation of sensory neuropeptide release may facilitate tissue repair *(54–56)*. Denervation, and specifically sensory denervation, may also ameliorate synovitis, another process in which angiogenesis is thought to play an important role *(57,58)*. Such data suggest stimulatory or permissive roles of nerves during angiogenesis, although other mechanisms such as vasodilatation and inflammatory cellular recruitment also may be important.

Several molecules known to be released by nerves have been tested for their ability to modulate angiogenesis in vivo, and aspects of the angiogenic process in vitro. Neuropeptides have attracted the most attention, particularly the sensory neuropeptide substance P, which stimulates angiogenesis in a variety of model systems (*see* below).

Calcitonin gene-related peptide (CGRP) colocalizes with substance P in sensory nerves. CGRP also may stimulate angiogenesis because it increases endothelial cell proliferation in vitro, and enhances ^{133}Xe clearance from subcutaneous sponge granulomas in rats *(3,4,24)*. Vasoactive intestinal polypeptide (VIP), which localizes to cholinergic nerves, also enhances angiogenesis in the sponge granuloma model, although no direct effect on endothelial-cell proliferation was observed in vitro (4,25). Neuropeptide Y, released by sympathetic nerves, most recently has been identified as a stimulator of angiogenesis (59).

Not all neuropeptides have angiogenic activity. NKA, and other agonists of its preferred receptor, the NK_2 receptor, have not been shown to increase angiogenesis in vivo (23), nor to increase endothelial-cell proliferation and migration in vitro (1,12). NKB, whose actions are largely restricted to the central nervous system (CNS), did not increase endothelial cell proliferation or migration (1,12). The sympathetic cotransmitter neuropeptide Y (NPY) also did not increase endothelial-cell proliferation (4). Negative data must always be treated with some caution. Some neuropeptides such as somatostatin and β-endorphin can inhibit angiogenesis (60,61), effects that may not be observed in standard stimulatory assays (62). Balanced angiogenic and anti-angiogenic actions mediated by different receptor subtypes may result in no overall effect, as revealed for angiotensin II (ANG II) (see below). Furthermore, neuropeptides may have little activity on their own, but synergize with other classes of angiogenic agent, as has been observed with substance P and interleukin-1α (IL-1α) (23).

Other nerve-derived factors may also regulate angiogenesis. Nitric oxide (NO), as well as being generated by vascular endothelium and inflammatory cells, is released from the peripheral terminals of unmyelinated sensory nerves in the lung following activation of a specific, neuronal isoform of nitric oxide synthase (nNOS). NO can stimulate endothelial-cell proliferation and migration in vitro, and contributes to the angiogenic activities of NK_1 receptor agonists and VEGF in vivo (2,8). Although endothelial NO is now recognized as an important modulator of angiogenesis, the role of neuronal NO remains more speculative.

The development of selective, metabolically stable receptor antagonists for neuronal factors, the cloning and targeted disruption of neuropeptide and neuropeptide-receptor genes, and the further characterization of additional neuronal factors should help us understand the molecular mechanisms underlying the neuronal modulation of angiogenesis revealed by functional denervation studies. In the next section, we discuss the angiogenic actions of substance P in detail, this being the most intensively investigated of candidate neuronal modulators of angiogenesis studied to date.

Stimulation of Vascular Growth by Substance P In Vivo

Substance P-impregnated pellets stimulate vascular growth in rabbit corneas (1,2). High doses of substance P induced both inflammation and angiogenesis, whereas lower doses induced angiogenesis in the absence of inflammatory-cell infiltration (1). At least part of the angiogenic activity of substance P therefore may be owing to direct effects on the vasculature. Corneal vascularization was also induced by NK_1 receptor agonists, and was stereoselectively blocked by L-NAME, suggesting mediation by NK_1 receptor activation of endothelial NOS (1,2).

Substance P also enhances angiogenesis in the subcutaneous sponge granuloma model in the rat (23,27). Polyether sponges were inserted beneath the dorsal skin of male Wistar rats, and pharmacological agents were administered daily into each sponge through an indwelling cannula, beginning 24 h after implantation. Angiogenesis was measured as increased fibrovascular growth and as an increase in blood flow, indicated by increased rates of [133]Xenon clearance from the sponge. Untreated sponges are progressively infiltrated by fibrovascular tissue during the 14 d after implantation. This granulation tissue contains macrophages, giant cells, myofibroblasts, and scattered lymphocytes (63).

Daily administration of 10 nmol substance P or NK_1 receptor agonists increased angiogenesis in sponge implants. A lower dose of substance P (1 nmol sponge^{-1} d^{-1}) synergistically enhanced ^{133}Xenon clearance in the presence of IL-1α (but not IL-6 or IL-8). Stimulation of angiogenesis by the combination of substance P and IL-1α was prevented by peptide antagonists of substance P receptors and by nonpeptide, selective NK_1 receptor antagonists, but not by the histamine-receptor antagonists mepyramine and cimetidine. Substance P-enhanced angiogenesis in this model appears, therefore, to be mediated by NK_1 receptors, rather than by release of histamine from mast cells. [^{125}I]Bolton Hunter-labeled substance P bound in sponge granulomas to sites that had characteristics of NK_1 receptors (63). These sites were localized to microvascular endothelium, and not to infiltrating macrophages or fibroblasts. Substance P-enhanced angiogenesis both in sponge granulomas and in rabbit corneas may therefore result from direct effects on vascular endothelium.

These studies demonstrate that substance P can stimulate angiogenesis in vivo, and that substance P-enhanced angiogenesis can be dissociated from inflammatory-cell infiltration. It is less clear, however, under which physiological or pathological conditions substance P actually does stimulate angiogenesis. NK_1 receptor antagonists did not inhibit basal angiogenesis in sponge granulomas, in contrast to the inhibition observed following administration of IL-1 receptor antagonist and combined immunoblockade of basic fibroblast growth factor (bFGF), IL-8, and TNF-α (64).

Modulation of angiogenesis by endogenous substance P requires an endogenous source for the peptide. The normal subcutaneous mesenchyme is richly supplied with perivascular substance P-immunoreactive nerves and endothelial NK_1 receptors, but the neovasculature within the sponge granuloma remains noninnervated during the period of increasing blood flow up to 14 d after implantation (63). Innervation occurs late during vascular maturation, several weeks after the initiation of the angiogenesis that follows osseous and cutaneous wounding (65,66). Perivascular substance P-containing nerves are also absent in other tissues undergoing rapid vascular turnover, such as the chronically inflamed synovium from patients with rheumatoid arthritis (RA) (67,68). Endogenous substance P may be not available to stimulate of angiogenesis under these circumstances. On the other hand, endothelial NK_1 receptors are expressed prior to innervation during vascular maturation (63). Indeed, recently formed capillaries can be more sensitive to acute pro-inflammatory effects of substance P than are mature capillaries (69). Mismatch between the sites of peptide release and receptor localization may explain why exogenous agonists can have effects even in the absence of endogenous ligand

Smith and Wolpert's pioneering studies on amphibian limb regeneration provide a clue as to how neuroregulatory systems, which are absent during sustained angiogenesis, may yet play important roles in initiating the angiogenic process (48). They showed that denervation prevented the initiation of angiogenesis, but that denervation after the initiation of limb regeneration did not prevent sustained angiogenesis in the growing limb bud. Substance P is released into peripheral tissues during the early stages of injury and inflammation (39,40,70). It increases blood flow by the generation of NO following activation of endothelial NK_1 receptors, and enhances plasma extravasation from postcapillary venules (71–73). Sensory nerves, and, particularly substance P, are therefore well placed to initiate angiogenesis following tissue injury.

The sponge granuloma model is one of sustained angiogenesis (74). Initiation results from the creation of a subcutaneous air pouch and implantation of the polyether sponge 24 h before pharmacological agents are administered. Other methodological approaches are required to investigate the role of substance P in initiation of angiogenesis. Stimulation of corneal vascularization by substance P suggests that this peptide can initiate angiogenesis *(1,2)*. We have found that expression of the proliferation marker, proliferating cell nuclear antigen (PCNA) by synovial vascular endothelium is increased 24 h after a single intra-articular injection of substance P (Fig. 2) *(75)*. Substance P-induced endothelial-cell proliferation in the synovium was preceded by joint swelling and followed by macrophage infiltration. Initiation of angiogenesis may be one component of the package of protective responses afforded by neurogenic inflammation immediately following tissue injury. Circumstances in which substance P contributes to acute inflammation, such as carrageenan-induced synovitis, should be fertile grounds for seeking the initiation of angiogenesis by substance P *(76)*.

A second role of nerves in angiogenesis was suggested by Smith and Wolpert's finding that denervation after the initiation of angiogenesis resulted in abnormalities of vascular structure. Innervation of neovasculature by substance P-immunoreactive nerves normally occurs during the phase of vascular maturation and reorganization *(63)*, and vascular beds that are persistently noninnervated are often persistently disorganized, with shunting of blood and mismatch between perfusion and metabolic demand. Such is the case in a variety of haemangiomata, in tumor vasculature, and in the chronically inflamed human synovium *(77–80)*. Effects on vascular structure in part may be mediated by proliferative actions of substance P on smooth-muscle cells *(81,82)*. However, mice homozygous for disrupted preprotachykinin-A (PPT-A) or NK_1 receptor genes develop apparently normal vasculatures, suggesting that this system is not essential for normal angiogenesis in the mammalian embryo *(83–85)*. These studies are still in their early stages; vascular structure and function has yet to be studied in great detail in these animals, and angiogenesis in mature "knockout" animals has not been investigated fully.

Stimulation of Angiogenic Processes by Direct Actions of Substance P on Vascular Endothelium

The stimulation of angiogenesis in the absence of inflammatory cells, and inhibition by antagonists of NK_1 receptors that are specifically localized to vascular endothelium, suggest that substance P-enhanced angiogenesis results, at least in part, from a direct action on vascular endothelial cells. Substance P has a variety of effects on endothelial cells in culture that may mediate its angiogenic activity in vivo.

Substance P increases proliferation of endothelial cells derived from bovine aorta, human umbilical vein, and coronary venules, as indicated by increased [^{3}H]-thymidine incorporation and cell number *(1,2)*. Substance P-enhanced endothelial-cell proliferation is mimicked by selective NK_1 receptor agonists *(1,2)*, and inhibited by peptide antagonists of neurokinin receptors *(1)*. Substance P and NK_1 agonists also enhance bovine aortic endothelial-cell migration, to a similar extent, as does bFGF *(12)*. Tissue-type plasminogen activator (t-PA) release by endothelial cells is also enhanced by substance P, further suggesting possible roles for substance P in the facilitation of endothelial-cell migration through tissue matrix *(86)*. Substance P also enhances capillary tube formation by endothelial cells grown on collagen gels, to an extent comparable with IL-8 *(16)*. The nanomolar concentrations of substance P effective in this study suggest a specific receptor-mediated activity, although inhibition by selective NK_1 receptor antagonists was not reported.

Enhanced NOS activity appears to mediate the stimulatory actions of substance P on endothelial-cell proliferation and migration. Each is stereoselectively blocked by inhibitors of NOS *(2)*. The NO donor sodium nitroprusside and substance P each upregulated bFGF expression by coronary venular endothelial cells, and inhibition of

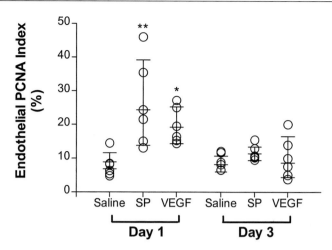

Fig. 2. Stimulation of endothelial cell proliferation by substance P and VEGF in rat knees. Substance P (SP) (10 nmol) or human recombinant VEGF (VEGF$_{167}$) (250 µg) in 100 µL of Normal saline were administered by single intra-articular injection into the right knees of male Wistar rats, and compared with control knees injected with 100 µL Normal saline. Synovium was removed at sacrifice after 24 or 72 h, and the proportion of endothelial cell nuclei displaying immunoreactivity for proliferating-cell nuclear antigen (endothelial PCNA index) was determined as previously described *(63,75)*. Endothelial-cell proliferation in the synovium was increased 24 h after injection of substance P or VEGF, consistent with induction of angiogenesis. Symbols represent individual cases, bars represent means ± 95% confidence intervals. $^*p < 0.05$, $^{**}p < 0.005$ compared with Normal saline-injected knees.

NOS prevented this effect of substance P *(87)*. Immunoblockade of bFGF inhibited substance P-induced endothelial-cell proliferation *(87)*. These data may indicate that substance P acts via NK$_1$ receptors to increase NO production, which stimulates endothelial cell proliferation by enhancing the autocrine production of bFGF.

Other factors may contribute to the in vivo angiogenic activity of substance P. Substance P-induced endothelial-cell proliferation is synergized by CGRP, which is co-released with substance P during sensory-nerve stimulation *(3)*. Substance P also synergizes with insulin, but not with platelet derived growth factor, nor platelet-derived endothelial-cell growth factor. As with the in vivo synergy with IL-1α, these observations suggest that the angiogenic activity of substance P is modulated by other factors in the vascular microenvironment.

Additional endothelium-dependent effects of substance P may contribute to its in vivo angiogenic activity. Substance P is well-recognized as an endothelium-dependent vasodilator and stimulator of plasma extravasation *(71,72)*. Increased blood flow and extravasated proteins such as fibrinogen are stimuli for angiogenesis *(88,89)*. Substance P also can enhance endothelial expression of intercellular adhesion molecule-1 (ICAM-1) *(90,91)*, which indirectly may enhance angiogenesis through the recruitment of inflammatory cells that in turn release angiogenic factors.

Angiogenic Actions of Substance P on Nonendothelial Cells

Substance P can stimulate nonendothelial cells to synthesize or release angiogenic factors. These include tumor necrosis factor-α (TNF-α), IL-1, -6, -8, and -10, and histamine. Substance P stimulates monocytes and macrophages to release TNF-α, IL-1, -6 and -10 *(92–94)*. It stimulates polymorphonuclear leukocytes to produce IL-8 *(95)*, enhances TNF-α and IL-1 release by neuroglia *(96)*, and IL-1 and IL-6 production by astrocytes *(97,98)*.

Substance P stimulates mast-cell release of TNF-α and histamine (99,100). Induction by substance P of endothelial e-selectin expression in vivo by substance P also is mediated by mast-cell degranulation (101). Mast-cell degranulation results from the direct activation of heterotrimeric G proteins by micromolar concentrations of substance P, an effect observed with other cationic substances including the wasp-venom constituent mastoparan (36). Blockade of in vivo enhancement of angiogenesis by NK_1 receptor antagonists, and not by the H_1 and H_2 histamine receptor antagonists mepyramine and cimetidine, suggests that substance P-enhanced angiogenesis in sponge implants is not mediated by mast-cell degranulation (23).

Effects of substance P on macrophages may complement direct angiogenic actions on vascular endothelium. Macrophages are well-recognized as mediators of angiogenesis through their release of a wide range of growth factors, and any factor that stimulates macrophage recruitment may be expected to have angiogenic activity in vivo (102). As well as stimulating adhesion-molecule expression by vascular endothelium (90,91,101,103), substance P can also induce monocyte chemotaxis even in the absence of endothelial cells (104). Furthermore, mononuclear cells are activated by substance P. TNF-α release by human monocytes is stimulated by nanomolar doses of substance P, and is inhibited by peptide neurokinin receptor antagonists and by the nonpeptide antagonist CP99,345, suggesting that this is an NK_1 receptor-mediated event (92,93,105). Receptor-like substance P binding sites have been demonstrated on cultured monocytes, but were not localized to tissue macrophages in in vitro autoradiographic studies of chronically inflamed synovia (44,106–108). This may indicate that NK_1 receptors are downregulated during maturation of tissue macrophages. NK_1 receptor-mediated cytokine production may be upregulated by tissue macrophages during some diseases, as demonstrated for TNF-α during *Clostridium difficile* toxin A enteritis in rats (109). Under these conditions, tissue macrophages may participate in substance P-enhanced angiogenesis in vivo.

In conclusion, peptides such as substance P are released by nerves, and are capable of stimulating angiogenesis through a variety of mechanisms. Sensory nerves are activated as an immediate response to tissue injury and may play an important role in the initiation of angiogenesis before other growth factors and their receptors have been upregulated. Innervation may be important for neovascular maturation and organization. Innervation, however, is a slow process, and other angiogenic factors must be present to sustain angiogenesis in a rapidly growing vascular bed.

ANGIOTENSIN II

Angiotensin II (ANG II) was one of the first vasoactive peptides found to have angiogenic activity in vivo (30). ANG II is generated from ANG I by angiotensin-converting enzyme (ACE), and subsequently cleaved by aminopeptidases to give ANG III, then ANG IV. ANG II has equal affinity for two subtypes of ANG II receptor in mammalian tissues, AT_1 and AT_2 (110). A further receptor (AT_4) has been pharmacologically characterized on vascular endothelium, which has high affinity and selectivity for ANG IV (111–114). Selective antagonists for AT_1, AT_2, and AT_4 receptors are now available (110,112), and AT_1 receptor antagonists such as losartan have entered clinical practice for hypertension. We shall discuss the evidence that ANG II can and does modulate angiogenesis, and explore conditions where ANG II-regulated angiogenesis may be important.

Stimulation of Vascular Growth by Angiotensin II In Vivo

Chronic administration of ANG II stimulates vascularization of rabbit corneas, chick chorioallantoic membranes (CAM), subcutaneous sponge granulomas, and carotid artery adventitia in rats and mice *(18,22,25,29,116)*. It also increases collateral formation following renal-artery ligation, and increases vascular density in the cremaster muscle of spontaneously hypertensive rats fed high-salt diets *(30,31)*. Coinfusion of ANG II (intravenous) and bFGF (intrapericardial) in rabbits induced greater increases in epicardial vascular density than did bFGF alone *(118)*. This last effect was attributed by the authors to ANG II-induced ventricular hypertrophy, although a more direct effect of ANG II on angiogenesis was not excluded. Neovascularization of cutaneous burns has been enhanced by topical application of ANG II *(118)*.

ANG II-enhanced angiogenesis in sponge granulomas is apparently mediated via AT_1 receptors because it is inhibited by the ANG II receptor antagonist saralasin, by selective AT_1 receptor antagonists losartan and Dup532, but is not mimicked by the AT_2 receptor agonist CGP 42112A, nor inhibited by the selective AT_2 receptor antagonists PD123319 *(25,63)*. ANG II-induced increases in cremaster muscle vascular density in rats on high-salt diets were also inhibited by the AT_1 receptor antagonist, losartan *(31)*. In contrast, neovascularization of the carotid-artery adventitia following 14 d of perivascular ANG II administration was attributed to AT_2 receptor activation *(29)*. Pharmacological classification of fowl ANG II receptors differs from that in rat and human. ANG II-stimulated angiogenesis in chick CAM is inhibited by the AT_2 receptor agonist CGP 42112A, but not by losartan or PD 123319 *(18)*. These last two ligands have very low affinity for fowl angiotensin binding sites (IC_{50} values >10 μM) *(19)*.

A further angiotensin receptor subtype has been implicated in angiotensin-induced angiogenesis in mammals. ANG IV has low affinity for both AT_1 and AT_2 receptors, and appears to exert biological effects through a distinct receptor subtype that has been partially characterized as an integral membrane glycoprotein *(119)*. ANG IV increases vascular density in the ischaemic rabbit heart *(118)*, and enhances endothelial cell proliferation in vitro *(113)*. ANG IV-induced vasodilatation is blocked by NOS inhibitors, raising the possibility that ANG IV, like substance P and VEGF, may belong to a family of NO-dependent vasodilators that can enhance angiogenesis *(120)*. Elucidation of the importance of active metabolites in the angiogenic activities of ANG II requires further study.

Modulation of Angiogenic Processes by Direct Actions of Angiotensin II on Vascular Endothelium

Despite the early demonstration that ANG II could be angiogenic in vivo, ANG I, ANG II, and ANG III, each administered alone, were not found to increase endothelial-cell proliferation in vitro *(5,6,121,122)*. The absence of proliferative effects of ANG II appears to be owing to expression of both AT_1 and AT_2 receptors by cultured endothelial cells *(5)*. ANG II binds to AT_1 and AT_2 receptor subtypes with approximately equal affinity *(110)*. AT_1 receptor activation can stimulate endothelial-cell proliferation, but this is masked in vitro by concurrent anti-mitogenic actions of AT_2 receptor-activation. AT_1 receptor mediated endothelial cell proliferation can be unmasked in the presence of a selective AT_2 receptor antagonist *(5)*.

Although ANG II administered alone did not stimulate proliferation and tube formation by retinal capillary endothelial cells, these angiogenic processes were enhanced by ANG II in the presence of VEGF *(6)*. This synergism appears to be owing to the AT_1 receptor-mediated upregulation by ANG II of the VEGF receptor, kinase domain-containing receptor (KDR). Further interactions between ANG II and VEGF are suggested by the finding of a losartan-sensitive increase in VEGF expression by rat-heart endothelial cells following exposure to ANG II *(123)*.

Despite the functional antagonism between AT_1 and AT_2 receptor activation on endothelial cell proliferation, endothelial-cell migration may be additively stimulated by both receptor subtypes *(12)*. ANG II-stimulated migration of bovine adrenal capillary endothelial-cells was partially inhibited by either AT_1 or AT_2 receptor antagonists, L-158,809 or PD123319, respectively, and completely inhibited by a combination of both AT_1 and AT_2 receptor antagonists. In the presence of the angiotensin-converting enzyme-inhibitor lisinopril, however, ANG II inhibited migration of bovine aortic endothelial cells *(121)*. Lisinopril and the subtype nonselective angiotensin-receptor antagonist saralasin each increased endothelial-cell migration and urokinase-like plasminogen-activator activity, possibly by increasing c-src expression *(121,124)*. Under differing conditions, therefore, ANG II may either stimulate or inhibit endothelial-cell migration. This variability in part may reflect differences between large- and small-vessel endothelial cells. Microvessels display higher densities of AT_1 receptors than do endothelia of larger arteries *(125)*. Furthermore, observations made using ACE inhibitors may result from complex interactions between different peptide systems, because ACE not only activates ANG II by cleavage of ANG I, but also inactivates bradykinin and substance P *(125)*.

ANG II therefore has direct effects on endothelial cells that may be expected to stimulate angiogenesis, but also can have anti-angiogenic activity. ANG II stimulates the production of other angiogenic factors such as VEGF, but also can stimulate the production of the angiogenesis inhibitors thrombospondin and TIMP-1 in endothelial cells *(127,128)*. AT_1 receptors may mediate both angiogenic and anti-angiogenic effects of ANG II, although, in some circumstances AT_1-mediated angiogenesis appears to be functionally antagonized by AT_2 receptor activation. The activity of ANG II as an angiogenic factor in vivo is likely to reflect a balance between angiogenic and anti-angiogenic effects.

Interactions Between AT_1 and AT_2 Receptors In Vivo

Consistent with effects on endothelial-cell proliferation in vitro, the AT_2 receptor antagonist PD123319 potentiated the ANG II-stimulated increase in vascular density in rat cremaster muscle *(31)*. However, AT_2 receptor agonists and antagonists had no effect on either basal or ANG II-enhanced angiogenesis in rat sponge granulomas *(25,26)*. In vitro autoradiographic studies using $[^{125}I](Sar^1, Ile^8)$ ANG II demonstrated dense AT_1 receptor-like binding sites within sponge implants, localized both to microvessels and to stromal cells, whereas AT_2 receptor-like binding sites were sparse and localized only to stromal cells *(26)*. In this model, lack of endothelial AT_2 receptor expression may result in a pure AT_1 receptor-mediated stimulation of angiogenesis by ANG II. AT_2 receptors are expressed at only low levels, if at all, in most mature tissues. They are upregulated during tissue repair, but not during the persistent inflammation of RA *(125,129,130)*. The sequential upregulation of AT_2 receptors after AT_1 receptors in sponge granulomas may indicate a role for AT_2 receptors in inhibiting angiogenesis during the late phases of tissue repair.

Modulation of Angiogenesis by Actions of Angiotensin II on Nonendothelial Cells

Specific receptors for ANG II are expressed by a wide variety of nonendothelial cells, including vascular smooth-muscle cells, pericytes, macrophages, and myofibroblasts *(63,131–134)*. Modulation of angiogenesis by ANG II therefore is unlikely to be solely mediated by actions on vascular endothelium.

ANG II stimulates the generation of angiogenic factors by vascular smooth-muscle cells, including VEGF, bFGF, transforming growth factor-β (TGF-β), endothelin-1, platelet-activating factor, and prostaglandin E_2 (135–139). On the other hand, ANG II stimulates vascular smooth-muscle synthesis of the angiogenesis inhibitor thrombospondin, and inhibits the cytokine induction of NOS (140,141). The roles of vascular smooth muscle-derived factors in angiogenesis remain ill-defined, but may be important particularly in the angiogenesis of atheromatous lesions.

Smooth-muscle cell proliferation and migration are essential for sustained angiogenesis and arterialization of newly formed vessels. ANG II increased the number and area of arteriolar arcades in chick CAM consistent with an in vivo effect on arterialization (142). Such an effect may be mediated by ANG II-enhanced proliferation and migration of vascular smooth-muscle cells (121,140). Smooth-muscle proliferation is mediated by AT_1 receptors, and is functionally antagonized by interactions between ANG II and AT_2 receptors (144,145). Parallels exist, therefore, for mitogenic and antimitogenic effects of ANG II receptor subtypes between vascular smooth-muscle and endothelial cells.

ANG II is a potent vasoconstrictor, acting via AT_1 receptors on vascular smooth-muscle cells (110). Reductions in blood flow may be expected to inhibit angiogenesis. However, new blood vessels, particularly tumor vasculature, are less responsive to the vasoconstrictor actions of ANG II than are mature vessels (110,146,147). Blood flow through tumors may actually be increased by ANG II, probably by diversion of blood flow to the immature tumor vasculature. This paradoxical increase in neovascular blood flow therefore may contribute to AT_1 receptor mediated angiogenesis in vivo.

In addition to its effects on vascular smooth muscle, ANG II may enhance recruitment and activation of macrophages. It stimulates adhesion of monocytes to vascular endothelium, and the release of TNF-α (148). ANG II-enhanced inflammatory-cell infiltration may partly be mediated by induced expression of adhesion molecules such as E-selectin by vascular endothelium (149). E-selectin itself may facilitate angiogenesis (150). Of potential relevance to angiogenesis in the corpus luteum, luteal cells are stimulated by ANG II to generate bFGF (151). Conversely, ANG II may inhibit production by other cell types of the potent angiogenic molecule hepatocyte growth factor (152). ANG II therefore may modulate angiogenesis in vivo through actions on a variety of cell types, as well as by direct actions on vascular endothelium.

Endogenous Angiotensin II and Angiogenesis In Vivo

Although it is now clear that AT_1 receptor activation by exogenous agonists can stimulate angiogenesis, enhancement of neovascularization by the endogenous renin-angiotensin system has yet to be demonstrated. Mice lacking the angiotensinogen gene cannot produce ANG II, but do not demonstrate gross abnormalities of vascular development, suggesting that ANG II is not essential for vasculogenesis, nor normal developmental angiogenesis (153–155). Similarly, double nullizygotes of the AT_{1A} and AT_{1B} genes display delayed maturity in glomerular growth, but no major defects in vasculogenesis (156). Mice lacking AT_2 receptors also develop normally (157). However, pathological angiogenesis has not been described yet in these animals.

Angiogenesis in sponge granulomas is modulated by ANG II receptor antagonists only if ANG II also is administered, and inhibition of endogenous ANG II production using ACE inhibitors has no effect in this model (26). Furthermore, in contrast to the inhibition of angiogenesis that may have been expected, the AT_1 receptor antagonists ZD 7155 and

ZD 8731 increased endoneurial vascular density in streptozocin-diabetic rats *(158,159)*. Similarly, losartan treatment after coronary-artery ligation in rats increased capillary density adjacent to the infarcted myocardium *(163)*. Losartan also increased arteriolar arcade formation in chick CAM *(142)*. Although these data may suggest inhibition of angiogenesis by endogenous AT_1 receptor agonists, inhibition of ANG II-enhanced stromal-cell hypertrophy and hyperplasia, and inhibitory effects of losartan on prostaglandins are alternative explanations.

The lack of modulation of angiogenesis by ANG II receptor antagonists in the absence of exogenous ANG II may indicate endogenous agonist was not available in those contexts that so far have been studied. A similar situation has been proposed above for substance P. ACE is downregulated by proliferating endothelial cells in vitro, its expression being a feature of maturation at confluence *(161)*. Correspondingly, ACE was not demonstrable within sponge granulomas during the period in which angiogenesis occurs *(26)*. ANG I is ineffective in stimulating angiogenesis in sponge granulomas, despite the angiogenic activity of ANG II, suggesting an inability to convert ANG I to ANG II within the sponge (Fig. 3). ACE is also focally absent from microvessels in human tissues undergoing angiogenesis, such as synovia from patients with RA *(46)*.

Vasoregulation by ANG II and by substance P is characteristic of a mature vascular bed. ANG II, acting via AT_1 receptors, may be important in the initiation of angiogenesis prior to the upregulation of other factors, in the same way as proposed earlier for substance P. ACE and AT_2 receptors are expressed before the neovasculature is innervated by substance P-containing nerves, and endogenous activation of AT_2 receptors could play a part in the switch between vascular growth and maturation.

BRADYKININ

Bradykinin is a well-characterized mediator of acute inflammation, generated during the extracellular cleavage of kininogens by kininogenases following tissue injury *(162)*. Bradykinin and Lys-bradykinin (kallidin) are further processed by carboxypeptidases, generating des-Arg^9-bradykinin and des-Arg^{10}-kallidin, respectively. Two major subtypes of kinin receptor have been cloned, B_1 and B_2 receptors *(163,164)*. B_2 receptors are constitutively expressed by vascular endothelium and smooth muscle, and mediate most actions of bradykinin in mature tissues. B_1 receptors are upregulated following tissue injury and inflammation and are selectively activated by the des-Arg kinins. During chronic inflammation, there is an increasing contribution of B_1 receptors to the plasma extravasation induced by kinins *(165)*.

Chronic administration of bradykinin enhanced ^{133}Xenon clearance from, and fibrovascular growth into subcutaneous sponge implants in rats, indicating angiogenic activity in vivo *(27)*. The sponge granuloma is a model of angiogenesis during inflammation, and, as expected, bradykinin-induced angiogenesis in this model appears to be mediated via the B_1 receptor subtype. It was inhibited by the selective B_1 receptor antagonist [Leu^8]des-Arg^9-bradykinin, but not by the B_2 receptor antagonist Ac-D-Arg-[Hyp^3, D-Phe^7,Leu^8]-bradykinin. IL-1α synergistically enhanced bradykinin-stimulated ^{133}Xenon clearance, further suggesting a role for bradykinin in inflammatory angiogenesis.

Whereas B_1 receptors may mediate bradykinin-enhanced angiogenesis in inflamed tissues, B_2 receptor activation may be more important in the absence of inflammation. The B_2 receptor antagonist icatibant inhibited the increase in cardiac capillary density induced by the ACE inhibitor ramipril in stroke-prone spontaneously hypertensive rats,

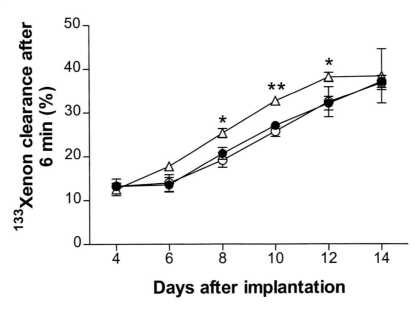

Fig. 3. Enhancement of [133]Xenon clearance from subcutaneous sponge implants following chronic administration of angiotensin II, but not following angiotensin I. Polyether sponges were subcutaneously implanted in male Wistar rats, peptides were administered daily via indwelling canulae, and [133]Xenon clearance measured as previously described *(26)*. Daily administration of 1 nmol angiotensin II (Δ) enhanced [133]Xenon clearance from 8–12 d compared with PBS injected sponges (●), whereas daily injection of 1 nmol angiotensin I was without effect (○). Exogenous ANG II stimulates angiogenesis, although angiotensin-converting enzyme is not available within sponge granuloma for the endogenous generation of ANG II *(26)*. Bars represent means ± S.E.M of 4–6 sponges. $^{*}p < 0.05$, $^{**}p < 0.01$.

suggesting mediation by endogenously generated bradykinin *(28)*. B_1 and B_2 receptors mediate similar actions of bradykinin on vasodilatation and plasma extravasation in inflamed and noninflamed tissues, respectively, in contrast to the functional antagonism observed between AT_1 and AT_2 receptors. However, the biological importance of switching from B_2 to B_1 receptor expression during inflammation remains enigmatic.

The mechanisms underlying bradykinin-enhanced angiogenesis in vivo may include both direct actions on vascular endothelium, and effects on other cell types. Bradykinin can stimulate proliferation of coronary venular endothelial cells *(9,10)*. Bradykinin-induced endothelial-cell proliferation appears to be mediated by the B_1 subtype of bradykinin receptors. It was mimicked by selective antagonists of B_1, but not B_2 receptors, and inhibited by antagonists of B_1, but not B_2 receptors. Bradykinin and bFGF displayed similar potencies in inducing endothelial-cell proliferation, and acted synergistically with each other *(9,10)*. On the other hand, another study found no effect of bradykinin on proliferation of bovine retinal or aortic endothelial cells *(122)*. These differences may reflect heterogeneity between endothelial cells from different sources, or differential expression of bradykinin-receptor subtypes during culture.

The mechanism by which bradykinin can stimulate endothelial-cell proliferation remains incompletely defined, but stimulation of protein kinase C (PKC) and NOS may each play a role *(166,167)*. Bradykinin also stimulates the release of other angiogenic factors by nonendothelial cells, including bFGF, IL-1, IL-6, histamine, and substance P *(168–172)*.

Stimulation of angiogenesis by bradykinin and substance P provide a possible link between acute inflammation and the initiation of angiogenesis. Bradykinin also may maintain angiogenesis during chronic inflammation. Bradykinin generation is sustained and B_1 receptors are upregulated in chronically inflamed tissues (165,173). On the other hand, a role for bradykinin in physiological angiogenesis has not been described, and mice genetically lacking B_2 receptors develop apparently normal vasculatures (174). Factors that regulate pathological, but not physiological angiogenesis, are attractive candidates for pharmacological intervention. More research is required, however, to determine which diseases may be driven by bradykinin-stimulated angiogenesis.

ANGIOTENSIN-CONVERTING ENZYME INHIBITION

The activities of regulatory peptides are modulated by membrane peptidases localized to sites of peptide generation and to sites at which peptides act. Peptide systems are thereby compartmentalized within a tissue, facilitating focal regulation of the vasculature. ACE is prominently expressed by microvascular endothelial cells, and is responsible for activating ANG II, and for inactivating bradykinin and substance P under a variety of circumstances in vivo (126). In particular, ACE inhibition can modulate the actions of each of these peptides (175,176). Modulation of angiogenesis by ACE inhibition provides strong evidence for a role of endogenous peptide systems in blood-vessel growth, although much work is still required to determine which specific peptides and receptor subtypes are responsible for the effects of ACE inhibition.

Chronic administration of ACE inhibitors including ramipril, spirapril, and zabicipril increased microvascular density in the hearts of spontaneously hypertensive rats, reducing capillary-diffusion distance, thereby facilitating oxygenation of the myocardium (28,177–179). Ramipril-enhanced angiogenesis was not mediated by its antihypertensive activity, because it was observed at doses of ramipril that were too low to prevent hypertension and left ventricular hypertrophy, and was not inhibited by the AT_1 receptor antagonist losartan (28,177). On the other hand, ramipril-increased vascular density was inhibited by the B_2 receptor antagonist icatibant, and was associated with inhibition of cardiac kininase activity. Ramipril enhanced myocardial blood flow also was inhibited by B_2 receptor antagonists (180). These data suggest that angiogenesis in this model is mediated by the increased levels of endogenous bradykinin that result from the inhibition of its local degradation by cardiac ACE. Inhibition of tissue ACE by quinaprilat was associated with increased angiogenesis in ischaemic rabbit limbs, indicating that ACE inhibitors may have a role in stimulating angiogenesis in a variety of pathologies that are characterized by arterial insufficiency (181).

Chronic ACE inhibition with lisinopril also increased capillary densities in the sciatic nerves of streptozotocin-diabetic rats (182). In diabetic animals (and probably humans), microangiopathy contributes to neural hypoxia and dysfunction, and chronic ACE inhibition improved sensory and motor-nerve conduction.

Some ACE inhibitors may have direct angiogenic activity on vascular endothelium because captopril and lisinopril can stimulate endothelial-cell migration in vitro (121,124,183). Further studies are required to determine whether this results from modulation of bradykinin levels in the culture medium, or from effects of these compounds, which are independent of their ability to inhibit ACE

Under other conditions, ACE inhibitors may have no effect, or inhibit, rather than enhance, angiogenesis (184). In contrast to its angiogenic activity when administered alone, captopril inhibited bFGF-enhanced endothelial-cell proliferation and migration, and corneal neovascularization *(12)*. Captopril also reduced the small arteriolar density in the cremaster muscle of both hypertensive and normotensive rats *(185)*. Part of the anti-angiogenic activity of captopril may be owing to inhibition of ACE activity, because lisinopril and enalopril also antagonized bFGF-enhanced endothelial-cell migration. Mechanisms other than ACE inhibition also have been suggested, because ANG II enhanced endothelial-cell migration was inhibited by captopril, but not by other ACE inhibitors. Inhibition of other metalloproteases that mediate angiogenesis is one possible mechanism.

Chronic enalapril treatment of immature rats reduced glomerular growth, suggesting inhibition of physiological angiogenesis during renal maturation *(186)*. Maternal use of ACE inhibitors during the second and third trimesters also is associated with renal dysfunction in human fetuses *(187)*. Perindopril, another ACE inhibitor, reduced that increase in microvessel density that is observed at the renal corticomedullary junction in diabetic rats *(188)*. Consistent with these teratogenic effects of ACE inhibition, mutant mice lacking ACE develop distorted vascular trees, with widened and thickened intrarenal arteries *(189)*. ACE therefore appears to be required for successful renal angiogenesis during growth and in disease, although no effect of ACE inhibition was observed on the mature kidneys of normal animals.

The various, but reproducible effects of ACE inhibition on angiogenesis perhaps best can be explained by involvement of different peptide-regulatory factors in different tissues under different experimental conditions. Where endogenous bradykinin is generated, inhibition of ACE may enhance angiogenesis by preventing bradykinin inactivation. Suppression of angiogenesis by ACE inhibition may point to an angiogenic role of ANG II. ACE is also responsible for the degradation of substance P released from perivascular sensory nerve fibers under some circumstances. However, a role for NK_1 receptor activation in ACE-enhanced angiogenesis has not been reported so far.

CONCLUSIONS

Vasoactive peptides play important roles in the regulation of blood flow in the mature vascular bed. In addition, they are increasingly being recognized as potent modulators of angiogenesis. Initiation of angiogenesis following tissue injury, and regulation of neovascular maturation are points in the process of angiogenesis where these peptides may have most influence. Vasoactive peptides that have not been discussed in detail in this chapter also may stimulate angiogenesis (Table 1), and more are likely to be discovered in the future. Endothelins have attracted considerable attention. Direct stimulatory effects on endothelial-cell proliferation and migration have been demonstrated in vitro (Table 1). Endothelins-1 and -3 also can stimulate endothelial cell proliferation and migration by increasing VEGF expression and release from vascular smooth-muscle cells *(190)*.

Peptides interact with other angiogenic factors in complex ways, and different peptides may regulate angiogenesis in different tissues, and in different conditions. Changes in the expression of receptor subtypes during development and disease necessitate the careful selection of animal models in which to test the therapeutic potential of angiogenesis inhibition using specific antagonists of receptor subtypes. The diversity of peptide regulatory systems offers hope for the specific targeting of that angiogenesis that is associated with particular diseases.

ACKNOWLEDGMENT

T.-P. D. F. thanks the British Heart Foundation and the Wellcome Trust for financial support.

REFERENCES

1. Ziche, M., Morbidelli, L., Pacini, M., Geppetti, P., Alessandri, G., and Maggi, C. A. (1990) Substance P stimulates neovascularization *in vivo* and proliferation of cultured endothelial cells. *Microvasc. Res.* **40,** 264–278.
2. Ziche, M., Morbidelli, L., Masini, E., Amerini, S., Granger, H. J., Geppetti, P., and Ledda, F. (1994) Nitric oxide mediates angiogenesis in vivo and endothelial cell growth and migration in vitro promoted by substance P. *J. Clin. Invest.* **94,** 2036–2044.
3. Villablanca, A. C., Murphy, C. J., and Reid, T. W. (1994) Growth-promoting effects of substance P on endothelial cells in vitro. Synergism with calcitonin gene-related peptide, insulin, and plasma factors. *Circ. Res.* **75,** 1113–1120.
4. Haegerstrand, A., Dalsgaard, C. J., Jonzon, B., Larsson, O., and Nilsson, J. (1990) Calcitonin gene-related peptide stimulates proliferation of human endothelial cells. *Proc. Natl. Acad. Sci. USA* **87,** 3299–3303.
5. Stoll, M., Steckelings, U. M., Paul, M., Bottari, S. P., Metzger, R., and Unger, T. (1995) The angiotensin AT_2–receptor mediates inhibition of cell proliferation in coronary endothelial cells. *J. Clin. Invest.* **95,** 651–657.
6. Otani, A., Takagi, H., Suzuma, K., and Honda, Y. (1998) Angiotensin II potentiates vascular endothelial growth factor-induced angiogenic activity in retinal microcapillary endothelial cells. *Circ. Res.* **82,** 619–628.
7. Ziche, M., Morbidelli, L., Donnini, S., and Ledda, F. (1995) ET_B receptors promote proliferation and migration of endothelial cells. *J. Cardiovasc. Pharmacol.* **26(Suppl. 3),** S284–S286.
8. Morbidelli, L., Chang, C.-H., Douglas, J. G., Granger, H. J., Ledda, F., and Ziche, M. (1996) Nitric oxide mediates mitogenic effect of VEGF on coronary venular endothelium. *Am. J. Physiol.* **270,** H411–H415.
9. Ziche, M., Parenti, A., Morbidelli, L., Meininger, C. J., Granger, H. J., and Ledda, F. (1992) The effect of vasoactive factors on the growth of coronary endothelial cells. Cardiologia **37,** 573–575.
10. Morbidelli, L., Parenti, A., Giovannelli, L., Granger, H. J., Ledda, F., and Ziche, M. (1998) B_1 receptor involvement in the effect of bradykinin on venular endothelial cell proliferation and potentiation of FGF–2 effects. *Br. J. Pharmacol.* **124,** 1286–1292.
11. Ziche, M, Morbidelli, L., Geppetti, P, Maggi, C. A., and Dolara, P. (1991) Substance P induces migration of capillary endothelial cells: a novel NK-1 selective receptor mediated activity. *Life Sci.* **48,** PL–7–11.
12. Volpert, O. V., Ward, W. F., Lingen, M. W., Chesler, L., Solt, D. B., Johnson, M. D., et al. (1996) Captopril inhibits angiogenesis and slows the growth of experimental tumors in rats. *J. Clin. Invest.* **98,** 671–679.
13. Morbidelli, L., Orlando, C., Maggi, C. A., Ledda, F., and Ziche, M. (1995) Proliferation and migration of endothelial cells is promoted by endothelins via activation of ET_B receptors. *Am. J. Physiol.* **269,** H686–H695.
14. Noiri, E., Hu, Y., Bahou, W. F., Keese, C. R., Giaever, I., and Goligorsky, M. S. (1997) Permissive role of nitric oxide in endothelin-induced migration of endothelial cells. *J. Biol. Chem.* **272,** 1747–1752.
15. Wren, A. D., Hiley, C. R., and Fan, T. P. (1993) Endothelin-3 mediated proliferation in wounded human umbilical vein endothelial cells. *Biochem. Biophys. Res. Commun.* **196,** 369–75.
16. Weidermann, C. J., Auer, B., Sitte, B., Reinisch, N., Schratzberger, P., and Kähler, C. M. (1996) Induction of endothelial cell differentiation into capillary-like structures by substance P. *Eur. J. Pharmacol.* **298,** 335–338.
17. Carlini, R. G., Reyes, A. A., and Rothstein, M. (1995) Recombinant human erythropoietin stimulates angiogenesis *in vitro. Kidney Intl.* **47,** 740–745.
18. le Noble, F. A., Hekking, J. W., Van Straaten, H. W., Slaaf, D. W., and Struyker-Boudier, H. A. (1991) Angiotensin II stimulates angiogenesis in the chorio–allantoic membrane of the chick embryo. *Eur. J. Pharmacol.* **195,** 305–306.
19. le Noble, F. A. C., Schreurs, N. H. J. S., Van Straaten, H. W. M., Slaaf, D. W., Smits, J. F. M., Rogg, H., and Struiyker-Boudier, H. A. J. (1993) Evidence for a novel angiotensin II receptor involved in angiogenesis in chick embryo chorioallantoic membrane. *Am. J. Physiol.* **264,** R460–R465.
20. Ribatti, D., Presta, M., Vacca, A., Ria, R., Giuliani, R., Dell'Era, P., et al. (1999) Human erythropoietin induces a pro-angiogenic phenotype in cultured endothelial cells and stimulates neovascularization in vivo. *Blood* **93,** 2627–2636.
21. Patel, P. C., Barrie, R., Hill, N., Landeck, S., Kurozawa, D., and Woltering, E. A. (1994) Postreceptor signal transduction mechanisms involved in octreotide-induced inhibition of angiogenesis. *Surgery* **116,** 1148–1152.

22. Fernandez L. A., Twickler J., and Mead A. (1985) Neovascularization produced by angiotensin II. *J. Lab. Clin. Med.* **105,** 141–145.

23. Fan, T.-P. D., Hu, D.-E., Guard, S., Gresham, G. A., and Watling, K. J. (1993). Stimulation of angiogenesis by substance P and interleukin–1 in the rat and its inhibition by NK_1 or interleukin–1 receptor antagonists. *Br. J. Pharmacol.* **110,** 43–49.

24. Fan, T.-P. D. and Hu, D.-E. (1991) Modulation of angiogenesis by inflammatory polypeptides. *Int. J. Radiat. Biol.* **60,** 71.

25. Hu, D. E., Hiley, C. R., and Fan, T. P. (1996) Comparative studies of the angiogenic activity of vasoactive intestinal peptide, endothelins-1 and -3 and angiotensin II in a rat sponge model. *Br. J. Pharmacol.* **117,** 545–551.

26. Walsh, D. A., Hu, D.-E., Wharton, J., Catravas, J. D., Blake, D. R., and Fan, T.-P. D. (1997) Sequential development of angiotensin receptors and angiotensin converting enzyme during angiogenesis in the rat subcutaneous sponge granuloma. *Br. J. Pharmacol.* **120,** 1302–1311.

27. Hu, D.-E. and Fan, T.-P. D. (1993) [Leu⁸]des–Arg⁹–bradykinin inhibits the angiogenic effect of bradykinin and interleukin–1 in rats. *Br. J. Pharmacol.* **109,** 14–17.

28. Gohlke, P., Kuwer, I., Schnell, A., Amann, K., Mall, G., and Unger, T. (1997) Blockade of bradykinin B2 receptors prevents the increase in capillary density induced by chronic angiotensin-converting enzyme inhibitor treatment in stroke-prone spontaneously hypertensive rats. *Hypertension* **29,** 478–482.

29. Scheidegger, K. J. and Wood, J. M. (1997) Local application of angiotensin II to the rat carotid artery induces adventitial thickening. *J. Vasc. Res.* **34,** 436–446.

30. Fernandez, L. A., Caride, J., Twickler, J., and Galardy, R. E. (1982). Renin-angiotensin and development of collateral circulation after renal ischemia. *Am. J. Physiol.* **243,** H869–H875.

31. Hernandez, I., Cowley, A. W., Lombard, J. H., and Greene, A. S. (1992) Salt intake and angiotensin II alter microvessel density in the cremaster muscle of normal rats. *Am. J. Physiol.* **263,** H664–H667.

32. Munzenmaier, D. H. and Greene, A. S. (1996) Opposing actions of angiotensin II on microvascular growth and arterial blood pressure. *Hypertension* **27,** 760–765.

33. Kato, H., Shichiri, M., Marumo, F., and Hirata, Y. (1997) Adrenomedullin as an autocrine/paracrine apoptosis survival factor for rat endothelial cells. *Endocrinology* **138,** 2615–2620.

34. Regoli, D., Boudon, A., and Fauchere, J. L. (1994) Receptors and antagonists for substance P and related peptides. *Pharmacol. Rev.* **46,** 551–599.

35. Devillier, P., Renoux, M., Giroud, J. P., and Regoli, D. (1985) Peptides and histamine release from rat peritoneal mast cells. *Eur. J. Pharmacol.* **117,** 89–96.

36. Mousli, M., Bronner, C., Landry, Y, Brockaert, J., and Rouot, B. (1990) Direct activation of GTP-binding regulatory proteins (G-proteins) by substance P and compound 48/80. *FEBS Lett.* **259,** 260–262.

37. White, D. M. and Helme, R. D. (1985) Release of substance P from peripheral nerve terminals following electrical stimulation of the sciatic nerve. *Brain Res.* **336,** 27–31.

38. Yaksh, T. L. (1988) Substance P release from knee joint afferent terminals: modulation by opioids. *Brain Res.* 458, 319–324.

39. Tissot, M., Pradelles, P., and Giroud, J. P. (1988) Substance P-like levels in inflammatory exudates. *Inflammation* **12,** 25–35.

40. O'Byrne, E., Blancuzzi, V., Wilson, D. E., Wong, M., and Jeng, A. Y. (1990) Elevated substance P and accelerated cartilage degradation in rabbit knees injected with interleukin-1 and tumor necrosis factor. *Arthritis Rheum.* **33,** 1023–1028.

41. Sigrist, S., Franco-Cereceda, A., Muff, R., Henke, H., Lundberg, J. M., and Fischer, J. A. (1986) Specific receptor and cardiovascular effects of calcitonin gene-related peptide. *Endocrinology* **119,** 381–389.

42. Lundberg, J. M., Hemsen, A., Rudehill, A., Harfstrand, A., Larsson, O., Sollevi, A., et al. (1988) Neuropeptide Y- and alpha-adrenergic receptors in pig spleen: localization, binding characteristics, cyclic amp effects and functional responses in control and denervated animals. *Neuroscience* **24,** 659–672.

43. Baraniuk, J. N., Lundgren, J. D., Okayama, M., Mullol, J., Merida, M., Shelhamer, J. H., and Kaliner, M. A. (1990) Vasoactive intestinal peptide in human nasal mucosa. *J. Clin. Invest.* **86,** 825–831.

44. Walsh, D. A., Mapp, P. I., Wharton, J., Rutherford, R. A. D., Kidd, B. L., Revell, P. A., et al. (1992) Localisation and characterisation of substance P binding to human synovium in Rheumatoid Arthritis. *Ann. Rheum. Dis.* **51,** 313–317.

45. Walsh D. A., Wharton J., Blake D. R., and Polak J. M. (1993). Species and tissue specificity of vasoactive regulatory peptides. *Int. J. Tissue Cell. Reactions* **15,** 109–124.

46. Walsh, D. A., Mapp, P. I., Wharton, J., Polak, J. M., and Blake, D. R. (1993) Neuropeptide degrading enzymes in normal and inflamed human synovium. *Am. J. Pathol.* **142,** 1610–1621.

47. Mapp, P. I., Walsh, D. A., Kidd, B. L., Cruwys, S. C., Polak, J. M., and Blake, D. R. (1992) Localisation of the enzyme neutral endopeptidase to the human synovium. *J. Rheumatol.* **19,** 1838–1844.

48. Smith, A. R., and Wolpert, L. (1975) Nerves and angiogenesis in amphibian limb regeneration. *Nature* **257,** 224–225.

49. Carr, R. W., Delaney, C. A., Westerman, R. A., and Roberts, R. G. (1993) Denervation impairs cutaneous microvascular function and blister healing in the rat hindlimb. *Neuroreport* **4,** 467–470.

50. Nordsletten, L., Madsen, J. E., Almaas, R., Rootwelt, T., Halse, J., Konttinen, Y. T., et al. (1994) The neuronal regulation of fracture healing. Effects of sciatic nerve resection in rat tibia. *Acta Orthop. Scand.* **65,** 299–304.

51. Kjartansson, J., Dalsgaard, C.-J., and Jonsson, C. E. (1987) Decreased survival of experimental critical flaps in rats after sensory denervation with capsaicin. *Plast. Reconst. Surg.* **79,** 218–221.

52. Tramontana, M., Renzi, D., Calabro, A., Panerai, C., Milani, S., Surrenti, C., and Evangelista, S. (1994) Influence of capsaicin-sensitive afferent fibers on acetic acid-induced chronic gastric ulcers in rats. *Scand. J. Gastroenterol.* **29,** 406–413.

53. Benrath, J., Zimmermann, M., and Gillardon, F. (1995) Substance P and nitric oxide mediate would healing of ultraviolet photodamaged rat skin: evidence for an effect of nitric oxide on keratinocyte proliferation. *Neurosci. Letts.* **200,** 17–20.

54. Kjartansson, J. and Dalsgaard, C.-J. (1987) Calcitonin gene-related peptide increases survival of a musculocutaneous critical flap in the rat. *Eur. J. Pharmacol.* **142,** 355–358.

55. Kang, J. Y., Teng, C. H., and Chen, F. C. (1996) Effect of capsaicin and cimetidine on the healing of acetic acid induced gastric ulceration in the rat. *Gut* **38,** 832–836.

56. Iinuma, T. and Sawada, Y. (1996) Topical application of capsaicin and flap survival. *Br. J. Plastic Surg.* **49,** 319–320.

57. Donaldson, L. F., McQueen, D. S., and Seckl, J. R. (1995) Neuropeptide gene expression and capsaicin-sensitive primary afferents: maintenance and spread of adjuvant arthritis in the rat. *J. Physiol.* **486,** 473–482.

58. Kidd, B. L., Cruwys, S. C., Garrett, N. E., Mapp, P. I., Jolliffe, V. A., and Blake, D. R. (1995) Neurogenic influences on contralateral responses during experimental rat monoarthritis. *Brain Res.* **688,** 72–76.

59. Zukowska-Grojec, Z., Karwatowska-Prokopczuk, E., Rose, W., Rone, J., Movafagh, S., Ji, H., et al. (1998) Neuropeptide Y: a novel angiogenic factor from the sympathetic nerves and endothelium. *Circ. Res.* **83,** 187–195.

60. Woltering, E. A., Barrie, R., O'Dorisio, T. M., Arce, D., Ure, T., Cramer, A., et al. (1991) Somatostatin analogues inhibit angiogenesis in the chick chorioallantoic membrane. *J. Surg. Res.* **50,** 245–251.

61. Pasi, A, Qu, B. X., Steiner, R., Senn, H. J., Bar, W., and Messiha, F. S. (1991) Angiogenesis: modulation with opioids. *Gen. Pharmacol.* **22,** 1077–1079.

62. Fischer, E. G., Stingl, A., and Kirkpatrick, C. J. (1990) Migration assay for endothelial cells in multwells. Application to studies on the effect of opioids. *J. Immunol. Methods* **128,** 235–239.

63. Walsh, D. A., Hu, D. E., Mapp, P. I., Polak, J. M., Blake, D. R., and Fan, T.-P. (1996) Innervation and neurokinin receptors during angiogenesis in the rat sponge granuloma. *Histochem. J.* **28,** 759–769.

64. Hu, D. E., Hori, Y., Presta, M., Gresham, G. A., and Fan, T. P. (1994) Inhibition of angiogenesis in rats by IL-1 receptor antagonist and selected cytokine antibodies. *Inflammation* **18,** 45–58.

65. Hukkanen, M., Konttinen, Y. T., Santavirta, S., Paavolainen, P., Gu, X. H., Terenghi, G., and Polak, J. M. (1993) Rapid proliferation of calcitonin gene-related peptide-immunoreactive nerves during healing of rat tibial fracture suggests neural involvement in bone growth and remodelling. *Neuroscience* **54,** 969–979.

66. Gu, X. H., Terenghi, G., Purkis, P. E., Price, D. A., Leigh, I. M., and Polak, J. M. (1994) Morphological changes of neural and vascular peptides in human skin suction blister injury. *J. Pathol.* **172,** 61–72.

67. Mapp, P. I., Kidd, B. L., Gibson, S. J., Terry, J. M., Revell, P. A., Ibrahim, N. B. N., et al. (1990) Substance P-, calcitonin gene-related peptide- and C-flanking peptide of neuropeptide Y-immunoreactive fibres are present in normal synovium but depleted in patients with rheumatoid arthritis. *Neuroscience* **37,** 143–153.

68. Walsh, D. A., Wade, M., Mapp, P. I., and Blake, D. R. (1998) Focally regulated endothelial proliferation and cell death in human synovium. *Am. J. Pathol.* **152,** 691–702.

69. Baluk, P., Bowden, J. J., Lefevre, P. M., and McDonald, D. M. (1997) Upregulation of substance P receptors in angiogenesis associated with chronic airway inflammation in rats. *Am. J. Physiol.* **273,** L565–L571.

70. Helme, R. D., Koschorke, G. M., and Zimmermann, M. (1986) Immunoreactive substance P release from skin nerves in the rat by noxious thermal stimulation. *Neurosci. Letts.* **63,** 295–299.

71. Lembeck, F. and Holzer, P. (1979) Substance P as a neurogenic mediator of antidromic vasodialtion and neurogenic plasma extravasation. *Naunyn-Schmiedeberg's Arch. Pharmacol.* **310**, 175–183

72. Rees, D. D., Palmer, R. M. J., Hodson, F., and Moncada, S. (1989) A specific inhibitor of nitric oxide formation from L-arginine attenuates endothelium-dependent relaxation. *Br. J. Pharmacol.* **96**, 418–424.

73. Lembeck, F., Donnerer, J., Tsuchiya, M., and Nagahisa, A. (1992) The non-peptide tachykinin antagonist, CP-96,345, is a potent inhibitor of neurogenic inflammation. *Br. J. Pharmacol.* **105**, 527–530.

74. Hu, D.-E., Hiley, C. R., Smither, R. L., Gresham, G. A., and Fan, T.-P. D. (1995) Correlation of ^{133}Xe clearance, blood flow and histology in the rat sponge model for angiogenesis; further studies with angiogenic modifiers. *Lab. Invest.* **72**, 601–610.

75. Walsh, D. A., Rodway, H. A., and Claxson, A. (1999) Vascular turnover during carrageenan synovitis in the rat. *Lab. Invest.* **78**, 1513–1521.

76. Lam, F. Y. and Ferrell, W. R. (1989) Inhibition of carrageenan induced inflammation in the rat knee joint by substance P antagonist. *Ann. Rheum. Dis.* **48**, 928–932.

77. Mitchell, B. S., Schumacher, U., and Kaiserling, E. (1994) Are tumors innervated? Immunohistological investigations using antibodies against the neuronal marker protein gene product 9. 5 (PGP 9. 5) in benign, malignant and experimental tumors. *Tumor Biol.* **15**, 269–274.

78. Rydh, M., Malm, M., Jernbeck, J., and Dalsgaard, C. J. (1991) Ectatic blood vessels in port-wine stains lack innervation: possible role in pathogenesis. *Plastic Reconstruct. Surg.* **87**, 419–422.

79. Naughton, D., Whelan, M., Smith, E. C., Williams, R., Blake, D. R., and Grootveld, M. (1993) An investigation of the abnormal metabolic status of synovial fluid from patients with rheumatoid arthritis by high field proton nuclear magnetic resonance spectroscopy. *FEBS Letts.* **317**, 135–138.

80. Chapman, J. D., Engelhardt, E. L., Stobbe, C. C., Schneider, R. F., and Hanks, G. E. (1998) Measuring hypoxia and predicting tumor radioresistance with nuclear medicine assays. *Radiotherapy Oncol.* **46**, 229–237.

81. Payan, D. G. (1985) Receptor-mediated mitogenic effects of substance P on cultured smooth muscle cells. *Biochem. Biophys. Res. Commun.* **130**, 104–109.

82. Hultgardh–Nilsson, A., Nilsson, J., Jonzon, B., and Dalsgaard, C. J. (1988) Coupling between inositol phosphate formation and DNA synthesis in smooth muscle cells stimulated with neurokinin A. *J. Cell. Physiol.* **137**, 141–145.

83. De Felipe, C., Herrero, J. F., O'Brien, J. A., Palmer, J. A., Doyle, C. A., Smith, A. J., et al. (1998) Altered nociception, analgesia and aggression in mice lacking the receptor for substance P. *Nature* **392**, 394–397.

84. Zimmer, A., Zimmer, A. M., Baffi, J., Usdin, T., Reynolds, K., Konig, M., et al. (1998) Hypoalgesia in mice with a targeted deletion of the tachykinin 1 gene. *Proc. Natl. Acad. Sci. USA* **95**, 2630–2635.

85. Bozic, C. R., Lu, B., Hopken, U. E., Gerard, C., and Gerard, N. P. (1996) Neurogenic amplification of immune complex inflammation. *Science* **273**, 1722–1725.

86. Tranquille, N. and Emeis, J. J. (1992) The involvement of products of the phospholipase pathway in the acute release of tissue–type plasminogen activator from perfused rat hindlegs. *Eur. J. Pharmacol.* **213**, 285–292.

87. Ziche, M., Parenti, A., Ledda, F., Dell'Era, P., Granger, H. J., Maggi, C. A., and Presta, M. (1997) Nitric oxide promotes proliferation and plasminogen activator production by coronary venular endothelium through endogenous bFGF. *Circ. Res.* **80**, 845–852.

88. Ando, J. and Kamiya, A. (1996) Flow–dependent regulation of gene expression in vascular endothelial cells. *Japn. Heart J.* **37**, 19–32.

89. van Hinsbergh, V. W. M., Koolwijk, P., and Hanemaaijer, R. (1997) Role of fibrin and plasminogen activators in repair-associated angiogenesis: *in vitro* studies with human endothelial cells, in *Regulation of Angiogenesis* (Goldberg, I. D. and Rosen, E. M., eds.), Birkhäuser Verlag, Basel, Switzerland, pp. 391–411.

90. Nakagawa, N., Iwamoto, I., and Yoshida, S. (1993) Effect of substance P on the expression of an adhesion molecule ICAM-1 in human vascular endothelial cells. *Regulatory Peptides* **46**, 223–224.

91. Nakagawa, N., Sano, H., and Iwamoto, I. (1995) Substance P induces the expression of intercellular adhesion molecule-1 on vascular endothelial cells and enhances neutrophil transendothelial migration. *Peptides* **1**, 721–725.

92. Lotz, M., Vaughan, J. H., and Carson, D. A. (1988) Effect of neuropeptides on production of inflammatory cytokines in human monocytes. *Science* **241**, 1218–1221.

93. Lee, H. R., Ho, W. Z., and Douglas, S. D. (1994) Substance P augments tumor necrosis factor release in human monocyte derived macrophages. *Clin. Diag. Lab. Immunol.* **1**, 419–423.

94. Ho, W. Z., Kaufman, D., Uvaydova, M., and Douglas, S. D. (1996) Substance P augments interleukin-10 and tumor necrosis factor–alpha release by human cord blood monocytes and macrophages. *J. Neuroimmunol.* **71,** 73–80.

95. Serra, M. C., Calzetti, F., Ceska, M., and Cassatella, M. A. (1994) Effect of substance P on superoxide anion and IL-8 production by human PMNL. *Immunology* **82,** 63–69.

96. Luber-Narod, J., Kage, R., and Leeman, S. E. (1994) Substance P enhances the secretion of tumor necrosis factor-alpha from neuroglial cells stimulated with lipopolysaccharide. *J. Immunol.* **152,** 819–824.

97. Martin, F. C., Charles, A. C., Sanderson, M. J., and Merrill, J. E. (1992) Substance P stimulates IL–1 production by astrocytes via intracellular calcium. *Brain Res.* **599,** 13–18.

98. Palma, C., Minghetti, L., Astolfi, M., Ambrosini, E., Silberstein, F. C., Manzini S., et al. (1997) Functional characterization of substance P receptors on cultured human spinal cord astrocytes: synergism of substance P with cytokines in inducing interleukin-6 and prostaglandin E2 production. *GLIA* **21,** 183–193.

99. Ansel, J. C., Brown, J. R., Payan, D. G., and Brown, M. A. (1993) Substance P selectively activates TNF–alpha gene expression in murine mast cells. *J. Immunol.* **150,** 4478–4485.

100. Lowman, M. A., Benyon, R. C., and Church, M. K. (1988) Characterization of neuropeptide-induced histamine release from human dispersed skin mast cells. *Br. J. Pharmacol.* **95,** 121–130.

101. Matis, W. L., Lavker, R. M., and Murphy, G. F. (1990) Substance P induces the expression of an endothelial–leucocyte adhesion molecule by microvascular endothelium. *J. Invest. Dermatol.* **94,** 492–495.

102. Polverini, P. J. (1997) Role of the macrophage in angiogenesis-dependent diseases, in *Regulation of Angiogenesis* (Goldberg, I. D. and Rosen, E. M., eds.), Birkhäuser Verlag, Basel, Switzerland, pp. 11–28.

103. Goebeler. M., Henseleit, U., Roth, J., and Sorg C. (1994) Substance P and calcitonin-gene related peptide modulate leukocyte infiltration to mouse skin during allergic contact dermatitis. *Arch. Dermatol. Res.* **286,** 341–346.

104. Weidermann, C. J., Wiedermann, F. J., Apperl, A., Kieselbach, G., Konwalinka, G., and Braunsteiner, H. (1989) In vitro human polymorphonuclear leukocyte chemokinesis and human monocyte chemotaxis are different activities of aminoterminal and carboxyterminal substance P. *Naunyn-Schmiedeberg's Arch. Pharmacol.* **340,** 185–190.

105. Ho, W. Z., Stavropoulos, G., Lai, J. P., Hu, B. F., Magafa, V., Anagnostides, S., and Douglas S. D. (1998) Substance P C-terminal octapeptide analogues augment tumor necrosis factor-alpha release by human blood monocytes and macrophages. *J. Neuroimmunol.* **82,** 126–132.

106. Hartung, H. P., Wolters, K., and Toyka, K. V. (1986) Substance P: binding properties and studies on cellular responses in guinea pig macrophages. *J. Immunol.* **136,** 3856–3863.

107. Jeurissen, F., Kavelaars, A., Korstjens, M., Broeke, D., Franklin, R. A., Gelfand, E. W., and Heijnen, C. J. (1994) Monocytes express a non-neurokinin substance P receptor that is functionally coupled to MAP kinase. *J. Immunol.* **152,** 2987–2994.

108. Walsh, D. A., Salmon, M., Mapp, P. I., Wharton, J., Garrett, N., Blake, D. R., Polak, J. M. (1993) Microvascular substance P binding to normal and inflamed rat and human synovium. *J. Pharmacol. Exp. Therapeut.* **267,** 951–960.

109. Castagliuolo, I., Keates, A. C., Qiu, B., Kelly, C. P., Nikulasson, S., Leeman, S. E., and Pothoulakis, C. (1997) Increased substance P responses in dorsal root ganglia and intestinal macrophages during Clostridium difficile toxin A enteritis in rats. *Proc. Natl. Acad. Sci. USA* **94,** 4788–4793.

110. Timmermans, P. B. M. W. M., Wong, P. C., Chiu, A. T., Herblin, W. F., Benfield, P., Carini, D. J., et al. (1993) Angiotensin II receptors and angiotensin II receptor antagonists. *Pharm. Rev.* **45,** 205–251.

111. Swanson, G. N., Hanesworth, J. M., Sardinia, M. F., Coleman, J. K., Wright, J. W., Hall, K. L., et al. (1992) Discovery of a distinct binding site for angiotensin II (3-8), a putative angiotensin IV receptor. *Regul. Peptides* **40,** 409–419.

112. Bernier, S. G., Servant, G., Boudreau, M., Fournier, A., and Guillemette G. (1995) Characterization of a binding site for angiotensin IV on bovine aortic endothelial cells. *Eur. J. Pharmacol.* **291,** 191–200.

113. Hall, K. L., Venkateswaran, S., Hanesworth, J. M., Schelling, M. E., and Harding, J. W. (1995) Characterization of a functional angiotensin IV receptor on coronary microvascular endothelial cells. *Regul. Peptides* **58,** 107–115.

114. Riva, L. and Galzin, A. M. (1996) Pharmacological characterization of a specific binding site for angiotensin IV in cultured porcine aortic endothelial cells. *Eur. J. Pharmacol.* **305,** 193–199.

115. Krebs, L. T., Kramar, E. A., Hanesworth, J. M., Sardinia, M. F., Ball, A. E., Wright, J. W., and Harding, J. W. (1996) Characterization of the binding properties and physiological action of divalinal-angiotensin IV, a putative AT4 receptor antagonist. *Regul. Peptides* **67,** 123–130.

116. Andrade, S. P., Cardoso, C. C., Machado, R. D., and Beraldo, W. T. (1996) Angiotensin-II-induced angiogenesis in sponge implants in mice. *Int. J. Microcirc. Clin. Exp.* **16,** 302–307.

117. Landau, C., Jacobs, A. K., and Haudenschild, C. C. (1995) Intrapericardial basic fibroblast growth factor induces myocardial angiogenesis in a rabbit model of chronic ischemia. *Am. Heart J.* **129,** 924–931.

118. Rodgers, K. E., DeCherney, A. H., St. Amand, K. M., Dougherty, W. R., Felix, J. C., et al. (1997) Histologic alterations in dermal repair after thermal injury effects of topical angiotensin II. *J. Burn. Care Rehab.* **18,** 381–388.

119. Bernier, S. G., Bellemare, J. M., Escher, E., and Guillemette, G. (1998). Characterization of AT_4 receptor from bovine aortic endothelium with photosensitive analogues of angiotensin IV. *Biochemistry* **37,** 4280–4287.

120. Coleman, J. K., Krebs, L. T., Hamilton, T. A., Ong, B., Lawrence, K. A., Sardinia, M. F., et al. (1998) Autoradiographic identification of kidney angiotensin IV binding sites and angiotensin IV-induced renal cortical blood flow changes in rats. *Peptides* **19,** 269–277.

121. Bell, L. and Madri, J. A. (1990) Influence of the angiotensin system on endothelial and smooth muscle cell migration. *Am. J. Pathol.* **137,** 7–12.

122. Porta, M., Dosso, A. A., Williams, F. M., Kanse, S., and Kohner, E. M. (1992) A study of the effects of angiogtensins 1,2,3 and bradykinin on the replication of bovine retinal capillary endothelial cells and pericytes. *Eur. J. Ophthalmol.* **2,** 21–26.

123. Chua, C. C., Hamdy, R. C., and Chua, B. H. (1998) Upregulation of vascular endothelial growth factor by angiotensin II in rat heart endothelial cells. *Biochim. Biophys. Acta.* **1401,** 187–194.

124. Bell, L., Luthringer, D. J., Madri, J. A., and Warren, S. L. (1992) Autocrine angiotensin system regulation of bovine aortic endothelial cell migration and plasminogen activator involves modulation of proto-oncogene pp60c-src expression. *J. Clin. Invest.* **89,** 315–320.

125. Walsh, D. A., Suzuki, T., Knock, G., Blake, D. R., Polak, J. M., and Wharton, J. (1994) AT_1 receptor characteristics of angiotensin analogue binding in human synovium. *Br. J. Pharmacol.* **112,** 435–442.

126. Kenny, A. J., Stephenson, S. L., and Turner, A. J. (1987) Cell surface peptidases, in *Mammalian Ectoenzymes* (Kenny, A. J. and Turner, A. J., eds.), Elsevier, Amsterdam, pp. 169–210

127. Chua, C. C., Hamdy, R. C., and Chua, B. H. (1996) Angiotensin II induces TIMP–1 production in rat heart endothelial cells. *Biochim. Biophys. Acta.* **1311,** 175–180.

128. Chua, C. C., Hamdy, R. C., and Chua, B. H. (1997) Regulation of thrombospondin-1 production by angiotensin II in rat heart endothelial cells. *Biochim. Biophys. Acta.* **1357,** 209–214.

129. Viswanathan, M. and Saavedra, J. M. (1992) Expression of angiotensin II AT_2 receptors in the rat skin during experimental wound healing. *Peptides* **13,** 783–786.

130. Nio, Y., Matsubara, H., Murasawa, S., Kanasaki, M., and Inada, M. (1995) Regulation of gene transcription of angiotensin II receptor subtypes in myocardial infarction. *J. Clin. Invest.* **95,** 46–54.

131. Whitebread, S., Mele, M., Kamber, B., and De Gasparo, M. (1989) Preliminary biochemical characterization of two angiotensin II receptor subtypes. *Biochem. Biophys. Res. Commun.* **163,** 264–291.

132. Millan, M. A., Carvallo, P., Izumi, S.-I., Zemel, S., Catt, K. J., and Aguilera, G. (1989) Novel sites of expression of functional angiotensin II receptors in the late gestation fetus. *Science* **244,** 1340–1342.

133. Thomas, D. W., and Hoffman, M. D. (1984) Identification of macrophage receptors for angiotensin; a potential role in antigen uptake for T lymphocyte responses? *J. Immunol.* **132,** 2807–2812.

134. Ferrari-Dileo, G., Davis, E. B., and Anderson, D. R. (1996) Glaucoma, capillaries and pericytes. 3. Peptide hormone binding and influence on pericytes. *Ophthalmologica* **210,** 269–275.

135. Kurtz, A., Pfeilschifter, J., Kuhn, K., and Koch, K. M. (1987) Cyclosporin A inhibits PGE2 release from vascular smooth muscle cells. *Biochem. Biophys. Res. Commun.* **147,** 542–549.

136. Scott-Burden, T., Resink, T. J., Hahn, A. W. A., and Vanhoutte, P. M. (1991) Induction of endothelin secretion by angiotensin II: effects on growth and synthetic activity of vascular smooth muscle cells. *J. Cardiovasc. Pharmacol.* **17(Suppl. 7),** S96–S100.

137. Itoh, H., Mukoyama, M., Pratt, R. E., Gibbons, G. H., and Dzau, V. J. (1993) Multiple autocrine growth factors modulate vascular smooth muscle cell growth response to angiotensin II. *J. Clin. Invest.* **91,** 2268–2274.

138. Tomlinson, P. R., Croft, K., Harris, T., and Stewart AG. (1994) Platelet-activating factor biosynthesis in rat vascular smooth muscle cells. *J. Vasc. Res.* **31,** 144–152.

139. Williams, B., Baker, A. Q., Gallacher, B., and Lodwick, D. (1995) Angiotensin II increases vascular permeability factor gene expression by human vascular smooth muscle cells. *Hypertension* **25,** 913–917.

140. Nakayama, I., Kawahara, Y., Tsuda, T., Okuda, M., and Yokoyama, M. (1994) Angiotensin II inhibits cytokine-stimulated inducible nitric oxide synthase expression in vascular smooth muscle cells. *J. Biol. Chem.* **269**, 11,628–11,633.

141. Green, R. S., Lieb, M. E., Weintraub, A. S., Gacheru, S. N., Rosenfield, C. L., Shah, S., et al. (1995) Identification of lysyl oxidase and other platelet-derived growth factor-inducible genes in vascular smooth muscle cells by differential screening. *Lab. Invest.* **73**, 476–482.

142. le Noble, F. A., Kessels-van Wylick, L. C., Hacking, W. J., Slaaf, D. W., oude Egbrink, M. G., and Struijker-Boudier, H. A. (1996) The role of angiotensin II and prostaglandins in arcade formation in a developing microvascular network. *J. Vasc. Res.* **33**, 480–488.

143. Campbell-Boswell, M. and Robertson, A. L. (1981) Effects of angiotensin II and vasopressin on human smooth muscle cells *in vitro*. *Exp. Mol. Pathol.* **35**, 265–276.

144. Sung, C.-P., Arleth, A. J., Storer, B. L., and Ohlstein, E. H. (1994) Angiotensin type 1 receptors mediate smooth muscle proliferation and endothelin biosynthesis in rat vascular smooth muscle. *J. Pharmacol. Exp. Therapeut.* **271**, 429–437.

145. Nakajima, M., Hutchinson, H. G., Fujinaga, M., Hayashida, W., Morishita, R., Zhang, L., et al. (1995) The angiotensin II type 2 (AT_2) receptor antagonizes the growth effects of the AT_1 receptor: gain-of-function study using gene transfer. *Proc. Natl. Acad. Sci. USA* **92**, 10,663–10,667.

146. Sasaki, Y., Imaoka, S., Hasegawa, Y., Nakano, S., Ishikawa, O., Ohigashi, H., et al. (1985) Changes in distribution of hepatic blood flow induced by intra-arterial infusion of angiotensin II in human hepatic cancer. *Cancer* **55**, 311–316.

147. Zlotecki, R. A., Baxter, L. T., Boucher, Y., and Jain, R. K. (1995) Pharmacological modification of tumor blood flow and interstitial fluid pressure in human tumor xenograft: network analysis and mechanistic interpretation. *Microvasc. Res.* **50**, 429–443.

148. Hahn, A. W., Jonas, U., Buhler, F. R., and Resink, T. J. (1994) Activation of human peripheral monocytes by angiotensin II. *FEBS Letts.* **347**, 178–180.

149. Grafe, M., Auch-Schwelk, W., Zakrzewicz, A., Regitz-Zagrosek, V., Bartsch, P., Graf, K., et al. (1997) Angiotensin II-induced leukocyte adhesion on human coronary endothelial cells is mediated by E-selectin. *Circ. Res.* **81**, 804–811.

150. Koch, A. E., Halloran, M. M., Haskell, C. J., Shah, M. R., and Polverini, P. J. (1995) Angiogenesis mediated by soluble forms of E-selectin and vascular cell adhesion molecule-1. *Nature* **376**, 517–519.

151. Stirling, D., Magness, R. R., Stone, R., Waterman, M. R., and Simpson, E. R. (1990) Angiotensin II inhibits luteinizing hormone-stimulated cholesterol side chain cleavage expression and stimulates basic fibroblast growth factor expression in bovine luteal cells in primary culture. *J. Biol. Chem.* **265**, 5–8.

152. Yo, Y., Morishita, R., Yamamoto, K., Tomita, N., Kida, I., Hayashi, S., et al. (1998) Actions of hepatocyte growth factor as a local modulator in the kidney: potential role in pathogenesis of renal disease. *Kidney Intl.* **53**, 50–58.

153. Tanimoto, K., Sugiyama, F., Goto, Y., Ishida, J., Takimoto, E., Yagami, K., et al. (1994) Angiotensinogen-deficient mice with hypotension. *J. Biol. Chem.* **269**, 31,334–31,337.

154. Niimura, F., Labosky, P. A., Kakuchi, J., Okubo, S., Yoshida, H., Oikawa, T., et al. (1995) Gene targeting in mice reveals a requirement for angiotensin in the development and maintenance of kidney morphology and growth factor regulation. *J. Clin. Invest.* **96**, 2947–2954.

155. Nagata, M., Tanimoto, K., Fukamizu, A., Kon, Y., Sugiyama, F., Yagami, K., et al. (1996) Nephrogenesis and renovascular development in angiotensinogen-deficient mice. *Lab. Invest.* **75**, 745–753.

156. Tsuchida, S., Matsusaka, T., Chen, X., Okubo, S., Niimura, F., Nishimura, H., et al. (1998) Murine double nullizygotes of the angiotensin type 1A and 1B receptor genes duplicate severe abnormal phenotypes of angiotensinogen nullizygotes. *J. Clin. Invest.* **101**, 755–760.

157. Hein, L., Barsh, G. S., Pratt, R. E., Dzau, V. J., and Kobilka, B. K. (1995) Behavioural and cardiovascular effects of disrupting the angiotensin II type-2 receptor in mice. *Nature* **377**, 744–747.

158. Maxfield, E. K., Cameron, N. E., Cotter, M. A., and Dines, K. C. (1993) Angiotensin II receptor blockade improves nerve function, modulates nerve blood flow and stimulates endoneurial angiogenesis in streptozotocin-diabetic rats and nerve function. *Diabetologia* **36**, 1230–1237.

159. Maxfield, E. K., Love, A., Cotter, M. A., and Cameron, N. E. (1995) Nerve function and regeneration in diabetic rats: effects of ZD-7155, an AT_1 receptor antagonist. *Am. J. Physiol.* **269**, E530–E537.

160. Sladek, T., Sladkova, J., Kolar, F., Papousek, F., Cicutti, N., Korecky, B., and Rakusan K. (1996) The effect of AT1 receptor antagonist on chronic cardiac response to coronary artery ligation in rats. *Cardiovasc. Res.* **31**, 568–576.

161. Shai, S. Y., Fishel, R. S., Martin, B. M., Berk, B. C., and Bernstein, K. E. (1992) Bovine angiotensin converting enzyme cDNA cloning and regulation. Increased expression during endothelial cell growth arrest. *Circ. Res.* **70,** 1274–1281.

162. Bhoola, K. D., Figueroa, C. D., and Worthy, K. (1992) Bioregulation of kinins: Kallikreins, kininogens, and kininases. *Pharmacol. Rev.* **44,** 1–80.

163. Hall, J. M. and Morton, K. M. (1997) The pharmacology and immunopharmacology of kinin receptors, in *The Kinin System* (Farmer, S. G., ed.), Academic, London, 1997, pp. 9–43.

164. Hess, J. F. (1997) Molecular Pharmacology of kinin receptors, in *The Kinin System* (Farmer, S. G. ed.), Academic, London, 1997, pp. 46–55.

165. Cruwys, S. C., Garrett, N. E., Perkins, M. N., Blake, D. R. and Kidd, B. L. (1994) The role of bradykinin B_1 receptors in the maintenance of intra-articular plasma extravasation in chronic antigen-induced arthritis. *Br. J. Pharmacol.* **113,** 940–944.

166. Mackie, K., Lai, Y., Nairn, A. C., Greengard, P., Pitt, B. R., and Lazo, J. S. (1986) Protein phosphorylation in cultured endothelial cells. *J. Cell. Physiol.* **128,** 367–374.

167. Schini, V. B., Boulanger, C., Regoli, D., and Vanhoutte, P. M. (1990) Bradykinin stimulates the production of cyclic GMP *via* activation of B_2 recpeptors in cultured porcine aortic endothelial cells. *J. Pharmacol. Exp. Ther.* **252,** 581–585.

168. Lowe, W. L., Jr., Yorek, M. A., Karpen, C. W., Teasdale, R. M., Hovis, J. G., Albrecht, B., and Prokopiou, C. (1992). Activation of protein kinase C differentially regulates insulin-like growth factor-I and basic fibroblast growth factor messenger RNA levels. *Mol. Endocrinol.* **6,** 741–752.

169. Tiffany, C. W. and Burch, R. M. (1989) Bradykinin stimulates tumor necrosis factor and interleukin-1 release from macrophages. *FEBS Lett.* **247,** 189–192.

170. Rehbock, J., Chondromatidou, A., Buchinger, P., Hermann, A., and Jochum, M. (1997) Bradykinin stimulates interleukin-6 and interleukin-8 secretion of human decidua derived cells. *Br. J. Obs. Gynaecol.* **104,** 495–499.

171. Bueb, J.-L., Mousli, M., Bronner, C., Rouot, B., and Landry, Y. (1990) Activation of G_i-like proteins, a receptor–independent effect of kinins in mast cells. *Mol. Pharmacol.* **38,** 816–822.

172. Geppetti, P., Del Bianco, E., Tramontana, M., Vigano, T., Folco, G. C., Maggi, C. A., Manzini, S., and Fanciullacci, M. (1991). Arachidonic acid and bradykinin share a common pathway to release neuropeptide form capsaicin-sensitive sensory nerve fibres of the guinea-pig heart. *J. Pharmacol. Exp. Ther.* **259,** 759–765.

173. Melmon, K. L., Webster, M. E., Goldfinger, S. E. and Seegmiller, J. E. (1967) The presence of a kinin in inflammatory synovial effusion from arthritides of varying etiologies. *Arthritis Rheum.* **10,** 13–20.

174. Borkowski, J. A., Ransom, R. W., Seabrook, E. R., Trumbauer, M., Chen, H., Hill, R. E., et al. (1995) Targeted disruption of a B_2 bradykinin receptor gene in mice eliminates bradykinin action in smooth muscle and neurons. *J. Biol. Chem.* **270,** 13,706–13,710.

175. Warren, J. B. and Loi, R. K. (1995) Captopril increases skin microvascular blood flow secondary to bradykinin, nitric oxide and prostaglandins. *FASEB J.* **9,** 411–418.

176. Cascieri, M. A., Bull, H. G., Mumford, R. A., Patchett, A. A., Thornberry, N. A., and Liang, T. (1984) Carboxyl-terminal tripeptidyl hydrolysis of substance P by purified rabbit lung angiotensin-converting enzyme and the potentiation of substance P activity *in vivo* by captopril and MK-422. *Mol. Pharmacol.* **25,** 287–293.

177. Unger, T., Mattfeldt, T., Lamberty, V., Bock, P., Mall, G., Linz, W., Schölkens, B. A., and Gohlke, P. (1992) Effect of early onset angiotensin converting enzyme inhibition on myocardial capillaries. *Hypertension* **20,** 478–482.

178. Olivetti, G., Cigola, E., Lagrasta, C., Ricci, R., Quaini, F., Monopoli, A., and Ongini, E. (1993) Spirapril prevents left ventricular hypertrophy, decreases myocardial damage and promotes angiogenesis in spontaneously hypertensive rats. *J. Cardiovasc. Pharmacol.* **21,** 362–370.

179. Bock, P. (1998) The arterial length-densities under preventive angiotensin-converting-enzyme inhibiting treatment in the myocardium of spontaneously hypertensive rats. *Basic Res. Cardiol.* **93,** 18–22.

180. Schölkens, B. A., Linz, W., and König, W. (1988) Effects of the angiotensin converting enzyme inhibitor ramipril, in isolated ischaemic rat heart are abolished by a bradykinin antagonist. *J. Hypertens.* **6(S4),** 25–28.

181. Fabre, J. E., Rivard, A., Magner, M., Silver, M., and Isner, J. M. (1999) Tissue inhibition of angiotensin-converting enzyme activity stimulates angiogenesis *in vivo. Circulation* **99,** 3043–3049.

182. Cameron, N. E., Cotter, M. A., and Robertson, S. (1992) Angiotensin converting enzyme inhibition prevents development of muscle and nerve dysfunction and stimulates angiogenesis in streptozotocin-diabetic rats. *Diabetologia* **35,** 12–18.

183. Kohama, Y., Oka, H., Murayama, N., Iida, K., Itoh, M., Ying, X., and Mimura, T. (1992) Increase of migration of cultured endothelial cells by angiotensin-converting enzyme inhibitor derived from tuna muscle. *J. Pharmacobio–Dyn.* **15,** 223–229.

184. Kalkman, E. A., van Haren, P., Saxena, P. R., and Schoemaker, R. G. (1999) Early captopril prevents myocardial infarction-induced hypertrophy but not angiogenesis. *Eur. J. Pharmacol.* **369,** 339–348.

185. Wang, D.-H. and Prewitt, R. L. (1990) Captopril reduces aortic and microvascular growth in hypertensive and normotensive rats. *Hypertension* **15,** 68–77.

186. Fogo, A., Yoshida, Y., Yared, A., and Ichikawa, I. (1990) Importance of angiogenic action of angiotensin II in the glomerular growth of maturing kidneys. *Kidney Intl.* **38,** 1068–1074.

187. Buttar, H. S. (1997) An overview of the influence of ACE inhibitors on fetal-placental circulation and perinatal development. *Mol. Cell. Biochem.* **176,** 61–71.

188. Vranes, D., Dilley, R. J., and Cooper, M. E. (1995) Vascular changes in the diabetic kidney: effects of ACE inhibition. *J. Diabetes Complic.* **9,** 296–300.

189. Hilgers, K. F., Reddi, V., Krege, J. H., Smithies, O., and Gomez, R. A. (1997) Aberrant renal vascular morphology and renin expression in mutant mice lacking angiotensin–converting enzyme. Hypertension **29,** 216–221.

190. Pedram, A., Razandi, M., Hu, R. M., and Levin, E. R. (1997) Vasoactive peptides modulate vascular endothelial cell growth factor production and endothelial cell proliferation and invasion. *J. Biol. Chem.* **272,** 17,097–17,103.

7

Angiogenesis in Wound Healing and Surgery

*Wayne A. Morrison, Geraldine M. Mitchell,
Jane E. Barker, Tamara Konopka,
and Alastair G. Stewart*

ANGIOGENESIS IN THE SURGICAL CONTEXT

Angiogenesis is fundamental to wound healing and tissue repair. Healing of lacerations, surgical incisions, burns, or ischaemic damage depends on a successful co-ordinated cascade of events that includes angiogenesis. Skin-graft "take" involves a process of serum imbibition followed by inosculation where the graft becomes pink. In this process, red blood cells enter the graft vessels by an actual realignment of capillary ends in the underlying vascular bed with those on the undersurface of the graft. After 24–48 h, new capillary buds commence growing across the gap and by 72 h the circulation has been established to secure graft survival *(1,2)*. Wounds do not heal and grafts do not revascularise in avascular sites where angiogenesis is impeded, such as scarred tissue beds or on bare tendon, bone, and cartilage. In contrast, in certain situations angiogenesis is excessive as in diabetic retinopathy, rheumatoid arthritis, haemangioma, and malignancy *(3–6)*.

In plastic surgery, the staged transfer of skin flaps from one site to another depends on adequacy of angiogenic connections at the new site before the original base attachment can be severed. The art and craft of plastic surgery depends on the skill of manipulating the angiogenic and vasculogenic processes within the tissues in a directional way to extend the potential area of flap survival. Techniques used to induce directional angiogenesis prior to flap transfer include ring-barking incisions to selectively exclude the circulation, partial severance, tourniquets, or vasoconstrictive injections at the base of the

From: *The New Angiotherapy*
Edited by: T.-P. D. Fan and E. C. Kohn © Humana Press Inc., Totowa, NJ

flap. These techniques are designed to induce controlled ischaemia that will in turn stimulate angiogenesis. Ischaemia is a potent stimulus to angiogenesis *(7)*, well-exemplified by the development of collateral branches and capillary networks in an attempt to compensate in response to chronic obstruction of coronary and limb vessels.

Angioplasty and coronary artery bypass have traditionally been used to treat coronary artery disease. However, the rate of restenosis following these procedures is unacceptably high. Recently, an alternative approach involving omentum and latissimus dorsi muscles being wrapped around the heart has been used to provide a new blood supply *(8)*. Angiogenic bridging occurs between the wrapped tissue and the underlying ischaemic heart. Vessels have been directly implanted into cardiac muscle to achieve the same purpose *(9)*. Ischaemic limbs and digits have been salvaged by tunneling vascularized omental or fascial flaps into the subcutaneous space of the ischaemic hand or foot *(10)*. A new capillary network buds out from the surface of the implanted tissue and invades the ischaemic areas *(11)*. Similarly, chronically scarred and ischaemic peripheral nerves can be revascularized by wrapping with living vascularized fascia or adipose tissue *(12)*. Necrotic bone has also been revascularizd by the implantation of vessel pedicle *(13)*. Gene transfer of vascular endothelial-cell growth factor (VEGF) into blood vessels or muscle is a therapeutically promising alternative method of induction of collateral sprouting in ischaemic tissue *(14–16)*.

VEGF is also likely to play a key role in wound healing-associated angiogenesis, because hypoxia is one of the better-characterized stimuli for the expression of VEGF *(17,18)*. However, excessive ischaemia encountered in some wounds may lead to impaired wound healing *(19)*. Impaired healing of burn wounds has been ascribed to a decreased production of angiogenic factors such as TNF-α *(20)*, which is both a pro-inflammatory and pro-angiogenic cytokine *(21)*. We have shown that hypoxia alone enhances TNF-α expression in human cultured monocytes, whereas a combination of hypoxia and glucose deprivation, which better mimics wound ischaemia, results in a decreased expression of TNF-α *(22)*, which may in part explain the diminished wound healing response. Hyperbaric oxygen, which corrects wound hypoxia, accelerates wound healing *(23)*. On the other hand, excessive angiogenesis may delay wound healing by preventing the wound-maturation process *(24)*. A model has been developed in which wound healing and angiogenesis can be measured simultaneously. The ear of the hairless mouse is subjected to a full dermal thickness wound to the cartilage, and epithelialization and neovascularization rates can be measured by intravital microscopy *(25)*.

Tissue engineering or prefabrication is a new and exciting field or surgery. In this process, large vascular pedicles are implanted into combinations of autogenous tissues, allografts, or synthetic biocompatible material, such as polytetrafluoroethylene *(26)*, silicone *(27)*, titanium, or hydroxyapatite. Matrices with implanted cells and growth factors may be used to enhance proliferation and differentiation. Angiogenic invasion into the construct from the implanted pedicle converts it into a living part or organ, which can then be transplanted by microvascular anastomosis to the desired site in the body. We have studied the process of prefabrication of skin flaps *(28)* and in a histological study using colored ink injections—blue for the pedicle and black for the skin *(29)*. These tracing studies indicated that capillary budding from the isolated vascular pedicle linked with budding from the canopy of vessels in the overlying skin. Once this delicate microvascular link is established, the whole flap can be cut free from its surrounding tissue and vascularized solely on the implanted vessel. Basic fibroblast growth factor (bFGF) enhances the rate of this process and therefore has the potential to make it clinically more acceptable *(29,30)*. Blood vessels *(31)*, skin flaps *(32,33)*, ears *(34)*, face *(35)*, and joints have been engineered based on these principles.

The next logical step in the development of tissue engineering, which is being undertaken in our laboratory, is to develop extracorporeal circulation upon which such parts will be engineered ex vivo in the laboratory and reimplanted into the body. Angiogenesis is the lynch pin for these processes and understanding the mechanisms that switch angiogenesis on or off, enhance or accelerate the process, or directionally guide it are fundamental to progress in tissue engineering. For this reason there have been many attempts to produce an ideal model of angiogenesis.

A MODEL OF FUNCTIONAL ANGIOGENESIS OF RELEVANCE TO WOUND HEALING AND PLASTIC AND RECONSTRUCTIVE SURGERY

The most commonly used in vivo models of angiogenesis involve direct measurements of new blood vessel growth into a previously avascular area. In the rabbit corneal model, slow release of angiogenesis stimulants and/or inhibitors is achieved by affixing a disc to the cornea. Similar methods are used in the chick chorioallantoic model (CAM) to examine the growth of new blood vessels into fetal tissue. Neither of these models is suitable for assessing the angiogenesis that occurs following a reconstructive surgical procedure. In the case of the cornea, the development of vessels is not occurring in response to the classic hypoxic stimulus and the vessels that do grow are not required to supply metabolic needs. These deficiencies are also true of the CAM model, with the additional *caveat* that the fetal angiogenic response may model a developmental rather than a wound healing-type angiogenic response. A number of other models of angiogenesis including the use of subcutaneous injections of the extracellular matrix, matrigel *(36)*, sponges *(37)*, and airpouches *(38)* have been used. These models are more closely aligned to an inflammatory-type angiogenic response, showing a pronounced leukocyte infiltrate. Thus, a new model of functional angiogenesis has been established in our laboratory *(39)* in which the angiogenesis is assessed by measuring the surviving area of a skin/muscle flap sustained by the new blood vessel growth. The first experimental study of spontaneously anastomosing small vessels was reported by Smahel and Jentsch *(40)*. Our model is a modification of a skin flap model in rats developed by Brown et al. *(41)*.

Through bilateral transverse groin crease incisions, the epigastric artery, vein, and nerve are dissected from the surrounding connective tissue, the nerve is excised and perivascular adventitia meticulously stripped from the artery and vein using the operating microscope. The artery and vein are separated and the isolated artery is subjected to diathermy centrally and resected at the mid-point of the coagulated region. The retraction of the sealed ends of the artery results in the formation of a 7-mm gap. The epigastric vein is left intact to minimize further separation of the artery ends (Fig. 1). Following wound closure, the rats were maintained for periods from 0–21 d, during which time an increasing amount of angiogenic growth occurred between the ends of the severed artery.

At the end of this period of 0–21 d, a 3 × 3 cm epigastric abdominal flap (skin and panniculus muscle) is cut out and severed from all supplying blood vessels, except the previously severed epigastric artery and accompanying vein. Thus, the only blood supply now reaching the flap is via the new blood vessels that have grown across the severed left epigastric artery (Fig. 1). The flap is then resutured into its original position. In the same operation, the right epigastric vascular pedicle is harvested for histologic assessment. The wounds are then closed and the rats housed for a further 5 d. During this 5-d period

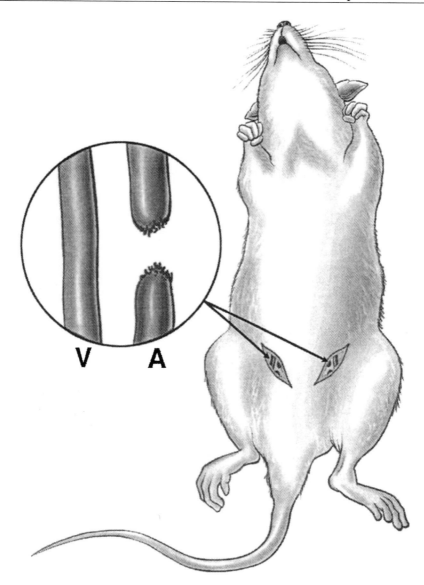

Fig. 1. In the initial stage of the model, bilateral groin incisions are made to expose the epigastric pedicle and the artery is cauterised to create a 7-mm gap (left hand side diagram). The wounds are closed and a variable period of time allowed for vessels to develop between the ends of the artery. A flap of skin is raised on this reconstituted vascular pedicle (right hand side diagram) and its survival is determined by skin blood flow 5 d after elevation. Reproduced with the permission from ref. *49.*

the skin flap would necrose, either partly or completely, if the angiogenic response had been insufficient to supply the metabolic needs of the tissue. The extent of any necrosis is determined after 5 d, by intralinguinal administration of fluorescein to delineate the portion of the skin flap with blood perfusion. As the period allowed for angiogenesis increased, so did flap survival, reaching a maximum at 14 d *(39).*

This model of angiogenesis has also been established in mice to allow the use of the ever-increasing array of relevant transgenic mice. The C57 BL6 mice underwent a slightly modified procedure: in the first operation the gap created in the epigastric artery was reduced to 4 mm; in the second operation the abdominal skin/muscle flap lifted on the left epigastric pedicle was 1.5×2.5 cm. A time-course of flap survival in C57 BL6 mice indicates that, as in rats, flaps lifted on the day of epigastric artery resection showed no survival, indicating that the vascular pedicle doesn't function as a venous flap. Flap survival then increased with the length of time allowed for angiogenesis with flap survival reaching a maximum after 21 d.

The surgical model described here in rats and mice establishes a functional model of angiogenesis where new vessel growth supplies a distinct skin flap, the area of which can be measured. Variations in flap survival indicate differences in the degree of new vessel growth. By determining a time-course of angiogenesis related to flap survival, and then selecting the period of angiogenesis that causes approx 50% flap survival, agents that may inhibit or promote angiogenesis can be administered systemically or locally to the pedicle to alter the rate of new vessel growth. This clinically relevant model has practical advantages over other commonly utilized in vivo models of angiogenesis, particularly because the model does not require measurement of blood vessel numbers, which is well-recognized to present methodological difficulties *(42)*. Using this model we have investigated the effects of manipulating nitric oxide (NO) production.

NITRIC OXIDE

Several groups have recognised that nitric oxide (NO) influences the intra- and extracellular signaling of angiogenesis. However, in contrast to the roles of NO in other physiological and pathophysiological processes such as blood-pressure regulation, neurotransmission, host-defense mechanism, and inflammation *(43)*, the role of NO in angiogenesis remains controversial. The net effect of manipulating NO levels appears to be dependent on both the model of angiogenesis being used and selectivity of inhibitors or type of NO donor used (*see* Table 1).

The Influence of NO in Surgically Induced Angiogenesis

We have tested whether selective inhibition of the isoforms of NOS can be used to influence the outcome of angiogenesis and functional survival of tissue dependent on that angiogenic response. In this model of bridging angiogenesis in the rat, the selective iNOS inhibitors, S-methylisothiourea, aminoethylthiourea, and aminoguanidine, reduced skin-flap survival. Nitro-L-arginine methyl ester (L-NAME), which has some selectivity for eNOS, enhanced flap survival, whereas the nonselective NOS inhibitor nitro-imino-L-ornithine had no effect on flap survival *(44)*. These findings were interpreted to suggest that NO derived from iNOS is pro-angiogenic and that conversely, NO derived from eNOS is anti-angiogenic.

Although iNOS-selective inhibitors consistently decreased the angiogenic responses in the rat, the available inhibitors had insufficient selectivity to make a definitive conclusion regarding the role of iNOS-derived NO. Thus, flap survival was compared in the iNOS knockout (iNOS KO) mouse with wild type, C57/BL6 mice wild-type. The iNOS KO mouse showed a delayed angiogenic response, and even after 21 d, flap survival was not significant. In contrast, the wild-type mice attained 50% flap survival by d 5. Further evidence for the opposing roles of eNOS and iNOS-derived NO was gained by the administration of L-NAME to the iNOS KO mice, which increased flap survival to a level comparable with that observed in normal wild-type mice *(44)*.

Table 1

Nitric Oxide Influences on Angiogenesis

Model	Findings	Conclusion	Reference
CAM	SNP ↓ angiogenesis	NO ↓ angiogenesis	(53)
Matrigel tube formation	SNP ↓ tube formation	NO ↓ angiogenesis	(53)
Corneal implant	L-NAME ↓ VEGF-angiogenesis	NO ↑ angiogenesis	(54)
Corneal implant	iNOS expressing tumor	iNOS ↑ angiogenesis	(50)
Surgical	iNOS KO ↓ flap survival	iNOS ↑ angiogenesis	(44)
	INOS inhibitors ↓ flap survival	iNOS ↑ angiogenesis	(44)
Melanoma (B-16 Tumor)	iNOS KO ↓ tumor growth	iNOS ↑ angiogenesis	(51)

Abbreviations: CAM, Chorioallantoic membrane of the chick embryo; SNP, sodium nitroprusside; iNOS KO, iNOS knockout.

Is There a Simple Explanation for the Complexity of the Role of NO in Angiogenesis?

Three genetically distinct isoforms of nitric oxide synthase (NOS) have been identified. The calcium-dependent endothelial NOS (eNOS) is constitutively expressed and produces relatively small (pM) amounts of NO. By contrast, iNOS produces large (up to μM) amounts of NO for prolonged periods, and can be expressed following cytokine stimulation in many cell types (43). In view of these marked functional differences in the isoforms of NOS, it has been suggested that the role of NO is dependent on the NOS isoform stimulated and the cellular location of the enzyme. iNOS is induced under conditions that also result in induction of superoxide anion generation favoring the formation of peroxynitrite. We have shown that low concentrations of peroxynitrite enhance mast-cell degranulation (45). Because mast cells contain angiogenic factors such as bFGF (46) enhancement of degranulation could result in increased availability of angiogenic factors. In contrast, exogenous NO inhibits mast cell degranulation responses (47). Thus, in a surgical model of angiogenesis, the diverse influence of NO may be related to the complex and opposing roles of NO derived from the different isoforms of NOS (44).

Importance of Nitric Oxide in Angiogenic-Associated Processes

iNOS knockout (KO) mice appear to have little phenotypic variation from their wild-type controls (48), suggesting that developmental angiogenesis is not profoundly influenced by iNOS knockout. The role of endogenous NO in angiogenesis appears to be limited to inflammatory or pathophysiological conditions. We have previously noted prolonged ulceration of scratch wounds in the iNOS KO mice, suggesting impaired wound healing (48). This observation was recently corroborated by Yamasaki et al. (49). Additionally, this group established the importance of iNOS by reversing the impairment of wound healing by the administration of an adenovirus containing cDNA for iNOS. These raise hopes for the use of iNOS as a clinically useful angiogenesis promoter.

In humans, the association of NOS in primary head and neck cancer with microvessel density (50) has suggested a role for NOS in tumor angiogenesis. Our own studies of B16 melanoma growth in mice indicate that host iNOS plays a role in the initial stage of tumor growth, because tumors inoculated into iNOS KO mice showed a bimodal size distribution with the smaller sized tumors being either undetectable or not larger than 100 mg after 14 d compared with those in wild-type mice having a unimodal distribution centring on a weight of about 1 g *(51)*. Several other studies have suggested a link between NOS activity and tumor growth including an elegant demonstration by Gallo and colleagues that iNOS expressing cells, isolated from human tumors, stimulate angiogenesis in the rabbit cornea model *(50)*. In a recent review on the role of NO in tumor growth, the potentially confounding influences of NO on tumor blood flow, angiogenesis, host defense and direct cytotoxicity were discussed *(52)*. Nevertheless, there does appear to be general agreement in the literature that NO promotes tumor growth.

CONCLUSIONS

Irrespective of the mechanism of iNOS-mediated angiogenesis, there is clinical potential for the manipulation of NOS in the regulation of angiogenesis. This could be applied to either tissue engineering or wound healing in which transfection with the iNOS gene or selective induction at the site of desired angiogenesis would be therapeutic. Conversely, selective inhibition of iNOS would limit tumor growth and reduce inflammation. We suggest that the exploitation of iNOS pathway in the clinical setting for wound healing and tissue engineering warrants further investigation.

REFERENCES

1. David, J. S. and Traut, H. F. (1925) Origin and development of the blood supply of whole thickness skin grafts. An experimental study. *Ann. Surg.* **82,** 87.
2. Birch, J. and Branemark, P. I. (1969) The vascularization of a free full thickness skin graft. I. A vital microscope study. *Scand. J. Plast. Reconstr. Surg.* **3,** 1–10.
3. Folkman, J. (1990) What is the evidence that tumors are aniogenesis dependent? *J. Natl. Cancer Inst.* **82,** 4–6.
4. Colville-Nash, P. R. and Scott, D. L. (1992) Angiogenesis and rheumatoid arthritis: pathogenic and therapeutic implications. *Ann. Rheum. Dis.* **51,** 919–925.
5. Roberts, A. B., Sporn, M. B., and Lefer, A. M. (1992) *Trends Cardiovasc. Med.* **3,** 77–81.
6. Gross, C. E., Bednar, M. M., Howard, D. B., and Sporn, M. B. (1993) Transforming growth factor-beta-1 reduces infarct size after experimental cerebral ischaemia in a rabbit model. *Stroke* **24,** 558–562.
7. Falanga, V., McKenzie, A., and Eaglestein, W. H. (1991) Heterogeneity in oxygen diffusion around venous ulcers. *J. Dematol. Surg. Oncol.* **17,** 336–339.
8. Mannion, J. D., Blood, V., Bailey, W., Bauer, T. L., Magno, M. G., DiMeo, F., et al. (1996) The effect of basic fibroblast growth factor on the blood flow and morphologic features of a latissimus dorsi cardiomyoplasty. *J. Thor. Cardiovasc. Surg.* **111(1),** 19–28.
9. Brown, D. M., Lantieri, L. A., Chung, S. H., and Khouri, R. K. (1994) Coronary artery bypass without a vascular anastomosis. Presented at the 39th Plastic Surgery Research Council Meeting, Ann Arbor, Michigan, June 4–7.
10. Colen, L. B. (1987) Limb salvage in the patient with severe peripheral vascular disease: the role of microsurgical free-tissue transfer. *Plast. Reconstr. Surg.* **79,** 389–395.
11. Morrison, W. A. and Cavallo, A. V. (1993) Revascularization of an ischaemic replanted thumb using a lateral fascial forearm free flap. *Ann. Plast. Surg.* **31,** 467–470.
12. Tham, S. K., Ireland, D. C., Riccio, M., and Morrison, W. A. (1998) Reverse radial artery fascial flap: a treatment for the chronically scarred median nerve in recurrent carpal tunnel syndrome. *J. Hand. Surg.* **21(5),** 849–854.
13. Hori, Y., Tamai, S., Okuda, H., Sakamoto, M., Takita, T., and Masuhara, K. (1979) Blood vessel transplantation to bone. *J. Hand Surg.* **4,** 23–33.
14. Tsurumi, Y., Takeshita, S., Chen, D., Kearney, M., Rossow, S. T., Passeri, J., et al. (1996) Direct intramuscular gene transfer of naked DNA encoding vascular endothelial growth factor augments collateral development and tissue perfusion. *Circulation* **94(12),** 3281–3290.
15. Majesky, M. W. (1996) A little VEGF goes a long way. Therapeutic angiogenesis by direct injection of vascular endothelial growth factor-encoding plasmid DNA. *Circulation* **94(12),** 3062–3064.

16. Bauters, C., Asahara, T., Zheng, L. P., et al. (1995) Site-specific therapeutic angiogenesis after systemic administration of vascular endothelial growth factor. *J. Vasc. Surg.* **21,** 314–324.
17. Schweiki, D., Itin, A., Sofler, D., and Keshet, E. (1992) Vascular endothelial growth factor induced by hypoxia may mediate hypoxia-initiated angiogenesis. *Nature* **359,** 843–845.
18. Schweiki, D., Neelman, M., Itin, A., and Keshet, E. (1995) Induiction of vascular endothelial growth factor expression by hypoxia mamnd by glucose deficiency in multicell spheroids: implications for tumor angiogenesis. *Proc. Natl. Acad. Sci. USA* **92,** 768–772.
19. Stephens, F. O. and Hunt, T. K. (1971) Effect of changes in inspired oxygen and carbon dioxide tensions on wound tensile strength: an experimental study. *Ann. Surg.* **173,** 515–519.
20. Pejnovic, N., lilic, D., Zunic, G., Colic, M., Kataranovski, M., and Dujic, A. (1995) Aberrant levels of cytokines within the healing wound after burn injury. *Arch. Surg.* **130,** 99–106.
21. Fajardo, L. F., Kwan, H. K., Kowalski, J., Prionas, S. D., and Allsion, A. C. (1992) Dual role of tumor necrosis factor-α in angiogenesis. *Am. J. Pathol.* **140,** 539–544.
22. Guida, E. and Stewart, A. (1998) Influence of hypoxia and glucose deprivation on tumor necrosis factor-alpha and granulocyte-macrophage colony-stimulating factor expression in human cultured monocytes. *Cell Physiol. Biochem.* **8,** 75–88.
23. Hammerlund, C. and Sundberg, T. (1994) Hyperbaric oxygen reduced the size of chronic leg ulcers. A randomised, double-blind study. *Plast. Reconstr. Surg.* **93,** 829–833.
24. Pierce, G. F., Tarpley, J. E., Yanagihara, D., Mustoe, T. A., Fox, G. M., and Thomason, A. (1992) Platelet-derived growth factor (BB homodimer), transforming growth factor-β1 and basic fibroblast growth factor in deraml wound healing. *Am. J. Pathol.* **140,** 1375–1388.
25. Kjolseth, D., Kim, M. K., Andresen, L. H., Morsing, A., Frank, J. M., Schuschke, D., et al. (1994) Direct visualisation and measurements of wound neovascularisation: application in microsurgery research. *Microsurgery* **15,** 390–398.
26. Walton, R. L. and Brown, R. E. (1993) Tissue engineering of composite reconstruction: An experimental model. *Ann. Plast. Surg.* **30,** 105–111.
27. Costa, H., Cunha, I., Guimaraes, I., Camba, S., Malta, A., and Lopes, A. (1993) Prefabricated flaps for the head and neck: a preliminary report. *Br. J. Plast. Surg.* **46,** 223.
28. Morrison, W. A., Dvir, E., Doi, K., Hurley, J. V., Hickey, M. J., and O'Brien, B. C. (1990) Prefabrication of thin transferable axial-pattern skin flaps: an experimental study in rabbits. *Br. J. Plast. Surg.* **43,** 645.
29. Hickey, M. J., Wilson, Y., Hurley, J. V., and Morrison, W. A. (1998) Mode of vascularization of control and basic fibroblast growth factor-stimulated prefabricated skin flaps. *Plast. Reconstr. Surg.* **101,** 1296–1306.
30. Bayati, S. and Russell, R. C. (1994) Angiogenic properties of basic fibroblast growth factor in prefabricated flaps. Presented at the 73rd Annual Meeting of the American Association of Plastic Surgeons, St. Louis, MO, May, 1–4.
31. L'Heureux, N., Pâquet, S., Labbé, R., Germain, L., and Auger, F. A. (1998) A completely biological tissue-engineered human blood vessel. *FASEB J.* **12,** 47–56.
32. Yao, S. T. (1982) Microvascular transplantation of a prefabricated free thigh flap. *Plast. Reconstr. Surg.* **69,** 568.
33. Morrison, W. A., Penington, A. J., Callan, P., and Kumta S. (1997) Clinical applications and technical limitations of prefabricated flaps. *Plast. Reconstr. Surg.* **99,** 378–385.
34. Sims, C. D., Butler, P. E. M., Cao, Y. L., Casanova, R., Randolph, M. A., Black, A., et al. (1998) Tissue engineering neocartilage using plasma derived polymer substrates and chondrocytes. *Plast. Reconstr. Surg.* **101,** 1580.
35. Baudet, J. (1991) Oral communication. 4th Annual Meeting of the American Society for Reconstructive Microsurgery, Orlando, FL, September. (Quoted in Khouri, R. K., Upton, J., and Shaw, W. W. (1992) Principles of flap prefabrication. *Clin. Plast. Surg.* **19,** 763.
36. Kibbey, M. C., Corcoran, M. L., Wahl, L. M., and Kleinman, H. K. (1994) Laminin SIKVAV peptide-induced angiogenesis in vivo is potentiated by neutrophils. *J. Cell Physiol.* **160,** 185–193.
37. Hu, D. E., Hiley, C. R., Smither, R. L., Gresham, G. A., and Fan, T.-P. D. (1995) Correlation of ^{133}Xe clearance, blood flow and histology in the rat sponge model for angiogenesis. Further studies with angiogenic modifiers. *Lab. Invest.* **72,** 601–610.
38. Appleton, I., Brown, N. J., Willis, D., Colvilie-Naash, P. R., Alam, C., Brown, J. R., and Willoughby, D. A. (1996) The role of vascular endothelial growth factor in a murine chronic granulomatous air pouch model of angiogenesis. *J. Pathol.* **180,** 90–94.
39. Theile, D. R. B., Kane, A. J., Romeo, R., Mitchell, G., Crowe, D., Stewart, A. G., and Morrison, W. A. (1998) A model of bridging angiogenesis in the rat. *Br. J. Plast. Surg.* **51,** 243–249.

40. Smahel, J. and Jentsch, B. (1984). Spontaneous anastomosis of vessels approximately 10 µm in diameter: an experimental study. *Br. J. Plast. Surg.* **37,** 236–240.

41. Brown, D. M., Hong, S. P., Farrell, C. L., Pierce, G. F., and Khouri, R. K. (1995) Platelet-derived growth factor BB induces functional vascular anastomoses in vivo. *Proc. Natl. Acad. Sci. USA* **92,** 5920–5924.

42. Jain, R. K., Schlenger, K., Hockel, M., and Yuan, F. (1997) Quantitative angiogenesis assays: Progress and problems. *Nature Med.* **3,** 1203–1208.

43. Moncada, S., Palmer, R. M., and Higgs, E. A. (1991) Nitric oxide: physiology, pathophysiology, and pharmacology. *Pharmacol. Rev.* **43,** 109–142.

44. Kane, A. J., Barker, L. E., Mitchell, G. M., et al. (2001) Inducible nitric oxide synthase (NOS$_2$) activity promotes ischaemic skin flap survival. *Br. J. Pharmcol.* (in press).

45. Barker, J. and Stewart, A. G. (1998) Differeing effects of nitric oxide compared with peroxynitrite on mast cell degranulation in vitro. *Br. J. Pharmacol.* **123,** 305P.

46. Qu, Z., Liebler, J. M., Powers, M. R., Galey, T., Ahmadi, P., Huang, X-N., et al. (1995) Mast cells are a major source of basic fibroblast growth factor in chronic inflammation and cutaneous hemangioma. *Am. J. Pathol.* **147,** 564–573.

47. Salvemini, D., Masini, E., Pistelli, A., Mannaioni, P. F., and Vane, J. (1991) Nitric oxide: a Regulatory mediator of mast cell reactivity. *J. Cardiovasc. Pharmacol.* 17(Suppl.) S258–S264.

48. Nathan, C. (1997) Inducible nitric oxide synthase: what difference does it make ? *J. Clin. Invest.* **100(10),** 2417–2423.

49. Yamasaki, K., Edington, H. D. J., McClosky, C., Tzeng, E., Lizonova, A., Kovesdi, I., et al. (1998) Reversal of wound repair in iNOS-deficient mice by topical adenoviral-mediated iNOS gene transfer. *J. Clin. Invest.* **101(5),** 967–971.

50. Gallo, O., Masini, E., Morbidelli, L., Franchi, A., Fini-Storchi, I., Vergari, W. A., and Ziche, M. (1998) Role of nitric oxide in angiogenesis and tumor progression in head and neck cancer. *J. Natl. Cancer Inst.* **90(8),** 587–596.

51. Konopka, T., Barker, J., Bamford, T., Guida, E., Anderson, R. L., and Stewart, A. G. (2001) Nitric Oxide synthase II gene disruption: implications for tumour growth and vascular endothelial growth factor production. *Cancer Research* (in press).

52. Lala, P. K. and Orucevic, A. (1998) Role of nitric oxide in tumor progression: lessons from experimental tumors. *Cancer Metast. Rev.* **17,** 91–106.

53. Pipili-Synetos, E., Sakkoula, A. E., Haralabopoulos, G., Andriopoulou, P., Peristeris, P., and Maragoudakis, M. E. (1994) Evidence that nitric oxide is an endogenous antiangiogenic mediator. *Br. J. Pharmacol.* **111,** 894–902.

54. Ziche, M., Morbidelli, L., Choudri, R., Zhang, H. T., Donnini, S., Granger, H. J., and Bicknell, R. (1997) Nitric oxide synthase lies down stream from vascular endothelial growth factor-induced but not basic fibroblast growth factor-induced angiogenesis. *J. Clin. Invest.* **99(11),** 2625–2634.

8

Angiogenesis and Vascular Endothelial Growth Factor (VEGF) in Reproduction

D. Stephen Charnock-Jones, Yulong He, and Stephen K. Smith

CONTENTS

INTRODUCTION

In the adult organism angiogenesis is generally rare and is usually confined to pathological conditions. However, one marked exception to this is the female reproductive tract. In both the ovary and the uterus, there is cyclic growth and regression of specialized tissues that necessitates the growth and regression of vascular structures. These events are coordinated by steroid hormones, but it is now increasingly recognized that local effectors mediate their actions. Thus the female reproductive tract permits the study of the cyclic growth and regression of blood vessels in a normal physiological setting. This is obviously of importance to reproductive biology, but is also relevant to the study of blood vessels generally.

Angiogenesis, the process by which new capillaries develop from pre-existing vessels, plays a major role in physiological as well as pathological conditions *(1)*. The development of a new capillary network is a complex process involving basement membrane degradation and extracellular matrix proteolysis, accompanied by the proliferation and migration of endothelial cells, formation of rudimentary vascular structures, and remolding of the extracellular matrix *(2–4)*. The regulation of angiogenesis is thought to occur via a balance between angiogenic inducers and inhibitors, many of which interact with specific receptors on target cells *(5)*. Several factors of both peptide and nonpeptide nature have been shown to induce angiogenesis in vivo: epidermal growth factor (EGF)

From: *The New Angiotherapy*
Edited by: T.-P. D. Fan and E. C. Kohn © Humana Press Inc., Totowa, NJ

(6), transforming growth factor-α (TGF-α) *(7)* and transforming growth factor-β (TGF-β) *(8,9)*, tumor necrosis factor-α (TNF-α, in vivo) *(10)*, angiogenin *(11)*, acidic and basic fibroblast growth factor (aFGF/bFGF) *(12,13)*, vascular endothelial growth factor (VEGF) *(14)*, PGE_2 and monobutyrin *(15–17)*. Inhibitors of angiogenesis have been identified ranging from complex steroids to polypeptides including thrombospondin *(18)*, platelet factor IV *(19)*, TNF-α (in vitro) *(20)*, TGF-β *(9)*, interferons *(21)*, angiostatin *(22)*, integrin $α_vβ_3$ inhibitors *(23)*, and 16-kDa prolactin *(24,25)*.

Endothelium is generally quiescent in the healthy adult organism. A marked exception is the female reproductive tract, where the need for additional vasculature is constantly imposed by the periodic evolution of transient structures and by the cyclic repair of damaged tissues. Widespread and profound disruption of the female reproductive pathways were recently described *(26)* in mice treated with the angiogenesis inhibitor AGM-1470. These also showed that ovarian and endometrial cyclicity could be abolished, rendering the animals infertile, and that decidualization and placentation were also disrupted by the systematic blockade of angiogenesis. It is most likely that the cyclic angiogenic events in the female reproductive system are coordinated by hormones, the actions of which may be mediated by angiogenic factors that are either directly or indirectly hormone inducable. Ovarian, uterine, and placental tissues have been shown to contain and produce angiogenic and anti-angiogenic factors. Among those various angiogenic factors, VEGF possesses several unique attributes that suggest it plays an important role in these tissues. Specifically it promotes mitogenesis of vascular endothelial cells and vascular permeability, and it also modulates production of a number of proteolytic enzymes involved in the process of neovascularization. Thus it is able to regulate all the steps of neovascularization and is likely to be important in physiological and pathological angiogenesis in the female reproductive tract and other tissues. VEGF binding sites are detected in many adult tissues *(27)*, indicating that VEGF is probably important not only in angiogenesis, but also in the maintenance of existing vessels. This is confirmed by studies in the eye where reduction in VEGF levels causes regression of existing vessels *(28)*.

The pivotal role of VEGF in the development of the vascular system is further emphasized by the recent data (reviewed recently by Risau, ref. *29*). Loss of a single VEGF allele leads to embryonic lethality *(30,31)*, which indicates that even a relatively modest reduction in VEGF level can have profound effects. Gene knockout studies have also demonstrated that Flt-1 and KDR (the receptors for VEGF) are essential for the development and differentiation of embryonic vasculature. Mice null for the Flk-1 gene lacked vasculogenesis and blood-island formation, resulting in death in utero between days 8.5 and 9.5 *(32)*. Mouse embryos homozygous for a targeted mutation in the Flt-1 locus died in utero at mid-somite stages *(33)*.

VEGF AND ITS RECEPTORS

Vascular endothelial growth factor (VEGF) is a heparin-binding, secreted homodimeric glycoprotein of 30–46 kDa, also known as vascular permeability factor. It is a potent mitogen for vascular endothelium *(14,34–36)*, possesses potent vascular permeability-enhancing activity, and modulates the expression of several proteolytic enzymes involved in angiogenesis *(37,38)* and also has a role in the maintenance of newly formed blood capillaries *(28)*.

Analysis of the *VEGF* gene has revealed that the protein coding regions are arranged in eight exons. By alternative splicing of the exons five different mRNAs for VEGF are generated, which have 121, 145, 165, 189, and 206 amino acids respectively ($VEGF_{121}$,

VEGF$_{145}$, VEGF$_{165}$, VEGF$_{189}$, VEGF$_{206}$). In most tissues the 121 and 165 amino acid forms predominate and the 145 amino acid form is generally the rarest. This form was initially described in human endometrial and placental tissue *(39)* and has recently been shown to have unique features not shared by other forms of VEGF *(40)*. Rodent and bovine VEGFs are predicted to be one amino acid shorter but are generally highly conserved. Recently several other proteins have been identified which show considerable homology with VEGF. These have been termed placenta growth factor (PlGF) *(41)*, VEGFB *(42)*, VEGFC *(43)*, and VEGFD *(44)*. It has been shown *(45)* that placenta growth factor can form heterodimers with VEGF and that these heterodimers can bind to one of the VEGF receptors. However, they are 20–50-fold less mitogenic than VEGF $_{165}$ homodimers.

VEGF acts through two tyrosine kinase family receptors that are c-fms-like tyrosine kinase (flt-1) *(46,47)* and the kinase domain insert containing receptor (KDR) *(48)*. Both flt-1 and KDR possess seven immunoglobulin (IG)-like loops in their extracellular domains, which are different from the previously described class III receptor tyrosine kinases, which have five. They also contain a single transmembrane region, and a consensus tyrosine kinase sequence that is interrupted by a kinase-insert region *(46,48–50)*. The second IG-like extracellular domain of Flt-1 is essential for ligand binding and specificity *(51,52)*. Both receptors have been shown to bind VEGF with high affinity. Flt-1 has the highest affinity for VEGF, with a kDa of 10–20 p*M* *(50)* and KDR has a lower kDa of 100–125 p*M* *(53,54)*. The murine homolog of KDR, fetal liver kinase-1 (Flk-1) has also been identified and shares 85% sequence identity with human KDR *(48)*. Both Flt-1 and KDR/Flk-1 mRNAs are predominantly expressed in vascular endothelial cells in both fetal and adult tissues *(14,27,47,54–56)*. They are also found on nonendothelial cells including peripheral blood monocytes *(57)*, malignant melanoma cell lines *(58)*, trophoblast-like choriocarcinoma cell line BeWo *(59)*, and peritoneal fluid macrophages. Flt-4 tyrosine kinase receptor is related to the VEGF receptors, flt-1, and KDR, but does not bind VEGF and its expression is restricted mainly to lymphatic endothelia during development. mRNAs for flt-1, KDR/Flk-1, and flt-4 have distinct expression patterns and certain endothelia lack one or two of the three receptor mRNAs, suggesting that the receptor tyrosine kinases encoded by this gene family may have different functions in the regulation of the growth/differentiation of blood vessels *(29)*.

There are also several endogenously encoded soluble flts that are generated by alternative splicing of the same pre-mRNA used to produce the full-length flt-1. The identified sflts possess six (flt-K) *(60)*, or five or four *(61)* N-terminal immunoglobulin (IG)-like extracellular ligand-binding domains, respectively, and all missing the membrane-proximal seventh IG-like domain, the transmembrane-spanning region, and the intracellular tyrosine kinase domains. They all can bind VEGF with high affinity and inhibit the binding of ^{125}I-VEGF to bovine aortic endothelial cells in vitro and so can act as specific high-affinity antagonists of VEGF.

When we performed ligand-binding studies with ^{125}I-VEGF to localize functional receptors in the placenta, we were surprised to find that the VEGF binding was confined exclusively to the endothelial cells. There was no detectable binding to the trophoblast cells. The explanation for this discrepancy between the *in situ* hybridization and the ligand binding results is that the trophoblast actually expresses the soluble form of the receptor. We confirmed this by *in situ* hybridization with a probe specific for the mRNA encoding the sflt-1. The secreted sflt-1 protein was readily detectable in villus conditioned media and in maternal serum. It was not detectable in the serum of nonpregnant women or males and we have made similar observation in mice *(62,63)*.

Owing to the initial *in situ* hybridization results, we and many others have sought to identify direct actions of VEGF on trophoblast. This has not been straightforward owing to the problems of culturing primary trophoblast. Given that these cells produce large amounts of sflt-1, which is a potent VEGF antagonist, this would seem a little unlikely.

CYCLIC ANGIOGENESIS IN THE OVARY

The ovarian cycle is characterized by the repeated growth and development of follicles, ovulation, the formation, and finally regression of corpus luteum. There is concomitant development of elaborate vascular networks in the ovary during the cycle (64). Preantral follicles embedded in the stromal cells have no independent vascular supply of their own and depend on stromal vessels for delivery of nutrients and hormones. As they develop into the antral phase, their thecal layers (theca interna) become highly vascularized. But their granulosa cell layers are avascular and are separated from thecal layers by the membrane propria. At the time of ovulation, the membrane propria degenerates and capillaries rapidly grow from the richly vascularized thecal layers into the avascular granulosa cell layers and later develop into a new and complex network of sinusoidal vessels that nourish the parenchma of the newly formed corpus luteum (CL) (65).

The precise control of angiogenesis during the cycle is crucial for ovarian function. Angiogenesis may play an important role in the selective growth of oocytes and follicles (66). There is a striking difference in the distribution of blood vessels to individual follicles in the mammalian ovary. The dominant follicles possess a more elaborate microvasculature within the thecal layer than other follicles and this increased capillary density results in preferential delivery of radiolabeled human chorionic gonadotropin (hCG) to the maturing follicle (67). Intrafollicular vascularization may be critical processes that might be used to predict ovulation and could possibly be modified to help achieve or avoid pregnancy. The granulosa layer remains avascular until the LH surge has subsided and maximum vascularization is achieved by the midluteal phase. Growth of capillary sprouts accounts for substantial angiogenesis in the developing CL (68). Enhanced angiogenesis may also contribute to the delivery of low-density lipoprotein-cholesterol to the CL during its progesterone biosynthesis (69). Endothelial-cell proliferation is unchanged throughout the follicular, early and midluteal phases, but decreases significantly in the late luteal. Angiogenic factors are clearly implicated in the regulation of angiogenesis during the ovarian cycle. Indeed systemic blockade of angiogenesis leads to a reduction in luteal number and size (26).

VEGF is expressed in the interstitial tissue of the mouse ovary and in the thecal layers of the follicle, but not in the inner granulosa at preantral and with small antrum stages (70). In normal ovaries of premenopausal women, VEGF is also localized to the thecal cell layer, with minimal VEGF peptide detected in the granulosa cell layer and with no VEGF expression in atretic follicles (71). Concomitant with further growth and maturation of follicles, the expression of VEGF is also found in cumulus cells engulfing the oocyte. In the granulosa compartment, high levels of VEGF mRNA are detectable only at the immediate preovulatory stage in the mouse, human and primate ovaries (72,73).

VEGF receptors are also detectable in capillaries arranged in the peripheral thecal layers of growing follicles, on the endothelium of large medullar vessels from which the thecal networks originate, and on cells interspersed in the stroma, which are probably the migrating endothelial cells (70). Therefore VEGF is ideally positioned to induce angiogenesis and later provoke the increased permeability of thecal blood vessels shortly before ovulation. VEGF expression is also found in the luminal epithelium of the fallo-pian tube as well as smooth-muscle cells and pericytes lining small and large blood vessels within the tube and hilum of the ovary, which suggest that VEGF may increase vascular permeability and modulate tubal luminal secretions *(71)*.

The role of VEGF in the ovarian angiogenesis is further confirmed by ovary transplan-tation. Expression of VEGF mRNAs increases by a 40- to 60-fold in immature rat ovary after autotransplantation, accompanying its vascular in growth. This may result partly from the ischemic hypoxia in the transplanted ovary *(74)*, and partly from the rapid increase in serum gonadotropin levels. Treatment with LHRH antagonist Nal-Glu LHRH can diminish the increase of VEGF gene expression *(75)*. GnRH agonist, D-Trp6 LHRH is also found to have a selective inhibition of VEGF expression in ovarian carcinoma cell lines *(76)*.

VEGF AND CORPUS LUTEUM FORMATION

After ovulation, the cells of the follicle differentiate to form the progesterone-produc-ing corpus luteum. This tissue is one of the most vascular tissues of the body and also has one of the greatest blood perfusion rates of any tissue *(77)*, but it is likely that factors able to regulate blood-vessel growth in the corpus luteum would have profound effects on its development and function.

Shortly after ovulation, as granulosa cells differentiate to form into the corpus luteum, the predominant site of VEGF expression is within the luteal cells *(70–72,78)* suggesting that VEGF expression at this stage may be important for the angiogenesis that accompanies corpus luteum formation. Luteal cells continue to express VEGF in the fully developed, functional CL in the rat *(78)*. Detailed immunohistology by Doraiswamy et al. *(79)* has suggested that VEGF expression is restricted to pericytes in the developing ovine corpus luteum. In the primate ovary, VEGF mRNAs are detectable in corpora lutea collected during the early luteal phase of the menstrual cycle, but not in the regressing corpora lutea. Treatment of monkeys with GnRH antagonist during the midluteal phase of the menstrual cycle brings about a significant reduction in the levels of mRNA for VEGF *(73)*, although this could be a consequence of luteolysis. Consistent with its role as a paracrine endothelial-cell mitogen, it has been shown that VEGF-binding activity is expressed on the endothelial cells comprising the vascular networks of the corpus luteum *(70)*.

Luteal cells differentiate from granulosa cells and the mRNAs for VEGF are also expressed by cultured bovine granulosa cells. TPA (19-0 tetradecaenoylphorbol 13 acetate) and forskolin can induce VEGF transcription, which act through distinct signal-transduction pathways, the first involving protein kinase C (PKC), and the second acti-vated by cAMP and involving protein kinase A (PKA). Lutenising hormone (LH), a known activator of adenylylcyclase, also induces VEGF transcription *(79)*. Luteinized human granulosa cells (GCs) also express VEGF mRNAs in vitro *(80)*, and the expres-sion is dose and time-dependently enhanced by hCG. VEGF protein is also produced by GCs. These results imply that granulosa cells may be a source of VEGF, which could play a role in the angiogenic process associated with ovulation and corpus luteum formation.

Compelling evidence for the importance of VEGF in luteal growth has been obtained by inhibition of its action during luteral growth. Ferrara et al. *(81)* have, using VEGF antagonists based on soluble receptor molecules *(60)*, blocked the actions of VEGF and prevented lutenization and progesterone production in the superovulated rat. These studdies show that VEGF is essential for early lutenization.

Other angiogenic factors also play a role in the development of the vasculature of the corpus luteum. For example, Doraiswamy et al. *(82)* have shown that in addition to VEGF playing a role, members of the FGF family are also important. Taken together, these data would suggest that endothelial-cell proliferation and maintenance is regulated by several factors and that although VEGF is essential early in this process, other factors may play a role at other stages of luteal development.

VEGF may also have a pathophysiological role in ovary. Prominent features of Ovarian hyperstimulation syndrome (OHSS) are an elevated risk of thromboembolism owing to enhanced production of von Willebrand factor (vWF) by endothelial cells and ascites, or pulmonary edema owing to increased vascular permeability followed by third-space fluid accumulation. The vWF glycoprotein is produced and released predominantly by vascular endothelial cells *(83)* and this can be enhanced by VEGF *(84)*. High concentrations of VEGF are found in ascites from OHSS patients *(85)*. VEGF is also overexpressed in the hyperthecotic ovarian stroma of Stein-Leventhal syndrome/polycystic ovary *(72)*.

CYCLIC ANGIOGENESIS OF ENDOMETRIUM

In concert with the cyclic changes of the ovarian function, the secretory activity and structure of endometrium and its blood vessel system also undergo cyclic changes. The rapid growth of the endometrium in preparation for blastocyst implantation requires dynamic tissue remodeling, which involves a variety of growth modulators, cytokines, prostanoids, and enzymes participating in the synchronous development of a receptive endometrium. The arteries that supply the stratum basale of the endometrium maintain the integrity of the basal layer through all phases of the cycle and appear to be unaffected by hormonal stimuli. In humans, endometrial microvascular density does not alter during the cycle *(86,87)*. However, the spiral arteries, which supply the stratum functionale, are extremely sensitive to the endocrine environment and undergo fluctuations in gross morphology and length under the influence of ovarian steroids. Specifically, after the partial destruction of the endometrium at the end of each cycle, the distal portion of the spiral arteries undergoes regeneration. The lengthening and coiling of arteries begin during the proliferative phase of the endometrium and continues during the secretory phase *(88)*, which lead to the development of a complex subepithelial capillary plexus.

VEGF IN THE ENDOMETRIUM

The initial stimulus for neovascularization is likely to be steroidal which may induce the expression of secreted angiogenic factors, which in turn, initiate a cascade of downstream responses that lead to the growth of new capillaries. Significant angiogenic activity has been demonstrated in the whole human endometrium, endometrial gland, and endometrial stromal-cell preparations in all phases of the cycle except for the late secretory phase. This suggests that human endometrium produces local angiogenic factors throughout the menstrual cycle and that these factors may decrease towards the end of the cycle *(89)*. aFGF and bFGF stimulate vascular endothelial-cell growth in vitro and angiogenesis in vivo *(90,91)* and are present in human endometrium. However, these angiogenic factors are unlikely to be principal regulators of cyclic endometrial neovascularization, as their expression does not change throughout the menstrual cycle and actually increases in atrophic menopausal endometrium *(92,93)*.

Recent studies show that VEGF may be a paracrine mediator of the effects of sex steroids on endometrial angiogenesis. Four species of mRNA encoding VEGFs (VEGF$_{121}$, VEGF$_{145}$,

VEGF$_{165}$, and VEGF$_{189}$) have been identified in human endometrium throughout the menstrual cycle *(39)*. VEGF is expressed by both stromal and epithelial glandular cells during the proliferative phase of the cycle, with greatly increased expression in the glands of the secretory endometrium. However, the highest expression level is in endometrial glands during menstruation, which may result from ischaemia that precedes menstruation owing to vaso-constriction of spiral arterioles, suggesting that VEGF is involved in angiogenesis following menstruation in the normal cycle. Indeed, endometrial adenocarcinoma cells cultured under hypoxic conditions are able to upregulate VEGF protein and RNA levels (unpublished date). These authors also found that treatment with estradiol could increase the steady-state level of VEGF mRNA in cultured adenocarcinomal cells (HEC-1A) *(39)*.

In the mouse, VEGF expression in the endometrium also shows a cycle-dependent pattern. At the early stage of estrous cycle, VEGF is found to be expressed in the estrogen-responsive, secretory columnar epithelium, lining both the oviducts and the uterus. However, under the influence of progesterone, the site of VEGF expression shifts to cells of the underlying stroma composing the functional endometrium, which may serve as a source of angiogenic activity that supports the extension of stromal vessels. Transcripts encoding VEGF are also detected in the uterus of the rat and the dominant forms are VEGF$_{164}$ and VEGF$_{120}$. Estrogen can rapidly induce an increase of the level of VEGF mRNAs, especially the two smaller transcripts, encoding VEGF$_{120}$ and VEGF$_{164}$. This does not require new protein synthesis, suggesting that VEGF is a primary reponse gene *(94,95)*. Therefore VEGF may mediate the estrogen-induced increase of microvascular permeability and proliferation of microvascular endothelial cells. The antiestrogens, tamoxifen, 4-OH tamoxifen, and nafoxidine can also elevate uterine VEGF mRNA expression, which can be inhibited by actinomycin D but not by puromycin, again suggesting direct transcriptional regulation of VEGF expression by antiestrogens *(96)*. Proges-terone was found to lead to an increase in levels of mRNAs encoding VEGF$_{164}$ and VEGF$_{120}$, but not that of VEGF$_{188}$ *(94)*. Consistent with these in vivo results, the treatment of isolated human endometrial stromal cells with estradiol (E2), medroxyprogesterone acetate (MPA), or E2 plus MPA significantly increase VEGF mRNAs expression *(97)*. However, those authors did not report on the effects of steroids on endometrial epithelial cells. VEGF gene expression is also found to be enhanced by the addition of estradiol to human endometrial carcinoma cell lines *(39)*. It seems likely that the relationship between VEGF expression and oestradiol and progesterone treatment in the endometrium is complex. In addition to the effects of oestradiol already described it appears that long-term treatment of endometrial cells with gestagen results in upregulation of VEGF expression by the decidualising endometrial stromal cells (Charnock-Jones, et al., unpublished data).

VEGF may also be involved in the pathological angiogenesis involving endometrium. Elevated levels of VEGF are found in peritoneal fluid of women with endometriosis, which show cyclic variations, with the VEGF concentration in proliferative phase being significantly higher than that in the secretory phase *(98)*.

NEOVASCULARIZATION DURING PLACENTA FORMATION

The mammalian placenta is derived from embryonic tissue and the earliest events that lead to endothelial-cell differentiation and vessel formulation is termed "vasculogenesis." In this process, so-called hemangioblasts differentiate to form angioblasts and haematopoietic precursors. VEGF is implicated in the process because embryos deficient in the VEGF receptor flk have defects in both cell lineages *(32)*. VEGF is also important for the formulation of intact patent vessels. This has been shown by studies of mice lacking the other VEGF receptor flt-1 *(33)*. Furthermore the critical role of VEGF in embryonic (and placental) vasculogenesis and angiogenesis is shown by "knock-out" studies in which mice lacking even a single VEGF die *in utero*.

Implantation and growth of the placenta requires extensive angiogenesis in the maternal decidua and neovascularization in the fetal villi to establish an anastomosing network of neovasculatures involved in the maternal-fetal exchange *(99)*. In humans the starting point is the attachment of the blastocyst to the uterine wall, and the invasion of the decidua by trophoblast derived from embryonic trophectoderm. The trophectoderm cells of the conceptus adhere to the luminal epithelial cells of the endometrium and induct the changes in the underlying endometrial stromal tissue such as the increased vascular permeability, which is followed by localized decidualization of the stroma and apoptosis of the luminal epithelium at the sites of blastocyst implantation *(100)*, facilitating invasion of trophoblast cells through the underlying basement membrane *(101)*. These processes are accompanied by remodeling of the extracellular matrix, widespread vascular expansion and reorganization in the stromal bed. The invasive extravillous trophoblast can modify the maternal spiral arteries leading to their transformation into high-flow, low-resistance vessels *(102)*, which supply the maternal contribution of the placenta. Simultaneously the growing conceptus develops its own blood vascular system and one or more highly vascularized regions of its extra-embryonic surface that interchanges materials with the corresponding specialized and vascularized areas in the maternal endometrial tissues. This zone of adjacent and highly vascularized contact between mother and conceptus is called the placenta, in which the two discrete circulations lie suffi-ciently close that rapid and efficient transfer of materials can occur between them. The establishment of a vascular network is crucial to the development of the placenta, which is tightly regulated to allow for the steady increase in fetoplacental blood flow necessary to sustain the growing fetus *(103)*.

The presence of angiogenic activity within the placenta has long been recognized *(104)*. The complex interactions that occur between the trophoblast and the maternal vessels in establishing the blood supply of the placenta may require the full range of angiogenic growth factors present in endometrium and trophoblast. However, rapid growth and vascularization of placenta are accomplished in an hypoxic environment. So hypoxia-induced angiogenesis may be of particular importance during placental growth, as suggested by Wheeler et al. *(105)*.

When the implantation process is initiated, there is an increased uterine vascular permeability at the sites of blastocyst apposition. In the mouse, this increased vascular permeability and attachment reactions first occur in the evening of day 4 of pregnancy *(106)*. Expression VEGF and its receptors have been shown to be temporally and spatially regulated in the mouse uterus around the time of implantation, suggesting that VEGF may participate in this increased vascular permeability and the angiogenesis that occurs in the uterine vascular bed during implantation *(107)*. VEGF receptors (flt-1 and flk-1) also show differential expression in the mouse developing placenta. flt-1 mRNA is detected in the spongiotrophoblast layer. This cellular compartment is located between the maternal and labyrinthine layers of the placenta, which both express VEGF. Flk-1 transcripts are present in endothelial cells within the labyrinthine layer *(108,109)*.

In human placenta, four species of mRNA encoding VEGF ($VEGF_{121}$, $VEGF_{145}$, $VEGF_{165}$, $VEGF_{189}$) are found to be expressed by villous trophoblast, fetal macrophages (Hofbauer cells) within the villi, glandular epithelium, and maternal macrophages in the decidua in first trimester. The strongest site of expression is in maternal macrophages adjacent to Nitabuch's stria, a zone of necrosis at the site of implantation (59). VEGF is highly expressed by cytotrophoblast cells during the first trimester (110). The production of VEGF by trophoblast cells in early pregnancy may be indicative of the trophoblast playing an active role in influencing the development of the villous vascular network. During the late pregnancy, VEGF mRNA and protein are localized to the syncytiotrophoblast (110), extravillous trophoblast, and Hofbauer cells (111,112), and also in extracellular matrix within the villous core (110,112).

As already stated, the principle target cell for VEGF is the endothelial cell, although there is increasing evidence of direct actions upon macrophages and monocytes (60). However, a striking observation made in the human placenta was that the trophoblast cells contain very large amounts of mRNA including one of the VEGF receptors (59,113). These authors suggested that locally produced VEGF could have direct actions upon trophoblast lineage in the placenta and indeed mild stimulation of proliferation was observed when BeWo cells, a trophoblast-like choriocarcinoma cell line was treated with VEGF. More recent work by these authors, however, has shown that the mRNA originally detected by the in situ hybridization experiments described earlier encodes for a soluble form of flt-1. Using a combination of ligand binding, crosslinking and affinity chromatography it has been shown that the trophoblast secretes large amounts of soluble VEGF receptor. In fact, this activity is readily in maternal circulation during pregnancy. Thus in addition to the VEGF produced locally the placenta also secretes a potent antagonist to VEGF. This is therefore another example of the fine control of blood-vessel growth being achieved by the balance of positive and negative regulatory factors (60,61).

Angiogenesis occurs as a cyclically regulated process in the ovary and the uterus, which is critical for the follicle development and ovulation, the formation of corpus luteum, and the preparation of uterus for the conceptus. Angiogenesis is also of paramount importance in the well-orchestrated sequence of events surrounding implantation and placentation. Recent data demonstrate that VEGF is an important mediator in this process. Further research into potentiation and inhibition of its role in the angiogenesis will provide novel ways to control reproduction and also for developing efficient therapies for some reproductive diseases that have an intimate relation with angiogenesis. Neutralizing antibody against VEGF and manipulation of the VEGF receptors have been used to control angiogenesis and have yielded promising results in model systems and further developments in this field may lead to new therapeutic strategies.

REFERENCES

1. Folkman, J. (1995) Angiogenesis in cancer, vascular, rheumatoid and other disease. Nature Med. 1, 27–31.
2. Schor, A. M. and Schor, S. L. (1983) Tumor angiogenesis. J. Pathol. 141, 385–413.
3. Folkman, J. (1985) Tumor angiogenesis. Adv. Cancer Res. 43, 175–203.
4. Gordon, J. D., Shifren, J. L., Foulk, R. A., Taylor, R. N., and Jaffe, R. B. (1995) Angiogenesis in the human female reproductive tract. Obstet. Gynaecol. Survey 50, 688–697.
5. Mustonen, T. and Alitalo, K. (1995) Endothelial receptor tyrosine kinases involved in angiogenesis. J. Cell Biol. 129, 895–898.
6. Nelson, K. G., Takahashi, T., Bossert, N. L., Walmer, D. K., and McLachlan, J. A. (1991) Epidermal growth factor replaces estrogen in the stimulation of female genital-tract growth and differentiation. Proc. Natl. Acad. Sci. USA 88, 21–25.
7. Schreiber, A. B., Winkler, M. E., Derynck, R. (1986) Transforming growth factor-alpha: a more potent angiogenic mediator than epidermal growth factor. Science 232, 1250–1253.

8. Roberts, A. B., Sporn, M. B., Assoian, R. K., et al. (1986) Transforming growth factor type beta: rapid induction of fibrosis and angiogenesis in vivo and stimulation of collagen formation in vitro. *Proc. Natl. Acad. Sci. USA* **83,** 4167–4171.

9. Pepper, M. S., Vassalli, J. D., Orci, L., et al. (1993) Biphasic effect of transforming growth factor-beta 1 on in vitro angiogenesis. *Exp. Cell Res.* **204,** 356–363.

10. Leibovich, S. J., Polverini, P. J., Shepard, H. M., et al. (1987) Macrophage-induced angiogenesis is mediated by tumor necrosis factor-alpha. *Nature* **329,** 630–632.

11. Fett, J. W., Strydom, D. J., Lobb, R. R., et al. (1985) Isolation and characterization of angiogenin, an angiogenic protein from human carcinoma cells. *Biochemistry* **24,** 5480–5486.

12. Esch, F., Ueno, N., Baird, A., et al. (1985) Primary structure of bovine brain acidic fibroblast growth factor (FGF). *Biochem. Biophys. Res. Commun.* **133,** 554–562.

13. Montesano, R., Vassalli, J. D., Baird, A., et al. (1986) Basic fibroblast growth factor induces angiogenesis in vitro. *Proc. Natl. Acad. Sci. USA* **83,** 7297–7301.

14. Ferrara, N. and Henzel, W. J. (1989) Pituitary follicular cells secrete a novel heparin-binding growth factor specific for vascular endothelial cells. *Biochem. Biophys. Res. Commun.* **161,** 851–858.

15. Folkman, J. and Klagsbrun, M. (1987) Angiogenic factors. *Science* (Wash.) **235,** 442–445.

16. Folkman, J. and Shing, Y. (1992) Angiogenesis. *J. Biol. Chim.* **267,** 10,931–10,934.

17. Klagsbrun, M. and D'Amore, P. A. (1991) Regulators of angiogendsis. *Annu. Rev. Physiol.* **53,** 217–239.

18. Good, D. J., Polverini, P. J., Rastinejad, F., et al. (1990) A tumor suppressor-dependent inhibitor of angiogenesis is immunologically and functionally indistinguishable from a fragment of thrombospondin. *Proc. Natl. Acad. Sci. USA* **87,** 6624–6628.

19. Maione, T. E., Gray, G. S., Petro, J., et al. (1990) Inbibition of angiogenesis by recombinant human platelet factor-4 and related peptides. *Science* **247,** 77–79.

20. Frater, S. M., Risau, W., Hallmann, R., et al. (1987) Tumor necrosis factor type alpha, a potent inhibitor of endothelial cell growth in vitro, is angiogenic in vivo. *Proc. Natl. Acad. Sci. USA* **84,** 5277–5281.

21. Tsuruoka, N., Sugiyama, M., Tawaragi, Y., et al. (1988) Inhibition of in vitro angiogenesis by lymphotoxin and interferon-gamma. *Biochem. Biophys. Res. Commun.* **155,** 429–435.

22. O'Reilly, M. S., Holmgren, L., Shing, Y., et al. (1994) Angiostatin: a novel angiogenesis inhibitor that mediates the suppression of metastases by a Lewis lung carcinoma. *Cell* **79,** 315–328.

23. Brooks, P. C., Montgomery, A. M., Rosenfeld, M., et al. (1994) Integrin alpha versus beta 3 antagonists promote tumor regression by inducing apoptosis of angiogenic blood vessels. *Cell* **79,** 1157–1164.

24. Ferrara, N., Clapp, C., and Weiner, R. (1991) The 16K fragment of prolactin specifically inhibits basal or fibroblast growth factor-stimulated growth of capillary endothelial cells. *Endocrinology* **129,** 896–900.

25. Clapp, C., Martial, J. A., Guzman, R. C., et al. (1993) The 16-kilodalton N-terminal fragment of human prolactin is a potent inhibitor of angiogenesis. *Endocrinology* **133,** 1292–1299.

26. Klauber, N., Rohan, R. M., Flynn, P., and D'Amato, R. J. (1997) Critical components of the female reproductive tract are suppressed by the angiogenesis inhibitor AGM-1470. *Nature Med.* **4,** 443–446.

27. Jakeman, L. B., Winer, J., Bennett, G. L., et al. (1992) Binding sites for vascular endothelial growth factor are localized on endothelial cells in adult rat tissues. *J. Clin. Invest.* **89,** 244–253.

28. Alon, T., Hemo, I., Itin, A., et. al. (1995) Vascular endothelial growth factor acts as a survival factor for newly formed retinal vessels and has implications for retinopathy of prematurity. *Nature Med.* **1,** 1024–1028.

29. Risau, W. (1997) Mechanisms of angiogenesis. *Nature* **386,** 671–674.

30. Carmeliet, P., et al. (1996) Abnormal blood vessel development and lethality in embryos lacking a single VEGF allele. *Nature* **380,** 435–439.

31. Ferrara, N., et al. (1996) Heterozygous embryonic lethality induced by targeted inactivation of the VEGF gene. *Nature* **380,** 439–442.

32. Shalaby, F., et al. (1995) Failure of blood-island formation and vasculogenesis in Flk-1-deficient mice. *Nature* **376,** 62–66.

33. Fong, G. H., Rossant, J., Gertsenstein, M., and Breitman, M. L. (1995) Role of the Flt-1 receptor tyrosine kinase in regulating the assembly of vascular endothelium. *Nature* **376,** 66–70.

34. Gospodarowicz, D., Abraham, J. A., and Schilling, J. (1989) Isolation and characterization of a vascular endothelial cell mitogen produced by pituitary-derived folliculostellate cells. *Proc. Natl. Acad. Sci. USA* **86,** 7311–7315.

35. Keck, P. J., Hauser, S. D., Krivi, G., et al. (1989) Vascular permeability factor, an endothelial cell mitogen related to PDGF. *Science* **246,** 1309–1312.

36. Leung, D., Cachianes, G., Kuang, W., et al. (1989) Vascular endothelial growth factor is a secreted angiogenic mitogen. *Science* **246,** 1306–1309.

37. Pepper, M., Ferrara, N., Orci, L., and Montesano, R. (1991) Vascular endothelial growth factor (VEGF) induces plasminogen activators and plasminogen activator inhibitor-1 in microvascular endothelial cells. *Biochem. Biophys. Res. Commun.* **181,** 902–906.

38. Unemori, E., Ferrara, N., Bauer, E., and Amento, E. (1992) Vascular endothelial growth factor induces interstitial collagenase expression in human endothelial cells. *J. Cell Physiol.* **153,** 557–562.

39. Charnock-Jones, D. S., et al. (1993) Identification and localization of alternately spliced mRNAs for vascular endothelial growth factor in human uterus and estrogen regulation in endometrial carcinoma cell lines. *Biol. Reprod.* **48,** 1120–1128.

40. Poltorak, Z., Cohen, T., Sivan, R., Kandelis, Y., Spira, G., Vlodavsky, I., et al. (1997) VEGF$_{145}$, a secreted vascular endothelial growth factor isoform that binds to extracellular matrix. *J. Biol. Chem. USA* **272,** 7151–7158.

41. Maglione, D., Guerriero, V., Viglietto, G., Ferraro, M. G., Aprelikova, O., Alitalo, K., et al. (1993) Two alternative mRNAs coding for the angiogenic factor, placenta growth factor (PlGF), are transcribed from a single gene of chromosome 14. *Oncogene* **8,** 925–931.

42. Olofsson, B., et al. (1996) Vascular endothelial growth factor B, a novel growth factor for endothelial cells. *Proc. Natl. Acad. Sci. USA* **93,** 2576–2581.

43. Joukov, V., Pajusola, K., Kaipainen, A., Chilov, D., Lahtinen, I., Kukk, E., et al. (1996) A novel vascular endothelial growth factor, VEGF-C, is a ligand for the Flt4 (VEGFR-3) and KDR (VEGFR-2) receptor tyrosine kinases. *EMBO J.* **15,** 290–298.

44. Yamada, Y., Nezu, J.-I., Shimane, M., and Hirata, Y. (1997) Molecular cloning of a novel vascular endothelial growth factor, VEGFD. *Genomics* **42,** 483–488.

45. Cao, Y., et al. (1996) Heterodimers of placenta growth factor/vascular endothelial growth factor: endothelial activity, tumor cell expression, and high affinity binding to Flk-1/KDR. *J. Biol. Chem.* **271,** 3154–3162.

46. Shibuya, M., Yamaguchi, S., Yamane, A., Ikeda, T., Tojo, A., Matsushime, H., and Sato, M. (1990) Nucleotide sequence and expression of a novel human receptor type tyrosine kinase (flt) closely related to the fms family. *Oncogene* **5,** 519–524.

47. Peters, K. G., DeVries, C., and Williams, L. T. (1993) Vascular endothelial growth factor expression during embryogenesis and tissue repair suggests a role in endothelial differentiation and blood vessel growth. *Proc. Natl. Acad. Sci. USA* **90,** 8915–8919.

48. Matthews, W., Jordan, C. T., Gavin, M., Jenkins, N. A., Copeland, N. G., and Lemischka, I. R. (1991) A receptor tyrosine kinase cDNA isolated from a population of enriched primitive hemopoietic cells and exhibiting close genetic linkage to c-kit. *Proc. Natl. Acad. Sci. USA* **88,** 9026–9030.

49. Terman, B. I., Carrion, M. E., Kovacs, E., Rasmussen, B. A., Eddy, R. L., and Shows, T. B. (1991) Identification of a new endothelial cell growth factor receptor tyrosine kinase. *Oncogene* **6,** 1677–1683.

50. de Vries, C., Escobedo, J. A., Ueno, H., Houck, K., Ferrara, N., and Williams, L. T. (1992) The fms-like tyrosine kinase, a receptor for vascular endothelial growth factor. *Science* **255,** 989–991.

51. Davis-Smyth, T., et al. (1996) The second immunoglobulin-like domain of the VEGF tyrosine kinase receptor Flt-1 determines ligand binding and may initiate a signal transduction cascade. *EMBO J.* **15,** 4919–4927.

52. Barleon, B., Totzke, F., Herzog, C., Blanke, S., Kremmer, E., Siemeister, G., et al. (1997) *J. Biol. Chem. USA* 10,382–10,388.

53. Terman, B. I., et al. (1992) Identifivation of the KDR tyrosine kinase as a receptor for vascular endothelial growth factor. *Biochem. Biophys. Res. Commun.* **34,** 1578–1586.

54. Millauer, B., Wizigmann-Voos, S., Schnurch, H., Martinez, R., Moller, N. P. H., Risau, W., and Ullrich, A. (1993) High affinity VEGF binding and developmental expression suggest Flk-1 as a major regulator of vasculogenesis and angiogenesis. *Cell* **72,** 835–846.

55. Connolly, D. T., Heuvelman, D. M., Nelson, R., et al. (1989) Tumor vascular permeability factor stimulates endothelial cell growth and angiogenesis. *J. Clin. Invest.* **84,** 1470–1478.

56. Quinn, T. P., Peters, K. G., DeVris, D., Ferrara, N., and Williams, L. T. (1993) Fetal liver kinase 1 is a receptor for vascular endothelial growth factor and is selectively expressed in vascular endothelium. *Proc. Natl. Acad. Sci. USA* **90,** 7533–7537.

57. Shen, H., Clauss, M., et al. (1993) Characterisation of vascular permeability factor/vascular endothelial growth factor receptors on mononuclear phagocytes. *Blood* **10,** 2767–2773.

58. Gitay-Goren, H., Halaban, R., and Neufeld, G. (1993) Human melanoma cells but not normal melanocytes express vascular endothelial growth factor receptors. *Biochem. Biophys. Res. Commun.* **190,** 702–708.

59. Charnock-Jones, D. S., et al. (1994) Vascular endothelial growth factor receptor localisation and activation in human trophoblast and choriocarcinoma cells. *Biol. Reprod.* **51,** 524–530.

60. Kendall, R. L. and Thomas, K. A. (1993) Inhibition of vascular endothelial cell growth factor activity by an endogenously encoded soluble receptor. *Proc. Natl. Acad. Sci. USA* **90,** 10,705–10,709.

61. Boocock, C. A., Charnock-Jones, D. S., Sharkey, A. M., McLaren, J., Baker, P. J., Wright, K. A., et al. (1995) Expression of vascular endothelial growth factor and its receptors flt and KDR in ovarian carcinoma. *J. Natl. Cancer Inst.* **87,** 506–516.

62. Clark, D. E., Smith, S. K., He, Y., Day, K. A., Licence, D. R., Corps, A. C., et al. (1998) A vascular endothelial growth factor antagonist is produced by the human placenta and released into the maternal circulation. *Biol. Reprod.* **59,** 1540–1548.

63. He, Y., Smith, S. K., Day, K. A., Clark, D. E., Licence, D. R., and Charnock-Jones, D. S. (1999) Alternative splicing of vascular endothelial growth factor (VEGF) - R1 (FLT-1) pre-mRNA is important for the regulation of VEGF activity. *Mol. Endocrinol.* **13,** 537–545.

64. Findlay, J. K. (1986) Angiogenesis in reproductive tissue. *J. Endocrinol.* **111,** 357–366.

65. Bassett, D. L. (1943) The changes in the vascular pattern of the ovary of the albino rat during the estrous cycle. *Am. J. Anat.* **73,** 251–291.

66. Miyamoto, Y., Nakayama, T., Haraguchi, S., Miyamoto, H., and Sato, E. (1996) Morphological evaluation of microvascular networks and angiogenic factors in the selective growth of oocytes and follicles in the ovaries of mouse fetuses and newborns. *Dev. Growth Differ.* **38,** 291–298.

67. Zeleznik, A. J., Schuler, H. M., Reichert, Jr., L. E. (1981) Gonadotropin-binding sites in the rhesus monkey ovary, role of the vasculature in the selective distribution of human chorionic gonadotropin to the preovulatory follicle. *Endocrinology* **109,** 356–362.

68. Meyer, G. T. and McGeachie, J. K. (1988) Angiogenesis in the developing corpus luteum of pregnant rats, A stereologic and autoradiographic study. *Anatom. Record* **222,** 18–25.

69. Carr, B. R., MacDonald, P. C., and Simpson, E. R. (1982) The role of lipoproteins in the regulation of progesterone secretion by the corpus luteum. *Fertil. Steril.* **38,** 303–311.

70. Shweiki, D., Itin, A., Neufeld, G., Gitay-Goren, H., and Keshet, E. (1993) Patterns of expression of vascular endothelial growth factor (VEGF) and VEGF receptors in mice suggest a role in hormonally regulated angiogenesis. *J. Clin. Invest.* **91,** 2235–2243.

71. Gordon, J. D., Mesiano, S., Zaloudek, C. J., and Jaffe, R. B. (1996) Vascular endothelial growth factor localization in human ovary and fallopian tubes, possible role in reproductive function and ovarian cyst formation. *J. Clin. Endocrinol. Metab.* **81,** 353–359.

72. Kamat, B. R., Brown, L. F., Manseau, E. J., et al. (1995) Expression of vascular permeability factor/vascular endothelial growth factor by human granulosa and theca lutein cells.Role in corpus luteum development. *Am. J. Pathol.* **146,** 157–165.

73. Ravindranath, N., Little-Ihrig, L., Phillips, H. S., Ferrara, N., and Zeleznik, A. J. (1992) Vascular endothelial growth factor messenger ribonucleic acid expression in the primate ovary. *Endocrinology* **131,** 254–260.

74. Koos, R. D. and Olson, C. E. (1991) Hypoxia stimulates expression of the gene for vascular endothelial growth factor (VEGF), a putative angiogenic factor,by granulosa cells of the ovarian follicle,a site of angiogenesis. *J. Cell Biol.* **115,** 421a (Abstract).

75. Dissen, G. A., Lara, H. E., Fahrenbach, W. H., Costa, M. E., and Ojeda, S. R. (1994) Immature rat ovaries become revascularized rapidly after autotransplantation and show a gonadotropin-dependent increase in angiogenic factor gene expression. *Endocrinology* **134,** 1146–1154.

76. Olson, T. A., Mohanraj, D., and Ramakrishnan, S. (1995) The selective inhibition of vascular permeability factor (VPF) expression in voarian carcinoma cell lines by a gonadotropin-releasing hormone (GnRH) agonist. *Intl. J. Oncol.* **6,** 905–910.

77. Ellinwood, W. E., Nett, T. N., Niswender, G. D., and Jones, R. E. (1978) Ovarian vasculature: structure and function, in *The Vertebrate Ovary,* (Jones, R. E., ed.), Blenheim, New York, pp. 583–614.

78. Phillips, H. S., Hains, J., Leung, D. W., and Ferrara, N. (1990) Vascular endothelial growth factor is expressed in rat corpus luteum. *Endocrinology* **127,** 965–967.

79. Doraiswamy, V., Moor, R. M., Dai, Y., Reynolds, L. P., and Redmer, D. A. (1997) Immunohistochemical localization of vascular endothelial growth factor (VEGF) in the ovine ovary during the periovulatory period. *Biol. Reprod.* **56(Suppl. 1),** 161.

79. Garrido, C., Saule, S., and Gospodarowicz, D. (1993) Transcriptional regulation of vascular endothelial growth factor gene expression in ovarian bovine granulosa cells. *Growth Factors* **8,** 109–117.

80. Yan, Z., Weich, H. A., Bernart, W., Breckwoldt, M., and Neulen, J. (1993) Vascular endothelial growth factor (VEGF) messenger ribonucleic acid (mRNA) expression in luteinized human granulosa cells in vitro. *J. Clin. Endocrinol. Metab.* **77,** 1723–1725.

81. Ferrara, N., Chen, H., Davis-Smith, T., Gerber, H. P., Nguyen, T. N., Peers, D., et al. (1998) Vascular endothelial growth factor is essential for corpus luteum angiogenesis. *Nature Med.* **4,** 336–340.

82. Doraiswamy, V., Grazul-Bilska, A. T., Ricke, W. A., Redmer, D. A., and Reynolds, L. P. (1995) Immunoneutralization of angiogenic activity from ovine corpora lutea with antibodies against fibroblast growth factor and vascular endothelial growth factor. *Biol. Reprod.* **52(Suppl. 1),** 112.

83. Handin, R. I. and Wagner, D. D. (1989) Molecular and cellular biology of von Willebrand factor, in *Progress in Hemostasis and Thrombosis,* vol. 9. (Coller, B. S., ed.). Saunders, Philadelphia, pp. 233–259.

84. Brock, T. A., Dvorak, H. F., and Senger, D. R. (1991) Tumor secreted vascular permeability factor increases cytosolic Ca2+ and von Willebrand factor release in human endothelial cells. *Am. J. Pathol.* **138,** 213–221.

85. McClure, N., Healy, D. L., Rogers, P. A. W., et al. (1994a) Vascular endothelial growth factor as capillary permeability agent in ovarian hyperstimulation syndrome. *Lancet* **344,** 255–236.

86. Hourihan, H. M., Sheppard, B. L., and Brosens, I. A. (1990) Endometrial haemostasis, in *Proceedings of Symposium on Contraception and Mechanisms of Endometrial Bleeding.* (D' Arcangues, C. D., Fraser, I. S., Newton, J. R., and Odlind, V., eds.), Cambridge University Press, Cambridge, UK, pp. 95–116.

87. Rogers, P. A. W., Au, C. L., and Affandi, B. (1993) Endometrial microvascular density during the normal menstrual cycle and following exposure to long-term levonorgestrel. *Hum. Reprod.* **8,** 1396–1404.

88. Christianes, G. C. M. L., Sixma, J. J., and Haspels, A. A. (1982) Hemostasis in menstrual endometrium, a review. *Obstet. Gynecol. Survey* **37,** 281–303.

89. Peek, M. J., Markham, R., and Fraser, I. S. (1995) Angiogenic activity in normal and dysfunctional uterinebleeding human endometrium; as measured by the chick chorioallantoic membrane assay. *Exp. Toxicol. Pathol.* **47,** 397–402.

90. Gospodarowicz, D., Ferrara, N., Schweigerer, L., and Neufeld, G. (1987) Structural characterization and biological functions of fibroblast growth factor. *Endocr. Rev.* **8,** 95–114.

91. Frederick, J., Shimanuke, T., and Di Zerega, G. (1984) Initiation of angiogenesis by human follicular fluid. *Science* **224,** 389–390.

92. Rusnati, M., Casarotti, G., Pecorelli, S., Ragnotti, G., and Presta, M. (1990) Basic fibroblast growth factor in ovulatory cycle and postmenopausal human endometrium. *Growth Factors* **3,** 299–307.

93. Ferriani, R., Charnock-Jones, D., Prentice, A., Thomas, E., and Smith, S. (1993) Immunohistochemical localization of acidic and basic fibroblast growth factors in normal human endometrium and endometriosis and the detection of their mRNA by polymerase chain reaction. *Human Reprod.* **8,** 11–16.

94. Cullinan-Bove, K. and Koos, R. D. (1993) Vascular endothelial growth factor/vascular permeability factor expression in the rat uterus, rapid stimulation by estrogen correlates with estrogen-induced increases in uterine capillary permeability and growth. *Endocrinology* **133,** 829–837.

95. Hyder, S. M., Stancel, G. M., Chiappetta, C., Murthy, L., Boettger-Tong, H. L., and Makela, S. (1996) Uterine expression of vascular endothelial growth factor is increased by estradiol and tamoxifen. *Cancer Res. USA* **56(17),** 3954–3960.

96. Salman, M., et al. (1996) Uterine expression of vascular endothelail growth factor is increased by estradiol and tamoxifen. *Cancer Res.* **56,** 3954–3960.

97. Shifren, J. L., et al. (1996) Ovarian steroid regulation of vascular endothelial growth factor in the human endometrium, Implications for angiogenesis during the menstrual cycle and in the pathogenesis of endometriosis. *J. Clin. Endocrinol. Metab.* **81,** 3112–3118.

98. McLaren, J., Prentice, A., Charnock-Jones, D. S., and Smith, S. K. (1996a) Vascular endothelial growth factor (VEGF) concentrations are elevated in peritoneal fluid of women with endometriosis. *Human Reprod.* **11,** 220–223.

99. King, B. F. (1987) Ultrastructural differentiation of stromal and vascular components in early macaque placental villi. *Am. J. Anat.* **136,** 190–203.

100. Parr, E. L., Tung, H. N., and Parr, M. B. (1987) Apoptosis as the mode of uterine epithelial cell death during embryo implantation in mice and rats. *Biol. Reprod.* **36,** 211–225.

101. Schlafke, S. and Enders, A. (1975) Cellular basis of interaction between trophoblast and uterus at implantation. *Biol. Reprod.* **12,** 41–65.

102. Benirschke, K. and Kaufmann, P. (1995) *Pathology of the Human Placenta.* Springer Verlag, London.

103. Kaufmann, P. and Scheffen, I. (1992) Placental development, in *Maternal-Fetal Physiology.* (Polin, R. A., Fox, W. W., eds.), WB Saunders, Philadelphia, pp. 47–55.

104. Eldad, A., Stark, M., Anais, D., et al. (1977) Amniotic membranes as a biological dressing. *S. Afr. Med. J.* **51,** 272–275.

105. Wheeler, T., Elcock, C. L., and Anthony, F. W. (1995) Angiogenesis and the placental environment. *Placenta* **16,** 289–296.

106. Das, S. K., Wang, X. N., Paria, B. C., Damm, D., Abraham, J. A., Klagsbrun, M., et al. (1994) Heparin-binding EGF-like growth factor gene is induced in the mouse uterus temporally by the blastocyst solely at the site of its apposition, a possible ligand for interaction with blastocyst EGF-receptor in implantation. *Development* **120,** 1071–1083.

107. Chakraborty, I., Das, S. K., and Dey, S. K. (1995) Differential expression of vascular endothelial growth factor and its receptor mRNAs in the mouse uterus around the time of implantation. *J. Endocrinol.* **147,** 339–352.

108. Breier, G., Clauss, M., and Risau, W. (1995) Coordinate expression of vascular endothelial growth factor receptor-1 (flt-1) and its ligand suggests a paracrine regulation of murine vascular development. *Dev. Dynamics* **204,** 228–239.

109. Dumont, D. J., Fong, G. H., Puri, M. C., Gradwohl, G., Alitalo, K., and Breitman, M. L. (1995) Vascularization of the mouse embryo: a study of flk-1, tek, tie, and vascular endothelial growth factor expression during development. *Dev. Dynamics* **203,** 80–92.

110. Jackaon, M. R., Carney, E. W., Lye, S. J., and Knox Ritchie, J. W. (1994) Localization of two angiogenic growth factors (PDECGF and VEGF) in human placentae throughout gestation. *Placenta* **15,** 341–353.

111. Sharkey, A. M., Charnock-Jones, D. S., Boocock, C. A., Brown, K. D., and Smith, S. K. (1993) Expression of mRNA for vascular endothelial growth factor in human placenta. *J. Reprod. Fertility* **99,** 609–615.

112. Cooper, J. C., Sharkey, A. M., McLaren, J., Charnock-Jones, D. S., and Smith, S. K. (1995) Localization of vascular endothelial growth factor and its receptor, flt, in human placenta and decidua by immunohistochemistry. *J. Reprod. Fertility* **105,** 205–213.

113. Clark, D. E., Smith, S. K., Sharkey, A. M., and Charnock-Jones, D. S. (1996) Localization of VEGF and expression of its receptors flt and KDR in human placenta throughout pregnancy. *Human Reprod.* **11,** 1090–1098.

9

Rheumatoid Arthritis

A Target For Anti-Angiogenic Therapy?

Ewa M. Paleolog and Jadwiga M. Miotla

Contents

INTRODUCTION

Rheumatic diseases are musculoskeletal and connective tissue disorders exhibiting chronicity, variability, and periods of exacerbation and remission. One of the best characterized rheumatic disorders is rheumatoid arthritis (RA), a systemic autoimmune disease of the joints affecting about 1% of the adult population in a female to male ratio of approx 3:1 *(1)*. RA is characterized by symmetric and erosive joint inflammation, which results in progressive joint destruction, deformity, disability, and premature death. Clinical involvement presents as pain, swelling, stiffness, and motion impairment. Any joint can be involved, but the preferential sites are the proximal interphalangeal and metacarpophalangeal joints of the hand and the wrist, as well as the metatarsophalangeal joint of the foot, the knee, and the joints of the shoulder, the ankle, and the hip. Systemic involvement may result in metabolic bone disorders such as osteoporosis, Sjogren's syndrome, and pleuro-pulmonary abnormalities. Soft tissue (subcutaneous nodules), muscles (weakness and atrophy), and blood vessels (vasculitis) may also be involved. The involvement in RA of at least four joints has resulted in the classification of RA as an "inflammatory polyarthritis" *(2)*. In this respect, RA appears to differ from other degenerative joint diseases such as osteoarthritis (OA), which, at least in the early stages, is generally associated with pathological changes at the large, weight-bearing joints of the lower extremities (hips and knees, i.e., four joints) and the absence of an inflammatory component.

From: *The New Angiotherapy*
Edited by: T.-P. D. Fan and E. C. Kohn © Humana Press Inc., Totowa, NJ

It is unclear whether RA should be considered as a single disease of unique etiology, or as a syndrome with a range of etiological factors, which initiate pathogenic mechanisms culminating in a similar spectrum of features. At present, it is thought that development of RA is triggered by environmental and infectious influences, leading to a systemic inflammatory response that predominantly targets the joints. Genetic associations have been identified, particularly with the major histocompatibility complex class II antigens. Furthermore, twin studies have shown a 30–50% concordance rate for monozygotic twins *(3)*. Approximately 70–80% of patients with RA have rheumatoid factor present in the blood, although its role remains unclear.

A feature of RA is an alteration in the density of sublining capillaries and postcapillary venules in the inflamed synovium, associated with marked new blood-vessel formation *(4)*. Synovial fluids from patients with RA and OA contain a low molecular-weight angiogenesis factor apparently identical with that derived from tumors, and cause morphological changes in human endothelial-cell cultures, including the formation of tubular networks resembling capillaries *(5)*. The number of blood vessels in the synovium has been found to correlate with other features of RA, namely synovial-cell hyperplasia, mononuclear-cell infiltration, and indices of joint tenderness *(6)*. The formation of new blood vessels in RA is thought to be important in the pathogenesis of RA, in that it may play a role in delivery of inflammatory cells and molecules to the arthritic lesion, leukocyte extravasation, and maintenance of the inflamed synovium *(7,8)*.

The development of the inflammatory and invasive synovium in RA can thus be viewed as the culmination of three interdependent processes, namely infiltration, inflammation, and neovascularization (Fig. 1). Current therapeutic strategies for the treatment of RA target these different processes that contribute to the development of the arthritic lesion. Some of these therapies (e.g., steroids) are in use in the clinic, whereas others (e.g., anti-cytokine and anti-adhesion molecule antibodies) have been used in clinical trials, with varying degrees of success. This chapter will focus on the mechanisms underlying the development of arthritis, with particular reference to the importance of new blood-vessel formation, and the presence of a pro-angiogenic phenotype in RA. We will also compare the different therapeutic strategies used to develop treatments for RA, and review the effects of these anti-arthritic therapies on new blood-vessel formation. Finally, we will address the possibility that angiotherapy may be beneficial in the treatment of RA.

MECHANISMS OF PATHOGENESIS OF ARTHRITIS
The Inflammatory Response

One of the characteristic features of RA is the inflammatory component of the disease *(9)*. Measurement of inflammation in RA consists of quantifying the classic symptoms of pain, swelling, heat, redness, and limitation of movement. Disease activity, as measured by acute episodes of pain, is associated with markers of the acute-phase response, including increased erythrocyte sedimentation rate (ESR) and acute-phase proteins such as serum amyloid A and C-reactive protein (CRP). For example, the mean serum concentration of CRP has been shown to correlate with disease activity and response to therapy, and with the rate of appearance of bony erosions in the early phase of RA *(10)*. To facilitate diagnosis of RA, the American College of Rheumatology identified a number of distinguishing criteria, which include pain or tenderness in at least one joint, radiographic changes of wrists and hands, and symmetrical joint swelling. Active RA is defined by the presence of six or more swollen joints plus at least three of four secondary criteria (duration of morning stiffness of at least 45 min, 6 or more tender or painful joints, ESR >28 mm/h, CRP >20 mg/L) *(11)*.

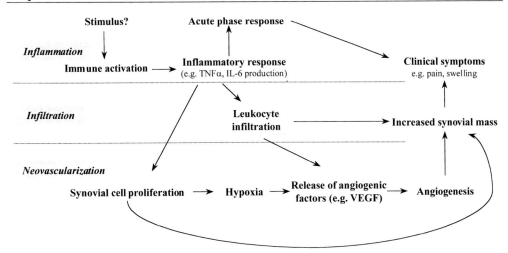

Fig. 1. The development of the destructive synovium in RA. The formation of RA pannus can be viewed as the culmination of three inter-dependent processes: infiltration, inflammation, and neovascularization.

The primary site of inflammation in RA is the synovium, which lines the closed spaces of the joints. The synovium is made up of proteoglycan matrix, within which are found macrophage- and fibroblast-like synovial cells, as well as a network of capillaries and lymphatics. Between the cartilage and synovium is the synovial fluid, which nourishes and lubricates the joint. The earliest abnormalities in RA consist of synovial cell proliferation and infiltration of the synovial membrane by cells recruited from the blood, predominantly activated memory CD4+ T cells and macrophages. The synovial fluid becomes rich in neutrophils, and increases in volume owing to edema, leading to joint swelling and pain. At later stages, the thickened and inflamed synovium (termed "pannus") extends across the cartilage surface, leading to destruction of cartilage and small bone erosions at the joint margin. Marginal and central erosions follow in advanced stages, and finally fibrous ankylosis, joint deformities, and fractures occur (1).

Regulation of the inflammatory and the immune responses in vivo is achieved by a family of endogenously produced pleiotropic proteins termed "cytokines" (Fig. 2). Many pro-inflammatory cytokines are expressed in RA, including molecules such as tumor necrosis factor-α (TNF-α) and interleukin (IL)-1 (12). The RA joint contains a wide variety of activated cell types, and this has lead to a number of studies involving enzymatically dissociated, unstimulated RA synovial membrane cell cultures. Research from our laboratory at the Kennedy Institute showed that, in the absence of any exogenous stimuli, cells isolated from RA synovial membranes spontaneously secrete both TNF-α and IL-1, as well as other pro-inflammatory cytokines such as IL-6, IL-8, and granulocyte-macrophage colony-stimulating factor (GM-CSF) (13–17). Immunohistochemical analyses have additionally revealed the presence in RA joints of a wide range of cytokines and growth factors, including chemokines, namely IL-8, RANTES, monocyte chemoattractant protein-1 (MCP-1), ENA-78, and Groα, as well as TNF-α (18). These cytokines can potentially play various roles in induction and perpetuation of the inflammatory state in RA. For example, IL-6 is a potent B-cell growth and differentiation factor, and induces acute-phase protein synthesis, whereas GM-CSF may activate synovial cells to express MHC

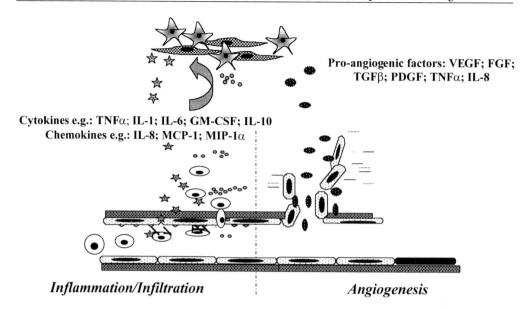

Pro-angiogenic factors: VEGF; FGF; TGFβ; PDGF; TNFα; IL-8

**Cytokines e.g.: TNFα; IL-1; IL-6; GM-CSF; IL-10
Chemokines e.g.: IL-8; MCP-1; MIP-1α**

Inflammation/Infiltration   *Angiogenesis*

Fig. 2. The role of growth factors, cytokines, and chemokines in the pathogenesis of RA. The RA synovium consists of macrophages, endothelial cells, fibroblasts, and T cells, all of which can contribute to infiltration, inflammation, and neovascularization, through the release of growth factors, cytokines, and chemokines, leading to a cascade of reactions that culminate in pannus formation.

class II. Other cytokines, such as TNF-α, IL-1, and members of the chemokine family might function to recruit leukocytes to the developing lesion, through the activation of leukocytes and/or induction of adhesion molecules on the vascular endothelium *(12)*.

Many of these cytokines are produced by cells of the monocyte/macrophage lineage, which form the predominant population (≥50%) of cells in the RA joint. The mechanisms involved in regulating monocyte/macrophage cytokine production are not fully understood, but are thought to involve both soluble factors and cell-cell contact. Production of TNF-α by monocytes has been shown to be induced by cytokine-activated fixed T cells, in the absence of T-cell receptor stimulation. Stimulation of monocyte TNF-α was markedly inhibited when T cells were physically separated from monocytes within the tissue culture well, confirming that T cell contact is necessary. Addition of interferon-γ (IFN-γ) or GM-CSF to the T cell-monocyte cultures enhanced T cell induction of monocyte TNF-α, suggesting that cytokine-stimulated T cells, interacting with macrophages in the RA synovial membrane, may contribute to the continuous excessive production of TNF-α observed in the RA joint *(19)*.

There is also evidence to indicate that homeostatic immunoregulatory mechanisms are present in the RA joint, and are in many cases upregulated (albeit insufficiently), in an attempt to oppose the inflammatory process. Cytokine inhibitors such as IL-1 receptor antagonist and soluble TNF-α receptors are markedly elevated in RA *(17)*, and immunomodulatory cytokines such as IL-10 and transforming growth factor-β (TGF-β) are both abundantly secreted by RA synovial cells. Addition of anti-IL-10 antibody to these cells significantly increased spontaneous release of TNF-α and IL-1. IL-10 also induces the release from cultured monocytes of soluble receptors for TNF-α, while downregulating surface expression, suggesting that IL-10 may act as an inhibitor of inflammation in RA *(20,21)*.

In summary, the balance in RA clearly favors the inflammatory state, in that the production of pro-inflammatory cytokines such as TNF-α appears to exceed the expression of immunomodulatory cytokines such as IL-10. This fosters many of the destructive immune and inflammatory processes in RA, in particular the ingress of leukocytes, which will be covered in greater detail in the subsequent section.

Leukocyte Infiltration as a Key Step in the Development of RA

The infiltration of the synovial membrane is one of the most profound changes that occur in RA. The infiltrating cells most probably play a role in the immune response seen in RA *(9)*. A number of cells can present antigens in RA, including macrophages, dendritic cells, B cells, and endothelial cells, which might explain the abundance in RA synovial membranes of CD4 cells, expressing activation markers such as CD45 RO, CD29, MHC class II, and IL-2 receptor (CD25). The relative proportion of T-cell subsets in joints compared to those in the peripheral blood indicates that specific T-cell populations actively enter the joint, through the selective expression of adhesion molecules. Cell adhesion must overcome the normal vascular mobility of the circulating cells and result in a localized arrest of leukocytes at relevant sites, a process that depends on a complex balance of pro- and anti-adhesive activities, expressed by endothelial cells as well as by other participating cells.

The vascular endothelial lining of blood vessels is one of the primary targets for the action of circulating and cell-bound cytokines, and as such acts as a focal point for the interplay and information exchange of cells and molecules during the development of the RA lesion. Endothelial cells have the capacity to respond to many cytokines expressed in RA, for example TNF-α and IL-1. In order to transmit a signal and hence exert an effect on endothelial cells, TNF-α must initially bind to specific high affinity cell surface receptors. We and others have shown expression of TNF-α receptors on human endothelial cells *(22)*. Using sections of RA synovial membranes, studies from our laboratory have also localized TNF-α and its receptors to endothelium *(14,23)*. Activation of endothelial cells by TNF-α and IL-1 increases the expression of several adhesion molecules for leukocytes *(24)*. Expression of E-selectin, which is now known to mediate the early phase of neutrophil binding, as well as binding eosinophils, basophils, monocytes, and certain subsets of T cells, has been documented in RA, predominantly on venules and capillaries *(25)*. In addition, RA synovial endothelial cells also express increased levels of vascular-cell adhesion molecule-1 (VCAM-1), as well as intercellular adhesion molecule (ICAM)-1 and -3. However, whereas E-selectin expression in RA synovial sections is endothelial cell-specific, staining for VCAM-1, ICAM-1, and ICAM-3 was also detectable on other cell types, including synovial tissue macrophages, fibroblasts, and some lymphocytes *(25–27)*. In terms of the counter-ligands for these molecules, the typical RA synovial infiltrate is rich in memory CD45RO+ T cells. Synovial membrane T cells display an enhanced capacity to interact with purified E-selectin and VCAM-1, relative to peripheral blood leukocytes from either the same patients or from healthy donors, owing to the presence on the T cells of increased levels of VLA-4α and relatively low levels of L-selectin *(28,29)*. RA synovial membrane T cells from patients express a high density of $\alpha_4\beta_7$, $\alpha_E\beta_7$ (a mucosal homing receptor), and VLA-1α, VLA-3α, VLA-5α, and VLA-6α, when compared to paired samples of peripheral blood leukocytes *(26)*. The RA synovium also exhibits features normally associated with peripheral lymphoid organs, including formation of high endothelial venules, which are probably important in mediating lymphocyte homing *(30)*. Taken together, these observations suggest that in RA the endothelium exists in an activated state, and that the accumulation of T cells in the RA lesion results from elevated expression of adhesion receptors on synovial microvascular endothelium. This leads to the selective emigration of monocytic cells and memory T lymphocytes, which may bear enhanced levels of ligands for these adhesion molecules as a result of a previous (and as yet unidentified) activation step. In addition, such cells may be retained at the inflammatory site because they also express raised levels of receptors that interact with other inflammatory cells (such as macrophages) and matrix proteins.

By their very ability to bind more than one leukocyte subset (for example cells that bind to E-selectin include neutrophils, monocytes, and T cells), adhesion molecules cannot themselves promote selective recruitment of leukocytes, such as the trafficking of memory T cells to arthritic joints. Additional intricate selectivity in terms of leukocyte recruitment is achieved by chemoattractant cytokines ("chemokines"), which target subsets of effector cells to specific tissue sites (Fig. 2). It may be hypothesized that as a leukocyte encounters different adhesion substrates such as endothelial cells, basement membrane, or extracellular matrix, the expression of chemokines by both the leukocyte and the substrate may be modulated to further regulate leukocyte recruitment. In RA, endothelial cells have been shown to express ENA-78, whereas RA synovial-fluid mononuclear cells produce RANTES, IL-8, Groα, MCP-1, MIP-1α, and MIP-1β, in contrast to peripheral blood mononuclear cells of RA patients and normal subjects (18,31–35). Chemokine receptors have also been shown to be differentially expressed on T-cell subsets, in that activated memory T cells express high levels of the CXCR3 and CCR5 receptors. The ligands for these receptors, IP-10 and Mig (CXCR3) and RANTES (CCR5) act predominantly on T cells of this phenotype, and it is interesting that immunostaining of T cells in RA synovial fluid demonstrated that virtually all T cells expressed CXCR3 and CCR5, representing a significant enrichment over levels of CXCR3[+] and CCR5[+] T cells in blood (36). This suggests that in Th1-type diseases such as RA, chemokine receptors CXCR3 and CCR5 identify subsets of T cells with a predilection for homing to the site of the arthritic lesion.

Thus, the combined action of adhesion molecules, chemokines, and cytokines ensures the efficient capture, activation, and retention in the developing lesion of T cells and monocytes, as well as proliferation of fibroblast-like synovial cells. These processes serve to promote the destruction of cartilage and bone through the production of degradative enzymes such as matrix metalloproteinases. However, the maintenance of the inflamed and infiltrated pannus requires supply of oxygen and nutrients, and it is in this context that formation of new blood vessels plays a particularly focal role in RA.

Angiogenesis in the Arthritic Lesion

Histological analyses have revealed that that the thickened and heavily infiltrated RA synovium is also rich in blood vessels, which exhibit an activated phenotype, in that the endothelial cells lining the blood vessels are cuboidal, rather than elongated in shape, similar to the high endothelial venules of peripheral lymphoid organs. Several studies have demonstrated that the oxygen consumption of the RA synovium (per unit weight of tissue) is increased, and that glucose is oxidized through the anaerobic, as opposed to aerobic, pathway, most probably owing to the excessive proliferative activity of the synovial cells (37). This hyperplasia of the synovium necessitates a compensatory increase in the number of blood vessels required to adequately nourish and oxygenate the tissue, and to deliver the inflammatory cells and molecules to the developing lesion. Endothelial cells lining the small blood vessels within RA synovium express cell cycle-associated antigens such as PCNA and Ki67 (38), as well as markers of angiogenesis such as integrin $\alpha_v\beta_3$. Interestingly, a recent report described increased markers of DNA fragmentation in RA, suggesting that vascular regression may also be increased in RA, relative to OA and noninflamed controls *(39)*.

However, despite this pro-angiogenic phenotype, there has been considerable debate as to whether the overall density of blood vessels in the arthritic synovium per unit area is increased, unchanged or even reduced. It may well be that the process of new blood-vessel formation does not keep pace with synovial-tissue proliferation, and hence the vessel density may, if anything, appear to be reduced. A study in 1991 suggested that capillaries in RA synovium are distributed more deeply, and are less densely arranged, than in normal synovial tissue (80/mm^2 in RA, 242/mm^2 in normal synovium) *(4)*. As a consequence, there may exist within the RA synovium regions of hypoperfusion and hypoxia, owing to insufficient delivery of oxygen to the areas of increased metabolic and proliferative activity. There have been many reports of reduced synovial-fluid PO_2 measurements in human arthritic joints. In a study of 40 patients with a variety of joint disorders, the lowest synovial-fluid PO_2 values were found in individuals with RA (mean PO_2 26 mm Hg, compared to 43 mm Hg in patients with OA and 63 mm Hg in individuals with traumatic joint exudates) *(40)*. A significant correlation between lactate and both pH and PO_2 led to suggestions that the anaerobic glycolysis by the hypoxic synovium may underlie the low PO_2 of the synovial fluid. Conversely, calculation of the ratio of regional blood flow to joint oxygen consumption demonstrated that blood flow in inflamed synovium is increased *(41)*. Taken together, these results suggest that the formation of new vessels and increased blood flow in RA are insufficient to meet the increased metabolic demands imposed by the proliferating synovium, leading to a state of relative hypoxia. Moreover, the large volume of fluid within the joints may increase intra-articular pressure and temporarily obliterate capillary flow in the synovium, compounding the hypoxic state *(42)*. The resting intra-articular pressure in inflamed joints has been found to be raised relative to normal joints, and this effect would be exarcebated during movement of joints. Thus, in RA, as in tumors, there may exist the apparently paradoxical situation of angiogenesis and concomitant hypoxia.

Whether or not the density of blood vessels per unit area is increased, unchanged, or decreased in the RA synovium, there is undoubtedly formation of new blood vessels in RA, as demonstrated by the expression of many pro-angiogenic mediators and molecules associated with angiogenic vasculature, such as integrin $\alpha_v\beta_3$. The subsequent section describes some of these mediators, and discusses their possible roles in mediating neovascularization in RA.

ANGIOGENIC MEDIATORS EXPRESSED IN ARTHRITIS

Although a pro-angiogenic phenotype prevails in RA, it is not known at present which of the many angiogenic mediators expressed in arthritic synovium play the major role in promoting new blood vessel formation. Indeed it is not even clear whether multi-functional cytokines such as fibroblast growth factor (FGF)-2, which exhibit other activities as wells as stimulation of endothelial-cell proliferation, actually modulate angiogenesis in RA. However, the presence of mRNA and protein for many factors capable of inducing angiogenesis in RA synovium is well-documented, and it is generally thought that an accumulation of signals (e.g., recurrent hypoxia, release of low/moderate levels of pro-angiogenic cytokines) may eventually breach the angiogenic "threshold," leading to disregulated vascular proliferation (Fig. 2). The angiogenic stimuli expressed in RA include various growth factors, chemokines, extracellular matrix proteins, adhesion molecules, and cytokines. This chapter does not aim to provide an exhaustive review of all of the regulators of angiogenesis expressed in RA, many of which have been described in detail elsewhere. The key molecules that may play a role in modulating angiogenesis in RA are listed in Table 1.

Vascular Endothelial Growth Factor

It has emerged over the last few years that one of the key players in the pathogenesis of angiogenesis-dependent diseases is vascular endothelial growth factor (VEGF) *(43)*. Many growth factors are pleiotropic in their effects, and promote proliferation of target cells other than endothelium. In contrast, VEGF appears to be the most endothelial-specific angiogenic factor described to date. The mechanisms whereby VEGF stimulates angiogenesis are both direct and indirect, in that VEGF not only stimulates microvascular endothelial cells to proliferate and migrate, but also renders these endothelial cells hyperpermeable, leading to alterations in the extracellular matrix that may favor angiogenesis. The VEGF family now comprises at least 6 related cytokines, of which the original member, VEGF, is probably the best-characterized. VEGF is secreted by various cell types in vitro, including keratinocytes, fibroblasts, osteoblasts smooth-muscle cells, macrophages, platelets, and lymphocytes. VEGF-induced effects are mediated through receptor tyrosine kinases, namely flt-1 and KDR, with the latter receptor thought to be predominantly responsible for mediating the mitogenic effects of VEGF.

Expression of VEGF is elevated in a range of angiogenesis-dependent disease states, such as malignancies (e.g., breast ovarian and colon carcinomas, angiosarcoma), diabetic retinopathy, psoriasis, AIDS-associated Kaposi's sarcoma, and RA *(43)*. The dual activities of VEGF as an endothelial mitogen and vascular permeability factor are both relevant in the pathogenesis of RA, because VEGF may potentially play role in both angiogenesis and edema observed in RA. Expression of VEGF mRNA and protein in RA synovial biopsy sections has been reported, with VEGF localized to the predominantly fibroblast-like lining layer cells and blood vessels *(44,45)*. Stimulation of endothelial-cell proliferation and chemotaxis by RA synovial fluids is partially blocked by anti-VEGF antibodies *(45)*. A recent study from our laboratory demonstrated that serum VEGF concentrations in patients with active RA are markedly increased relative to nonarthritic individuals, and correlate with levels of CRP, a conventional marker of inflammation and disease activity *(46)*. It is noteworthy that serum VEGF levels are elevated in patients with a variety of cancers, and it has been suggested that a high pre-treatment level of VEGF may be associated with a poor clinical outcome *(47)*. By analogy, serum VEGF levels could be a useful prognostic marker of disease progression in arthritis. For example, high serum VEGF concentrations in patients with RA of less than 1 yr duration might be associated with rapid progression to more aggressive disease. If this were the case, measurement of serum VEGF prior to commencement of therapy might allow more rational therapeutic intervention, and this is currently under investigation in our laboratory. One caveat in this context is the demonstration of the existence of a soluble form of the high-affinity VEGF receptor flt-1, which might neutralize any pro-angiogenic effects of serum VEGF. It would be of interest to measure soluble flt-1 in RA and in other angiogenesis-dependent pathologies, to determine whether it may be the balance between VEGF and its soluble receptor, which is important in determining the progression to a pro-angiogenic state.

The stimuli responsible for induction/upregulation of VEGF expression in pathological states such as RA are at present unclear. Pro-inflammatory cytokines such as TNF-α and

Table 1
Mediators of Angiogenesis in RA

	Endothelial proliferation	Endothelial migration	Angiogenesis in vivo	Expressed in RA
VEGF	+	+	+	+
FGF-1	+	+	+	+
FGF-2	+	+	+	+
HGF		+	+	+
PDGF	+	+	+	+
PD-ECGF	+	+	+	+
TGF-β	+/–	+	+	+
EGF	+			+
IGF-1	+			+
IL-8	+	+	+	+
Groα	–		–	+
ENA-78	+		+	+
Soluble E-selectin	+	+	+	+
Soluble VCAM-1	+	+	+	+
$\alpha_v\beta_3$			+	+
TNF-α	+/–	+/–	+	+
TSP-1	+/–		–	+
Angiogenin	+		+	+

(+), Stimulatory; (–), Inhibitory; (+/–), Both reported.

IL-1 may directly upregulate VEGF expression in RA. We have found that incubation of RA synovial membrane cells in the presence of inhibitors of cytokine bio-activity (a combination of anti-TNF-α antibody and IL-1 receptor antagonist) markedly downregulated release of VEGF by these cells *(46)*. However, a significant component of VEGF release by these cells was not sensitive to inhibition of TNF-α and IL-1 action, suggesting that other stimuli may additionally contribute to VEGF production in RA. One of the most potent signals for upregulation of VEGF expression in vitro and in vivo is low PO_2. VEGF mRNA levels are dramatically increased within a few hours of exposing cell cultures to hypoxia and return to background levels when normal oxygen supply is resumed. The increase in the levels of VEGF mRNA in response to hypoxic stress is owing to both transcriptional activation and an increase in mRNA stability *(48)*. The hypoxic state in the RA joint suggests that formation of new blood vessels in the pannus may be driven by hypoxia-induced expression of VEGF. Studies from our own group and from other laboratories have shown that cells that may be capable of producing VEGF in RA (e.g., monocytic cells and fibroblasts) release increased levels of VEGF protein under hypoxic conditions. We have also demonstrated that incubation of enzymatically dissociated, unstimulated RA synovial membrane cells (which are a heterogeneous population of monocytic, lymphocytic, and fibroblast cells) in hypoxic conditions leads to a significant upregulation of VEGF secretion. In contrast, production of IL-1β and IL-8 was unaffected *(46)*.

There have been some reports of VEGF expression by endothelium, especially by cells derived from the microvasculature *(49)*. This latter observation is somewhat controversial, in that endothelial cells are considered to be a target, but not a source, of VEGF. Immunohistochemical analyses of RA synovial biopsies have revealed VEGF expression by endothelial cells lining small blood vessels within the pannus *(44)*. Clearly binding of anti-VEGF antibody to endothelial cells in RA synovial sections may reflect either synthesis of VEGF by endothelium or VEGF bound to cell-surface receptors, and indeed microvascular endothelial cells in the vicinity of VEGF-positive cells in RA synovium have been found to express mRNA for both VEGF receptor sub-types flt-1 and KDR. However, our own unpublished observations of release of biologically active VEGF by an SV40-immortalized dermal microvascular cell line in response to TNF-α nonetheless support the view that there may exist an autocrine pathway to augment endothelial-cell proliferation. More recently we have demonstrated that untransformed microvascular endothelial cells express VEGF mRNA, and that hypoxia further enhances VEGF mRNA levels in these cells.

Growth Factors

In addition to VEGF, several other heparin-binding growth factors have been detected in RA. Both acidic fibroblast growth factor (aFGF; FGF-1) and basic fibroblast growth factor (bFGF; FGF-2), which are broad-range mitogens, have been reported to be present in human disease and in animal models of arthritis *(50,51)*. Synovial tissue from patients with both RA and degenerative joint diseases such as OA have been shown to express FGF-1, with staining present in the lining layer and at the pannus-cartilage interface, suggesting that FGF-1 may play a role in synovial hyperplasia and joint destruction. In contrast, FGF-2 staining appears to be more extensive and intense in the synovium of RA patients relative to individuals with OA. The targets of FGFs, apart from endothelial cells, include fibroblasts and chondrocytes, and as such, it is not clear to what extent these growth factors are involved in angiogenesis during the course of RA. Interestingly, FGF-2 synergises with VEGF in promoting endothelial-cell proliferation, and may additionally exert at least part of its angiogenic effect through the induction of VEGF release by target cells such as synovial fibroblasts *(52)*. These observations suggest that the effects of the FGFs in terms of induction of angiogenesis during the development of RA may be both direct and indirect. Another heparin-binding growth factor expressed in synovium is hepatocyte growth factor (HGF) or scatter factor, so called owing its ability to disperse cohesive epithelial colonies. HGF, which induces both directed (chemotactic) and random migration of endothelial cells, as well as many epithelial-cell types, has been found in RA and OA synovial fluids, although levels of HGF were higher in RA compared to OA. Anti-HGF antibody partially neutralized the chemotactic activity for endothelial cells found in RA synovial fluids, suggesting that HGF may contribute to endothelial migration and angiogenesis in RA *(53)*.

Other growth factors expressed in RA include platelet-derived growth factor (PDGF) and platelet-derived endothelial-cell growth factor (PD-ECGF). Immunostaining of RA synovium with anti-PDGF antibody showed predominant localization of this mitogen to macrophage-like cells, with the extent and intensity of PDGF staining correlating with mononuclear-cell infiltration. However, PDGF receptors have been demonstrated to be strongly expressed by synovial lining cells of the fibroblastic type, suggesting that PDGF may play a more important role in stimulating fibroblast, as opposed to endothelial, proliferation *(50)*. Recent studies have also suggested that PDGF may modulate angiogenesis indirectly, by inducing release from synovial fibroblasts of more endothelial cell-specific angiogenic cytokines such as VEGF. PD-ECGF, now known to be identical with the enzyme thymidine phosphorylase, has been detected in RA synovial fluids and in serum, with serial measurements of serum PD-ECGF levels reflecting changes in the disease activity during the clinical course of RA *(54)*.

The immunomodulatory cytokine TGF-β plays a complex role in angiogenesis and arthritis. In terms of its effects on new blood-vessel formation, TGF-β inhibits proliferation of endothelial cells in vitro, but paradoxically in vivo TGF-β is a powerful pro-angiogenic agent. This may be owing to the ability of TGF-β to induce VEGF gene expression and secretion in fibroblast and epithelial-cell lines, and indeed TGF-β has been found to be the most powerful inducer of VEGF secretion by human synovial fibroblasts (55). TGF-β immunolocalizes to macrophages and fibroblasts in the RA synovial-lining layer (20). Systemic administration of TGF-β was protective in an experimental model of arthritis (56), but in contrast intra-articular injection of neutralizing anti-TGF-β antibody ameliorated arthritis (57). It is thus difficult to comment on the role of TGF-β in modulating angiogenesis during the development of RA lesions, although it seems likely that TGF-β may exert some pro-angiogenic effects through stimulation of VEGF production by cells present in the synovium such as fibroblasts and endothelial cells.

Chemokines

Members of the chemokine family also modulate angiogenesis, in addition to playing important roles in leukocyte recruitment in RA (18). For example, IL-8 is present in synovial fluids of RA patients and is produced by synovial cells and monocytes (31,58). We have shown that blockade of TNF-α and IL-1 activity in cultures of RA synovial membrane cells decreases the production of IL-8, suggesting that this cytokine lies downstream of TNF-α and IL-1 (59). It has also been reported that the angiogenic activity present in the conditioned media of human RA synovial-tissue macrophages was partially blocked by antibodies to IL-8. Anti-angiogenic chemokines, including the neutrophil chemoattractant Groα have been reported to be present in human arthritic synovial fluids and tissue (35). The contribution made by these chemokines to angiogenesis during RA are complicated by their leukocyte chemoattractant and activating activities. It is perhaps most likely that these chemokines primarily play a role in monocyte and lymphocyte recruitment to and retention within the leukocytic aggregates present in RA synovium. Additional effects might be activation of these cells to release other well-known mediators of angiogenesis, as opposed to direct stimulation of endothelial proliferation.

TNF-α

As discussed in an earlier section, the importance of TNF-α in the inflammatory processes that occur during the development of RA is now widely acknowledged (12). The effects of TNF-α on angiogenesis are both stimulatory and inhibitory, depending on the experimental system. TNF-α inhibits basal and FGF-2-stimulated endothelial cell proliferation and migration in vitro. In contrast, in the rabbit cornea, a high dose of TNF-α stimulates neovascularization (60). This apparent discrepancy may be related to the dose of TNF-α used and the time of exposure. A recent study demonstrated that brief exposure to TNF-α can induce release from endothelial cells of VEGF, IL-8, and FGF-2. In addition, antibodies against VEGF and IL-8 blocked TNF-α-mediated angiogenesis in the rabbit corneal assay in vivo (49). Prolonged exposure of microvascular cells to TNF-α inhibits capillary-like structure formation in vitro with associated morphological changes from a cobblestone-like appearance into a disordered array of elongated, spindle-shaped cells (61). In terms of the effects of TNF-α on angiogenesis in RA, it is likely that this cytokine may exert either direct or indirect effects on blood-vessel formation in addition to its pro-inflammatory effects. Certainly production by synovial-joint cells of angiogenic cytokines such as VEGF is at least in part induced by TNF-α, as shown by the ability of anti-TNF-α antibody to reduce VEGF release by synovial cells in culture *(46)*. The role of TNF-α in the stimulation of angiogenesis by synovial fluids of patients with RA has also been studied in a mouse in vivo model. New blood vessel formation in response to synovial fluids of patients with RA but not with OA was partially inhibited by monoclonal antibodies (MAbs) against TNF-α, suggesting that angiogenesis observed in rheumatoid synovitis may be owing, at least in part, to the angiogenic effect of locally produced TNF-α *(62)*. However, as yet there is no definitive evidence to prove that TNF-α affects new blood vessel formation in RA.

Other Angiogenic Mediators

Another molecule with apparently discrepant actions on angiogenesis is thrombospondin-1 (TSP-1). TSP-1 is a large (approx 450kDa) disulphide-bonded trimer composed of three identical polypeptide chains, and the size and structure of TSP-1 enables it to interact with a wide variety of matrix and plasma proteins. TSP-1 is released from platelet alpha granules, and is synthesized by smooth-muscle cells, endothelial cells, and macrophages. Although TSP-1 is actively synthesized by endothelial cells, the synthesis is downregulated as the endothelial cells organize into vessel-like structures. Stable transfection of endothelial cells with TSP-1 anti-sense mRNA resulted in greatly enhanced chemotaxis and capillary formation. However, TSP-1, probably by virtue of its adhesive interactions, has also been shown to promote angiogenesis and the progression of metastatic disease. In RA, TSP-1 is generally found in the matrix of synovial vessels, although immunoreactivity for TSP-1 was also seen associated with macrophages in synovium and in the synovial-lining layer *(63)*. It is possible that TSP-1 plays both an inductive and inhibitory role on angiogenesis in RA, depending on the context within which the endothelium is exposed to TSP-1, and may also function as an adhesive glycoprotein in RA, facilitating intercellular interactions.

A variety of other molecules have been proposed to play a role in neovascularization during RA. For example, the heparin-binding proteins angiogenin and midkine have been found to be expressed in RA. Midkine, which is functional similarity to members of the FGF has family, has been detected in synovial fluid, synoviocytes, and endothelial cells of new blood vessels in RA and OA. Normal synovial fluid and noninflammatory synovial tissue did not contain detectable midkine *(64)*. Angiogenin has been found to be present at relatively high levels in synovial fluids from RA and OA patients, and to co-localize with FGF-2 in synovial membranes. Synovial-lining cells, macrophages, endothelial cells, and vascular smooth-muscle cells were immunopositive for angiogenin. Interestingly, angiogenin levels did not appear to be higher in RA vs OA fluids and tissues, and it may be that angiogenin plays a role in the physiology of normal synovium *(18)*. In addition, certain adhesion molecules and extracellular matrix proteins may be important in regulating new blood-vessel formation. Adhesion molecules expressed on endothelial cells are important in the inflammatory and infiltrating phases of RA, in that these molecules bind circulating cells such as leukocytes, prior to their extravasation into underlying tissue. It has also been proposed that circulating forms of E-selectin and VCAM-1 may promote angiogenesis. Serum levels of E-selectin and VCAM-1 are elevated in the serum of patients with RA *(65)*. Soluble E-selectin and VCAM-1 were shown to promote endothelial-cell chemotaxis, and promoted angiogenesis in a rat cornea assay. The chemotactic activity of RA synovial fluid for endothelial cells, and also its angiogenic activity, were blocked by antibodies to either soluble E-selectin or soluble VCAM-1 *(66)*. These observations provide a possible link between leukocyte adhesion and new blood-vessel formation, which may be of relevance in the development of inflammatory states such as RA, although the mechanism whereby E-selectin and VCAM-1 modulate angiogenesis is unclear.

The integrins, which function in cell-cell and cell-matrix interactions, have been implicated in angiogenesis by virtue of their anti-apoptotic effects (67). Integrin $\alpha_v\beta_3$, which binds matrix proteins including vitronectin and fibronectin, was identified as a marker of angiogenic vascular tissue, and showed an increase in expression during angiogenesis in the chick chorioallantoic membrane. Administration of $\alpha_v\beta_3$ antibody prevented the growth of human tumors transplanted into mice, suggesting that $\alpha_v\beta_3$ antagonists may provide an effective anti-angiogenic approach for the treatment of human cancer. The mechanism whereby $\alpha_v\beta_3$ functions in angiogenesis is thought to involve apoptosis, because endothelial cells become apoptotic in response to $\alpha_v\beta_3$ antagonists of integrin, leading to the regression of angiogenic blood vessels (68). A second integrin, $\alpha_v\beta_5$, is also involved in new blood-vessel development. Integrin $\alpha_v\beta_3$ appears to mediate angiogenesis induced by FGF-2 and TNF-α, whereas responses initiated by VEGF may be $\alpha_v\beta_5$-dependent (69). Integrin $\alpha_v\beta_3$ has recently been demonstrated to be expressed in a rabbit model of arthritis resembling human RA, and our own data indicates that blood vessels in RA synovium also express integrin $\alpha_v\beta_3$.

In summary, many growth factors and cytokines may potentially induce/upregulate angiogenesis in arthritis. It is not known yet which is the most important angiogenic molecule, although VEGF does appear to play a very significant role. VEGF receptors may also be upregulated, and indeed it could be hypothesized that the synovium may exhibit temporal and spatial expression of VEGF and its receptors, in a manner comparable to that seen in tumors. For example, the lowest *PO2* may be observed at the invasive edge of the synovium (the area of cartilage-pannus junction), leading to upregulation of VEGF expression and angiogenesis. At areas distal to the pannus, where mature blood vessels already exist, VEGF production may be shut down. Such a speculative model would certainly fit with the observations that pannus is frequently hypoperfused. This would drive VEGF expression and angiogenesis, but at the same time favor further synovial proliferation, thus creating a positive feedback loop to further amplify lesion development.

THERAPEUTIC TARGETS FOR THE DEVELOPMENT OF ANTI-ARTHRITIC THERAPIES

Although RA is a chronic disease, this condition responds well to therapeutic intervention. Nonsteroidal anti-inflammatory drugs have been shown to reduce joint pain, tenderness, and inflammation. Local corticosteroid use is common, but long-term use may lead to potentially serious adverse events. Steroids probably act via suppression of the functions of activated monocyte/macrophages, including the release of TNF-α. The primary treatment for RA, however, is disease-modifying anti-rheumatic drug (DMARD) therapy, with an increasing emphasis on the use of combination therapy. The DMARDs include gold, methotrexate, sulphasalazine, and penicillamine, and reduce the symptoms of inflammatory synovitis, such as the tender and swollen joint count. Nevertheless, even with relatively aggressive use of DMARDs, the majority of patients develop erosions. However, all of these therapies aim to reduce pain and joint inflammation, minimize disability, and alter the course of disease by reducing the progression of joint damage. A more attractive approach is to directly target processes that play a role in the disease, such as the pro-inflammatory cytokine cascade or infiltration of the synovium by cells migrating from the blood. Therapeutic strategies can be broadly divided into (a) anti-cytokine, (b) anti-lymphocyte, and (c) anti-adhesion therapy.

Because of its central role in the pathogenesis of RA, TNF-α has been proposed to be a primary target for anti-cytokine therapy. Much of the evidence for the key role of TNF-α has emerged from research led by the Kennedy Institute. For example, it was shown that addition of antibodies to block the activity of TNF-α abolished the secretion by RA synovial cells of IL-1, IL-6, IL-8, and GM-CSF, suggesting that TNF-α is a prime cytokine in fostering this destructive cascade of cytokines in the RA joint *(59,70)*. This hypothesis was successfully tested in animal models, in which anti-TNF-α antibody, injected into DBA/1 mice with collagen-induced arthritis, decreased inflammatory joint damage. These studies provided the rationale for clinical trials of anti-TNF-α therapy in patients with long-standing RA. Several clinical trials using a chimeric (human IgG1κ, mouse Fv) anti-TNF-α monoclonal antibody have shown marked clinical benefit. Randomized clinical trials with a single cycle of neutral-izing anti-TNF-a antibody showed substantial benefit in the majority of patients, with marked reduction in CRP lasting several weeks *(71)*. The mechanism of action of anti-TNF-α antibody has been studied in detail in our laboratory. We have shown that treatment with anti-TNF-α decreased soluble E-selectin and ICAM-1 levels, with a concomitant rapid and sustained increase in circulating lymphocytes *(65)*. As a consequence, we proposed that decreased serum levels of adhesion molecules reflect diminished activation of endothelial cells in the synovial microvasculature, leading to reduced migration of leukocytes into synovial joints. This was supported by a parallel study showing a significant reduction in expression of adhesion molecules and in synovial-tissue cellularity, and by more recent data showing reduced chemotactic cytokine gradients and decreased ^{111}In-labeled leukocyte trafficking to joints following anti-TNF-α therapy *(72)*.

Alternative approaches to anti-cytokine therapy have involved the use of soluble TNF-α receptor fusion proteins. For example, a p75 receptor fusion protein has been shown in placebo-controlled trials to significantly improve the signs and symptoms of RA *(73)*. The application of gene therapy for the treatment of RA and other articular diseases is also being explored to overcome current limitations with delivery of therapeutics to joint tissues. Gene products that have therapeutic efficacy in animal models of RA include IL-1 receptor antago-nist, soluble TNF-α receptors and immunomodulatory cytokines such as IL-10 and TGF-β, and these studies are currently in progress. Finally, use of immunomodulatory cytokines such as IL-11 and IL-10 has been considered. IL-10 is an important immunoregulatory component in the cytokine network of RA, in that neutralization of endogenously produced IL-10 in RA synovial-membrane cultures results in an increase in the levels of pro-inflammatory cytokines such as TNF-α and IL-1 *(21)*. IL-10 can ameliorate arthritis in the collagen-induced arthritis model of RA, indicating a potential therapeutic role for IL-10 in RA *(74)*. Similarly, IL-11 has been found in RA synovial membranes and synovial fluids. Blockade of endogenous IL-11 resulted in an increase in TNF-α production by synovial cells, which was further enhanced if endogenous IL-10 was also blocked, suggesting that exogenous IL-11 may have therapeutic activity in RA *(75)*.

Targeting the infiltrating lymphocytes has also been utilized for the evolution of novel treatments for RA. Anti-lymphocyte MAbs have also produced long-lasting disease suppression in animal models of disease. Anti-CD4 treatment caused some reduction in paw-swelling in the murine collagen-induced arthritis model, but did not significantly prevent joint erosion, although addition of anti-CD4 plus suboptimal anti-TNF-α antibody significantly reduced paw-swelling, limb involvement, and joint erosion *(76)*. In RA, the use of depleting anti-lymphocyte MAbs has been disappointing as these antibodies did not penetrate the synovial joint in sufficient quantity to suppress disease without producing severe and protracted peripheral blood lymphopenia *(77)*. In contrast, clinical trials of nondepleting anti-CD4 MAbs appear more promising. In recent trials, anti-CD4 was well-tolerated at the doses used and saturation of CD4 receptors in peripheral blood could be routinely obtained for over 1 wk with a single infusion of antibody *(78)*. In addition, several studies have investigated the possible use of anti-ICAM-1 antibody in RA. A single course of therapy with an anti-ICAM-1 MAb was associated with clinical improvement in patients with RA. Unfortunately, a second course of therapy in patients who previously received anti-ICAM-1 was associated with adverse effects suggestive of immune-complex formation *(79)*. Repeated courses of therapy with a murine antibody to ICAM-1 would thus probably not be a useful therapeutic strategy in patients with RA, probably because of its immunogenicity.

In summary, current treatments improve symptoms of RA such as pain, and regulate synovial inflammation and infiltration. There is little evidence for significant reduction of joint damage, and as a consequence many cases of RA have a poor eventual outcome. MAb treatment, although expensive, may in future be useful to treat flares of disease in combination with conventional DMARDs such as methotrexate. There is undoubtedly scope for new therapeutic advances, such as anti-angiogenic therapies, and these will be discussed in the next section.

IS ARTHRITIS A POTENTIAL TARGET FOR ANTI-ANGIOGENIC THERAPY?

Therapeutic agents are being devised to either interrupt or inhibit one or more of the pathogenic steps involved in the process of neovascularization, and blockade of angiogenesis has been effective in many tumor models. It is not unreasonable to suggest that targeting the newly formed vasculature of the RA pannus may lead to a more persistent reduction in pannus volume and hence in the clinical symptoms of disease.

The most commonly studied anti-angiogenic agent is O-(chloroacetyl-carbamoyl) fumagillol or TNP-470, also known as AGM-1470, a semi-synthetic analog of the antibiotic fumagillin. This compound has been demonstrated to exhibit anti-proliferative effects in vitro and in vivo, and to block the progression of a variety of tumors in animal models. TNP-470 has been used in animal models of arthritis to demonstrate the importance of new blood-vessel formation in the maintenance arthritic disease. Disease was induced in rats by injection of heterologous collagen, resulting in synovitis and joint erosion, associated with neovascularization, in a manner comparable to that observed in human RA. Administration of TNP-470, or the microtubule stabilizing agent Taxol, was found to prevent onset of arthritis and significantly suppressed established disease, in parallel with marked inhibition of pannus formation. Histological analyses showed an absence of neovascularization in joint sections from animals who received angiogenesis inhibitors *(80,81)*. A concomitant reduction in circulating VEGF levels was also observed *(82)*. A polysaccharide Streptococcal toxin named CM101, an anti-neovascularization agent, which has been shown to exhibit anti-tumor activity, has also been reported to inhibit arthritis in the murine collagen-induced arthritis model. More recently, specific antagonists of $\alpha_v\beta_3$ antagonist were used in a rabbit model resembling human RA. Arthritis was induced by bilateral knee injection of ovalbumin and FGF-2, and treatment consisted of intra-articular injections of $\alpha_v\beta_3$ antagonist or control. Angiogenesis inhibition was assessed by quantifying synovial endothelial-cell density, and arthritis severity assessed by measuring multiple macroscopic and histological parameters. Treatment with $\alpha_v\beta_3$ antagonist (LM609) decreased vascularity in the arthritic synovium, and was associated with a significant decrease in all arthritic parameters including joint swelling, synovitis, and synovial hypertrophy (83).

It is also noteworthy that many of the anti-rheumatic drugs currently in clinical use or in trials apparently exert effects on the vasculature. For example, anti-rheumatic drugs such as indomethacin, methotrexate, and corticosteroids inhibit angiogenesis in in vitro assays. Methotrexate, at doses that are attained in the serum of RA patients treated with this drug, inhibited both basal and stimulated endothelial proliferation in vitro (84). Thiol-containing and gold compounds, also used therapeutically in RA, may modulate neovascularization indirectly by inhibiting the production of angiogenic activity by macrophages (85,86). In addition, as discussed earlier, we have previously shown that treatment of human RA with MAb to TNF-α results in amelioration of disease symptoms, associated with improvements in clinical and laboratory disease parameters. Based on the upregulation by TNF-α of VEGF expression by cells such as monocytes and endothelial cells, we hypothesized that a possible mechanism of action of anti-TNF-α could be decreased angiogenesis in vivo, mediated by cytokines such as VEGF. We therefore investigated whether elevated serum VEGF concentrations in RA could be altered by anti-TNF-α therapy, and observed that treatment of RA patients with anti-TNF-a significantly reduced serum VEGF in a time- and dose-dependent manner. The reduction in serum VEGF concentrations correlated with alterations in disease parameters such as CRP levels and swollen joint counts. In a subsequent trial of multiple infusions of anti-TNF-α, alone or with methotrexate, the reduction in serum VEGF levels was more prolonged in patients who received anti-TNF-α with methotrexate, relative to patients who were treated with anti-TNF-α alone, and was maintained until the end of the trial period, more than 10 wk after the final anti-TNF-α infusion (Fig. 3). These observations correlated well with the clinical observations, in that combination therapy with anti-TNF-α and methotrexate was effective in 70–80% patients (46). These findings suggested that the clinical benefits of anti-TNF-α antibody therapy are associated with a reduction in circulating VEGF levels, which may lead to decreased joint vascularity and swelling (possibly owing to reduced vascular permeability). However, further studies are clearly required to demonstrate that anti-TNF-α actually reduces synovial vascularity, and these are currently underway in our laboratory.

FUTURE PERSPECTIVES

Based on the close association of angiogenesis and VEGF in arthritic disease, a hypothesis could also be made that suppression of VEGF activity should be an effective therapy in RA. VEGF inhibition has been effective in models of other diseases with pathogenic neovascularization. For example, growth of tumors in mice is blocked by anti-VEGF antibody and by administration of a dominant-negative form of KDR (87). Humanized anti-VEGF-IgG1 constructs, which bind VEGF with affinities very similar to those of the original murine antibody, have been described and are currently in clinical trials for the treatment of solid tumors and other disorders in humans (88). Soluble VEGF receptor chimeras have been shown to suppress VEGF-induced retinal neovascularization, and antisense to VEGF suppressed human glioblastoma angiogenicity and tumorigenicity (89,90). Interruption of downstream effects, such as the tyrosine kinases linked to VEGF receptors,

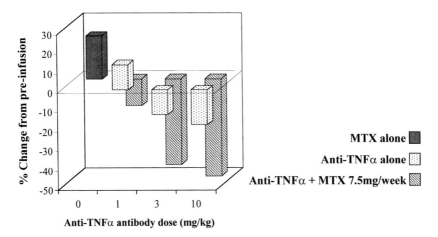

Fig. 3. VEGF levels in RA patients are reduced by anti-TNF-α antibody treatment. Patients with active RA were enrolled in a clinical trial of a human/murine chimeric monoclonal IgGlk antibody, with specificity for recombinant and natural human TNF-α. Treatment was either placeo tablets or methotrexate at a dose of 7.5 mg/wk, and multiple infusions of either 0, 1, or 10 mg/kg anti-TNF-α antibody on weeks 0, 2, 6, 10, and 14. Data are % change relative to pre-infusion values, 20 wk after the commencement of the trial.

may also be effective, and inhibitors have been generated that are more specific for VEGF receptor tyrosine kinases than for other receptor tyrosine kinases (e.g., EGF and FGF receptors). The prospect of anti-VEGF therapy in RA is an exciting one, and it is to be hoped that in the not too distant future clinical trials of VEGF-targeted therapies in malignancies might be followed by similar trials in arthritis.

ACKNOWLEDGMENTS

The authors gratefully acknowledge the support of the Arthritis and Rheumatism Council of Great Britain, and Zeneca Pharmaceuticals (J.M.M.).

REFERENCES

1. Harris, E. D., Jr. (1986) Pathogenesis of rheumatoid arthritis. *Am. J. Med.* **80,** 4–10.
2. Grassi, W., De Angelis, R., Lamanna, G., and Cervini, C. (1998) The clinical features of rheumatoid arthritis. *Eur. J. Radiol.* **27(Suppl. 1),** S18–S24.
3. Reveille, J. D. (1998) The genetic contribution to the pathogenesis of rheumatoid arthritis. *Curr. Opin. Rheumatol.* **10,** 187–200.
4. Stevens, C. R., Blake, D. R., Merry, P., Revell, P. A., and Levick, J. R. (1991) A comparative study by morphometry of the microvasculature in normal and rheumatoid synovium. *Arthritis Rheum.* **34,** 1508–1513.
5. Brown, R. A., Weiss, J. B., Tomlinson, I. W., Phillips, P., and Kumar, S. (1980) Angiogenic factor from synovial fluid resembling that from tumors. *Lancet* **1(8170),** 682–685.
6. Rooney, M., Condell, D., Quinlan, W., Daly, L., Whelan, A., Feighery, C., and Bresnihan, B. (1988) Analysis of the histologic variation of synovitis in rheumatoid arthritis. *Arthritis Rheum.* **31,** 956–963.
7. Paleolog, E. M. (1996) Angiogenesis: a critical process in the pathogenesis of RA: a role for VEGF? *Br. J. Rheumatol.* **35,** 917–919.
8. Koch, A. E. (1998) Review: angiogenesis: implications for rheumatoid arthritis. *Arthritis Rheum.* **41,** 951–962.
9. Feldmann, M., Brennan, F. M., and Maini, R. N. (1996) Rheumatoid arthritis. *Cell.* **85,** 307–310.
10. Emery, P. and Luqmani, R. (1993) The validity of surrogate markers in rheumatic disease. *Br. J. Rheumatol.* **32(Suppl. 3),** 3–8.

11. Arnett, F. C., Edworthy, S. M., Bloch, D. A., McShane, D. J., Fries, J. F., Cooper, N. S., et al. (1988) The American Rheumatism Association 1987 revised criteria for the classification of rheumatoid arthritis. *Arthritis Rheum.* **31**, 315–324.

12. Feldmann, M., Brennan, F. M., and Maini, R. N. (1996) Role of cytokines in rheumatoid arthritis. *Ann. Rev. Immunol.* **14**, 397–440.

13. Buchan, G., Barrett, K., Turner, M., Chantry, D., Maini, R. N., and Feldmann, M. (1988) Interleukin-1 and tumor necrosis factor mRNA expression in rheumatoid arthritis: prolonged production of IL-1α. *Clin. Exp. Immunol.* **73**, 449–455.

14. Chu, C. Q., Field, M., Feldmann, M., and Maini, R. N. (1991) Localization of tumor necrosis factor alpha in synovial tissues and at the cartilage-pannus junction in patients with rheumatoid arthritis. *Arthritis Rheum.* **34**, 1125–1132.

15. Haworth, C., Brennan, F. M., Chantry, D., Turner, M., Maini, R. N., and Feldmann, M. (1991) Expression of granulocyte-macrophage colony-stimulating factor in rheumatoid arthritis: regulation by tumor necrosis factor-alpha. *Eur. J. Immunol.* **21**, 2575–2579.

16. Chu, C. Q., Field, M., Allard, S., Abney, E., Feldmann, M., and Maini, R. N. (1992) Detection of cytokines at the cartilage/pannus junction in patients with rheumatoid arthritis: implications for the role of cytokines in cartilage destruction and repair. *Br. J. Rheumatol.* **31**, 653–661.

17. Deleuran, B. W., Chu, C. Q., Field, M., Brennan, F. M., Katsikis, P., Feldmann, M., and Maini, R. N. (1992) Localization of interleukin-1 alpha, type 1 interleukin-1 receptor and interleukin-1 receptor antagonist in the synovial membrane and cartilage/pannus junction in rheumatoid arthritis. *Br. J. Rheumatol.* **31**, 801–809.

18. Hosaka, S., Akahoshi, T., Wada, C., and Kondo, H. (1994) Expression of the chemokine superfamily in rheumatoid arthritis. *Clin. Exp. Immunol.* **97**, 451–457.

19. Parry, S. L., Sebbag, M., Feldmann, M., and Brennan, F. M. (1997) Contact with T cells modulates monocyte IL-10 production: role of T cell membrane TNF-alpha. *J. Immunol.* **158**, 3673–3681.

20. Chu, C. Q., Field, M., Abney, E., Zheng, R. Q., Allard, S., Feldmann, M., and Maini, R. N. (1991) Transforming growth factor-beta 1 in rheumatoid synovial membrane and cartilage/pannus junction. *Clin. Exp. Immunol.* **86**, 380–386.

21. Katsikis, P. D., Chu, C. Q., Brennan, F. M., Maini, R. N., and Feldmann, M. (1994) Immunoregulatory role of interleukin 10 in rheumatoid arthritis. *J. Exp. Med.* **179**, 1517–1527.

22. Paleolog, E. M., Delasalle, S. A., Buurman, W. A., and Feldmann, M. (1994) Functional activities of receptors for tumor necrosis factor-α on human vascular endothelial cells. *Blood* **84**, 2578–2590.

23. Deleuran, B. W., Chu, C. Q., Field, M., Brennan, F. M., Mitchell, T., Feldmann, M., and Maini, R. N. (1992) Localization of tumor necrosis factor receptors in the synovial tissue and cartilage-pannus junction in patients with rheumatoid arthritis. Implications for local actions of tumor necrosis factor alpha. *Arthritis Rheum.* **35**, 1170–1178.

24. Cines, D. B., Pollak, E. S., Buck, C. A., Loscalzo, J., Zimmerman, G. A., McEver, R. P., et al. (1998) Endothelial cells in physiology and in the pathophysiology of vascular disorders. *Blood* **91**, 3527–3561.

25. Koch, A. E., Burrows, J. C., Haines, G. K., Carlos, T. M., Harlan, J. M., and Leibovich, S. J. (1991) Immunolocalization of endothelial and leukocyte adhesion molecules in human rheumatoid and osteoarthritic synovial tissues. *Lab. Invest.* **64**, 313–320.

26. Johnson, B. A., Haines, G. K., Harlow, L. A., and Koch, A. E. (1993) Adhesion molecule expression in human synovial tissue. *Arthritis Rheum.* **36**, 137–146.

27. Szekanecz, Z., Haines, G. K., Lin, T. R., Harlow, L. A., Goerdt, S., Rayan, G., and Koch, A. E. (1994) Differential distribution of intercellular adhesion molecules (ICAM-1, ICAM-2, and ICAM-3) and the MS-1 antigen in normal and diseased human synovia. Their possible pathogenetic and clinical significance in rheumatoid arthritis. *Arthritis Rheum.* **37**, 221–231.

28. Kohem, C. L., Brezinschek, R. I., Wisbey, H., Tortorella, C., Lipsky, P. E., and Oppenheimer-Marks, N. (1996) Enrichment of differentiated CD45RBdim,CD27- memory T cells in the peripheral blood, synovial fluid, and synovial tissue of patients with rheumatoid arthritis. *Arthritis Rheum.* **39**, 844–854.

29. Postigo, A. A., Garcia-Vicuna, R., Diaz-Gonzalez, F., Arroyo, A. G., De Landazuri, M. O., Chi-Rosso, G., et al. (1992) Increased binding of synovial T lymphocytes from rheumatoid arthritis to endothelial-leukocyte adhesion molecule-1 (ELAM-1) and vascular cell adhesion molecule-1 (VCAM-1). *J. Clin. Invest.* **89**, 1445–1452.

30. Jalkanen, S., Steere, A. C., Fox, R. I., and Butcher, E. C. (1986) A distinct endothelial cell recognition system that controls lymphocyte traffic into inflamed synovium. *Science* **233**, 556–558.

31. Koch, A. E., Polverini, P. J., Kunkel, S. L., Harlow, L. A., DiPietro, L. A., Elner, V. M., et al. (1992) Interleukin-8 as a macrophage-derived mediator of angiogenesis. *Science* **258**, 1798–1801.

32. Koch, A. E., Kunkel, S. L., Harlow, L. A., Johnson, B., Evanoff, H. L., Haines, G. K., et al. (1992) Enhanced production of monocyte chemoattractant protein-1 in rheumatoid arthritis. *J. Clin. Invest.* **90,** 772–779.

33. Koch, A. E., Kunkel, S. L., Harlow, L. A., Mazarakis, D. D., Haines, G. K., Burdick, M. D., et al. (1994) Epithelial neutrophil activating peptide-78: a novel chemotactic cytokine for neutrophils in arthritis. *J. Clin. Invest.* **94,** 1012–1018.

34. Snowden, N., Hajeer, A., Thomson, W., and Ollier, B. (1994) RANTES role in rheumatoid arthritis. *Lancet* **343,** 547–548.

35. Koch, A. E., Kunkel, S. L., Shah, M. R., Hosaka, S., Halloran, M. M., Haines, G. K., et al. (1995) Growth-related gene product alpha. A chemotactic cytokine for neutrophils in rheumatoid arthritis. *J. Immunol.* **155,** 3660–3666.

36. Qin, S., Rottman, J. B., Myers, P., Kassam, N., Weinblatt, M., Loetscher, M., et al. (1998) The chemokine receptors CXCR3 and CCR5 mark subsets of T cells associated with certain inflammatory reactions. *J. Clin. Invest.* **101,** 746–754.

37. Stevens, C. R., Williams, R. B., Farrell, A. J., and Blake, D. R. (1991) Hypoxia and inflammatory synovitis: observations and speculation. *Ann. Rheum. Dis.* **50,** 124–132.

38. Ceponis, A., Konttinen, Y. T., Imai, S., Tamulaitiene, M., Li, T. F., Xu, J. W., et al. (1998) Synovial lining, endothelial and inflammatory mononuclear cell proliferation in synovial membranes in psoriatic and reactive arthritis: a comparative quantitative morphometric study. *Br. J. Rheumatol.* **37,** 170–178.

39. Walsh, D. A., Wade, M., Mapp, P. I., and Blake, D. R. (1998) Focally regulated endothelial proliferation and cell death in human synovium. *Am. J. Pathol.* **152,** 691–702.

40. Lund-Olesen, K. (1970) Oxygen tension in synovial fluids. *Arthritis Rheum.* **13,** 769–776.

41. Falchuk, K. H., Goetzl, E. J., and Kulka, J. P. (1970) Respiratory gases of synovial fluids. An approach to synovial tissue circulatory-metabolic imbalance in rheumatoid arthritis. *Am. J. Med.* **49,** 223–231.

42. Blake, D. R., Merry, P., Unsworth, J., Kidd, B. L., Outhwaite, J. M., Ballard, R., et al. (1989) Hypoxic-reperfusion injury in the inflamed human joint. *Lancet* **1(8633),** 289–293.

43. Brown, L. F., Detmar, M., Claffey, K., Nagy, J. A., Feng, D., Dvorak, A. M., and Dvorak, H. F. (1997) Vascular permeability factor/vascular endothelial growth factor: a multifunctional angiogenic cytokine. *EXS* **79,** 233–269.

44. Fava, R. A., Olsen, N. J., Spencer-Green, G., Yeo, K. T., Yeo, T. K., Berse, B., et al. (1994) Vascular permeability factor/endothelial growth factor (VPF/VEGF): accumulation and expression in human synovial fluids and rheumatoid synovial tissue. *J. Exp. Med.* **180,** 341–346.

45. Koch, A. E., Harlow, L. A., Haines, G. K., Amento, E. P., Unemori, E. N., Wong, W. L., et al. (1994) Vascular endothelial growth factor. A cytokine modulating endothelial function in rheumatoid arthritis. *J. Immunol.* **152,** 4149–4156.

46. Paleolog, E. M., Young, S., Stark, A. C., McCloskey, R. V., Feldmann, M., and Maini, R. N. (1998) Modulation of angiogenic vascular endothelial growth factor (VEGF) by TNF-α and IL-1 in rheumatoid arthritis. *Arthritis Rheum.* **41,** 1258–1265.

47. Salven, P., Teerenhovi, L., and Joensuu, H. (1997) A high pre-treatment serum vascular endothelial growth factor concentration is associated with poor outcome in non-Hodgkin's lymphoma. *Blood* **90,** 3167–3172.

48. Shweiki, D., Itin, A., Soffer, D., and Keshet, E. (1992) Vascular endothelial growth factor induced by hypoxia may mediate hypoxia-initiated angiogenesis. *Nature* **359,** 843–845.

49. Yoshida, S., Ono, M., Shono, T., Izumi, H., Ishibashi, T., Suzuki, H., and Kuwano, M. (1997) Involvement of interleukin-8, vascular endothelial growth factor, and basic fibroblast growth factor in tumor necrosis factor alpha-dependent angiogenesis. *Mol. Cell Biol.* **17,** 4015–4023.

50. Sano, H., Engleka, K., Mathern, P., Hla, T., Crofford, L. J., Remmers, E. F., et al. (1993) Coexpression of phosphotyrosine-containing proteins, platelet-derived growth factor-B, and fibroblast growth factor-1 *in situ* in synovial tissues of patients with rheumatoid arthritis and Lewis rats with adjuvant or streptococcal cell wall arthritis. *J. Clin. Invest.* **91,** 553–565.

51. Qu, Z., Huang, X. N., Ahmadi, P., Andresevic, J., Planck, S. R., Hart, C. E., and Rosenbaum, J. T. (1995) Expression of basic fibroblast growth factor in synovial tissue from patients with rheumatoid arthritis and degenerative joint disease. *Lab. Invest.* **73,** 339–346.

52. Pepper, M. S., Ferrara, N., Orci, L., and Montesano, R. (1992) Potent synergism between vascular endothelial growth factor and basic fibroblast growth factor in the induction of angiogenesis in vitro. *Biochem. Biophys. Res. Commun.* **189,** 824–831.

53. Koch, A. E., Halloran, M. M., Hosaka, S., Shah, M. R., Haskell, C. J., Baker, S. K., et al. (1996) Hepatocyte growth factor. A cytokine mediating endothelial migration in inflammatory arthritis. *Arthritis Rheum.* **39,** 1566–1575.

54. Waguri, Y., Otsuka, T., Sugimura, I., Matsui, N., Asai, K., Moriyama, A., and Kato, T. (1997) Gliostatin/platelet-derived endothelial cell growth factor as a clinical marker of rheumatoid arthritis and its regulation in fibroblast-like synoviocytes. *Br. J. Rheumatol.* **36,** 315–321.

55. Pertovaara, L., Kaipainen, A., Mustonen, T., Orpana, A., Ferrara, N., Saksela, O., and Alitalo, K. (1994) Vascular endothelial growth factor is induced in response to transforming growth factor-beta in fibroblastic and epithelial cells. *J. Biol. Chem.* **269,** 6271–6274.

56. Kuruvilla, A. P., Shah, R., Hochwald, G. M., Liggitt, H. D., Palladino, M. A., and Thorbecke, G. J. (1991) Protective effect of transforming growth factor beta 1 on experimental autoimmune diseases in mice. *Proc. Natl. Acad. Sci. USA* **88,** 2918–2921.

57. Wahl, S. M., Allen, J. B., Costa, G. L., Wong, H. L., and Dasch, J. R. (1993) Reversal of acute and chronic synovial inflammation by anti-transforming growth factor beta. *J. Exp. Med.* **177,** 225–230.

58. Brennan, F. M., Zachariae, C. O., Chantry, D., Larsen, C. G., Turner, M., Maini, R. N., et al. (1990) Detection of interleukin 8 biological activity in synovial fluids from patients with rheumatoid arthritis and production of interleukin 8 mRNA by isolated synovial cells. *Eur. J. Immunol.* **20,** 2141–2144.

59. Butler, D. M., Maini, R. N., Feldmann, M., and Brennan, F. M. (1995) Modulation of proinflammatory cytokine release in rheumatoid synovial membrane cell cultures. Comparison of monoclonal anti TNF-alpha antibody with the interleukin-1 receptor antagonist. *Eur. Cytokine Netw.* **6,** 225–230.

60. Frater-Schroder, M., Risau, W., Hallmann, R., Gautschi, P., and Bohlen, P. (1987) Tumor necrosis factor type alpha, a potent inhibitor of endothelial cell growth in vitro, is angiogenic in vivo. *Proc. Natl. Acad. Sci. USA* **84,** 5277–5281.

61. Mawatari, M., Kohno, K., Mizoguchi, H., Matsuda, T., Asoh, K., Van Damme, J., et al. (1989) Effects of tumor necrosis factor and epidermal growth factor on cell morphology, cell surface receptors, and the production of tissue inhibitor of metalloproteinases and IL-6 in human microvascular endothelial cells. *J. Immunol.* **143,** 1619–1627.

62. Lupia, E., Montrucchio, G., Battaglia, E., Modena, V., and Camussi, G. (1996) Role of tumor necrosis factor-alpha and platelet-activating factor in neoangiogenesis induced by synovial fluids of patients with rheumatoid arthritis. *Eur. J. Immunol.* **26,** 1690–1694.

63. Koch, A. E., Friedman, J., Burrows, J. C., Haines, G. K., and Bouck, N. P. (1993) Localization of the angiogenesis inhibitor thrombospondin in human synovial tissues. *Pathobiology* **61,** 1–6.

64. Takada, T., Toriyama, K., Muramatsu, H., Song, X. J., Torii, S., and Muramatsu, T. (1997) Midkine, a retinoic acid-inducible heparin-binding cytokine in inflammatory responses: chemotactic activity to neutrophils and association with inflammatory synovitis. *J. Biochem. (Tokyo)* **122,** 453–458.

65. Paleolog, E. M., Hunt, M., Elliott, M. J., Feldmann, M., Maini, R. N., and Woody, J. N. (1996) Deactivation of vascular endothelium by monoclonal anti-tumor necrosis factor alpha antibody in rheumatoid arthritis. *Arthritis Rheum.* **39,** 1082–1091.

66. Koch, A. E., Halloran, M. M., Haskell, C. J., Shah, M. R., and Polverini, P. J. (1995) Angiogenesis mediated by soluble forms of E-selectin and vascular cell adhesion molecule-1. *Nature* **376,** 517–519.

67. Brooks, P. C. (1996) Role of integrins in angiogenesis. *Eur. J. Cancer* **32A,** 2423–2429.

68. Brooks, P. C., Montgomery, A. M., Rosenfeld, M., Reisfeld, R. A., Hu, T., Klier, G., and Cheresh, D. A. (1994) Integrin alpha v beta 3 antagonists promote tumor regression by inducing apoptosis of angiogenic blood vessels. *Cell* **79,** 1157–1164.

69. Friedlander, M., Brooks, P. C., Shaffer, R. W., Kincaid, C. M., Varner, J. A., and Cheresh, D. A. (1995) Definition of two angiogenic pathways by distinct alpha v integrins. *Science* **270,** 1500–1502.

70. Brennan, F. M., Chantry, D., Jackson, A., Maini, R., and Feldmann, M. (1989) Inhibitory effect of TNF-α antibodies on synovial cell interleukin-1 production in rheumatoid arthritis. *Lancet* **2,** 244–247.

71. Elliott, M. J., Maini, R. N., Feldmann, M., Kalden, J. R., Antoni, C., Smolen, J. S., et al. (1994) Randomised double-blind comparison of chimeric monoclonal antibody to tumor necrosis factor alpha (cA2) versus placebo in rheumatoid arthritis. *Lancet* **344,** 1105–1110.

72. Tak, P. P., Taylor, P. C., Breedveld, F. C., Smeets, T. J., Daha, M. R., Kluin, P. M., et al. (1996) Decrease in cellularity and expression of adhesion molecules by anti- tumor necrosis factor alpha monoclonal antibody treatment in patients with rheumatoid arthritis [see comments]. *Arthritis Rheum.* **39,** 1077–1081.

73. Moreland, L. W., Baumgartner, S. W., Schiff, M. H., Tindall, E. A., Fleischmann, R. M., Weaver, A. L., et al. (1997) Treatment of rheumatoid arthritis with a recombinant human tumor necrosis factor receptor (p75)-Fc fusion protein. *N. Engl. J. Med.* **337,** 141–147.

74. Walmsley, M., Katsikis, P. D., Abney, E., Parry, S., Williams, R. O., Maini, R. N., and Feldmann, M. (1996) Interleukin-10 inhibition of the progression of established collagen- induced arthritis. *Arthritis Rheum.* **39,** 495–503.

75. Hermann, J. A., Hall, M. A., Maini, R. N., Feldmann, M., and Brennan, F. M. (1998) Important immunoregulatory role of interleukin-11 in the inflammatory process in rheumatoid arthritis. *Arthritis Rheum.* **41,** 1388–1397.
76. Williams, R. O., Mason, L. J., Feldmann, M., and Maini, R. N. (1994) Synergy between anti-CD4 and anti-tumor necrosis factor in the amelioration of established collagen-induced arthritis. *Proc. Natl. Acad. Sci. USA* **91,** 2762–2766.
77. Choy, E. H., Kingsley, G. H., and Panayi, G. S. (1998) Monoclonal antibody therapy in rheumatoid arthritis. *Br. J. Rheumatol.* **37,** 484–490.
78. Moreland, L. W., Haverty, T. P., Wacholtz, M. C., Knowles, R. W., Bucy, R. P., Heck, L. W., Jr., and Koopman, W. J. (1998) Nondepleting humanized anti-CD4 monoclonal antibody in patients with refractory rheumatoid arthritis. *J. Rheumatol.* **25,** 221–228.
79. Kavanaugh, A. F., Davis, L. S., Jain, R. I., Nichols, L. A., Norris, S. H., and Lipsky, P. E. (1996) A phase I/II open label study of the safety and efficacy of an anti- ICAM-1 (intercellular adhesion molecule-1; CD54) monoclonal antibody in early rheumatoid arthritis. *J. Rheumatol.* **23,** 1338–1344.
80. Peacock, D. J., Banquerigo, M. L., and Brahn, E. (1992) Angiogenesis inhibition suppresses collagen arthritis. *J. Exp. Med.* **175,** 1135–1138.
81. Oliver, S. J., Banquerigo, M. L., and Brahn, E. (1994) Suppression of collagen-induced arthritis using an angiogenesis inhibitor, AGM-1470, and a microtubule stabilizer, taxol. *Cell Immunol.* **157,** 291–299.
82. Oliver, S. J., Cheng, T. P., Banquerigo, M. L., and Brahn, E. (1995) Suppression of collagen-induced arthritis by an angiogenesis inhibitor, AGM-1470, in combination with cyclosporin: reduction of vascular endothelial growth factor (VEGF). *Cell Immunol.* **166,** 196–206.
83. Storgard, C. M., Stupack, D. G., and Cheresh, D. A. (1997) Angiogenesis inhibition with aVb3 antagonist ameliorates early and chronic arthritis. *Arthritis Rheum.* **40,** S97.
84. Hirata, S., Matsubara, T., Saura, R., Tateishi, H., and Hirohata, K. (1989) Inhibition of *in vitro* vascular endothelial cell proliferation and *in vivo* neovascularization by low-dose methotrexate. *Arthritis Rheum.* **32,** 1065–1073.
85. Koch, A. E., Cho, M., Burrows, J., Leibovich, S. J., and Polverini, P. J. (1988) Inhibition of production of macrophage-derived angiogenic activity by the anti-rheumatic agents gold sodium thiomalate and auranofin. *Biochem. Biophys. Res. Commun.* **154,** 205–212.
86. Koch, A. E., Burrows, J. C., Polverini, P. J., Cho, M., and Leibovich, S. J. (1991) Thiol-containing compounds inhibit the production of monocyte/macrophage-derived angiogenic activity. *Agents Actions* **34,** 350–357.
87. Millauer, B., Longhi, M. P., Plate, K. H., Shawver, L. K., Risau, W., Ullrich, A., and Strawn, L. M. (1996) Dominant-negative inhibition of Flk-1 suppresses the growth of many tumor types in vivo. *Cancer Res.* **56,** 1615–1620.
88. Presta, L. G., Chen, H., O'Connor, S. S., Chisholm, V., Meng, Y. G., Krummen, L., et al. (1997) Humanization of an anti-vascular endothelial growth factor monoclonal antibody for the therapy of solid tumors and other disorders. *Cancer Res.* **57,** 4593–4599.
89. Aiello, L. P., Pierce, E. A., Foley, E. D., Takagi, H., Chen, H., Riddle, L., Ferrara, N., et al. (1995) Suppression of retinal neovascularization *in vivo* by inhibition of vascular endothelial growth factor (VEGF) using soluble VEGF-receptor chimeric proteins. *Proc. Natl. Acad. Sci. USA* **92,** 10,457–10,461.
90. Cheng, S. Y., Huang, H. J., Nagane, M., Ji, X. D., Wang, D., Shih, C. C., et al. (1996) Suppression of glioblastoma angiogenicity and tumorigenicity by inhibition of endogenous expression of vascular endothelial growth factor. *Proc. Natl. Acad. Sci. USA* **93,** 8502–8507.

10 Diagnostic and Prognostic Significance of Tumor Angiogenesis

Stephen B. Fox and Adrian L. Harris

CONTENTS

INTRODUCTION

The significance of tumor angiogenesis has been recognized for many centuries. Fallopio in the 1600s stated "cancers have dilated swollen veins resembling the legs of a crab, and this I single out from many signs since if its cure is undertaken the man nevertheless dies of the same cancer." However, it has only been since the turn of the century that continual and widespread research has been been performed, and it was not until the 1970s when Folkman and colleagues aroused interest in pathological angiogenesis that the first attempt was made to generate a systematic method for quantifying angiogenesis. The score was based on the assessment of several morphological parameters of "endothelial cell regeneration" stained by routine histological methods. Named the MAGS score (Microscopic Angiogenesis Grading System), it assessed the number of vessels, the degree of endothelial-cell hyperplasia, and the cytology of the tumor endothelium *(1)*. The aim was to develop an objective method for quantifying the tumor neovasculature that could be used as a standard for angiogenesis reasearch, to compare with other clinicopathological characteristics and be useful in the development and assessment of efficacy of anti-angiogenic agents and vascular targeting therapies *(2)*. However, many of the difficulties that still impede the clinical utility of angiogenesis quantitation systems today, including problems of tissue-sample selection, inter- and intraobserver variation, were such that the technique was not adopted. Further attempts to assess tumor angiogenesis were carried out using a variety of nonspecific endothelial markers but it has been only in the last five years, with the advent of highly specific endothelial markers *(3–5)* that can be used in histological archival tissues, that quantitation studies have been performed. As indicated earlier, there are still limitations to the current

From: *The New Angiotherapy*
Edited by: T.-P. D. Fan and E. C. Kohn © Humana Press Inc., Totowa, NJ

methodologies for measuring tumor angiogenesis but new methods are continually being assessed (*see* below). Furthermore, many of these mght have potential supplementary clinical uses such as in diagnosis, prediction of treatment response, and monitoring of disease status. Such methods might also be applied to other common and debilitating diseases such as psoriasis, rheumatoid arthritis (RA), atherosclerosis, and diabetic retin-opathy where angiogenesis is central to the pathological process.

The majority of studies on quantifying tumor angiogenesis have followed the method of Weidner et al. *(6)* and used anti-endothelial cell antibodies and a variety of immunohis-tochemical techniques to highlight the tumor vasculature. Briefly, the three areas contain-ing the maximum number of discrete microvessels are identified by scanning the tumor at low power. Individual microvessels are then counted on high-power objectives. Any immunoreactive endothelial cell(s) that is separate from adjacent microvessels is consid-ered a countable vessel. Vascular lumina are not a requirement to be included in the count and the vessels within any central sclerotic area of the tumor are not included. Most of these studies have shown that an increased microvessel density as a measure of angiogenesis is a powerful prognostic tool in many human tumor types (*see* below). Nevertheless, despite the initial confirmatory publications, numerous reports are now appearing in the literature that fail to show a positive association between increasing tumor vascularity and reduced patient outcome and caution as to the clinical utility of tumor angiogenesis is being urged *(7,8)*. However many of these negative studies are owing to significant differences in methodologies originally recognized by Brem et al. with the MAGS score *(1)* and demon-strate that the quantitation of tumor angiogenesis is still limited by the methods used for capillary identification and quantitation. There are several major considerations to take into account when quantifying tumor angiogenesis in histological sections using immunohis-tochemistry. These include the method used to identify the tumor vasculature, the represen-tative tumor area measured, the vascular parameter and the counting technique selected, and the cut-off used in the statistical analysis to derive the method.

VARIABLES IN THE QUANTIATION OF TUMOR ANGIOGENESIS
Methods to Identify the Tumor Vasculature

Studies vary in their method used to highlight tumor capillaries. Early studies used tinc-torial stains and morphology to identify the tumor vasculature. Many of these such as Masson's Tricrome *(9)* highlight the basement membrane of the microvessels. Other studies have used nonspecific endothelial cell markers such as alkaline phosphatase *(3)*, vimentin *(10)*, anti-lectin antibodies *(4,5,11,12)*, and type IV collagen *(13–15)*. Tinctorial stains and the latter antibody only pick up a small proportion of the total tumor vasculature because these highlight basement membrane, which is often discontinuous and has abnormal proportions of laminins and collagens. Nonspecific endotheial-cell markers also suffer because their sensitivity is below that of the newer endothelial-cell markers of which factor VIII related antigen, CD31 (PECAM) and CD34 are preferred. Specific anti-endothelial antibodies have their own prob-lems, not only owing to their distribution of expression (Table 1), but owing to significant heterogeneity between endothelia of different tissues *(16–18)*. Nevertheless it is a testament to the power of the technique that many using suboptimal markers have demonstrated a significant correlation between increasing angiogenesis and poor patient outcome. After assessing numerous endothelial-cell markers in our labortatory *(19)*, we selected an anti-CD31 antibody which in our hands is most sensitive and gives reliable microvessel immunostaining in routinely handled formalin-fixed, paraffin-embedded tissues *(19–22)*.

Table 1
Examples of Different Classes of Endothelial-Cell Markers

	Antigen	Distribution	Reference
Constitutive			
CD13	Aminopeptidase-n	Many cell types; brain endothelium	(195)
CD31	PECAM	Endothelium; plasma cells	(20)
CD34	Sialomucin	Endothelium; fibroblasts	(196)
CD36	Glycoprotein IV	Most endothelium	(197)
CD54	ICAM-1	Endothelium; leukocytes	(198)
CD 63	Lysosomal protein	Many cell types	(199)
CD102	ICAM-2	Most endothelium; leukocytes	(200)
FVIII RA	Von Willebrand factor	Most endothelium; platelets	(201)
Inducible			
CD62 P	P-selectin	endothelium; platelets	(199)
CD62 E	E-selectin	Activated endothelium	(198)
CD106	VCAM-1	Activated endothelium; leukocytes	(201)
Tumor-associated			
CD105	Endoglin	Tumor > normal vessels	(28)
FB5	Endosialin	Most tumor vessels	(202)
EN 7/44	p30.5 kD	Stains, tumors and inflammation	(203)
PAL-E	Unknown	Normal small vessels and tumor	(204)
4A11	Blood group	Preferential tumor and Inflammation	(205)

Nevertheless, where different antibodies have been compared, many have provided prognostic information (19,23–25). Furthermore, there is a significant correlation between the mean and median microvessel counts (19,23,26,27), suggesting that the negative findings in some studies (Table 2) is mostly owing to the differences in methodology for measuring tumor vascularity.

Several groups have investigated the use of antibodies that do not highlight all endothelium but selectively identify only the tumor-associated vasculature. This might not only more accurately measure tumor angiogenesis but might be useful as a objective for anti-angiogenesis and/or vascular-targeting strategies (28). Several antibodies have been generated that identify epitopes that are induced on tumor-associated endothelium and are largely absent or show highly restricted expression in normal tissues (Table 1). Thus, E-9, an anti-endoglin antibody is reported to be upregulated on tumor-associated endothelium, whereas anti-CD31, a more standard endothelial-cell marker, is negative (29). Similarly other restricted epitopes, such as a fetal fibronectin splice variant, are highly expressed on tumor-associated vessels (in up to 78% of breast cancers) compared to normal adult tissues (30). However, to date no quantification studies assessing the prognostic utlity of these markers have been performed.

The Selection of the Representative Tumor Area

Studies examining different tumor areas have shown significant heterogeneity between different tumor regions. The edge of the tumor is the most active area of angiogenesis (31,32) with little or no endothelial-cell proliferation occurring within its body (31). This is reflected in the microvessel density, which is usually highest at the periphery. Thus the particular tumor area that is measured will have profound effects on the data derived.

Table 2
Summary of Published Series Reporting the Relationship Between Quantitative Tumor Angiogenesis and Prognosis in Breast Cancer

Author (Ref. No.)	Year	n	Follow-up (months)	Magnification	Microscope field area mm²	Antibody	Cut-off	N° fields	Vessels/mm²	Univariate RFS	Univariate OS	Multivariate RFS	Multivariate OS
FOR													
Weidner et al. (26)	(1992)	165	51	×200	0.7386	FVIII	<34; 34–67; 68–100; >100	3	76	p < 0.001	p < 0.001	p < 0.001	p < 0.001
Horak et al. (19)	(1992)	103	30	×400	0.196	CD31	Median	3	100	p < 0.004	p < 0.04	p < 0.028	
Bosari et al. (49)	(1992)	120	108 min	×200	-	FVIII	Mean node- & recurrence	3	84^	p < 0.004	p < 0.008		
Toi et al. (23)	(1993)	125	62	×200	-	FVIII/CD31	100/150	3	99^	p < 0.01	-	p < 0.0226	
Visscher et al.[a] (13)	(1993)	58	-	×50	-	collagen IV	-	All tumor	19	p < 0.001			p < 0.019
Fox et al. (22)	(1994)	109 (N−)	5.3	×250	0.196	CD31	Median	3	53 (CC)	p < 0.01	p < 0.028	p < 0.039	
Lipponen et al. (169)	(1994)	173	120	×40	0.49	collagen IV	40	6	86.3 (CC)	NS	p < 0.0054	NS; significant in some models	
Fregone et al. (206)	(1994)	316	94	×400	0.19	FVIII	<25; 25–75; >75 centiles	1	-	p = 0.02		p < 0.0000011	p < 0.009
Toi et al. (166)[b]	(1995)	328	-	×200	-	FVIII	100	3	84	p < 0.00001			
Fox et al. (37)	(1995)	211	42	×250	0.196	CD31	Thirds	3	5.7 (CC)				
Bevilcqua et al. (207)	(1995)	211 (N−)	78	×200	0.74	CD31	Continuous variable	3	-	p < 0.000	p < 0.018	p < 0.0033	p < 0.044
Ogawa et al. (208)	(1995)	155	82	×200	0.785	FVIII	Mean	3	67.5	p < 0.025	p < 0.01	p < 0.002	p < 0.001
Obermair et al. (209)	(1995)	230	74	×200	0.25	FVIII	40	1	51	p < 0.0001		p < 0.004	
Barbareschi et al. (39)[a]	(1995)	91	66.3	×200	0.74	CD31	66	3	84	p < 0.002			
Kohlberger et al. (210)[a]	(1996)	60	79	×200	0.25	FVIII	Median	4	52.5	p < 0.024		p < 0.002 (N+)	p < 0.002 (N+)
Simpson et al. (211)[a]	(1996)	178	71	×20	0.74	CD34	Vessel area and number	1	142	NS	p < 0.023	p < 0.04	
Heinmann et al. (212)	(1996)	167	184	×400	0.1452	CD34	<15 per field	3 (<10)	138	p < 0.018			
AGAINST													
Hall et al. (34)	(1992)	87	-	×400	0.1256	FVIII	-	5	13	p < 0.92	0.05		
Van Hoef et al. (33)	(1993)	93 (N−)	151	×200	0.1225	FVIII	<68; 68–100; >100	4	245	NS	p < 0.99		
Siitonen et al. (24)	(1995)	77 (N−)	84 max	×200	0.739	CD34/FVIII	Highest/upper tertile	3	44/64				
Axelsson et al. (38)	(1995)	220-	136	×250	0.37	FVIII	Median	3	184 (N−/N+)	NS	NS	p < 065	p < 0.67
Goulding et al. (213)	(1995)	141	144 min	×250	0.37	CD31	Median	3	64	p < 0.06	p < 0.05	NS	NS
Costello et al. (53)	(1995)	87	114 max	×200	0.22	FVIII	≤75; 76–100:	3	186	NS	NS		
Morphopoulos et al. (214)	(1996)	160	61.2	×200	0.785	FVIII	>101–125; >126	3	139	NS			

The number of vessels/mm and follow-up times are median; boldface indicates median; max, maximal; min, minimal; NS, not significant. [a] image analysis; - not stated in paper; ^ per field area; [b] an undate of the 1993 paper; CC-Chalkley count (a CC of 6 equates to a 100 vessels/mm² at ×250); N−/N+, node negative/positive. Adapted with permission from ref. (28).

However, it is still remarkable that assessment of only one representative section can give a useful measure of tumor angiogenesis, because it has been estimated that one tissue section accounts for only 1/1000 of the total tumor mass.

Many tumors demonstrate significant heterogeneity within the tumor periphery with the presence of so-called vascular "hot spots." Although studies have measured random fields *(9)* and average vascularity *(4,11)*, most have assessed these hot spots, acknowledging that these are the areas that are likely to be biologically important in tumor-cell growth and metastases *(6,26)*. However, there is little agreement as to the optimal number of hot spots to assess, which currently ranges from 1–5 *(6,12,26,33–36)*. This number also has important bearings on the efficacy of the method because tumors have a limited number of identifiable hot-spots. Counting a large number of tumor fields will tend to diminish the power of the hot spot technique because there will be a tendency to reduce the average tumor vascularity the more fields that are assessed.

The tumor field area, determined by the microscopic magnification and particular objectives used, will also significantly effect the vascular index. A higher magnification gives an increased resolution, which enables more microvessels to be identified but to the detriment that all fields at too higher magnification become an angiogenic hot spot *(19)*. Conversely a low magnification with its lower resolution will identify a smaller number of vessels and will dilute out the "hot spot." We have demonstrated that measurements within magnification $\times 200$–400 over a range of 0.12–0.74 mm^2 give comparable information *(37)*.

The Vascular Parameter and the Counting Technique

Most studies quantifying tumor angiogenesis have measured microvessel density as a measure of tumor angiogenesis *(see* Tables 2 and 3). However, the vascular perimeter might be a better measure of angiogenesis than microvessel density because it may reflect the endothelial surface area available for interaction with the tumor, thereby increasing the likelihood of dissemination and metastasis. Similarly, the vascular surface area might give an indication of blood volume from which the tumor can derive nutrients in exchange for its waste products. We have examined the vascular parameters, microvessel density, luminal area, and perimeter *(37)* and have observed significant correlations between all, suggesting that these indices are equivalent for quantifying tumor vascularity.

In addition to the conceptual difficulties of microvessel density, there are several practical considerations making it unsuitable for a diagnostic pathology service. Microvessel counting is time-consuming, particularly when the tumor is of high vascularity and there is significant inter- and intraobserver variation, even when accounting for possible variations in microvessel criteria. In a confirmatory study, two pathologists trained by Weidner assessed microvessel density in 220 breast carcinoma patients with an extended period of follow-up *(38)*. No correlation between microvessel density and clinicopathological variables including patients survival, was observed. These findings are probably owing to the experience of the observers. It has been demonstrated that experienced observers differ significantly from trainee observers in quantifying tumor angiogenesis in breast tumors *(39)*. Nevertheless, in our experience, highly trained observers also occasionally disagreed on counts even with strict adherence to guidelines.

Owing to the aforementioned problems together with the additional conceptual difficulty of adjacent microvessels with significantly different vascular parameters assuming equal importance with the set criteria *(6,26)*, we and others have explored the use of a number of different techniques with the aim of developing a rapid and objective method for quantifying tumor angiogenesis.

Table 3
Some of the Published Series Showing the Relationship Between Quantitative Tumor Angiogenesis and Prognosis in Various Human Tumors

Author (Ref. No)	Year	n	Follow-up (mo)	Magnification/ field area	Antibody	Cut-off	N fields	Vessles/ mm^2	Analysis Univariate RFS	Univariate OS	Multivariate RFS	Multivariate OS
Bladder												
Dickinson et al. (21)	(1994)	45	37	×400/0.155	CD31	>7	3	6.3 (CC)		p = 0.019		p = 0.026
Bochner et al. (215)	(1995)	164	80	×200/-	CD34	≤64:65–99 ≥100	3	–	p = 0.0001	p = 0.0007	p = 0.0001	p = 0.0001
Philip et al. (216)	(1996)	113	>144	×160/-	CD31	–	12	–		p = 0.01		p = 0.04 (+ stage)
Prostate												
Vesalainen et al. (15)	(1994)	325	142.8	×400.49	Collagen IV	≤26:27–55 ≥55	5	50		p = 0.02		NS
Hall et al. (34)	(1994)	25	44	×200/0.754	FVIII	79.6	1	72.4	0.0003 (treated with radiotherapy)			
Kidney												
MacLennan et al. (217)	(1995)	97	90	×400/0.1855	FVIII	–	1	741.2		p = 0.05		
Colorectal												
Frank et al. (218)	(1995)	105	78	×100/-	FVIII	28	3	27.9^a	p = 0.0009	p = 0.004		
Bossi et al. (219)	(1995)	178	>60	×200/0.9	CD31	115/quantiles	3	115^a	NS	NS	NS	
Takebayashi et al. (220)	(1996)	166	76	×400/-	FVIII	65.3	1	65.3^a	p = 0.001	p = 0.03		p = 0.007
Lindmark et al. (221)	(1996)	212	55	×125/-	FVIII	≤5:6–10≥11	5	–		p = 0.007 (longer survival)		
Engel et al. (222)	(1996)	35	42	×400/0.152	CD31	>65	3	–	p = 0.0035		p = 0.0783	
Stomach												
Maeda et al. (179)	(1995)	124	>60	×200/0.785	FVIII	16	5	22	p = 0.05	p = 0.05	p = 0.05	p = 0.05
Tanigawa et al. (223)	(1996)	107	57	×200/-	FVIII/CD34	155	5	131(143)^a		p = 0.0001		p = 0.0001
Esophagus												
Tanigawa et al. (25)	(1997)	43	37	×200/-	FVIII/CD34	45/145	5	–	p = 0.05			
Cervix												
Rutgers et al. (224)	(1995)	70	24.5	×400/-	FVIII	–	3	56^a	p = 0.65			
Wiggins et al. (171)	(1995)	29	>14	×200/-	FVIII	–	1	–	4 relapsed all with high MVD			
Kainz et al. (225)	(1995)	43	–	×200/0.74	FVIII	>40	2	–	p = 0.01 (longer survival)			
Endometrium												
Kirschner et al. (226)	(1996)	45	75	×400/-	FVIII	≥10	–	–	NS	p = 0.02		
Ovary												
Van Diest (227)	(1995)	49	–	×250	ULEX	–	4	49.4/21.5^a		NS		
Hollingsworth et al. (173)	(1995)	43	30	×200/40/–0	CD34	16–44:≥45	3	48	p = 0.05	p = 0.034		NS
Gasparini et al. (228)	(1996)	112	90	×200/0.74	CD31	Continuous	1	–				
Lung												
Yamazaki et al. (229)	(1994)	42	>60	×200/0.723	FVIII	≤30:31–60: 61–90≥91	1	60^a	NS			
Macchiarini et al. (230)	(1994)	28	42	×200/-	FVIII	≥6	1	6^a	p = 0.0011	p = 0.0005	p = 0.008	
Mattern et al. (231)	(1995)	204	–	×250/-	FVIII	>9.6	1	9.6^a		NS		
Fontanini et al. (232)	(1995)	94	16	×250/0.41	FVIII	>61	1	61		p = 0.00067		p = 0.00046
Giatromanolaki et al. (232)	(1996)	107	45	×250/0.155	CD31	High vs low/medium	3	VG		p = 0.0004		p = 0.007

Table 3 (cont.)
Some of the Published Series Showing the Relationship Between Quantitative Tumor Angiogenesis and Prognosis in Various Human Tumors

Author (Ref. No)	Year	n	Follow-up (mo)	Magnification/ field area	Antibody	Cut-off	N° fields	Vessels/ mm²	Analysis Univariate		Analysis Multivariate	
									RFS	OS	RFS	OS
Bladdergeletti et al. (233)	(1996)	96	24	×200/0.78	FVIII	>31	1	31		$p = 0.00076$		$p = 0.02$
Harpole et al. (234)	(1996)	275	>68	×200/– (10)	FVIII	>4(>25)	1	4/16[a]		$p = 0.006$ (0.046)		$p = 0.021$ (NS)
Head and Neck												
Gasparini et al. (183)	(1993)	70	16	×250/0.384	CD31	>25	1	36 (**37.42**)	9/10 relapses>25			
Williams et al. (44)	(1994)	66	**48**	×400	FVIII	>10%	1	area	$p = 0.0001$	$p = 0.0766$		
Leedy et al. (182)	(1994)	57	**52**	×200/0.82	FVIII	>27	1	28	NS	NS		
Dray et al. (236)	(1995)	106	**53.2**	×200/–	FVIII	<33: 34–66: 67–100:>100	–	–	NS	NS	NS	NS
Roychowdhury et al. (237)	(1996)	30	44	×200/0.739	FVIII	>60	–	–	$p = 0.05$	$p = 0.02$		
Shpitzer et al. (238)	(1996)	25	>30	×250/–	FVIII	–	4	–	$p = 0.05$			
Melanoma												
Srivastava et al. (4)	(1988)	20	>60	×160/400	UEA-1	–	3–18	–	$p = 0.025$ (area only; 0.76–4.0 mm lesions)			
Carnochan et al. (11)	(1991)	107	>60	×200/–	UEA-1	–	3	–	NS (0.85–1.25 mm lesions)			
Graham et al. (239)	(1994)	10	≥120	×250/–	FVIII/CD34	–	1	–	$p = 0.05$	$p = 0.05$ (< 0.76 mm lesions)		
Busam et al. (240)	(1995)	120	**106.8**	×400/–	UEA-1	–	5	–	NS			

The number of vessels/mm and follow-up times are median; boldface indicates mean: NS, not significant; [a] per field area; VG, vascular grade; CC, Chalkley count (a CC of 6 equates to a 100 vessels/mm² at ×250); MVD, microvessel density.

In an attempt to automate the procedure, improve reproducibity and overcome the variations associated with "manual" counting, computer-image analysis systems have been assessed *(4,10,13,37,39–46)*. Using similar endothelial markers and vascular parameters, these reports have confirmed the findings of the manual studies and shown that quantitative angiogenesis gives independent prognostic information. However, in a manner similar to manual counting, these computer systems have their own general and specific problems, above their capital and running costs. An endothelial marker that will give a high signal-to-noise ratio is essential. This is important because the softwear employed to analyze the staining, unlike the human eye, is unable to determine specific from nonspecific immunoreactivity. The systems are not usually automated and require a high degree of operator interaction and will reproduce what the operator observes. To date, no software is available for identifying hot spots, although, partially automated systems with area and shape filters using defined color tolerances are available, which require reduced human control. In our experience, computer-image analysis system is more costly, time-consuming, unsuited to routine diagnostic practice, and no more accurate than a trained observer *(47)*.

To overcome the time and observer variation associated with microvessel density, we have assessed a method based on a point-counting method. The tumor section is scanned at low power (×10–100) to identify the three most vascular fields, before, at high power (×250), a 25-point Chalkley point eyepiece graticule is placed over each hot spot *(48)*. The eyepiece graticule is oriented so the maximum number of points are on or within areas of highlighted vessels, thereby bypassing interpretation difficulties of microvessel counting and reducing observer bias to the selection of the tumors area. This technique gives independent prognostic information for breast *(22,37)* and bladder carcinomas *(21)*.

To simplify the procedure further, and analgous to assessing tumor differentiation, we have explored the use of a vascular grading system based on the subjective appraisal by trained observers over a conference microscope. This method is significantly correlated with both microvessel density and Chalkley count and we have also shown it to be related to the presence of bone marrow micrometastasis in breast cancer patients (*see* below).

Statistical Analysis

There is considerable variation in cut-offs and types of analyses performed on angiogenesis data (Table 2). This alone can determine whether a particular angiogneic index correlates with other clinicopathological characteristics and/or will give prognostic information. Studies have used a variety of stratification indices including the highest and/or average microvessel density, the mean, the mean count in node-negative patients with recurrence *(49)*, or variable cut-offs given as a function of tumor area *(26,33)* or microscope magnification *(9,23,35,50–52)*. We and others have used the median *(19,21,22,53)* or tertile groups *(37)* because these stratifications avoid making any assumption regarding the relationship between tumor vascularity and other variables including survival.

ADDITIONAL METHODS FOR MEASURING TUMOR ANGIOGENISIS ACTIVITY

Tumor angiogenesis a complex pathway involving extracellular matrix remodeling, endothelial-cell migration and proliferation, capillary differentiation, and anastomosis *(54–56)*. There has been a huge increase in our knowledge over the past 15 yr facilitated by improvements in cell culture, molecular, and immunological teachniques that have identified many regulators of, and molecules involved in executing these events. Alternative strategies using these newly identified molecules as indices of tumor angiogenesis are being pursued and in due course these might complement or supercede vascular counts as angiogenic markers.

Angiogenic Factors and Receptors

In adult tissues, angiogenesis is actively suppressed such that new vessel formation only occurs during female reproductive cycle and wound healing. Tumor neovascularization results from the loss of this supression by altering the balance of angiogenic stimulators to inhibitors. Thus the tumor usurps the normal physiological angiogenic molecules for its own benefit, appropriating them to promote vessel growth. There is evidence that the switch to an angiogenic phenotype can occur before neoplastic transformation because many hyperplastic lesions demonstrate angiogenic activity; this has implications for the identification of clinical lesions, which are likely to progress (see below).

Upregulation of angiogenic factors and their receptors such as vascular endothelial growth factor A (VEGF-A), basic fibroblast growth factor (bFGF), and thymidine phosphorylase (TP) both at the mRNA and protein level has been reported in a range of histological tumor types (57–72). In lung (73), cervix (70), germ cell (74), and breast tumors (75) a significant relationship between microvessel density and VEGF has been observed. In gliomas (76), bladder (77), gastric (78), esophageal (79), lung, and breast cancers (80), VEGF expression is significantly higher in tumors that relapse compared to those that do not recur and in the latter tumor, VEGF gives independent prognostic information (75). Recently high expression of KDR, a VEGF receptor, has also been correlated with high vessel counts and advanced-stage colon carcinomas (57). Furthermore, TP expression in breast carcinomas has also been shown to correlate with tumor vascularity in breast (81) and colon cancers (82,83), although not all studies in breast carcinomas have confirmed this observation (84) TP is expressed not only in the neoplastic tumor epithelium, but is also present in stromal fibroblasts, macrophages, and endothelium (84). Thus a tumor unable to express this angiogenic factor in its neoplastic component might still be able to raise total tumor TP by upregulating this angiogenic factor in ancilliary cells such as macophages and fibroblasts. Indeed in colon cancers where TP expression rarely occurs in the neoplastic epithelium, the intensity of staining in tumor infiltrating cells correlates with tumors vascularity (82).

Angiogenic factors have been measured in cancer patients' serum (85,86), urine (77,87), and cerebrospinal fluid (88). These have shown that although angiogenic factors are expressed more highly with advancing tumor grade and stage, there is considerable overlap with controls and elevated levels are likely to be prominant in other pathological processes such as inflammation. Soluble tyrosine kinase receptors such as flt-1 (89) as well as angiogenic receptor ligands might also give an index of angiogenic activity of a tumor.

An alternative and more perhaps profitable strategy would be to identify diferent angiogenic pathways that might indicate the clinical behavior of particular tumors. Thus superficial and invasive bladder carcinomas are characterized by different angogenic pathways defined by high VEGF and low TP (and vice versa) (77). Similarly, in colorectal carcinomas those tumors with high vessel counts but low VEGF are distinguished by high TP (82).

The identification of several naturally occuring negative regulators of angiogenesis (90–93) raises the question as to their role in determining the angiogenic activity of tumors. In animal models, angiostatin, a 38kD plasminogen fragment generated within the primary tumor that actively suppresses angiogenesis, induces tumor dormancy by increasing tumor-cell apoptosis, such that it balances tumor-cell proliferation (93). However, to date, no clinical studies in carcinoma-bearing patients have been reported. Similarly, there is little human data on thrombospondin-1 (TSP-1) another powerful inhibitory angiogenic factor. In tumor-cell lines, angiogenesis is associated with low TSP-1 expression (94,95) and in Li-Fraumeni patients, p53 inhibits angiogenesis through regulation of TSP-1 (96). The identification of other naturally occuring inhibitors that might be useful in assessing tumor angiogenesis, such as TSP-2 (97) and an angiogenic inhibitor isolated from gliomas (92), suggests that more negative angiogenic regulators will be characterized.

Considerable improvements in specificity and sensitivity of the current techniques are necessary to accurately assess the angiogenic activity of a tumor. Angiogenic factors can be secreted by any of the tumor elements and can act directly by stimulating endothelial cells and/or indirectly via other stromal cells. Further modulation can result from cleaving matrix-bound growth factors (98) and receptors (99) by enzymes secreted by the tumor. Thus study of the expression of individual tumor compartments might give a better understanding of the origin of angiogenic factors and the contribution that ancilliary cells have in determining the vascularity of the tumors. Therefore the measurement of an angiogenic profile derived from a variety of assays will give a more reliable quantiative index and be clinically useful.

Although there are numerous potent angiogenic molecules, for many little is known about their role in different stages of the development of the tumor vasculature. It is difficult for some such as bFGF to dissect out their precise effect on angiogenesis because they have a number of effects on many cell types (71,100). Similarly, the mechanism of action of others, e.g., TP, is unknown. Continuing research will overcome shortcomings in our understanding and help give a more complete picture of the role of many candidate angiogenic pathways in human tumor angiogenesis, permitting their use in the quantitation of tumor angiogenesis.

Endothelial-Cell Proliferation

The current methods for measuring EC proliferation are cumbersome (31), but it is feasible that in the future, a rapid and technically robust measure might give an index of the angiogenic activity of a tumor. This particular measurement might have more utility in identifying which patients might benefit from those anti-angiogenic agents that effect EC proliferation than other aspects of the angiogenic pathway (see below).

Proteolytic Enzymes

The proteolytic systems such as the plasminogen activators (101) and the matrix metalloproteinases (102) that are important in tumor-cell invasion are also used for remodeling the existing vasculature during angiogenesis. Elevated levels of uPA and PAI-1 are associated with a poor prognosis in several tumor types, including breast (103–109) and colon (110). A significant correlation between microvessel density and both uPA and PAI-1 has been observed in breast-cancer patients (31,111) with expression of uPA, uPAR, and PAI-1 concentrated at the endothelial-tumor interface where angiogenic remodeling is most prominent (31,32). This suggests that the reduction in patient survival in patients with high levels of uPA and PAI-1 is partly owing to the angiogenic activity of these tumors, the expression of the latter having a protective rather than inhibitory effect.

Thus measurement of proteases particularly the urokinase system might give an indication of the angiogenic activity of a tumor. Currently, assays using homogenates of primary tumor have shown potential, but measurement of the components of this system in the serum of cancer-bearing patients might also be a possibility.

Cell-Adhesion Molecules

Endothelial-cell adhesion molecules (CAMs) of the immunoglobulin, selectin *(112–114)*, and integrin *(115–123)* superfamilies, which have physiological roles in immune and inflammatory trafficking and tumor metastasis, also play a major role in angiogenesis *(32,124)* and tumor stroma formation *(125,126)* In melanoma patients, upregulation of E and P selectins on the tumor endothelium is significantly associated with a shorter survival *(128)* and soluble CAMs are readily identified in sera of cancer-bearing patients *(128,129)*. Furthermore, in addition to the use of CAMs as a prognostic marker, they might be also serve as a traget for anti-angiogenic or vascular-targeting therapies *(119,120)*. Several integrins have also been shown to be expressed selectively during angiogenesis and are critical in the formation of capillaries through their effects on cell-cell and cell-matrix interactions. In vivo, the same integrins are important in mediating endothelial integrity ($\alpha_2\beta_1$ and $\alpha_5\beta_1$), whereas others effect endothelial-cell migration and tube formation ($\alpha_2\beta_1$ and $\alpha_v\beta_3$) *(113,114,116,129,130)*, the effects of particular growth factors being dependent on different integrins. bFGF is dependent on $\alpha_v\beta_3$, whereas VEGF is dependent on $\alpha_v\beta5$ *(131)*. In vivo angiogenesis is severly perturbed by interruption of $\alpha_v\beta_3$ integrin function *(118,119)*, underlining the importance of these adhesion molecules in new vessel growth.

Tumor Vascular Architecture

Newly formed vessels are abnormal in several respects: the capillaries are dilated, saccular, sinusoidal, and tortuous, and there are multiple bifurcations, loops, and blind-ending sprouts *(132)*. The vascular architecture of tumors varies not only within different anatomical sites *(133,134)* but also within tumors of similar and different histological types *(132)*. It has been suggested that the morphological assessment of particular vascular patterns might distinguish benign from malignant lesions *(135,136)* and act as a prognostic indicator (e.g., a closed back-to-back loop vascular pattern in occular malignant melanomas) *(137)*.

In Vivo Measurement of Tumor Angiogenesis

The aforementioned methods for assessing tumor angiogenic activity are mostly invasive techniques. The single and/or repeated measurement of in vivo tumor angiogenesis has many potential uses particularly in appraising the efficacy of anti-angiogenic agents and in designing appropriate treatment strategies.

Like the vascular architecture of tumors, tumor blood flow also shows significant variation with arterio-venous shunting, accounting for up to 30% of blood flow in human head and neck tumors. In addition, bloodflow is intermittent, with periods of reverse flow or stasis *(138,139)*. The high interstitial pressure and abnormal vascular architecture further compromise bloodflow *(139,140)*. These physical characteristics together with a lack of innervation *(141)* and abnormal responses to vasoactive stimuli result in perfusion indices for some tumors below that of the normal tissue counterpart *(142)*.

Nevertheless, studies investigating bloodflow using the imaging techniques of color Doppler *(143)* and magnetic resonance (MRI), particularly in breast *(144,145)* and gynecological lesions, have reported differences between benign and malignant lesions (although overlap is observed) *(61,146,147)*. Although these techniques have a high specificity, they suffer from a low sensitivity *(148)*. Further use of contrast agents significantly improves the sensitivity of these techniques, allowing imaging of tumor vessels not assessable at the baseline level *(149)*. However, not all studies have shown these noninvasive methods to be related to microvessel density *(144,145,150)*, which probably reflects the technical difficulties in directly comparing the radiological and histological planes. Nevertheless, these methods do give complementary data on the angiogenic activity of a tumor demonstrated by the significant correlation in ovarian tumors between bloodflow and tumor TP mRNA expression *(61)*. Indeed it has been suggested that the magnetic resonance contrast enhancement observed in ductal carcinoma *in situ* of the breast *(151)* is owing to the increased vascularity in the stroma between effected ducts *(152,153)*.

Other techniques that have not been fully evaluated include positron emmission spectroscopy, magnetic resonance spectroscopy, and thermography *(154)*. These techniques are experimental and have not been validated in serial monitoring of cancers, limiting their current use. Although no human data are reported, oxygen tension can be measured with an Eppendorf oximeter, and this has shown the degree of tumor hypoxia relates to tumor behaviour. Studies to date are promising, with tumor oxygenation being a prognostic factor in advanced cervical carcinoma *(155)* and soft-tissue sarcomas *(156)*. Indeed hypoxia is one epigenetic mechanism by which tumors upregulate angiogenic factors such as VEGF *(157)* and scanning patients for angiogenic factors such as VEGF and/or their receptors might be a useful noninvasive technique to assess the angiogenic activity of particular tumors. Monitoring tumor oxygen tension might also play a role in assessing suitablility for bioreductive drugs.

CLINICAL APPLICATIONS OF TUMOR ANGIOGENESIS
Diagnosis

Early studies using bioassays examining the angiogenic activity of normal, hyperplastic, and neoplastic breast lesions demonstrated a progressive increase in angiogenic activity during the transition from hyperplasia to carcinoma with a proportion of hyperplastic lesions able to elicit an angiogenic response *(158,159)*; similar angiogenic actitivy has been reported for pre-neoplastic bladder lesions *(160)*. The measurement of this angiogenic switch before neoplastic transformation might therefore give an indication of the likelihood of the progression of individual proliferative lesions

There is some evidence to support this premise: the risk of developing breast cancer is higher in those patients with fibrocystic disease and an elevated microvessel density *(50)*. Studies have also shown that the increase in vascularity in benign breast disease *(161)* over controls is proportional to the degree of epithelial proliferation *(162)*. Moreover, even after neoplastic transformation, like its invasive counterpart, vascular density might give clinically useful information. Particular patterns of vascularity in comdeo-type ductal carcinoma in situ (DCIS) identifies a subset of lesions that are at increased risk of progression to invasive disease *(152,153,162)*; a similar increase in microvessel density has been reported for the transition from normal to neoplastic prostatic tissues *(163,164)*.

Many of the aforementioned measures of angiogenesis, particularly those techniques suitable for in vivo use, might not only be useful for this determining which benign or *in situ* lesions are likely to progress, but with complementary investigations help in screening programs such as those for breast and ovary, increasing the ability to detect progressing disease.

Table 4
Quantitative Angiogenesis Studies in Other Miscellaneous
Human Tumors

Author (ref.)	Tumor type
Leon et al (241)	Brain
Li et al. (86)	Brain
Wesseling et al. (242)	Brain
Ito et al. (243)	Brain metastasis
Foss et al. (244)	Uveal melanoma
Folberg et al. (137)	Uveal melanoma
Ohsawa et al. (186)	Sarcoma
Pluda and Parkinson (245)	Pancreas
Hellstrom et al. (246)	Fallopian tube
Liu et al. (247)	Phaeochromocytomas
Sulh et al. (248)	Giant-cell tumors of bone
Meitar et al. (249)	Neuroblastoma
Vacca et al. (250)	Myeloma
Segal et al. (251)	Thyroid
Fontanini et al. (252)	Thyroid
Staibano et al. (253)	Basal-cell carcinoma

Prognostic Marker

Initial studies in breast cancer by Weidner et al. (6) showed that the number of vessels in lymph-node positive tumors had a significantly higher microvessel density than lymph-node negative tumors. Several groups using a similar technique subsequently showed that microvessel density was an independent prognostic factor in breast cancer (19,26,49). Then, there have been numerous papers examining the relationships between quantiative tumor angiogenesis and survival in numerous human tumor types. Although there is significant variation in patient populations and techniques used, most studies have demonstrated in a variety tumor types—including breast (19,26,49,165–169), female (170–173), and male genitourinary (10,41,51,174,175), brain (88), bladder (21,176), lung (177,178), gastro-intestinal (5,179,180), head and neck (44,181–185) and soft tissue (186)—that tumors of high vascularity are associated with lymph-node metastasis and a poor prognostic phenotype (Tables 2–4). The negative studies have usually resulted from using methodologies that have significantly strayed from the original technique of Weidner et al. (see Tables 2 and 3); also reviewed in refs. 6,187).

Staging

Despite appropriate surgical treatment, many early-stage breast cancer patients will die from metastastic disease that is undetected by conventional methods at presentation. Because immunohistochemically identified bone marrow micrometastasis at primary surgery has predicted disease progression, it has been suggested that procedure would be useful staging procedure and help to define who would benefit from adjuvant therapy. However the methods are technically difficult, the sensitivity relying on the number of sites and volume of marrow examined together with the antibody and detection system used (188–190). We have shown a significant association between high angiogenesis in primary breast tumors measured by vascular grading and the presence of bone marrow micrometastasis, suggesting that quantitative angiogenesis might be useful as a surrogate marker for the capacity of a tumor to metastasize.

Treatment Stratification and Disease Monitoring

Quantitative tumor angiogenesis can potentially identify a subgroup of patients with have poor prognoses who might benefit from adjuvant therapy. Patients with estrogen-receptor positive tumors that are highly angiogenic have a significant reduction in relapse-free survival despite tamoxifen treatment *(191)*. These patients could be offered more aggressive therapeutic options. At present, this is limited to high-dose chemotherapy and stem-cell rescue, but as anti-angiogenic and vascular targeting agents become available, the angiogenic activity of tumors might be used to stratify patients for these novel anti-cancer therapies. Particular measures of angiogensis might also give an indication as to which anti-angiogenic/vascular targeting strategies would be most effective.

These same angiogenesis assays also might help in several additional aspects of patient management, including monitoring immediate patient response, refining treatment, and identifying and treating relapses.

Prediction of Response to Therapy

Tumor vascularity might not only be useful in stratifying patients for different treatment regimes, but there is some evidence to suggest that they might be useful in predicting patient response to chemotherapy. Protopapa et al. *(9)* showed that high vascular counts are predictive of response to chemotherapy in a small series of breast carcinomas, although other studies have not confirmed this observation *(192)*. We have shown that tumor expression of TP is associated with a significant increase in survival in node-positive patients treated with cyclophosphamide, methotrexate, and 5-fluorouracil (5-FU) *(193)*. This might be owing to the enzymatic action of this angiogenic factor converting 5-FU to its active metabolite, in addition to preventing thymidine salvage of the methotrexate block *(193)*. Thus in additon to the use of TP as a predictive marker, it might also be helpful in stratifying patients for chemotherapy.

Trials Using Conventional and Antiangiogenic/Vascular Targeting Agents

The problems of assessing angiogenic agents in clinical trials are not unique to these drugs, but apply to many novel agents. In Phase I trials, the conventional endpoints are assessment of toxicity and development of a dose that will be tolerable for Phase II trials. Although encouraging, response to treatment is not an end-point in Phase I. However, it is desirable to show some therapeutic modification of the target, because it may be the only time a dose-response effect can be studied. Serial biopsies (trucut or fine-needle aspirates), conventional systemic markers (aFP, CA125, and PSA), together with assessment of angiogenesis (methods discussed earlier) can be used to monitor patients. These in vivo effects must be considered in advance as many potentially useful drugs will be discarded because assays are unavailable for the planned trial start date, thereby losing a major opportunity for drug assessment. A close partnership of clinical researchers with basic laboratories and the pharmaceutical industry is therefore essential for the testing of novel agents.

Although less common than patients with visceral metastases, skin, or superficial lymph-node metastases are readily studied. Direct intralesional drugs can be administered, the effect monitored by MRI, color Doppler, and thermography, combined with invasive techniques to quantify drug levels, study target enzymes, or receptors and changes in angiogenic mRNA levels.

CONCLUSIONS

Histological quantitation of tumor angiogenesis gives independent prognostic information in many tumor types. However, standardization of the technique using optimal endothelial markers, a reproducible method for microvessel quantitation and a standard cut-off for patient stratification is required that, when applied to a randomized prospective study, will establish the true value of tumor angiogenesis as a clinical marker in routine practice. Newer assays like growth factor or protease profiles might complement or supercede histological measures and in the future, the use of molecular techniques on samples derived from biopsies, fine-needle aspirations, serum, urine, or CSF will establish the angiogenic activity of tumor and help in the selection of particular drugs. The advances in basic angiogenesis research, which are now being transfered to clinical trials *(194)*, might, in the not -too-distant future, be applied to routine practice.

REFERENCES

1. Brem, S., Cotran, R., and Folkman, J. (1972) Tumor angiogenesis: a quantitative method for histological grading. *J. Natl. Cancer Inst.* **48,** 34–356.
2. Folkman, J. (1971) Tumor angiogenesis: therapeutic implications. *N. Engl. J. Med.* **285,** 82–86.
3. Mlynek, M., van Beunigen, D., Leder, L.-D., and Streffer, C. (1985) Measurement of the grade of vascularisation in histological tumor tissue sections. *Br. J. Cancer* **52,** 945–948.
4. Svrivastava, A., Laidler, P., Davies, R., Horgan, K., and Hughes, L. (1988) The prognostic significance of tumor vascularity in intermediate thickness (0.76–4.0mm thick) skin melanoma. *Am. J. Pathol.* **133,** 419–423.
5. Porschen, R., Classen, S., Piontek, M., and Borchard, F. (1994) Vascularization of carcinomas of the esophagus and its correlation with tumor proliferation. *Cancer Res.* **54,** 587–91.
6. Weidner, N., Semple, J. P., Welch, W. R., and Folkman, J. (1991) Tumor angiogenesis and metastasis—correlation in invasive breast carcinoma. *N. Engl. J. Med.* **324,** 1–8.
7. Page, D. L. and Dupont, W. D. (1992) Breast cancer angio-histogenesis: through a narrow window [editorial; comment]. *J. Natl. Cancer Inst.* **84,** 1850–1851.
8. Page, D. and Jensen, R. (1995) Angiogenesis in human breast carcinoma. *Human Pathol.* **26,** 1173–1174.
9. Protopapa, E., Delides, G. S., and Revesz, L. (1993) Vascular density and the response of breast carcinomas to mastectomy and adjuvant chemotherapy. *Eur. J. Cancer.* **29A,** 1141–1145.
10. Wakui, S., Furusato, M., Itoh, T., Sasaki, H., Akiyama, A., Kinoshita, I., et al. (1992) Tumor angiogenesis in prostatic carcinoma with and without bone marrow metastases: a morphometric study. *J. Pathol.* **168,** 257–262.
11. Carnochan, P., Briggs, J. C., Westbury, G., and Davies, A. J. (1991) The vascularity of cutaneous melanoma: a quantitative histological study of lesions 0.85–1.25 mm in thickness. *Br. J. Cancer* **64,** 102–107.
12. Barnhill, R. L., Fandrey, K., Levy, M. A., Mihm, M. J., and Hyman, B. (1992) Angiogenesis and tumor progression of melanoma. Quantification of vascularity in melanocytic nevi and cutaneous malignant melanoma. *Lab. Invest.* **67,** 331–337.
13. Visscher, D., Smilanetz, S., Drozdowicz, S., and Wykes, S. (1993) Prognostic significance of image morphometric microvessel enumeration in breast carcinoma. *Anal. Quant. Cytol.* **15,** 88–92.
14. Visscher, D., DeMattia, F., and Boman, S. (1994) Technical factors affecting image morphometric microvessel density counts in breast carcinomas. *Lab. Invest.* **70,** 168A (abstract).
15. Vesalainen, S., Lipponen, P., Talja, M., Alhava, E., and Syrjanen, K. (1994) Tumor vascularity and basement membrane structure as prognostic factors in T1-2M0 prostatic adenocarcinoma. *Anticancer Res.* **14,** 709–714.
16. Kuzu, I., Bicknell, R., Harris, A. L., Jones, M., Gatter, K. C., and Mason, D. Y. (1992) Heterogeneity of vascular endothelial cells with relevance to diagnosis of vascular tumors. *J. Clin. Pathol.* **45,** 143–148.
17. Schlingemann, R. O., Rietveld, F. J., Kwaspen, F., van, d. K. P., de, W. R., and Ruiter, D. J. (1991) Differential expression of markers for endothelial cells, pericytes, and basal lamina in the microvasculature of tumors and granulation tissue. *Am. J. Pathol.* **138,** 1335–1347.
18. Page, C., Rose, M., Yacoub, M., and Pigott, R. (1992) Antigenic heterogeneity of vascular endothelium. *Am. J. Pathol.* **141,** 673–683.

19. Horak, E. R., Leek, R., Klenk, N., LeJeune, S., Smith, K., Stuart, N., et al. (1992) Angiogenesis, assessed by platelet/endothelial cell adhesion molecule antibodies, as indicator of node metastases and survival in breast cancer. *Lancet* **340,** 1120–1124.

20. Parums, D., Cordell, J., Micklem, K., Heryet, A., Gatter, K., and Mason, D. (1990) JC70: a new monoclonal antibody that detects vascular endothelium associated antigen on routinely processed tissue sections. *J. Clin. Pathol.* **43,** 752–757.

21. Dickinson, A. J., Fox, S. B., Persad, R. A., Hollyer, J., Sibley, G. N., and Harris, A. L. (1994) Quantification of angiogenesis as an independent predictor of prognosis in invasive bladder carcinomas. *Br. J. Urol.* **74,** 762–766.

22. Fox, S., Leek, R., Smith, K., Hollyer, J., Greenall, M., and Harris, A. (1994) Tumor angiogenesis in node negative breast carcinomas-relationship to epidermal growth factor receptor and survival. *Breast Cancer Res. Treat.* **29,** 109–116.

23. Toi, M., Kashitani, J., and Tominaga, T. (1993) Tumor angiogenesis is an independent prognostic indicator in primary breast carcinoma. *Int. J. Cancer.* **55,** 371–374.

24. Siitonen, S., Haapasalo, H., Rantala, I., Helin, H., and Isola, J. (1995) Comparison of different immunohistochemical methods in the assessment of angiogenesis: lack of prognostic value in a group of 77 selected node-negative breast carcinomas. *Mod. Pathol.* **8,** 745–752.

25. Tanigawa, N., Matsumura, M., Amaya, H., Kitaoka, A., Shimomatsuya, T., Lu, C., et al. (1997) Tumor vascularity correlates with the prognosis of patients with esophageal squamous carcinoma. *Cancer* **79,** 220–225.

26. Weidner, N., Folkman, J., Pozza, F., Bevilacqua, P., Allred, E. N., Moore, D. H., et al. (1992) Tumor angiogenesis: a new significant and independent prognostic indicator in early-stage breast carcinoma. *J. Natl. Cancer Inst.* **84,** 1875–1887.

27. Weidner, N., Gasparini, G., Bevilacqua, P., Maluta, S., Palma, P., Caffo, O., et al. (1994) Tumor microvessel density, p53 expression, and tumor size are relevant prognostic markers in node negative breast carcinomas. *Lab. Invest.* **70,** A24 (abstract).

28. Burrows, F. J. and Thorpe, P. E. (1994) Vascular targeting: a new approach to the therapy of solid tumors. *Pharmacol. Ther.* **64,** 155–174.

29. Wang, J. M., Kumar, S., Pye, D., Haboubi, N., and Al-Nakib, L. (1994) Breast carcinoma: comparative study of tumor vasculature using two endothelial cell markers. *J. Natl. Cancer Inst.* **86,** 386–388.

30. Kaczmarek, J., Castellani, P., Nicolo, G., Spina, B., Allemanni, G., and Zardi, L. (1994) Distribution of oncofetal fibronectin isoforms in normal, hyperplastic and neoplastic human breast tissues. *Int. J. Cancer* **58,** 11–16.

31. Fox, S., Gatter, K., Bicknell, R., Going, J., Stanton, P., Cooke, T., and Harris, A. (1993) Relationship of endothelial cell proliferation to tumor vascularity in human breast cancer. *Cancer Res.* **53,** 9161–9163.

32. Fox, S., Turner, G., Gatter, K., and Harris, A. (1995) The increased expression of adhesion molecules ICAM-3, E and P selectin on breast cancer endothelium. *J. Pathol.* **177,** 369–376.

33. Van Hoef, M. E., Knox, W. F., Dhesi, S. S., Howell, A., and Schor, A. M. (1993) Assessment of tumor vascularity as a prognostic factor in lymph node negative invasive breast cancer. *Eur. J. Cancer* **29A,** 1141–1145.

34. Hall, N. R., Fish, D. E., Hunt, N., Goldin, R. D., Guillou, P. J., and Monson, J. R. (1992) Is the relationship between angiogenesis and metastasis in breast cancer real? *Surg. Oncol.* **1,** 223–229.

35. Sahin, A., Sneige, N., Singletary, E., and Ayala, A. (1992) Tumor angiogenesis detected by Factor-VIII immunostaining in node-negative breast carcinoma (NNBC): a possible predictor of distant metastasis. *Mod. Pathol.* **5,** 17A (abstract).

36. Sightler, H., Borowsky, A., Dupont, W., Page, D., and Jensen, R. (1994) Evaluation of tumor angiogenesis as a prognostic marker in breast cancer. *Lab. Invest.* **70,** 22A (abstract).

37. Fox, S. B., Leek, R. D., Weekes. M P, Whitehouse, R. M., Gatter, K. C., and Harris, A. L. (1995) Quantitation and prognostic value of breast cancer angiogenesis: comparison of microvessel density, Chalkley count and computer image analysis. *J. Pathol.* **177,** 275–283.

38. Axelsson, K., Ljung, B., Moore II, D., Thor, A., Chew, K., Edgerton, S., et al. (1995) Tumor angiogenesis as a prognostic assay for invasive ductal breast carcinoma. *J. Natl. Cancer Inst.* **87.**

39. Barbareschi, M., Weidner, N., Gasparini, G., Morelli, L., Forti, S., Eccher, C., et al. (1995) Microvessel quantitation in breast carcinomas. *Appl. Immunochem.* **3,** 75–84.

40. Simpson, J., Ahn, C., Battifora, H., and Esteban, J. (1994) Vascular surface area as a prognostic indicator in invsasive breast carcinoma. *Lab. Invest.* **70,** 22A.

41. Brawer, M. K., Deering, R. E., Brown, M., Preston, S. D., and Bigler, S. A. (1994) Predictors of pathologic stage in prostatic carcinoma. The role of neovascularity. *Cancer* **73,** 678–687.

42. Furusato, M., Wakui, S., Sasaki, H., Ito, K., and Ushigome, S. (1994) Tumor angiogenesis in latent prostatic carcinoma. *Br. J. Cancer* **70,** 1244–1246.

43. Bigler, S., Deering, R., and Brawer, M. (1993) Comparisons of microscopic vascularity in benign and malignant prostate tissue. *Human Pathol.* **24,** 220–226.

44. Williams, J. K., Carlson, G. W., Cohen, C., Derose, P. B., Hunter, S., and Jurkiewicz, M. J. (1994) Tumor angiogenesis as a prognostic factor in oral cavity tumors. *Am. J. Surg.* **168,** 373–380.

45. Wesseling, P., Vandersteenhoven, J. J., Downey, B. T., Ruiter, D. J., and Burger, P. C. (1993) Cellular components of microvascular proliferation in human glial and metastatic brain neoplasms. A light microscopic and immunohistochemical study of formalin-fixed, routinely processed material. *Acta. Neuropathol. (Berl.)* **85,** 508–514.

46. Charpin, C., Devictor, B., Bergeret, D., Andrac, L., Boulat, J., Horschowski, N., et al. (1995) CD31 Quantitative immunocytochemical assays in breast carcinomas. *Am. J. Clin. Pathol.* **103,** 443–448.

47. Fox, S., Turner, G., Leek, R., Whitehouse, R., Gatter, K., and Harris, A. (1995) The prognostic value of quantitative angiogenesis in breast cancer and role of adhesion molecule expression in tumor endothelium. *Br. Cancer Res. Treat.* **36,** 219–226.

48. Chalkley, H. (1943) Method for the quantative morphological analysis of tissues. *J. Natl. Cancer Inst.* **4,** 47–53.

49. Bosari, S., Lee, A. K., DeLellis, R. A., Wiley, B. D., Heatley, G. J., and Silverman, M. L. (1992) Microvessel quantitation and prognosis in invasive breast carcinoma. *Hum. Pathol.* **23,** 755–761.

50. Guinebretiere, J. M., Le, M. G., Gavoille, A., Bahi, J., and Contesso, G. (1994) Angiogenesis and risk of breast cancer in women with fibrocystic disease [letter]. *J. Natl. Cancer Inst.* **86,** 635–636.

51. Olivarez, D., Ulbright, T., DeRiese, W., Foster, R., Reister, T., Einhorn, L., and Sledge, G. (1994) Neovascularization in clinical stage A testicular germ cell tumor: prediction of metastatic disease. *Cancer Res.* **54,** 2800–2802.

52. Bundred, N., Bowcott, M., Walls, J., Faragher, E., and Knox, F. (1994) Angiogenesis in breast cancer predicts node metastasis and survival. *Br. J. Surg.* **81,** 768 (Abstract).

53. Costello, P., McCann, A., Carney, D. N., and Dervan, P. A. (1995) Prognostic significance of microvessel density in lymph node negative breast carcinoma. *Hum. Pathol.* **26,** 1181–1184.

54. Paweletz, N. and Knierim, M. (1989) Tumor-related angiogenesis. *Crit. Rev. Oncol. Hematol.* **9,** 197–242.

55. Blood, C. H. and Zetter, B. R. (1990) Tumor interactions with the vasculature: angiogenesis and tumor metastasis. *Biochim. Biophys. Acta.* **1032,** 89–118.

56. Bicknell, R. and Harris, A. L. (1991) Novel growth regulatory factors and tumor angiogenesis. *Eur. J. Cancer* **27,** 781–785.

57. Takahashi, Y., Kitadai, Y., Bucana, C. D., Cleary, K. R., and Ellis, L. M. (1995) Expression of vascular endothelial growth factor and its receptor, KDR, correlates with vascularity, metastasis and proliferation of human colon cancer. *Cancer Res.* **55,** 3964–3968.

58. Brown, D. M., Hong, S. P., Farrell, C. L., Pierce, G. F., and Khouri, R. K. (1995) Platelet-derived growth factor BB induces functional vascular anastomoses in vivo. *Proc. Natl. Acad. Sci. USA* **92,** 5920–5924.

59. Moghaddam, A., Zhang, H. T., Fan, T. P., Hu, D. E., Lees, V. C., Turley, H., et al. (1995) Thymidine phosphorylase is angiogenic and promotes tumor growth. *Proc. Natl. Acad. Sci. USA* **92,** 998–1002.

60. Anandappa, S. Y., Winstanley, J. H., Leinster, S., Green, B., Rudland, P. S., and Barraclough, R. (1994) Comparative expression of fibroblast growth factor mRNAs in benign and malignant breast disease. *Br. J. Cancer* **69,** 772–776.

61. Reynolds, K., Farzaneh, F., Collins, W. P., Campbell, S., Bourne, T. H., Lawton, F., et al. (1994) Association of ovarian malignancy with expression of platelet-derived endothelial cell growth factor. *J. Natl. Cancer Inst.* **86,** 1234–1238.

62. Garver, R. J., Radford, D. M., Donis, K. H., Wick, M. R., and Milner, P. G. (1994) Midkine and pleiotrophin expression in no.mal and malignant breast tissue. *Cancer* **74,** 1584–1590.

63. Janot, F., el, N. A., Morrison, R. S., Liu, T. J., Taylor, D. L., and Clayman, G. L. (1995) Expression of basic fibroblast growth factor in squamous cell carcinoma of the head and neck is associated with degree of histologic differentiation. *Int. J. Cancer* **64,** 117–123.

64. Gomm, J. J., Smith, J., Ryall, G. K., Ballic, R., Turnbull, L., and Coombes, R. C. (1991) Localisation of basic fibroblast growth factor and transforming growth factor b1 in the human mammary gland. *Cancer Res.* **51,** 4685–4692.

65. Zarnegar, R. and DeFrances, M. C. (1993) Expression of HGF-SF in normal and malignant human tissues. *Exs.* **65,** 181–199.

66. Daa, T., Kodama, M., Kashima, K., Yokoyama, S., Nakayama, I., and Noguchi, S. (1993) Identification of basic fibroblast growth factor in papillary carcinoma of the thyroid. *Acta Pathol. Jpn.* **43,** 582–589.

67. Wong, S. Y., Purdie, A. T., and Han, P. (1992) Thrombospondin and other possible related matrix proteins in malignant and benign breast disease. *Am. J. Pathol.* **140,** 1473–1482.

68. Schultz-Hector, S. and Haghayegh, S. (1993) B-Fibroblast growth factor expression in human and murine squamous cell carcinomas and its relationship to regional endothelial cell proliferation. *Cancer Res.* **53,** 1444–1449.

69. Alvarez, J. A., Baird, A., Tatum, A., Daucher, J., Chorsky, R., Gonzalez, A. M. and Stopa, E. G. (1992) Localisation of basic fibroblast growth factor and vascular endothelial cell growth factor in human glial neoplasms. *Mod. Pathol.* **5,** 303–307.

70. Guidi, A. J., Abu, J. G., Berse, B., Jackman, R. W., Tognazzi, K., Dvorak, H. F., and Brown, L. F. (1995) Vascular permeability factor (vascular endothelial growth factor) expression and angiogenesis in cervical neoplasia. *J. Natl. Cancer Inst.* **87,** 1237–1245.

71. Zagzag, D., Brem, S., and Robert, F. (1988) Neovascularization and tumor growth in the rabbit brain. A model for experimental studies of angiogenesis and the blood-brain barrier. *Am. J. Pathol.* **131,** 361–372.

72. Visscher, D. W., DeMattia, F., Ottosen, S., Sarkar, F. H., and Crissman, J. D. (1995) Biologic and clinical significance of basic fibroblast growth factor immunostaining in breast carcinoma. *Mod. Pathol.* **8,** 665–670.

73. Mattern, J., Koomagi, R., and Volm, M. (1996) Association of vascular endothelial growth factor expression with intratumoral microvessel density and tumor cell proliferation in human epidermoid lung carcinoma. *Br. J. Cancer* **73,** 931–934.

74. Viglietto, G., Romano, A., Maglione, D., Rambaldi, M., Paoletti, I., Lago, C., et al. (1996) Neovascularisation in human germ cell tumors correlates with a marked increase in the expression of the vascular endothelial growth factor but not the placenta growth factor. *Oncogene* **13,** 577–587.

75. Toi, M., Hoshina, S., Takayanagi, T., and Tominaga, T. (1994) Association of vascular endothelial growth factor expression with tumor angiogenesis and with early relapse in primary breast cancer. *Jpn. J. Cancer Res.* **85,** 1045–1049.

76. Takano, S., Yoshii, Y., Kondo, S., Suzuki, H., Maruno, T., Shira, S., and Nose, T. (1996) Concentration of vascular endothelial growth factor in the serum and tumor tissue of brain tumor patients. *Cancer Res.* **56,** 2185–2190.

77. O'Brien, T., Cranston, D., Fuggle, S., Bicknell, R., and Harris, A. L. (1995) Different angiogenic pathways characterize superficial and invasive bladder cancer. *Cancer Res.* **55,** 510–513.

78. Maeda, K., Chung, Y. S., Ogawa, Y., Kang, S., Takatsuka, S., Ogawa, M., Sawada, T., and Sowa, M. (1996) Prognostic value of vascular endothelial growth factor expression in gastric carcinoma. *Cancer* **77,** 858–863.

79. Inoue, K., Ozeki, Y., Suganuma, T., Sugiura, Y., and Tanaka, S. (1996) Vascular endothelial growth factor expression in primary esophageal squamous cell carcinoma-assocation with angiogenesis and tumor progression. *Cancer* **79,** 206–213.

80. Ohta, Y., Endo, Y., Tanaka, M., Shimizu, J., Oda, M., Hayashi, Y., et al. (1996) Significance of vascular endothelial growth factor messenger RNA expression in primary lung cancer. *Clin. Cancer Res.* **2,** 1411–1416.

81. Toi, M., Hoshina, S., Taniguchi, T., Yamamoto, Y., Ishitsuka, H., and Tominaga, T. (1995) Expression of platelet derived endothelial cell growth factor/thymidine phosphorylase in human breast cancer. *Int. J. Cancer* **64,** 79–82.

82. Takahashi, Y., Bucana, C., Liu, W., Yoneda, J., Kitadai, Y., Cleary, K. R., and Ellis, L. M. (1996) Platelet-derived endothelial cell growth factor in human colon angiogenesis: role of infiltrating cells. *J. Natl. Cancer Inst.* **88,** 1146–1151.

83. Takebayashi, Y., Akiyama, S., Akiba, S., Yamada, K., Miyadera, K., Sumizawa, T., et al. (1996) Clinicpathologic and prognostic significance of an angiogenic factor, thymidine phosphorylase, in human colorectal carcinoma. *J. Natl. Cancer Inst.* **88,** 1110–1117.

84. Fox, S. B., Westwood, M., Moghaddam, A., Comley, M., Turley, H., Whitehouse, R. M., et al. (1996) The angiogenic factor platelet-derived endothelial cell growth factor/thymidine phosphorylase is up-regulated in breast cancer epithelium and endothelium. *Br. J. Cancer* **73,** 275–280.

85. Fujimoto, K., Ichimori, Y., Kakizoe, T., Okajima, E., Sakamoto, H., Sugimura, T., and Terada, M. (1991) Increased serum levels of basic fibroblast growth factor in patients with renal cell carcinoma. *Biochem. Biophys. Res. Comm.* **180,** 386–392.

86. Kondo, S., Asano, M., Matsuo, K., Ohmori, I., and Suzuki, H. (1994) Vascular endothelial growth factor/vascular permeability factor is detectable in the sera of tumor-bearing mice and cancer patients. *Biochim. Biophys. Acta* **1221,** 211–214.

87. Nguyen, M., Watanabe, H., Budson, A. E., Richie, J. P., Hayes, D. F., and Folkman, J. (1994) Elevated levels of an angiogenic peptide, basic fibroblast growth factor, in the urine of patients with a wide spectrum of cancers. *J. Natl. Cancer Inst.* **86,** 356–361.

88. Li, V., Folkerth, R., Watanabe, H., Yu, C., Rupnick, M., Barnes, P., et al. (1994) Microvessel count and cerebrospinal fluid basic fibroblast growth factor in children with brain tumors. *Lancet* **344,** 82–86.

89. Kendall, R. L. and Thomas, K. A. (1993) Inhibition of vascular endothelial cell growth factor activity by an endogenously encoded soluble receptor. *Proc. Natl..Acad. Sci. USA* **90,** 10,705–10,709.

90. Good, D. J., Polverini, P. J., Rastinejad, F., Le, B. M., Lemons, R. S., Frazier, W. A., and Bouck, N. P. (1990) A tumor suppressor-dependent inhibitor of angiogenesis is immunologically and functionally indistinguishable from a fragment of thrombospondin. *Proc. Natl. Acad. Sci. USA* **87,** 6624–6628.

91. Rastinejad, F., Polverini, P. J., and Bouck, N. P. (1989) Regulation of the activity of a new inhibitor of angiogenesis by a cancer suppressor gene. *Cell* **56,** 345–355.

92. Van Meir, E. G., Polverini, P. J., Chazin, V. R., Su Huang, H. J., de Tribolet, N., and Cavenee, W. K. (1994) Release of an inhibitor of angiogenesis upon induction of wild type p53 expression in glioblastoma cells. *Nat. Genet.* **8,** 171–176.

93. O'Reilly, M. S., Holmgren, L., Shing, Y., Chen, C., Rosenthal, R. A., Moses, M., et al. (1994) Angiostatin: a novel angiogenesis inhibitor that mediates the suppression of metastases by a Lewis lung carcinoma. *Cell* **79,** 315–328.

94. Zabrenetzky, V., Harris, C. C., Steeg, P. S., and Roberts, D. (1994) Expression of the extracellular matrix molecule thrombospondin inversely correlates with malignant progression in melanoma, lung and breast carcinoma cell lines. *Int. J. Cancer* **59,** 191–195.

95. Weinstat-Saslow, D. L., Zabrenetzky, V. S., Van, H. K., Frazier, W. A., Roberts, D. D., and Steeg, P. S. (1994) Transfection of thrombospondin 1 complementary DNA into a human breast carcinoma cell line reduces primary tumor growth, metastatic potential, and angiogenesis. *Cancer Res.* **54,** 6504–6511.

96. Dameron, K. M., Volpert, O. V., Tainsky, M. A., and Bouck, N. (1994) Control of angiogenesis in fibroblasts by p53 regulation of thrombospondin-1. *Science* **265,** 1582–1584.

97. Volpert, O., Tolsma, S., Pellerin, S., Feige, J., Chen, H., Mosher, D., and Bouck, N. (1995) Inhibition of angiogenesis by thrombospondin-2. *Biochim. Biophys. Res. Comm.* **217,** 326–332.

98. Vlodavsky, I., Korner, G., Ishai, M. R., Bashkin, P., Bar, S. R., and Fuks, Z. (1990) Extracellular matrix-resident growth factors and enzymes: possible involvement in tumor metastasis and angiogenesis. *Cancer Metastasis Rev.* **9,** 203–226.

99. Hanneken, A., Maher, P., and Baird, A. (1995) High affinity immunoreactive FGF receptors in the extracellular matrix of vascular endothelial cells-implications for the modulation of FGF-2. *J. Cell Biol.* **128,** 1221–1228.

100. Friesel, R. E. and Maciag, T. (1995) Molecular mechanisms of angiogenesis: fibroblast growth factor signal transduction. *FASEB J.* **9,** 919–925.

101. Pepper, M. and Montesano, R. (1990) Proteolytic balance and capillary morphogenesis. *Cell Diff. Dev.* **32,** 319–328.

102. Fisher, C., Gilbertson, B. S., Powers, E. A., Petzold, G., Poorman, R., and Mitchell, M. A. (1994) Interstitial collagenase is required for angiogenesis in vitro. *Dev. Biol.* **162,** 499–510.

103. Grondahl-Hansen, J., Christensen, I. J., Rosenquist, C., Brunner, N., Mouridsen, H. T., Dano, K., and Blichert, T. M. (1993) High levels of urokinase-type plasminogen activator and its inhibitor PAI-1 in cytosolic extracts of breast carcinomas are associated with poor prognosis. *Cancer Res.* **53,** 2513–2521.

104. Janicke, F., Schmitt, M., Pache, L., Ulm, K., Harbeck, N., Hofler, H., and Graeff, H. (1993) Urokinase (uPA) and its inhibitor PAI-1 are strong and independent prognostic factors in node-negative breast cancer. *Breast Cancer Res. Treat.* **24,** 195–208.

105. Foekens, J. A., Schmitt, M., van, P. W., Peters, H. A., Bontenbal, M., Janicke, F., and Klijn, J. G. (1992) Prognostic value of urokinase-type plasminogen activator in 671 primary breast cancer patients. *Cancer Res.* **52,** 6101–6105.

106. Duffy, M. J., Reilly, D., O'Sullivan, C., O'Higgins, N., Fennelly, J. J., and Andreasen, P. (1990) Urokinase-plasminogen activator, a new and independent prognostic marker in breast cancer. *Cancer Res.* **50,** 6827–6829.

107. Schmitt, M., Janicke, F., Moniwa, N., Chucholowski, N., Pache, L., and Graeff, H. (1992) Tumor-associated urokinase-type plasminogen activator: biological and clinical significance. *Biol. Chem. Hoppe Seyler* **373,** 611–622.

108. Spyratos, F., Martin, P. M., Hacene, K., Romain, S., Andrieu, C., Ferrero, P. M., et al. (1992) Multiparametric prognostic evaluation of biological factors in primary breast cancer. *J. Natl. Cancer Inst.* **84,** 1266–1272.

109. Sumiyoshi, K., Serizawa, K., Urano, T., Takada, Y., Takada, A., and Baba, S. (1992) Plasminogen activator system in human breast cancer. *Int. J. Cancer* **50,** 345–348.

110. Ganesh, S., Sier, C. F. M., Heerding, M. M., Griffioen, G., Lamers, C. B. H. W., and Verspaget, H. W. (1994) Urokinase receptor and colorectal cancer survival. *Lancet* **344,** 401–402.

111. Hildenbrand, R., Dilger, I., Horlin, A., and Stutte, H. J. (1995) Urokinase plasminogen activator induces angiogenesis and tumor vessel invasion in breast cancer. *Pathol. Res. Pract.* **191,** 403–409.

112. Nguyen, M., Strubel, N. A., and Bischoff, J. (1993) A role for sialyl Lewis-X/A glycoconjugates in capillary morphogenesis. *Nature* **365,** 267–269.

113. Kaplanski, G., Farnarier, C., Benoliel, A., Foa, C., Kaplanski, S., and Bongrand, P. (1994) A novel role for E- and P-selectins: shape of endothelial cell monolayers. *J. Cell Sci.* **107,** 2449–2457.

114. Koch, A., Halloran, M. M., Haskell, C. J., Shah, M. R., and Polverini, P. J. (1995) Angiogenesis mediated by soluble forms of E-selectin and vascular cell adhesion molecule-1. *Nature* **376,** 517–519.

115. Leavesley, D. I., Schwartz, M. A., Rosenfeld, M., and Cheresh, D. A. (1993) Integrin beta 1- and beta 3-mediated endothelial cell migration is triggered through distinct signaling mechanisms. *J. Cell Biol.* **121,** 163–170.

116. Davis, C. M., Danehower, S. C., Laurenza, A., and Molony, J. L. (1993) Identification of a role of the vitronectin receptor and protein kinase C in the induction of endothelial cell vascular formation. *J. Cell Biochem.* **51,** 206–218.

117. Bauer, J., Margolis, M., Schreiner, C., Edgell, C. J., Azizkhan, J., Lazarowski, E., and Juliano, R. L. (1992) In vitro model of angiogenesis using a human endothelium-derived permanent cell line: contributions of induced gene expression, G-proteins, and integrins. *J. Cell Physiol.* **153,** 437–449.

118. Luscinskas, F. W. and Lawler, J. (1994) Integrins as dynamic regulators of vascular function. *FASEB J.* **8,** 929–938.

119. Brooks, P. C., Clark, R. A., and Cheresh, D. A. (1994) Requirement of vascular integrin alpha v beta 3 for angiogenesis. *Science* **264,** 569–571.

120. Brooks, P. C., Montgomery, A. M., Rosenfeld, M., Reisfeld, R. A., Hu, T., Klier, G., and Cheresh, D. A. (1994) Integrin alpha v beta 3 antagonists promote tumor regression by inducing apoptosis of angiogenic blood vessels. *Cell* **79,** 1157–1164.

121. Brooks, P. C., Stromblad, S., Klemke, R., Visscher, D., Sarkar, F. H., and Cheresh, D. A. (1995) Antiintegrin $\beta_3\alpha_v$ blocks human breast cancer growth and angiogenesis in human skin. *J. Clin. Invest.* **96,** 1815–1822.

122. Gamble, J. R., Matthias, L. J., Meyer, G., Kaur, P., Russ, G., Faull, R., et al. (1993) Regulation of in vitro capillary tube formation by anti-integrin antibodies. *J. Cell Biol.* **121,** 931–943.

123. Jackson, C. J., Knop, A., Giles, I., Jenkins, K., and Schrieber, L. (1994) VLA-2 mediates the interaction of collagen with endothelium during in vitro vascular tube formation. *Cell Biol. Int.* **18,** 859–867.

124. Zocchi, M. R. and Poggi, A. (1993) Lymphocyte-endothelial cell adhesion molecules at the primary tumor site in human lung and renal cell carcinomas [letter]. *J. Natl. Cancer Inst.* **85,** 246–247.

125. Dvorak, H. F. (1987) Thrombosis and cancer. *Hum. Pathol.* **18,** 275–284.

126. Palabrica, T., Lobb, R., Furie, B. C., Aronovitz, M., Benjamin, C., Hsu, Y. M., et al. (1992) Leukocyte accumulation promoting fibrin deposition is mediated in vivo by P-selectin on adherent platelets. *Nature* **359,** 848–851.

127. Schadendorf, D., Heidel, J., Gawlik, C., Suter, L., and Czarnetzki (1995) Association with clinical outcome of expression of VLA-4 in primary cutaneous malignant melanoma as well as P-selectin and E-selectin on intratumoral vessels. *J. Natl. Cancer Inst.* **87,** 366–371.

128. Kageshita, T., Yoshii, A., Kimura, T., Kuriya, N., Ono, T., Tsujisaki, M., et al. (1993) Clinical relevance of ICAM-1 expression in prmary lesions and serum of patients with malignant melanoma. *Cancer Res.* **53,** 4927–4932.

129. Banks, R. E., Gearing, A. J., Hemingway, I. K., Norfolk, D. R., Perren, T. J., and Selby, P. J. (1993) Circulating intercellular adhesion molecule-1 (ICAM-1), malignancies. *Br. J. Cancer* **68,** 122–124.

130. Bauer, H. C., Steiner, M., and Bauer, H. (1992) Embryonic development of the CNS microvasculature in the mouse: new insights into the structural mechanisms of early angiogenesis. *Exs* **61,** 64–68.

131. Gamble, J. R., Khew, G. Y., and Vadas, M. A. (1993) Transforming growth factor-beta inhibits E-selectin expression on human endothelial cells. *J. Immunol.* **150,** 4494–4503.

132. Warren, T., Keck, P. J., Hauser, S. D., Krivi, G., Sanzo, K., Feder, J., Connolly, D. T. (1989) Vascular permeability factor, an endothelial cell mitogen related to PDGF. *Science* **246,** 1309–1312.

133. Paku, S. and Lapis, K. (1993) Morphological aspects of angiogenesis in experimental liver metastases. *Am. J. Pathol.* **143,** 926–936.

134. Lauk, S., Zietman, A., Skates, S., Fabian, R., and Suit, H. D. (1989) Comparative morphometric study of tumor vasculature in human squamous cell carcinomas and their xenotransplants in athymic nude mice. *Cancer Res.* **49,** 4557–4561.

135. Smolle, J., Soyer, H. P., Hofmann-Wellenhof, Smolle-Juettner, F. M., and Kerl, H. (1989) Vascular architecture of melanocytic skin tumors. *Path. Res. Pract.* **185,** 740–745.

136. Cockerell, C. J., Sonnier, G., Kelly, L., and Patel, S. (1994) Comparative analysis of neovascularisation in primary cutaneous melanoma and Spitz nevus. *Am. J. Dermatopathol.* **16,** 9–13.

137. Folberg, R., Rummelt, V., Ginderdeuren, R.-V., Hwang, T., Woolson, R., Pe'er, J., and Gruman, L. (1993) The prognostic value of tumor blood vessel morphology in primary uveal melanoma. *Ophthalmology* **100,** 1389–1398.

138. Jain, R. K. (1994) Barriers to drug delivery in solid tumors. *Sci. Am.* **271,** 58–65.

139. Vaupel, P., Kallinowski, F., and Okunieff, P. (1990) Blood flow, oxygen consumption and tissue oxygenation of human tumors. *Adv. Exp. Med. Biol.* **277,** 895–905.

140. Jain, R. K. (1990) Vascular and interstitial barriers to delivery of therapeutic agents in tumors. *Cancer Metastasis Rev.* **9,** 253–266.

141. Mitchell, B. S., Schumacher, U., and Kaiserling, E. (1994) Are tumors innervated? Immunohistological investigations using antibodies against the neuronal marker protein gene product 9.5 (PGP 9.5) in benign, malignant and experimental tumors. *Tumor Biol.* **15,** 269–274.

142. Nystrom, C., Forssman, L., and Roos, B. (1969) Myometrial blood flow studies in carcinoma of the corpus uteri. *Acta Radiol. Ther.* **8,** 193–198.

143. Kurjak, A., Salihagic, A., Kupesic, U. S., and Predanic, A. (1992) Clinical value of the assessment of gynaecological tumour angiogenesis by transvaginal colour Doppler. *Ann. Med.* **24,** 97–103.

144. Frouge, C., Guinbretiere, J., Contesso, G., di Paola, R., and Blery, M. (1994) Correlation between contrast enhancement in dynamic magnetic resonance imaging of the breast and tumor angiogenesis. *Invest. Radiol.* **29,** 1043–1049.

145. Lee, W. J., Chu, J. S., Houng, S. J., Chung, M. F., Wang, S. M., and Chen, K. M. (1995) Breast cancer angiogenesis: a quantitative morphologic and Doppler imaging study. *Ann. Surg. Oncol.* **2,** 246–251.

146. Antonic, J. and Rakar, S. (1995) Colour and pulsed doppler US and tumor marker CA125 in differentiation between benign and malignant ovarian masses. *Anticancer Res.* **15,** 1527–1532.

147. Wu, C. C., Lee, C. N., Chen, T. M., Shyu, M. K., Hsieh, C. Y., Chen, H. Y., and Hsieh, F. J. (1994) Incremental angiogenesis assessed by color Doppler ultrasound in the tumorigenesis of ovarian neoplasms. *Cancer* **73,** 1251–1256.

148. Carter, J., Lau, M., Saltzman, A., Hartenbach, E., Chen, M., Johnson, P., et al. (1994) Gray scale and color flow Doppler characterization of uterine tumors. *J. Ultrasound Med.* **13,** 835–840.

149. Ernst, H., Hahn, E., Balzer, T., Schlief, R., and Heyder, N. (1996) Color doppler ultrasound of liver lesions: signal enhancement after intravenous injection of the ultrasound contrast agent Levovist. *J. Clin. Ultrasound.* **24,** 31–35.

150. Huang, S. C., Yu, C. H., Huang, R. T., Hsu, K. F., Tsai, Y. C., and Chou, C. Y. (1996) Intratumoral blood flow in uterine myoma correlated with a lower tumor size and volume, but not correlated with cell proliferation or angiogenesis. *Obstet. Gynecol.* **87,** 1019–1024.

151. Gilles, R., Zafrani, B., Guinebretiere, J. M., Meunier, M., Lucidarme, O., Tardivon, A. A., et al. (1995) Ductal carcinoma in situ: MR imaging-histopathologic correlation. *Radiology* **196,** 415–419.

152. Guidi, A., Fischer, L., Harris, J., and Schnitt, S. (1994) Microvessel density and distribution in ductal carcinoma *in situ* of the breast. *J. Natl. Cancer Inst.* **86,** 614–619.

153. Engels, K., Fox, S. B., Gatter, K. C., and Harris, A. L. (1995) Distinct angiogenenic patterns are associated with high grade in-situ ductal carcinoma of breast. *J. Pathol.* **181,** 207–212.

154. Sterns, E., Zee, B., SenGupta, S., and Saunders, F. (1996) Thermography: its relation to pathologic characteristics, vascularity, proliferation rate and survival of patinets with invasive ductal carcinoma of the breast. *Cancer* **77,** 1324–1328.

155. Hockel, M., Schlenger, K., Aral, B., Mitze, M., Schaffer, U., and Vaupel, P. (1996) Association between tumor hypoxia and malignant progression in advance cancer of the uterine cervic. *Cancer Res.* **56,** 4509–4515.

156. Brizel, D., Scully, S., Harrelson, J., Layfield, L., Beach, J., Prosnitz, L., and Dewhitst, M. (1996) Tumor oxygenation profiles for the likelihood of distant metastases in human soft tissue sarcomas. *Cancer Res.* **56,** 941–943.

157. Shweiki, D., Neeman, M., Itin, A., and Keshet, E. (1995) Induction of vascular endothelial growth factor expression by hypoxia and by glucose deficiency in multicell spheroids: implications for tumor angiogenesis. *Proc. Natl. Acad. Sci. USA* 92, 768–772.

158. Brem, S. S., M., J. H. and Gullino, P. M. (1978) Angiogenesis as a marker of pre-neoplastic lesions of the human breast. *Cancer* **41**, 239–248.

159. Jensen, H. M., Chen, I., DeVault, M. R., and Lewis, A. E. (1982) Angiogenesis induced by "normal" human breast tissue: a probable marker for precancer. *Science* **218**, 293–295.

160. Chodak, G. W., Haudenschild, C., Gittes, R. F., and Folkman, J. (1980) Angiogenic activity as a marker of neoplastic and preneoplastic lesions of the human bladder. *Ann. Surg.* **192**, 762–771.

161. Fregene, T. A., Kellog, C., and Pienta, K. J. (1994) Microvessel quantitation as a measure of angiogenic activity in benign breast tissues lesions: a marker for precancerous disease? *Int. J. Oncol.* **4**, 1199–1202.

162. Heffelfinger, S., Yassin, R., Miller, M., and Lower, E. (1996) Vascularity of proliferative breast disease and carcinoma in situ correlates with histological features. *Clin. Cancer Res.* **2**, 1873–1878.

163. Montironi, R., Galluzzi, C., Diamanti, L., Taborro, R., Scarpelli, M., and Pisani, E. (1993) Prostatic intra-epithelial neoplasia. Qualitative and qualitative analysis of the blood capillary architecture. *Path. Res Pract.* **189**, 542–548.

164. Deering, R. E., Bigler, S. A., Brown, M., and Brawer, M. K. (1995) Microvascularity in benign prostatic hyperplasia. *Prostate* **26**, 111–115.

165. Fox, S. B., Leek, R. D., Smith, K., Hollyer, J., Greenall, M., and Harris, A. L. (1994) Tumor angiogenesis in node-negative breast carcinomas: relationship with epidermal growth factor receptor, estrogen receptor, and survival. *Breast Cancer Res. Treat.* **29**, 109–116.

166. Toi, M., Inada, K., Suzuki, H., and Tominaga, T. (1995) Tumor angiogenesis in breast cancer: its importance as a prognostic indicator and the association with vascular endothelial growth factor expression. *Breast Cancer Res.Treat.* **36**, 193–204.

167. Ogawa, Y., Chung, Y., Nakata, B., Takatsuka, S., Maeda, K., Sawada, T., et al. (1995) Microvessel quantitation in invasive breast cancer by staining for factor VIII-related antigen. *Br. J. Cancer* **71**, 1297–1301.

168. Gasparini, G. and Harris, A. L. (1994) Does improved control of tumor growth require an anti-cancer therapy targeting both neoplastic and intratumoral endothelial cells? *Eur. J. Cancer* **30A**, 201–206.

169. Lipponen, P., Ji, H., Aaltomaa, S., and Syrjanen, K. (1994) Tumor vascularity and basement membrane structure in breast cancer as related to tumor histology and prognosis. *J. Cancer Res. Clin. Oncol.* **120**, 645–650.

170. Smith-McCune, K. and Weidner, N. (1994) Demonstration and characterization of the angiogenic properties of cervical dysplasia. *Cancer Res.* **54**, 800–804.

171. Wiggins, D. L., Granai, C. O., Steinhoff, M. M., and Calabresi, P. (1995) Tumor angiogenesis as a prognostic factor in cervical carcinoma. *Gynecol. Oncol.* **56**, 353–356.

172. Palczak, R. and Splawinski, J. (1989) Angiogenic activity and neovascularization in adenocarcinoma of endometrium. *Int. J. Gynaecol. Obstet.* **29**, 343–357.

173. Hollingsworth, H. C., Kohn, E. C., Steinberg, S. M., Rothenberg, M. L., and Merino, M. J. (1995) Tumor angiogenesis in advanced stage ovarian carcinoma [see comments]. *Am. J. Pathol.* **147**, 33–41.

174. Weidner, N., Carroll, P. R., Flax, J., Blumenfeld, W., and Folkman, J. (1993) Tumor angiogenesis correlates with metastasis in invasive prostate carcinoma. *Am. J. Pathol.* **143**, 401–409.

175. Hall, M. C., Troncoso, P., Pollack, A., Zhau, H. Y., Zagars, G. K., Chung, L. W., and von, E. A. (1994) Significance of tumor angiogenesis in clinically localized prostate carcinoma treated with external beam radiotherapy. *Urology* **44**, 869–875.

176. Jaeger, T., Weidner, N., Chew, K., Moore, D., Kerschman, R., Waldman, F., and Carrol, P. (1995) Tumor angiogenesis correlates with lymph node metastasis in invasive bladder cancer. *J. Urol.* **154**, 69–71.

177. Macchiarelli, G., Nottola, S. A., Vizza, E., Kikuta, A., Murakami, T., and Motta, P. M. (1991) Ovarian microvasculature in normal and hCG stimulated rabbits. A study of vascular corrosion casts with particular regard to the interstitium. *J. Submicrosc. Cytol. Pathol.* **23**, 391–395.

178. Giatromanolaki, A., Koukourakis, O'Byrne, K., Fox, S., Whitehouse, R., Talbot, D., et al. (1995) Prognostic value of angiogenesis in operable non-small cell lung cancer. *J. Pathol.* **179**, 80–88.

179. Maeda, K., Chung, Y. S., Takatsuka, S., Ogawa, Y., Sawada, T., Yamashita, Y., et, al. (1995) Tumor angiogenesis as a predictor of recurrence in gastric carcinoma. *J. Clin. Oncol.* **13**, 477–481.

180. Saclarides, T. J., Speziale, N. J., Drab, E., Szeluga, D. J., and Rubin, D. B. (1994) Tumor angiogenesis and rectal carcinoma. *Dis. Colon. Rectum.* **37**, 921–926.

181. Klijanienko, J., El-Naggar, A., de Braud, F., Rodriguez-Peralto, J., Rodriguez, R., Itzhaki, M., et al. (1995) Tumor vascularisation, mitotic index, histopathological grade, and DNA ploidy in the assessment of 114 head and neck squamous cell carcinomas. *Cancer* **75**, 1649–1656.

182. Leedy, D. A., Trune, D. R., Kronz, J. D., Weidner, N., and Cohen, J. I. (1994) Tumor angiogenesis, the p53 antigen, and cervical metastasis in squamous carcinoma of the tongue. *Otolaryngol. Head Neck Surg.* **111,** 417–422.

183. Gasparini, G., Weidner, N., Maluta, S., Pozza, F., Boracchi, P., Mezzetti, M., et al. (1993) Intratumoral microvessel density and p53 protein: correlation with metastasis in head-and-neck squamous-cell carcinoma. *Int. J. Cancer* **55,** 739–744.

184. Zatterstrom, U., Brun, E., Willen, R., Kjellen, E., and Wennerberg, J. (1995) Tumor angiogenesis and prognosis in squamous carcinoma of the head and neck. *Head Neck* **17,** 312–318.

185. Albo, D., Granick, M., Jhala, N., Atkinson, B., and Solomon, M. (1994) The relationship of angiogenesis to biological activity in human squamous cell carcinomas of the head and neck. *Ann. Plast. Surg.* **32,** 558–594.

186. Ohsawa, M., Tomita, Y., Kuratsu, S., Kanno, H., and Aozasa, K. (1995) Angiogenesis in malignant fibrous histiocytoma. *Oncology* **52,** 51–54.

187. Weidner, N. (1995) Intratumoral microvessel density as a prognostic factor in cancer. *Am. J. Pathol.* **147,** 9–19.

188. Dearnaley, D., Sloane, J., Ormerod, M., Steele, K., Coombes, R., Clink, H., et al. (1981) Increased setection of mammary carcinoma cells in marrow smears using antisera to epithelial membrane antigen. *Br. J. Cancer* **44,** 85–90.

189. Osborne, M. P., Wong, G. Y., Asina, S., Old, L. J., Cote, R. J., and Rosen, P. P. (1991) Sensitivity of immunocytochemical detection of breast cancer cells in human bone marrow. *Cancer Res.* **51,** 2706–2709.

190. Pantel, K., Schlimok, G., Angstwurm, M., Weckermann, D., Schmaus, W., Gath, H., et al. (1994) Methodological analysis of immunocytochemical screening for disseminated epithelial tumor cells in bone marrow. *J. Hematother.* **3,** 165–173.

191. Gasparini, G., Fox, S., Verderio, P., E., B., Bevilacqua, P., Borrachi, P., Dante, S., et al. (1996) The determination of angiogenesis adds information to estrogen receptor status in predicting the efficacy of adjuvant tamoxifen in node positive breast cancer patients. *Clin. Cancer Res.* **2,** 1191–1198.

192. Gasparini, G. and Harris, A. L. (1995) Clinical importance of the determination of tumor angiogenesis in breast carcinoma: much more than a new prognostic tool. *J. Clin. Oncol.* **13,** 765–782.

193. Fox, S., Engels, K., Comley, M., Whitehouse, R., Turley, H., Gatter, K., and Harris, A. (1997) Relationship of elevated tumor thymidine phosphorylase in node positive breast carcinomas to the effects of adjuvant CMF. *Ann. Oncol.* **8,** 271–275.

194. Larsen, N. S. (1993) Angiogenesis research yields new approaches to cancer treatment and prognosis [news]. *J. Natl. Cancer Inst.* **85,** 1629–1630.

195. Dixon, J., Kaklamanis, L., Turley, H., Hickson, I. D., Leek, R. D., Harris, A. L., and Gatter, K. C. (1994) Expression of aminopeptidase-n (CD13) in normal tissues and malignant neoplasms of epithelial and lymphoid origin. *J. Clin. Pathol.* **47,** 43–47.

196. Fina, L., Molgaard, H. V., Robertson, D., Bradley, N. J., Monaghan, P., Delia, D., et al. (1990) Expression of the CD34 gene in vascular endothelial cells. *Blood* **75,** 2417–2426.

197. Silverstein, R. L., Baird, M., Lo, S. K., and Yesner, L. M. (1992) Sense and antisense cDNA transfection of CD36 (glycoprotein IV) in melanoma cells. Role of CD36 as a thrombospondin receptor. *J. Biol. Chem.* **267,** 16,607–16,612.

198. Wellicome, S. M., Thornhill, M. H., Pitzalis, C., Thomas, D. S., Lauchbury, J. S., Panayi, G. S., and Haskard, D. O. (1990) A monoclonal antibody that detects a novel antigen on endothelial cells that is induced by tumor necrosis factor, IL-1, or lipopolysaccharide. *J. Immunol.* **144,** 2558–2565.

199. Metzelaar, M. J., Schuurman, H. J., Heijnen, H. F., Sixma, J. J., and Nieuwenhius, H. K. (1991) Biochemical and immunohistochemical characteristics of CD62 and CD63 monoclonal antibodies. Expression of GMP-140 and LIMP-CD63 (CD63 antigen) in human lymphoid tissues. *Virchows Arch. B Cell. Pathol.* **61,** 269–277.

200. de Fougerolles, A., Stacker, S. A., Schwarting, R., and Springer, T. A. (1991) Characterization of ICAM-2 and evidence for a third counter-receptor for LFA-1. *J. Exp. Med.* **174,** 253–267.

201. Kuzu, I., Bicknell, R., Fletcher, C. D., and Gatter, K. C. (1993) Expression of adhesion molecules on the endothelium of normal tissue vessels and vascular tumors. *Lab. Invest.* **69,** 322–328.

202. Rettig, W. J., Garin, C. P., Healey, J. H., Su, S. L., Jaffe, E. A., and Old, L. J. (1002) Indentification of endosialin, a cell surface glycoprotein of vascular endothelial cells in human cancer. *Proc. Natl. Acad. Sci. USA* **89,** 10,832–10,836.

203. Hagemeier, H. H., Vollmer, E., Goerdt, S., Schulze, O. K., and Sorg, C. (1986) A monoclonal antibody reacting with endothelial cells og budding vessels in tumors and inflammatory tissues, and non-reactive with normal adult tissues. *Int. J. Cancer* **38,** 481–488.
204. Schlingemann, R. O., Dingjan, G. M., Emeis, J. J., Blok, J., Warnaar, S. O., and Ruiter, D. J. (1985) Monoclonal antibody PAL-E specific for endothelium. *Lab. Invest.* **52,** 71–76.
205. Koch, A. E., Harlow, L. A., Haines, G. K., Amento, E. P., Unemori, E. N., Wong, W. L., et al. (1994) Vascular endothelial growth factor. A cytokine modulating endothelial function in rheumatoid arthritis. *J. Immunol.* **152,** 4149–4156.
206. Fregene, T. A., Khanuja, P. S., Gimotty, P. A., Kellogg, C., George, J., and Pienta, K. J. (1994) The relationship of microvessel counts to tumor size, estrogen receptor status, lymph node metastasis, and disease-free survival in patients with stage I and II breast cancer. *Int. J. Oncol.* **5,** 1437–1445.
207. Bevilacqua, P., Barbareschi, M., Verderio., P., Boracchi, P., Caffo, O., Dalla Palma, P., et al. (1994) Prognostic value of intratumoral microvessel density, a measure of tumor angiogenesis, in node-negative breast carcinoma-results of a multiparametric study. *Breast Cancer Res. Treat.* **36,** 205–217.
208. Ogawa, Y., Chung, Y., Nakata, B., Takatsuka, S., Maeda, K., et al. (1994) An evaluation of angiogenesis in breast cancer with factor VIII related antigen staining. *Proc. Am. Assoc. Cancer Res.* **35,** 186(Abstract 1113).
209. Obermair, A., Kurz, C., Czerwenka, K., Thoma, M., Kaider, A., and Wagner, T. (1995) Microvessel density and vessel invasion in lymph-node-negative breast cancer: effect on recurrence-free survival. *Int. J. Cancer* **62,** 126–131.
210. Kohlberger, P., Obermair Sliutz, G., Heinzl, H., Koelbl, H., Breitenecker, G., Gitsch, G., and Kainz, C. (1996) Quantitive immunohistochemistry of factor VIII-related antigen in breast carcinoma. *Am. J. Clin. Pathol.* **105,** 705–710.
211. Simpson, J., Ahn, C., Battifora, H., and Esteban, J. (1996) Endothelial area as a prognostic indicator for invasive breast carcinoma. *Cancer* **77,** 2077–2085.
212. Heinman, R., Ferguson, D., Powers, C., Recant, W., Weichselbaum, R., and Hellman, S. (1996) Angiogenesis as a predictor of long term survival for patients wit node-negative breast cancer. *J. Natl. Cancer Inst.* **88,** 1764–1769.
213. Goulding, H., Abdul, R. N., Robertson, J. F., Bell, J. A., Elston, C. W., Blamey, R. W., and Ellis, I. O. (1995) Assessment of angiogenesis in breast carcinoma: an important factor in prognosis? *Hum. Pathol.* **26,** 1196–1200.
214. Morphopoulos, G., Pearson, M., Ryder, W., Howell, A., and Harris, M. (1996) Tumor angiogenesis as a prognostic marker in infiltrating lobular carcinoma of the breast. *J. Pathol.* **180,** 44–49.
215. Bochner, B., Cote, R., Groshen, S., Esrig, D., Freeman, J., Weidner, N., et al. (1995) Tumor angiogenesis is an independent prognostic indicator in invasive transitional cell carcinoma of the bladder. *J. Urol.* **153,** 456A(Abstract 909).
216. Philip, E., Stephenson, T., and Reed, M. (1996) Prognostic significance of angiogenesis in transitional carcinoma of the human urinary bladder. *Br. J. Urol.* **77,** 352–357.
217. MacLennan, G. and Bostwick, D. (1995) Microvessel density in renal cell carcinoma: lack of prognostic significance. *Urology* **46,** 27–30.
218. Frank, R. E., Saclarides, T. J., Leurgans, S., Speziale, N. J., Drab, E. A., and Rubin, D. B. (1995) Tumor angiogenesis as a predictor of recurrence and survival in patients with node-negative colon cancer [see comments]. *Ann. Surg.* **222,** 695–699.
219. Bossi, P., Viale, G., Lee, A. K., Alfano, R., Coggi, G., and Bosari, S. (1995) Angiogenesis in colorectal tumors: microvessel quantitation in adenomas and carcinomas with clinicopathological correlations. *Cancer Res.* **55,** 5049–5053.
220. Takebayashi, Y., Akiyama, S., Yamada, K., Akiba, S., and Aikou, T. (1996) Angiogenesis as an unfavorable prognostic factor in human colorectal carcinoma. *Cancer* **78,** 226–231.
221. Lindmark, G., Gerdin, B., Sundberg, C., Pahlman, L., Bergstrom, R., and Glimelius, B. (1996) Prognostic significance of the microvessel count in colorectal cancer. *J. Clin. Oncol.* **14,** 461–466.
222. Engel, C., Bennett, S., Chambers, A., Doig, G., Shimomatsuya, T., Horiuchi, T., et al. (1996) Tumor angiogenesis predicts recurrence in invasive colorectal cancer when controlled for Dukes staging. *Am. J. Clin. Pathol.* **20,** 1260–1265.
223. Tanigawa, N., Amaya, H., Matsumura, M., Shimomatsuya, T., Horiuchi, T., Muraoka, R., and Iki, M. (1996) Extent of tumor vascularization correlates with prognosis and hematogenous metastasis in gastric carcinoma. *Cancer Res.* **56,** 2671–2676.
224. Rutgers, J. L., Mattox, T. F., and Vargas, M. P. (1995) Angiogenesis in uterine cervical squamous cell carcinoma. *Int. J. Gynecol. Pathol.* **14,** 114–118.

225. Kainz, C., Speiser, P., Wanner, C., Obermair, A., Tempfer, C., Sliutz, G., et al. (1995) Prognostic value of tumour microvessel density in cancer of the uterine cervix stage IB and IIB. *Anticancer Res.* **15,** 1549–1552.

226. Kirschner, C., Alanis-Amerzcua, J., Martin, V., Luna, N., Morgan, E., Yang, J., and Yordan, E. (1996) Angiogenesis factor in endometrial carcinoma: a new prognastic indicator? *Am. J. Obstet. Gynecol.* **174,** 1879–1884.

227. Van Diest, P., Zevering, L., and Baak, J. (1995) Lack of prognostic value of microvessel density counts in FIGO 3 and 4 cisplatinum treated ovarian cancer patients. *Pathol. Res. Pract.* **191,** 25–30.

228. Gasparini, G., Bonoldi, E., Viale, G., Verderio, P., Boracchi, P., Panizzoni, G., et al. (1996) Prognostic and predictive value of tumor angiogenesis in ovarian carcinomas. *Int. J. Cancer* **69,** 205–211.

229. Yamazaki, K., Abe, S., Takekawa, H., Sukoh, N., Watanabe, N., Ogura, S., et al. (1994) Tumor angiogenesis in human lung adenocarcinoma. *Cancer* **74,** 2245–2250.

230. Macchiarini, P., Fontanini, G., Dulmet, E., de Montepreville, V., Chapelier, A., Cerrina, J., et al. (1994) Angiogenesis: an indicator of metastasis in non-small cell lung cancer invading the thoracic inlet. *Ann. Thor. Surg.* **57,** 1534–1539.

231. Mattern, J., Koomagi, R., Volm, M. (1995) Vascular endothelial growth factor expression and angiogenesis in non-small cell lung carcinomas. *Int. J. Oncol.* **6,** 1059–1062.

232. Fontanini, G., Bigini, D., Vignati, S., Basolo, F., Mussi, A., Lucchi, M., et al. (1995) Microvessel count predicts metastatic disease and survival in non-small cell lung cancer. *J. Pathol.* **177,** 57–63.

233. Angeletti, C., Lucchi, M., Fontanini, G., Mussi, A., Chella, A., Ribechini, A., et al. (1996) Prognostic significance of tumoral angiogenesis in completely resected late stage lung carcinoma (stage IIIA-N2). *Cancer* **78,** 409–415.

234. Harpole, D. J., Richards, W. G., Herndon, J. N., and Sugarbaker, D. J. (1996) Angiogenesis and molecular biologic substaging in patients with stage I non-small cell lung cancer. *Ann. Thorac. Surg.* **61,** 1470–1476.

235. Carrau, R., Barnes, E., Snyderman, C., Petruzzelli, G., Kachman, K., Rueger, R., et al. (1995) Tumor angiogenesis as a predictor of tumor aggressiveness and metastatic potential in squamous carcinomas of the head and neck. *Inv. Metastasis* **15,** 197–202.

236. Dray, T., Hardin, N., Sofferman, R. (1995) Angiogenesis as a prognostic marker in early head and neck cancer. *Ann. Otol. Rhinol. Laryngol.* **104,** 724–729.

237. Roychowdhury, D., Tseng, A., Fu, K., Weinberg, V., and Weidner, N. (1996) New prognostic factors in nasopharyngeal carcinoma: tumor angiogenesis and c-erbB-2 expression. *Cancer* **77,** 1419–1226.

238. Shpitzer, T., Chaimoff, M., Gal, R., Stern, Y., Feinmesser, R., and Segal, K. (1996) Tumor angiogenesis as a prognostic factor in early oral tongue cancer. *Arch. Otolaryngol. Head Neck Surg.* **122,** 865–868.

239. Graham, C., Rivers, J., Kerbel, R., Stankiewicz, K., and White, W. (1994) Extent of vascularization as a prognostic indicator in thin (< 0.76 mm) malignant melanomas. *Am. J. Pathol.* **145,** 510–514.

240. Busam, K., Berwick, M., Blessing, K., Fandrey, K., Kang, S., Karaoli, T., et al. (1995) Tumor vascularity is not a prognostic factor for malignant melanoma. *Am. J. Pathol.* **147,** 1049–1956.

241. Leon, S., Folkerth, R., and Black, P. (1996) Microvessel density is a prognostic indicator for patients with astroglial brain tumors. *Cancer* **77,** 362–372.

242. Wesseling, P., Ruiter, D. J., Burger, P. C., et al. (1994) Quantitative immunohistolgical analysis of the microvasculature in untreated human glioblastoma mutliforme. Computer-assisted image analysis of whole-tumor sections. *J. Neurosurg.* **81,** 902–909.

243. Ito, T., Kitamura, H., Nakamura, N., Kameda, Y., and Kanisawa, M. (1993) A comparative study of vascular proliferation in brain metastasis of lung carcinomas. *Virchows Arch. A Pathol. Anat. Histopathol.* **423,** 13–17.

244. Foss, A., Alexander, R., Jefferies, L., Hungerford, J., Harris, A., and Lightman, S. (1996) Microvessel count predicts survival in uveal melanoma. *Cancer Res.* **56,** 2900–2903.

245. Pluda, J. and Parkinson, D. (1996) Clinical implications of tumor-assicited neovascularization and current anti-angiogenic strategies for the treatment of malignancies of pancreas. *Cancer* **78,** 680–687.

246. Hellstrom, A., Frankendal, B., Nilsson, B., Pettersson, F., Silfversward, C., and Auer, C. (1996) Primary fallopian tube carcinoma-the prognostic impact of stage, histopathology, and biological parameters. *Int. J. Gynecol Cancer* **6,** 456–462.

247. Liu, Q., Djuricin, G., Staren, E., Gattuso, P., Gould, V., and Shen, J. (1996) Tumor angiogenesis in phaeochromocytomas and paragangliomas. *Surgery* **120,** 938–942.

248. Sulh, M., Greco, M., Jiang, T., Goswani, S., Present, D., and Steiner, G. (1996) Proliferation index and vascular density of giant cell tumors of bone. *Cancer* **77,** 2044–2051.

249. Meitar, D., Crawford, S., Rademaker, A., and Cohn, S. (1996) Tumor angiogenesis correlates with metastatic disease, n-myc amplification and poor outcome in human neuroblastoma. *J. Clin. Oncol.* **14,** 405–414.
250. Vacca, A., Ribatti, D., Roncali, L., Ranieri, G., Serio, G., Silvestris, F., and Dammacco, F. (1994) Bone marrow angiogenesis and progression in multiple myeloma. *Br. J. Haematol.* **87,** 503–508.
251. Segal, K., Shpitzer, T., Feinmesser, M., Stern, Y., and Feinmesser, R. (1996) Angiogenesis in follicular tumors of the thyroid. *J. Surg. Oncol.* **63,** 95–98.
252. Fontanini, G., Vignati, S., Pollina, L., and Basolo, F. (1996) Microvessel count: an indicator of poor outcome in medullary thryroid carcinoma, but not in other types of thyroid carcinoma. *Mod. Pathol.* **9,** 636–841.
253. Staibano, S., Boscaino, A., Salvatore, G., Orabona, P., Palombini, L., and De Rosa, G. (1996) The prognostic significance of tumor angiogenesis in nonaggessive and aggressive basal cell carcinoma of the human skin. *Human Pathol.* **27,** 695–700.

III STIMULATION OF ANGIOGENESIS [THERAPEUTIC ANGIOGENESIS]

11

Hyaluronan Oligosaccharides Promote Wound Repair

Its Size-Dependent Regulation of Angiogenesis

David C. West and Tai-Ping D. Fan

CONTENTS

INTRODUCTION
THE ANTIANGIOGENIC NATURE OF MACROMOLECULAR HYALURONAN
HYALURONAN- OLIGOSACCHARIDES AND ANGIOGENESIS
CONCLUSIONS
ACKNOWLEDGMENTS
REFERENCES

INTRODUCTION

Hyaluronan (HA, previously called hyaluronic acid or hyaluronate) is a high-molecular weight linear polysaccharide, a member of the glycosaminoglycan family, composed of repeating 1,4- linked disaccharide units of 1,3- linked glucuronic acid and N-acetylglucosamine (Fig.1). It is present in the extracellular matrix of most animal tissues, occurring at greatest concentration in adult connective tissues. Several factors, including its ubiquitous distribution, the high concentration in cartilage and synovial fluid, the capacity to bind large amounts of water, and its simple structure, led to the general belief that its function was essentially that of an inert viscoelastic lubricant, or space-filling molecule (1,2). Furthermore, its viscoelastic properties, chemical simplicity, and lack of immunogenicity have made it the basis for biomaterials used in viscosurgery, tissue engineering, and drug delivery systems (3). However, in recent years, a growing number of reports have appeared indicating that HA has profound effects on the behavior of various cell-types, apparently mediated by several surface receptors (4,5).

A transient HA-rich matrix develops during embryogenesis and adult tissue regeneration, or remodeling, coincident with rapid-cell proliferation and migration. Subsequent tissue differentiation, with vasculogenesis and angiogenesis, occurs concomitantly with a decrease in tissue HA levels (6). Localized accumulation also occurs in association with tissue damage, organ rejection, and many inflammatory diseases, notably psoriasis and

From: *The New Angiotherapy*
Edited by: T.-P. D. Fan and E. C. Kohn © Humana Press Inc., Totowa, NJ

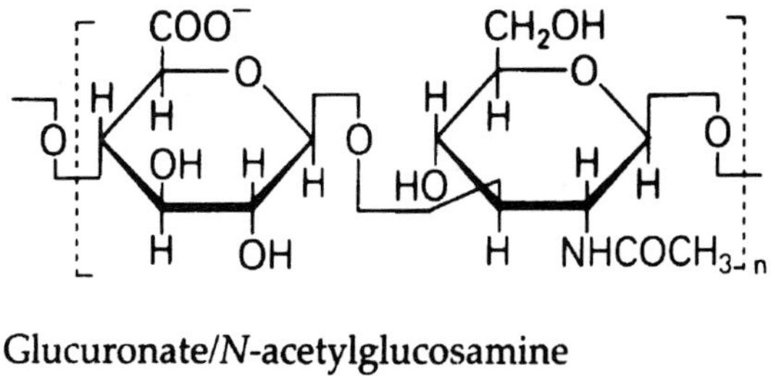

Glucuronate/N-acetylglucosamine

Fig. 1. A schematic representation of the disaccharide unit of hyaluronan.

distribution of HA during embryogenesis, and tissue remodeling, suggests that the synthesis and degradation of HA plays an important regulatory role in these processes, and certain pathological conditions such as tumor growth.

In this chapter, we will review the evidence for the regulatory role of HA in angiogenesis and summarize our current studies on HA oligosaccharides in wound healing and their mechanism of action.

THE ANTIANGIOGENIC NATURE OF MACROMOLECULAR HYALURONAN

The Effect of Exogenous HA on Wound Healing and Development

The high concentration of HA found in avascular tissues, such as cartilage and vitreous humour, and at relatively avascular sites, including the desmoplastic region of invasive tumors, suggests that extracellular matrix HA can inhibit angiogenesis (9,10). In vivo studies indicate that implantation of high concentrations of macromolecular hyaluronan inhibits granulation tissue and associated blood-vessel formation (11–15), in a concentration and size-dependent manner (16–18), and induces regression of the capillary plexus in the developing chick limb bud (19) (Table 1).

HA and Angiogenesis in Normal Adult and Fetal Wound Healing

Determination of excisional wound HA in adult animal models indicates that an increase in tissue HA occurs shortly after injury (20–22). Although the exact source of this HA is obscure, it binds strongly to extravasated fibrinogen/fibrin to form the early wound matrix (23–25). Chemoattractants, released by trapped platelets, promote the rapid invasion of this primary matrix by inflammatory cells and fibroblasts. In vitro studies suggest that, under the direction of inflammatory cytokines, fibroblasts synthesize large amounts of HA, further increasing tissue HA. However, reports on the effects of HA on inflammatory cells indicate that increased levels of high-molecular weight HA may reduce leukocyte chemotaxis, or migration, and also their level of activation and scavenging ability.

In our studies on the relationship between angiogenesis and tissue HA metabolism, we have employed a rat polyether sponge-implant wound-healing model (26), monitoring vascularization by ^{133}Xe clearance and vessel counting (Fig. 2). The results suggest granulation tissue vascularization is closely linked with the degradation of matrix hyaluronan, evidenced by a rapid fall in tissue HA size (2×10^3 to 550 kDa), content (600–200 µg/g tissue), and increased tissue hyaluronidase levels (27). No discernible increase in inflammatory cells, especially macrophages, accompanied these changes. The addition of exogenous HA

Table 1

Anti-Angiogenic Properties of High-Molecular-Weight Hyaluronan

In vivo:
- Inhibits granulation tissue formation and vascularization *(11)*,
- Inhibits vascularization of implanted fibrin gels *(14,36)*,
- Causes regression of the capillary plexus in chick limb buds *(19)*, and
- Endogenous HA inhibits angiogenic activity of human wound fluids in CAM assay *(9)*.

In vitro:
- Inhibits endothelial cell proliferation *(33)*,
- migration *(35,36,49)* and
- Cell-cell adhesion *(33)*, at physiological relevant concentrations, i. e., 100–200 mg/mL.

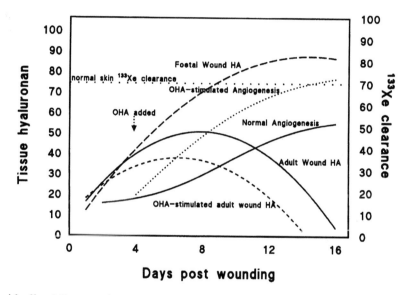

Fig. 2. An idealized diagram showing the relative differences in hyaluronan in early fetal wounds, late fetal or adult wounds, and adult wounds stimulated with exogenous OHA, 50 µg/d between day 4 and day 8 postwounding. Also show is the relative changes in wound vascularization in normal and OHA-treated wounds.

oligonucleotides (OHA) accelerated both the onset and rate of HA degradation (*see* below), in parallel with angiogenesis, supporting the hypothesis that macromolecular HA is an important inhibitory regulator of angiogenesis.

In the fetal wound, the addition of exogenous streptomyces hyaluronidase decreases wound HA content and increases both fibroplasia and capillary formation *(28)*. A similar change, from fetal regenerative healing to an adult fibrotic type of healing, occurs in late gestation (Fig. 2). In sheep, this change occurs between 100 and 120 d gestation and is associated with both an increase in hyaluronidase activity and a decrease in hyaluronan concentration and size *(29)*. Interestingly, macromolecular HA has been reported to inhibit transforming growth factor α_1 (TGF-α_1; *30*), a promoter of tissue angiogenesis and extracellular matrix synthesis. Furthermore, it appears to stimulate the secretion of tissue inhibitors of metalloproteinases (TIMP; *31*), known inhibitors of angiogenesis, at concentrations similar to those reported to be present in the early wound. Both of these latter studies found the effects to be size dependent, decreasing significantly with the size of the HA. Such reports imply that HA degradation must precede the onset of vascularization.

In Vitro Effects on Vessel Formation

In vitro studies on cultured endothelial cells have shown that macromolecular HA inhibits endothelial proliferation and migration *(9,32–34)* and disrupts newly formed monolayers, at physiologically relevant concentrations (≥ 100 µg/mL), i.e., concentrations found in the avascular phase of tissue remodeling and in adult avascular connective tissues. The inhibitory effect of HA decreases with reducing size, and the HA- mediated inhibition can not be reversed by addition of exogenous growth factors, such as basic fibroblast growth factor (bFGF; *9,34*). We, together with Watanabe et al. *(35)*, have recently confirmed these findings in a three-dimensional collagen-gel culture system. Furthermore, high concentrations (1 mg/mL) of HA have been reported to inhibit the migration of human adipose-tissue capillary endothelial cells into fibrin gels, in vitro, and vascularization of fibrin gels implanted subcutaneously in guinea pigs *(14,36)*.

Degradation of Hyaluronan

The antiangiogenic nature of macromolecular HA, both in vitro and in vivo, suggests that the levels of hyaluronan found in adult and embryonic wounds *(27,29)* and tumors *(8)* should substantially inhibit their neovascularization. This is difficult to equate with the vascularization seen in both adult and late embryonic wounds, and also the increased angiogenesis reported for many tumors, especially metastatic tumors. In the wound-healing studies outlined earlier, there appears to be a close temporal relationship between tissue HA level and size, "lysosomal" hyaluronidase activity and angiogenesis, suggesting that tissue HA is degraded through the action of hyaluronidase. This is supported by our recent finding that metastatic tumors, which are highly vascularized, have very low levels of HA. However, cultured cell lines from these and other metastasizing tumors produce large amounts of mainly low molecular-weight HA. These cells also have high levels of acidic "lysosomal" hyaluronidase activity, either cell-associated or secreted in to the medium *(37–40)*. These data appeared to support previous studies that indicate that HA degradation occurs exclusively intracellularly, in the lysosomal system, after receptor-mediated internalization. Catabolism appears to go to completion in the hepatocytes, kupffer cells, and sinusoidal endothelial cells, yielding acetate, ammonia, and water *(41,42)*. Initial extracellular depolymerization of HA or proteoglycan complexes appears to be a necessary prerequisite for internalization, and has been reported to be mediated by either oxygen-derived free radicals or proteinases.

Although this may be the case for circulating HA, our analysis of HA in wound tissues, tumors, and cultured tumor cell lines suggests that a large scale, sequential degradation takes place, involving essentially the whole population of HA molecules. Furthermore, the extent of HA depolymerization appears to increase with increasing hyaluronidase levels. The most likely explanation of these data being that, in many tissues, HA degradation is mainly extracellular and is catalyzed by extracellular hyaluronidase(s).

Until recently, only one such enzyme had been reported, the glycosylphosphatidylinositol (GPI)-anchored, sperm PH-20 hyaluronidase, whose distribution is restricted to the testes *(43)*. Interestingly, Liu et al. *(43)* have recently reported the presence of a potential "neutral" surface-associated hyaluronidase, similar to the (GPI)-anchored sperm PH-20 hyaluronidase, expressed by angiogenic tumor cell-lines. We have recently examined several tumor cell-lines for PH-20, using Northern blotting and polymerase chain reaction (PCR) techniques. In most cell-lines PH-20 expression was related to the cells "lysosomal" hyaluronidase activity and inversely related to the size of HA present in both the culture medium and on the cell-surface of each cell line. In a series of related human colon carcinoma cell lines, increasing PH-20 expression was also accompanied by an increase in both angiogenic activity and metastasis. Initial studies have shown the presence of GPI-anchored "neutral" surface-associated hyaluronidase on these cells. The expression of PH-20 hyaluronidase, by cells other than sperm, may eventually be shown to be limited to transformed cells. However, the recent finding that normal serum hyaluronidase—which differs from the tumor enzyme *(44)*—also contains the GPI-anchor suggests that cell-surface hyaluronidase(s) are present on many cell-types *(45)*. In the case of wound healing, it is difficult to identify the cell-type responsible for the degradation of matrix HA, as macrophages, fibroblasts, and endothelial cells have all been reported to express hyaluronidase activity *(46–48)*, but the strongest candidate is probably the macrophage *(48)*.

HYALURONAN- OLIGOSACCHARIDES AND ANGIOGENESIS

In Vivo Angiogenic Activity

In contrast to the effects of macromolecular HA outlined earlier, we have found that low molecular-weight HA-oligosaccharides (OHA; 2–8 kDa or 4–20 disaccharides in length) stimulate angiogenesis in the CAM assay *(9,33,49)*. Also, Hirata et al. *(50)*, using the rabbit corneal assay, independently confirmed the angiogenic activity of this size-range of OHA (Table 2). The hexa- and tetra- saccharide products of HA digestion appear to be inactive, at least in the CAM assay.

In an early study we implanted methylcellulose pellets, containing 0–100 µg of OHA, subcutaneously at various sites in the rabbit. After 3 d, a definite local increase in vascularity was evident on visual and microscopic examination (Kumar and West, unpublished results; *48*). In more quantitative studies, we have examined the angiogenic effect of topical OHA *(56)* and also that of subcutaneous implants of slow-release OHA, in an impaired full- thickness skin-graft model *(57)*. Twice-daily application of citrate-buffered, pH 3.5, radiolabeled OHA to the skin of adult rats, over 5 d, showed that by day 8 the OHA had penetrated to a depth of 800 µm beneath the epidermis. The oligosaccharides did not alter the general morphology of the skin, but quantitative histological analysis of vessel number showed a small, but significant, increase in the vascularity of treated skin. In the latter model, revascularization of full-thickness skin autografts in rats was delayed by sublethal cryoinjury prior to grafting. The effect of an OHA fraction (1.5–4 kDa, 4–10 disaccharides) was compared with that of a nonangiogenic HA fraction (33 kDa), in both the cryoinjured model and in a noninjured graft model. 100 µg/ graft of the oligosaccharides was applied in "ELVAX" slow-release pellets, placed under the outer edge of the graft. Revascularization of the graft over the next 10 d was determined by blood-flow measurements, using both ^{133}Xe clearance and laser Doppler flowmetry, and by vessel counts. The revascularization of the cryoinjured grafts was significantly slower than the normal grafts, but did not ultimately decrease graft survival. The OHA implants had little effect on the vascularization of the noninjured grafts, but significantly increasing both blood flow and vessel density in the cryoinjured model. The 33 kDa HA had no effect in either model, confirming earlier results in the CAM assay. Interestingly, histological localization of

Table 2
Angiogenic Nature of OHA (4–20 disaccharides)

In vitro:
Stimulates endothelial:
- Proliferation *(16,33)*,
- Migration *(49,56)*,
- Migration into collagen/fibrin gels *(51,52)*, and
- Tube formation *(50,53)*.
Induces synthesis of:
- Proliferation-/activation-associated proteins *(9)*,
- Type VIII collagen *(54)*, and
- UPA and PAI-1 *(51)*
In vivo:
Induces angiogenesis in:
- The CAM *(49,55)*,
- The rabbit corneal assay *(50)*,
- Rat skin on topical application *(56)*, and
- Rabbit after subcutaneous implantation (Kumar and West, unpublished; *58*).
Stimulates angiogenesis in:
- An impaired rat skin-graft model *(57)*,
- A rat polyvinyl sponge-implant model *(27)*, and

tissue HA, using a specific biotinylated HA-binding protein, revealed that in both the cryoinjured and normal grafts, there was a transient loss of HA during the period of maximal vascularization.

A study of the effect of exogenous HA preparations on the healing of full-thickness skin wounds in pigs has also revealed differences between OHA, intermediate-sized HA oligosaccharides (100 kDa), and macromolecular 1,000 kDa HA *(16)*. Laser Doppler measurements at 3 and 7 d after wounding showed that, at day 3, OHA-treated wounds had a significantly higher blood flow than those treated with intermediate and macromolecular HA. However, by day 7, all treatments had elevated wound blood flow, or vascularization. Differences were also apparent between the HA preparations with respect to wound contraction and wound fracture strength. OHA inhibited early wound contraction, at day 3, and the intermediate and macromolecular HA preparations decreased wound strength, presumably owing to inhibition of fibril formation or collagen synthesis. However, no gross histological differences were apparent in any of the treatment groups. These data suggest that the main effect of OHA in this model is to increase early wound vascularization.

To investigate in more detail the effect of OHA on wound healing, we have employed a rat polyether sponge-implant wound-healing model *(26)*, monitoring vascularization by ^{133}Xe clearance and vessel counting (*see* above). Introduction of 5 µg/ sponge of OHA on days 4–8 after implantation rapidly induced sponge neovascularization. A significant increase in ^{133}Xe clearance already apparent by day 6, as compared with day 9 in the control group. In addition, the accelerated neovascularization continued until day 16, 8 d after addition of OHA had ceased. Thus treated sponges attained normal levels of blood flow, or vascularization, on day 13 compared with day 20 in control sponges. Sponge wet weight, protein, and DNA content were also increased. Local levels of the eicosanoids,

PGE2, 6-keto-PGF1α, TxB2, and LTB4, were not altered by application of OHA and, furthermore, immunohistochemical staining for tissue macrophages showed that there was no change in their numbers between the treated and control groups. Thus the OHA stimulation of sponge angiogenesis does not seem to be driven by the inflammatory reaction that always accompanies adult wound healing.

As outlined earlier, high molecular-weight HA inhibits angiogenesis and cellulose acetate electrophoresis indicated that HA was the major component in the early sponge tissue. Analysis of HA in the control sponges showed a decrease in both HA size and content closely linked to, if not preceding, angiogenesis. Similar examination of OHA-treated sponges showed an earlier onset and more extensive degradation of tissue HA. Here again, both the timing and extent of degradation mimicked that of angiogenesis. An increase in tissue hyaluronidase levels coincided with this degradation, at least in the control group, and it is probable that one of the early consequences of OHA treatment is an induction of hyaluronidase, although the source is not clear.

In Vitro Effects of OHA

Our own studies have shown that OHA (4–20 disaccharides) specifically stimulate both proliferation, and to a lesser extent migration, of both bovine and human endothelial cells (16,33,49). Hirata et al. (50), and more recently Rahmanian et al. (53), reported that angiogenic OHA markedly stimulated endothelial tube formation, on "matrigel." Furthermore, two recent studies, and our own preliminary studies, have shown that OHA (4–20 disaccharides in length) stimulate angiogenesis in three-dimensional collagen and fibrin matrices (Burbridge and West; unpublished results; 51,52). Trouchon et al. (52) have also confirmed that the HA hexasaccharide is not angiogenic.

Mechanism of Action of Angiogenic HA-Oligosaccharides

Several workers, including ourselves, have reported that endothelial cells possess high-affinity HA-binding proteins, or receptors, on their cell surface, that both bind and internalize HA (33,53, 59–61). Initially, using macromolecular HA (10^6 Da), we detected 2,000 receptors/cell, with a Kd of 10^{-12} M. Similar values have been obtained by other groups, using high molecular-weight HA (53,61). More recently, we have repeated this study using a defined 42 kDa HA fraction, and have found approx 10^5 receptors/cell and a Kd of 10^{-12} M, the disparity owing to steric exclusion of large HA molecules from the cell surface (59,60). Sodium dodecyl sulfate-polyacrylamide gel electrophoresis (SDS-PAGE) analysis, of HA-affinity purified human and bovine endothelial I^{125}- labeled cell-surface proteins, identified five major cell-surface HA- binding proteins, between 90 and 125 kDa, with two minor bands at 78 and 46 kDa (34,59). Western blotting with anti-CD44 and anti-ICAM-1 antibodies, together with reverse transcription (RT-PCR) determination of CD44 splice-variants, indicates that the 78–125 kDa proteins are forms of nonvariant CD44, differing in their glycosylation, and ICAM-1 isoforms (West, unpublished results). Using affinity-isolation techniques similar to our own, McCourt et al. (62) identified ICAM-1 as a HA-receptor on rat-liver sinusoidal endothelial cells, but a recent publication from the same group (63) suggests that ICAM-1 is binding to the hydrophobic spacer arm and is not a HA-receptor. However, using a modified HA-affinity resin, they have identified two putative liver endothelial-cell surface HA-binding proteins of 200 and 400 kDa (63), similar to those reported earlier by Yannariello-Brown et al (64). Other cell-surface HA-receptors, such as RHAMM and hyaluronectin, have been characterized, but antibodies to these do not interact with either human or bovine endothelial cells.

Anti-CD44 antibodies have been reported to inhibit the migration and tube formation of bovine and porcine endothelial cells in vitro (52,65) suggesting that CD44 plays an important role in angiogenesis. However, CD44 binds the hexamer, which is not angiogenic (52,55), and is unlikely to be the primary "angiogenic" receptor for the active oligosaccharides.

Recently we compared the effect of vascular endothelial growth factor (VEGF), bFGF, and OHA on endothelial-cell expression of CD44, ICAM-1, and E-Selectin. All three angiogenic agents increased CD44 expression by around 75%. In agreement with Melder et al. (66), we also found that VEGF increased both ICAM-1 and E-Selectin expression, whereas bFGF upregulated ICAM-1 expression but had only a marginal effect on E-selectin. OHA greatly increased E-Selectin, but surprisingly downregulated ICAM-1 expression. Initially, this suggested that ICAM-1, possibly with bound HA-oligosaccharide, was being phagocytosed by the activated endothelial cells and that ICAM-1 may mediate the angiogenic activity of these oligosaccharides. However, inhibition of endothelial-cell ICAM-1 expression using the ISIS 1939 antisense oligonucleotide (67) failed to inhibit the upregulation of E-selectin and CD44 by OHA, indicating that CD44 interactions are responsible for at least part of the endothelial activation by OHA (West, preliminary data). OHA also rapidly increases IL-8 mRNA levels (West and Noble, preliminary data), which, together with the upregulation of E-selectin, indicates that an early result of OHA-CD44 interaction is the activation of the NFκB transcription factor. Similar inflammatory gene activation has been reported by Noble et al. (68–70), who have shown that HA-oligosaccharides, between the hexasaccharide and 440 kDa, rapidly induce and activate NFκB and reduce IκBα expression in cultured macrophages. In an earlier study, they found that the binding of HA (80 kDa in size) to CD44 induced TNF-α and IL-1β expression within 1 h, and IGF-1 after 12 h (69). More recently, they have shown that a discrete 35 kDa HA fraction has similar effects (70), which suggests that OHA's effect on wound macrophages may contribute little to its angiogenic effect, especially in the cryoinjured graft model (see above). It is difficult to imagine why there should be this difference in the size distribution of HA-oligosaccharides that activate macrophages and those that induce angiogenesis, if only CD44 is induced. The regulation of CD44 is complex and has many cell-specific features (71), such as the density of CD44 on the cell surface and its interaction with RHAMM.

Montesano et al. (51) have recently reported that angiogenic OHA acts synergistically with VEGF, arguably the main angiogenic cytokine in tumors, but not bFGF. However our own preliminary results, using rat aorta cultured in a serum-free collagen-gel matrix (72), indicate that although both VEGF and OHA stimulate microvessel growth in this model, their combined effect is at best additive and not synergistic (Burbridge and West, unpublished results). In contrast, we have recently found that OHA does upregulate VEGF receptor expression by cultured human endothelial cells (West, in preparation), so the jury remains out in this case.

Deed et al. (73) recently reported that OHA induces the immediate early response genes c-fos, c-jun, jun-B, Krox-20, and Krox-24 in bovine aortic endothelial cells, whereas high molecular-weight HA did not. The authors also point out that chronic or sustained treatment with OHA was necessary for activation of cell proliferation. Activation of NFκB, and to a lesser extent the AP-1 transcription factor, has previously been reported in response to 12(R)-hydroxyeicosatrienoic acid, an angiogenic arachidonic acid metabolite (74).

CONCLUSIONS

Studies on high molecular-weight HA suggest that it is inhibitory to new blood vessel formation and that its degradation is a necessary component of adult wound healing. Recent reports, largely from tumor studies, has identified at least two GPI-linked cell-surface hyaluronidases whose expression coincides with matrix HA degradation. The action of these same, or similar, enzymes appear responsible for HA breakdown, and thus regulate wound angiogenesis. OHA stimulates angiogenesis in vitro and in many in vivo models, including several wound healing models. Present evidence indicates that, although OHA can stimulate macrophages, the stimulation of wound angiogenesis is probably by direct action on the vasculature. This appears to involve binding to CD44, with subsequent rapid activation of the NFκB and AP-1 transcription factors.

ACKNOWLEDGMENTS

D. C. W. thanks the North West Cancer Research Fund and the MRC (DCW, DMS) for their support. T.–P. D. F. thanks the British Heart Foundation and the Wellcome Trust for financial support.

REFERENCES

1. Scott, J. E. (1995) Extracellular matrix, supramolecular organization and shape. *J. Anat.* **187,** 259–269.
2. Jackson, R. L., Busch, S. J., and Cardin, A. D. (1991) Glycosaminoglycans: Molecular properties, protein interactions, and role in physiological processes. *Physiol. Rev.* **71,** 481–538.
3. Prestwich, G. D., Marecak, D. M., Marecek, J. F., Vercruysse, K. P., and Ziebell, M. R. (1997) Chemical modification of hyaluronic acid for drug delivery, biomaterials, and biochemical probes, in *The Chemistry, Biology, and Medical Applications of Hyaluronan and its Derivatives* (Laurent, T. C. and Balazs, E. A., eds.), Portland Press, London, pp. 43–62.
4. Entwistle, J., Hall, C. L., and Turley, E. A. (1996) HA Receptors: regulators of signalling to the cytoskeleton. *J. Cell. Biochem.* **61,** 569–577.
5. Knudson, C. B. and Knudson, W. (1993) Hyaluronan- binding proteins in development, tissue homeostasis, and disease. *FASEB J.* **7,** 1233–1241.
6. Toole, B. P. (1982) Glycosaminoglycans in morphogenesis, in *Cell Biology of the Extracellular Matrix* (Hay, E. D., ed.), Plenum, New York, pp. 259–294.
7. Laurent, T. C. and Fraser, J. R. E. (1992) Hyaluronan. *FASEB J.* **6,** 2397–2404.
8. Knudson, W., Biswas, C., Li, X.-Q., Nemec, R. E., and Toole, B. P. (1989) The role and regulation of tumor-associated hyaluronan, in *The Biology of Hyaluronan* (Evered, D. and Whelan, J. eds.), Ciba Foundation Symposium 143, John Wiley and Sons, Chichester, UK, pp. 150–169.
9. West, D. C. and Kumar, S. (1989) Hyaluronan and angiogenesis, in *The Biology of Hyaluronan* (Evered, D. and Whelan, J. eds.), Ciba Foundation Symposium 143, John Wiley and Sons, Chichester, UK, pp. 187–207.
10. Barsky, S. H., Nelson, L. L., and Levy, V. A. (1987) Tumor demoplasia inhibits angiogenesis. *Lancet* **2,** 1336–1337.
11. Balazs, E. A. and Darzynkiewcz, Z. (1973) The effect of hyaluronic acid on fibroblasts, mononuclear phagocytes and lymphocytes, in *Biology of the fibroblast* (Kulonen, E. and Pikkarainen J., eds.), Academic, New York, pp. 237–252.
12. Rydell, N. (1970) Decreased granulation tissue reaction after installment of hyaluronic acid. *Acta Orthop. Scand.* **41,** 307–311.
13. Trabucchi, A., Preis- Baurffaldi, F., Baratti, C., and Montorsi, W. (1986) Topical treatment of experimental skin lesion in rats: macroscopic, microscopic and scanning electron microscopic evaluation of the healing process. *J. Tissue React.* **8,** 533–544.
14. Dvorak, H. F., Harvey, S., Estralla, P., Brown, L. F., McDonagh, J., and Dvorak, A. M., (1987) Fibrin containing gels induce angiogenesis. *Lab. Invest.* **57,** 673–686.
15. Lebel, L. and Gerdin, B. (1991) Sodium hyaluronate increases vascular ingrowth in rabbit ear chamber. *Int. J. Exp. Pathol.* **72,** 111–118.

16. Arnold, F., Jia, C. Y., He, C. F., Cherry, G. W., Carbow, B., Meyer-Ingold, W., Bader, D., and West, D. C. (1995) Hyaluronan, heterogeneity and healing: the effects of ultra-pure hyaluronan of defined molecular size on the repair of full thickness pig skin wounds. *Wound Rep. Reg.* **3**, 10–21.

17. King, S. R., Hickerson, W. L., and Proctor, K. G. (1991) Beneficial actions of exogenous hyaluronic acid on wound healing. *Surgery* **109**, 76–84.

18. Borognoni, L., Reali, U. M., and Santucci, M. (1996) Low-molecular-weight hyaluronic acid induces angiogenesis and modulation of the cellular infiltrate in primary and secondary healing wounds. *Eur. J. Dermatol.* **6**, 127–131.

19. Feinberg, R. N. and Beebe, D. C. (1983) Hyaluronate in vasculogenesis. *Science* **220**, 1177–1179.

20. Dunphy, J. E. and Upuda, K. N. (1955) Chemical and histochemical sequences in the normal healing wounds. *N. Engl J. Med.* **253**, 847–851.

21. Bently, J. P. (1967) Rate of chondroitin sulphate formation in wound healing. *Ann. Surg.* **165**, 186–191.

22. Bertolami, C. N., Berg, S., and Freymiller, E. G. (1992) Glycosaminoglycan processing during tissue repair: Degradation of hyaluronic acid, in: *Fetal Wound Healing* (Adzick, N. S. and Longaker, M. T., eds.), Elsevier, New York, pp. 215–226.

23. Weigel, P. H., Fuller, G. M., and Le Boeuf, R. D. (1986) A model for the role of hyaluronic acid and fibrin in the early events during the inflammatory response and wound healing. *J. Theor. Biol.* **119**, 219–234.

24. Weigel, P. H., Frost, S. J., McGary, C. T., and LeBoeuf, R. D. (1988) The role of hyaluronic acid in inflammation and wound healing. *Int. J. Tissue React.* **10**, 355–365.

25. Weigel, P. H., Frost, S. J., LeBoeuf, R. D., and McGary, C. T. (1989) The specific interaction between fibrin(ogen) and hyaluronan: possible consequences in haemostasis, inflammation and wound healing, in *The Biology of Hyaluronan* (Evered, D. and Whelan, J., eds.), Ciba Foundation Symposium 143, John Wiley and Sons, Chichester, UK, pp. 248–261.

26. Andrade, S. P., Fan, T-P. D., and Lewis, G. P. (1987) Quantitative in vivo studies on angiogenesis in a rat sponge model. *Br. J. Exp. Path.* **68**, 755–766.

27. West, D. C., Smither, R. L., Shaw, D. M., Joyce, M., Kumar, S., and Fan, T-P. D. (2000) Stimulation of wound repair by angiogenic oligosaccharides of hyaluronan: correlation between hyaluronan degradation and angiogenesis in a rat wound healing model. *Lab. Invest.*, submitted.

28. Mast, B. A., Haynes, J. H., Krummel, T. M., Diegelman, R. F., and Cohen, I. K. (1992) In vivo degradation of fetal wound hyaluronic acid results in increased fibroplasia, collagen deposition, and neovascularization. *Plastic Reconstr. Surgery* **89**, 503–509.

29. West, D. C., Shaw, D. M., Lorenz, P., Adzick, N. S., and Longaker, M. (1997) Fibrotic healing of adult and late gestation fetal wounds correlates with increased hyaluronidase activity and removal of hyaluronan. *Int. J. Biochem. Cell Biol.* **29**, 201–210.

30. Locci, P., Marinucci, L., Lilli, C., Martinese, D., and Becchetti, E. (1995) Transforming growth factor beta 1- hyaluronic acid interaction. *Cell Tissue Res.* **281**, 317–324.

31. Yasui, T., Akatsuka, M., Tobetto., K, Umemoto, J., Ando, T., Yamashita, K., and Hayakawa, T. (1992) Effects of hyaluronan on the production of stromelysin and tissue inhibitor of metalloproteinase-1 (TIMP-1) in bovine articular chondrocytes. *Biomed. Res.* **13**, 343–348.

32. West, D. C. and Kumar, S. (1988) Endothelial proliferation and diabetic retinopathy. *Lancet* **1**, 715–716.

33. West, D. C. and Kumar, S. (1989) The effect of hyaluronate and its oligosaccharides on endothelial proliferation and monolayer integrity. *Exp. Cell Res.* **183**, 179–196.

34. West, D. C. and Kumar, S. (1991) Tumor-associated hyaluronan: a potential regulator of tumor angiogenesis. *Int. J. Radiol.* **61/62**, 55–60.

35. Watanabe, M., Nakayasu, K., and Okisaka, S. (1993) The effect of hyaluronic acid on proliferation and differentiation of capillary endothelial cells. *Nippon Ganka Gakkai Zasshi.* **97**, 1034–1039.

36. Fournier, N. and Doillon, C. J. (1992) In vitro angiogenesis in fibrin matrices containing fibronectin or hyaluronic acid. *Cell. Biol. Int. Reports* **16**, 1251–1263.

37. Kumar, S., West, D. C., Ponting, J., and Gattamaneni, H. R. (1989) Sera of children with renal tumor contain low molecular mass hyaluronic acid. *Int. J. Cancer* **44**, 445–448.

38. Shaw, D. M. (1996) Ph.D. Hyaluronan metabolism in wound healing and in tumor growth. Thesis, University of Liverpool.

39. Shaw, D. M., West, D. C., and Hamilton, E. (1994) Hyaluronidase and hyaluronan in tumors and normal tissues, quantity and size distribution. *Int. J. Exp. Pathol.* **75**, A67.

40. West, D. C. and Shaw, D. M. (1998) Tumor hyaluronan in relationship to angiogenesis and metastasis, in *The Chemistry, Biology and Medical Applications of Hyaluronan and its Derivatives* (Laurent, T. C. and Balazs, E. A., eds.), Portland Press, London. pp. 227–233.

41. Fraser, J. R. E. and Laurent, T. C. (1989) Turnover and metabolism of hyaluronan, in *The Biology of Hyaluronan* (Evered, D. and Whelan, J. eds.), Ciba Foundation Symposium 143, John Wiley and Sons, Chichester, UK, pp. 41–59.

42. Fraser, J. R. E., Brown, T. J., and Laurent, T. C. (1998) Catabolism of hyaluronan, in *The Chemistry, Biology and Medical Applications of Hyaluronan and its Derivatives* (Laurent, T. C. and Balazs, E. A., eds.), Portland Press, London, pp. 85–92.

43. Liu, D., Pearlman, E., Diaconu, E., Guo, K., Mori, H., Haqqi, T., Markowitz, S., Willson, J., and Sy, M.-S., (1996) Expression of hyaluronidase by tumor cells induces angiogenesis in vivo. *Proc. Natl. Acad. Sci. USA* **93**, 7832–7837.

44. Podyma, K. A., Yamagata, S., Sakata, K., and Yamagata, Y. (1997) Differences of hyaluronidase produced by human tumor cell lines with hyaluronidase present in human serum as revealed by zymography. *Biochem. Biophys. Res. Comm.* **241**, 446–452.

45. Frost, G. I., Csoka, T., and Stern, R. (1997) Purification, cloning and expression of human plasma hyaluronidase. *Biochem. Biophys. Res. Comm.* **236**, 10–15.

46. Frost, G. I., Csoka, T., and Stern, R. (1996) The hyaluronidases: a chemical, biological and clinical overview. *Trends Glycosci. Glycotechnol.* **8**, 419–434.

47. Schwartz, D. M., Jumper, M. D., Lui, G-M., Dang, S., Schuster, S., and Stern, R. (1997) Corneal endothelial hyaluronidase: A role in anterior chamber hyaluronic acid catabolism. *Cornea* **16**, 188–191.

48. Fiszer-Szafarz, B., Rommain, M., Brossard, C., and Smets, P. (1988) Hyaluronic acid-degrading enzymes in rat alveolar macrophages and in alveolar fluid: Stimulation of enzyme activity after oral treatment with the immunomodulator RU41740. *Biol. Cell.* **63**, 355–360.

49. Sattar, A., Kumar, S., and West D. C. (1992) Does hyaluronan have a role in endothelial cell proliferation of the synovium. *Semin. Arthritis Rheum.* **21**, 43–49.

50. Hirata, S., Akamarsu, T., Matsubara, T., Mizuno, K., and Ishikawa, H. (1993) In vitro angiogenesis induced by oligosaccharides hyaluronic acid. *Arthritis Rheum.* **36**, S247.

51. Montesano, R., Kumar, S., Orci, L., and Pepper, M. S. (1996) Synergistic effect of hyaluronan oligosaccharides and vascular endothelial growth factor on angiogenesis in vitro. *Lab. Invest.* **75**, 249–262.

52. Trouchon, V., Mabilat, C., Bertrand, P., Legrand, Y., Smadia-Joffe, F., Soria, C., et al. (1996) Evidence of involvement of CD44 in endothelial cell proliferation, migration and angiogenesis in vitro. *Int. J. Cancer* **66**, 664–668.

53. Rahmanian, P., Pertoft, H., Kanda, S., Christofferson, R., Claesson-Welsh, L., and Heldin, P. (1997) hyaluronan oligosaccharides induce tube formation of brain endothelial cell line *in vitro. Exp. Cell Res.* **237**, 223–230.

54. Rooney, P., Wang, M., Kumar, P., and Kumar, S. (1993) Angiogenic oligosaccharides of hyaluronan enhance the production of collagen by endothelial cells. *J. Cell Sci.* **105**, 213–218.

55. West, D. C., Hampson, I. N., Arnold, F., and Kumar, S. (1985) Angiogenesis induced by degradation products of hyaluronic acid, *Science* **228**, 1324–1328.

56. Sattar, A., Rooney, P., Kumar, S., Pye, D., West, D.C., Scott, I., and Ledger, P. (1994) Application of angiogenic oligosaccharides of hyaluronan increase blood vessel numbers in rat skin. *J. Invest. Dermatol.* **103**, 576–579.

57. Lees, V. C., Fan, T.-P. D., and West, D. C. (1995) Angiogenesis in a delayed revascularization model is accelerated by angiogenic oligosaccharides of hyaluronan, *Lab. Invest.* **73**, 259–266.

58. Kumar, S., Kumar, P., Ponting, J. M., Sattar, A., Rooney, P., Pye, D., and Hunter, R. D. (1992) Hyaluronic acid promotes and inhibits angiogenesis, in *Angiogenesis in Health and Disease* (Maragoudakis, M. E., Leikes, P., and Gullino, P. M., eds.), Plenum Press, New York, pp. 253–253.

59. West, D. C. (1993) Hyaluronan receptors on human endothelial cells: the effect of cytokines, in *Vascular Endothelium: Physiological Basis of Clinical Problems II* (Catravas, J. D., ed.), Plenum Press, New York, pp. 209–210.

60. Smedrod, B., Pertoft, H., Eriksson, S., Fraser, J. R. E., and Laurent, T. (1984) Studies in vitro on the uptake and degradation of sodium hyaluronate by rat liver endothelial cells. *Biochem J.* **223**, 617–626.

61. Madsen, K., Schenholm, M., Jahnke, G., and Tengblad, A. (1989) Hyaluronate binding to intact corneas and cultured endothelial cells. *Invest. Opth. Vis. Sci.* **30**, 2132–2137.

62. McCourt, P. A. G., Ek, B., Fosberg, N., and Gustafson, S. (1994) Intracellular adhesion molecule-1 is a cell surface receptor for hyaluronan. *J. Biol Chem.* **269**, 30,081–30,084.

63. McCourt, P. A. G. and Gustafson, S. (1997) On the adsorption of hyaluronan and ICAM-1 to modified hydrophobic resins. *Int. J. Biochem. Cell Biol.* **29**, 1179–1189.

64. Yannariello-Brown, J., Frost, S. J., and Wiegel, P. H. (1992) Identification of the Ca^{2+}-independent endocytic hyaluronan receptor in rat liver sinusoidal endothelial cells using a photoaffinity cross-linking reagent. *J. Biol. Chem.* **267,** 20,451–20,456.

65. Banerjee, S. D. and Toole, B. P. (1992) Hyaluronan-binding protein in endothelial morphogenesis. *J. Cell Biol.* **119,** 643–652.

66. Melder, R. J., Koenig, G. C., Witwer, B. P., Safabakhsh, N., Munn, L. L., and Jain, R. K. (1996) During angiogenesis, vascular endothelial growth factor and basic fibroblast growth factor regulate natural killer cell adhesion to tumor endothelium. *Nature Med.* **2,** 992–997.

67. Bennett, C. F., Condon, T. P., Grimm, S., Chan, H., and Chiang M.-Y. (1994) Inhibition of endothelial cell adhesion molecule expression with antisense oligonucleotides. *J. Immunol.* **152,** 3530–3540.

68. Noble, P. W., McKee, C. M., Cowman, M., and Shin, H. S. (1996) Hyaluronan fragments activate an NFκB/IkBα autoregulatory loop in murine macrophages. *J. Exp Med.* **186,** 2373–2378.

69. Noble, P. W., Lake, F. R., Henson, P. M., and Riches, D. W. H. (1993) Hyaluronate activation of CD44 induces insulin-like growth factor-1 expression by tumor necrosis factor-α-dependent mechanism in murine macrophages. *J. Clin. Invest.* **91,** 2368–2377.

70. Noble, P. W., McKee, C. M., and Horton, M. R. Induction of inflammatory gene expression by low-molecular-weight hyaluronan fragments in macrophages, in *The Chemistry, Biology, and Medical Applications of Hyaluronan and its Derivatives* (Laurent, T. C. and Balazs, E. A., eds.), Portland Press, London, pp. 219–225.

71. Lesley, J. (1998) Hyaluronan binding function of CD44, in *The Chemistry, Biology, and Medical Applications of Hyaluronan and its Derivatives* (Laurent, T. C. and Balazs, E. A., eds.), Portland Press, London, pp. 123–134.

72. Nicosia, R. F. and Ottinetti, A, (1990) Growth of microvessels in serum-free matrix culture of rat aorta. *Lab. Invest.* **63,** 115–122.

73. Deed, R., Rooney P., Kumar, P., Norton, J. D., Smith, J., Freemont, A. J., and Kumar, S. (1997) Early-response gene signalling is induced by angiogenic oligosaccharides of hyaluronan in endothelial cells. Inhibition by non-angiogenic, high-molecular-weight hyaluronan. *Int. J. Cancer* **71,** 251–256.

74. Laniado-Schwartzman, M., Lavrovsky, Y., Stoltz, R. A., Conners, M. S., Falck, J. R., Chauhan, K., and Abraham, N. G. (1994) Activation of nuclear factor κB and oncogene expression by 12 (R)-hydroxyeicosatrienoic acid, an angiogenic factor in microvessel endothelial cells. *J. Biol. Chem.* **269,** 24,321–24,327.

12 Role of Thymic Peptides in Wound Healing

Hynda K. Kleinman, Derrick S. Grant, and Katherine M. Malinda

INTRODUCTION

Wound repair requires the concerted action of numerous cells and factors. The inflammation, proliferation, and remodeling phases of wound healing occur in a highly coordinated cascade. Angiogenesis, the formation of new blood vessels, is one of the critical steps in the proliferative phase of wound repair *(1–5)*. Like wound healing, angiogenesis requires cell migration, proliferation, and extracellular matrix synthesis and assembly. New vessels provide nutrients to support the repair cells, promote granulation tissue formation, and facilitate the clearance of debris. Granulation tissue is mainly composed of blood vessels that also supply the necessary oxygen to stimulate repair. Wound angiogenesis is a complex multistep process that involves many mediators. Despite a detailed knowledge about many angiogenic factors present in the wound, little progress has been made in defining the source of these factors and the regulatory events involved in their production *(1–9)*. Further complicating the understanding of wound angiogenesis and repair is the fact that the mechanisms and mediators involved in repair likely vary depending on the depth of the wound, type of wound (burn, trauma, etc.), and the location (muscle, skin, bone, etc.). The condition and age of the patient (diabetic, paraplegic, on steroid therapy, elderly vs infant, etc) can also determine the rate of repair and response to angiogenic factors. Furthermore, the sex of the patient and hormonal status (premenopausal, postmenopausal, etc.) may also influence the repair mechanisms and responses. Impaired wound healing particularily affects the elderly and many of the 14 million diabetics in the United States and reduced angiogenesis is often a causative agent for wound-healing problems in these patient populations.

From: *The New Angiotherapy*
Edited by: T.-P. D. Fan and E. C. Kohn © Humana Press Inc., Totowa, NJ

A number of angiogenic stimulators have been identified in wound fluids (1,3–5,7). The majority, but not all, of the stimulators in wound fluids are growth factors known to increase endothelial-cell migration and proliferation in vitro. Some of these factors act directly on endothelial cells, such as vascular endothelial growth factor (VEGF), fibroblast growth factor FGF, and thymosin β4, which promote endothelial cell migration, whereas others, such as prostaglandin E$_2$ (PGE$_2$), epidermal growth factor (EGF), transforming growth factor-β (TGF-β), and tumor necrosis factor-α (TNF-α), regulate the inflammatory phase of wound healing and may not directly affect angiogenesis (10–30). It is likely that the angiogenic stimulators act via different signaling mechanisms. For example, in addition to promoting endothelial-cell migration, VEGF promotes proliferation also, but has no effect on the formation of capillary-like structures (tube formation) on the basement membrane matrix matrigel (11). In contrast, thymosin β4 has no effect on proliferation but promotes tube formation (18). FGF can promote both proliferation and tube formation (12).

This chapter will deal with two new low molecular angiogenic molecules originally isloated from the thymus that are involved in wound repair. Thymosin α1 and β4 are potent mediators of endothelial cell migration and angiogenesis (18,31–33). Thymosin β4 has been found in wound fluid and its highest concentration in the body is in the platelets, which are the first cells to arrive at the wound. Platelets release mediators that affect the remainder of the repair process. Patients with impaired platelet function do not heal wounds well supporting an important regulatory role for the initial mediators released by these cells. Thymosin α1 is present in serum that is present in the early phase of wound healing (34). Thus, both thymic peptides could be normal physiological mediators of wound repair.

WOUND HEALING

The cascade of wound healing has been arbitrarily divided into three phases: clotting/inflammation, proliferation, and remodeling (Table 1) (35). These phases of wound healing can overlap and last many days or even months. The initial clotting step, which can last up to 5 d, involves platelet aggregation and clot formation and results in the release of many chemoattractants, which recruit the repair cells involved in the removal of the debris (neutrophils and monocytes) and restoration of the tissue (endothelial cells and fibroblasts). The inflammatory period is very important, with various studies demonstrating the key role macrophages have in repair. During debris removal by macrophages, the repair phase begins with cell proliferation and deposition of matrix. Macrophages are rich in chemoattractants, which regulate the subsequent repair process (8). Extracts of macrophages and macrophages themselves have been used to accelerate repair in animal models and in elderly humans with impaired healing (7,10). Furthermore, animals with low levels of macrophages exhibit delayed and impaired wound healing (36). During the proliferative phase of wound healing, which can last from 2 d to 3 wk, granulation tissue forms. Approximately 60% of the granulation tissue mass is new blood vessels, which supply the nutrients needed for repair. Patients with an impaired ability to form blood vessels suffer from poor wound healing. For example, interferons have been shown to reduce angiogenesis. Animals and patients treated with interferons experience an inhibition of wound healing (37; Cid, unpublished observations). During this phase, collagen deposition begins, the wound contracts and re-epithelialization occurs. In the final remodeling phase of wound healing, which can last from 3 d to years, wound contraction continues and the collagen fibrils mature into a highly crosslinked matrix.

Table 1
Wound-Healing Stages

Inflammation	Proliferation	Remodeling
Clot formation	Granulation tissue	Clot lysis
Vasoconstriction	Angiogenesis	Collagen crosslinking
Platelet aggregation	Collagen deposition	Contraction continues
Chemoattractant release	Wound contraction	Scar tissue matures
Neutrophils/monocytes remove debris	Reepithelialization	

ANGIOGENESIS

The formation of new blood vessels involves a highly ordered cascade of events that is regulated all or in part by angiogenic factors *(38,39)*. Initially the basement membrane underlying the endothelial cells is degraded. Several proteases, including metalloproteinases and the plasminogen system, have been shown to be involved in this degradation *(40)*. The cells then migrate through spaces in the basement-membrane matrix into the underlying connective tissue. Various agents, including many growth factors (which are small diffusable molecules that are active at very low concentrations), have been found to trigger cell migration *(1–3)*. In a wound, these growth factors could be coming from the serum, platelets, macrophages, the phagocytosed debris, and/or even the degraded basement-membrane matrix, which is highly enriched in both growth and angiogenic factors. Basement membrane contains several known angiogenic stimulators, such as FGF, EGF, TGF-α and platelet-derived growth factor (PDGF), as well as proteases that could facilitate cell migration *(41)*. In addition, certain sequences from laminin-1 have been found to be highly angiogenic and one (ser-ile-lys-val-la-val: SIKVAV) also induces protease activity *(42)*. With degradation of the basement membrane, such active sequences may become more available and be physiologically important. Endothelial cells located in the original vessel proliferate to generate new migratory cells. Proliferation is also induced mainly by growth factors, but these molecules may be active for proliferation at a different concentration than that required for migration. The final step in angiogenesis occurs when the endothelial cells form tubular structures and the basement membrane matrix is resynthesized by the endothelial cells. It is not clear what initiates this process but it may be related to the cessation of cell migration. Inhibitors of collagen IV (basement-membrane collagen) synthesis have been found to affect tube formation in vitro and angiogenesis in vivo, demonstrating the importance of matrix synthesis in angiogenesis *(43)*.

ANGIOGENIC THYMIC PEPTIDES: THYMOSIN α1 AND THYMOSIN β4

When endothelial cells are plated in vitro on a basement-membrane matrix (matrigel), they attach, migrate, secrete proteases, and form capillary-like structures with a lumen in 18 hours *(44)*. This in vitro tube assay has been used reliably to characterize many angiogenic and antiangiogenic factors. Using subtractive cDNA cloning, we have identified a small 43 amino acid thymic peptide, thymosin β4, as a gene that is induced some fivefold at 4 h after plating on matrigel (Table 2A) *(31)*. Thymosin β4 was originally isolated from the thymus and found to be important in T-cell differentiation *(33)*. It also binds to G-actin and is an active actin-sequestering protein *(45)*. Thymosin β4 has a

Table 2
Characteristics of Thymic Peptides

A. Thymosin β4
43 amino acids, 4.9 kD, highly conserved among mammals
Ubiquitous, found at high concentrations in blood platelets (560 μM) and in the brain
Binds to G-actin and is an actin-sequestering protein
Influences T-cell differentiation (induces deoxynucleotidyl transferase)
Important in cell differentiation

B. Thymosin α1
28 amino acids, 3.1 kD It is the N terminus of a 113 amino acid precursor,
     prothymosin α1. The C terminus has a nuclear-targeting sequence.
Found in blood (690 pg/mL), brain, and spleen
Affects maturation and function of T cells
Affects proliferation of estrogen-treated breast-cancer cells and synergizes with EGF
     to stimulate fibroblast proliferation
Clinical trials suggest it increases the immune response

---

number of biological effects on endothelial cells demonstrating that it is important in angiogenesis (Table 3A) (18). Antisense oligonucleotides block tube formation on matrigel and either transfection of the gene or exogenous addition of thymosin β4 results in increased and more rapid cell migration and tube formation. Thymosin β4 promotes endothelial-cell migration but does not influence the migration of smooth-muscle cells, neutrophils, monocytes, fibroblasts, or tumor cells (18). Another family member, thymosin β15, has recently been found to be elevated in prostate cancer and to be important in tumor-cell migration (46). Thymosin β4 is active at the ng level for endothelial-cell migration (Fig. 1A). Sprouting from aortic rings in vitro is also induced by thymosin β4, confirming its activity for endothelial-cell tube formation (Grant, unpublished observations). In vivo, it is highly angiogenic and has been found to promote angiogenesis in a subcutaneous implant model (18). It is also present in mature vessels, suggesting it may have a role in stabilization of the differentiated phenotype (31).

When tested in a punch biopsy model of wound repair (Table 4), thymosin β4 stimulates healing. When given topically on at the time of wounding and on the second day, the wound gap is significantly reduced at day 7 (Fig. 2; Table 5). Likewise, if the rats are treated every other day with intraperitoneal injections of thymosin β4, the wound gap is reduced. These data suggest that thymosin β4 is an effective wound-healing agent. It is likely that owing to its small size it can rapidly diffuse to the tissue surrounding the wound and stimulate enodthelial-cell migration and angiogenesis.

Another thymic peptide thymosin α1 is highly angiogenic and has been found to promote wound healing (32). Thymosin α1 is a 28 amino acid N terminal fragment of the 113 amino acid prothymosin alpha 1 (Table 2B). Thymosin α1 is an immune modulator that promotes the maturation and function of T cells (47). It is present in serum and can regulate the proliferation of some cells. It has been used in the treatment of certain infectious diseases because it can increase the immune repsonse. Recently its role in angiogenesis and wound healing has been demonstrated (Table 3B). Thymosin α1 promotes endothelial-cell migration with activity also in the ng range (Fig. 1B) (32). The activity is highly specific with monocytes showing some response at certain doses but smooth-muscle cells, neutrophils, fibroblasts, and tumor cells showing no response. It has no effect on endothelial-cell proliferation. In vivo thymosin α1 promotes angiogenesis in a subcutaneous matrigel implant model.

Table 3
Angiogenic Activities of Thymic Peptides

A. Thymosin β4

Increases mRNA during endothelial-cell tube formation on matrigel

Increases rates and amount of tube formation on matrigel

Antisense oligo to thymosin β4 blocks tube formation on matrigel

Transiently transfected endothelial cells form tubes faster on matrigel

Increases vessel sprouting from aortic rings

Increases endothelial-cell migration (but not the migration of neutrophils, monocytes, fibroblasts, smooth muscle cells, or tumor cells)

Increases angiogenesis in subcutaneous matrigel implants

Increases wound angiogenesis and repair in full thickness wounds in rats

B. Thymosin α1

Increases endothelial-cell tube formation on matrigel

Increases endothelial-cell migration and monocyte migration (but does not effect fibroblasts, neutrophils, or tumor cells)

Increases vessel sprouting from aortic rings

Increases angiogenesis in subcutaneous matrigel implants

Increases wound angiogenesis and repair in full thickness wounds in rats

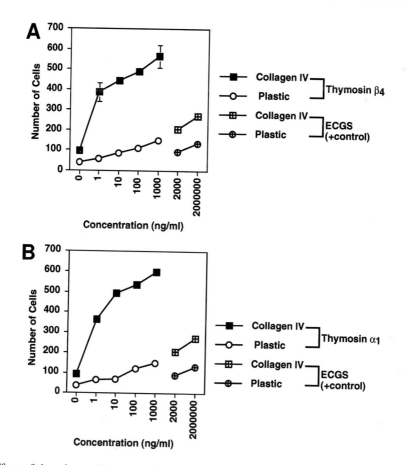

Fig. 1. Effect of thymic peptides on cell migration in the Boyden chamber assay. $p = 0.0006$ for all doses of the thymic peptides.

Table 4
Skin Punch Wound Model in Rats[a]

Rats	8-mm punch wounds on back
	6 punch wounds per rat
	3 rats per test group
Topical testing	9 wounds are treated topically with 5 µg/50 µL at time 0 and at 48 h
	9 control wounds receive 50 µL saline at time 0 and at 48 h
Intraperitoneal testing	3 rats (18 wounds) receive intraperitoneal injections of
	60 µg/0.3 mL every other day
	3 rats (18 wounds) receive intraperitoneal injections of 0.3 mL
	saline every other day

[a]Each experiment is done twice.

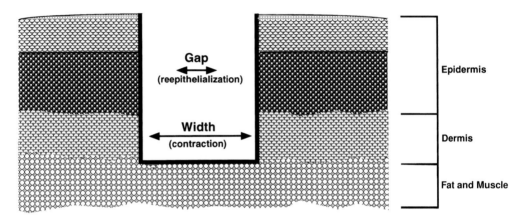

Fig. 2. Schematic diagram of a punch wound.

Table 5
Effect of Thymosin β4 on Wound Closure in Vivo

| | Wound Gap at Day 7[a] | |
	IP treatment	Topical
Control	1669 ± 293	1883 ± 305
Thymosin β4	659 ± 1778	720 ± 394

[a]Data are expressed as gap length (µm).

Thymosin α1 is also a potent promoter of wound repair and wound angiogenesis *(32)*. When given topically at day 0 and day 2 after wounding on 8-mm punch biopsies, repair is accelerated. A significant increase in epithelial-gap closure, collagen content, wound contraction, and wound angiogenesis is observed (Fig. 3). Wound repair is also accelerated with intraperitoneal injections given every other day.

We conclude that small diffusable factors, such as the thymic peptides described here, are important modulators of angiogenesis and may have clinical uses in the treatment of patients with impaired healing. Their role in disease processes, such as impaired healing and tumor growth, is not known at this time.

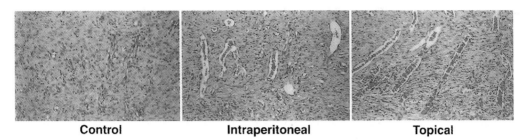

Fig. 3. Appearance of punch wounds after 7 d with thymosin α1. Data are from *(32)* with permission. Wounds of 8-mm were made in 200 gm rats and treated either topically at the time of wounding and 48 h later or intraperitoneally every other day. At 7 d, the animals were sacrificed and histological sections were made of the wounds.

SUMMARY

Wound healing appears to involve a process more complex than simple angiogenesis and tissue growth. A variety of stimulators of inflammation, repair, and angiogenesis are expressed temporally in wounds in a highly specific manner. Two new low molecular-weight angiogenic peptides have been identified that can affect angiogenesis and wound repair. These thymic peptides either alone or in combination with each other and with other factors may be useful in treating chronic wounds that have not been responsive to the growth and angiogenic factors tested to date. Topical fibroblast growth factor (FGF) had no effect. Topical platelet-derived growth factor-BB trials have required large amounts for only a modest effect on wound healing in diabetic ulcers with no effect on pressure ulcers *(48)*. It is possible that the large amount of proteases present in the wounds degrades the added factors. These data suggest that a single growth factor will likely not be able to effect complete wound healing and that a combination of specific factors for each type of wound may be needed along with protease inhibitors.

REFERENCES

1. DiPietro, L. A. and Nissen, N. N. (1998) Angiogenic mediators in wound healing, in *Angiogenesis: Models, Modulators and Clinical Applications* (Maragoudakis, M. E., ed.), Plenum Press, NY.
2. Coleville-Nash, P. R. and Willoughby, D. A. (1997) Growth factors in angiogenesis: current interest and therapeutic potential. *Mol. Med. Today* **January,** 14–23.
3. Bennett, N. T. and Schultz, G. S. (1993) Growth factors and wound healing: Part II. role in normal and chronic wound healing. *Am. J. Surg.* **166,** 74–81.
4. Arnold, F., West, D. C., Schofield, P. F., and Kumar, S. (1987) Angiogenic activity in human wound fluid. *Int. J. Microcirc. Clin. Exp.* **5,** 381–386.
5. Dvonch, V. M., Murphy, R. J., Matsuoka, J., and Grotendorst, G. (1992) Changes in growth factor levels in human wound fluid. *Surgery* **112,** 18–23.
6. Hunt, T. K., Knighton, D. R., Thakral, K. K., Goodson, W. H., III, and Andrew, W. S. (1984) Studies on inflammation and wound healing:angiogenesis and collagen synthesis stimulated in vivo by resident and activated wound macrophages. *Surgery* **96,** 48–54.
7. Rapollee, D. A., Mark, D., Banda, M. J., and Werb, Z. (1988) Wound macrophages express TGF-alpha and other growth factors in vivo: analysis by RNA phenotyping. *Science* **241,** 708–712.
8. Poverini, P. and DiPietro, L. A. (1992) Role of macrophages in the regulation of physiological and patholgoical angiogenesis, in *Angiogenesis in Health and Disease* (Maragoudkis, M. E., ed.), Plenum Press, NY pp. 43–53.
9. Liebovich, S. J. and Ross, R. (1974) The role of the macrophage in wound repair: a study with hydrocortisone and antimacrophage serum. *Am. J. Pathol.* **78,** 81–84.

10. Danon, D., Madjar, J., Edinov, E., Knyszynski, A., Brill, S., Dimanmtishtein, L., and Shinar, E. (1997) Treament of human ulcers by application of macrophages prepared from a blood unit. *Exp. Gerontol.* **32,** 633–641.

11. Ferrara , N., Houck, K., Jakeman L., and Leung, D. (1992) Molecular and biological properties of the vascular endothelial growth factor family of proteins. *Endocr. Rev.* **13,** 18–23.

12. Gospodarowicz, D., Ferrara, N., Schweiger, L., and Neufeld, G. (1987) Structural characterization and biological functions of fibroblast growth factor. *Endocrinol. Rev.* **8** 95–114.

13. Xu, X., Weinstein, M., Li, C., Naski, M., Cohen, R. I., Ornitz, D.M., Leder, P., and Deng, C. (1998). Fibroblast frowth factor receptor 2 (FGFR2)-mediated reciprocal regulation loop between FGF8 and FGF10 is essential for limb induction. *Development* **125,** 753–765.

14. Knighton, D. R., Phillips, G. D., and Fiegel, V. D. (1990) Wound healing angiogenesis:indirect stimulation by basic fibroblast growth factor. *J. Trauma* **30,** 134–144.

15. Nissen, N. N., Poverini , P. D., Gamelli, R. L., and DiPietro, L. A. (1996) Basic fibroblast growth factor mediates angiogenic activity in early surgical wounds. *Surgery* **119,** 457–465.

16. Okumura, M., Okuda,T., Nakamura, T., and Yajima, M. (1996) Acceleration of wound healing in diabetic mice by basic fibroblast growth factor. *Biol. Pharm. Bull.* **19,** 530–535.

17. Greenhalgh, D., G., Sprugel, K. H., Murray, M. J., and Ross, R. (1990) PDGF and FGF stimulate wound healing in the genetically diabetic mouse. *Am. J. Pathol.* **136,** 1235–1245.

18. Malinda, K. M., Goldstein, A. L., and Kleinman, H. K. (1997) Thymosin β4 stimulates directional migration of human umbilical vein endothelial cells. *J. Immunol.* **11,** 474–481.

19. Knighton, D. R., Ciresi, K., Fiegel, V. D., Schuermerth, S., Butler, E., and Cerra, F. (1990) Stimulators of repair in chronic, non healing, cutaneous ulcers using platelet-derived wound healing formula. *Surg. Gynecol. Obstet.* **170,** 50–60.

20. Szabo, S. (1994) Accelerated wound healing of duodenal ulcers by oral administration of a mutein of basic fibroblast growth factor. *Gastroenterology* **106,** 1106–1111.

21. Arnold, F., West, D., and Kumar, S. (1987) Wound healing: the effect of macrophage and tumor derived angiogenic factors on skin graft vascularization. *Br. J. Exp. Pathol.* **68,** 569–574.

22. Eppley, B. L., Doucet , M., Connolly, D. T., and Feder, J. (1988) Enhancement of angiogenesis by bFGF in mandibular bone graft healing in the rabbit. *J. Oral Maxillo. Fac. Surg.* **46,** 391–398.

23. Joyce, M. E., Roberts, A. B., Sporn, M. B., and Bolander, M. E. (1990) Transforming growth factor beta and initiation of chondrogenesis and osteogenesis in the femur. *J. Cell Biol.* **110,** 2195–2207.

24. Kurita, Y., Tsuboi, R., Uiki, R., Rifkin, D. B., and Ogawa, H. (1992) Immunohistomchemical localization of basic fibroblast growth factor in wound healing site of mouse skin. *Arch. Dermatol. Res.* **284,** 193–197.

25. Bashkin, P., Doctrow, S., Klagsbrun, M., Svahn, C. M., Folkman, J., and Vlodavsky, I. (1989) Basic fibroblast growth factor binds to subendothelial extracellular matrix and is released by heparitinase and heparin-like molecules. *Biochemistry* **28,** 1737–1743.

26. Uhl, E., Rosken, F., and Messmer, K. (1997) Transdermal administration of platelet-derived growth factor for improved wound healing in local ischemia and diabetes mellitus. *Langenbecks Arch. Chir. Suppl. Kongress* **114,** 705–708.

27. Malchereck, P., Schultz, G., Wingren, U., and Franzen, L. (1994) Formation of healing tissue and angiogenesis in repair of connective tissue stimulated by epidermal growth factor. *Scand. J. Plast. Reconstr. Hand Surg.* **28,** 1–7.

28. Brown, L. F., Yeo, K. T., Berse, B., Yeo, T. K., Senger, D. R., Dvorak, H. F., and Van Der Water, L. (1992) Expression of vascular permeability factor (vascular endothelial growth factor) by epidermal keratinocytes during wound healing. *J. Exp. Med.* **176,** 1375–1381.

29. Nissen, N. N., Poverini, P. J., Koch, A. E., Volin, M. V., Gamelli, R. L., and DiPietro, L. A. (1998) Vascular endothelial growth factor mediates angiogenic activity during the proliferative phase of wound healing. *Am. J. Pathol.* **152,** 1445–1452.

30. Chegni, N. (1997) The role of growth factors in peritoneal healing; transforming growth factor beta. *Eur. J. Surg.* **577,** 17–23.

31. Grant, D. S., Kinsella, J. L., Kibbey, M. C., LaFlamme, S., Burbelo, P. D., Goldstein, A. L., and Kleinman, H. K. (1995) Matrigel induces thymosin beta 4 in differentiating endothelial cells. *J. Cell Sci.* **108,** 3685–3694.

32. Malinda, K. M., Sidhu, G. S., Banaudha, K. K., Gaddipati, J. P., Maheshwari, R. K., Goldstein, A. L., and Kleinman, H. K. (1998) Thymosin alpha 1 stimulates endothelial cell migration, angiogenesis and wound healing. *J. Immunol.* **160,** 1001–1006.

33. Oates, K. and Goldstein, A.L. (1995) Thymosin, in *Biological Therapy of Cancer* (DeVita , V. T., Hellman, S., and Rosenberg, R. A., eds.), J. B. Lippincott Co, PA, pp. 841–853.

34. Yokoi, H., Saitoh, T., Nakazawa, U., and Ohno, H. (1996) An immunoradiometric assay for thymosin α1. *J. Immunoassay* **17,** 85–88.
35. Clark, A. F. (1996) Wound repair: an overview and general considerations, in *The Molecular and Cellular Biology of Wound Repair* (Clark, A. F., ed.), Plenum Press, New York, pp. 1–50.
36. Danon, D., Kovatch, M. A ., and Rogh, G. S. (1989) Promotion of wound repair in old mice by local injections of macrophages. *PNAS* **86,** 2018–2020.
37. Stout, A. J., Gusser, I., and Thompson, W., D. (1993) Inhibition of wound healing in mice by local interferon α/β injection. *Int. J. Pathol.* **74,** 79–85.
38. Folkman, J. and Shing, Y. (1992) Angiogenesis. *J. Biol. Chem.* **267,** 10,931–10,934.
39. Sephel, G. C., Kennedy, R., and Kudav, S. (1996) Expression of capillary basement membrane components during sequential phases of wound angiogenesis. *Matrix Biol.* **15,** 263–279.
40. Moscatelli, D. and Rifkin, D. B. (1988) Membrane and matrix localization of proteases: a common theme in tumor cell invasion and angiogenesis. *Biochem. Biophys. Acta* **948,** 67–85.
41. Vukecivic, S., Kleinman, H. K., Luyten, F. P., Roberts, A. B., Roche, N. S., and Reddi, A. H. (1992) Identification of multiple active growth factors in basement membrane matrigel suggests caution in interpretation of cellular activity related to extracellular matrix components. *Exp. Cell Res.* **202,** 1–8.
42. Grant, D. S., Kinsella, J. L., Fridman, R., Auerbach, R., Piasecki, B. A., Yamada, Y., et al. (1992) Interaction of endothelial cells with a laminin A chain peptide (SIKVAV) in vitro and induction of angiogenic behavior in vivo. *J. Cell. Physiol.* **153,** 614–625.
43. Haralabopoulos, G. C., Grand, D. S., Kleinman, H. K, Lelkes, P. I., Papaionnou, S. P., and Maragoudakis, M. E. (1994) Inhibitors of basement membrane collagen synthesis prevent endothelial cell alignment in matrigel in vitro and angiogenesis in vivo. *Lab. Invest.* **71,** 575–582.
44. Kubota, Y., Kleinman, H. K., Martin, G. R., and Lawley, T. J. (1988) Role of laminin and basement membrane in the differentiation of human endothelial cells into capillary-like structures. *J. Cell Biol.* **170,** 1589–1597.
45. Safer, D. and Nachamias, V. T. (1994) Beta thymosins as actin binding proteins. *BioEssays* **16,** 473–479.
46. Bao, L., Loda, M., Janmey, P. A., Stewart, R., Anand-Apte, B., and Zetter, B. R. (1996) Thymosin beta 15 : a novel regulator of tumor cell motility upregulated in metastatic prostate cancer. *Nature Med.* **2,** 1322–1328.
47. Goldstein, A. L. (1994) Clinical applications of thymosin α1. *Cancer Invest.* **12,** 545–560.
48. Robson, M. C., Mustoes, T. A., Hunt, T. K. (1998) The future of recombinant growth factors in wound healing. *Am. J. Surg.* **176,** 80S–82S.

13 Angiogenesis and Growth Factors in Ulcer Healing

Sandor Szabo, Yuen Shing, M. Judah Folkman,
Aron Vincze, Zoltan Gombos, Xiaoming Deng,
Tetayana Khomenko, and Masashi Yoshida

INTRODUCTION

Angiogenesis, i.e., endothelial-cell proliferation and tube formation in postembryonic tissue, is a crucial element in granulation tissue production. The formation of granulation tissue, i.e., angiogenesis followed by proliferation of fibroblasts and deposition of collagen, on the other hand, is a rate-limiting step in the repair of major tissue injury (e.g., after the loss of cardiac or smooth muscle). Only in certain organs such as the liver, adrenal and renal cortex, the regeneration involves the proliferation of original parenchymal cells that fast replace the lost tissue.

The healing of external (e.g., skin) and internal (e.g., gastrointestinal) wounds usually need granulation tissue, which forms the basis for proliferating and migrating epithelial cells to complete the healing process. Namely, migrating epithelial cells cannot grow over necrotic tissue, unless it is gradually replaced by angiogenesis-dependent granulation tissue. Thus, stimulation of only epithelial-cell proliferation is counter-productive in the healing of internal and external wounds, unless it is accompanied by the expansion of a loose or solid granulation tissue, which provides the basis and physical framework for the migration of epithelial cells to complete the healing process.

Superficial mucosal lesions such as erosions that do not penetrate the muscularis mucosae usually do not require granulation tissue and heal fast. The healing of deep ulcers that reach or penetrate the muscularis propria, on the other hand, almost always requires initial angiogenesis and proliferation of other elements of granulation tissue.

From: *The New Angiotherapy*
Edited by: T.-P. D. Fan and E. C. Kohn © Humana Press Inc., Totowa, NJ

Because cell proliferation (i.e., angiogenesis) and granulation production are stimulated by growth factors, these peptides represent a new molecular tool to gain insights into the mechanisms of ulcer healing *(1,2)*. The angiogenesis-targeted tissue repair is thus a novel cellular and molecular approach to ulcer healing, which until recently has been stimulated only indirectly *(1,2)*. Namely, by reduction or elimination of endogenous and exogenous aggressive factors such as acid, pepsin, *H. pylori*, nonsteroidal anti-inflammatory drugs (NSAID) ulcers have been left alone to heal themselves. Our approach, on the other hand, has always been to stimulate directly ulcer healing by growth factors, which preferentially affect angiogenesis and granulation tissue production *(2,3)*.

We thus review here our initial and recent pharmacologic experiments as well as the emerging pathophysiologic role of endogenous growth factors in the natural healing of gastrointestinal (GI) ulcers.

PHARMACOLOGY OF ANGIOGENESIS AND GI ULCERS

Growth factors, such as, epidermal growth (EGF), basic fibroblast growth factor (bFGF), platelet-derived growth factor (PDGF), and more recently vascular endothelial growth factor (VEGF) have been used extensively to heal experimental gastric, duodenal, and colonic ulcers in animal models *(3–9)*. Among these, only EGF has an effect on gastroduodenal secretion, whereas the other peptides stimulate virtually all the cellular elements of ulcer healing (Table 1).

The table demonstrates that the most consistent common effect of these growth factors in ulcer healing is the stimulation of cell proliferation, especially angiogenesis. The molar potency of bFGF, PDGF, and VEGF is 2–7 million times higher than that of cimetidine in the healing of cysteamine-induced chronic duodenal ulcer in rats (Table 2). Because VEGF apparently has no relevant effect other than stimulation of angiogenesis, it is probably safe to conclude that enhancement of angiogenesis that is accompanied by granulation-tissue production is the most important cellular event leading to ulcer healing. Apparently spontaneous proliferation and migration of epithelial cells over dense granulation tissue then complete the healing process.

In most countries of the world, duodenal ulcer is the most prevalent form of "peptic ulcers." For that reason, we first used animal models of duodenal ulcers to test the hypothesis that angiogenic peptides like bFGF might accelerate the healing of chronic duodenal ulcers. Our laboratories were the first to investigate the effects of bFGF, PDGF, and most recently VEGF and their derivates on ulcer healing. In these studies, we focused on investigating the role of angiogenesis and its modulation in the natural healing of GI ulceration. Specific studies were devoted to characterize the role of vascular factors such as angiogenesis in the mechanism of action of sucralfate, which stimulates ulcer healing without decreasing gastric acidity *(10–13)*. Namely our in vitro studies revealed that sucralfate and its water-soluble component sucrose octasulfate are structurally very similar to heparin, and bind bFGF more strongly than heparin *(11,12)*.

bFGF

Chronic Duodenal Ulcer

Because duodenal ulcer disease is still the most prevalent form of peptic ulcer, we first tested the effect of bFGF in the most widely used animal models of duodenal ulcer in rats. We used the modified model of chronic duodenal ulcer induced by cysteamine *(3,4,14)*.

Table 1
Comparative Effect of Growth Factors on Gastroduodenal Secretion,
Cell Proliferation, and Angiogenesis

Peptides	Gs-acid	Du-bicarb.	Epith.↑	Fibrobl.↑	Angiogenesis
EGF	↓	↑	++	+/–	+/–
bFGF	–/↑	–	+	++	++
PDGF	–	–	+	++	+
VEGF	–	NT	–	–	++

+, mild; ++, strong; –, no effect; NT, not tested.

Table 2
The Major Comparison of Antiulcerogenic Doses of bFGF, PDGF, VEGF, and Cimetidine
in the Rat Model of Cysteamine-Induced Chronic Duodenal Ulcer

	bFGF	PDGF	VEGF	Cimetidine
Antiulcerogenic dose(/100 g)	100 ng	500 ng	1 µg (1,000 ng)	10 mg (10^{10} pg)
Molecular weight	18,000	34,000	45,000	252
1 pmole	18 ng	34 ng	45 ng	252 pg
Antiulcerogenic dose in pmole/100g	5.6	14.7	22.2	39,682,540.0
Molar comparison	7,086,168	2,699,492	1,787,502	1

In this model, bFGF was found to be about seven million times more potent on a molar basis in its antiulcerogenic effect than cimetidine in the healing of chronic duodenal ulcer *(3,7)*. These studies demonstrated that *per os* treatment with either naturally occurring bFGF or its acid-resistant mutein, in which the second and third cysteines are replaced by serine residues *(15)*, bFGF-CS23 (100 ng/100 g twice daily) accelerated the healing of cysteamine-induced chronic duodenal ulcer *(3,4)*. This effect was more potent than the oral administration of cimetidine (10 mg/100 g, twice a day for 3 wk), however, only the treatment with acid-resistant mutein bFGF-CS23 (100 ng/100 g twice a day for 3 wk) significantly decreased both size ($p < 0.01$ vs control) and prevalence ($p < 0.05$ vs control) of the remaining chronic ulcers.

Secretory studies showed that a single dose of bFGF had no effect on gastric output of acid and pepsin, whereas daily treatment for 2 or 3 wk resulted in enhanced outputs of both products *(3,7,16)*.

To test both the direct and indirect mode of action of antiulcer drugs we compared cimetidine (10 mg/100 g) and bFGF (50 ng/100 g) alone and in combination in the healing of cysteamine-induced chronic duodenal ulcers. We found that the ulcer size in the combination group was significantly lower (2.0 ± 0.6 mm^2, $p < 0.05$) than in the group that received cimetidine alone (7.5 ± 2.1 mm^2). Histologic evaluation showed that the combination treatment reduced the extent of necrosis and inflammation in the ulcer crater *(17,18)*.

In the cysteamine-induced duodenal ulcer model we found that *per os* administration of sucralfate elevated local levels of bFGF in the ulcer crater. Based on these and previous in vitro findings on the binding of bFGF to sucralfate, we postulated that the locally accumulated angiogenic bFGF may contribute to the ulcer-healing properties of sucralfate, and this peptide might be one of the key endogenous mediators of ulcer healing by sucralfate *(10–13)*.

Novel derivatives of human recombinant (hr) bFGF were also tested in treatment of experimental chronic duodenal ulcer in rats *(19)*, e.g., Ser 78,96-hrbFGF, which is bioequivalent to rbFGF-CS23, CMC-hrbFGF, a carboxymethyl cysteine derivate of hrbFGF and PEG-hrbFGF, a polyethylene glycol (PEG) derivate of hrbFGF. Oral administration of these novel derivates for 3 wk accelerated the healing of cysteamine-induced chronic duodenal ulcer, stimulated angiogenesis and PEG-hrbFGF was more active than the other analogs.

The antiulcerogenic effect of bFGF was recently confirmed in preliminary human studies, which demonstrated that previously therapy-resistant duodenal and antral ulcers healed within 4 wk after oral treatment with bFGF-CS23, without any adverse effect or systemic absorption *(20)*. Subsequently, the potent ulcer-healing effect of bFGF-CS23 was confirmed only in NSAID-induced gastric and duodenal ulcers *(21,22)*.

Chronic Gastric Ulcer

In the studies performed by H. Satoh, a former coworker of ours, *per os* administration of a mutein of rhbFGF twice a day for 2 wk, significantly accelerated the healing of acetic acid-induced gastric ulcer in rats; size of the ulcers decreased while the regeneration of the mucosa was enhanced *(23)*. The same mutein of rhbFGF had no effect on the development of ethanol-induced acute gastric erosions when given to the rats prior to ethanol administration *(23)*. These results suggest that a mucosal protective effect may not be involved in the healing effect of bFGF. Furthermore bFGF, the aforementioned mutein of hrbFGF, was shown to be able to prevent the indomethacin-induced relapse of acetic acid-induced gastric ulcer in rats that were given in either prior to or with indomethacin *(24)*.

In the cryoprobe-induced experimental gastric ulcer the interaction of indomethacin with bFGF and omeprazole was investigated *(25)*. Contrary to omeprazole, bFGF accelerated healing only in the late phase (d 10–15). Omeprazole reversed all indomethacin-induced effects, e.g., angiogenesis, cell proliferation, maturation of granulation tissue, and ulcer-healing rate, whereas bFGF, despite stimulation of angiogenesis did not reverse indomethacin-induced delay in ulcer healing.

The involvement of bFGF in gastric-ulcer was also studied using an experimental gastric ulcer model of mice *(26)* with acetic anhydride applied to the serosal surface of the stomach. Electron microscopic immunohistochemical studies of stomach tissues for bFGF were performed at 5 and 21 d after the treatment. bFGF was localized in fibroblasts in the ulcer bed with distribution throughout the cytoplasm excluding organelles involved in the usual secretory system, such as rough endoplasmic reticulum, Golgi apparatus, and secretory vacuoles, but it was present also in the nucleus. Three weeks after the treatment, when the surface of the lesion was covered by regenerated epithelium, the samples were immunohistochemically negative for bFGF. Nevertheless, untreated normal stomach tissues were also negative for bFGF. This suggests the participation of bFGF in gastric-ulcer healing.

Besides the ulcer healing and angiogenic actions, bFGF was found to promote the reinervation of the newly formed microvessels, regeneration of autonomic nerves in the granulation tissue in the experimental gastric ulcer induced by acetic acid in rats *(27)*. One of the few human studies tested the efficacy and safety of bFGF-CS23 *(28)* for healing of NSAID-associated gastric ulcers, which were resistant to or relapsed after conventional treatment. Five patients with nine ulcers were treated *per os* and after 4 wk, four ulcers had healed and there was significant reduction in the area of others.

Chronic Gastritis

Inflammatory GI diseases such as chronic gastritis are more frequent than duodenal ulcer in certain countries (e.g., Japan). Unfortunately, contrary to the plethora of models of acute gastric erosions and ulcers there has been no appropriate animal model of diffuse acute and chronic gastritis. Based on previous investigations on the role of sulfhydryls (SH) compounds as gastroprotective agents *(29,30)*, our laboratory developed a new model for gastritis: ingestion of low concentrations of SH alkylators (e.g., 0.1% [w/v] iodoacetamide) in drinking water induced severe, diffuse acute and chronic gastritis in rats *(31,32)*.

We investigated the effect of bFGF and sucralfate in this animal model. After the induction of gastritis by the SH alkylator iodoacetamide in drinking water for 1 wk, at the beginning of the second week rats were randomized to receive: native bFGF-w; acid-stable bFGF-CS23; sucralfate in low dose; or combinations of these agents by gavage twice daily. Untreated rats received vehicle and the rats remained on drinking water containing iodoacetamide for one more week. At the autopsy on the 14th day, macroscopic and microscopic signs of inflammation were evaluated and wet and dry weights of stomach were measured. The results demonstrate that only acid-resistant bFGF was effective in accelerating the healing of chronic chemically induced gastritis. Neither native bFGF-w nor sucralfate had any effect at low doses on chronic gastritis. However, both native bFGF and the acid-resistant mutein in combination with sucralfate at low dose were more efficient in the repair of mucosal injury and significantly ($p < 0.001$) more effective than either of these agents alone. Thus, bFGF and sucralfate may act synergistically in healing chronic erosive gastritis.

INFLAMMATORY BOWEL DISEASE (IBD)

The effect of bFGF was also studied in animal models of IBD. As in experimental gastritis (*see* above), these experiments were also mainly performed with new animal models of IBD induced by SH alkylators *(33,34)*. Rats were given the SH alkylator iodoacetamide (6%) *per rectum* once to initiate IBD-like lesions. From the second day animals were treated daily with bFGF *per rectum*. bFGF was found to accelerate the healing of iodoacetamide-induced ulcerative colitis and reduced the extent of necrosis and inflammation *(33)*.

Immunohistochemically bFGF was shown to be most prominent in the extracellular matrix of inflammatory lesions. The expression of fibrogenic cytokines increased in rat small intestine after irradiation *(35)*, most probably owing to inflammatory reaction caused by radiation.

The development of colitis and rectosigmoiditis is a well-known side effect of abdominal irradiation for the treatment of certain malignant neoplasms. This so-called radiation colitis or enterocolitis or rectosigmoiditis is a major clinical problem and it is relatively unresponsive to the usual therapy. Hence, new animal models of radiation have been developed to study the pathogenesis, prevention, and treatment of these lesions *(36,37)*. Most recently, we adapted and simplified an animal model of radiation-induced enterocolitis in our laboratory *(40)*. Groups of rats after receiving 20 Gy gamma radiation on abdominal parts were given sucralfate (10, 20, and 50 mg/100 g) or bFGF-CS23 (100 or 500 ng/100 g) by intragastric gavage twice daily from the second day of experiment. Autopsy was performed on the 10th day when the area of the ileal and colonic lesions as well as the wet weight of the ileum and colon were measured. All clinical signs and parameters were dose-dependently decreased by sucralfate. bFGF-CS23, in the small doses used, exerted a beneficial effect only on a few parameters of enterocolitis. Light microscopic examination of inflamed bowel sections revealed that the lesions were reduced in irradiated and sucralfate or bFGF-treated rats, e.g., the submucosal edema was absent and the necrotic-mucosa was replaced mainly by proliferating granulation tissue, which was covered by flat epithelium.

Thus, these results suggest a beneficial effect of sucralfate and bFGF in radiation-induced enterocolitis, but extended animal studies and clinical confirmation are essential to explore the full therapeutic benefit of these agents in this application.

PDGF

CHRONIC DUODENAL ULCER

After bFGF, PDGF was the second growth factor tested in our laboratories to accelerate the healing of experimental duodenal ulcers. Duodenal ulcer was induced by cysteamine as in the previous experiments with bFGF, and after 3 wk *per os* treatment with PDGF, rats were killed when the ulcer size was evaluated macroscopically and with stereomicroscopic planimetry. Administration of PDGF-BB (100 and 500 ng/100 g, twice daily for 3 wk) significantly accelerated the healing of chronic cysteamine-induced ulcer: ulcer sizes were 2.5 ± 1.1 mm^2 ($p < 0.05$) and 2.0 ± 1.4 mm^2 ($p < 0.05$), respectively, vs 16.9 ± 6.8 mm^2 in the control group. It is important to stress that gastric-acid secretion was not influenced by any of the doses of PDGF *(41)*.

As a follow-up to our studies, the effect of bFGF and PDGF was investigated on the migration and proliferation of cultured rabbit gastric epithelial cells *(42)*. Although any dose of bFGF had virtually no effect on the epithelial cells, PDGF significantly increased the migration of cultured epithelial cells in a dose-dependent manner. The action of PDGF-BB was investigated in addition to the confluent rabbit gastric epithelial cells after wounding *(43)*. PDGF-BB dose-dependently accelerated the migration and proliferation of cultured cells. Therefore, PDGF-BB may have a role in gastric epithelial cell restoration during the healing of gastric ulcers.

CHRONIC GASTRIC ULCER

In our gastroprotective studies, PDGF was tested first for the prevention of acute ethanol-induced gastric erosions, and subsequently for the acceleration of healing of indomethacin-induced gastric ulcers *(44)*. In our studies, groups of fasted rats were given PDGF at doses of 500 ng/100 g, 1 or 2.5 µg/100 g subcutaneously or by intragastric gavage, 30 min prior to the *per os* administration of 1 mL 75% ethanol. As a positive control, an additional group of rats received SH-containing taurine (50 mg/100 g). All of the animals were killed 1 h after receiving ethanol and the area of hemorrhagic mucosal lesions in the glandular stomach was measured by computerized stereomicroscopic planimetry. The results indicated that only 2.5 µg/100 g of PDGF administered intragastrically reduced the area of acute mucosal lesions at the borderline of statistical significance ($p = 0.095$), whereas pretreatment with taurine resulted in about 50% reduction of gastric damage ($p = 0.027$).

It was also reported that PDGF-BB accelerated the repair of gastric mucosa after indomethacin-induced damage, without influencing gastric-acid secretion *(44)*.

CHRONIC GASTRITIS

We found as a follow-up to our investigation on the gastroprotective role of SH *(29,30)* that the ingestion of low concentrations of SH alkylators (e.g., 0.1% iodoacetamide) in drinking water induced severe diffuse acute and chronic erosive gastritis in rats *(31)*. We used this new animal model of gastritis to investigate the possible beneficial effect of bFGF and PDGF.

After the induction of gastritis using 0.1% iodoacetamide in drinking water for 1 wk rats were treated with PDGF in doses of 500 ng/100 g or 2.5 µg/100g *per os* twice daily. At autopsy on the 14th day, macroscopic and histologic involvement of gastric glandular mucosa was quantified and wet weights of the stomach were obtained. Oral treatment with PDGF dose-dependently decreased the severity of gastritis induced by iodoacetamide as exemplified by the dose-dependent decrease in the wet weight of the stomach *(45)*.

IBD

We used our previously developed new ulcerative-colitis model to test the effect of PDGF on the healing of colonic ulcers and inflammation. Colitis-like lesions were induced in rats by giving 6% iodoacetamide solution *per rectum* once on the first day *(34)*. From the second day PDGF-BB was given to the rats *per rectum* twice daily at doses of 100 ng/ 100g and 500 ng/100g *(46,47)*. PDGF dose-dependently decreased the wet weight of the colon, the lesion area, and the severity of colonic lesions, as well as the extent of adhesions after 10 d of treatment. All parameters were significantly improved in the high PDGF-dose group. Histologically, the ulcer size was smaller, the signs of inflammation were reduced, and in the majority of cases extensive re-epithelization was seen.

VEGF/VPF

CHRONIC DUODENAL ULCER

The list of growth factors that stimulate angiogenesis (e.g., bFGF, acidic FGF [aFGF], PDGF) has been extended by the recent availability of VEGF for pharmacologic studies. Also, there is a potent synergism between VEGF and bFGF in the induction of angiogenesis in vitro and probably also in vivo *(48)*.

Our previous studies demonstrated that bFGF and PDGF, which stimulate angiogenesis and granulation-tissue production, accelerated experimental duodenal ulcer healing that was 2–7 million times more potent on molar basis than the similar effect of cimetidine (Table 2). Because VEGF is highly specific for endothelial cells, we have recently tested the hypothesis that stimulation of angiogenesis alone is sufficient for chronic-ulcer healing *(49)*. To induce chronic duodenal ulcers, groups of rats were given cysteamine-HCl on the first day, as in previous experiments with bFGF and PDGF. To randomize rats with equally severe penetrating or perforated duodenal ulcers, the animals were anesthetized and laparotomized on the third day when treatment started with vehicle saline or rhVEGF-165, 1 µg/100 g once daily by gavage for 21 d. At autopsy, the size of duodenal ulcers was measured, evaluated by stereomicroscopic planimetry, and histologic sections taken. The results revealed that the size of duodenal ulcers in controls was 7.4 ± 1.6 mm^2 whereas in the VEGF group 1.9 ± 0.9 mm^2 ($p < 0.05$), histologically accompanied by complete healing or prominent angiogenesis and granulation tissue production. The density of blood vessels per ×400 magnification field in the granulation tissue at the ulcer edge was 8.0 ± 0.5 in controls, and 16.9 ± 1.9 ($p < 0.001$) in the VEGF-treated rats.

More recently, we also demonstrated a potent ulcer healing effect of VEGF, administered rectally in the aforementioned rat model of IBD induced by iodoacetamide *(50)*. Conceptually, the potent ulcer-healing effect of VEGF in the upper and lower GI tract is very important because it demonstrates that stimulation of vascular factors alone, i.e., angiogenesis is sufficient for ulcer healing, probably because epithelial cells proliferate and migrate spontaneously over dense granulation tissue to complete the healing process.

Thus, the molecular and cellular basis of ulcer healing remains a productive research area *(1)*, and previous pharmacologic studies with bFGF and PDGF are now greatly expanded with VEGF.

THE PATHOPHYSIOLOGY OF ENDOGENOUS GROWTH FACTORS AND ANGIOGENESIS

After learning about the potent ulcer healing effect of growth factors whose main cellular target seems to be angiogenesis (Table 1), we wanted to investigate whether bFGF, PDGF, and VEGF might have a role in the pathophysiology, i.e., natural history of GI ulceration, especially in the healing stage. Namely, years of investigations in our laboratories and others revealed several biochemical and functional pathways leading to gastroduodenal ulceration *(51–53)*. Most of these studies were focused on the initiation and prevention of early GI lesions with little attention to healing. On the other hand, it has been a common clinical observation that artificial gastric ulcers (e.g., after biopsy) heal rapidly, thus placing a special emphasis on the lack of or inappropriate healing. With the availability of tools of modern cellular and molecular biology (e.g., Western and Northern blots, *in situ* hybridization, enzyme-linked immunosorbent assay [ELISA]), it was tempting to look into the possible physiologic role of these growth factors in angiogenesis-dependent GI ulcer-healing.

The first surprising role of angiogenesis in spontaneous ulcer healing became evident in our initial ulcer-healing studies with bFGF. Namely, we found that the density of small blood vessels (e.g., mostly capillaries) in the base of spontaneously healing experimental duodenal ulcers was about 50% lower than in the adjacent normal duodenal mucosa (Fig. 1) *(3,7,17)*. We actually proposed that this hypovascular ulcer base is one of the reasons of poor quality of ulcer healing and the high ulcer-relapse rate after discontinuation of treatment with antisecretory drugs or antacids *(1,7)*. Namely, the poorly vascularized loose granulation tissue, partly or completely covered by epithelium, may be more susceptible for new ulceration. Treatment of rats having cysteamine-induced duodenal ulcers with acid-resistant bFGF-CS23 not only corrected the poorly vascularized ulcer base, but actually increased ulcer angiogenesis by about 10-fold (Fig. 1) *(3,7)*. Thus, angiogenesis, which is susceptible to bFGF and probably to other growth factors, seems to be an important pathogenetic element in ulcer healing.

bFGF

The role of endogenous bFGF, a heparin-binding growth factor, was also investigated because of the structural similarity between heparin and sucralfate. Namely, bFGF avidly binds not only to heparin but sucralfate as well both in vitro and in vivo *(11,12)* in the in vivo experiments, sucralfate was tested in rats at an effective and an ineffective dose, alone and in combination with the naturally occurring bFGF-wild. After duodenal-ulcer induction, rats were randomized into groups treated with either vehicle or sucralfate and/or bFGF by gavage twice daily for 3 wk. An additional group of rats received only bFGF-w at the same dose, which is a partially effective anti-ulcer dose of this growth factor, based on our previous dose-response studies. The results showed that the addition of a small dose of bFGF markedly potentiated the ulcer-healing effect of sucralfate.

Other data support the physiologic role of endogenous bFGF in ulcer healing. Endogenous bFGF was visualized by immunostaining techniques in the normal rat duodenum after administration of the duodenal ulcerogen cysteamine, and bFGF immunoreactivity was time-dependently reduced in the mucosa, submucosa, and muscularis propria *(18,55,56)*. Western-blot analysis of rat duodenal mucosa revealed a rapid depletion of mucosal cytoplasmic 18 kDa bFGF and increased synthesis of nuclear 21–25 kDa bFGF in cysteamine-induced ulceration in rats. At 12 h, we found a two- to threefold increase in nuclear forms of bFGF with a 50% decrease in the cytoplasmic form, whereas 48 h after administration of cysteamine the samples showed a trend toward the pattern seen in the control rats.

The physiologic importance of endogenous bFGF in ulcer healing seems to be further supported by the results showing significantly delayed healing of cysteamine-induced duodenal ulcer after administration of neutralizing IgG antibody against bFGF *(57)*.

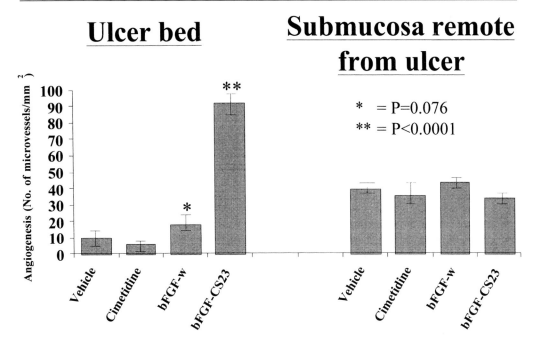

Fig.1. Angiogenesis in experimental duodenal ulcer and in adjacent normal duodenum 21 d after administration of duodenal ulcerogen cysteamine in rats. Adapted with permission from ref. *(7)*.

Because the mechanism of delayed ulcer healing in the presence of *H. pylori* in humans is only partially understood, we postulated that decreased local bioavailability of growth factors (e.g., owing to proteolytic degradation of peptides and/or receptors) might be one of the mechanisms of poor healing of *H. pylori*-positive ulcers. Indeed, *H. pylori* unlike other Gram-negative bacterial lysates and supernatants decreased the bioavailability of bFGF and PDGF *(58,59)*. Pretreatment with nontoxic concentrations of the supernatants abolished the proliferative response of NIH 3T3 fibroblasts not only to bFGF, but also PDGF *(60)*. Because fibroblasts are key elements in ulcer healing, the *H. pylori*-induced impairment of proliferation and a decreased bioactivity of growth factors in the presence of the bacteria may be an important mechanism of interference of bacterial infection with ulcer healing.

Others examined the effects of lansoprazole and famotidine on gastric bFGF levels and ulcer healing in patients with gastric ulcer *(61)*. Patients were examined endoscopically during the treatment to assess periodically the ulcer healing and to measure the level of bFGF in the stomach. Cumulative healing rates and bFGF levels were significantly lower in the famotidine group than in the lansoprazole group. Apparently, lansoprazole increases the tissue bFGF levels, thus promotes gastric ulcer healing in humans.

A very recent clinical study was designed to investigate whether chronic duodenal -ulcer disease is a consequence of disturbed mucosal turnover and growth-factor expression, before, during, and after endoscopic healing with lansoprazole or sucralfate *(62)*. Before treatment, gastric fundal and antral mucosal protein turnover rates were higher in patients than controls, without parallel increases in growth factors. Both forms of therapy produced similar changes, with overall increases in duodenal mucosal turnover and transforming growth factor-α (TGR-α) and epidermal growth factor receptor (EGF-r) levels. Measurements after healing showed persistent elevations of mucosal turnover in the antrum and duodenum and depressions of bFGF in gastric fundal and duodenal mucosa. The authors concluded that mucosal turnover was abnormally high in patients with chronic duodenal-ulcer disease and the failure of lansoprazole and sucralfate to normalize rates, despite endoscopic healing, may explain the high ulcer relapse rates in non-*H. pylori*-eradicated patients *(62)*.

Thus, in addition to the possible pharmacologic role of bFGF in ulcer therapy and prevention, endogenous bFGF may also have a physiologic role in ulcer healing. Results from animal experiments and human studies indicate that the proton-pump inhibitors might stimulate ulcer healing at least in part, via local increase of bFGF levels. However, comprehensive and controlled clinical investigations are needed to elucidate these possibilities.

PDGF

In addition to the pharmacologic use of exogenous growth factors, we demonstrated that endogenous PDGF and bFGF play a role in the healing of both duodenal and gastric ulcer *(57)*. Administration of the anti-PDGF and anti-bFGF neutralizing antibodies delayed the healing of duodenal ulcers. During the natural history of experimental duodenal ulcers, the levels of mucosal PDGF and bFGF were elevated only in the duodenum and not stomach, suggesting a local duodenum-specific role of growth factors in duodenal ulceration.

VEGF

The role of endogenous VEGF, the most specific angiogenic factor so far identified, is being investigated in our laboratory, which had been the first to report that intragastric administration of VEGF in rats caused acute gastroprotection and stimulated chronic duodenal-ulcer healing *(49,50)*. After these pharmacologic experiments we wanted to test whether endogenous VEGF levels might be altered in duodenal ulceration and the modulation of bioavailability of endogenous VEGF might influence the natural history of spontaneous healing of experimental duodenal ulcers.

In the first series of experiments *(63)*, groups of rats had unlimited access to food and water, and were given cysteamine-HCl (25 mg/100 g by gavage ×1 or ×3 with 4-h intervals) and were killed 0.5, 1, 2, and 6 h after single dose, or 12 and 24 h after 3 doses of the duodenal ulcerogen. Mucosal scrapings of proximal duodenum were homogenized for the measurement of VEGF by ELISA (Human VEGF Immunoassay Kit, R&D Systems). The duodenal VEGF concentrations (pg/mg protein) in controls were 0.84 ± 0.3, and 0.79 ± 0.13, 0.93 ± 0.38, 0.81 ± 0.44, 0.85 ± 0.42, 1.39 ± 0.88, and 1.10 ± 0.74 at 0.5, 1, 2, 6, 12, and 24 h after cysteamine, respectively. Although these studies are still in progress, we concluded that experimental duodenal ulceration was preceded by an early increase in VEGF concentration in the duodenal mucosa, preceding the first morphologic signs of healing, such as angiogenesis and granulation tissue production in the ulcer base.

In the second series of experiments, groups of rats with cysteamine-induced acute duodenal ulcers (*see* above) were given neutralizing anti-VEGF monoclonal antibody (MAb) either i.v. twice on third and fifth day after cysteamine or daily i.m. for 1 wk when the animals were killed and size of duodenal ulcers measured. Control rats receiving saline or nonspecific IgG had ulcers almost completely healed (3.3 ± 0.5 or 4.8 ± 2.9 mm^2 respectively), while after administration of neutralizing anti-VEGF i.m. or i.v. were markedly increased (39.5 ± 17.3 or 63.6 ± 21.6 mm^2, respectively). Actually, some of the duodenal ulcers in the latter groups of rats were so large (e.g., reaching 15–19 mm in diameter) that even in humans, these lesions would qualify as "giant duodenal ulcers."

Thus, the most recent studies with VEGF seem to provide the most direct evidence that angiogenesis and its molecular regulators are key elements in the natural healing of

Table 3
VEGF and Duodenal Ulceration: Direct Evidence for the Role of Angiogenesis in Ulcer-Healing

Studies	Parameter
Treatment with VEGF	Acceleration of ulcer healing
Treatment with neutralizing anti-VEGF	Delayed ulcer healing
VEGF ELISA	Release in duodenal mucosa before morphologic evidence of healing

duodenal ulcers (Table 3). Thus, in addition to the previously demonstrated pharmacologic role of VEGF in ulcer healing, endogenous VEGF may also play a role in the pathogenesis of duodenal ulceration.

SUMMARY

Recent pharmacologic, biochemical, morphologic, and molecular biologic studies with PDGF, bFGF, and VEGF, in increasing order of specificity to stimulate angiogenesis demonstrated not only that administration of these peptides accelerated the healing of experimental chronic duodenal, gastric, and colonic ulcers, but that these growth factors play a role in the natural history of spontaneous ulcer healing. We also found that the base of spontaneously healed experimental duodenal ulcers is hypovascular, which can be corrected by oral treatment with bFGF. The poor angiogenesis and loose granulation tissue, especially in *H. pylori*-infected ulcers, might be one of the mechanisms of poor ulcer healing and high rate of ulcer recurrence. We thus conclude that stimulation of cell proliferation is the most consistent mechanism of ulcer healing by growth factors. Furthermore, enhancement by VEGF of angiogenesis and granulation tissue production is sufficient for ulcer healing. Hence, growth factors are potent, endogenously derived antiulcer agents that directly stimulate ulcer healing in which angiogenesis seems to be the most important process.

REFERENCES

1. Szabo, S., Kusstatscher, S., Sandor, Z., et al. (1995) Molecular and cellular basis of ulcer healing. *Scand. J. Gastroenterol.* **30(Suppl. 208)**, 3–8.
2. Szabo, S., Kusstatcher, S., Sakoulas, G., Sandor, Z., Vincze, A., and Jadus, M. (1995) Growth factors: "new endogenous drugs" for ulcer healing. *Scand. J. Gastroenterol.* **30(Suppl. 210)**, 15–18.
3. Szabo, S., Folkman, J., Vattay, P., et al. (1991) Duodenal ulcerogens: the effect of FGF on cysteamine-induced duodenal ulcer, in *Mechanism of Peptic Ulcer Healing.* (Halter, F., Garner, A., and Tytgat, G. N. J., eds.), Kluwer Academic Publishers, London, pp. 139–150.
4. Poulsen, S. S., Olsen, K. S., and Kierkegaard, P. (1985) Healing of cysteamine-induced duodenal ulcers in rats. *Dig. Dis. Sci.* **30**, 161–167.
5. Garner, A. (1989) Strategies for the development of novel anti-ulcer drugs, in *Advances in Drug Therapy of Gastrointestinal Ulceration.* (Garner, A. and Whittle, B. J. R., eds.), A Wiley-Interscience Publication, New York, pp. 275–288.
6. Konturek, S. J., Brzozowski, T., Dembinski, A., Warzecha, Z., and Yamazaki, J. (1989) Gastric protective and ulcer-healing action of epidermal growth factor, in *Advances in Drug Therapy of Gastrointestinal Ulceration.* (Garner, A. and Whittle, B. J. R., eds.), A Wiley-Interscience Publication, New York, pp. 261–273.
7. Szabo, S., Folkman, J., Vattay, P., et al. (1994) Accelerated healing of duodenal ulcers by oral administration of a mutein of fibroblast growth factor in rats. *Gastroenterology* **106**, 1106–1111.
8. Szabo, S., Sandor, Z. s. (1996) Basic fibroblast growth factor and PDGF in GI diseases. *Bailliere's Clin. Gastroenterol.* **10**, 97–112.

9. Szabo, S., Vincze, A., Jadus, M., Gombos, Z., Pedram, A., et al. (1998) Vascular approach to gastroduodenal ulceration. New studies with endothelins and VEGF. *Dig. Dis. Sci.* **43**, 40S–45S.
10. Szabo, S. (1991) The mode of action of sucralfate: the 1x1x1 mechanism of action. *Scand. J. Gastroenterol.* **26(Suppl. 185),** 7–12.
11. Folkman, J., Szabo, S., and Shing, Y. (1990) Sucralfate affinity for fibroblast growth factor. *J. Cell Biol.* **111,** 223a.
12. Folkman, J., Szabo, S., Stovroff, M., et al. (1991) Duodenal ulcer: discovery of a new mechanism and development of angiogenic therapy which accelerates healing. *Ann. Surg.* **214,** 414–426.
13. Szabo, S., Vattay, P., Scarborough, E., et al. (1991) Role of vascular factors, including angiogenesis in the mechanism of action of sucralfate. *Am. J. Med.* **91(Suppl. 2A),** S158–S160.
14. Szabo, S. (1978) Animal model of human disease: duodenal ulcer disease. Animal model: cysteamine-induced acute and chronic duodenal ulcer in the rat. *Am. J. Pathol.* **93,** 273–276.
15. Seno, K., Sasada, R., Iwane, K., et al. (1988) Stabilizing basic fibroblast growth factor using protein engineering. *Biochem. Biophys. Res. Comm.* **151,** 701–708.
16. Konturek, S. J., Brzozowski, T., Majka, J., et al. (1993) Fibroblast growth factor in gastroprotection and ulcer healing: interaction with sucralfate. *Gut* **34,** 881–887.
17. Kusstatscher, S., Nagy, L., Morales, R. E., and Szabo, S. (1993) Additive effect of basic fibroblast growth factor (bFGF) and cimetidine on chronic duodenal ulcer healing in rats. *Gastroenterology* **102,** A104.
18. Szabo, S., Sakoulas, G., Kusstatscher, S., et al. (1993) Effects of endogenous and exogenous basic fibroblast growth factor in ulcer healing. *Eur. J. Gastroenterol.* **5(Suppl. 3),** S53–S57.
19. Kusstatscher, S., Sandor, Z., Szabo, S., et al. (1995) Different molecular forms of basic fibroblast growth factor (bFGF) accelerate duodenal ulcer healing in rats. *J. Pharmacol. Exp. Ther.* **275,** 456–461.
20. Wolfe, M. M., Bynum, T. E., Parson, W. G., et al. (1994) Safety and efficacy of an angiogenic peptide, basic fibroblast growth factor (bFGF), in treatment of gastroduodenal ulcers: a preliminary report. *Gastroenterology* **106,** A212.
21. Syngal, S., Bynum, T. E., Folkman, J., et al. (1996) Randomized, double-blind placebo-controlled trial of basic fibroblast growth factor (bFGF) in the healing of gastroduodenal ulcers. *Gastroenterology* **100,** A267.
22. Hull, M. A., Knifton, A., Filipowicz, B., et al. (1996) Basic fibroblast growth factor reduces indomethacin-induced relapse in a human model of gastric ulceration. *Gastroenterology* **110,** A138.
23. Satoh, H., Shino, A., Inatomi, N., et al. (1991) Effect of rhbFGF mutein CS23 (TGP-580) on the healing of gastric ulcers induced by acetic acid in rats. *Gastroenterology* **100,** A155.
24. Satoh, U., Shino, A., Sato, F., et al. (1992) Role of endogenous and exogenous bFGF in the healing of gastric ulcers in rats. *Gastroenterology* **102,** A159.
25. Schmassman, A., Tarnawski, A., Peskar, B. M., et al. (1995) Influence of acid and angiogenesis on kinetics of gastric ulcer healing in rats: interaction with indomethacin. *Am. J. Physiol.* **286,** G267–G285.
26. Yabu, M., Shinomura, Y., Minami, T., et al. (1993) Immunohistochemical localization of basic fibroblast growth factor in the healing stage of mouse gastric ulcer. *Histochemistry* **100,** 409–413 .
27. Nakamura, M., Oda, M., Inoue, J., et al. (1995) Effect of basic fibroblast growth factor on reinervation of gastric microvessels. Possible relevance to ulcer recurrence. *Dig. Dis. Sci.* **40,** 1451–1458.
28. Hull, M. A., Cullen, D. J., Hudson, N., et al. (1995) Basic fibroblast growth factor treatment for non-steroidal anti-inflammatory drug associated gastric ulceration. *Gut* **37,** 610–612.
29. Szabo, S., Trier, J. S., and Frankel, P. W. (1981) Sulphydryl compounds may mediate gastric cytoprotection. *Science* **214,** 200–202.
30. Dupuy, D., Raza, A., and Szabo, S. (1989) The role of endogenous nonprotein and protein sulfhydryls in gastric mucosal injury and protection, in *Ulcer Disease: New Aspects of Pathogenesis and Pharmacology.* (Szabo, S. and Pfeiffer, C. J., eds.). CRC Press, Boca Raton, pp. 421–434.
31. Szabo, S., Trier, J. S., Brown, A., et al. (1984) Sulfhydryl blockers induce severe inflammatory gastritis in the rat. *Gastroenterology* **86,** A271.
32. Stovroff, M., Vattay, P., Marino, B., et al. (1991) Healing of experimental gastritis by oral fibroblast growth factor. *Surg. Forum.* **42,** 174–175.
33. Satoh, H. and Szabo, S. (1990) New animal model of ulcerative colitis induced by sulfhydryl blockers in the rat. *Gastroenterology* **98,** A202.
34. Sandor, Z., Nagata, M., Kusstatscher, S., and Szabo, S. (1994) New animal model of ulcerative colitis associated with depletion of glutathione and protein SH alkylation. *Gastroenterology* **106(4),** A766.
35. Langberg, C. W., Martin, H. J., Sung, C. C., et al. (1994) Expression of fibrogenic cytokines in rat small intestine after fractionated irradiation. *Radiother. Oncol.* **32,** 29–36.
36. Saclarides, T. J., King, D. G., Franklin, J. L., and Doolas, A. (1996) Formalin instillation for refractory radiation-induced hemorrhagic proctitis. *Dis. Col. Rect.* **39,** 196–199.

37. Henriksson, R., Frazen, L., and Littbrand, B. (1992) Prevention and therapy of radiation-induced bowel discomfort. *Scand. J. Gastroenterol.* **191,** 7–11.
38. Dubray, B. M. and Thames, H. D. (1994) Chronic radiation damage in the rat rectum: an analysis of the influences of fractionation, time and volume. *Radiother. Oncol.* **33,** 41–47.
39. Delaney, J. P., Kimm, G. E., and Bonsack, M. E. (1992) The influence of lumenal pH on the severity of acute radiation enteritis. *Int. J. Radiat. Biol.* **61,** 381–386.
40. Sandor, Z. s., Vincze, A., Gombos, Z., et al. The effect of sucralfate and basic fibroblast growth factor (bFGF) in a model of radiation-induced enterocolitis in rats. *J. Gastroenterol.,* in press.
41. Vattay, P., Gambier, E., Morales, R. E., et al. (1991) Effect of orally administered platelet-derived growth factor (PDGF) on healing of chronic duodenal ulcers and gastric secretion in rats. *Gastroenterology* **100,** A180.
42. Watanabe, S., Maehiro, K., Hirose, M., et al. (1994) Modulation of gastric mucosal restoration by growth factors in a culture cell model. *Gastroenterology* **106,** A209.
43. Watanabe, S., Wang, X. E., Hirose, M., et al. (1996) Platelet-derived growth factor accelerates gastric epithelial restoration in a rabbit cultured cell model. *Gastroenterology* **110,** 775–779.
44. Guglietta, A., Hervada, T., Nardi, R. V., et al. (1992) Effect of platelet-derived growth factor-BB on indomethacin-induced gastric lesions in rats. *Scand. J. Gastroenterol.* **27,** 673–676.
45. Kusstatscher, S. and Szabo, S. (1993) Effect of platelet derived growth factor (PDGF) on the healing of chronic gastritis in rats. *Gastroenterology* **104,** A125.
46. Sandor, Z., Szeli, D., Charette, M., and Szabo, S. (1995) Platelet-derived growth factor (PDGF) accelerates the healing of experimental ulcerative colitis in rats. *Gastroenterology* **108(4),** A887.
47. Sandor, Z., Kusstatscher, S., Szeli, D., and Szabo, S. (1995) Effect of platelet-derived growth factor in experimental colitis in rats. *Orvosi Hetilap.* **136,** 1059–1061.
48. Pepper, M. S., Ferrara, N., Orci, L., et al. (1992) Potent synergism between vascular endothelial growth factor and basic fibroblast growth factor in the induction of angiogenesis in vitro. *Biochem. Biophys. Res. Comm.* **189,** 824–829.
49. Szabo, S., Folkman, J., Vincze, A., Sandor, Z. s., and Gombos, A. (1997) Modulation of vascular factors by VEGF/VPF (vascular endothelial cell growth factor/vascular permeability factor) is sufficient for chronic ulcer healing and acute gastroprotection. *Gastroenterology* **112,** A303.
50. Sandor, Z. s., Singh, G., and Szabo, S. (1998) The effect of vascular endothelial growth factor (VEGF) on experimental ulcerative colitis in rats. *Gastroenterology* **114,** G4403.
51. Szabo, S. (1984) Biology of disease. Pathogenesis of duodenal ulcer disease. *Lab. Invest.* **51,** 121–147.
52. Szabo, S. and Cho, C. H. (1988) From cysteamine to MPTP: structure-activity studies with duodenal ulcerogens. *Toxicol. Pathol.* **16,** 205–212.
53. Szabo, S. (1991) Gastroduodenal mucosal injury – acute and chronic: pathways, mediators, and mechanisms. *J. Clin. Gastroenterol.* **13(Suppl. 1),** S1–S8.
54. Gallagher, J. T. (1994) Heparin sulphates as membrane receptors for the fibroblast growth factors. *Eur. J. Clin. Chem. Clin. Biochem.* **32,** 239–247.
55. Kusstatscher, S., Bishop, J., Brown, L., et al. (1993) Basic fibroblast growth factor (bFGF) immunolocalization in duodenum of normal rats after duodenal ulcer induction. *Gastroenterology* **104,** A125.
56. Sakoulas, G., Kusstatscher, S., Ku, P. T., et al. (1993) Role of endogenous basic fibroblast growth factor in duodenal ulceration. *Dig. Dis. Sci.* **38,** A11.
57. Kusstatscher, S., Sandor, Z., Satoh, H., and Szabo, S. (1994) Inhibition of endogenous basic fibroblast growth factor (bFGF) delays duodenal ulcer healing in rats: implications for a physiologic role of bFGF. *Gastroenterology* **106,** A113.
58. Szabo, S., Shing, Y., Fox, J., et al. (1994) Inactivation of basic fibroblast growth factor (bFGF) by gastric helicobacters and not by *E. coli. Gastroenterology* **106,** A190.
59. Vincze, A., Wyle, F. A., Domek, M. J., et al. (1996) Helicobacter pylori supernatants interfere with growth and proliferative response of fibroblasts to bFGF and PDGF. *Gastroenterology* **110,** A286.
60. Vincze, A., Domek, M. J., Gombos, Z., et al. (1997) Inhibition of cell proliferation by Helicobacter pylori supernatants and lysates might be a mechanism in delayed ulcer healing. *Gastroenterology* **112,** A323.
61. Tsuji, S., Kawano, S., Higashi, T., et al. (1995) Gastric ulcer healing and basic fibroblast growth factor: effects of lansoprazole and famotidine. *J. Clin. Gastroenterol.* **20,** S1–S4.
62. Zhang, T., O'Keefe, S. J. D., Winter, T., Marks, I. N., and Ogden, J. (1998) Effect of chronic duodenal ulceration and its treatment with lanzoprazole or sucralfate on gastroduodenal mucosal protein turnover and TGF-α, bFGF, and EGF receptor expression in humans. *Dig. Dis. Sci.* **43,** 2764–2770.
63. Deng, X., Szabo, S., Khomenko, T., Yoshida, M., and Florsheim, W. (1999) Changes in endogenous vascular endothelial growth factor (VEGF) in duodenal ulceration. *Gastroenterology,* in press.

14 Angiogenesis in Skeletal and Cardiac Muscle

Role of Mechanical Factors

Margaret D. Brown and Olga Hudlická

CONTENTS

INTRODUCTION

The role that mechanical factors deriving from blood flow play in the growth of blood vessels was most probably mentioned for the first time by John Hunter in his "Treatise on the Blood Flow, Inflammation and Gunshot Wounds," published in 1794. Hunter was an anatomist who kept a deer herd in Richmond Park. He described enlargement of the carotid arteries in deer, coincident with the development of new antlers, which is known to involve intensive vascular growth. Almost a century later, Thoma *(1)* demonstrated that ontogenetic growth of vessels is caused by a combination of hemodynamic forces — increased blood flow, blood pressure, and wall tension — and mechanical stretch of vessels owing to the growth of the surrounding tissue. The importance of flow for capillary development was later shown in tadpole tails by Clark *(2)*, who exposed to observation under the microscope the same site over many days, and in wound healing in the rabbit ear chamber *(3)*. Today, the roles in angiogenesis of mechanical factors such as shear stress, circumferential stress, stretch, or physical forces owing to modification of the extracellular matrix are widely studied in tissue culture.

From: *The New Angiotherapy*
Edited by: T.-P. D. Fan and E. C. Kohn © Humana Press Inc., Totowa, NJ

The importance of mechanical forces in growth of vessels in tumors is also increasingly being acknowledged (e.g., ref. 4), but evidence of the mechanisms by which these factors induce vessel growth in normal adult tissues is still very inadequate.

In this chapter, we will first examine the individual mechanical and physical factors that could be signals to angiogenesis and the possible pathways by which they could promote angiogenesis. Secondly, we will review the evidence for involvement of these factors in vessel growth in skeletal and cardiac muscle under both physiological and pathological conditions to elucidate the circumstances in which specific mechanical factors may be operative.

MECHANICAL FACTORS INVOLVED IN ANGIOGENESIS

The growth of new blood vessels begins with mitotic activity of existing endothelium and development of capillaries, from which larger vessels may subsequently differentiate (*see* ref. 5). It is generally accepted that the fundamental pattern of new blood vessel growth follows the same pattern in vivo as in vitro:- degradation of existing basement membrane by locally released proteases, followed by endothelial cell (EC) migration, proliferation, sprout/tube formation, followed by production of new basement membrane by endothelial cells themselves with the involvement of fibroblasts and pericytes *(6,7)*. In the adult organism, angiogenesis is strictly controlled in most tissues, although it does occur in, e.g., female reproductive organs, in response to tissue injury (wound healing), and during tumor growth.

The main sources from which mechanical forces with the potential for involvement in angiogenesis derive are related to the physical effects of blood flow and external forces from surrounding tissues that impact directly on endothelial cells. These are: 1) increased fluid/blood flow leading to elevated shear stress in both in vivo and in vitro models of angiogenesis and altered hematocrit and vessel-wall tension in vivo; 2) increased pressure/ blood flow leading to stretch of either endothelial or smooth-muscle cells in vitro and in vivo; and 3) changes in the substratum in vitro and mechanical distortion of the surrounding tissue in vivo, that apply forces to endothelial and smooth-muscle cells (Fig. 1).

The transduction pathways by which these forces stimulate cellular proliferation or expansion leading to angiogenesis have been studied primarily in vitro and were reviewed recently *(8,9)*. Intracellular events that can be triggered by mechanical forces include activation of protein kinase C (PKC), tyrosine kinases, and phosphatases leading to phosphorylation of proteins, breakdown of the nuclear envelope and a sequence of nuclear, cytoplasmic, and ultimately cellular division. The steps initiating these processes are multiple and share similarities with transduction mechanisms for other processes such as changes in the vascular tone (e.g., 10) or cell-to-cell adhesion, but in the case of angiogenesis, the initial stimulus may be different depending on which surface of a blood vessel it acts from — luminal or abluminal — and transduction pathways may vary according to which mechanical factor is operating — shear stress, stretch, or changes in the extracellular matrix. These will be examined in more detail in turn.

Shear Stress

Shear stress (τ) is directly proportional to the velocity of flow and viscosity (η) and, when measured in tubes or vessels, indirectly to the radius. Studies in tissue cultures show that shear stress leads to proliferation of endothelial cells *(11–13)* and enhances synthetic activity of endothelial cells in perfused rabbit aorta *(14)*. In vitro, steady laminar shear stress was found not to disturb the contact inhibition between endothelial-cells but turbulent flow increased endothelial cell turnover *(12,15)*. However, laminar shear stress

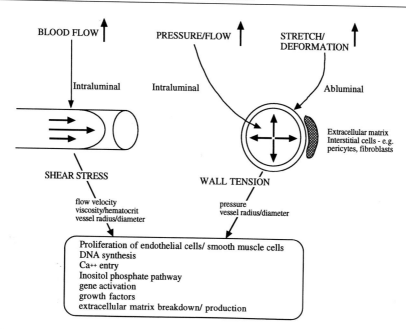

Fig. 1. Schematic representation of mechanical forces acting on endothelial and smooth-muscle cells that could play a role in angiogenesis and possible signal-transduction pathways (*see* text for details).

at levels as low as 1–2 dyn.cm^2, but not turbulent flow, induced synthesis of nitric oxide (NO) *(16,17)*, and because NO promotes DNA synthesis in endothelial cells *(18)*, shear stress could cause endothelial-cell proliferation by this mechanism. Shear stress also triggers an inward rectifying K$^+$-selective current *(19)* that increases Ca^{2+} entry into endothelial cells, thus providing conditions for nuclear division, causing perturbation of the endothelial cell membrane and phospholipids *(20)*, and activating phophatidyl inositol-specific phospholipase C with consequent hydrolysis of phosphatidylinositol 4,5 diphosphate into inositol triphosphate (IP3) and diacyl glycerol *(21)*.

Shear stress can also activate number of genes in endothelial cells. Brown *(22)* described increased mRNA for metalloproteinases and Resnick and Gimbrone *(23)* summarized the effects of shear stress on endothelial cells in terms of changes that can take seconds or minutes (activation of ion channels, release of NO and prostaglandins [PGs], increases in cytosolic Ca^{2+}), those that take minutes to hours (increase in endothelial-cell NO synthase [ecNOS], early immediate genes, e.g., c-fos, some growth factors, and cell replication), or those occurring after hours or even days (changes in cell shape and extracellular matrix remodeling). Changes in cell shape lead to reorganization of the cytoskeleton, which could affect the extracellular matrix by creating focal adhesion sites *(24)*, which can then modify endothelial-cell migration and proliferation. Finally, perturbation of the endothelial-cell surface in tissue cultures by flow, and thus shear stress, inhibits synthesis of fibronectin *(25)*, the first extracellular-matrix component to provide an environment facilitating migration of endothelial-cell precursors in the chick chorioallantoic membrane (CAM) *(26)* and in developing heart *(27)*.

Stretch

Stretch in vivo can arise either because of increased vessel diameter and/or pressure and hence wall tension (wall tension T = P.r where r = vessel radius, P = pressure) or by stretch of the adjacent tissues. The latter is particularly important during development, where it is imposed on vessels by the expansion of surrounding tissue, but it can also play a role in the heart during enlargement of the ventricular volume or in skeletal muscle, where stretch is induced by artificial lengthening (e.g., by overloading with springs or extirpation of the agonist muscles). In tissue cultures, stretch has been imposed on endothelial or vascular smooth-muscle cells by growing them on a flexible substratum undergoing cyclic (repeated elongation and relaxation) or prolonged continuous stretch. In either of these situations, DNA synthesis and endothelial-cell division were increased within 5–7 d *(28)* and this may have involved the inositol phosphatide pathway since levels of IP3 were elevated *(29)*. It also upregulated the expression of some growth factors in endothelial cells *(30)* and proto-oncogene expression and phosphoinositide turnover in smooth-muscle cells *(31)*. Likewise, cells exposed to cyclic strain showed increased production of the prostacyclin PGI_2 *(32)* and tissue plasminogen activator (tPA) production *(33)*, both of which factors have been shown to be involved in angiogenesis *(34,35)*.

The highest incorporation of ^{3}H-thymidine was found in the thinnest endothelial cells of those grown on hydrogel, which promoted spreading *(36)*, and in those grown on substrata which ensured greater spreading, e.g., collagen IV *(37)*. Stretch may increase intracellular calcium ion concentration, a prerequisite for cell proliferation, via stretch-activated ion channels *(38)*. Furthermore, stretch inhibits collagen production *(39)*, which may weaken the basement membrane of existing vessels and lead to its disruption, considered to be a prerequisite for angiogenesis *(40)*.

In vivo, stretch owing to increased pressure has been known to stimulate hypertrophy and hyperplasia of vascular smooth muscle in resistance arteries of varying sizes *(41,42)* and in veins *(43)*. However, it was recently shown that this depends more on the phenotype of the smooth-muscle cells than to a generalized effect of stretch, because smooth-muscle cells isolated from human saphenous arteries exposed to stretch proliferated whereas those from the aorta did not *(44)*.

Extracellular Matrix

An intact basement membrane and extracellular matrix (ECM) limit endothelial-cell and thus capillary growth. The disturbance of basement membrane, which consists of collagen Type IV, laminin, and fibronectin *(45)*, is thought to be the first step in angiogenesis, enabling cell migration and division *(46)*. Endothelial cells secrete both extracellular matrix-related proteins and metalloproteinases (MMPs) and tissue inhibitors of metalloproteinases (TIMPs) *(47,48)*, thus keeping in balance the enzymes capable of disturbing and protecting the basement membrane. In tissue culture, extracellular matrix molecules dictate whether endothelial cells will proliferate, differentiate, or undergo involution. For example, the A chain of laminin is involved in the initial attachment of endothelial cells, whereas the B1 chain mediates cellular reorganization and reorientation within hollow tubes *(49)*, and appears during development before Type IV collagen *(50,51)*, a temporal sequence that is thought to be important for the regulation and coordination of vessel growth *(52)*.

The role of extracellular matrix during vasculogenesis and angiogenesis in vivo has also recently been examined by Rongish et al. *(27)*. Concomitant staining with lectins and for CD31 to demonstrate vessels and for fibronectin, laminin, and collagens I, III, and IV to identify components of the extracellular matrix enabled the authors to follow the sequence of vessel development and evaluate the role of individual ECM component in migration, proliferation, and tube formation. The presence of fibronectin preceded vasculogenesis and provided an environment that facilitated cell migration, while the appearance of laminin coincided with tube formation and maturation, closely followed by appearance of type IV collagen and the newly forming basement membrane. Collagen I and III were not related to tube formation but were an important component of arteriolar and venular adventitia. A similar sequence has been described in the CAM *(53)*.

When cells start to migrate, they express mRNA for urokinase (uPA), a proteolytic enzyme that helps to disrupt the extracellular matrix and create space for newly formed capillaries *(35,54)*. Migration of endothelial cells was inhibited when matrix protease activity was blocked by TIMP-1 *(55)*. The ECM also regulates endothelial-cell growth by changing cell response to growth factors. Binding of ECM molecules to trans-membrane integrin receptors has been shown to activate the Na^+/H^+ antiport, which stimulates DNA synthesis *(56)*. The role of integrins in angiogenesis has been recently reviewed by Strömblad and Cheresh *(57)*, who demonstrated that disruption of $\alpha_v\beta_3$ binding to ECM prevented vessel formation on CAM, whereas both $\alpha_v\beta_3$ and $\alpha_v\beta_5$ were shown to be involved in growth factor-induced angiogenesis in the cornea *(58)*. Moreover, integrins caused induction of the early growth genes such as c jun and cMyc.

The influence of different growth factors on the ECM has been established by several groups (see refs. *56,57*), but although Woessner *(59)* postulated that physical factors are important in ECM remodeling, the mechanism has so far not been fully clarified.

Pericytes

Pericytes lie closely apposed to capillaries and have been shown to exhibit an inhibitory effect on endothelial-cell growth in co-cultures by Orlidge and D'Amore *(60)*, in the diabetic retina by Kuwabara and Cogan *(61)* and in wound healing by Crocker et al. *(62)*, which is thought to be mediated via transforming growth factor β1 (TGF-β1) *(60,63)*. Endothelial proliferation starts when pericytes retract and Sims *(64)* showed that apposition of pericytes to newly formed capillaries terminates proliferation, but pericytes can also play a positive role in angiogenesis by acting as scaffolding for migrating endothelial cells *(7,65)*. Reduced contact surfaces between pericytes and endothelial cells was observed in developmental angiogenesis *(66)* and our own work has shown that in chronically stimulated skeletal muscles that show capillary growth after 7 d, pericyte coverage of capillaries was significantly reduced prior to this *(67)*, possibly indicating removal of inhibitory influence.

METHODOLOGICAL CRITERIA FOR ASSESSMENT OF ANGIOGENESIS IN SKELETAL AND CARDIAC MUSCLE

Most of the mechanisms involved in angiogenesis referred to earlier have been studied in tissue cultures of endothelial and vascular smooth-muscle cells of differing origin and the different types of growth were reviewed recently *(68)*. Here we would like to describe methods relevant to studies of angiogenesis in skeletal and cardiac muscle, with respect to growth of capillaries and larger vessels.

Angiogenesis **In Situ**

The advantages of studying angiogenesis *in situ* are that it is possible to observe the whole sequence of events from capillary sprouting to formation of new vascular networks and to assess the appearance of vessel growth quantitatively and qualitatively in relation to mechanical stimuli. The use of immunohistochemistry or *in situ* hybridization techniques enables investigation of cellular mechanisms. The greatest disadvantage is the difficulty encountered in attempting to elucidate signal transduction on a molecular basis and to quantify precisely the mechanical factors involved.

INTRAVITAL OBSERVATIONS

The growth pattern of small vessels — arterioles, venules and capillaries — can be investigated by intravital microscopic observations in living organisms (e.g., 2). Rhodin and Fujita (7) combined intravital observations of vessels with electron microscopy in the rat mesentery during early postnatal development to provide a classical description of growth of the microcirculation. Originating from arteriolar-venular arcades, solid sprouts of endothelial cells lengthened by migration while a lumen developed between the ECs. Fibroblasts approached and settled down on the sprouts and were converted to pericytes that reinforced the wall of the delicate new capillary. Perivascular cells surrounding the arteriole feeding the capillary network represented precursors of smooth-muscle cells, which would later be apposed to the newly formed capillaries.

Intravital observations can provide data on vessel diameters and lengths and quantification of changes in vascular branching pattern in thin, flat skeletal muscles such as spinotrapezius, tenuissimus, or cremaster, or on the surface of bulkier muscles such as tibialis anterior and extensor digitorum longus, and they allow measurements of flow velocity and vessel diameters for estimation of wall shear stress and tension, thereby enabling the involvement of mechanical factors in the initiation of angiogenesis to be determined. However, observations in the living heart are technically much more difficult because of its beating and there are only a few studies that have successfully achieved this.

ASSESSMENT OF MICROCIRCULATORY GROWTH

Angiogenesis in the adult organism occurs primarily by capillary growth and the specificity of markers for microvessels becomes crucial because the majority of quantitation is based on examination and counting of vessels under the light microscope. Examples of methods commonly used to identify capillaries in skeletal and cardiac muscle are staining of basement membrane with the periodic acid-Schiff/amylase method; silver methenamine, or antibodies to laminin, fibronectin, or Type IV collagen; and staining for enzymatic markers of the capillary endothelium such as alkaline phosphatase, ATPase, serine protease, or carbonic anhydrase, which are ideal for use on frozen tissue sections. However, it should be noted that these enzyme reactions are not necessarily consistent among species, between organs, during ontogenetic development, or in certain pathological conditions (69) so that each method should be validated by comparison with electron microscopy. Other endothelial markers such as antibodies to Factor VIII-related antigen and von Willebrand Factor (vWF) are used particularly for human tissues, and lectin staining of the sugar residues of cell-surface glycoproteins are very useful, with specific lectins being suitable for particular species. For example, lectin Ulex europeaus is most widely used to depict capillaries in human tissues, whereas Griffonia simplicifolia reacts with vessels in many animal tissues.

The co-localization of EC markers with labeling of cells undergoing proliferation is an important tool for the study of angiogenesis because it enables not only quantitation of angiogenesis, but also the spatio-temporal involvement of other factors in relation to angiogenic locations. In addition to incorporation of ^{3}H-thymidine, widely used to study development of coronary collateral circulation, and its analog bromodeoxyuridine (BrdU), antibodies are available to nuclear components specific to other time-points of the cell-division cycle, such as Ki-67 antigen or proliferating cell nuclear antigen (PCNA), which has been used in the heart (70).

Once capillaries have been detected by a suitable marker, evaluation of the anatomical extent of the capillary bed can be made on the basis of simple vessel counts as capillary density (CD), or by the ratio of numbers of vessels to units of tissue area, e.g., capillary/fiber ratio (C/F) in skeletal or cardiac muscle. Length density, Jv, which evaluates the length of capillaries per unit volume of tissue, enables the impact of vessel tortuousity to be estimated, which is important for such anisotropic tissues as cardiac and skeletal muscle. If capillary dimensions are known, capillary volume and surface densities can be calculated from the product of Jv and capillary cross-sectional area and perimeter, respectively *(71)*.

Electron microscopy can be used for low-power quantification of capillary morphology and to demonstrate the presence of capillary sprouts and initial stages of capillary angiogenesis, identified from signs of EC activation, EC proliferation, and other changes in fine structure, such as breakage of the basal lamina. The great advantage is the high magnification, which enables unequivocal identification of the cell types undergoing proliferation and the nature of interaction between ECs and perivascular cell types such as pericytes. Because of the small areas examined, such studies should be combined with analysis of larger sample areas under the light microscope to confirm angiogenesis.

ASSESSMENT OF LARGE VESSEL GROWTH

The growth of larger vessels has been studied by methods that identify structural features of the vascular bed, e.g., angiography; vascular casts; standard histological techniques to depict arteries/arterioles or veins/venules, and labeling of proliferating components, endothelial, or smooth-muscle cells, in the vessel walls. Analysis of vascular topology has been made from vascular casts in both skeletal muscles and heart, although three-dimensional reconstruction and quantification of such casts is difficult. The total cast volume as a proportion of total organ volume gives some indication of changes in vascular supply, but it is difficult to partition any growth that occurs among the various vessel categories.

Although standard histological techniques and light microscopy do not always allow unequivocal discrimination between arterial and venous vessels, staining of vascular endothelium in larger vessels with lectins, provided that the staining characteristics of a particular lectin in vessels of a particular tissue are well-documented, can be used quantitatively to ascribe growth to one or other size class of either arterial or venous vessels. Immuno-staining for alpha-smooth muscle actin can distinguish arterial vessels down to quite small sizes and has been successfully used to show arteriolar growth in skeletal muscles subjected to electrical stimulation *(72)* or chronic vasodilatation *(73)*. Nevertheless, larger vessels such as arterioles occur with a relatively low density compared to that of capillaries, so a large enough sample area should be used.

In ischemic tissue, larger vessels grow predominantly as part of the collateral vascular tree (*see* ref. *74*). This has been studied in considerable detail in the heart in response to either abrupt or gradual occlusion of a major coronary artery *(75)* using incorporation of ^{3}H-thymidine to locate proliferation in smooth muscle and endothelial cells of both large and small vessels, although it is still difficult to assess whether proliferation is owing to expansion of pre-existent vessels or to *de novo* synthesis. An index of growth of arterioles and conduit arteries can also be derived in vivo by the functional measure of maximal vascular conductance (maximal blood flow/blood pressure) because resistance to flow is located primarily within these vessels. This approach has been used to ascertain that there is growth of the larger vessels in the myocardium in response to endurance exercise training and in skeletal muscles where angiogenesis was induced by chronic electrical stimulation *(74)*. In ischemic myocardium, there was a good correlation between the increase in arteriolar density and cross-sectional area and rise in maximum conductance over time *(76)*.

MECHANICAL FACTORS INVOLVED IN ANGIOGENESIS IN SKELETAL AND CARDIAC MUSCLE

Growth of vessels in skeletal and cardiac muscle has been described as a result of endurance training and administration of long-term dilatation (*see* ref. *74*). Both conditions are linked with a long-term increase in blood flow and thus potentially high shear stress and/or wall tension. Increased blood flow also occurs in skeletal and cardiac muscle, particularly in the right ventricle, in animals exposed to chronic hypoxia *(77)*. In addition, growth of capillaries occurs in skeletal muscles as a result of overload hypertrophy, whereas in the heart, size of the vascular bed may or may be not increased with stretch of muscle fibers resulting from either physiological (training) or pathological (pressure or volume overload) hypertrophy. In this section, we will review evidence for the participation of individual mechanical factors previously identified as playing a role in angiogenesis in relation to the growth of capillaries in skeletal muscle and heart.

Shear Stress

As already mentioned, shear stress τ is related by the formula $\tau = \eta$ (4Vrbc/r) to blood viscosity η (and thus hematocrit), velocity of flow (which in vivo means primarily the velocity of red blood cells, Vrbc) and vessel radius r. In skeletal muscles, although there are numerous measurements of Vrbc in capillaries during or shortly after acute muscle contractions (e.g., *78–80*), there are no data on shear stress in skeletal muscles with training-induced capillary growth. In lower hindlimb muscles that were chronically activated by imposition of low-frequency indirect stimulation for 8 h/d, capillary growth was evident from a 20% increase in C/F ratio after 7 d of stimulation. The velocity of flow was higher than in control muscles even at rest and, together with a relatively small increase in capillary diameter, shear stress was calculated (taking viscosity as 0.02cP) to have increased by 46% *(81)* (Fig. 2).

It is known that hematocrit also increases during muscle dilatation *(82)*, and we therefore attempted to ascertain what proportion of the response to chronic stimulation could be attributed to increased hematocrit as a component of shear stress. In experiments where systemic hematocrit was increased from 45 to 60% by repeated $CoCl_2$ injections, Vrbc, capillary diameters, and shear stress were similar to those in control animals and there was no evidence of capillary growth *(81)*. In contrast, in animals treated with α_1 antagonist prazosin, which caused long-lasting vasodilation in skeletal muscles, Vrbc was increased by ~75% and because capillary diameters were slightly smaller than in control animals, shear stress was ~90% higher (Fig. 2) and C/F ratio 20% higher than in control muscles *(81)*.

Although the experiments of Dawson and Hudlická *(81)* do not implicate increased hematocrit in capillary growth in skeletal muscles, it is possible that increased shear stress resulting from increased blood viscosity could explain some of the capillary growth in skeletal muscle during long-term exposure to cold in mammals *(83–85)* and fish *(86,87)*. Increased hematocrit may also play a role in increased capillary supply in the heart described in several studies on animals exposed to high-altitude hypoxia (*see* ref. *74*).

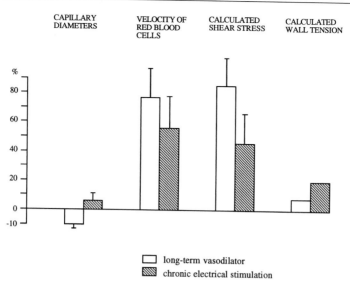

Fig. 2. Percentage changes from control values (= 100%) in capillary diameters and velocity of red blood cells measured in skeletal muscles after either long-term treatment with the vasodilator prazosin or chronic electrical stimulation (10 Hz, 8 h/d, 7 d) based on data from Dawson and Hudlicka, *(81)*, and calculated changes in vessel shear stress and wall tension. Both treatments increase shear stress, but the increase in capillary wall tension was greater with stimulation than the vasodilator.

However, a systemic increase in hematocrit has very little effect on viscosity in tubes as small as capillaries *(88)*. Moreover, the change in viscosity appears systemically but Turek et al. *(89)* found increased capillary density in the right but not in the left ventricle, whereas Pietschman and Bartels *(90)* found no additional capillary growth in the hearts of growing animals exposed to high-altitude hypoxia.

In the heart, capillary growth has been achieved by long-term administration of different coronary vasodilators *(91–93)* (Table 1). It has been calculated, based on available data for Vrbc in myocardial capillaries and capillary diameters after treatment with the vasodilator dipyridamole *(94)*, that capillary shear stress was significantly increased *(95)*, which could act as a stimulus for angiogenesis (Fig. 3). Although it is possible that an increase in myocardial capillary supply could occur via longitudinal splitting of existing vessels, Mandache et al. *(96)* showed incorporation of ³H-thymidine in capillary nuclei in rats trained by swimming, indicative of capillary proliferation. The exact mechanisms of capillary growth in the heart have yet to be elucidated in the same detail as for skeletal muscle because it has not even been shown whether growth occurs by sprouting.

The mechanism by which shear stress may initiate capillary growth has been discussed in the Shear Stress section primarily on the basis of experimental evidence from in vitro studies. We have shown that in vivo in chronically stimulated skeletal muscles, shear stress resulting from an increase in blood flow disturbs the glycocalyx on the endothelial luminal surface of capillaries at a time prior to the increase in capillary numbers *(97)* (Fig. 4). This could possibly start a cascade of events including, e.g., activation of mRNA for MMPs *(22)*, leading to proliferation of endothelial cells, which was observed in stimulated muscles *(98)* at the same time as the luminal surface disruption.

Table 1
Mechanical Factors as Stimuli and Capillary Growth in the Heart[a]

Intervention	Ref.	Blood flow of Contraction	Stretch/Force	Duration of Intervention (wk)	Effect on capillary supply
Heart rate reduction					
Rabbit	(112)	No change	SV ↑ ~70%, Stroke work ↑ 55%	4	↑ 34%
Pig	(114)	No change	SV ↑~30%, Stroke work ↑ 42%	4	↑ 26%
Rat	(115)	Decreased	SV ↑ ~34%, dP/dt decreased	5	↑19%
Vasodilator treatment					
Rabbit					
Adenosine	(93)	↑ 38%	No change	3–5	↑ 39%
Propentofylline	(93)	↑ 41%	No change	3–5	↑ 34%
Inotrope treatment					
Rabbit					
Dobutamine	(130)	Slight increase	SV↑ 30%, dP/dt ↑24%	2	↑ 25%

[a]Changes in coronary blood flow, stroke volume (SV), stroke work, or left ventricular dP/dt that occurred during acute application of the interventions (bradycardia by pacing or drugs, vasodilator, or inotrope treatment) are shown in relation to values in the control state. These changes represent the stimuli present during long-term application of the intervention for the durations as shown and the long-term effects on capillary supply (capillary density) are shown as % increases above control.

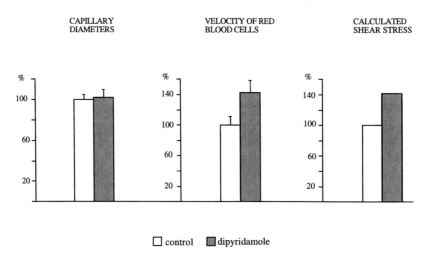

Fig. 3. Percentage changes from control values (= 100%) in coronary capillary diameters and velocity of red blood cells with dipyridamole administration based on data from Tillmanns et al. (94) and calculated shear stress (95). Shear stress is increased ~40%, but data on pressure measurements (108,109) suggest that wall tension would not be altered.

However, our recent work suggests that shear stress may also lead to capillary growth in skeletal muscles in the absence of endothelial cell proliferation. Animals treated with the α_1 antagonist prazosin had a similar increase in C/F ratio to that found in the stimulated muscles without any increase in the labeling index for BrdU in capillary-linked nuclei (99). Electron microscopic studies showed that the increase in capillarization seemed to be achieved by longitudinal splitting of existing vessels without any evidence for disturbance of the basement membrane (100), a mechanism similar to that described

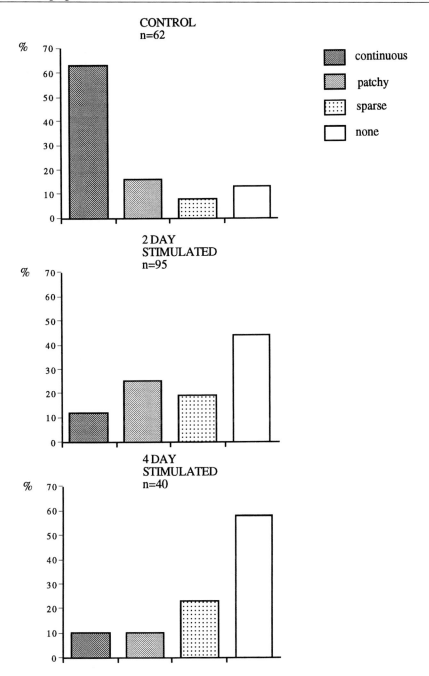

Fig. 4. Categorization of electron microscopic appearance of endothelial-cell luminal glycocalyx in capillaries of skeletal muscles (extensor hallucis proprius) after 2 and 4 d electrical stimulation (10 Hz, 8 h/d, n = number of capillaries examined), based on data from Brown et al.*(97).* The majority of control capillaries have a full luminal covering of glycocalyx. In stimulated muscles, in which capillary growth is not yet evident, the glycocalyx is already disrupted or absent in more capillaries.

in the developing heart *(101).* Thus, the same mechanical factor — shear stress — is associated with quite different forms of angiogenesis in different in vivo models.

Increased shear stress is known to release several dilating and constricting factors from the endothelium, the most commonly investigated being nitric oxide (NO), prostaglandins, and endothelins. Although endothelins may stimulate growth of vascular smooth muscle, there is no evidence for their involvement in growth of endothelial cells and hence capillaries. On the other hand, both prostaglandins and NO have been implicated in growth of endothelial cells in vitro (18,102). We have also shown that in chronically stimulated muscles capillary growth and the increase in labeling index for BrdU in capillary-linked nuclei can be attenuated by concomitant administration of either indomethacin (103) or the NO inhibitor L-NNA (104).

Whether hypoxia leads to capillary growth is not clear because it results in release of metabolites and vasodilation, which of themselves may act as stimuli for angiogenesis (see ref. 74). In addition, exposure to hypoxia was shown to produce vasodilatation in skeletal muscle by release of prostaglandins (105), which could thus be a mechanism involved in capillary growth — if it exists — under these conditions.

Capillary-Wall Tension

A long-term increase in blood flow, whether achieved by chronic muscle contractions owing to increased electrically evoked activity or exercise training, or long-term administration of vasodilators, results in increased capillary pressure. Capillary pressure was estimated in resting muscles as 16 mmHg rising to 32 mmHg during muscle contractions (106), while Fronek and Zweifach (107) measured a pressure of 25 mmHg in muscles maximally dilated by papaverine. Using these data for capillary pressure and our own measured data for capillary diameters in chronically stimulated and prazosin-treated animals (81), we calculate that capillary tension was slightly increased in prazosin-treated animals and almost doubled in capillaries in chronically stimulated muscles (see Fig. 2). Such an increase in capillary-wall tension may contribute to disturbance of the basement membrane, which was observed by electron microscopy in some capillaries in muscles stimulated for 4 d (72).

In the heart, dipyridamole administration, which induces capillary growth, did not alter capillary diameters but venular diameters were increased while venular pressures remained unchanged (108). Thus, even in the presence of moderate dilatation in terminal arterioles (20%) (109), it is possible to assume that the capillary pressure and hence wall tension were not increased and that stretch of the capillary wall is probably not an important factor initiating capillary growth in hearts exposed to the effects of long-term dilatation.

The most extensive increase in myocardial capillary supply was induced by long-term bradycardial pacing. It has long been known (110,111) that "athletic" animals such as a hare or wild rat have a higher capillary density and a lower heart rate than their more sedentary counterparts such as rabbit or laboratory rat. When heart rate in the rabbit was decreased to about half of the normal frequency by long-term pacing-induced bradycardia, capillary density (112) and capillary/fiber ratio (113) were increased on average by 25% and up to 70% after 60 d of pacing. An increase in capillarization was also achieved by bradycardial pacing in pig hearts (114) and by a specific negative chronotropic drug alinidine in rat hearts (115) (Table 1), the increase in capillarization being proportional to the decrease in heart rate.

In all these experiments, average coronary blood flow was no different from that in control hearts, although it was slightly increased on a per beat basis because of the lower heart rate (116), except by alinidine where contractility was somewhat depressed at the same time (Table 1). The duration of diastole per cardiac cycle was doubled with the degree of bradycardia achieved *(95)* and capillaries have been observed to be wider during diastole than during systole with a lower Vrbc *(117)* and hence lower calculated shear stress (Fig. 5). Consequently, the aggregate shear stress over time with a lower heart rate is not likely to increased *(95)* and can be discounted as a stimulus for angiogenesis in this situation. However, the wider capillaries are exposed to a pressure that is only slightly lower during diastole than systole, and thus calculated capillary-wall tension is higher by around 50% *(95)* (Fig. 5). Increased capillary-wall tension will stretch the endothelial cells, which could disturb their basement membrane or release of some growth factors stored in it. Stretched endothelial cells may also be more sensitive to soluble circulating growth factors, as demonstrated in tissue cultures by Folkman and Moscona *(118)*, or to soluble adhesion molecules such as E selectins, which have been shown to take part in angiogenesis *(119)*.

Stretch Induced by Abluminal Forces

Capillary growth in skeletal muscles can be elicited by long-term stretch induced either by extirpation of agonist muscles *(120–123)* or by stretch of muscles using weights or springs *(124,125)*. Because blood flow under these conditions was not increased *(123,126)*, the stimulus for growth is more likely to be as a result of the disturbance of the extracellular matrix required to accommodate increased sarcomere length *(127)* and thus alterations of the capillary tethering to muscle fibers. The pattern of capillary growth in this situation is different from that found either in prazosin-treated *(128)* or chronically stimulated muscles *(72)* with numerous abluminal sprouts and no luminal protrusions *(128)*.

In the heart, stretch of muscle fibers should obviously be considered as a factor contributing to capillary growth in cases of long-term bradycardia where the prolongation of diastole results obviously in greater end-diastolic filling and stretching of muscle fibers (Table 1). This leads to an increase in stroke volume, which precedes capillary growth by several days *(112)*. Capillaries are more tortuous during systole than in diastole (*see* ref. *129*) and the repeated stretching, with its ensuing more vigorous contraction, may act in a similar way as stretch or repeated contractions in skeletal muscles. In order to elucidate the role of contractile forces in the contribution to angiogenesis in the heart, we administered to rabbits dobutamine, a drug with a positive inotropic effect, which resulted in an increase in stroke volume and increased dP/dt without higher coronary blood flow. This treatment caused an increase in capillary density *(130)* that was similar to that achieved by bradycardial pacing (Table 1).

Role of Pericytes in Capillary Growth in Skeletal and Cardiac Muscle

As described previously for other tissues, pericytes may play a dual role in capillary growth in skeletal muscle and the heart. We have found smaller coverage of the capillary circumference by pericytes in both tissues in conjunction with capillary growth elicited by chronic stimulation in skeletal muscle and bradycardial pacing in the heart *(67)*. This retraction of pericytes could facilitate disturbance of the vessel wall, enabling endothelial-cell migration. Moreover, modification of the capillary basement membrane in the vicinity of pericytes in chronically stimulated muscles *(72)* suggests that pericytes may alter ECM, perhaps by secretion of metalloproteinases or by a phenotypic change in the type of collagen secreted, as suggested by in vitro studies on retinal pericytes *(63)*. However, the presence of pericytes in capillaries with a slit-like lumen, which may represent capillary sprouts *(72)*, indicates that pericytes in stimulated muscles could also act by forming scaffolding for sprouts as suggested in the mesentery *(7,65)*.

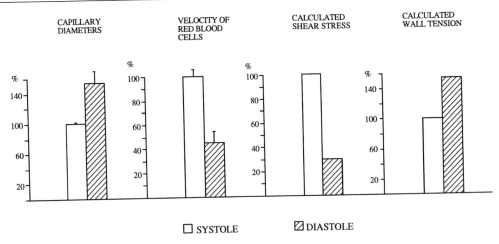

Fig. 5. Relative changes in coronary capillary diameter and red blood cell velocity between systole (= 100%) and diastole, based on data from Tillmanns et al. *(117)*, and calculated shear stress and wall tension *(95)*. Shear stress decreases ~70% during diastole while wall tension increases nearly 50%.

CAPILLARY GROWTH IN SKELETAL AND CARDIAC MUSCLE INDUCED BY EXERCISE TRAINING

Skeletal Muscle

Athletic animals have a considerably higher capillary supply in comparable skeletal muscles than sedentary animals of related species. This has been demonstrated by comparison of the hare with the rabbit *(131)* and greyhounds with other dog species and thoroughbreds with other horses *(132)*. Thus greater muscular activity is linked with higher capillary supply. It is acknowledged that training results in capillary growth in skeletal muscle but the extent of this growth varies with the length and types of training *(133)*. Because muscle fiber diameters change with different types of training, e.g., greater hypertrophy in strength than endurance training, it is more appropriate to concentrate on the findings on C/F ratio, which is less dependent on fiber size.

An increased C/F ratio was found in men undergoing endurance training *(134,135)* but took 5–6 wk to achieve significance, and equally long periods were required to stimulate capillary growth in other studies both in men and in animals. Capillary growth in endurance training has been described in both men and women *(see 74,133,136)*, even in older people *(137)* and is specific to the muscles being activated by the particular exercise, e.g., vastus lateralis in cyclists *(138)*, deltoid muscle in swimmers *(139)* or rowers *(140)*. The importance of activity was clearly demonstrated in cross-country skiers, where EMG recording showed greater activity in the triceps brachii than in vastus lateralis, with a greater increase in capillary supply in the former than in the latter *(141)*, and in rats undergoing swimming exercise, where capillary growth occurred in their hind-limb muscles *(142)*.

There is a limit to the maximal capillary supply inducible by training because it is difficult to achieve growth in muscles where capillary density is already high. This may explain the lack of training effect in wood mice *(143)* or foxhounds *(144)*. However, increased capillarization in response to endurance training occurs first in the vicinity of slow and fast oxidative fibers both in animals *(145)* and men *(146)* and these are already surrounded by more capillaries than fast glycolytic fibers *(147,148)*. This can be readily be explained if it is assumed that increased blood flow, and hence shear stress, plays a crucial role in capillary growth. Laughlin and Armstrong (149) demonstrated a preferential increase in blood flow in slow and fast oxidative muscle during exercise, whereas flow in fast glycolytic muscles, which rely on anaerobic metabolism and are recruited only during exhaustive exercise, is usually not increased by endurance training (150). By the same token, it is understandable that training for speed (151P) or heavy resistance training (152–155) did not lead to capillary growth. Gute et al. (156) showed the specificity of C/F increase in response to changes in blood flow in training which activated either primarily white or oxidative muscle fibers in rats (Fig. 6).

Unfortunately, there is no direct evidence for capillary growth with training using, for instance, labeling index of endothelial cells for ^{3}H-thymidine, but because all data in the preceding papers were based on either electron microscopy or staining specific for capillary endothelium to demonstrate all capillaries present, the evidence of increased capillary density or C/F ratio clearly demonstrates capillary growth.

Cardiac Muscle

The concept that exercise performed to sufficient intensity and for long enough would lead to increased myocardial capillary density would follow from observations that the hearts of athletic animals have higher capillary density than their more sedentary counterparts (see section on Capillary-Wall Tension). However, the evidence on capillary growth in the heart with training, recently reviewed by Laughlin and McAllister (157) and Tomanek (158), indicates that it is somewhat limited and occurs mainly in young animals. Several studies have shown increased capillary density or C/F ratio in young rats (e.g., ref. 159), whereas others found that it occurred specifically in young but not older animals trained by running (160) or swimming (142). The intensity and duration of training may also be significant factors. Moderate training of young animals increased myocardial capillary density but vigorous training of rats, pigs, or dogs (see refs. 157,158) decreased capillary supply; either capillary density or C/F ratio. Early reports also showed a direct relationship between increased capillarization and the total distance and/or speed of running and reports of differential changes across the ventricular wall with training vary from higher values in subepi- than subendocardium, with no difference or decreased density in both regions (for reviews, see refs. 5,74)

If capillary density does not change, it would not necessarily indicate lack of capillary growth. Training results in a mild heart hypertrophy and thus larger fibers and maintenance of capillary density implies that some growth must have occurred. The relative lack of capillary growth with training may also be owing to the already very high capillary density in the myocardium. However, unlike in skeletal muscle, capillary growth in the heart after training has been unequivocally proven by studies of incorporation of ^{3}H-thymidine into nuclei of capillary endothelial cells using electron microscopy with autoradiography (96).

Mechanical Factors Involved in Capillary Growth During Training

There is no doubt that blood flow is increased both in the heart and skeletal muscles during muscle contractions. Therefore factors related to increased blood flow such as shear stress or increased capillary-wall tension should be considered as triggers for capillary growth. Evidence so far supports the concept that shear stress is more likely to be important in skeletal muscle, whereas in the heart, on the basis that the increase in

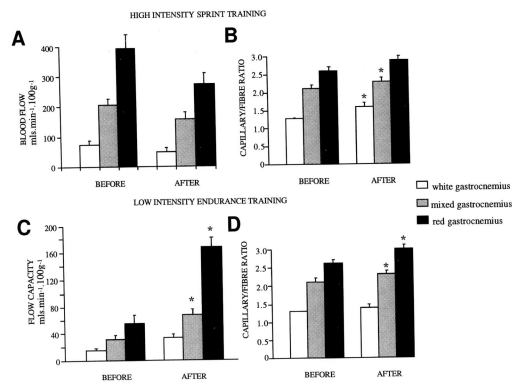

Fig. 6. Blood flow and capillary supply in muscles of different fiber-type composition in rats before and after 2–3 mo of high-intensity training: **(A)** Blood flow measured in conscious animals by microspheres and **(B)** C/F ratios before and after 2–3 mo of low-intensity endurance training: **(C)** Flow capacity measured in isolated hindquarters and **(D)** C/F ratios. Blood-flow capacity is increased by endurance but not sprint training, whereas C/F ratio is increased in the muscle type specifically activated by the training. Asterisks indicate significance at 5% level vs values before training. Adapted with permission from ref. *156*.

coronary blood flow in conjunction with bradycardia is not great enough to compensate for the increased diameter of capillaries, wall tension is more important (see section on Capillary-Wall Tension). In addition to blood flow, stretch and relaxation of skeletal muscle and stretch of cardiac myocytes in conjunction with bradycardia present factors acting from the abluminal side of capillaries by disturbing the ECM and possibly the basement membrane. However, there is no direct evidence based on either electron microscopy or intravital observation, which would confirm the expected steps in angiogenesis — disturbance of the basement membrane, migration and proliferation of endothelial cells, and formation of sprouts in any kind of endurance training, either in the heart or in skeletal muscle.

Exercise training upregulated mRNA for ecNOS in arterioles in skeletal muscle *(161)* and enhanced production of NO in coronary arteries *(162)*. Thus the role of NO either as a factor enhancing dilatation in arterioles, and thereby increasing flow in capillaries, or as a direct stimulus for the growth of endothelial cells should be considered.

CAPILLARY GROWTH IN SKELETAL MUSCLE WITH INCREASED ACTIVITY RESULTING FROM CHRONIC ELECTRICAL STIMULATION AND OVERLOAD

Increasing skeletal muscle activity by electrical stimulation as an stimulus for capillary growth and improvement of performance is becoming increasingly important in the context of cardiomyoplasty. In this procedure, skeletal muscles are conditioned so as to make them less fatiguable and therefore suitable as auxiliary hearts to provide pump support in cases of heart failure. Because the only cure for severe heart failure is heart transplantation, and the number of donors is severely limited, the possibility of "wrapping" a nonfatiguable skeletal muscle around the myocardium to help cardiac function has been widely explored. Alternatively, skeletal muscles are wrapped around the aorta to create "secondary" ventricle (163).

The original work investigating the effect of chronic electrical stimulation on capillary growth in skeletal muscle was based on the findings of Adrian and Bronk (164), who recorded electrical activity from nerves to slow and fast muscles. They established that while slow postural muscles were continuously activated by low-frequency (10 Hz), activity in nerves to fast muscles occurred in short bursts at 60–100 Hz. This finding was utilized by Salmons and Vrbova (165) to transform fast into slow muscles by stimulating the supplying nerves continuously at 10 Hz. It was this frequency and lower (5 Hz) activity that, when applied for 8 h/d, was subsequently shown to increase C/F ratio by 20% within 4 d, with a 50% increase in muscles stimulated for 14 d and doubling of the capillary supply within 28 d (166). It was then demonstrated that capillary growth starts within 2 d in the vicinity of fast glycolytic fibers, which, in contrast to natural exercise, are activated first during stimulation (167), and that this growth was preceded by increased capillary perfusion (168), indicating the role of flow and, as confirmed later, shear stress as a stimulus for capillary growth. However, even higher frequencies of stimulation (40 Hz) also caused increased capillarization, albeit later (after 14 d), possibly because the resultant tetanic contractions did not cause such an increase in flow as 10Hz continuous stimulation (168).

Since these original findings, alternative durations of stimulation and patterns of frequencies for transforming skeletal muscles to serve as cardiac support have been investigated, mainly using the latissimus dorsi in rabbits, dogs, sheep, or goats (e.g., 169). Because higher frequencies stimulate capillary growth, albeit with a delay, to the same extent as low frequency (170) and preserve or even enhance tension (171), they seem to be more successful for the purposes of myoplasty (172). Alternating low and high frequencies would also be a good choice, but it should be recognized that disturbance of vascular supply during transposition of the muscle could cause degeneration (173,174). We have indeed found that even 10 Hz applied for intervals of 2 h for 6 h/d to muscles with limited blood supply is detrimental to muscle performance and does not stimulate growth of capillaries (175). Similarly, uninterrupted stimulation (24 h/d) eventually causes muscle degeneration even though the muscles become less fatigable (176,177). An important feature of the procedure is that chronic stimulation actually enhanced formation of collateral flow from the latissimus dorsi to the heart (178).

It has been mentioned that capillary growth can also be elicited by muscle overload (stretch), also resulting in improved muscle resistance to fatigue (123). Frischknecht and Vrbova (179) showed that a combination of chronic stimulation and stretch results in virtually unfatiguable muscles. Moreover, stretch increases the levels of mRNA for c-fos and c-jun (180) and in combination with stimulation activates protein synthesis and increases the muscle mass (181). Although there is no information to date on the use of stretched and stimulated muscles and capillary growth and possible collateralization of the heart, this seems a promising avenue for improvement of the technique of cardiomyoplasty.

ANGIOGENESIS UNDER PATHOLOGICAL CONDITIONS

Growth of capillaries in skeletal and cardiac muscle may or may not occur in cases of overload hypertrophy and reparative injury (healing) such as regeneration in skeletal muscle and infarction in the heart. Although by the nature of the insult it is more likely that growth factors are involved as stimuli for capillary growth, and this has indeed been established, we would like to consider the possible involvement of mechanical factors.

Skeletal Muscle

The role of mechanical factors in capillary growth in muscles hypertrophied as a result of overload, particularly with respect to reorganization of the extracellular matrix has been discussed in the section on Stretch Induced by Abluminal Forces. Surprisingly, there is apparently capillary growth in some cases of muscle atrophy, although this might be misleading since during denervation or immobilization atrophy, muscle fibers become smaller or gradually disappear while the vascular bed is retained, and thus the relative increase in C/F ratio or capillary density does not really indicate growth (see ref. 74). One reason for the maintenance of the relatively intact capillary bed is the fact that blood flow in atrophic muscles is comparatively high (182,183), perhaps owing to metabolites released by degenerating muscle fibers, and thus mechanical factors linked with increased blood flow contribute to the maintenance and even growth (120) of capillaries. Increased capillarization was described in dystrophic mice (184) and some human dystrophies (185), but the causes of his growth are not understood.

In contrast, in regenerating muscle grafts, blood flow does not play any role because it is only re-established after the vascular bed has been assembled from endothelial cells remaining in the graft, not from the original supplying vessels. However, capillaries were observed sometimes to grow into channels created by the basal lamina of the degenerating muscle fibers and in this sense, mechanical factors would help to establish the final vascular network (186).

The Heart

Cardiac hypertrophy occurs in response to both physiological (training) and pathological (pressure or volume overload) stimuli and has been described in the remaining viable tissue of infarcted hearts. Recent reviews of capillary supply in hypertrophic hearts (129,187,188) summarize the relevant literature in this field and the following section will consider the mechanical factors involved.

HYPERTROPHY

Pressure Overload. Hypertrophy resulting from pressure overload owing to spontaneous or renal hypertension is usually associated with decreased capillary density, particularly in the subendocardial region, in rats (189), pigs (190), and dogs (191). However, the duration of pressure overload, the age at which it is initiated, and the mode of its origin may contribute to variations in the extent of capillarization observed. In renal hypertension of longer duration, capillary adaptation was found to be adequate in dogs (192), and White et al. (193) also reported an increase in vascular supply in right ventricular pressure overload hypertrophy in pigs and demonstrated ^{3}H-thymidine incorporation in arterial and capillary vessels, indicating proliferative capacity. The age at which the growth stimulus of hypertrophy occurs is an important factor because hypertrophy owing to both exercise and hypertension is accompanied by appropriate capillary growth in the young animal (194–196). Capillary growth was also observed in young spontaneously hypertensive rats as an increased labeling index for ^{3}H-thymidine incorporation *(197)* or morphometric capillary supply *(198)*, and in children with congenital aortic stenosis *(195)*, but in the majority of studies on adult onset pressure overload hypertrophy, either animal *(see 196)* or human *(195)*, angiogenesis is insufficient at capillary level *(199)*. All capillaries are perfused at rest in hypertrophic hearts *(200,201)*, so even if capillary density was not lower there would be no reserve for recruitment in emergency. Thus lack of capillary growth and increased intercapillary distances with larger capillary domains *(202)* together with absence of a vasodilator reserve produces hypoxia, particularly in subendocardial regions, leading eventually in most types of pressure overload hypertrophy to decreased protein synthesis *(203)* and heart failure.

Volume Overload. Increases in capillary density were reported in the right ventricle of hearts with volume-overload hypertrophy owing to high-altitude hypoxia *(89)*, but when volume-overload was owing to cold alone *(204)*, capillary density was unchanged. Decreased capillary density was reported in volume overload hypertrophy induced by aorto-caval fistula *(205–207)*, or aortic-valve lesion *(208,209)*. In contrast, volume overload elicited by anemia from iron deficiency *(210)* or iron and copper deficiency *(211)* led to increased capillary density and 60% greater total length of capillaries, respectively. However, the increase in heart size in anemia is owing to hyperplasia rather than hypertrophy of individual fibers *(210,212)* and growth of capillaries occurred concomitant with that of new fibers.

After myocardial infarction, the remaining viable noninfarcted tissue undergoes hypertrophy to compensate for increased work load, and this too is not accompanied by adequate capillary growth *(213)*, leading to impaired tissue oxygenation. The increase in myocyte size was greater and the decrease in capillary length per ventricle greater (30%) with infarcts affecting 50% left of the left ventricle than with smaller infarcts (23%) where capillary length decreased 19% *(214)*. In hypertrophy of the right ventricle after left coronary artery ligation, capillary density was 30% lower than in control animals *(215)*. On the other hand, in pathological hypertrophy resulting from increased stroke volume owing to bradycardia caused by heart block, proliferation of vessels was shown by increased incorporation of labeled thymidine *(216)*.

Interventions to Stimulate Capillary Growth. The many attempts to prevent capillary loss in either pressure or volume-overload heart hypertrophy have in general not been successful. Swimming training of rats with hypertrophy induced by aortic or renal artery constriction, which increased incorporation of ^{3}H-thymidine into capillary endothelial nuclei in normal hearts, failed to stimulate capillary growth *(217,218)*. The decrement in capillary density in spontaneously hypertensive rats was not reversed by treadmill running *(219)* but when treated with alpha-methyldopa from the time of weaning, this strain had a normal capillary supply at 20 wk of age *(220)*. Capillary density was also increased by hydroxydopamine *(220)* or captopril *(221)* and nifedipine normalized capillary density in spontaneously *(222)* and renal hypertensive *(223)* rats. Although none of these treatment resulted in an increase in capillarization above the values found in normal heart, administration of a relatively specifically negative chronotropic drug alinidine to rats with renal pressure-overload hypertrophy increased C/F ratio above the levels found in hypertrophic and control hearts *(224)*. Long-term bradycardia also stimulated capillary growth in hearts with volume overload *(209)*. Pacing-induced bradycardia commencing 1 mo after aortic-valve lesion increased capillary density by 60% in comparison with unpaced hypertrophic hearts, and by 20% in comparison with control hearts from animals of similar body weight with a slightly greater increase in the subendo- than subepicardial region. The explanation of this effect may be similar to the effect of bradycardial pacing in normal hearts: a combination of increased capillary-wall tension and positive inotropic effect of the prolonged diastolic filling and subsequent contraction.

MYOCARDIAL INFARCTION

Myocardial infarction seldom involves a discrete region of tissue owing to the existent collaterals, which enable some perfusion of the ischemic area via the numerous interdigitations between capillary beds (225), the extent of which varies between species. Impairment of capillary perfusion occurs because of capillary endothelial-cell swelling (226) and trapping of red blood cells (227). However, despite impaired capillary perfusion and oxygen supply, and hence hypoxia, at the border of an infarct, there is little anatomical evidence for proliferation of capillaries. Capillary growth may occur as a healing response to tissue damage, and proliferating vessels were described within the infarct border zone in rats (228) and demonstrated by labeling index for ^{3}H-thymidine in capillaries in pigs (229,230), but careful morphological studies in rats showed that in this region, C/F ratio was actually decreased (231). Przyklenk and Groom (232) used histochemical methods to demonstrate a border zone around infarct scar in rat hearts extending up to 525 mm laterally from the edge of necrosis, where capillary density was reduced by 23%.

MECHANICAL FACTORS IN PATHOLOGICAL CORONARY ANGIOGENESIS

Overall, these studies show that despite marked increases in ventricular mass occur- ring in response to different types of functional overload by pressure or work, capillary growth is limited and takes place, if at all, only after the increased myocyte mass has been established for some time. In contrast is the observation that myocardial hypertrophy resulting from treatment with thyroid hormones was accompanied by significant increases in capillary supply (233,234). It is thus possible to have myocardial hypertrophy with (e.g., thyroxine-induced) or without (hypertensive) capillary growth. The exact nature of the stimulus that promotes capillary growth in some hypertrophied hearts but not others, e.g. adult-onset pressure-overload hypertrophy, is therefore not clear, because it cannot solely be myocyte enlargement and the physical stretch this would impose.

Increased Coronary Blood Flow. Increased blood flow is a potent stimulus to myocardial capillary growth in the absence of hypertrophy and could explain the increased capillarization seen in the right ventricular hypertrophied during long-term exposure to low pO$_2$ (89) where the heart does increased work against higher pulmonary resistance (77). Increased coronary blood flow may also be a stimulus to capillary growth in animals exposed to thyroxine, high-altitude hypoxia, or cold or anemia, when cardiac work and hence coronary flow would also be increased. However, during pressure-overload hyper- trophy, blood flow is not necessarily increased and despite increased diffusion distances and hypoxia, there is no good evidence for the presence of various growth factor that could stimulate growth of endothelial cells. Hypoxia itself has been considered a potent stimulus for coronary angiogenesis, particularly in relation to development of collateral circulation (235,236) and functional collateral blood flow was increased by ischemia in the absence of pressure differences across vessels during anemia (237,238). Although hypoxia stimulates endothelial-cell proliferation in cultures (239), it is much more difficult to establish a role for hypoxia in vivo because it causes metabolic vasodilatation and hence increased blood flow.

Stretch and the Extracellular Matrix. Because it is possible to induce coronary capillary growth in the absence of significant changes in blood flow, the stimulus of stretch of myocytes owing to increased stroke volume, or an increase in force of myocyte contraction or both combined, imparting mechanical forces to capillary endothelial cells must be considered. The conditions under which this occurs in order to induce angiogenesis must be very specific, because otherwise the rhythmic contraction of each cardiac cycle would represent a stimulus. Also, neither volume overload of the heart nor exercise, which increase stroke volume, nor myocardial infarction, which leads to global chamber dilatation *(240)*, are very effective for angiogenesis. A significant difference between these situations and the experimental conditions under which capillary growth has been observed, e.g., chronic heart-rate reduction, vasodilator or inotrope treatment, is that none of the latter caused any increase in heart/body-weight ratios, whereas hypertrophy is a feature of the other functional overload situations. It is possible, then, that adaptive alterations in myocardial structure in response to work load may inhibit the effect of mechanical stresses on endothelial cells. In this respect, an important aspect is the role of the extracellular matrix in determining how endothelial cells respond to stimuli.

The interstitium of the heart — mainly the collagen network — is responsible for support and alignment of myocytes and capillaries, and represents a major determinant of myocardial stiffness, undergoing extensive remodeling of itself during heart hypertrophy. Loss of the fibrillar collagen network, which provides structural integrity to the myocardium *(241)*, leads to ventricular dilatation, whereas its excess results in fibrosis and reduced compliance *(242)*. Structural disruption of the collagen network was observed when left ventricular pressure was increased *(243)*, and was very rapid during ischemia *(244–247)*. Collagen content also increased as pressure overload persisted with either renal hypertension *(242)* or aortic stenosis *(248)*, and after coronary-artery ligation, collagen-gene expression was enhanced *(249)* in both the infarcted and noninfarcted region *(250)*. Because a prerequisite for endothelial migration during angiogenesis is that cells are able to invade the extracellular matrix, an enhanced collagen content in hypertrophied/infarcted myocardium would be obstructive to this process. Indeed, in culture, newly formed vessels were smaller when the collagen presence was greater *(251)* and collagen-gene expression was found to be inversely proportional to the proliferative state of endothelial cells *(39)*. Also, in two examples of hypertrophy where capillary growth does occur, volume-overload and thyroxine-induced hypertrophy, collagen content/fibrosis is not increased *(252)* and collagen gene expression is actually decreased *(253)*, respectively. Also, hypertrophic fibrosis regressed following treatment with captopril *(254)*, while capillary density increased *(221)*. It has been suggested that cardiac fibroblasts, not myocytes, are responsible for synthesis of extracellular-matrix collagen *(255)* and although these cells are known to be involved in developmental angiogenesis *(7)*, possibly contributing to production of new vessel basement membrane, and/or differentiating into pericytes or vascular smooth musle cells, their role in capillary growth in the heart should be investigated in relation to specific stimuli such as mechanical stretch or blood flow.

On a structural basis, the extracellular matrix components could be responsible for imparting specific mechanical forces to capillary walls; remodeling of the extracellular matrix itself could therefore contribute to pathological changes in the myocardium in such a way as to alter mechanical load, not only on myocytes but also on vessels. Collagen Types I and III also form "struts," described by Caulfied and Borg *(256)* and Robinson et al. *(257)*, which tether capillaries to myocytes and adopt different angular configurations depending on whether the heart was arrested in systole or diastole. It was suggested *(256)* that these struts are important for supporting capillary walls and maintaining patency during systolic contractions, and as such would be mechanical couplers between myocytes and vessels signaling mechanical forces to endothelial cells. How these structures respond to mechanical loads and what impact this has on capillary-vessel walls has not been investigated.

Fibronectin is another extracellular matrix component located close to vessels (228), forming the initial matrix for collagen deposition and adhering fibrillar collagen to myocytes (258). Fibronectin content increased within hours of coronary-artery occlusion (228) with increased gene expression (249), in advance of any changes observed in collagen. Likewise, it increased before collagen during cardiac pressure overload (248). Cultured endothelial cells synthesize fibronectin and its gene expression and production were suppressed by increased blood flow and high shear stress (25). At the same time, binding of endothelial cells to fibronectin is necessary for their growth and leads to cell and nuclear spreading with increased DNA synthesis (56) and microvessel elongation (259). Fibronectin is also thought to be located at the interface between capillary walls and pericytes and could be involved in communicating physical stresses to endothelial cells (260) and therefore play a role in myocardial angiogenesis in response to mechanical stimuli.

Capillary growth is also limited by the presence of intact basement membrane, the disturbance of which is considered the first step in angiogenesis, enabling cell migration and division (46). Breakdown of basement membrane components such as collagen Type IV, laminin, and fibronectin is controlled by plasminogen activators and matrix metalloproteinases (MMPs) and their interaction with modulatory inhibitors. A low molecular-weight endothelial-cell stimulating angiogenic factor (ESAF), which has been isolated from many vascular tissues (261), is the only factor known to activate all three MMPs involved in basement-membrane breakdown (262). Our studies have shown a positive relationship between levels of ESAF and increased capillary density in bradycardially paced rabbit and pig hearts (263), suggesting that ESAF may be involved in capillary growth stimulated by mechanical factors connected with either increased wall tension and stretch of the basement membrane and surrounding tissues.

GROWTH OF LARGER VESSELS
Skeletal Muscle

Although there is abundant evidence for capillary growth as a result of exercise training, data on growth of larger vessels is somewhat scarce. Higher maximal blood flow and conductance, indicators of the size of the whole vascular bed, have been reported in endurance-trained men (e.g., 264–266). Laughlin and colleagues have demonstrated enhanced vascular-transport capacity in rat hindlimbs after training by low-, but not high-intensity running (e.g., 150) (Fig. 6) and the density of arterioles was reported to be increased in spinotrapezius but not gracilis muscles in trained rats (267).

When muscle activity was increased by chronic electrical stimulation, the size of the feed arteries was increased after 4 wk (268) and maximal conductance after 2 wk (269) (Fig. 7). However, the total size of the vascular bed estimated by casts was already enlarged after only 1 wk of stimulation (270), although this was not yet reflected in altered blood flow capacity (Fig. 7). This was probably owing to an increased density of the small alpha smooth-muscle actin-positive arterioles demonstrated by histochemical staining at the same time (271). A similar increase in the arteriolar network was described in muscles of animals

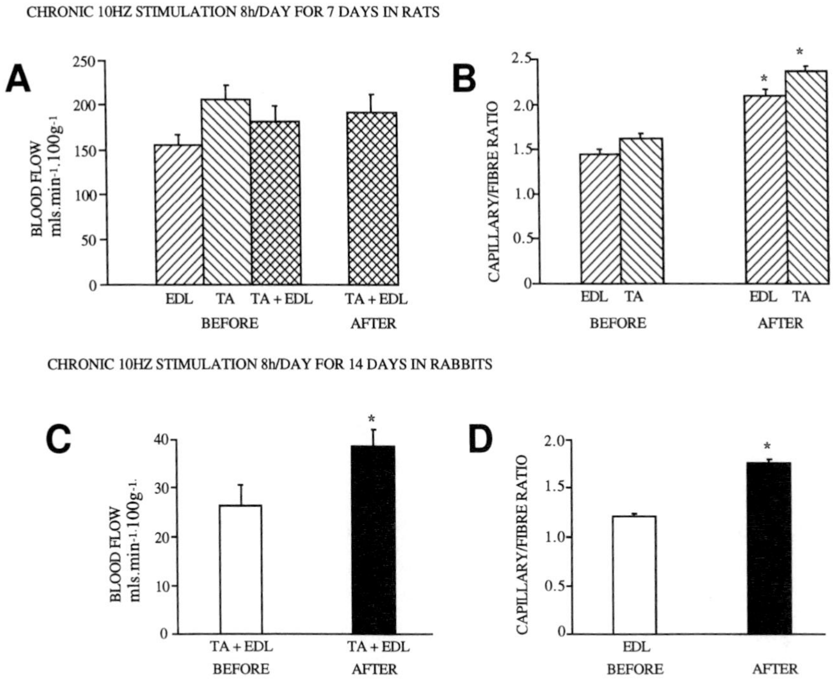

Fig. 7. Blood flow and capillary supply in hindlimb muscles (TA - tibialis anterior, EDL - extensor digitorum longus) in response to 10 Hz chronic electrical stimulation for 7 d in rats and 14 d in rabbits. C/F ratios are increased by 7 d but blood flow capacity is only increased after 14 d. Asterisks indicates significance at 5% level vs pre-training value. Adapted with permission from refs. *69,70.*

treated with the vasodilator prazosin *(73)* or the beta-blocker salbutamol *(272).* It was attributed to "arteriolarization" of capillaries and suggested that it is owing mainly to increased blood flow and shear stress *(273)* and a similar explanation may be true for the increased arteriolar density in chronically stimulated muscles and maybe trained muscles, but the forces that transform capillaries into arterioles are still poorly understood.

Heart

Whereas capillary growth in the normal adult heart as a result of training is questionable, growth of arterioles and even conduit vessels has been demonstrated by several authors. Recent reviews describe large vessel growth on the basis of vascular casts, greater maximal coronary blood flow, increased conductance and larger main coronary arteries in both animals and humans following various training regimes *(157,158,274).* Increased maximal blood flow after training is likely to be owing to changes in conduit and resistance arterioles and does not seem to be linked with capillary growth. For example, Breisch et al. *(275)* found higher coronary blood flow and increased arteriolar density but a lower capillary density in trained pig hearts. White and Bloor *(276)* also recently demonstrated an increase in the number of arterioles starting after 3 wk of training in pigs. However, after a full 16 wk of training, the increase in the numerical density of arterioles accounted for only 11% out of 50% increase in the total cross-sectional area of the vascular bed, the rest being owing to the increase in diameter of existing vessels, thus complementing previous findings.

Which factors are involved in the growth of arterioles or enlargement of conduit vessels, as opposed to growth of capillaries, is not understood. It is certainly not higher blood flow because neither long-term administration of vasodilating drugs *(93)* nor sympathectomy *(277)* led to increased maximal coronary blood flow. Also, maximal coronary blood flow was not increased in bradycardially paced hearts or hearts in animals treated with dobutamine, procedures that stimulated growth of capillaries. It is therefore a challenge to establish why procedures that stimulate capillary growth do not affect growth of larger vessels whereas those that do not stimulate capillary growth do.

Measurement of total coronary vascular reserve is indicative of changes in large vessels and arterioles in pressure-overload hypertrophy and is reported to be decreased in most species examined *(see 74,188)*. This could be owing to loss of arterioles, but Tomanek *(197)* did not find any decrease in the number of arterioles in dogs, although a reduced number of medium-size arterioles (20–40 µm) was described in rats *(278)*. A decrement in coronary vascular reserve could also be owing to thickening of the vessel wall or periarteriolar fibrosis restricting vasodilator capacity *(279)*, or impaired function of endothelium *(242)*.

In contrast to pressure-overload hypertrophy, there was no impairment of the minimal coronary vascular resistance in volume-overload hypertrophy *(280)* and growth of collaterals seemed to be enhanced in cardiomegaly owing to anemia *(281)*. Villari et al. *(282)* described enlargement of the left anterior descending coronary artery in a patient with aortic-valve insufficiency, that regressed after valve replacement. During development of collateral circulation after either abrupt or gradual occlusion of a coronary artery, vascular proliferation has been shown by thymidine incorporation studies in all classes of vessels in dogs and pigs *(75)*, although it is always difficult in such studies to differentiate between expansion of pre-existent vessels and *de novo* formation. Endothelial cells, and to a lesser extent, smooth-muscle cells, were also labeled in large arteries and there was a considerable increase (43%) in arteriolar density with very thin walls *(283)*. DeBrabande et al. *(229)* showed proliferation of all classes of arterial and venous vessels in a pig model of gradual coronary-artery occlusion and ^{3}H-thymidine labeling was also increased within the area at risk in contrast to dogs *(75)*. In human hearts the response was similar to pigs *(75)*. Collaterals are also reported to be more numerous at the onset on myocardial infarction in patients with preinfarction angina *(236)*.

CONCLUSIONS

It is clear that mechanical factors such as shear stress, wall tension, and stretch of vessels are as important in in vivo angiogenesis in skeletal muscle and heart as they have been shown to be in vitro and our understanding of the circumstances under which they operate has developed considerably. However, in order to be able to use this knowledge for effective regulation of vessel growth — either promotion or inhibition — there are questions that must still be answered. Increased shear stress resulting from increased blood flow is important for angiogenesis in both skeletal muscle and the heart, but in the former, the mechanism of vessel growth appears to be different depending on whether blood flow/shear is increased by a vasodilator or by functional hyperemia, and in the latter, even our understanding of how capillary growth takes place is as yet incomplete. The exact sequence of events that follows an elevation of shear stress therefore remains to be determined in terms of luminal signals to endothelial cells, possible changes to the glycocalyx, and subsequent intracellular activation.

The significance of the extracellular matrix and interstitial cells for either guiding vessel growth or restricting it also requires further investigation, particularly in situations of pathological angiogenesis, where the tissue itself may be undergoing remodeling and complex endothelial/smooth-muscle cell – matrix interactions are taking place. This could help to explain why capillary growth is evident in the heart in some models of cardiac hypertrophy (e.g., thyroxine-induced) but not in others (pressure-overload), and why the stimulus of increased coronary blood flow *per se* is not always sufficient to remedy the decrement in capillary supply in the hypertrophied heart, whereas long-term bradycardia is the most effective intervention yet.

There are also questions to be answered regarding tissue-specific responses. A case in point is exercise training, which provides the same factors capable of initiating angiogenesis — increased blood flow and shear stress, altered mechanical forces in vessel walls — to heart (*see* ref. *157*) as to skeletal muscle, yet in the former growth of larger vessels is the predominant response with little, if any, growth of capillaries, whereas in the latter, capillary growth occurs more readily than large vessel growth. Investigations of the complex nature of interactions between luminal and abluminal mechanical factors in relation to other angiogenic stimuli such as hypoxia and growth factors will therefore be needed to fully define the role of mechanical factors in in vivo angiogenesis.

REFERENCES

1. Thoma, R. (1893) *Untersuchungen uber die Histogenese und Histomechanik des Gefssystems.* Enkeverlag, Stuttgart.
2. Clark, E. R. (1918) Studies on the growth of blood vessels in the tail of the frog. *Am. J. Anat.* **23**, 37–88.
3. Clark, E. R. and Clark, E. L. (1940) Mircroscope observation of the extraendothelial cells of living mammalian blood vessels. *Am. J. Anat.* **66**, 1–49.
4. Folkman, J. and Shing, Y. (1992) Angiogenesis. *J. Biol. Chem.* **267**, 10,931–10,934.
5. Hudlická, O. and Tyler, K. R. (1986) *Angiogenesis: The Growth of the Vascular System.* Academic, London.
6. D'Amore, P. A. and Thompson, R. W. (1987) Mechanisms of angiogenesis. *Ann. Rev. Physiol.* **49**, 453–464.
7. Rhodin, J. A. G. and Fujita, H. (1989) Capillary growth in the mesentery of normal young rats. Intravital video and electron microscope analyses. *J. Submicrosc. Cytol. Pathol.* **21**, 1–34.
8. Sumpio, B. F. (1991) Haemodynamic forces and the biology of endothelium: signal transduction pathways in endothelial cells subjected to physical forces in vitro. *J. Vasc. Surg.* **13**, 744–746.
9. Patrick, C. W., Jr. and McIntire, L. V. (1995) Shear stress and cyclic strain modulation of gene expression in vascular endothelial cells. *Blood Purific.* **13**, 112–124.
10. Wolin, M. S. (1996) Reactive oxygen species and vascular signal transduction mechanisms. *Microcirculation* **3**, 1–17.
11. Dewey, C. F., Jr., Bussolari, S. R., Gimbrone, M. A. Jr., and Davies, P. F. (1981) The dynamic response of vascular endothelial cells to fluid shear stress. *J. Biochem. Eng.* **103**, 177–185.
12. Davies, P. F., Remuzzi, A., Gordon, E. J., Dewey, C. F., and Gimbrone, M. A. (1986) Turbulent fluid shear stress induces vascular endothelial cell turnover in vitro. *Proc. Natl. Acad. Sci. USA* **83**, 2114–2117.
13. Ando, J., Nomura, H., and Kamiya, A. (1987) The effect of fluid shear stress on the migration and proliferation of cultured endothelial cells. *Microvasc. Res.* **33**, 62–70.
14. De Forrest, J. M. and Hollis, T. M. (1980) Relationship between low intensity shear stress, antihistamine formation and aortic albumin uptake. *Exp. Mol. Pathol.* **32**, 217–225.
15. Davies, P. F. (1989) How do vascular endothelial cells respond to flow? *NIPS* **4**, 22–25.
16. Hecker, M., Mülsch, A., Bassenge, E., and Busse, R. (1993) Vasoconstriction and increased flow: two principal mechanisms of shear stress-dependent endothelial autacoid release. *Am. J. Physiol.* **265**, H828–H833.
17. Noris, M., Morigi, M., Donadelli, R., Aillo, S., Foppolo, M., Todeschini, M., et al. (1995) Nitric oxide synthesis of cultured endothelial cells is modified by flow conditions. *Circ. Res.* **76**, 536–543.

18. Ziche, M., Morbidelli, L., Masini, E., Granger, H., Geppetti, P., and Ledda, F. (1993) Nitric oxide promotes DNA synthesis and cyclic GMP formation in endothelial cells from postcapillary venules. *Biochem. Biophys. Res. Commun.* **192,** 1198–1203.

19. Olesen, S. P., Clapham, D. E., and Davies, P. F. (1988) Haemodynamics shear stress activates a K+ current in vascular endothelial cells. *Nature* **331,** 168–170.

20. Berthiaume, F. and Frangos, J. A. (1990) Fluid flow causes membrane perturbation in cultured human umbilical vein endothelial cells (HUVECs). *FASEB J.* **4,** A835.

21. Nollert, M. U., Eskin, S. G., and McIntire, L. V. (1990) Shear stress increases inositol triphosphate levels in human endothelial cells. *Biochem. Biophys. Res Commun.* **170,** 281–282.

22. Brown, L. C., Messick, F. C., Koki, M. P., Hamilton, I. G., and Girard, P. R. (1995) Fluid flow stimulates metalloproteinase production and deposition into extracellular matrix of endothelial cells. *FASEB J.* **9,** A617.

23. Resnick, N. and Gimbrone, M. A. (1995) Hemodynamic forces are complex regulators of endothelial gene expression. *FASEB J.* **9,** 874–882.

24. Davies, P. F. (1995) Flow-mediated endothelial mechanotransduction. *Physiol. Rev.* **75,** 519–560.

25. Gupte, A. and Frangos J. A. (1990) Effects of flow on the synthesis and release of fibronectin by endothelial cells. *In Vitro* **26,** 57–60.

26. Ausprunck, D. H., Dethlefsen, S. M., and Higgins, E. R. (1991) Distribution of fibronectin, calcium and type IV collagen during development of blood vessels in the chick chorioallantoic membrane, in T*he Development of the Vascular System* (Feinberg, R. N., Scherer, G.-K., and Auerbach, R., eds.), Karger, Basel, pp. 93–108.

27. Rongish, B. J., Hinchman, G., Doty, M. K., Baldwin, S., and Tomanek, R. J. (1996) Relationship of the extracellular matrix to coronary neovascularization during development. *J. Mol. Cell. Cardiol.* **28,** 2203–2215.

28. Sumpio, B. F., Banes, A. J., Levin, A. G., and Johnson, G. (1987) Mechanical stress stimulates aortic endothelial cells to proliferate. *J. Vasc. Surg.* **6,** 252–256.

29. Sumpio, B., Du, W., Gallagher, G., Gimbrone, M., and Resnick, N. (1995) Regulation of PDGF ß promotor in endothelial cells. *FASEB J.* **9,** A272.

30. Widmann, M. D., Letsou, G. V., Phan, S., Baldwin, J. C., and Sumpio, B. E. (1992) Isolation and characterization of rabbit cardiac endothelial cells: response to cyclic strain and growth factors in vitro. *J. Surg. Res.* **53,** 331–334.

31. Lyall, F., Deehan, M. R., Greer, I. A., Boswell, F., Brown, W. C., and McInnes, G. T. (1994) Mechanical stretch increases proto-oncogene expression and phosphoinositide turnover in vascular smooth muscle cells. *J. Hypert.* **12,** 1139–1145.

32. Iba, T., Maitz, S., Furbert, T., Rosales, O., Widmann, M. D., Spillane, B., et al. (1991) Effect of cyclic stretch on endothelial cells from different vascular beds. *Circ. Shock.* **35,** 193–198.

33. Iba, T., Sain, T., Sonoda, T., Rosales, O., and Sumpio, B. E. (1991). Stimulation of endothelial secretion of tissue- type plasminogen activator by repetitive stretch. *J. Surg. Res.* **50,** 457–460.

34. Gullino, P. M., Alessandri, G., and Ziche, M. (1990) Regulatory events in angiogenesis. *Front. Diabetes* **9,** 175–182.

35. Pepper, M. S., Montesano, R., Mandriota, S. J., Orci, L., and Vassalli, J. D. (1996) Angiogenesis: a paradigm for balanced extracellular proteolysis during cell migration and morphogenesis. *Enzyme Protein* **49,** 138–162.

36. Haudenschild, C. C. (1980) Growth control of endothelial cells in atherogenesis and tumor angiogenesis, in *Advances in Microcirculation*, vol. 9. (Altura, B. M., ed.), Karger, Basel, pp. 226–251.

37. Ingber, D. E. and Folkman, J. (1987) Regulation of endothelial growth factor action - solid state control of extracellular matrix. *Prog. Clin. Biol. Res.* **249,** 273–282.

38. Lansman, J. B. and Hallam, T. J. (1987) Single stretch-activated ion channels in vascular endothelial cells as mechanotransducers? *Nature* **325,** 811–812.

39. Sumpio, B. F., Banes, A. J., Link, G. W., and Iba, T. (1990) Modulation of endothelial cell phenotype by cyclic stretch: inhibition of collagen production. *J. Surg. Res.* **48,** 415–420.

40. D'Amore, P. A. and Orlidge, A. (1988) Growth factors and pericytes in microangiography. *Diabete Metab.* **14,** 495–504.

41. Folkow, B. (1982) Physiological aspects of primary hypertension. *Physiol. Rev.* **62,** 347–504.

42. Mulvany, M. J. and Aaalkjaer, C. (1990) Structure and function of small arteries. *Physiol. Rev.* **70,** 921–962.

43. Liebow, A. A. (1963) Situations which lead to changes in vascular patterns. in *Handbook of Physiology, Circulation, vol. 2*, American Physiolical Society, Bethesda, MD, pp. 1258–1259.

44. Dethlefsen, S. M., Shepro, D., and D'Amore, P. A. (1996) Comparison of the effects of mechanical stimulation on venous and arterial smooth muscle cells. *J. Vasc. Res.* **33**, 405–413.

45. Speiser, B., Riess, C. F., and Schaper, J. (1991) The extracellular matrix in human myocardium: Part 1: Collagens I, III, IV and VI. *Cardioscience* **2**, 225–232.

46. Glaser, B. M., Kalebic, T., Garbisa, S., Connor, T. B., Jr., and Liotta, L. A. (1983) Degradation of basement membrane components by vascular endothelial cells: role in neovascularisation, in *Development of the Vascular System*, Ciba Foundation Symposium 100, Pitman, London, pp. 150–162.

47. Unemori, E. N., Bouhana, K. S., and Werb, E. (1990) Vectorial secretion of extracellular matrix proteins, matrix degrading proteinases and tissue inhibitor of metalloproteinases by endothelial cells. *J. Biol. Chem.* **265**, 445–451.

48. Moscatelli, D. and Rifkin, D. B. (1988) Membrane and matrix localisation of proteases: a common theme in tumor invasion and angiogenesis. *Biochem. Biophys. Acta* **948**, 67–85.

49. Ingber, D. E. and Folkman, J. (1989b) How does extracellular matrix control capillary morphogenesis? *Cell* **58**, 803–805.

50. Form, M. D., Pratt, B. M., and Madri, J. A. (1986) Endothelial cell proliferation during angiogenesis: in vitro modulation by basement membrane components. *Lab. Invest.* **55**, 521–530.

51. Hausman, G. J., Wright, J. T., and Thomas, G. B. (1991) Vascular and cellular development in fetal adipose tissue: lectin binding studies and immunocytochemistry for laminin and Type IV collagen. *Microvasc. Res.* **41**, 111–125.

52. Maragoudakis, M. E., Tsopanoglou, N. E., Bastaki, M., and Haralabopoulos, G. (1992) Evaluation of promotors and inhibitors of angiogenesis using basement membrane biosynthesis as an index, in *Angiogenesis in Health and Disease*, (Maragoudakis, M. E., Gullino, P., and Lelkes, P. I., eds.), Plenum, NY, pp. 275–285.

53. Ausprunck, D. H., Dethlefsen, S. M., and Higgins, E. R. (1991) Distribution of fibronectin, calcium and type IV collagen during development of blood vessels in the chick chorioallantoic membrane, in *The Development of the Vascular System*, (Feinberg, R. N., Scherer, G.-K., and Auerbach, R., eds.), Karger, Basel, pp. 93–108.

54. Pepper, M. S., Vassalli, J. D., Montesano, R., and Orci, L. (1987) Urokinase-type plasminogen activator is induced in migrating capillary endothelial cells. *J. Cell. Biol.* **105**, 2535–2541.

55. Johnson, M. D., Kim, H. R. C., Chesler, L., Tsaowu, G., Bouck, N., and Polverini, P. J. (1994) Inhibition of angiogenesis by tissue inhibior of metalloproteinase. *J. Cell. Physiol.* **160**, 194–202.

56. Ingber, D. (1991) Extracellular matrix and cell shape: potential control points for inhibition of angiogenesis. *J. Cell. Biochem.* **47**, 236–241.

57. Strömblad, A. and Cheresh, D. A. (1996) Cell adhesion and angiogenesis. *Trends Cell Biol.* **6**, 462–467.

58. Friedlander, M., Brooks, P. C., Shaffer, R. W., Kincaid, C. M., Varner, J. A., and Cheresh D. A. (1995) Definition of two angiogenic pathways by distinct αv integrins. *Science* **270**, 1500–1502.

59. Woessner, J. F., Jr. (1991) Matrix metalloproteinases and their inhibitors in connective tissue remodeling. *FASEB J.* **5**, 2145–2154.

60. Orlidge, A. and D'Amore, P. A. (1987) Inhibition of capillary endothelial cell growth by pericytes and smooth muscle cells. *J. Cell. Biol.* **105**, 1455–1462.

61. Kuwabara, T. and Cogan, D. G. (1963) Retinal vascular patterns. VI. Mural cells of the retinal capillaries. *Archs. Ophthal.* **69**, 492–502.

62. Crocker, D. J., Murad, T. M., and Geer, J. P. (1970) Role of pericyte in wound healing. An ultrastructural study. *Exp. Mol. Path.* **13**, 51–65.

63. Sato, Y. and Rifkin, D. B. (1989) Inhibition of endothelial cell movement by pericytes and smooth muscle cells: activation of a latent transforming growth factor-β1 like molecule by plasmin co-culture. *J. Cell Biol.* **109**, 309–315.

64. Sims, D. E. (1986) The pericyte: a review. *Tissue Cell* **18**, 153–174.

65. Nehls, V., Denzer, K., and Drenckhahn, D. (1992) Pericyte involvement in capillary sprouting during angiogenesis in situ. *Cell Tissue Res.* **270**, 469–474.

66. Diaz, F. L., Gutierrez, R., and Varela, H. (1992) Behaviour of postcapillary venule pericytes during postnatal angiogenesis. *J. Morphol.* **213**, 33–45.

67. Egginton, S., Hudlická, O., Brown, M. D., Graciotti, L., and Granata, A.-L. (1996) In vivo pericyte-endothelial cell interaction during angiogenesis in adult cardiac and skeletal muscle. *Microvasc. Res.* **51**, 213–228.

68. Lelkes, P. I., Manolopoulos, V., Silverman, M., Zhang, S., Karmiol, S., and Unsworth, B. R. (1996). On the possible role of endothelial cell heterogeneity in angiogenesis, in *Molecular, Cellular and Clinical Aspects of Angiogenesis*, (Maragoudakis, M., ed.), Plenum Press, New York, pp. 1–17.

69. Hudlická, O., Brown, M. D., and Egginton, S. (1997) Angiogenesis - basic concepts and methodology, in *Proceedings of An Introduction to Vascular Biology* London, in press.

70. Heron, M. I. and Rakusan, K. (1995) Proliferating cell nuclear antigen (PCNA) detection of cellular proliferation in hypothyroid and hyperthyroid rat hearts. *J. Mol. Cell. Cardiol.* **27**, 1393–1703.

71. Egginton, S. (1990) Morphometric analysis of tissue capillary supply. *Adv. Comp. Environ. Physiol.* **6**, 73–141.

72. Hansen-Smith, F. M., Hudlická, O., and Egginton, S. (1996) In vivo angiogenesis in adult rat skeletal muscle: early changes in capillary network architecture and ultrastructure. *Cell Tissue Res.* **286**, 123–136.

73. Price, R. J. and Skalak, T. C. (1996) Chronic alpha 1-adrenergic blockade stimulates terminal and arcade arteriolar development. *Am. J. Physiol.* **271**, H752–H759.

74. Hudlická, O., Brown, M. D., and Egginton, S. (1992) Angiogenesis in skeletal and cardiac muscle. *Physiol. Rev.* **72**, 369–417.

75. Schaper, W., Görge, G., Winkler, B., and Schaper, J. (1988) The collateral circulation of the heart. *Prog. Cardiovasc. Dis.* **31**, 57–77.

76. White, F. C. and Bloor, C. M. (1992) Coronary vascular remodeling and coronary resistance during chronic ischemia. *Am. J. Cardiovasc. Pathol.* **4**, 193–202.

77. Kasalicky, J., Ressl, J., Urbanova, D., Widimsky, J., Ostadal, B., Pelouch, V., et al. (1977) Relative organ blood flow in rats exposed to intermittent high altitude hypoxia. *Pflügers Arch.* **368**, 111–115.

78. Tyml, K. (1991) Heterogeneity of microvascular flow in rat skeletal muscle is reduced by contraction and by hemodilution. *Int. J. Microcirc. Clin. Exp.* **10**, 75–86.

79. Berg, B. R. and Sarelius, I. H. (1995) Functional capillary organization in striated muscle. *Am. J. Physiol.* **268**, H1215–H1222.

80. Anderson, S. I., Hudlická, O., and Brown M. D. (1997) Capillary red blood cell flow and activation of white blood cells in chronic muscle ischemia in the rat. *Am. J. Physiol.*, in press.

81. Dawson, J. M. and Hudlická, O. (1993) Can changes in microcirculation explain capillary growth in skeletal muscle? *Int. J. Exp. Pathol.* **74**, 65–71.

82. Duling, B. R. and Desjardins, C. (1987) Capillary hematocrit: what does it mean? *NIPS* **2**, 66–69.

83. Heroux, O. and Pierre, J. S. (1957) Effect of cold acclimation on vascularisation of ears, heart, liver and muscles of white rats. *Am. J. Physiol.* **188**, 163–168.

84. Sillau, A. H., Aquin, L., Lechner, A. J., and Bui, M. V. (1980) Increased capillary supply in skeletal muscle of guinea pigs acclimated to cold. *Respir. Physiol.* **42**, 233–245.

85. Wickler, S. J. (1981) Capillary supply of skeletal muscles from acclimatized white-footed mice *Peromyseus. Am. J. Physiol.* **241**, R357–R361.

86. Johnston, I. A. (1982) Capillarisation, oxygen diffusion distances and mitochondrial content of carp muscles following acclimation to summer and winter temperatures. *Cell Tissue Res.* **222**, 325–337.

87. Egginton, S. and Hoofd, L. (1994) Effects of low temperature on calculated intracellular oxygen tension in fish skeletal muscle. *J. Physiol.* **479P**, 6.

88. Folkow, B. and Neil, E. (1971) *Circulation.* Oxford University Press, New York, London.

89. Turek, Z., Grandtner, M., and Kreuzer, F. (1972) Cardiac hypertrophy, capillary and muscle fiber density, muscle fiber diameter, capillary radius and diffusion distance in the myocardium of growing rats adapted to a simulated altitude of 3500m. *Pflügers Arch.* **335**, 19–28.

90. Pietschmann, M. and Bartels, H. (1985) Cellular hyperplasia and hypertrophy, capillary proliferation and myoglobin concentration in the heart of newborn and adult rats at high altitude. *Respir. Physiol.* **59**, 347–360.

91. Tornling, G. (1982) Capillary neoformation in the heart of dipyridamole treated rats. *Acta Pathol. Microbiol. Scand. sec A.* **90**, 269–271.

92. Mattfeldt, T. and Mall, G. (1983) Dipyrimadole-induced capillary endothelial proliferation in the rat heart: a morphometric investigation. *Cardiovasc. Res.* **17**, 229–237.

93. Ziada, A. M. A. R., Hudlická, O., Tyler, K. R., and Wright A. J. A. (1984) The effect of long term vasodilation on capillary growth and performance in rabbit heart and skeletal muscle. *Cardiovasc. Res.* **18**, 724–732.

94. Tillmanns, H., Steinhausen, M., Leinberger, H., Thederan, H., and Kübler, W. (1982) The effect of coronary vasodilators on the microcirculation of the ventricular myocardium, in *Microcirculation of the Heart* (Tillmanns, H., Kübler, W., and Zebe, H., eds.), Springer Verlag, Berlin, Heidelberg, pp. 305–312.

95. Hudlická, O. (1994) Mechanical factors involved in the growth of the heart and its blood vessels. *Cell. Mol. Biol. Res.* **40**, 143–152.

96. Mandache, E., Unge, G., Appelgren, L. E., and Ljungqvist, A. (1973) The proliferation activity of the heart tissues in various forms of experimental cardiac hypertrophy studied by electron microscope autoradiography. *Virchow's Arch. Cell. Pathol.* **12**, 112–122.

97. Brown, M. D., Egginton, S., and Hudlická, O. (1996) Appearance of the capillary endothelial glycocalyx in chronically stimulated rat skeletal muscles in relation to angiogenesis. *Exp. Physiol.* **81,** 1043–1046.

98. Pearce, S., Hudlická, O., and Egginton, S. (1995) Early stages in activity-induced angiogenesis in rat skeletal muscles: incorporation of bromodeoxyuridine into cells of the interstitium. *J. Physiol.* **483,** 146P.

99. Brown, M. D., Hudlická, O., Weiss, J. B., Bate, A., and Silgram, H. (1996) Prazosin-induced capillary growth in rat skeletal muscle: link with endothelial-cell-stimulating angiogenic factor. *Int. J. Microcirc. Clin. Exp.* **16,** 207.

100. Zhou, A.-L., Egginton, S., and Hudlická, O. (1996) Ultrastructural evidence for a novel mechanism of capillary growth in rat skeletal muscle. *J. Physiol.* **491,** 28P.

101. van Groningen, J. P.,Weninck, A. C., and Testers, L. H. (1991). Myocardial capillaries increase in number by splitting of existing vessels. *Acta Embryologica* **184,** 65–70.

102. Gullino, P. M. (1992) Microenvironment and angiogenic response. *EXS* **61,** 125–128.

103. Pearce, S. C. and Hudlická, O. (1995) Possible involvement of prostaglandins in capillary growth in chronically stimulated skeletal muscles. *Microcirculation* **2,** 98.

104. Hudlická, O., Brown, M. D., and Silgram, H. (1996) Role of nitric oxide in capillary proliferation in chronically stimulated rat skeletal muscle. *Int. J. Microcirc. Clin. Exp.* **16(Suppl. 1),** 92.

105. Messina, E. J., Sun, D., Koller, A., Wolin, M. S., and Kaley, G. (1992) Role of endothelium derived prostaglandins in hypoxia-elicited arteriolar dilation in rat skeletal muscle. *Circ. Res.* **71,** 790–796.

106. Maspers, M.. Bjornberg, J., and Mellander, S. (1990) Relation between capillary pressure and vascular tone over the range from maximum dilatation to maximum constriction in cat skeletal muscle. *Acta Physiol. Scand.* **140,** 73–83.

107. Fronek, K. and Zweifach, B. W. (1975) Microvascular pressure distribution in skeletal muscle and the effect of vasodilation. *Am. J. Physiol.* **228,** 791–796.

108. Tillmanns, T. H., Steinhausen, M., Therderan, H., and Parekh, N. (1977) In vivo microscopic studies of the ventricular microcirculation of the rat heart. *J. Mol. Cell Cardiol.* **9(Suppl.),** 57–58.

109. Tillmanns, T. H., Dart, A. M., Parekh, N., Neumann, F. J., Moller, P., Zimmerman, R., et al. (1984) Calcium antagonists (nifedipine) and coronary vasodilators (dipyridamole) - different effects on small coronary resistance vessels. *Int. J. Microcirc. Clin. Exp.* **3,** 342.

110. Wachtlová, A., Rakusan, K., and Poupa, O (1965) The coronary terminal vascular bed in the heart of the hare *(Lepidus europeus)* and the rabbit *(Orytolagus domesticus). Physiol. Bohemoslov* **14,** 328–331.

111. Wachtlová, M., Rakusan, K., Roth, Z., and Poupa, O. (1967) The terminal bed of the myocardium in the wild rat *(Rattus Norvegicus)* and the laboratory rat *(Rattus Norvegicus Lab.). Physiol. Bohemoslov* **16,** 548–554.

112. Wright, A. J. A. and Hudlická, O. (1981) Capillary growth and changes in heart performance induced by chronic bradycardial pacing in the rabbit. *Circ. Res.* **49,** 469–478.

113. Hudlická, O., Wright, A. J. A., Hoppeler, H., and Uhlmann, E. (1988) The effect of chronic bradycardial pacing on the oxidative capacity in rabbit hearts. *Respir. Physiol.* **72,** 1–12.

114. Brown, M. D., Davies, M. K., Hudlická, O., and Townsend, P. (1994) Long-term bradycardia by electrical pacing: a new method for studying heart rate reduction. *Cardiovasc. Res.* **28,** 1774–1779.

115. Brown, M. D. and Hudlická, O. (1992) Capillary growth in the heart. *EXS* **61,** 389–394

116. Hudlická, O., West, D., Kumar, S., El Khelly, F., and Wright, A. J. A. (1989) Can growth of capillaries in the heart and skeletal muscle be explained by the presence of an angiogenic factor? *Br. J. Exp. Path.* **70,** 237–246.

117. Tillmanns, T., Ikeda, S., Hansen, H., Samara, J. S., Fauvel, J. H., and Bing, R. J. (1974) Microcirculation in the ventricule of the dog and turtle. *Circ. Res.* **34,** 561–569.

118. Folkman, J. and Moscona, A. (1978) Role of cell shape in growth control. *Nature* **273,** 345–349.

119. Koch, A. E., Halloran, M., Haskell, C. J., Shah, M. R., and Polerini, P. J. (1995) Angiogenesis mediated by soluble forms of E selectin and vascular cell adhesion molecule-1. *Nature* **376,** 517–519.

120. Hassler, O. and Stroinska-Kusinova, B. (1976) The angioarchitecture of normal, hypertrophic and denervated muscle. A study in the rat, using microangiography and the scanning electron microscope. *Pathol. Eur.* **11,** 57–61.

121. James, N. T. (1981) A stereological analysis of capillaries in normal and hypertrophic muscle. *J. Morph.* **168,** 43–49.

122. Degens, H., Turek, Z., Hoofd, L. J. C., Van de Hoff, M. A., and Binkhorst, R. A. (1992) The relationship between capillarisation and fibre types during compensatory hypertrophy of the plantaris muscle in the rat. *J. Anat.* **180,** 455–463.

123. Egginton S., and Hudlická, O. (1992) Effect of long-term overload on capillary supply, blood flow and performance in rat fast muscle. *J. Physiol.* **454,** 9P.

124. Holly, R. G., Barnett, J. G., Ashmore, C. R., Taylor, R. G., and Mole, P. A. (1980) Stretch induced growth in chicken wing muscles: a new model of stretch hypertrophy. *Am. J. Physiol.* **238,** C62–C71.

125. Snyder, G. K. and Coelho, J. R. (1989) Microvascular development in chick anterior latissimus dorsi following hypertrophy. *J. Anat.* **162,** 215–224.

126. Armstrong, R. B., Ianuzzo, C. D., and Laughlin, M. H. (1986) Blood flow and glycogen use in hypertrophied rat muscles during exercise. *J. Appl. Physiol.* **61,** 685–687.

127. Egginton, S., Hudlická, O., Walter, H., Brown, M. D., Weiss, J. B., and Bate, A. (1997) Is angiogenesis in stretch-overloaded rat skeletal muscle linked with increased blood flow and performance? (manuscript in preparation).

128. Zhou, A.-L. and Egginton, S. (1997) Capillary growth in overloaded rat skeletal muscle: an ultrastructural study. *J. Physiol.* **499,** 39P.

129. Hudlická, O. and Brown, M. D. (1994) Growth of blood vessels in normal and diseased hearts. *Therap. Res.* **15,** 93–145.

130. Brown, M. D. and Hudlická, O. (1991) Capillary supply and cardiac performance in the rabbit after chronic dobutamine treatment. *Cardiovasc. Res.* **25,** 909–915.

131. Wachtlová, M. and Parizková, J. (1972) Comparison of capillary density in skeletal muscles of animals differing in respect of their physical activity: the hare *(Lepus europaeus)*, the domestic rabbit *(Oryctolagus domesticus)*, the brown rat *(Rattus norvegicus)* and the trained and untrained rat. *Physiol. Bohemoslov* **21,** 489–495.

132. Gunn, H. M. (1981) Potential blood supply to muscles in horses and dogs and its relation to athletic ability. *Am. J. Vet. Res.* **42,** 679–684.

133. Hudlická, O. (1990) The response of muscle to enhanced and reduced activity. *Bailliere's Clin. Endocrinol. Metab.* **4,** 417–439.

134. Hermansen, L. and Wachtlova, M. (1971) Capillary density of skeletal muscle in well-trained and untrained men. *J. Appl. Physiol.* **30,** 860–863.

135. Andersen, P. and Henriksson, J. (1977) Capillary supply of the quadriceps femoris muscle of man: adaptive response to exercise. *J. Physiol.* **270,** 677–690.

136. Saltin, B. and Gollnick, P. D. (1983) Skeletal muscle adaptability: significance for metabolism and performance, in *Handbook of Physiology* (Peachey, L. D., Adrian, R. H., and Geiger, S. R., eds.), American Physiological Society, Bethesda, MD, pp. 555–631.

137. Denis, C., Chatard, J. C., Dormois, D., Linossier, M. T., Geyssant, A., and Lacour, J. R. (1986) Effects of endurance training on capillary supply of human skeletal muscles in two age groups (20 and 60 years). *J. Physiol.* **81,** 379–385.

138. Zumstein, A., Mathieu, O., Howald, H., and Hoppeler, H. (1983) Morphometric analysis of the capillary supply in skeletal muscles of trained and untrained subjects - its limitations in muscle biopsies. *Pflügers Arch.* **397,** 277–283.

139. Nygaard, E. (1982) Skeletal muscle fibre characteristics in young women. *Acta Physiol. Scand.* **112,** 299–304.

140. Larsson, L. and Forsberg, A. (1980) Morphological muscle characteristics in rowers. *Can. J. Sports Sci.* **5,** 239–244.

141. Schantz, P., Henriksson, J., and Jansson, E. (1983) Adaption of human skeletal muscle to endurance training of long duration. *Clin. Physiol.* **3,** 141–151.

142. Ljungqvist, A., Tornling, G., Unge, G., Jurdahl, B., and Larsson, B. (1984) Capillary growth in the heart and skeletal muscle during dipyridamole treatment and exercise. *Prog. Appl. Microcirc.* **4,** 9–15.

143. Hoppeler, H., Lindstedt, S. L., Uhlmann, E., Niesel, A., Cruz-Orive, L. M., and Weibel, E. R. (1984) Oxygen consumption and the composition of skeletal muscle tissue after training and inactivation in the european woodmouse *(Apodemus Sylvaticus)*. *J. Comp. Physiol. B.* **155,** 51–61.

144. Parson, D., Musch, T. I., Moore, R. L., Hailet, G. C., and Ordway, G. A. (1985) Dynamic exercise training in foxhounds II. Analysis of skeletal muscle. *J. Appl. Physiol.* **59,** 190–197.

145. Mai, J. V., Edgerton, V. R., and Barnard, R. J. (1970) Capillarity of red, white and intermediate muscle fibres in trained and untrained guinea-pigs. *Experientia* **26,** 1222–1223.

146. Ingjer, F. (1979) Effects of endurance training on muscle fibre ATPase activity, capillary supply and mitochondria in man. *J. Physiol.* **294,** 419–432.

147. Romanul, F. C. (1965) Capillary supply and metabolism of muscle fibres. *Arch. Neurol.* **12,** 497–509.

148. Gray, S. D. and Renkin, E. M. (1978) Microvascular supply in relation to fiber metabolic type in mixed skeletal muscles of rabbits. *Microvasc. Res.* **16,** 406–425.

149. Laughlin, M. H. and Armstrong, R. B. (1982) Muscular blood flow distribution patterns as a function of running speed in rats. *Am. J. Physiol.* **243,** H296–H306.
150. Sexton, W. L. and Laughlin, M. H. (1994) Influence of endurance exercise training on distribution of vascular adaptations in rat skeletal muscle. *Am. J. Physiol.* **266,** H483–H490.
151. Daub, W. D., Green, H. Y., Houston, M. E., Thomson, J. A., Fraser, I. G., and Ranney, D. A. (1982) Cross-adaptive responses to different forms of leg training: skeletal muscle biochemistry and histochemistry. *Can. J. Physiol. Pharmacol.* **60,** 628–635.
152. Schantz, P. (1982) Capillary supply in hypertrophied human skeletal muscle. *Acta Physiol. Scand.* **114,** 635–637.
153. Schantz, P. (1983) Capillary supply in heavy-resistance trained non-postural human skeletal muscle. *Acta Physiol. Scand.* **117,** 153–156.
154. Tesch, P. A., Thorsson, A., and Kaiser, P. (1984) Muscle capillary supply and fiber type characteristics in weight and power lifters. *J. Appl. Physiol.* **56,** 35–38.
155. Luthi, J. M., Howald, H., Claasen, H., Rosler, K., Voek, P., and Hoppeler, H. (1986) Structural changes in skeletal muscle tissue with heavy resistance exercise. *Int. J. Sports Med.* **7,** 123–127.
156. Gute, D., Laughlin, M. H., and Amann, J. F. (1994) Regional changes in capillary supply in skeletal muscle of interval-trained-sprint and low-intensity, endurance-trained rats. *Microcirculation* **1,** 183–193.
157. Laughlin, M. H. and McAllister, R. M. (1992) Exercise training-induced coronary vascular adaptation. *J. Appl. Physiol.* **73,** 2209–2225.
158. Tomanek, R. J. (1994) Exercise-induced coronary angiogenesis: a review. *Med. Sci. Sports Exerc.* **26,** 1245–1251.
159. Anversa, P., Levicky, V., Beghi, C., McDonald, S. L., and Kikkawa, Y. (1983) Morphometry of exercise-induced right ventricular hypertrophy in the rat. *Circ. Res.* **52,** 57–64.
160. Tomanek, R. J. (1970) Effects of age on the extent of the myocardial capillary bed. *Anat. Rec.* **167,** 55–62.
161. Zhou, J. Sun, D., Kaley, G., and Kumar, A. (1996) Endothelial nitric oxide synthase gene expression is up-regulated by chronic exercise in rat microvessels. *FASEB J.* **10,** A39.
162. Shen, W., Zhang, X. Ÿ., Zhao, G., Wolin, M. S., Sessa, W., and Hintze, T. H. (1995) Nitric oxide production and NO synthase gene expression contribute to vascular regulation during exercise. *Med. Sci. Sports Exerc.* **27,** 1125–1134.
163. Greer, K. A., Anderson, D. R., Hammond, R. L., and Stephenson, L. W. (1996) Skeletal muscle as a myocardial substitute. *Proc. Soc. Exp. Biol. Med.* **211,** 297–305.
164. Adrian, E. D. and Bronk, D. A. (1929) The discharge of impulses in motor nerve fibres. *J. Physiol.* **67,** 119–151.
165. Salmons, S. and Vrbová, G. (1969) The influence of activity on some contractile characteristics of mammalian fast and slow muscles. *J. Physiol.* **210,** 535–549.
166. Brown, M. D., Cotter, M. A., Hudlická, O., and Vrbova, G. (1976) The effects of different patterns of muscle activity on capillary density, mechanical properties and structure of slow and fast rabbit muscles. *Pflügers Arch.* **361,** 241–250.
167. Hudlická, O., Dodd, C., Renkin, E. M., and Gray, S. D. (1982) Early changes in fiber profiles and capillary density in long-term stimulated muscles. *Am. J. Physiol.* **243,** H528–H535.
168. Hudlická, O., Tyler, K. R., Wright, A. J. A., and Ziadam A. M. A. R. (1984) Growth of capillaries in skeletal muscles. *Progr. Appl. Microcirc.* **5,** 44–61.
169. Salmons, S., Jarvis, J. C., Sutherland, H., Gilroy, S. J., and Kwende, M. M. N. (1996) Optimizing the properties of fuctional skeletal muscle grafts. *J. Muscle Res. Cell Motil.* **17,** 97.
170. Hudlická, O. and Tyler, K. R. (1984) The effect of long-term intermittent high frequency stimulation on capillary density and fibre profiles in rabbit fast muscles. *J. Physiol.* **353,** 435–445.
171. Hudlická, O., Tyler, K. R., Srihari, T., Heilig, A., and Pette, D. (1982) The effect of different patterns of long-term stimulation on contractile properties and myosin light chains in rabbit fast muscles. *Pflügers Arch.* **393,** 164–170.
172. Lucas, C. M., Havenith, M. G., Vandervenn, F. H., Habets, J., Vandernagel, T., Schrijversvanschendel, J. M., et al. (1992) Changes in canine latissimus dorsi muscle during 24-wk of continuous electrical stimulation. *J. Appl. Physiol.* **72,** 828–835.
173. Eloakley, R. M., Jarvis, J. C., Barman, D., Greenhalgh, D. L., Currie, J., Downham, D. Y., et al. (1995) Factors affecting the integrity of latissimus dorsi muscle grafts: implications for cardiac assistance from skeletal muscle. *J. Heart Lung Transplant.* **14,** 359–365.
174. Ianuzzo, C. D., Lanuzzo, S. E., Carson, N., Feild, M., Locke, M., Gu., J., et al. (1996) Cardiomyoplasty-degeneration of the assisting skeletal muscle. *J. Appl. Physiol.* **80,** 1205–1213.

175. Hudlická, O., Egginton, S., Brown, M. D., and Okyayuz-Baklouti, I. (1994) effect of torbafylline on muscle blood flow, performance and capillary supply in ischemic muscles subjected to varying levels of activity. *Can. J. Physiol. Pharm.* **72,** 811–817.
176. Pette, D., Muller, W., Leisner, E., and Vrbova, G. (1976) Time dependent effects on contractile properties, fibre population, myosin light chains and enzymes of energy metabolism in intermittently and continuously stimulated fast twitch muscles of the rabbit. *Pflugers Archiv.* **364,** 103–112.
177. Lexell, J., Jarvis, J., Downham, D., and Salmons, S. (1992) Quantitative morphology of stimulation - induced damage in rabbit fast-twitch skeletal muscles. *Cell Tissue Res.* **269,** 195–204.
178. Bailey, W. F., Magno, M. G., Buckman, P. D., Dimeo, F., Langan, T., Armenti, V. T., and Mannion, J. D. (1993) Chronic stimulation enhances extramyocardial collateral blood flow after a cardiomyplasty. *Ann. Thorac. Surg.* **56,** 1045–1053.
179. Frischknecht, R. and Vrbová, G. (1991) Adaptation of rat extensor digitorum longus to overload and increased activity. *Pflügers Arch.* **419,** 319–326.
180. Osbaldeston, N. J., Lee, D. M., Cox, V. M., Hesketh, J. E., Morrison, J. F. J., Blair, G. E., and Goldspink, D. F. (1995) The temporal and cellular expression of c-fos and c-jun in mechanically stimulated rabbit latissimus dorsi muscle. *Biochem. J.* **308,** 465–471.
181. Goldspink, D. F., Cox, V. M., Smith, S. K., Eaves, L. A., Osbaldeston, N. J., Lee, D. M., and Mantle, D. (1995) Muscle growth in respone to mechanical stimuli. *Am. J. Physiol.* **31,** E288–E297.
182. Hudlická, O. (1967) Blood flow and oxygen consumption in muscles after section of ventral roots. *Circ. Res.* **20,** 570–577.
183. Hudlická, O. and Renkin, E. M. (1968) Blood flow and blood tissue diffusion of 86Rb in denervated and tenotomized muscle udergoing atrophy. *Microvasc. Res.* **1,** 147–157.
184. Atherton, G. W., Cabric, M., and James, N. T. (1982) Stereological analyses of capillaries in muscles of dystrophic mice. *Virchows Arch. A Pathol. Anat.* **397,** 347–382.
185. Carry, M. R., Ringel, S. P., and Starcevich, J. M. (1986) Distribution of capillaries in normal and diseased human skeletal muscle. *Muscle Nerve* **9,** 445–454.
186. Hansen-Smith, F. M., Carlson, B. M., and Irwin, K. L. (1980) Revascularization of the freely grafted extensor digitorum longus muscle in the rat. *Am. J. Anat.* **158,** 65–82.
187. Tomanek, R. J. (1990) Response of the coronary vasculature to myocardial hypertrophy. *J. Am. Coll. Cardiol.* **15,** 528–533.
188. Hudlická, O. and Brown, M. D. (1996) Postnatal growth of the heart and its blood vessels. *J. Vasc. Res.* **33,** 266–287.
189. Wiener, J., Giacomelli, F., Loud, A. V., and Anversa, P. (1979) Morphometry of cardiac hypertrophy induced by experimental renal hypertension. *Am. J. Cardiol.* **44,** 919–929.
190. Breisch, E. A., White, F. C., Nimmo, L. E., and Bloor, C. M. (1986) Cardiac vasculature and flow during pressure-overload hypertrophy. *Am. J. Physiol.* **251,** H1031–H1037.
191. Tomanek, R. J., Palmer, P. J., Peiffer, G. L., Schreiber, K. L., Eastham, C. L., and Marcus, M. L. (1986) Morphometry of canine coronary arteries, arterioles and capillaries during hypertension and left ventricular hypertrophy. *Circ. Res.* **58,** 38–46.
192. Tomanek, R. J., Wessel, T. J., and Harrison, D. G. (1991) Capillary growth and geometry during long-term hypertension and myocardial hypertrophy in dogs. *Am. J. Physiol.* **261,** H1011–H1018.
193. White, F. C., Nakatini, Y., Nimmo, L., and Bloor, C. M. (1992) Compensatory angiogenesis during progressive right ventricular hypertrophy. *Am. J. Cardiovasc. Pathol.* **4,** 51–68.
194. Crisman, R. P., Rittman, B., and Tomanek, R. J. (1985) Exercise induced myocardial capillary growth in the spontaneously hypertensive rat. *Microvasc. Res.* **30,** 185–194.
195. Rakusan, K., Flanagan, M. F., Geva, T., Southern, J., and Vanpraagh, R. (1992) Morphometry of human coronary capillaries during normal growth and the effect of age in left ventricular pressure-overload hypertrophy. *Circulation* **86,** 38–46.
196. Tomanek, R. J. (1992) Age as a modulator of coronary capillary angiogenesis. *Circulation* **86,** 320–321.
197. Tomanek, R. J., Searls, J. C., and Lachenbruch, P. A. (1982) Quantitative changes in the capillary bed during developing peak and stabilized hypertrophy in a spontaneously hypertensive rat. *Circ. Res.* **51,** 295–304.
198. Anversa, P., Melissari, M., Beghi, C., and Olivetti, G. (1984) Structural compensatory mechanisms in rat heart in early spontaneous hypertension. *Am. J. Physiol.* **246,** H739–H746.
199. Rakusan, K. (1987) Microcirculation in the stressed heart, in *The Stressed Heart* (Legato, M. J., ed.), Martinus Nijhoff, Boston, pp. 107–123.
200. Henquell, L., Odoroff, C. L., and Honig, C. R. (1977) Intercapillary distance and capillary reserve in hypertrophied rat hearts beating in situ. *Circ. Res.* **41,** 400–408.

201. Marsicano, T. H., Duran, W. N., Edwards, C. H., and Anderson, R. W. (1977) Effect of left ventricular hypertrophy on myocardial capillary perfusion. *Surg. Forum* **28,** 240–241.
202. Batra, S., Rakusan, K., and Campbell, S. E. (1991) Geometry of capillary networks in hypertrophied rat heart. *Microvasc. Res.* **41,** 29–40.
203. Bucher, F. (1971) Qualitative morphology of heart failure. *Methods Achiev. Exp. Pathol.* **5,** 60–120.
204. Kayar, S. R. and Banchero, N. (1985) Volume overload hypertrophy elicited by cold and its effects on myocardial capillarity. *Resp. Physiol.* **59,** 1–14.
205. Rakusan, K., Moravec, B., and Hatt, P. Y. (1980) Regional capillary supply in the normal and hypertrophied rat heart. *Microvasc. Res.* **20,** 319–326.
206. Thomas, D. P., Phillips, St. J., and Bove, A. A. (1984) Myocardial morphology and blood flow distribution in chronic volume overload hypertrophy in dogs. *Basic Res. Cardiol.* **79,** 379–388.
207. Camilleri, J. P., Michel, J. B., Ossondo, M., and Barres, D. (1984) Morphometric analysis of the perfused capillary bed in the rat subendocardial myocardium during carbochrome induced dilatation and developing cardiac hypertrophy. *Int. J. Microcirc. Clin. Exper.* **3,** 428.
208. Shipley, R. A., Shipley, L. J., and Wearn, J. T. (1937) Capillary supply in normal and hypertrophied hearts of rabbits. *J. Exp. Med.* **65,** 29–42.
209. Wright, A. J. A., Hudlická, O., and Brown, M. D. (1989) Beneficial effect of chronic bradycardial pacing on capillary growth and heart performance in volume overload heart hypertrophy. *Circ. Res.* **64,** 1205–1212.
210. Poupa, O., Korecky, B., Kroftta, K., Rakusan, K., and Prochazka, J. (1964) The effect of anaemia during the early postnatal period on vascularisation of the myocardium and its resistance to anoxia. *Physiol. Bohemoslov* **13,** 281–287.
211. Olivetti, G., Lagrasta, C., Quaini, F., Ricci, R., Moccia, G., Capasso, J. M., and Anversa, P. (1989) Capillary growth in anaemia induced ventricullar wall remodelling in the rat heart. *Circ. Res.* **65,** 1182–1192.
212. Rakusan, K., Korecky, B., and Mezl, V. (1983) Cardiac hypertrophy and/or hyperplasia. *Persp. Cardiovasc. Res.* **7,** 103–109.
213. Anversa, P., Capasso, J. M., Sonnenblick, E. H., and Olivetti, G. (1990) Mechanisms of myocyte and capillary growth in the infarcted heart. *Eur. Heart J.* **11(Suppl. B),** 123–132.
214. Anversa, P., Beghi. C., Kikkawa, Y., and Olivetti, G. (1986) Myocardial infarction in rats. Infarct size, myocyte hypertrophy, and capillary growth. *Circ. Res.* **58,** 26–37.
215. Turek, Z., Grandtner, M., Kubat, K., Ringnalda, B. E., and Kreuzer, F. (1978) Arterial blood gases, muscle fibre diameters and intercapillary distance in cardiac hypertrophy of rats with an old myocardial infarction. *Pflügers Arch.* **376,** 209–215.
216. Wüsten, B., Flameng, W., Turschmann, W., and Schaper, W. (1975) [Coronary dilation reserve in experimental cardiac hypertrophy]. [German] *Verhandlungen der Deuts. Gesellsch. fur Kreislauff.* **41,** 136–139.
217. Ljungqvist, A. and Unge, G. (1973) The proliferative activity of the myocardial tissue in various forms of experimental cardiac hypertrophy. *Acta Pathol. Microbiol. Scand. sec A.* **81,** 235–240.
218. Rakusan, K., Wicker, P., Samad, A., Healy, B., and Turek Z. (1987) Failure of swimming exercise to improve capillarisation in cardiac hypertrophy of renal hypertensive rats. *Circ. Res.* **61,** 641–647.
219. Tomanek, R. J., Gisolfi, C. V., Bauer, C. A., and Palmer, P. J. (1988) Coronary vasodilator reserve, capillarity and mitochondria in trained hypertensive rats. *J. Appl. Physiol.* **64,** 1179–1185.
220. Tomanek, R. J. (1989) Sympathetic nerves modify mitochondrial and capillary growth in normotensive and hypertensive rats. *J. Mol. Cell Cardiol.* **21,** 755–764.
221. Canby, C. A. and Tomanek, R. J. (1989) Role of lowering arterial pressure on maximal coronary flow with and without regression of cardiac hypertrophy. *Am. J. Physiol.* **257,** H1110–H1118.
222. Amann, K., Greber, D., Gharehbaghi, H., Wiest, G., Lange, B., Ganten, U., et al. (1992) Effects of nifedipine and monoxidine on cardiac structure in spontaneously hypertensive rats. Stereological studies on myocytes, capillaries, arteries and cardiac interstitium. *Am. J. Hypertens.* **5,** 76–83.
223. Turek, Z., Kubat, K., Kazda, S., Hoodf, L., and Rakusan, K. (1987) Improved myocardial capillarization in spontaneously hypertensive rats treated with nifedipine. *Cardiovasc. Res.* **21,** 725–729.
224. Brown, M. D., Cleasby, M. J., and Hudlická, O. (1990) Capillary supply of hypertrophied rat hearts after chronic treatment with the bradycardic agent alinidine. *J. Physiol.* **427,** 40P.
225. Hearse, D. J. and Yellon, D. M. (1982) The three-dimensional geometry of regional myocardial ischemia: the role of the coronary microcirculation in determining patterns of injury, in *Microcirculation of the Heart* (Tillmanns, H., Kubler, W., and Zebe, Z., eds.), Springer-Verlag, Berlin, pp. 149–161.

226. Jennings, R. B., Kloner, R. A., Ganote, C. E., Hawkins, H. K., and Reimer, K. A. (1982) Changes in capillary fine structure and function in acute myocardial ischemic injury, in *Microcirculation of the Heart* (Tillmanns, H., Kubler, W., and Zebe, Z., eds.), Springer-Verlag, Berlin, pp. 87–95.

227. Reynolds, J. M. and McDonagh, P. F. (1989) Early in reperfusion, leukocytes alter perfused coronary capillarity and vascular resistance. *Am. J. Physiol.* **256**, H982–H989,

228. Casscells, W., Kimura, H., Sanchez, J. A., Yu, Z. X., and Ferrans, V. J. (1990) Immunohistochemical study of fibronectin in experimental myocardial infarction. *Am. J. Pathol.* **137**, 801–810.

229. DeBrabander, M., Schaper, W., and Verheyen, F. (1973) Regenerative changes in the porcine heart after gradual and chronic coronary artery occlusion. *Beitr. Path. Bd.* **149**, 170–185.

230. Weihrauch, D., Mohri, M., Schaper, W., and Schaper, J. (1992) Neovascularization in ischemic myocardium. *J. Mol. Cell. Cardiol.* **24(Suppl V)**, S75.

231. Olivetti, G., Ricci, R., Beghi, C., Guideri, G., and Anversa, P. (1986) Respone of the border zone to myocardial infarction in rats. *Am. J. Pathol.* **125**, 476–483.

232. Przyklenk, K. and Groom, A. C. (1983) Microvascular evidence for a transition zone around a chronic myocardial infarct in the rat. *Can. J. Physiol. Pharmacol.* **61**, 1516–1522.

233. Chilian, W. H., Wangler, R. D., Peters, K. G., Tomanek, R. J., and Marcus, M. L. (1985) Thyroxine-induced left ventricular hypertrophy in the rat: anatomical and physiological evidence for angiogenesis. *Circ. Res.* **57**, 591–598.

234. Breisch, E. A., White, F. C., Hammond, H. K., Flynn, S., and Bloor, C. M. (1989) Myocardial characteristics of thyroxine stimulated hypertrophy. A structural and functional study. *Basic Res. Cardiol.* **84**, 345–358.

235. Schaper, W. (1971) *The Collateral Circulation of the Heart.* North Holland Publishing Co., Amsterdam.

236. Sasayama, S. and Fujita, M. (1992) Recent insights into coronary collateral circulation. *Circulation* **85**, 1197–1204.

237. Scheel, K. W. and Williams, S. E. (1985) Hypertrophy and coronary and collateral vascularity in dogs with severe chronic anaemia. *Am. J. Physiol.* **249**, H1031–H1037.

238. Chilian, W. M., Mass, H. J., Williams, S. E., Layne, S. M., Smith, E. E., and Scheel, K. W. (1990) Microvascular occlusions promote coronary collateral growth. *Am. J. Physiol.* **258**, H1103–H1111.

239. Smith, P. (1989) Effect of hypoxia upon the growth and sprouting activity of cultured aortic endothelium from the rat. *J. Cell Sci.* **92**, 505–512.

240. Olivetti, G., Capasso, J. M., Sonnenblick, E. H., and Anversa, P. (1990) Side-to-side slippage of myocytes participates in ventricular wall remodelling acutely after myocardial infarction in rats. *Circ. Res.* **67**, 23–34.

241. Eghbali, M. and Weber, K. T. (1990) Collagen and the myocardium: fibrillar structure, biosynthesis and degradation in relation to hypertrophy and its regression. *Mol. Cell. Biochem.* **96**, 1–14.

242. Weber, K. T., Anversa, P., Armstrong, P. W., Brilla, C. G., Burnett, J. C., Cruickshank, J. M., et al. (1992) Remodeling and reparation of the cardiovascular system. *J. Am. Coll. Cardiol.* **20**, 3–16.

243. Factor, S. M., Flomenbaum, M., Zhao, M. J., Eng, C., and Robinson, T. F. (1988) The effects of acutely increased ventricular cavity pressure on intrinsic myocardial connective tissue. *J. Am. Coll. Cardiol.* **12**, 1582–1589.

244. Sato, S., Ashraf, M., Millard, R. W., Fujiwara, H., and Schwartz, A. (1983) Connective tissue changes in early ischemia of porcine myocardium: an ultrastructural study. *J. Mol. Cell. Cardiol.* **15**, 261–275.

245. Zhao, M. J., Zhang, H., Robinson, T. F., Factor, S. M., Sonnenblick, E. H., and Eng, C. (1987) Profound structural alterations of the extracellular collagen matrix in postischemic dysfunctional ("stunned") but viable myocardium. *J. Am. Coll. Cardiol.* **10**, 1322–1334.

246. Whittaker, P., Boughner, D. R., and Kloner, R. A. (1989) Analysis of healing after myocardial infarction using polarized light microscopy. *Am. J. Pathol.* **143**, 879–893.

247. Whittaker, P., Boughner, D. R., and Kloner, R. A. (1991) Role of collagen in acute myocardial infarct expansion. *Circulation* **84**, 2123–2134.

248. Contard, F., Koteliansky, V., Marotte, F., Dubus, I., Rappaport, L., and Samuel, J. L. (1991) Specific alterations in the distribution of extracellular matrix components within rat myocardium during the development of pressure overload. *Lab. Invest.* **64**, 65–75.

249. Knowlton, A. A., Connelly, C. M., Romo, G. M., Mamuya, W., Apstein, C. S., and Breche, R. (1992) Rapid expression of fibronection in the rabbit heart after myocardial infarction with and without reperfusion. *J. Clin. Invest.* **89**, 1060–1068.

250. Cleutjens, J. P. M., Smits, J. F. M., and Daemen, M. J. A. P. (1992) Type I and III collagen mRNA and protein increase in the infarcted and non-infarcted rat heart after myocardial infarction. *J. Mol. Cell. Cardiol.* **24(Suppl. V),** S50.

251. Nicosia, R. F., Belser, P., Bonanno, E., and Diven, J. (1991) Regulation of angiogenesis in vitro by collagen metabolism. *In Vitro Cell Dev. Biol.* **27A,** 961–966.

252. Michel, J. B., Salzmann, J. L., Ossondo-Nlom, M., Bruneval, P., Barres, D., and Camilleri, J. P. (1986) Morphometric analysis of collagen network and plasma perfused capillary bed in the myocardium of rats during evolution of cardiac hypertrophy. *Basic Res. Cardiol.* **81,** 142–154.

253. Yao, J. and Eghbali, M. (1992) Decreased collagen gene expression and absence of fibrosis in thyroid hormone-induced myocardial hypertrophy. Response of cardiac fibroblasts to thyroid hormone in vitro. *Circ. Res.* **71,** 831–839.

254. Rossi, M. A. and Peres, L. C. (1992) Effect of captopril on the prevention and regression of myocardial cell hypertrophy and interstitial fibrosis in pressure overload hypertrophy. *Am. Heart J.* **124,** 700–709.

255. Zeydel, M., Puglia, K., Eghbali, M., Fant, J., Seifer, S., and Blumenfeld, O. O. (1991) Properties of heart fibroblasts of adult rats in culture. *Cell Tissue Res.* **265,** 353–359.

256. Caulfield, J. B. and Borg, T. K. (1979) The collagen network of the heart. *Lab. Invest.* **40,** 364–372.

257. Robinson, T. F., Cohen-Gould, L., Factor, S. M., Eghbali, M., and Blumenfeld, O. O. (1988) Structure and function of connective tissue in cardiac muscle: collagen types I and III in endomysial struts and pericellular fibres. *Scann. Electron. Microsc.* **2,** 1005–1015.

258. Villareal, F. J. and Dillmann, W. F. (1992) Cardiac hypertrophy-induced changes in mRNA levels for TGF-beta 1, fibronectin and collagen. *Am. J. Physiol.* **262,** H1861–H1866.

259. Nicosia, R. F., Bonnano, E., and Smith, M. R. (1992) Fibronectin-mediated elongation of microvessels during angiogenesis in vitro. *In Vitro Cell Dev. Biol.* **28,** 151A.

260. Courtoy, P. J. and Boyles, J. (1983) Fibronectin in the microvasculature: localization in the in the pericyte-endothelial interstitium. *J. Ultrastruct. Res.* **83,** 258–273.

261. Odedra, R. and Weiss, J. B. (1991) Low molecular weight angiogenesis factors. *Pharmac. Ther.* **49,** 111–124.

262. Weiss, J. B. and McLaughlin, B. (1992) Involvement of low molecular mass angiogenic factors (ESAF) in the activation of latent matrix metalloproteinases, in *Angiogenesis in Health and Disease* (Maragondakis, M. E., Gullino, P., and Lelkes, P. L., eds.), Plenum, New York, pp. 243–252.

263. Hudlická, O., Brown, M. D., Walter, H., Weiss, J. B., and Bate, A. (1995) Factors involved in capillary growth in the heart. *Mol. Cell. Biochem.* **147,** 57–68.

264. Clausen, J. P. (1977) Effect of physical training on cardiomuscular adjustments to exercise. *Physiol. Rev.* **57,** 779–815.

265. Snell, P. G., Martin, W. H., Buckey J. C., and Blomqvist, C. G. (1987) Maximal vascular leg conductance in trained and untrained men. *J. Appl. Physiol.* **62,** 606–610.

266. Sinoway, L. I., Shenberger, J., Wilson, J., McLaughlin, D., Musch, T., and Zelis, R. (1987) A 30-day forearm work protocol increases maximal forearm blood flow. *J. Appl. Physiol.* **62,** 1063–1067.

267. Lash, J. M. and Bohlen, H. G. (1992) Functional adaptations of rat skeletal muscle arterioles to aerobic exercise training. *J. Appl. Physiol.* **72,** 2052–2062.

268. Adair, T. H., Hang, J., Wells, M. L., Magee, F. D., and Montani, J. P. (1995) Long-term electrical stimulation of rabbit skeletal muscle increases growth of paired arteries and veins. *Am. J. Physiol.* **269,** H717–H724.

269. Brown, M. D. and Hudlická, O. (1995) Vascular conductance and capillary supply in heart and skeletal muscle in response to altered activity. *Microcirculation* **2,** 98.

270. Dawson, J. D. and Hudlická, O. (1989) The effect of long-term activity on the microvasculature of rat glycolytic skeletal muscle. *Int. J. Microcirc. Clin. Exp.* **8,** 53–69.

271. Hansen-Smith, F. M., Egginton, S., Owens, G. K., and Hudlická, O. (1995) Growth of arterioles in chronically stimulated muscles. *J. Physiol.* **489,** 165P.

272. Dusseau, J. W. and Hutchins, P. M. (1979) Stimulation of arteriolar number by salbutamol in spontaneously hypertensive rats. *Am. J. Physiol.* **236,** H134–H140.

273. Skalak, T. C. and Price, R. J. (1996) The role of mechanical stresses in microvascular remodeling. *Microcirculation* **3,** 143–165.

274. Brown, M. D. and Hudlická, O. (1997) Exercise, training and coronary angiogenesis, in *Coronary Angiogenesis* (Rakusan, K., ed.), Jai Press Inc., CT, in press.

275. Breisch, E. A., White, F. C., Nimmo, L. E., McKirnan, M. D., and Bloor, C. M. (1986) Exercise-induced cardiac hypertrophy: a correlation of blood flow and microvasculature. *J. Appl. Physiol.* **60,** 1259–1267.

276. White, F. C. and Bloor, C. M. (1995) Coronary growth, not angiogenesis, is the dominant response increasing coronary vascular bed cross-sectional area induced by exercise training. *FASEB J.* **9,** A909.

277. Torry, R. J., Connell, P. M., O'Brien, D. M., Chilian, W. M., and Tomanek, R. J. (1991) Sympathectomy stimulates capillary but not precapillary growth in hypertrophic hearts. *Am. J. Physiol.* **260,** H1515–H1521.

278. Anversa, P. and Capasso, J. M. (1991) Loss of intermediate-sized coronary arteries and capillary proliferation after left ventricular failure in rats. *Am. J. Physiol.* **260,** H1552–H1560.

279. Schwartzkopf, B., Motz, W., Frenzel, H., Vogt, M., Knauer, S., and Strauer, B. E. (1993) Structural and functional alterations of the intermyocardial coronary arterioles in patients with arterial hypertension. *Circulation* **88,** 993–1003.

280. Tomanek, R. J. and Torry, R. J. (1994). Growth of the coronary vasculature in hypertrophy. *Cell. Mol. Biol. Res.* **40,** 129–136.

281. Pepler, W. and Meyer, B. (1960) Interarterial coronary anasomoses and coronary artery pattern; a comparative study of South African Bantu and European hearts. *Circulation* **22,** 14–23.

282. Villari, B., Hess, O. M., Meier, C., Pucillo, A., Gaglione, A., Turina, M., and Krayenbuehl, H. P. (1992) Regression of coronary artery dimensions after succesful aortic valve replacement. *Circulation* **85,** 972–978.

283. White, F. C., Roth, D. M., and Bloor, C. M. (1990) Coronary vascular remodelling during chronic ischaemia. *Circulation* **82(Suppl. IV),** 378.

15

Therapeutic Angiogenesis for the Treatment of Cardiovascular Disease

Jeffrey M. Isner and Takayuki Asahara

CONTENTS

INTRODUCTION

The development of blood vessels may be considered in several contexts. Vasculogenesis and angiogenesis are the processes responsible for the development of the circulatory system, the first functional unit in the developing embryo *(1)*. Pathologic angiogenesis includes the role of post-natal neovascularization in the pathogenesis of arthritis, diabetic retinopathy, and, most notably, tumor growth and metastasis *(2)*. Therapeutic angiogenesis involves the development of collateral blood vessels supplying ischemic tissues, either endogenously or in response to administered growth factors. The purpose of this review is to consider the mechanisms responsible for therapeutic angiogenesis, which develops endogenously, as well as novel strategies, which have been devised to augment this response. Because recapitulation of the embryonic paradigm forms the conceptual basis for therapeutic, as well as pathologic angiogenesis, selected aspects of embryonic blood-vessel development are included. While pathologic angiogenesis is beyond the scope of the current paper, certain principles which have emerged from studies of pathologic neovascularization are considered for the implications they may have for cardiovascular disease.

VASCULOGENESIS AND ANGIOGENESIS

Vasculogenesis refers to the in situ formation of blood vessels from progenitor endothelial cells (ECs), or angioblasts *(3)*. It is necessary to distinguish between vascular development which takes place in the yolk sac of the embryo from that which occurs in the embryo proper. Extraembryonic vasculogenesis begins as a cluster formation, or blood island. Growth and fusion of multiple blood islands in the yolk sac of the embryo

From: *The New Angiotherapy*
Edited by: T.-P. D. Fan and E. C. Kohn © Humana Press Inc., Totowa, NJ

ultimately give rise to the yolk-sac capillary network *(4)*; after the onset of blood circulation, this network differentiates into an arteriovenous vascular system *(5)*. The integral relationship between the elements which circulate in the vascular system — the blood cells — and the cells that are principally responsible for the vessels themselves — ECs — is implied by the composition of the embryonic blood islands. The cells destined to generate hematopoietic cells are situated in the center of the blood island and are termed hematopoietic stem cells (HSCs). Endothelial progenitor cells, or angioblasts, are located at the periphery of the blood islands. In addition to this spatial association, HSCs and angioblasts share certain antigenic determinants, including Flk-1, Tie-2, and CD-34. These progenitor cells have consequently been considered to derive from a common precursor, putatively termed a hemangioblast *(6–8)*.

Vasculogenesis, which occurs within the embryo proper, is currently considered to involve differentiation of so-called "solitary" angioblasts, i.e., angioblasts which are not intimately associated with concomitantly differentiating HSCs *(3)*. These angioblasts may migrate and fuse with other angioblasts and capillaries or form vessels *in situ*. In contrast to in situ differentiation of progenitor cells required to establish the primordial vascular network, extension of the primitive vasculature involves angiogenesis, i.e., sprouting of new capillaries from the pre-existing network; by definition, this implicates differentiated ECs as the responsible cellular element. Full development of the circulatory system involves recurrent remodeling as some vessels regress, presumably by apoptosis, and others branch and/or are invested with a multilayer architecture characteristic of medium to large arteries and veins. The extensive EC proliferative activity, which constitutes the basis for angiogenesis in the embryo, contrasts with extraordinary EC quiescence in the adult, where the interval for EC turnover is estimated to be >1000 d *(9)*.

Classic Paradigm for Angiogenesis

Until recently (vide infra), vasculogenesis was considered restricted to the embryo, while new blood-vessel formation in adult species was inferred to be the exclusive consequence of angiogenesis. The full paradigm for angiogenesis has been suggested to begin with "activation" of ECs within a parent vessel, followed by disruption of the basement membrane, and subsequent migration of ECs into the interstitial space, possibly in the direction of an ischemic stimulus *(10)* (Fig. 1). Concomitant and/or subsequent EC proliferation, intracellular-vacuolar lumen formation, pericyte "capping," and production of a basement membrane complete the developmental sequence.

During angiogenesis, migration always precedes proliferation by approx 24 h *(11)*. Sholley et al *(12)* documented the critical if not exclusive roles of migration and redistribution of pre-existing ECs in the commencement of neovascularization. Subsequent studies have established the critical role played by plasmin and other proteases in promoting migration through pre-existing matrix *(13,14)*.

In contrast to these in vivo inflammatory and in vitro organ-culture models, angiogenesis which develops in response to experimental vascular obstruction, i.e., collateral vessel development, has been shown by several previous investigators to involve proliferation of not only ECs, but SMCs as well. Peak EC proliferation which contributes to naturally occurring collateral development in the setting of vascular occlusion varies from 2.6–3.5 % in the canine coronary circulation *(15,16)*; from 5–6 % in the rodent renal vasculature *(17)*; and is < 1% in swine coronaries *(18)*. Proliferation of SMCs, the additional requisite cell type for the formation of larger blood vessels, is an implicit

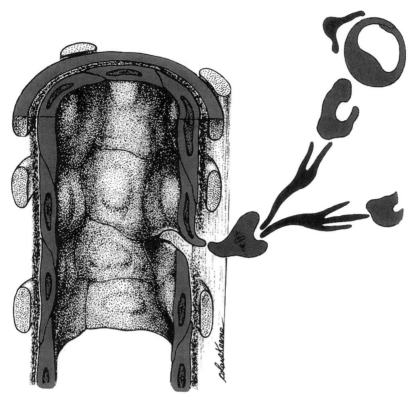

Fig. 1. Classic paradigm for angiogenesis. ECs break free from their basement membrane and surrounding extracellular matrix, migrate, proliferate, and remodel (i.e., form a lumen), thus generating new blood vessels or "sprouts" from the parent vessel. Adapted with permission from ref. *10.*

component of angiogenesis, regardless of animal species or circulatory site. Schaper et al in fact speculated nearly 25 yr ago that "... it is tempting to assume that EC proliferation not only serves the purpose of forming the endothelium of a finally larger artery but rather actively participates in the development of the tunica media" *(19).* Proliferative activity — for SMCs as well as ECs — is highest at the level of the smallest-diameter collateral vessels, the so-called midzone collateral segments *(15,16,20,21).* Fifth, while evidence of EC and SMC proliferation alone does not necessarily distinguish new vessel development from an increase in the size of pre-existing vessels, adjunctive data regarding increased capillary density *(22,23)* support the notion that proliferative activity does in fact reflect true angiogenesis.

Ligand-Receptor Systems Modulate Vasculogenesis and Angiogenesis

A series of gene targeting studies have elucidated the role of certain ligands and/or their receptors in vasculogenesis and angiogenesis. The phenotypic characteristics of these "knockout" mice are relevant to adult cardiovascular disease because of the implications they may have for the role played by these same ligand-receptor systems in promoting post-natal angiogenesis.

As indicated above, KDR (the murine equivalent is known as flk-1 or VEGFR-2), the principal receptor for vascular endothelial growth factor (VEGF), is expressed by both angioblasts and HSCs. It is perhaps not surprising, therefore, that mice deficient in this gene die in utero between 8.5 and 9.5 d postcoitum owing to an early defect in the development of hematopoietic and ECs. Yolk-sac blood islands were absent at 7.5 d, organized blood vessels could not be observed in the embryo and yolk sac at any stage, and hematopoietic progenitors were severely reduced *(24)*. Markers of early endothelial precursors such as flt-1, flt-4, and tie-2 were expressed, but a marker of later endothelial development, tie-2, could not be detected, indicating a deficiency of mature ECs *(24)*. Expression of CD34, a marker of HSCs, was greatly reduced as well. The absence of blood islands and blood vessels in these mice established that the flk-1 signalling pathway is required very early in the development of endothelial lineage, and may be important for blood cell development as well.

Findings in the flk-1 knockout mouse predicted what was to be found when the ligand, VEGF, was deficient. Mice deficient in even one of two VEGF alleles die in utero between days 10.5 and 12. Both blood-island formation (vasculogenesis) and vascular sprouting from pre-existing vessels (angiogenesis) were again impaired *(25,26)*. The failure of blood-vessel ingrowth was accompanied by apoptosis and disorganization of neuroepithelial cells. The heterozygous lethal phenotype was interpreted as evidence for tight dose-dependent regulation of embryonic vessel development by VEGF. Parenthetically, the aortas of VEGF-deficient mice have been noted to be hypoplastic, similar to that observed in mice deficient in endothelial nitric oxide synthase (NOS) (P. Huang, personal communication). It is interesting to speculate that this may reflect the role of NO in VEGF-modulation of EC function (vide infra).

The tyrosine kinase flt-1 receptor (VEGF-R1) constitutes a second high-affinity binding receptor for VEGF. Mouse embryos homozygous for a targeted mutation in the flt-1 locus formed fully differentiated ECs in both embryonic and extra-embryonic regions, but assembled these cells into abnormal vascular channels and died in utero *(27)*. Blood islands, for example, were disorganized, consisting of intermixed angioblasts and HSCs. In the head mesenchyme, instead of progressive development of individual small vessels, large fused vessels were seen which contained internally localized groups of ECs. These findings were interpreted as evidence that the flt-1 signalling pathway may regulate normal EC cell-cell or cell-matrix interactions during vascular development.

Tie-1 and tie-2 *(28)* comprise a second family of receptor tyrosine kinases, other than the VEGF family, in which expression is nearly specific for ECs. Mice embryos deficient in tie-1 fail to establish structural integrity of otherwise differentiated ECs *(29)*; consequently, erythrocytes extravasate through the blood-vessel EC (but not between ECs) leading to death immediately after birth with widespread hemorrhage. Embryos homozygous mutant for tie-2 die earlier (d 10.5 in utero) with dilated vessels lacking distinction between small and large vessels; absence of ordered branching has been inferred as evidence of disordered angiogenesis. Vasculogenesis per se was not disrupted.

Successful disruption of the ligand for tie-2, angiopoietin-1 *(30,31)*, resulted in embryonic lethality by day 12.5 with defects similar to those seen in the tie-2 receptor knockout. These included defects in organized branching, so that vessels remained dilated and almost syncitial. There was no change, however, in the total number of ECs.

The critical roles played by VEGF and its receptors in governing vasculogenesis and angiogenesis, and the tie receptor/ligand family in maturation of the vascular network, have implications for the roles of these EC mitogens in promoting angiogenesis under circumstances of tissue ischemia in adults. In contrast to the lethal consequences of

VEGF and tie deficiencies, it is interesting to note that mice in which gene targeting has been used to disrupt the gene for basic fibroblast growth factor survive to maturity with no apparent phenotypic abnormalities of either the vascular or hematopoietic systems (G. Dorn and T. Deutschman, personal communication).

Remodeling

Remodeling in angiogenesis refers to the formation of a vascular lumen. Whereas multiple cell types, including ECs, grown in vitro on a collagen-matrix gel will form cords, the presence of a lumen distinguishes vessels, or tubes, from solid cords. The presence of a lumen is clearly fundamental to the function of the circulatory system; yet the mechanisms responsible for tube formation are perhaps the least well-understood aspect of angiogenesis (32). As Risau has pointed out, because isolated ECs may combine to form a lumen in vitro (33), lumen formation must represent an intrinsic feature or differentiation program of these cells (3). Mechanisms which have been discussed include the joining of polarized ends of capillary ECs in a ring-like fashion, or alternatively, simple deletion of a portion of the cell (vacuole formation) (34). Adding further to the complexity is the requirement to form qualitatively differing luminal and abluminal surfaces. Finally, it is inferred that remodeling comprises a coordinated process of lumen formation and vessel extension with fusion of individual cells and their lumina via cell-cell adhesion molecules. The specific molecules responsible for vessel extension remain ambiguous. It is presumed that this aspect of vessel formation is subject to the regulatory factors responsible for vascular development in the embryo, as discussed earlier. In this respect, it is interesting to note that VEGF, for example, upregulates gap-junction expression (specifically connexin 43) in ECs (35).

Nascent Vessels

Capillary growth rates (i.e., the velocity of neovascularization) range from 0.23–0.8 mm/d, depending on the experimental system used and/or the type of tumor (36). The light microscopic features of newly formed vessels have been distinguished from those of native vessels (37). Whereas a histologic section of a capillary blood vessel in the normal brain reveals one or two ECs per lumen, in a brain tumor such as a glioblastoma, 5–10 ECs may occupy one lumen. Tumor-induced vessels often appear dilated and saccular. Moreover, tumors may contain giant capillaries and arteriovenous shunts without intervening capillaries, so that blood may even flow from one venule to another.

Ultrastructural analysis of newly formed vessels has focussed on features potentially responsible for augmented permeability. Dvorak et al. (38,39), for example, found that vascular leakage could not be attributed to passage of molecules through inter-endothelial cell junctions or injured tumor endothelium, but instead involved transendothelial transport via a novel cytoplasmic organelle which they termed the vesicular-vacuolar organelle (VVO). Others (40) have reported VEGF-induced ultrastructural features consistent with endothelial fenestration.

Matrix-Integrin Interactions

Activated or proliferative ECs have been shown to express high levels of $\alpha_v\beta_3$ (41,42). In non-human primates subjected to focal cerebral ischemia, for example, microvascular expression of $\alpha_v\beta_3$ was noted in ischemic, but not nonischemic, tissues (43). Ligation of $\alpha_v\beta_3$ on proliferating ECs promotes a critical adhesion-dependent cell-survival signal leading to inhibition of p53 activity, decreased expression of p21$^{WAF1/CIP1}$ and suppression of the bax cell death pathway (44). The intra-cellular molecular conflict that results from blocking $\alpha_v\beta_3$ thus leads to unscheduled apoptosis and the abrogation of angiogenesis (42,44,45). Failure to ligate $\alpha_v\beta_3$ may therefore inhibit the ability of actively cycling cells to ligate extracellular matrix proteins including fibronectin, vitronectin, fibrinogen, and osteopontin, thereby influencing adhesion, migration, and ultimately survival of these cells (46).

Consistent with this notion, the integrin $\alpha_v\beta_3$ has been shown to be required for angiogenesis in vivo (41) and antagonists of this integrin have been shown to inhibit angiogenesis by inducing apoptosis (42). Basic FGF, which has been shown to protect ECs from apoptosis (47), is known to modulate integrin expression by ECs (48–50). VEGF, by up-regulation of both the β_3 integrin and fibronectin, may similarly inhibit apoptosis by enhancing EC adhesion to matrix proteins (51). This notion is thus consistent with the concept that VEGF may exert a survival effect on ECs (41,42,52–54). These findings suggest that the net increase in EC viability following VEGF administration is not limited to the mitogenic effects of VEGF on ECs, but is supplemented by the potential for VEGF to inhibit apoptosis.

Vasculogenesis in the Adult

Postnatal neovascularization has been previously considered to result exclusively from the proliferation, migration, and remodeling of fully differentiated ECs derived from preexisting blood vessels, i.e., angiogenesis (3,4,9). The formation of blood vessels from EC progenitors, or angioblasts — i.e., vasculogenesis — has been considered restricted to embryogenesis (5,55).

We reasoned, however, that the use of HSCs derived from peripheral blood in lieu of bone marrow to provide sustained hematopoietic recovery constituted inferential evidence for circulating stem cells (56). Given the common ancestry of HSCs and angioblasts, we investigated the hypothesis that stem cells circulating in peripheral blood might under selected circumstances differentiate into ECs (57,58). Flk-1 and a second antigen, CD-34, shared by angioblasts and HSCs (24,59–69) were used to isolate putative angioblasts from the leukocyte fraction of peripheral blood. In vitro, these cells differentiated into ECs. In animal models of ischemia, heterologous, homologous, and autologous EC progenitors incorporated into sites of active angiogenesis (Fig. 2). These findings thus suggest that circulating EC progenitors may contribute to neoangiogenesis in adult species, consistent with vasculogenesis.

Parenthetically, these findings may have implications for augmenting collateral vessel growth to ischemic tissues (therapeutic angiogenesis, vide infra) and for delivery of anti- or pro-angiogenic agents, respectively, to sites of pathologic or utilitarian angiogenesis. A potentially limiting factor in strategies designed to promote neovascularization of ischemic tissues (70) is the resident population of ECs that is competent to respond to administered angiogenic cytokines (71). This issue may be successfully addressed with autologous EC transplants. The fact that progenitor ECs home to foci of angiogenesis suggests potential utility as autologous vectors for gene therapy. For anti-neoplastic therapies, MB^{CD34+} could be transfected with or coupled to anti-tumor drugs or angiogenesis inhibitors. For treatment of regional ischemia, angiogenesis could be amplified by transfection of MB^{CD34+} to achieve constitutive expression of angiogenic cytokines and/ or provisional matrix proteins (72).

ANGIOGENIC CYTOKINES

Beginning a little over a decade ago *(73)*, a series of polypeptide growth factors (Table 1) were purified, sequenced, and demonstrated to be responsible for natural as well as pathologic angiogenesis. These angiogenic cytokines all share in common the ability to act as mitogens for ECs.

Among the various growth factors which have been shown to promote angiogenesis, VEGF *(74)*, also known as vascular permeability factor (VPF) *(75)* and vasculotropin (VAS) *(76)*, is an EC-specific mitogen. Moreover, a plethora of studies have documented upregulation of VEGF in various cell types following exposure to other angiogenic cytokines. VEGF may thus be considered a prototypical angiogenic cytokine and for this reason will be discussed here in further detail. Specific aspects of the remaining angiogenic cytokines in Table 1 may be found in the accompanying lists of citations.

Four homodimeric species of VEGF have been identified, each monomer having 121, 165, 189, or 206 amino acids, respectively *(77)*. The secretion pattern of the four isoforms differs markedly. $VEGF_{121}$ is a weakly acidic polypeptide that does not bind to heparin, and is freely soluble in the conditioned medium of transfected cells. The heparin-binding capabilities of the remaining three isoforms are progressively augmented as the result of a step-wise enrichment in basic residues. Thus $VEGF_{165}$, the predominant form secreted by a variety of normal and transformed cells *(38)*, is a basic heparin-binding glycoprotein with an isoelectric point of 8.5; while secreted, a significant portion remains bound to the cell surface or extracellular matrix. The $VEGF_{189}$ isoform includes 24 additional amino acids and has been shown not to be freely secreted, but instead remains nearly completely bound to the cell surface and/or extracellular matrix *(78)*. $VEGF_{206}$ is a rare isoform so far identified only in a human fetal liver cDNA library.

Fig. 2. (*See* color plate 1 appearing after page 262). *(see next pages)* Heterologous (**A–L**), homologous (**M**), or autologous (**N and O**) EC progenitors incorporate into sites of angiogenesis in vivo. (A and B) CD34+ mononuclear peripheral blood cells (MB^{CD34+}) (red, arrows), labeled with the flourscent dye DiI, between skeletal myocytes (M), including necrotic (N) myocytes 1 week after injection; most are co-labeled with CD31 (green, arrows). Note pre-existing artery (small A), identified as CD31 positive, but DiI-negative. (**C and D**) Evidence of proliferative activity among several DiI-labeled MB^{CD34+} derived cells (red, arrows), indicated by coimmunostaining for Ki67 antibody (green). Proliferative activity is also seen among DiI negative, Ki67 positive capillary ECs (arrowhead); both cell types comprise neovasculature. (**E**) DiI (red) and CD31 (green) in capillary ECs (arrows) between skeletal myocytes, photographed through double filter 1 wk after DiI-labeled MB^{CD34+} injection. (**F**) Single green filter shows CD31 (green) expression in DiI-labeled capillary ECs, integrated into capillary with native (DiI negative, CD31 positive) ECs (arrowheads). (**G**) Immunostaining 1 wk after MB^{CD34+} injection showing capillaries comprised of DiI-labeled MB^{CD34+} derived cells expressing Tie-2 receptor (green). Several MB^{CD34+}-derived cells (arrow) are Tie-2 positive and are integrated with some Tie-2 positive host capillary cells (arrowhead) identified by the absence of red fluorescence. (**H**) Phase contrast photomicrograph of same tissue section shown in **G** indicates corresponding DiI-labeled (arrows) and -unlabeled (arrowheads) capillary ECs. (**I and J**) Six weeks after administration, MB^{CD34+} derived cells (red) colabel for CD31 in capillaries between preserved skeletal myocytes. (**K and L**) One week after injection of MB^{CD34-}, isolated MB^{CD34-} derived cells (red, arrows) are observed between myocytes, but do not express CD31. (**M**) Immunostaining of β-galactosidase in tissue section harvested from ischemic muscle of B6,129 mice 4 wk after administration of MB^{Flk-1+} isolated from transgenic mice constitutively expressing β-gal. (Flk-1 cell isolation was used for selection of EC progenitors owing to lack of a suitable anti-mouse CD34 antibody.) Cells overexpressing β-gal (arrows) have been incorporated into capillaries and small arteries; these cells were identified as ECs by anti-CD31 and anti-BS-1 lectin. (**N and O**) Sections of muscles harvested from rabbit ischemic hindlimb 4 wk after administration of autologous MB^{CD34+}. Red fluorescence indicates localization of MB^{CD34+}-derived cells in capillaries, seen (arrows) in phase-contrast photomicrograph (**O**). Each scale bar indicates 50 µm. Adapted with permission from ref. 56.

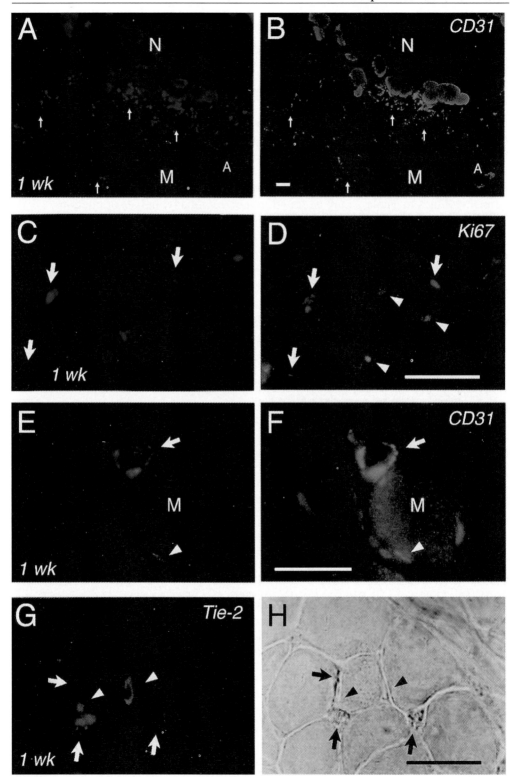

Figure 2

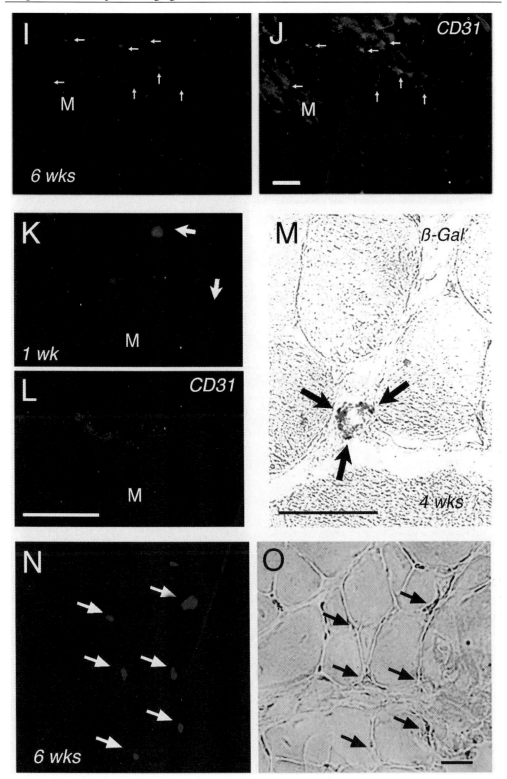

Figure 2

Table 1
Angiogenic Cytokines

Acidic fibroblast growth factor (aFGF) *(124,160,162,167,168)*
Angiopoietin *(30,31)*
Basic fibroblast growth factor (bFGF) *(98,125,126,135,157,161,164,169–172)*
Heparin-binding epidermal growth factor (HB-EGF) *(101)*
Insulin-like growth factor (IGF) *(173)*
Placental growth factor (PlGF) *(89)*
Platelet derived growth factor (PDGF) *(173)*
Scatter factor (hepatocyte growth factor, HGF) *(117)*
Transforming growth factor-beta (TGF-beta) *(101)*
Vascular endothelial growth factor (VEGF) *(23,25,26,70,127,128,158,159,169,172–174,163,175)*

The possibility of hierarchial efficacy among these three isoforms by performing arterial gene transfer of phVEGF$_{121}$, phVEGF$_{165}$, and phVEGF$_{189}$ was investigated in the rabbit ischemic hindlimb model *(79)*. Remarkably, no differences with regard to anatomic or physiologic evidence of angiogenesis could be demonstrated - although all three isoforms yielded statistically significant improvement in every parameter measured compared to the LacZ controls. Moreover, separate experiments performed using 100, 200, and 400 µg of each plasmid failed to disclose a differential dose-response curve among the three isoforms with respect to angiographic score, calf blood-pressure ratio, resting/maximum flow, or capillary/myocyte ratio (Y. Tsurumi, unpublished data).

These findings may be interpreted to support the observation made previously by Houck et al. *(78)* regarding the proteolytically clipped VEGF species which result from the action of plasmin on the 165 and 189 isoforms. The size of the resulting monomers, which in each case are mitogenic for ECs and enhance vascular permeability in a Miles assay *(80)*, is similar to the size of the intact 121 isoform. It is therefore possible that the proteolytic cascade of plasminogen activation, a key step during angiogenesis *(14)*, cleaves the longer forms of VEGF, releasing a soluble VEGF$_{121}$-like species that is the final common mediator of angiogenesis in vivo.

Besides VEGF, also referred to as VEGF-1 or VEGF-A, two additional proteins with particular abundance in heart and skeletal muscle, VEGF-2 or VEGF-C *(81)* and VEGF-3 or VEGF-B *(82)* have been isolated. In contrast to the widespread distribution of these VEGFs, the fourth member of the VEGF-family, placenta growth factor (PlGF) *(83)* appears to be restricted in vivo to placenta and certain tumors *(84,85)*. All four proteins share structural homology among themselves as well as with the platelet-derived growth factor A and B polypeptides (PDGF-A and -B), in particular a conserved motif, including eight cysteine residues in the putative receptor-binding domain *(86)*. Similar to the a nd b chains of PDGF, VEGF-1/VEGF-A and PlGF can form heterodimers with biological activity *(87–89)*. VEGF-3/VEGF-B is also able to heterodimerize with VEGF-1/VEGF-A in cells expressing both factors *(82)*. Although not shown thus far, it seems reasonable to assume that VEGF-2/VEGF-C, by virtue of its shared homology to the other members of the VEGF family, can form heterodimers in a similar manner, therefore adding another level of complexity to processes related to angiogenesis.

Whereas VEGF-1/VEGF-A is a high-affinity ligand for the receptors flt-1 and KDR/flk-1, VEGF-2/VEGF-C was shown to bind to another recently identified endothelial specific receptor tyrosine kinase, flt-4, as well as to flk-1/KDR, but not to flt-1 *(81,90)* (Fig. 3). PlGF was shown to bind with high affinity to flt-1, but not to flk-1/KDR *(89)* or flt-4 *(91)*. The receptor(s) for VEGF-3/VEGF-B *(82)* have not yet been characterized.

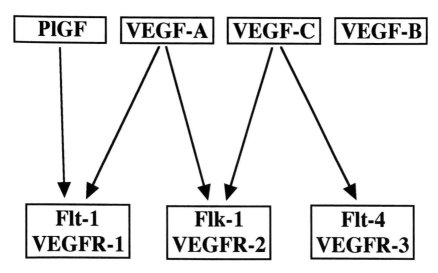

Fig. 3. Ligand-receptor relationships for placental growth factor (PlGF) and proteins encoded for by the three vascular endothelial growth factor (VEGF) genes. (VEGFR = vascular endothelial growth factor receptor; alternative receptor nomenclature is shown directly above). Adapted with permission from ref. *90*.

The constitutive coexpression of all three VEGF types in many adult tissues *(81,82,92)* suggests an interactive or at least redundant capacity of the VEGF members to regulate angiogenesis and modulate EC function. Data regarding the bioactivity of VEGF-2/VEGF-C and VEGF-3/VEGF-B, however, are currently limited. In vitro, both factors exhibit mitogenic activity *(81,82,92)*, and VEGF-2/VEGF-C stimulated EC outgrowth in a collagen gel assay *(81)*. In contrast, the fact that expression of PlGF is restricted to placental tissue and certain tumors *(84,85)* suggests that this protein plays a minor role in the maintenance of vascular integrity.

Autocrine Loop as a Feature of Angiogenic Cytokines

Certain angiogenic cytokines, notably aFGF and bFGF, lack a secretory signal sequence *(93,94)*. This prompted previous investigators to study the possibility that these cytokines act via an alternative pathway. Indeed, several groups established evidence to support the notion that aFGF and bFGF can indeed modulate EC behavior via an autocrine pathway *(95–98)*.

Evidence for a similar autocrine pathway in the case of VEGF was established by Namiki et al. *(99)*. Under quiescent conditions, VEGF mRNA was not detected in either HUVECs or human microvascular ECs (HMECs). Because ECs also express the high-affinity VEGF receptors, flt-1 and KDR, these cells in humans appear to include the requisite elements for an autocrine pathway. The finding that hypoxia induces activation of KDR in HUVECs is consistent with an external autocrine pathway *(100)* given that all VEGF isoforms include a secretory signal sequence.

The extent to which such an autocrine pathway may complement endogenous production of VEGF from SMCs, macrophages and tumor cells, or facilitate the response to exogenous administration of VEGF remains to be determined. With regard to the latter, it has been recognized that single bolus administration of VEGF may stimulate development of new collateral vessels over a period of several days, despite the fact that the circulating half-life of VEGF is <3 min. One explanation for this observation is that as VEGF is rapidly cleared from the circulation, it binds avidly to heparan sulfate proteoglycans present on the luminal surface of the vascular endothelium. Experimental evidence to support this concept in the case of bFGF has been previously reported by Fuks et al. *(47)*. Alternatively, an autocrine loop, activated under hypoxic conditions known to stimulate angiogenesis, might also serve to amplify and thereby protract the response in ECs stimulated by exogenously administered VEGF (Fig. 4). Such autocrine amplification may in fact represent a common motif shared by angiogenic cytokines in general.

Direct vs Indirect Cytokines

Certain stimuli capable of inducing the development of neovessels in vivo, specifically certain cytokines *(101–104)* and hypoxia, fail to stimulate EC proliferation in vitro, suggesting a role for additional mediators and/or cell types. We considered whether these so-called indirect angiogenic growth factors might stimulate vascular SMCs to express genes encoding direct EC mitogens. Such a sequential cascade would provide a mechanism by which growth factors which are otherwise nonmitogenic or frankly inhibitory for EC proliferation in vitro could instead stimulate angiogenesis in vivo.

Although PDGF BB, for example, can directly stimulate proliferation of selected populations of microvascular ECs in vitro *(105–107)*, ECs from most vascular districts do not respond to treatment with PDGF BB *(108)*. Nonetheless, in vivo PDGF BB has been clearly demonstrated to induce supportive angiogenesis in both a wound healing model *(102)* and chorioallantoic membrane assay *(103)*. Furthermore, microvascular ECs isolated from rat epididymal fat pads and not directly responsive to PDGF BB stimulation, when co-cultured with myofibroblasts from the same tissue source form capillary chords in the presence of PDGF BB *(104)*. The angiogenic action of PDGF BB documented in this way was attributed to production of soluble EC mitogen(s) by myofibroblasts in response to stimulation with PDGF BB.

We demonstrated that PDGF BB treatment of human vascular SMCs concurrently induces VEGF and bFGF mRNA species *(109)*. This finding indicates that PDGF BB, a known mitogen for SMCs, could also stimulate SMCs to produce direct angiogenic factors and thereby promote angiogenesis.

Likewise, the plurality of mechanisms that contribute to the angiogenic activity of transforming growth factor-β1 (TGF-β1) *(110)* has been the subject of controversy. Although clearly inhibiting growth and migration of subconfluent ECs in vitro *(111)*, TGF-β1 facilitates capillary formation in vivo *(110)*. Furthermore, TGF-β1 modulates the composition of the extracellular matrix *(112)* and may therefore act in part by locally creating a pro-angiogenic environment. While TGF-β1 directly inhibits EC proliferation *(111)*, it may nevertheless direct organization of ECs into tube-like structures, depending on conditions of culture tested *(113)*. TGF-β1 in high concentrations was found to inhibit the formation of capillary-like structures in an in vitro model of angiogenesis, whereas low doses were observed to potentiate VEGF- or bFGF-induced neovessel formation in the same assay system *(111)*. This phenomenon was interpreted by Pepper et al. as an example of "contextual" angiogenesis to indicate that the angiogenic response to a given cytokine is dependent upon the presence and concentration of other mediators in the peri-cellular environment of the target ECs. Winkles et al. have also observed that TGF-β1 stimulates bFGF expression by SMCs, thus supporting the notion that direct angiogenic mediators *(114)* might contribute in part to TGF-β1-induced angiogenesis. Our finding *(109)* that TGF-β1 stimulation induces VEGF as well as bFGF gene expression, in concert with the above-described mechanisms, suggests that both EC mitogens are likely instrumental for mediating the indirect angiogenic effects of TGF-β1 in vivo.

Subsequently this same motif has been demonstrated for insulin-like growth factor (IGF *[115]*), bFGF *(116)*, and scatter factor (hepatocyte growth factor) *(117)*. bFGF and scatter

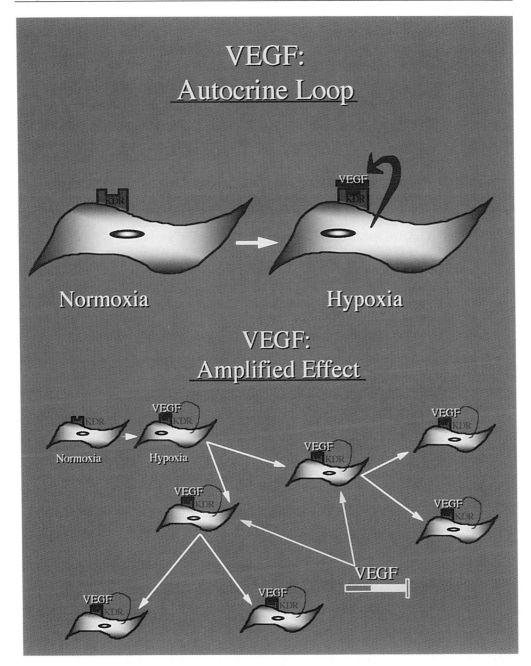

Fig. 4. Under conditions of hypoxia, ECs upreglate VEGF, which, once secreted, may then interact with its receptor. Such an autocrine loop provides the basis for amplification of any given VEGF secreted or administered into an ischemic territory. ECs simtulated to proliferate in response to VEGF may then serve as additional sources of VEGF synthesis, thus amplifying the effect of the initial dose of VEGF.

factor, however, are further distinguished by the fact that they exert a direct effect on EC proliferation and migration, in addition to upregulating VEGF synthesis in vascular SMCs.

In the context of factors which upregulate VEGF expression, it is important to empha-size the critical role played by hypoxia, because this explains at least in part the clinical observation that tissue ischemia is a fundamental stimulus for angiogenesis. Increased expression of VEGF has been documented at the periphery of necrotic foci of certain neoplasms, as well as hypoxia-stimulated induction of VEGF in cultured cells from glial tumor and rat skeletal muscle *(118)*. We have shown that low O_2 tension selectively modulates VEGF but not bFGF in vascular SMCs *(109)*. This observation is intriguing in light of homology between a sequence in the VEGF promoter *(77)* and a nucleotide sequence in the erythropoietin promoter identified as a binding site for a hypoxia-specific transcription factor (HIF-1) *(109)*. It is now clear that although transcriptional upregulation of VEGF does occur in response to hypoxia, post-translational mechanisms constitute the dominant basis for hypoxia-induced synthesis of VEGF protein *(120–123)*.

Site-Specific Effects of Angiogenic Cytokines

From a teleologic perspective, it would appear critical that EC mitogens not promote angiogenesis in an indiscriminate fashion; it is clearly preferable for the survival of the organism that angiogenesis be limited to sites of wound healing and tissue ischemia where it may have facilitatory effects. There is in fact evidence to indicate that this is the case. Studies in a variety of animal models using aFGF *(124)*, bFGF *(125,126)*, VEGF *(23,127,128)*, and scatter factor *(117)* have shown that systemic administration of angio-genic cytokines selectively produces neovascularization in the ischemic limb *(129)*; neither in the contralateral normal limb nor in any other organs were foci of neovascularization observed. In fact, when rhVEGF was injected into the normal or ischemic limb of rabbits with unilateral hindlimb ischemia, angiogenesis was observed only in the ischemic limb.

Furthermore, patients with peripheral vascular disease have been shown to have detectable levels of circulating bFGF *(130)*, yet evidence of angiogenesis appeared limited in these patients to collateral vessel development in the ischemic lower extremities. More recently, following intramuscular injection of the gene encoding VEGF, we have docu-mented circulating levels of VEGF (I. Baumgartner and J. Isner, unpublished data, vide infra), yet, again, evidence of angiogenesis was limited to the ischemic limb.

There is evidence to suggest that regional ischemia is the principal factor responsible for localization of angiogenesis. In rabbits, for example, treated with rhVEGF, the magnitude of augmented collateral development is inversely related to the extent of hindlimb collateral arteries seen prior to rhVEGF therapy *(23)*. The same is true for blood flow in the ischemic limb *(131)*. Thus, if a paucity of angiograpically visible collaterals and reduced blood flow are indicative of limb ischemia, then it would appear that the extent to which angiogenesis is enhanced is related to the severity of ischemia.

Experiments performed on ECs in vitro suggest that the basis for localized bioactivity of angiogenic cytokines such as VEGF is owing to upregulation of the VEGF receptor in response to hypoxia. In certain types of ECs, notably bovine retinal ECs, this may occur as a direct response to hypoxia *(132)*; in our experience, direct upregulation of receptor expression does not occur in human umbilical vein ECs (HUVECs) or microvas-cular ECs. The difference in these observations may be because of the fact that bovine retinal ECs possess three-fold more VEGF receptors *(132)*.

In the case of HUVECs and microvascular ECs, receptor upregulation appears to occur indirectly in response to hypoxia (Fig. 5). Specifically, we observed an increase in KDR mRNA levels in HUVECs treated for 3 h with conditioned medium from

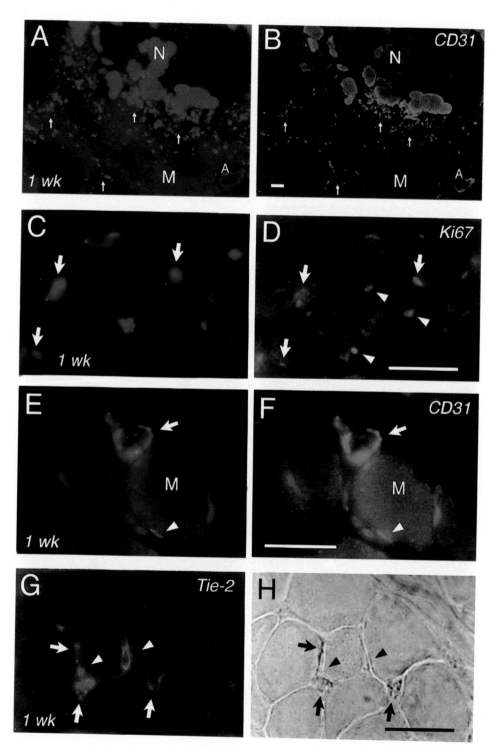

Plate 1. (Part 1) Heterologous (**A–H**) EC progenitors incorporate into sites of angiogenesis in vivo (*see* figure and full caption on pages 255–257).

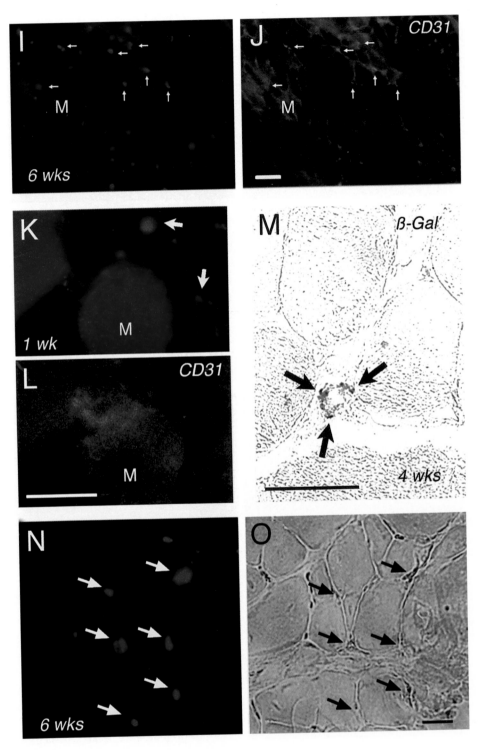

Plate 1. (Part 2) Heterologous (**I–L**), homologous (**M**), or autologous (**N** and **O**) EC progenitors incorporate into sites of angiogenesis in vivo (*see* figure and full caption on pages 255–257).

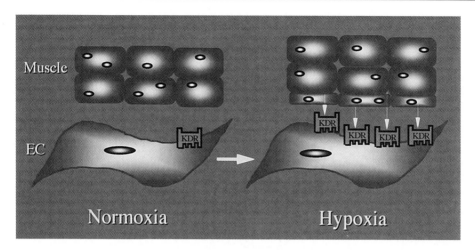

Fig. 5. Factors secreted by hypoxic myocytes upregulate VEGF receptor expression on ECs within the hypoxic milieu. Such localized receptor expression may explain the finding that angiogenesis does not occur indiscriminately, but rather at sites of tissue ischemia. Adapted with permission from ref. *176.*

hypoxic myoblasts, as compared to KDR mRNA levels of HUVECs treated for the same time with conditioned medium from normoxic myoblasts *(133)*. Such increase suggests new receptor synthesis, in conjunction with mobilization of preformed receptors from the cellular pool. Scatchard analysis of ^{125}I-VEGF binding indicated no substantial change in affinity of the KDR receptor in HUVECs treated with myoblast medium conditioned either in normoxia or hypoxia. Thus, increased binding observed using hypoxia-CM was owing to a 13-fold increase in the number of KDR receptors. These data suggest that a "factor" secreted from hypoxic myocytes in ischemic tissues upregulates VEGF receptor expression on adjacent ECs; consequently the ECs in these ischemic tissues act as a magnet for circulating VEGF.

THERAPEUTIC ANGIOGENESIS

The therapeutic implications of angiogenic growth factors were identified by the pioneering work of Folkman and colleagues over two decades ago *(134)*. Their work documented the extent to which tumor development was dependent on neovascularization and suggested that this relationship might involve angiogenic growth factors that were specific for neoplasms.

More recent investigations have established the feasibility of using recombinant formulations of such angiogenic growth factors to expedite and/or augment collateral artery development in animal models of myocardial and hindlimb ischemia. This novel strategy for the treatment of vascular insufficiency has been termed "therapeutic angiogenesis" *(23)*. The angiogenic growth factors first employed for this purpose comprised members of the FGF family. Baffour et al administered bFGF in daily intramuscular (IM) doses of 1 or 3 μg to rabbits with acute hindlimb ischemia; at the completion of 14 d of treatment, angiography and necropsy measurement of capillary density showed evidence of augmented collateral vessels in the lower limb, compared to controls *(126)*. Pu et al used aFGF to treat rabbits in which the acute effects of surgically-induced hindlimb ischemia were

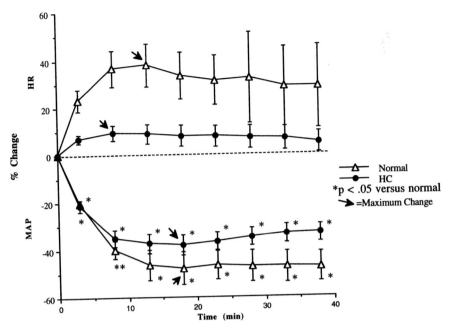

Fig. 6. (A) Administration of rhVEGF to normal and hypercholesterolemic (HC) rabbits leads to prompt reduction in mean arterial pressure (MAP), with compensatory increase in heart rate (HR). The magnitude and duration (≥ 40 min) of hypotension are not significantly different in HC vs normal rabbits. **(B)** MAP does not drop below baseline when administration of VEGF is preceded by administration of an inhibitor of nitric oxide synthase (L-NNA).

allowed to subside for 10 d before beginning a 10-d course of daily 4-mg IM injections; at the completion of 30 d follow-up, both angiographic and hemodynamic evidence of collateral development was superior to ischemic controls treated with IM saline *(124)*. Yanagisawa-Miwa et al likewise demonstrated the feasibility of bFGF for salvage of infarcted myocardium, but in this case growth factor was administered intra-arterially at the time of coronary occlusion, followed 6 h later by a second intra-arterial bolus *(135)*.

Evidence that VEGF stimulates angiogenesis in vivo had been developed in experiments performed on rat and rabbit cornea *(136,137)*, the chorioallantoic membrane *(74)*, and the rabbit bone graft model *(136)*. The finding that VEGF could be employed to achieve angiogenesis that was therapeutic was first demonstrated by Takeshita et al *(23)*. The 165-amino acid isoform of VEGF (VEGF$_{165}$) was administered as a single intra-arterial bolus to the internal iliac artery of rabbits in which the ipsilateral femoral artery was excised to induce unilateral hindlimb ischemia. The severity of hindlimb ischemia in this animal model has been shown in previous studies to include reduced TcO$_2$ *(126)*, increased femoral venous lactate *(138)*, and skeletal muscle necrosis *(126)*. Doses of 500-1,000 µg of VEGF produced statistically significant augmentation of angiographically visible collateral vessels (Fig. 7), and histologically identifiable capillaries (Fig. 8); consequent amelioration of the hemodynamic deficit in the ischemic limb was significantly greater in animals receiving VEGF than in nontreated controls (calf blood-pressure ratio = 0.75 ± 0.14 vs. 0.48 ± 0.19, *p* < 0.05). Serial (baseline, as well as 10 and 30 d post-VEGF) angiograms disclosed progressive linear extension of the collateral artery of origin (stem artery) to the distal point of parent-vessel (reentry artery) reconstitution in 7 of 9 VEGF-treated animals. Similar results were achieved in a

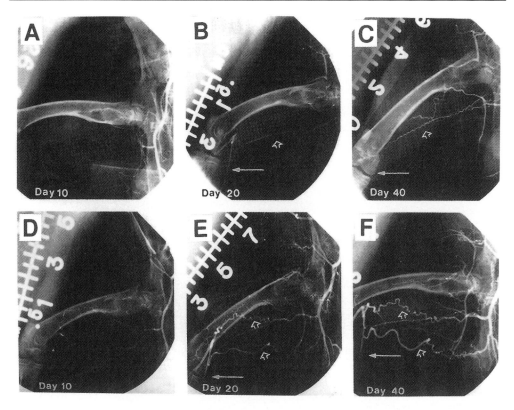

Fig. 7. Angiogenesis at level of medium-sized arteries.Selective internal iliac angiography of control rabbit witrh unilateral hindlimb ischemia performed at (**A**) day 10 (baseline), (**B**) day 20, and (**C**) day 40, and of VEGF-treated rabbit at (**D**) day 10 (baseline), (**E**) day 20, and (**F**) day 40. The angiograms shown here yielded angiographic scores of (**A**) 0.10, (**B**) 0.11, (**C**) 0.17, (**D**) 0.12, (**E**) 0.36, and (**F**) 0.41. Distal reconstitution, barely apparent in control group (B, C, arrows), was evident in the VEGF-treated group (**E**, **F**, arrows). Direct and linear extension of internal iliac artery to popliteal and/or saphenous arteries was also more evident in VEGF -treated group (B, C, **E**, **F**, open arrows). Adapted with permission from ref. *151*.

separate series of experiments in which VEGF was administered by an IM route daily for 10 d *(128)*. By 30 d post-VEGF$_{165}$, flow at rest, as well as maximum flow velocity and maximum blood flow provoked by 2 mg papaverine were all significantly higher in the VEGF-treated group *(131)*. These findings thus established proof of principle for the concept that the angiogenic activity of VEGF is sufficiently potent to achieve therapeutic benefit.

Therapeutic Angiogenesis Preserves Vasomotor Reactivity of Collateral Vessels

Abnormal vascular reactivity may limit the facilitatory effects of collateral vessels on tissue perfusion *(139–143)*. Previous studies have established that chronic perfusion through native coronary collateral vessels produces endothelial dysfunction in the recipient, downstream reconstituted vasculature *(139,142)*. Therapeutic angiogenesis may promote recovery of endothelium-dependent flow. In the rabbit model of hindlimb ischemia, endothelium-independent and endothelium dependent hindlimb blood flow were essentially restored 30 d following administration of a single intra-arterial bolus of VEGF *(144)*.

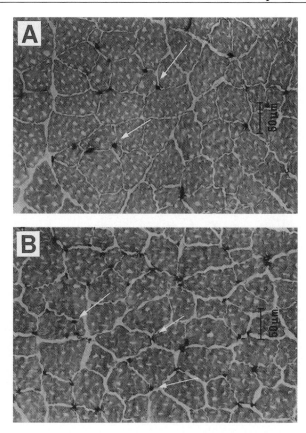

Fig. 8. Angiognesis at the capillary level. Alkaline phosphatase staining of rabbit ischemic hindlimb muscle harvested at day 40. (**A**) Control group and (**B**) VEGF-treated group. Dark blue dots indicate capillaries (arrows). (Counterstained with eosin) Adapted with permission from ref. *153*.

At least three mechanisms could explain an improvement in endothelium-dependent flow responses of the collateral-dependent limb after VEGF therapy. The first possibility relates to the characteristics of flow and perfusion pressure in arterioles distal to collaterals. We have previously demonstrated that VEGF therapy produces a significant increase in the calf blood-pressure of the ischemic limb *(23)*; it is entirely possible that such improved perfusion pressure may lead to repair of dysfunctional endothelium in the collateral-perfused distal vasculature. A second and intriguing possibility relates to a direct improvement of endothelial function by VEGF. In the case of bFGF, for example, in vitro studies have recently demonstrated that endothelial function in the coronary micro-circulation perfused via collateral vessels is preserved by chronic administration of this EC mitogen *(145)*. The fact that VEGF may also modulate qualitative aspects of EC function *(146)* suggests that it too may directly repair ECs presumed damaged by protracted ischemia in the collateral-dependent limb, and thereby restore normal endothelium-dependent flow. Third, the possibility that the documented improvement in endothelium-dependent flow is the result of the newly formed, VEGF-induced collateral vessels, cannot be discounted.

The finding that angiogenic growth factors restore the responses of the ischemic hindlimb to endothelium-dependent vasodilators may have important clinical implications. The hypersensitivity to serotonin of the collateral circulation is not limited to animal models. Platelet activation releases vasoactive quantities of serotonin in vitro (147), and the S_2-receptor antagonist ketanserin dilates limb collaterals in over 50% of human patients with advanced atherosclerosis (148). Ketanserin has also been reported to improve limb perfusion in selected patients with peripheral artery disease (149), suggesting that abnormal reactivity may largely limit the beneficial consequences of collaterals in humans.

Therapeutic Angiogenesis Achieved by Arterial Gene Transfer

No recombinant protein formulation of any of the three principal VEGF isoforms or any other angiogenic cytokine is currently approved or available for human clinical application. Arterial gene transfer constitutes an alternative strategy for accomplishing therapeutic angiogenesis in patients with limb ischemia. In the case of VEGF this is a particularly appealing strategy because, as indicated previously, the VEGF gene encodes a signal sequence that permits the protein to be naturally secreted from intact cells (77). Previous studies from our laboratory (150,151) indicated that arterial gene transfer of cDNA encoding for a secreted protein could potentially yield meaningful biological outcomes in spite of a low transfection efficiency. We therefore performed pre-clinical animal studies to establish the feasibility of site-specific gene transfer of phVEGF$_{121}$, phVEGF$_{165}$, and phVEGF$_{189}$ applied to the hydrogel polymer coating of an angioplasty balloon (152), and delivered percutaneously to the iliac artery of rabbits in which the femoral artery had been excised to cause unilateral hindlimb ischemia (138).

Site-specific transfection of phVEGF$_{165}$ was confirmed by analysis of the transfected internal iliac arteries using reverse transcriptase-polymerase chain reaction (RT-PCR) (153) and then sequencing the RT-PCR product. Augmented development of collateral vessels was documented by serial angiograms in vivo, and increased capillary density at necropsy. Consequent amelioration of the hemodynamic deficit in the ischemic limb was documented by improvement in the calf blood pressure ratio (ischemic/normal limb) to 0.70 ± 0.08 in the VEGF-transfected group vs. 0.50 ± 0.18 in controls ($p < 0.05$). Similar findings were achieved with the 121 and 189 VEGF isoforms (79). These findings thus established that site-specific arterial gene transfer can be used to achieve physiologically meaningful therapeutic modulation of vascular disorders, including therapeutic angiogenesis.

The relevance of these findings in the rabbit ischemic hindlimb model is supported by recent clinical application of arterial gene therapy (154). Using a dose-escalating design, treatment was initiated with 100 μg of phVEGF. Three patients presenting with rest pain (but no gangrene) and treated with 1000 μg were subsequently shown at 1-yr follow-up to have improved blood flow to the ischemic limb and remain free of rest pain. With the increase in dose of phVEGF$_{165}$ to 2000 μg, angiographic (Fig. 9) and histologic evidence of new blood-vessel formation became apparent (70) (Fig. 10). Subsequently, the use of intramuscular gene transfer, employed initially as a means of treating patients in whom vascular disease in the ischemic limb was too extensive to permit an intra-arterial approach, resulted in circulating levels of VEGF detectable by ELISA assay, as well as reproducible hemodynamic and angiographic improvement (I. Baumgartner and J. Isner, unpublished observations). In at least one case, therapeutic angiogenesis administered in this fashion accomplished genuine limb salvage (Fig. 11). The clinical reproducibility of these findings may ultimately be influenced by certain features of host diversity, including the extent of native VEGF and VEGF receptor expression among patients with peripheral and/or myocardial ischemia.

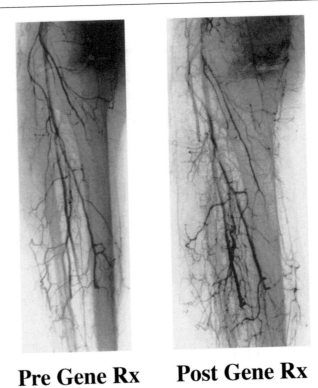

Pre Gene Rx   Post Gene Rx

Fig. 9. Selective digital subtraction angiograms performed in patient with critical limb ishemia due to occlusion of all three infrapopliteal vessels at mid-calf level. (**A**) immediately prior to, and (**B**) 1 mo post-gene therapy with 2000 μg of naked DNA encoding VEGF. The latter angiogram disclosed plethora of new collateral vessels in ischemic limb. Adapted with permission from ref. *177.*

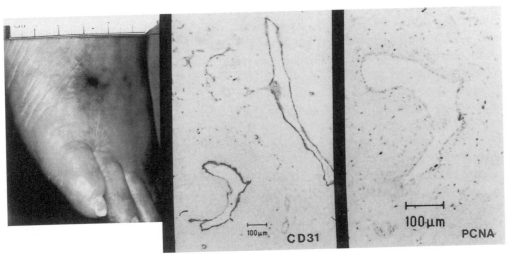

Fig. 10. One of three spider angiomata that developed approx 1 wk post-gene therapy in distal portion of ischemic limb of a patient. Photomicrographs of tissue sections immunostained with antibody to endothelial antigen CD31 indicate vascularity of lesion, while immunostain of adjacent section for proliferating cell nuclear antigen (PCNA) indicates extent of proliferative activity among ECs in lesion. Adapted with permission from ref. *177.*

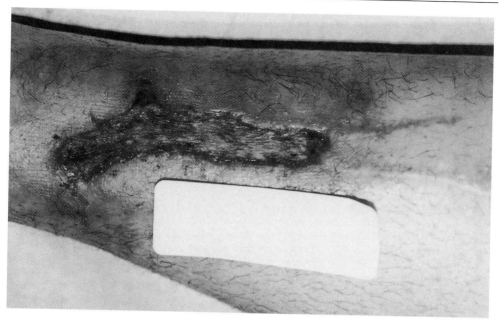

Fig. 11. Successful placement of split-thickness skin graft in first patient treated with intramuscular (IM) administration of naked DNA encoding VEGF (phVEGF$_{165}$). Following two IM injections of 2000 µg of phVEGF$_{165}$, patient's ankle-brachial index increased from 0.28 to 0.55, angiography disclosed new collateral vessels in ischemic limb, and 9×3cm wound at site of vein harvest in medial calf healed sufficiently to permit successful grafting.

Recombinant Protein vs Gene Therapy

There is now abundant data in animal models to support the potential utility of both recombinant protein therapy and arterial gene transfer for myocardial angiogenesis *(135,145,155–161)*. The same is true for lower extremity vascular insufficiency *(23,117,124–128,162–164)*. It is therefore reasonable to ask why, if the recombinant protein has or can be manufactured, consider transferring the gene encoding that protein (i.e., gene therapy)? There are at least four issues to consider in this regard. First, and perhaps most critical in the case of arterial gene therapy, is the potential requirement to maintain an optimally high and local concentration over time. In the case of therapeutic angiogenesis, for example, it may be preferable to deliver a lower dose over a period of several days or more from an actively expressing transgene in the ischemic limb, rather than a single or multiple bolus doses of recombinant protein. Second, there is the matter of economics; namely, which therapy would ultimately cost more to develop, implement, and reimburse, particularly for those indications requiring multiple or even protracted treatment? Third, in certain species — namely rats, rabbits, and swine — both rhbFGF and rhVEGF have been shown to produce varying degrees of systemic hypotension, even in the setting of hypercholesterolemia *(21,158,165,166)*. And fourth, the route of administration may be a factor depending on the target site for neovascularization. For example, the ready access to ischemic skeletal muscle together with the promising results of IM gene therapy make this approach eminently suitable for the treatment of lower extremity vascular insufficiency. In contrast, IM administration for myocardial angiogenesis cannot be accomplished as readily, and may therefore be more amenable to recombinant protein therapy.

Resolution of these issues will almost certainly require the empirical experience of human clinical trials. Recombinant bFGF and VEGF are now being investigated in human clinical trials for patients with lower extremity vascular disease and myocardial ischemia respectively, so that the magnitude of bioactivity that can be achieved with either of these should be ultimately clarified.

REFERENCES

1. Gilbert, S. F. (1997) *Developmental Biology,* 4th ed. Sinauer Associates, Inc., Sunderland, MA, pp. 342.
2. Folkman, J. (1995) Angiogenesis in cancer, vascular, rheumatoid and other disease. *Nature Med.* **1,** 27–30.
3. Risau, W. (1995) Differentiation of endothelium. *FASEB J.* **9,** 926–933.
4. Risau, W. and Flamme, I. (1995) Vasculogenesis. *Ann. Rev. Cell Dev. Biol.* **11,** 73–91.
5. Risau, W., Sariola, H., Zerwes, H-G., Sasse, J., Ekblom, P., Kemler, R., and Doetschman, T. (1988) Vasculogenesis and angiogenesis in embryonic stem cell-derived embryoid bodies. *Development* **102,** 471–478.
6. Flamme, I. and Risau, W. (1992) Induction of vasculogenesis and hematopoiesis in vitro. *Development* **116,** 435–439.
7. His, W. (1900) Leoithoblast und angioblast der wirbelthiere. *Abhandl. K. S. Ges. Wiss. Math. Phys.* **22,** 171–328.
8. Weiss, M. and Orkin, S. H. (1996) In vitro differentiation of murine embryonic stem cells: new approaches to old problems. *J. Clin. Invest.* **97,** 591–595.
9. Folkman, J. and Shing, Y. (1992) Angiogenesis. *J. Biol. Chem.* **267,** 10,931–10,934.
10. D'Amore, P. A. and Thompson, R. W. (1987) Mechanisms of angiogenesis. *Annu. Rev. Physiol.* **49,** 453–464.
11. Ausprunk, D. H. and Folkman, J. (1977) Migration and proliferation of endothelial cells in preformed and newly formed blood vessels during tumor angiogenesis. *Microvasc. Res.* **14,** 53–65.
12. Sholley, M. M., Ferguson, G. P., Seibel, H, R., Montour, J. L., and Wilson, J. D. (1984) Mechanisms of neovascularization: vascular sprouting can occur without proliferation of endothelial cells. *Lab. Invest.* **51,** 624–634.
13. Pepper, M. S., Ferrara, N., Orci, L., and Montesano, R. (1991) Vascular endothelial growth factor (VEGF) induces plasminogen activators and plasminogen activator inhibitor-1 in microvascular endotehlial cells. *Biochem. Biophys. Res. Comm.* **181,** 902–906.
14. Pepper, M. S. and Montesano, R. (1990) Proteolytic balance and capillary morphogenesis. *Cell Differ. Dev.* **32,** 319–328.
15. Pasyk, S., Schaper, W., Schaper, J., Pasyk, K., Miskiewicz, G., and Steinseifer, B. (1982) DNA synthesis in coronary collaterals after coronary artery occlusion in conscious dog. *Am. J. Physiol.* **242,** H1031–H1037.
16. Schaper, W., Brahander, M. D., and Lewi, P. (1971) DNA synthesis and mitoses in coronary collateral vessels of the dog. *Circ. Res.* **28,** 671–679.
17. Ilich, N., Hollenberg, N. K., Williams, D. H., and Abrams, H. L. (1979) Time course of increased collateral arterial and venous endotehlial cell turnover after renal artery stenosis in the rat. *Circ. Res.* **45,** 579–582.
18. White, F. C., Carroll, S. M., Magnet, A., and Bloor, C. M. (1992) Coronary collateral development in swine after coronary artery occlusion. *Circ. Res.* **71,** 1490–1500.
19. Schaper, W., Schaper, J., Xhonneux, R., and Vandesteene, R. (1969) The morphology of intercoronary anastomoses in chronic coronary artery occlusion. *Cardiovasc. Res.* **3,** 315–323.
20. Bucay, M., Nguy, J. H., Barrios, R., Kerns, S. A., and Henry, P. D. (1992) Impaired macro- and microvascular growth in hypercholesterolemic rabbits. *J. Am. Coll. Cardiol.* **19,** 151A. (Abstract.)
21. Cuevas, P., Carceller, F., Ortega, S., Zazo, M., Nieto, I., and Gimenez-Gallego, G. (1991) Hypotensive activity of fibroblast growth factor. *Science* **254,** 1208–1210.
22. Graham, A. M., Baffour, R., Burdon, T., DeVarennes, B., Ricci, M. A., Common, A., et al. (1989) A demonstration of vascular proliferation in response to arteriovenous reversal in the ischemic canine hind limb. *J. Surg. Res.* **47,** 341–347.
23. Takeshita, S., Zheng, L. P., Brogi, E., Kearney, M., Pu, L. Q., Bunting, S., et al. (1994) Therapeutic angiogenesis: A single intra-arterial bolus of vascular endothelial growth factor augments revascularization in a rabbit ischemic hindlimb model. *J. Clin. Invest.* **93,** 662–670.

24. Shalaby, F., Rossant, J., Yamaguchi, T. P., Gertsenstein, M., Wu, X.-F., Breitman, M. L., and Schuh, A. C. (1995) Failure of blood-island formation and vasculogenesis in Flk-1 deficient mice. *Nature* **376,** 62–66.

25. Carmeliet, P., Ferreira, V., Breier, G., Pollefeyt, S., Kieckens, L., Gertsenstein, M., et al. (1996) Abnormal blood vessel development and lethality in embryos lacking a single VEGF allele. *Nature* **380,** 435–439.

26. Ferrara, N., Carver-Moore, K., Chen, H., Dowd, M., Lu, L., O'Shea, K. S., et al. (1996) Heterozygous embryonic lethality induced by targeted inactivation of the VEGF gene. *Nature* **380,** 439–442.

27. Fong, G.-H., Rossant, J., Gersenstein, M., and Breitman, M. L. (1995) Role of the Flt-1 receptor tyrosine kinase in regulating the assembly of vascular endothelium . *Nature* **376,** 66–70.

28. Sato, T. N., Qin, Y., Kozak, C. A., and Audus, K. L. (1993) *Tie-1* and *tie-2* define another class of putative receptor tyrosine kinase genes expressed in early embryonic vascular system. *Proc. Natl. Acad. Sci. USA* **90,** 9355–9358.

29. Sato, T. N., Tozawa, Y., Deutsch, U., Wolburg-Buchholz, K., Fujiwara, Y., Gentron-Maguire, M., et al. (1995) Distinct roles of the receptor tyrosine kinases Tie-1 and Tie-2 in blood vessel formation. *Nature* **376,** 70–74.

30. Davis, S., Aldrich, T. H., Jones, P. F., Acheson, A., Compton, D. L., Jian, V., et al. (1996) Isolation of angiopoetin-1, a ligand for the TIE2 receptor by secretion-trap expression cloning. *Cell* **87,** 1161–1169.

31. Suri, C., Jones, P. F., Patan, S., Bartunkova, S., Maisonpierre, P. C., Davis, S., Sato, T., and Yancopoulos, G. D. (1996) Requisite role of angiopoetin-1, a ligand for the TIE2 receptor, during embryonic angiogenesis. *Cell* **87,** 1171–1180.

32. Ingber, D. E. and Folkman, J. (1989) How does extracellular-matrix control capillary morphogenesis. *Cell* **58,** 803–805.

33. Folkman, J. and Haudenschild, C. (1980) Angiogenesis in vitro. *Nature* **288,** 551–556.

34. Bar, T., Guldner, F.-H., and Wolff, J. R. (1984) "Seamless" endothelial cells of blood capillaries. *Cell Tissue Res.* **235,** 99–106.

35. Saffitz, J. E., Sullivan, A., and Isner, J. M. (1996) Regulation of endothelial cell connexin expression by vascular endothelial growth factor. *Circulation* **94,** I–238. (Abstract.)

36. Folkman, J. (1975) Tumor angiogenesis, in: *Cancer Biology*, (Becker, F. F., ed.), Plenum, New York, NY, Plenum Press, pp. 355–388.

37. Jain, R. K. (1988) Determinants of tumor blood flow. *Canc. Res.* **48,** 2641–2647.

38. Dvorak, H. F., Brown, L. F., Detmar, M., and Dvorak, A. M. (1995) Vascular permeability factor/vascular endothelial growth factor, microvascular hyperpermeability, and angiogenesis. *Am. J. Pathol.* **146,** 1029–1039.

39. Kohn, S., Nagy, J. A., Dvorak, H. F., and Dvorak, A. M. (1992) Pathways of macromolecular tracer transport across venules and small veins. Structural basis for the hyperpermeability of tumor blood vessels. *Lab. Invest.* **67,** 596–607.

40. Roberts, W. G. and Palade, G. E. (1995) Increased microvascular permeability and endothelial fenestration induced by vascular endothelial growth factor. *J. Cell Sci.* **108,** 2369–2379.

41. Brooks, P. C., Clark, R. A. F., and Cheresh, D. A. (1994) Requirement of vascular integrin alpha-v-beta-3 for angiogenesis. *Science* **264,** 569–571.

42. Brooks, P. C., Montgomery, A. M. P., Rossenfeld, M., Reisfeld, R. A., Hu, T., Killer, G., and Cheresh, D. A. (1994) Integrin alpha-v-beta-3 antagonists promote tumor regression by inducing apoptosis of angiogenic blood vessels. *Cell* **79,** 1157–1164.

43. Okada, Y., Copeland, B. R., Hamann, G. F., Koziol, J. A., Cheresh, D. A., and del Zoppo, G. J. (1996) Integrin alpha-v-beta-3 is expressed in selected microvessels after focal cerebral ischemia. *Am. J. Pathol.* **149,** 37–44.

44. Stromblad, S., Becker, J. C., Yebra, M., Brooks, P. C., and Cheresh, D. A. (1996) Suppression of p53 activity and p21^{WAF1CIP1} expression by vascular cell integrin alpha-v-beta-3 during angiogenesis. *J. Clin. Invest.* **98,** 426–433.

45. Breier, G., Albrecht, U., Sterrer, S., and Risau, W. (1992) Expression of vascular endothelial growth factor during embryonic angiogenesis and endothelial cell differentiation. *Development* **114,** 521–532.

46. Ruoslahti, E. and Reed, J. C. (1994) Anchorage dependence, integrins, and apoptosis. *Cell* **77,** 477–478.

47. Fuks, Z., Persaud, R. S., Alfieri, A., McLoughlin, M., Ehleiter, D., Schwartz, J. L., et al. (1994) Basic fibroblast growth factor protects endothelial cells against radiation–induced programmed cell death in vitro and in vivo. *Canc. Res.* **54,** 2582–2590.

48. Defilippi, P., Silengo, L., and Tarone, G. (1993) Regulation of adhesion receptors expression in endothelial cells. *Microbiol. Immunol.* **184,** 87–98.

49. Enenstein, J., Walsh, N. S., and Kramer, R. H. (1992) Basic FGF and TGF-β differentially modulate integrin expression of human microvascular endothelial cells. *Exp. Cell Res.* **203,** 499–503.

50. Klein, S., Giancotti, F. G., Presta, M., Albelda, S. M., Buck, C. A., and Rifkin, D. B. (1993) Basic fibroblast growth factor modulates integrin expression in microvascular endothelial cells. *Mol. Biol. Cell* **4,** 973–982.

51. Spyridopoulos, I., Brogi, E., Kearney, M., Sullivan, A. B., Cetrulo, C., Isner, J. M., and Losordo, D. W. (1997) Vascular endothelial growth factor inhibits endothelial cell apoptosis induced by tumor necrosis factor–alpha: balance between growth and death signals. *J. Mol. Cell Cardiol.* **29,** 1321–1330.

52. Alon, T., Hemo, I., Itin, A., Pe'er, J., Stone, J., and Keshet, E. (1995) Vascular endothelial growth factor acts as a survival factor for newly formed retinal vessels and has implications for retinopathy of prematurity. *Nature Med.* **1,** 1024–1028.

53. Friedlander, M., Brooks, P. C., Shaffer, R. W., Kincaid, C. M., Varner, J. A., and Cheresh, D. A. (1995) Definition of two angiogenic pathways by distinct alpha$_v$ integrins. *Science* **270,** 1500–1502.

54. Katoh, O., Tauchi, H., Kawaishi, K., Kimura, A., and Satow, Y. (1995) Expression of the vascular endothelial growth factor (VEGF) receptor gene *KDR*, in hematopoietic cells and inhibitory effect of VEGF on apoptotic cell death caused by ionizing radiation. *Canc. Res.* **55,** 5687–5692.

55. Pardanaud, L., Altman, C., Kitos, P., and Dieterien-Lievre, F. (1989) Relationship between vasculogenesis, angiogenesis and haemopoiesis during avian ontogeny. *Development* **105,** 473–485.

56. Asahara, T., Murohara, T., Sullivan, A., Silver, M., van der Zee, R., Li, T., et al. (1997) Isolation of putative progenitor endothelial cells for angiogenesis. *Science* **275,** 965–967.

57. Shi, Q., Wu, M. H., Hayashida, N., Wechezak, A. R., Clowes, A. W., and Sauvage, L. R. (1994) Proof of fallout endothelialization of impervious dacron grafts in the aorta and inferior vena cava of the dog. *J. Vasc. Surg.* **20,** 546–556.

58. Wu, M. H–D., Shi, Q. Wechezak, A. R., Clowes, A. W., Gordon, I. L., and Sauvage, L. R. (1995) Definitive proof of endothelialization of a Dacron arterial prosthesis in a human being. *J. Vasc. Surg.* **21,** 862–867.

59. Andrews, R. G., Singer, J. W., and Bernstein, I. D. (1986) Monoclonal antibody 12-8 recognizes a 115-kd molecular present on both unipotent and multipotent hematopoietic colony-forming cells and their precursors. *Blood* **67,** 842–845.

60. Civin, C. I., Banquerigo, M. L., Strauss, L. C., and Loken, M. R. (1987) Antigen analysis of hematopoiesis. VI. Flow cytometric characterization of My-10-positive progenitor cells in normal human bone marrow. *Exp. Hematol.* **15,** 10–17.

61. deVries, C., Escobedo, J. A., Ueno, H., Houck, K., Ferrara, N., and Williams, L. T. (1992) The *fms*-like tyrosine kinase, a receptor for vascular endothelial growth factor. *Science* **255,** 989–991.

62. Fina, J., Molgard, H. V., Robertson, D., Bradley, N. J., Managhan, P. D., Sutherland, D. R., et al. (1990) Expression of the CD34 gene in vascular endothelial cells. *Blood* **75,** 2417–2426.

63. Ito, A., Nomura, S., Hirota, S., Suda, T., and Kitamura, Y. (1995) Enhanced expression of CD34 messenger RNA by developing endothelial cells of mice. *Lab. Invest.* **72,** 532–538.

64. Katz, F., Tindle, R. W., Sutherland, D. R., and Greaves, M. D. (1985) Identification of a membrane glycoprotein associated with hemopoietic progenitor cells. *Leuk. Res.* **9,** 191–198.

65. Matthews, W., Jordan, C. T., Gavin, M., Jenkins, N. A., Copeland, N. G., and Lemischka, I. R. (1991) A receptor tyrosine kinase cDNA isolated from a population of enriched primitive hematopoietic cells and exhibiting close genetic linkage to c-kit. *Proc. Natl. Acad. Sci. USA* **88,** 9026–9030.

66. Millauer, B., Wizigmann-Voos, S., Schnurch, H., Martinez, R., Moller, N. P. H., Risau, W., and Ulrich, A. (1993) High affinity VEGF binding and developmental expression suggest *Flk*-1 as a major regulator of vasculogenesis and angiogenesis. *Cell* **72,** 835–846.

67. Soligo, D., Delia, D., Oriani, A., Cattoretti, G., Orazi, A., Bertolli, V., et al. (1991) Identification of CD34$^+$ cells in normal and pathological bone marrow biopsies by OBEND10 monoclonal antibody. *Leukemia* **5,** 1026–1030.

68. Terman, B. I., Carrion, M. E., Kovacs, E., Rasmussen, B. A., Eddy, R. L., and Shows, T. B. (1991) Identification of a new endotheelial cell growth factor receptor tyrosine kinase. *Oncogene* **6,** 1677–1683.

69. Yamaguchi, T. P., Dumont, D. J., Conlon, R. A., Breitman, M. L., and Rossant, J. (1993) *flk*–1, and *flt*–related receptor tyrosine kinase is an early marker for endothelial cell precursors. *Development* **118,** 489–498.

70. Isner, J. M., Pieczek, A., Schainfeld, R., Blair, R., Haley, L., Asahara, T., et al. (1996) Clinical evidence of angiogenesis following arterial gene transfer of phVEGF$_{165}$. *Lancet* **348,** 370–374.

71. Tschudi, M. R., Barton, M., Bersinger, N. A., Moreau, P., Cosentino, F., Noll, G., et al. (1996) Effect of age on kinetics of nitric oxide release in rat aorta and pulmonary artery. *J. Clin. Invest.* **98,** 899–905.

72. Senger, D. R., Ledbetter, S. R., Claffey, K. P., Papadopoulos-Sergiou, A., Perruzzi, C. A., and Detmar, M. (1996) Stimulation of endothelial cell migration by vascular permeability factor/vascular endothelial growth factor through cooperative mechanisms involving the αvβ3 integrin, osteopontin, and thrombin. *Am. J. Pathol.* **149,** 293–305.

73. Shing, Y., Folkman, J., Sullivan, J., Butterfield, R., Murray, J., and Klagsbrun, M. (1984) Heparin-afinity purification of a tumor-derived capillary endothelial cell growth factor. *Science* **223,** 1296–1299.

74. Ferrara, N. and Henzel, W. J. (1989) Pituitary follicular cells secrete a novel heparin-binding growth factor specific for vascular endothelial cells. *Biochem. Biophys. Res. Commun.* **161,** 851–855.

75. Keck, P. J., Hauser, S. D., Krivi, G., Sanzo, K., Warren, T., Feder, J., and Connolly, D. T. (1989) Vascular permeability factor, an endothelial cell mitogen related to PDGF. *Science* 246, 1309–1312.

76. Plouet, J., Schilling, J., and Gospodarowicz, D. (1989) Isolation and characterization of a newly identified endothelial cell mitogen produced by AtT–20 cells. *EMBO J.* **8,** 3801–3806.

77. Tischer, E., Mitchell, R., Hartmann, T., Silva, M., Gospodarowicz, D., Fiddes, J., and Abraham, J. (1991) The human gene for vascular endothelial growth factor: multiple protein forms are encoded through alternative exon splicing. *J. Biol. Chem.* **266,** 11,947–11,954.

78. Houck, K. A., Leung, D. W., Rowland, A. M., Winer, J., and Ferrara, N. (1992) Dual regulation of vascular endothelial growth factor bioavailability by genetic and proteolytic mechanisms. *J. Biol. Chem.* **267,** 26,031–26,037.

79. Takeshita, S., Tsurumi, Y., Couffinhal, T., Asahara, T., Bauters, C., Symes, J. F., et al. (1996) Gene transfer of naked DNA encoding for three isoforms of vascular endothelial growth factor stimulates collateral development in vivo. *Lab. Invest.* **75,** 487–502.

80. Miles, A. A. and Miles, E. M. (1952) Vascular reactions to histamine, histamine liberators or leukotoxins in the skin of the guinea pig. *J. Physiol.* **118,** 228–257.

81. Joukov, V., Pajusola, K., Kaipainen, A., Chilov, D., Lahtinen, I., Kukk, E., et al. (1996) A Novel vascular endothelial growth factor, VEGF-C, is a ligand for the Flt4 (VEGFR-3) and KDR (VEGFR-2) receptor tyrosine kinases. *EMBO J.* **15,** 290–298.

82. Olofsson, B., Pajusola, K., Kaipainen, A., vonEuler, G., Joukov, V., Saksela, O., et al. (1996) Vascular endothelial growth factor B, a novel growth factor for endothelial cells. *Proc. Natl. Acad. Sci. USA* **93,** 2576–2581.

83. Maglione, D., Guerriero, V., Viglietto, G., Delli–Bovi, P., and Persico, M. G. (1991) Isolation of a human placenta cDNA coding for a protein related to the vascular permeability factor. *Proc. Natl. Acad. Sci. USA* **88,** 9267–9271.

84. Hauser, S., and Weich, H. A. (1993) A heparin-binding form of placenta growth factor (PlGF-2) is expressed in human umbilical vein endothelial cells and in placenta. *Growth Factors* **9,** 259–268.

85. Maglione, D., Guerriero, V., Viglietto, G., Ferraro, M. G., Aprelikova, O., Alitalo, K., et al. (1993) Two alternative mRNAs coding for the angiogenic factor, placenta growth factor (PlGF), are transcribed from a single gene of chromosome 14. *Oncogene* **8,** 925–931.

86. Park, J. E., Keller, G.-A., and Ferrara, N. (1993) The vascular endothelial growth factor (VEGF) isoforms: differential deposition into the subepithelial ECM and bioactivity of ECM–bound VEGF. *Mol. Biol. Cell* **4,** 1317–1326.

87. Cao, Y., Linden, P., Shima, D., Browne, F., and Folkman, J. (1996) In vivo angiogenic activity and hypoxia induction of heterodimer of placenta growth factor/vascular endothelial growth factor. *J. Clin. Invest.* **98,** 2507–2511.

88. DiSalvo, J., Bayne, M. L., Conn, G., Kwok, P. W., Trivedi, P. G., Soderman, D. D., et al. (1995) Purification and characterization of a naturally occuring vascular endothelial growth factor. Placenta growth factor heterodimer. *J. Biol. Chem.* **270,** 7717–7723.

89. Park, J. E., Chen, H. H., Winer, J., Houck, K. A., and Ferrara, N. (1994) Placenta growth factor: potentiation of vascular endothelial growth factor bioactivity, in vitro and in vivo, and high affinity binding to *Flt-1* but not to *Flk-1*/KDR. *J. Biol. Chem.* **269,** 25,646–25,654.

90. Carmeliet, P. and Collen, D. (1997) Gene targeting studies of angiogenesis. *Am. J. Physiol.* in press.

91. Pajusola, K., Aprelikova, O., Pelicci, G., Weich, H., Claesson, Welsh, L., and Alitalo, K. (1994) Signaling properties of FLT4, a proteolytically processed receptor tyrosine kinase related to two VEGF receptors. *Oncogene* **9,** 3545–3555.

92. Lee, J., Gray, A., Yuan, J., Luoh, S., Avraham, H., and Wood, W. I. (1996) Vascular endothelial growth factor–related protein: a ligand and specific activator of the tyrosine kinase receptor Flt4. *Proc. Natl. Acad. Sci. USA* **93,** 1988–1992.

93. Jaye, M., Lyall, R. M., Mudd, R., Schlessinger, J., and Sarver, N. (1988) Expression of acidic fibroblast growth factor cDNA confers growth advantage and tumorigenesis to Swiss 3T3 cells. *EMBO J.* **7,** 963–969.

94. Mignatti, P., Morimoto, T., and Rifkin, D. B. (1991) Basic fibroblast growth factor released by single, isolated cells stimulates their migration in an autocrine manner. *Proc. Natl. Acad. Sci. USA* **88**, 11,007–11,011.

95. Bensaid, M., Malecaze, F., Prats, H., Bayard, F., and Tauber, J. P. (1989) Autocrine regulation of bovine retinal capillary endothelial cell (BREC) proliferation by BREC-derived basic fibroblast growth factor. *Exp. Eye Res.* **48**, 801–813.

96. Myoken, Y., Okamoto, T., Kan, M., Sato, D., and Takada, K. (1994) Release of fibroblast growth factor–1 by human squamous cell carcinoma correlates with autocrine cell growth. *In Vitro Cell Dev. Biol.* **30A**, 790–795.

97. Schweigerer, L., Neufeld, G., Friedman, J., Abraham, J. A., Fiddes, J. C., and Gospodarowicz, D. (1987) Capillary endothelial cells express basic fibroblast growth factor, a mitogen that promotes their own growth. *Nature* **325**, 257–259.

98. Villaschi, S. and Nicosia, R. F. (1993) Angiogenic role of endogenous basic fibroblast growth factor released by rat aorta after injury. *Am. J. Pathol.* **143**, 181–190.

99. Namiki, A., Brogi, E., Kearney, M., Wu, T., Couffinhal, T., Varticovski, L., and Isner, J. M. (1995) Hypoxia induces vascular endothelial growth factor in cultured human endothelial cells. *J. Biol. Chem.* **270**, 31,189–31,195.

100. Sporn, M. B., and Roberts, A. B. (1992) Autocrine secretion: 10 years later. *Ann. Int. Med.* **117**, 408–414.

101. Klagsbrun, M. and D'Amore, P. A. (1991) Regulators of angiogenesis. *Annu. Rev. Physiol.* **53**, 217–239.

102. Pierce, G. F., Tarpley, J. E., Yanagihara, D., Mustoe, T. E., Fox, G. M., and Thomason, A. (1992) Platelet derived growth factor (BB homodimer), transforming growth factor–beta1, and basic fibroblast growth factor in dermal wound healing. *Am. J. Pathol.* **140**, 1375–1388.

103. Risau, W., Drexler, H., Mironov, V., Smits, A., Siegbahn, A., Funa, K., and Heldin, C.-H. (1992) Platelet-derived growth factor is angiogenic in vivo. *Growth Factors* **7**, 261–266.

104. Sato, N., Beitz, J. G., Kato, J., Yamamoto, M., Clark, J. W., Calabresi, P., and Frackelton, Jr., R. A. (1993) Platelet–derived growth factor indirectly stimulates angiogenesis in vitro. *Am. J. Pathol.* **142**, 1119–1130.

105. Bar, R. S., Boes, M., Booth, B. A., Dake, B. L., Henley, S., and Hart, M. N. (1989) The effects of platelet–derived growth factor in cultured microvessel endothelial cells. *Endocrinology* **124**, 2021–2025.

106. Beitz, J. G., Kim, I. S., Calabresi, P., and Frackelton, A. R. (1991) Human microvascular endothelial cells express receptors for platelet-derived growth factor. *Proc. Natl. Acad. Sci. USA* **88**, 2021–2025.

107. Smits, A., Hermansson, M., Nister, M., Karnushina, I., Heldin, C.-H., and Oberg, K. (1989) Rat brain capillary endothelial cells express functional PDGF B-type receptors. *Growth Factors* **2**, 1–8.

108. D'Amore, P. and Smith, S. R. (1993) Growth factor effects on cells of the vascular wall: a survey. *Growth Factors* **8**, 61–75.

109. Brogi, E., Wu, T., Namiki, A., and Isner, J. M. (1994) Indirect angiogenic cytokines upregulate VEGF and bFGF gene expression in vascular smooth muscle cells, while hypoxia upregulates VEGF expression only. *Circulation* **90**, 649–652.

110. Roberts, A. B., Sporn, M. B., Assoian, R. K., Smith, J. M., Roche, N. S., Wakefield, L. M., et al. (1986) Transforming growth factor type-beta: rapid induction of fibrosis and angiogenesis in vivo and stimulation of collagen formation in vitro. *Proc. Natl. Acad. Sci. USA* **83**, 4167–4171.

111. Pepper, M. S., Vassalli, J. D., Orci, L., and Montesano, R. (1993) Biphasic effect of transforming growth factor-β1 on in vitro angiogenesis. *Exp. Cell Res.* **204**, 356–363.

112. Chen, J. K., Hoshi, H., and McKeehan, W. L. (1987) Transforming growth factor type β specifically stimulates synthesis of proteoglycans in human adult arterial smooth muscle cells. *Proc. Natl. Acad. Sci. USA* **84**, 5287–5291.

113. Madri, J., Pratt, B., and Tucker, A. (1988) Phenotypic modulation of endothelial cells by transforming growth factor-beta depends upon the composition and organization of the extracellular matrix. *J. Cell Biol.* **106**, 1375–1382.

114. Winkles, J. A. and Gay, C. G. (1991) Serum, phorbol ester, and polypeptide mitogens increase class 1 and 2 heparin binding (acidic and basic fibroblast growth factor) gene expression in human vascular smooth muscle cells. *Cell Growth Differ.* **2**, 531–540.

115. Warren, R. S., Yuan, H., Matli, M. R., Ferrara, N., and Donner, D. B. (1996) Induction of vascular endothelial growth factor by insulin-like growth factor 1 in colorectal carcinoma. *J. Biol. Chem.* **271**, 29,483–29,488.

116. Stavri, G. T., Zachary, I. C., Baskerville, P. A., Martin, J. F., and Erusalimsky, J. D. (1995) Basic fibroblast growth factor upregulates the expression of vascular endothelial growth factor in vascular smooth muscle cells: synergistic interaction with hypoxia. *Circulation* **92**, 11–14.

117. Witzenbichler, B., Van Belle, E., Chang, L., and Schwall, R. (1996) Scatter factor (SF) induces vascular endothelial growth factor (VEGF) expression in vascular smooth muscle cells (VSMC) and acts synergistic to VEGF on endothelial cell (EC) migration in vitro. *Circulation* **94,** I–593–I–594 (Abstract).

118. Shweiki, D., Itin, A., Soffer, D., and Keshet, E. (1992) Vascular endothelial growth factor induced by hypoxia may mediate hypoxia-initiated angiogenesis. *Nature* **359,** 843–845.

119. Wang, G. L. and Semenza, G. L. (1993) Characterization of hypoxia-inducible factor 1 and regulation of DNA binding activity by hypoxia. *Blood* **268,** 21,513–21,518.

120. Goldberg, M. A. and Schneider, T. J. (1994) Similarities between the oxygen-sensing mechanisms regulating the expression of vascular endothelial growth factor and erythropoietin. *J. Biol. Chem.* **269,** 4355–4359.

121. Levy, A. P., Levy, N. S., Wegner, S., and Goldberg, M. A. (1995) Transcriptional regulation of the rat vascular endothelial growth factor gene by hypoxia. *J. Biol. Chem.* **270,** 13,333–13,340.

122a. Levy, N. S., Levy, A. P., Goldberg, M. A., and Koren, G. (1994) Regulation of vascular endothelial growth factor isoforms by hypoxia and identification of a novel truncated vascular endothelial growth factor isoform in cardiac myocytes. *Circulation* **90,** I–521. (Abstract.)

122. Pepper, M. S., Ferrara, N., Orci, L., and Montesano, R. (1992) Potent synergism between vascular endothelial growth factor and basic fibroblast growth factor in the induction of angiogenesis in vitro. *Biochem. Biophys. Res. Comm.* **189,** 824–831.

123. Shima, D. T., Deutsch, U., and D'Amore, P. A. (1995) Hypoxic induction of vascular endothelial growth factor (VEGF) in human epithelial cells is mediated by increases in mRNA stability. *FEBS Lett* **370,** 203–208.

124. Pu, L. Q., Sniderman, A. D., Brassard, R., Lachapelle, K. J., Graham, A. M., Lisbona, R., and Symes, J. F. (1993) Enhanced revascularization of the ischemic limb by means of angiogenic therapy. *Circulation* **88,** 208–215.

125. Asahara, T., Bauters, C., Zheng, L. P., Takeshita, S., Bunting, S., Ferrara, N., et al. (1995) Synergistic effect of vascular endothelial growth factor and basic fibroblast growth factor on angiogenesis in vivo. *Circulation* **92,** II–365–II–371.

126. Baffour, R., Berman, J., Garb, J. L., Rhee, S. W., Kaufman, J., and Friedmann, P. (1992) Enhanced angiogenesis and growth of collaterals by in vivo administration of recombinant basic fibroblast growth factor in a rabbit model of acute lower limb ischemia: dose-response effect of basic fibroblast growth factor. *J. Vasc. Surg.* **16,** 181–191.

127. Bauters, C., Asahara, T., Zheng, L. P., Takeshita, S., Bunting, S., Ferrara, N., et al. (1995) Site-specific therapeutic angiogenesis following systemic administration of vascular endothelial growth factor. *J. Vasc. Surg.* **21,** 314–325.

128. Takeshita, S., Pu, L.-Q., Zheng, L., Ferrara, N., Stein, L. A., Sniderman, A. D., Isner, J. M., and Symes, J. F. (1994) Vascular endothelial growth factor induces dose–dependent revascularization in a rabbit model of persistent limb ischemia. *Circulation* **90,** II–228–II–234.

129. Berkman, R. A., Merrill, M. J., Reinhold, W. C., Monacci, W. T., Saxena, A., Clark, W. C., et al. (1993) Expression of the vascular permeability factor/vascular endothelial growth factor gene in central nervous system neoplasms. *J. Clin. Invest.* **91,** 153–159.

130. Rohovsky, S., Kearney, M., Pieczek, A., Rosenfield, K., Schainfeld, R., D'Amore, P. A., and Isner, J. M. (1996) Elevated levels of basic fibroblast growth factor in patients with limb ischemia. *Am. Heart J.* **132,** 1015–1019.

131. Bauters, C., Asahara, T., Zheng, L. P., Takeshita, S., Bunting, S., Ferrara, N., et al. (1994) Physiologic assessment of augmented vascularity induced by VEGF in ischemic rabbit hindlimb. *Am. J. Physiol.* **267,** H1263–H1271.

132. Thieme, H., Aiello, L. P., Takagi, H., Ferrara, N., and King, G. L. (1995) Comparative analysis of vascular endothelial growth factor receptors on retinal and aortic vascular endothelial cells. *Diabetes* **44,** 98–103.

133. Brogi, E., Schatteman, G., Wu, T., Kim, E. A., Varticovski, L., Keyt, B., and Isner, J. M. (1996) Hypoxia-induced paracrine regulation of VEGF receptor expression. *J. Clin. Invest.* **97,** 469–476.

134. Folkman, J. (1971) Tumor angiogenesis: therapeutic implications. *N. Engl. J. Med.* **285,** 1182–1186.

135. Yanagisawa-Miwa, A., Uchida, Y., Nakamura, F., Tomaru, T., Kido, H., Kamijo, T., et al. (1992) Salvage of infarcted myocardium by angiogenic action of basic fibroblast growth factor. *Science* **257,** 1401–1403.

136. Connolly, D. T., Hewelman, D. M., Nelson, R., Olander, J. V., Eppley, B. L., Delfino, J. J., et al. (1989) Tumor vascular permeability factor stimulates endothelial cell growth and angiogenesis. *J. Clin. Invest.* **84,** 1470–1478.

137. Levy, A. P., Tamargo, R., Brem, H., and Nathans, D. (1989) An endothelial cell growth factor from the mouse neuroblastoma cell line NB41. *Growth Factors* **2**, 9–19.

138. Pu, L. Q., Jackson, S., Lachapelle, K. J., Arekat, Z., Graham, A. M., Lisbona, R., et al. (1994) A persistent hindlimb ischemia model in the rabbit. *J. Invest. Surg.* **7**, 49–60.

139. Harrison, D. G. (1992) Neurohumoral and pharmacologic regulation of collateral perfusion, in *Collateral Circulation*, (Schaper, W., and Schaper, J., eds.), Kluwer, Boston, MA, pp. 329–343.

140. Hollenberg, N. K. (1992) Collateral arterial growth and reactivity: lessons from the limb and renal blood supply, in *Collateral Circulation*, (Schaper, W., and Schaper, J., eds.), Kluwer, Boston, MA, pp. 1–15.

141. McFadden, E. P., Clarke, J. C., Davis, G. J., Kaski, J. C., Haider, A. W., and Maseri, A. (1991) Effect of intracoronary serotonin on coronary vessels in patients with stable and patients with variant angina. *N. Engl. J. Med.* **324**, 648–654.

142. Orlandi, C., Blackshear, J. L., and Hollenberg, N. K. (1986) Specific increase in sensitivity to serotonin of the canine hindlimb collateral arterial tree via the 5-hydroxytrptamine-2 receptor. *Microvasc. Res.* **32**, 121–130.

143. Sellke, F. W., Kagaya, Y., Johnson, R. G., Shafique, T., Schoen, F. J., Grossman, W., and Weintraum, R. M. (1992) Endothelial modulation of porcine coronary microcirculation perfused via immature collaterals. *Am. J. Physiol.* **262**, H1669–H1675.

144. Bauters, C., Asahara, T., Zheng, L. P., Takeshita, S., Bunting, S., Ferrara, N., et al. (1995) Recovery of disturbed endothelium-dependent flow in the collateral-perfused rabbit ischemic hindlimb after administration of vascular endothelial growth factor. *Circulation* **91**, 2802–2809.

145. Sellke, F. W., Wang, S. Y., Friedman, M., Harada, K., Edelman, E. R., Grossman, W., and Simons, M. (1994) Basic FGF enhances endothelium-dependent relaxation of the collateral-perfused coronary microcirculation. *Am. J. Physiol.* **267**, H1303–H1311.

146. Peters, K. G., deVries, C., and Williams, L. T. (1993) Vascular endothelial growth factor receptor expression during embryogenesis and tissue repair suggests a role in endothelial differentiation and blood vessel growth. *Proc. Natl. Acad. Sci. USA* **90**, 8915–8919.

147. Cohen, R. A., Shepherd, J. T., and Vanhoutte, P. M. (1983) Inhibitory role of the endothelium in the response of isolated coronary arteries to platelets. *Science* **221**, 273–274.

148. Janicek, M. J., Meyerovitz, M., Harrington, D. P., and Hollenberg, N. K. (1992) Arterial response to ketanserin and aspirin in patients with advanced peripheral atherosclerosis. *Invest. Radiol.* **27**, 415–421.

149. DeCree, J., Leempoels, J., Geukens, H., and Verhaegen, H. (1984) Placebo-controlled double blind trial of ketanserin in intermittent claudication. *Lancet* **2**, 775–779.

150. Losordo, D. W., Pickering, J. G., Takeshita, S., Leclerc, G., Gal, D., Weir, L., et al. (1994) Use of the rabbit ear artery to serially assess foreign protein secretion after site specific arterial gene transfer in vivo: evidence that anatomic identification of successful gene transfer may underestimate the potential magnitude of transgene expression. *Circulation* **89**, 785–792.

151. Takeshita, S., Losordo, D. W., Kearney, M., and Isner, J. M. (1994) Time course of recombinant protein secretion following liposome-mediated gene transfer in a rabbit arterial organ culture model. *Lab. Invest.* **71**, 387–391.

152. Riessen, R., Rahimizadeh, H., Blessing, E., Takeshita, S., Barry, J. J., and Isner, J. M. (1993) Arterial gene transfer using pure DNA applied directly to a hydrogel–coated angioplasty balloon. *Hum. Gene Ther.* **4**, 749–758.

153. Takeshita, S., Weir, L., Chen, D., Zheng, L. P., Riessen, R., Bauters, C., et al. (1996) Therapeutic angiogenesis following arterial gene transfer of vascular endothelial growth factor in a rabbit model of hindlimb ischemia. *Biochem. Biophys. Res. Comm.* **227**, 628–635.

154. Isner, J. M., Walsh, K., Symes, J., Pieczek, A., Takeshita, S., Lowry, J., et al. (1996) Arterial gene transfer for therapeutic angiogenesis in patients with peripheral artery disease. *Human Gene Ther.* **7**, 959–988.

155. Banai, S., Jaklitsch, M. T., Shou, M., Lazarous, D. F., Scheinowitz, M., Biro, S., et al. (1994) Angiogenic-induced enhancement of collateral blood flow to ischemic myocardium by vascular endothelial growth factor in dogs. *Circulation* **89**, 2183–2189.

156. Giordano, F. J., Ping, P., McKirnan, D., Nozaki, S., DeMaria, A. N., Dillmann, W. H., et al. (1996) Intracoronary gene transfer of fibroblast growth factor-5 increases blood flow and contractile function in an ischemic region of the heart. *Nature Med.* **2**, 534–539.

157. Harada, K., Grossman, W., Friedman, M., Edelman, E. R., Prasad, P. V., Keighlcy, C. S., et al. (1994) Basic fibroblast growth factor improves myocardial function in chronically ischemic porcine hearts. *J. Clin. Invest.* **94**, 623–630.

158. Hariawala, M., Horowitz, J. R., Esakof, D., Sheriff, D. D., Walter, D. H., Chaudhry, G. M., et al. (1996) VEGF improves myocardial blood flow but produces EDRF-mediated hypotension in porcine hearts. *J. Surg. Res.* **63,** 77–82.

159. Pearlman, J. D., Hibberd, M. G., Chuang, M. L., Harada, K., Lopez, J. J., Gladston, S. R., et al. (1995) Magnetic resonance mapping demonstrates benefits of VEGF-induced myocardial angiogenesis. *Nature Med.* **1,** 1085–1089.

160. Selke, F. W., Jianyi, L., Stamler, A., Lopez, J. J., Thomas, K. A., and Simons, M. (1996) Angiogenesis induced by acidic fibroblast growth factor as an alternative method of revascularization for chronic myocardial ischemia. *Surgery* **120,** 182–188.

161. Unger, E. F., Banai, S., Shou, M., Lazarous, D. F., Jaklitsch, M. T., Scheinowitz, M., et al. (1994) Basic fibroblast growth factor enhances myocardial collateral flow in a canine model. *Am. J. Physiol.* **266,** H1588–H1595.

162. Tabata, H., Silver, M., and Isner, J. M. (1997) Arterial gene transfer of acidic fibroblast growth factor for therapeutic angiogenesis in vivo: critical role of secretion signal in use of naked DNA. *Cardiovasc. Res.* in press.

163. Walder, C. E., Errett, C. J., Ogez, J., Heinshon, H., Bunting, S., Lindquist, P., et al. (1996) Vascular endothelial growth factor (VEGF) improves blood flow and function in a chronic ischemic hind limb model . *J. Cardiovasc. Pharmacol.* **27,** 91–98.

164. Yang, H. T., Deschenes, M. R., Ogilvie, R. W., and Terjung, R. L. (1996) Basic fibroblast growth factor increases collateral blood flow in rats with femoral arterial ligation. *Circ. Res.* **79,** 62–69.

165. Horowitz, J., Hariawala, M., Sheriff, D. D., Keyt, B., and Symes, J. F. (1995) In vivo administration of vascular endothelial growth factor is associated with EDRF–dependent systemic hypotension in porcine and rabbit animal models. *Circulation* **92,** I–630–I–631. (Abstract.)

166. Yang, R., Bunting, S., Ko, A., Keyt, B., and Jin, H. (1995) Hemodynamic effects of vascular endothelial growth factor in conscious rats. *Circulation* **92,** I–659. (Abstract.)

167. Muhlhauser, J., Pili, R., Merrill, M., Maeda, H., Passaniti, A., Crystal, R., and Capogrossi, M. C. (1995) In vivo angiogenesis induced by recombinant adenovirus vectors coding either for secreted or nonsecreted forms of acidic fibroblast growth factor. *Human Gene Ther.* **6,** 1457–1465.

168. Nabel, E. G., Yang, Z. Y., Plautz, G., Forough, R., Zhan, X., Haudenschild, C. C., Maciag, T., and Nabel, G. J. (1993) Recombinant fibroblast growth factor-1 promotes intimal hyperplasia and angiogenesis in arteries *in vivo. Nature* **362,** 844–846.

169. Goto, F., Goto, K., Weindel, K., and Folkman, J. (1993) Synergistic effects of vascular endothelial growth factor and basic fibroblast growth factor on the proliferaion and cord formation of bovine capillary endothelial cells within collagen gels. *Lab. Invest.* **69,** 508–517.

170. Lyons, M. K., Anderson, R. E., and Meyer, F. B. (1991) Basic fibroblast growth factor promotes in vivo cerebral angiogenesis in chronic forebrain ischemia. *Brain Res.* **558,** 315–320.

171. Mignatti, P., Tsuboi, R., Robbins, E., and Rifkin, D. B. (1989) In vitro angiogenesis on the human amniotic membrane: requirement for basic fibroblast growth factor–induced proteinases. *J. Cell Biol.* **108,** 671–682.

173. Nicosia, R. F., Nicosia, S. V., and Smith, M. (1994) Vascular endothelial growth factor, platelet-derived growth factor, and insulin-like growth factor-1 promote rat aortic angiogenesis in vitro. *Am. J. Pathol.* **145,** 1023–1029.

174. Leung, D. W., Cachianes, G., Kuang, W. J., Goeddel, D. V., and Ferrara, N. (1989) Vascular endothelial growth factor is a secreted angiogenic mitogen. *Science* **246,** 1306–1309.

175. Walter, D. H., Hink, U., Asahara, T., Van Belle, E., Horowitz, J., Tsurumi, Y., et al. (1996) The in vivo bioactivity of vascular endothelial growth factor/vascular permeability factor is independent of N-linked glycosylation. *Lab. Invest.* **74,** 546–556.

176. Horowitz, J. R., Rivard, A., van der Zee, R., Hariawala, M. D., Sheriff, D. D., Esakof, D. D., et al. (1997) Vascular endothelial growth factor/vascular permeability factor produces nitric oxide-dependent hypotension. *Arterioscler. Thromb. Vasc. Biol.* in press.

177. Isner, J. M. and Feldman, L. (1994) Gene therapy for arterial disease. *Lancet* **344,** 1653–1654.

16 Therapeutic Angiogenesis for the Heart

Johannes Waltenberger and Vinzenz Hombach

CONTENTS

INTRODUCTION

Angiogenesis takes place in many different organ systems and circumstances. Angiogenesis can be an essential part of a physiological process or it may contribute to pathological processes, as extensively described in other chapters of this book. In the developing heart, angiogenesis is — in addition to vasculogenesis, the formation of vascular structures out of angioblasts — an important process providing this highly perfused organ with a sufficient vascular network in order to fulfill its high metabolic requirements. Not only in the developing heart, but also in the adult heart, vascular growth, i.e. proliferation of vascular cells, can be observed as well, as demonstrated by the pioneering work of Schaper and coworkers (1). Angiogenesis contributes to the formation of collaterals as does the process of arteriogenesis, i.e., the formation of arteries out of pre-existing arterioles (2).

If a coronary stenosis is severe enough to result in regional myocardial ischemia, compensatory mechanisms are being activated to salvage that part of the myocardium. This includes changes in the metabolism of the myocardium resulting in hibernation and stunning (3), but also structural changes, such as the induction of collateralization, take place (Fig. 1) (4). Morphologically, different variations of the angiogenic process can be discriminated, which will be discussed later. In functional terms, however, newly formed capillaries are enhancing the regional myocardial blood flow, and the extent of existing collaterals is an important denominator for the functional resistance to regional myocardial ischemia. The functional importance of a coronary collateral circulation has long been realized (5,6); however, it was not until recently, when methods were developed to functionally assess the role of these collaterals (7–10). Moreover, recent efforts have

From: *The New Angiotherapy*
Edited by: T.-P. D. Fan and E. C. Kohn © Humana Press Inc., Totowa, NJ

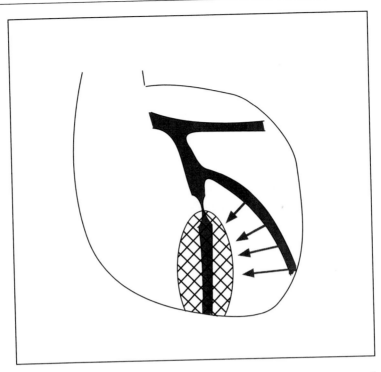

Fig. 1. Induction of collateral formation between two major coronary-artery branches secondary to regional myocardial ischemia (distal to high-grade coronary-artery stenosis).

been undertaken to stimulate the formation of coronary collaterals in experimental settings *(11)* as well as in the human situation *(12)*. This concept has been denominated "therapeutic angiogenesis" or "molecular bypass grafting" and is being developed as an alternative mode of myocardial revascularization.

It is the purpose of this chapter to highlight the functional significance and clinical importance of angiogenesis and arteriogenesis in the coronary circulation, to discuss the molecular and cellular basis of the formation of coronary collaterals, and to review the various strategies of therapeutic angiogenesis in the heart.

MYOCARDIAL ISCHEMIA
Scope of the Clinical Problem

Myocardial ischemia is a major cause of morbidity and mortality in the Western world. About half of all deaths in our society are directly or indirectly caused by myocardial ischemia and its sequelae, i.e., congestive heart failure and sudden cardiac death secondary to sustained ventricular arrhythmias. Recent efforts have resulted in the development of diagnostic tools covering both noninvasive as well as invasive means to detect myocardial ischemia. Moreover, substantial insights have been obtained into the mechanisms leading to the underlying atherosclerotic process *(13)*, clinical risk factors have been recognized, and strategies for preventing and decelerating this process have been developed. On the other hand, major advances in the development of therapeutic approaches have been made both in terms of options to treat acute and chronic myocardial ischema, as well as to prevent progression of the underlying atherosclerotic process and to reduce the likelihood of another recurring event.

Under certain circumstances, an evolving myocardial infarction may be regarded as a consequence of insufficient collateralization, and therefore of insufficient angiogenesis and arteriogenesis. It is interesting to note that the likelihood of developing a myocardial infarction is strictly dependent on the species, as is the ability to induce a collateral circulation, and there are species that do not develop a myocardial infarction at all; in these cases, a well developed collateral circulation can be found in normal hearts.

Options and Limitations of Current Therapeutic Approaches

Current modes and modalities of enhancing myocardial perfusion in the situation of acute and chronic myocardial ischemia are based on mechanical interventions: percutaneous transluminal coronary angioplasty (PTCA) (14), coronary-artery bypass surgery [15,16]), thrombolytic therapy (17), pharmacological modulation of vascular tone, and pharmacological modulation of the hemodynamic conditions affecting preload and afterload of the heart.

These conventional methods have clear limitations. Especially in diffusely narrowed epicardial coronary arteries, where both PTCA and the placement of coronary-artery bypass grafts is impossible and where medical treatment has become inefficient, alternative procedures such as cardiomyopexy or transmyocardial laser revascularization remain the only therapeutic options. Such procedures have been successfully applied. At least part of their beneficial effect is based on the induction of angiogenesis. These approaches will be discussed below (see section on Alternative Therapeutic Modalities).

THE CORONARY COLLATERAL CIRCULATION
Functional Impact of Coronary Collaterals

The functional importance of the coronary collateral circulation has been the subject of intense studies for almost a century (5,6,18–24), and these studies were initiated at times when the knowledge about its morphological basis was still rather poor. The important observation was made that the presence of coronary collaterals in patients is a reliable indicator of severe coronary-artery disease. When patients with angiographically documented coronary-artery disease were studied, those patients that developed collateral vessels had a higher prevalence of myocardial ischemia compared to those without collateral vessels (6), indicating that ischemia is the trigger for developing collaterals.

It is important to note that the presence of coronary collaterals may be of prognostic significance for the outcome of coronary events. The existence of an adequate collateral circulation supplying a coronary bed at risk may limit the infarct size following coronary occlusion (25) and may even result in a survival benefit (6,26,27). Therefore, the outcome and clinical presentation of an acute coronary occlusion is dependent on the existence and extent of preformed collaterals. Sasayama has summarized data obtained from studies of intracoronary thrombolysis and has drawn the following conclusions (28): (1) Myocardial ischemia is important for the development of a collateral circulation; (2) collaterals can perfuse the infarcted myocardium; and (3) the presence of collaterals prevents the left ventricular aneurysm formation following acute myocardial infarction, even when the amount of salvaged tissue is small. In the situation of stable angina pectoris, coronary collaterals can reduce the duration of exercise-induced ischemia by allowing a faster recovery (29). The collateral circulation limits myocardial ischemia (30) and reduces infarct size (31).

Recently, when methods were developed to functionally assess the role of these collaterals (8,9), the basis for a more detailed analysis of the individual status of the collateral circulation were set. It could already be shown that coronary collaterals are functionally regulated similar to small arteries (32).

Because exercise is regarded as a denominator of collateral formation *(33)*, efforts are being undertaken to stimulate collateral formation in patients at risk by enrolling them in coronary sport/exercise programs.

Development of Coronary Collaterals

Experimental models to stimulate coronary collateral development exist (reviewed in ref. *34*). Most of our current knowledge about the development of coronary collaterals was derived from these models. A well-established approach to induce regional myocardial ischemia in the animal model is to provoke the formation of coronary collaterals by the use of constrictor devices that are placed around a segment of an epicardial coronary artery during a surgical procedure. The most widely distributed device is the ameroid constrictor *(35)*, which—by progressive swelling—induces a continuous narrowing of the artery with total occlusion to be reached after a period of approx 2–3 wk. As an alternative to the ameroid constrictor, microembolization, i.e., injection of microspheres with a diameter of 25 µm into a defined region of the coronary circulation, has been shown to produce focal areas of myocardial ischemia without alteration of the pressure gradient between large coronary arteries *(36)*. Such an approach represents a sufficient stimulus to induce coronary collateral development *(37)*. Unlike ameroid constrictors and microspheres, inflatable cuff devices *(38)* carry the advantage that repeated episodes of ischemia can be generated. They also have been used successfully to induce a functional coronary collateral circulation *(39)*. Physical exercise is supporting this process *(40–42)*.

Using an ameroid-constrictor model, pioneering work by Schaper and coworkers was able to prove that regional myocardial ischemia was sufficient to induce the development of new coronary collaterals. Based on an active process of cellular growth involving active DNA synthesis, endothelial cells start to proliferate followed by smooth-muscle cell replication *(1)*. These findings represent a milestone in the establishment of the concept that coronary collateral development represents vascular growth and involves true angiogenesis, i.e., the formation of capillaries out of pre-existing capillaries *(43,44)*. Others have been able to reproduce these findings in a number of other species *(39,45)*.

It is important to note that the morphology of coronary collaterals varies strongly between different species: although the dog is a good model for studying the growth of large epicardial collaterals, pigs produce abundant small intramyocardial collaterals distributed over the entire area at risk *(44,46)*. This process of vascular growth in the porcine heart can be regarded as true angiogenesis, i.e., formation of new capillaries out of existing ones resulting in an increase of capillary density. On the other hand, the development of epicardial collaterals by remodeling of pre-existing arterioles into muscular distribution vessels can be observed in dogs. Historically, this process been regarded as a form of vasculogenesis, which is being recapitulated *(4)*, with vasculogenesis in its original sense describing the development of new vessels from angioblasts *in situ*, as normally observed during embryonic development *(47)*. More recently, the term "arteriogenesis" has been suggested and appears more appropriate for the process of the formation of muscular arteries out of small arterioles *(48)*. In the clinical context, this process has previously been described as the recruitment of preformed collaterals. In functional terms, arteriogenesis is responsible for the appearance of visible epicardial vessels with a diameter of about 100–200 µm. In the human heart, both mechanisms of angiogenesis and arteriogenesis contribute to the process of collateralization. Because of the fairly large diameter and flow capacity of true collaterals, the process of arteriogenesis represents an important mechanism of collateralization.

Although some cellular processes of collateral formation in the heart are well-understood, the mediators of this process are not well-defined yet; the functional impact of various candidate molecules remains to be established. Good candidates are the peptide growth factors acidic fibroblast growth factor (aFGF), basic fibroblast growth factor (bFGF), vascular endothelial growth factor-A (VEGF-A), insulin-like growth factor-1 (IGF-1), and platelet-derived growth factor (PDGF) (reviewed by Schaper and Ito, ref. *4*). These molecules and their functional cellular receptors have been shown to be present in the heart. VEGF-A has even been shown to be functionally active in the coronary circulation *(49)*, is strongly upregulated in the ischemic myocardium *(50)*, and its serum level is elevated following myocardial infarction in humans *(51)*. In addition, the mRNA expression of the VEGF receptor-1 (flt-1) and of the VEGF receptor-2 (KDR/flk-1) have been shown to be upregulated in a myocardial infarction model *(52)*. The same is true for KDR protein in the dog heart *(53)*. Data derived from cell-culture studies suggest that hypoxia seems to be the relevant stimulus leading to the upregulation of VEGF-A *(54)* and to the upregulation of its receptor KDR, the latter of which is upregulated both on the transcriptional level *(55)* as well as on the post-transcriptional level *(56)*. Because of an increased endothelial response under hypoxic conditions, VEGF-A may be called a survival factor for hypoxic endothelium. In the ischemic heart, monocytes and macrophages have been implied to contribute to the angiogenic process *(57)*. A number of inflammatory cytokines such as transforming growth factor-β (TGF-β), interleukin-1β (IL-1β) and IL-6 are capable of inducing the expression of angiogenic factors such as VEGF-A *(58,59)*. The potential of VEGF-A for playing a central role in this process is further supported by the recent observation that monocytes express a functional VEGF-receptor *(60)*. Besides the involvement of growth factors, local physical forces acting on the endothelial-cell membrane may be of importance in initiating and maintaining the angiogenic process in the coronary circulation *(44)*.

Although peptide growth factors are involved in both angiogenesis and arteriogenesis, a novel mechanism for the induction of arteriogenesis has recently been revealed. Using a model of rabbit hindlimb ischemia, Ito et al. *(2)* were able to show that the processes of angiogenesis and arteriogenesis are spatially dissociated with arteriogenesis taking place in the upper thigh, while angiogenesis can be observed in the lower thigh closely associated with tissue hypoxia. The observation was made that monocytes are being recruited and activated during arteriogenesis *(61)*. Finally, the hypothesis of the functional importance of monocytes for arteriogenesis could be proven by stimulating monocyte recruitment, which was achieved using monocyte chemoattractant protein-1 (MCP-1) *(62)*. The stimulation of arteriogenesis with MCP-1 is based on the release of various growth factors that are present in monocytes including VEGF-A, bFGF, endothelial growth factor (EGF), and TGF-β *(13)*. Stimulation of arteriogenesis using MCP-1 represents a novel conceptual approach. The feasibility of its therapeutic potential awaits to be proven in the ischemic and nonischemic heart.

According to our own, most recent findings, VEGF-A might well play an active role during the process of arteriogenesis *(63)*. We could demonstrate that VEGF-A induced migration of monocytes is significantly reduced in patients with diabetes mellitus. This finding provides first evidence that the loss of VEGF-A inducible migratory activity of monocytes may result in impaired arteriogenesis and collateral formation. The fact that diabetic patients develop significantly less collaterals has indeed been observed recently *(64)*.

There are two principle modes of the induction of coronary collateral formation: (1) Secondary to chronic regional ischemia or repeated episodes of ischemia, local mechanisms are being activated leading to the development of compensatory angiogenesis or arteriogenesis. This process is taking place within days and weeks after initiation. Therefore, these processes are not sufficient for the rapid generation of collaterals in the case of acute and complete regional ischemia, i.e., during the acute phase of myocardial infarction. Compensatory angiogenesis is being regarded as a functional repair mechanism resulting in the functional adaptation to a locally reduced myocardial blood flow, i.e., regional myocardial ischemia. In a number of circumstances, compensatory angiogenesis or arteriogenesis are inadequate to restore fully adequate tissue perfusion in time. Although a number of molecular promoters of this process have been identified as described earlier, the essential mediator (e.g., a specific growth factor or a combination of several growth factors) of collateral formation in the human heart is currently unknown. (2) Application of angiogenic and arteriogenic agents to accelerate and or intensify the induction of collaterals, i.e., therapeutic angiogenesis (see below).

THERAPEUTIC ANGIOGENESIS/THERAPEUTIC ARTERIOGENESIS IN THE HEART

Experimental Therapeutic Angiogenesis: Application of Growth Factors

The German gynecologist Michael Hoeckel was the first to create the expression "therapeutic angiogenesis" in 1989 to describe the stimulation of neovascularization aiming to treat or prevent local hypoperfusion. He has used this term in the context of wound healing and tissue regeneration (65). Following this pioneering work, a large number of studies were performed to treat regional ischemia (see below and Table 1). It is important to note, however, that angiogenesis (growth of capillaries) can only partly improve tissue perfusion owing to the limited flow capacity in these tiny vessels. Larger vessels such as arterioles and arteries (diameter > 100 µm) are required to transport relevant amounts of blood, as they are created by the process of arteriogenesis (growth of arteries out of arterioles/preformed collaterals) (48). This is why we suggest using the term "Therapeutic arteriogenesis" to describe the therapeutically induced growth of preformed collaterals for the treatment of regional ischemia.

The application of a variety of angiogenic agents, i.e., angiogenic growth factors (such as members of the FGF family or VEGF-A), to the heart has been performed in various laboratories and different animal models, mostly porcine or canine, starting in the early 1990s. These studies have proven the concept of the development of functional collaterals in the ischemic myocardium in response to the therapeutic application of an angiogenic factor (Table 1). The experimental work to stimulate angiogenesis in the heart has been performed in analogy to experiments done in other organs such as the peripheral circulation, where most of the data available for therapeutic angiogenesis have been obtained, providing valuable information about basics and principles of therapeutic angiogenesis (66).

It is important to note that the induction of angiogenesis is a process that takes place within days to weeks. One general problem of the different angiogenic molecules used so far is the short half-life of the known angiogenic proteins (67). Although there are data from animal experiments suggesting a single bolus of growth factor protein to be sufficient for the induction of collateral growth, most investigators have applied the angiogenic stimulus over a prolonged period of time. Efforts have been made to develop sustained-delivery approaches (see below).

Pioneering work on therapeutic angiogenesis in the heart was done using bFGF in the setting of acute myocardial ischemia. The application of an intracoronary bolus was

TABLE 1
Therapeutic Angiogenesis in the Heart

Growth factor	Species	Mode of Application	Results	Ref.
bFGF	Dog	2 × i.c. bolus	Capillary density (+) myocardial function (EF) (+)	(68)
bFGF	Pig	Slow-release bFGF i.c. bovine brain bFGF	Microvessel count (+)	(97)
bFGF	Pig	Slow-release polymer extravascular	Myocardial function (EF) (+) Left ventricular infarct size (−)	(98)
bFGF	Dog	Single bolus in pericardial cavity	Coronary blood flow (+) Vascular density (+) Infarct size (−)	(99)
bFGF	Dog	i.c.; daily bolus for 4 weeks	Density of distribution vessels (+) Collateral blood flow (+)	(100)
bFGF	Dog	Systemic; daily bolus for 4 weeks	Accelerated collateral development Collateral density (+) Maximal collateral flow (+)	(101)
bFGF	Rat	Slow-release matrix perivascular	Induction of a dense capillary Network by epicardial application in normal hearts	(102)
aFGF	Dog	Slow-release sponge perivascular	No angiogenic response	(103)
aFGF	Pigs	t1/2 mutated protein perivascular	Coronary blood flow (+) Myocardial function (EF) (+)	(70)
aFGF	Dog	Recombinant protein slow release device periadventitial	Myocardial perfusion in collateral dependent area (+)	(104)
FGF-5	Pig	Adenoviral vector encoding FGF-5	Regional myocardial blood flow (+) Regional contractile function (+)	(71)
VEGF-A	Dog	Chronic i.c.	Capillary density (+) Collateral blood flow (+) Density of intramyocardial Distribution vessels (+)	(71) (105)
VEGF-A	Pig	Chronic perivascular	Myocardial function (EF) (+) Left ventricular infarct size (−)	(106)
VEGF-A	Pig	Chronic perivascular	Collateral vessel density (+) Myocardial blood flow (+) Myocardial function (+)	(107)

Application of different growth factors/angiogenic factors can induce angiogenesis in different animal models of regional myocardial ischemia. Most of these studies demonstrate a functional benefit of this treatment for the perfusion of the ischemic myocardium and for the function of the whole heart. (+), stimulation; (−), reduction; i.c., intracoronary.

sufficient to find evidence for angiogenesis resulting in the improvement of myocardial function secondary to the reduction of infarct size (68). The induction of angiogenesis may be related to the decrease in infarct size, however, alternative mechanisms are likely to contribute to this functional benefit, because angiogenesis takes weeks rather than hours to contribute functionally to an improvement of tissue perfusion. One such mechanism might be the bFGF-induced improvement of ischemia-resistance of the myocardium, as suggested by a recent study (69). bFGF as well as VEGF-A have been successfully applied in models of chronic myocardial ischemia, generally provoked by the use of an ameroid constrictor (see earlier text).

A successful approach was the prolonged delivery of recombinant protein using various sustained-delivery approaches. They have been realized by the repeated application of recombinant protein, by continuous catheter-based delivery to the coronary artery or to the left atrium (intravascular approach). Alternatively, the epicardial or intrapericardial application of growth-factor protein, matrix-associated formulations such as sustained-release polymers or growth factor-saturated matrices is feasible (extravascular approach). An interesting novel approach is to modulate the half-life of the angiogenic protein itself by introducing a mutation into the recombinant protein (70).

An alternative approach to realize the sustained availability of an angiogenic factor is to use gene therapy. The first reported successful gene therapy-based approach to stimulate angiogenesis in the porcine heart was reported using an adenoviral construct encoding FGF-5, a member of the FGF family. The authors reported the stimulation of angiogenesis, enhancement of myocardial blood flow, and improvement of contractile function of the heart (71).

Clinical trials had been initiated to evaluate the feasibility of therapeutic angiogenesis in the human heart prone to coronary-artery disease. The study by Schumacher et al. (72) is a good example. Evidence for induction of angiogenesis in the heart has been presented before, but this is the first published study involving data obtained in human beings suffering from coronary-artery disease. Recombinant human fibroblast growth factor-1 (FGF-1, also denominated acidic FGF or aFGF) generated in *Escherichia coli* was injected into a defined area of the myocardium of 20 patients that underwent coronary artery bypass surgery. A total of 0.01 mg/kg body weight of FGF-1 were applied in each patient. Twelve weeks after the injection of the angiogenic agent, a part of the coronary circulation was visualized by injection of a contrast agent into the "feeding" bypass artery and using quantitative digital subtraction angiography. In the patients treated with FGF-1, accumulation of contrast medium was reported to be visible at the former site of injection and was associated with the presence of a capillary network. In the control group that received heat inactivated FGF-1, no such effect could be observed.

In the late 1990s, a number of different phase I/phase II trials have been initiated and reported, all of which — as far as there are data available to date — have all shown the feasibility of growth-factor application to the ischemic heart. These studies include the intracoronary application of recombinant bFGF (performed at the NIH, quoted in [73]), the extravascular application of recombinant bFGF vs placebo, where — at the time of bypass surgery — a slow-release polymer is applied locally to the extravascular surface of a coronary artery that could not be revascularized otherwise (73,74). In another study, recombinant human VEGF-A$_{165}$ was applied intracoronary as a single bolus, however, no beneficial effect of this approach over the negative control could be found after several months of follow-up (75). Several other studies have been initiated aiming in the realization of a gene-transfer approach. One study makes use of an adenoviral construct of FGF-4 that is injected into the coronary artery (Collateral Therapeutics, San Diego, CA). Adenoviral-based gene transfer approaches have also been initiated to induce coronary angiogenesis by intramyocardial injection of VEGF-A$_{121}$ during coronary-artery bypass surgery *(76)*. Finally, another strategy is based on the intramyocardial injection of a plasmid containing the gene for VEGF- A_{165} as the sole therapy of end-stage coronary-heart disease *(77)*. Again, this approach seems feasible. The lack of a control group, however, does not yet allow estimation the efficiency of this strategy.

Alternative Therapeutic Modalities to Stimulate Angiogenesis in the Human Heart

A number of established or novel approaches aiming at the revascularization of chronic ischemic myocardium are able to induce angiogenesis in the heart (or are believed to or claimed to do so).

An interesting surgical approach is a variant of cardiomyopexy *(78–81)*, i.e., transplantation of a perfused skeletal muscle onto the epicardium of an ischemic region of the heart. This procedure has already been introduced into clinical practise. Based on an intense contact between the epicardium of the ischemic area on one hand and the transplanted muscle on the other hand, functional new collaterals are developing providing evidence for the induction of angiogenesis, as shown in a canine model *(82)*. This process might be further enhanced by the intravascular application of bFGF *(83)*.

One of the oldest approaches for myocardial revascularization is the Vineberg procedure *(84)*, already introduced in 1945, at a time before the surgery of coronary anastomoses had been realized. The Vineberg procedure shows some similarities to cardiomyopexy *(85)*. The internal mammary artery is placed into the myocardium for additional blood supply. Unfortunately, this procedure had significant bleeding complications. It had never been systematically evaluated in terms of its exact functional mechanisms, including the induction of functional collaterals. It might have been worthwhile, however *(86)*.

During the past decade, transmyocardial laser revascularization (TMLR) *(87)* and more recently percutaneous myocardial (laser) revascularization (PMR), also called direct myocardial revascularization (DMR) *(88,89)*, have been developed to treat severe forms of ischemic heart disease, especially if there are no remaining options for classical forms of revasularization such as coronary-artery bypass grafting or angioplasty. The methodology to induce localized and small scars within the partially ischemic tissue may represent an alternative mode of inducing angiogenesis in the heart. There is good evidence for angiogenesis being induced in the heart secondary to the laser treatment *(90,91)*. Its functional significance, however, is subject to further investigation.

SUMMARY AND PERSPECTIVES

There is strong evidence for the functional relevance of coronary collaterals in myocardial perfusion. Regional myocardial ischemia and hypoxia have been found to induce the expression of angiogenic molecules and to activate mechanisms that enhance the formation of coronary collaterals. The concept of therapeutic angiogenesis, i.e., the application of angiogenic factors to induce angiogenesis in vivo, has been proven in a number of independent models of regional ischemia. The feasibility of the induction of "therapeutic angiogenesis" and "therapeutic arteriogenesis" in the human heart seems to be in reach. In fact, several phase I/phase II trials are currently under way to evaluate side effects of the administration of angiogenic factors, their cDNAs or viral constructs. The central question will be, however, whether beneficial effects of therapeutic angiogenesis could be shown in ischemic heart disease in man.

POTENTIAL LIMITATIONS AND OPEN QUESTIONS

So far, successful therapeutic stimulation of angiogenesis and/or arteriogenesis in the human heart that leads to a documented improvement of myocardial perfusion or myocardial function has not been achieved yet. There is evidence for angiogenesis in surgically induced collaterals on the basis of transplantation of a muscle flap (cardiomyopexy). Approaches to apply angiogenic factors have been initiated and prove of principle has been demonstrated recently *(72)*. One has to be aware that there are substantial differences in the diseased human heart as compared to the various animal models tested so far. The latter ones are based on inducing either a total and acute or a progressive and chronic myocardial ischemia in a previously healthy heart. It is currently unknown, whether the pre-existing coronary-artery disease will have significant impact on the ability to induce functional collaterals in these hearts. In fact, the transfer of the preclinical data into the human situation will be critical for the concept of therapeutic angiogenesis and therapeutic arteriogenesis. Currently, several different modes and routes of application are being evaluated for getting the angiogenic stimulus to where it is needed, including catheter-based strategies of local or regional application; surgical approaches, including adjunct measures to bypass surgery; as well as adjunct measures to surgical or percutaneous transmyocardial laser revascularization.

The best mode of application of the angiogenesis-promoting factor (the one that finally might work best in the human situation) remains to be defined. Both local and systemic applications have been tried: intravascular and extravascular ones, continuous, repeated, or prolonged applications of recombinant protein, matrix-bound sustained-delivery approaches; genetically modified proteins with different pharmacokinetics; as well as gene therapy-based approaches.

Although there is only a limited experimental basis at the moment, there is an interesting perspective for systemic therapeutic angiogenesis in the heart, which would greatly facilitate treatment protocols for patients: because the VEGF receptor KDR is upregulated under hypoxic conditions in vitro *(55,56)*, the ischemic area and its border zone, i.e., the area of interest, is likely to respond better to the angiogenic stimulus VEGF-A. In addition, there is experimental in vivo evidence that systemic therapeutic angiogenesis may be feasible *(92)*.

An interesting aspect of collateral formation in patients are (putative) denominators of the extent of the angiogenic and arteriogenic response. The functional response to VEGF-A is impaired in vitro in the presence of elevated glucose concentrations *(93)*, raising the interesting hypothesis of whether the response of therapeutic angiogenesis may be attenuated in diabetic patients.

Finally, angiogenic treatment has potential side effects. These include the stimulation of neointima formation and therefore progression of the atherosclerotic process *(94,95)* as suggested in the case of bFGF, which can directly stimulate smooth muscle-cell proliferation. This effect could not be found in a canine model *(96)*, which may be different from the human situation, because dogs normally do not develop atherosclerosis or atherosclerosis-like changes in the vessel wall. In this model, however, VEGF-A, which is mostly acting on endothelial cells, caused vascular remodeling. This issue is controversial and currently unresolved. Of potential clinical importance is the fact that angiogenic factors have been shown to contribute to tumor angiogenesis. Therefore, another potential side effect of angiogenic therapy could be the stimulation of tumor angiogenesis and therefore the activation and promotion of malignancies. Still, this concern is hypothetical and no experimental evidence for its occurrence has been found so far.

REFERENCES

1. Schaper, W., DeBrabander, M., and Lewi, P. (1971) DNA-synthesis and mitoses in coronary collateral vessels in the dog. *Circ. Res.* **28,** 671–679.
2. Ito, W. D., Arras, M., Scholz, D., Winkler, B., Htun, P., and Schaper, W. (1997) Angiogenesis but not collateral growth is associated with ischemia after femoral artery occlusion. *Am. J. Physiol.* **42,** H1255–H1265.
3. Heusch, G. (1991) The relationship between regional blood flow and contractile function in normal, ischemic, and reperfused myocardium. *Basic Res. Cardiol.* **86,** 197–218.
4. Schaper, W. and Ito, W. D. (1996) Molecular mechanisms of coronary collateral vessel growth. *Circ. Res.* **79,** 911–919.
5. Geninsi, G. G. and DaCosta, B. C. (1969) The coronary collateral circulation in living man. *Am. J. Cardiol.* **24,** 394–400.
6. Helfant, R. H., Vokonas, P. S., and Gorlin, R. (1971) Functional importance of the human coronary collateral circulation. *N. Engl. J. Med.* **284,** 1277–1281.
7. Rentrop, K. P., Feit, F., Sherman, W., and Thornton, J. C. (1989) Serial angiographic assessment of coronary artery obstruction and collateral flow in myocardial infarction. Report from the second Mount Sinai - New York University Reperfusion Trial. *Circulation* **80,** 1166–1175.
8. Sabia, P. J., Powers, E. R., Ragosta, M., Sarembock, I. J., Burwell, L. R., and Kaul, S. (1992) An association between collateral blood flow and myocardial viability in patients with recent myocardial infarction. *N. Engl. J. Med.* **327,** 1825–1831.
9. Bach, R. G., Donohue, T. J., Caracciolo, E. A., Wolford, T., Aguirre, F. V., and Kern, M. J. (1996) Quantification of collateral blood flow during PTCA by intravascular ultrasound. *Eur. Heart J.* **16(Suppl. J),** 74–77.
10. Piek, J. J., van Liebergen, R. A. M., Koch, K. T., Peters, R. J. G., and David, G. K. (1997) Clinical, angiographic and hemodynamic predictors of recruitable collateral flow assessed during balloon angioplasty coronary occlusion. *J. Am. Coll. Cardiol.* **29,** 275–282.
11. Waltenberger, J. (1997) Modulation of growth factor action. Implications for the treatment of cardiovascular diseases. *Circulation* **96,** 4083–4095.
12. Waltenberger, J. (1998) Therapeutic angiogenesis in the heart using peptide growth factors: Angiogenesis research entering clinical trials. *Angiogenesis* **2,** 115–117.
13. Ross, R. (1993) The pathogenesis of atherosclerosis: a perspective for the 1990s. *Nature* **362,** 801–809.
14. Landau, C., Lange, R. A., and Hillis, L. D. (1994) Medical progress: percutaneous transluminal coronary angioplasty. *N. Engl. J. Med.* **330,** 981–993.
15. Favaloro, R. G. (1969) Saphenous vein graft in the surgical treatment of coronary artery disease. *J. Thorac. Cardiovasc. Surg.* **41,** 178–185.
16. Kolessov, V. I. (1967) Mammary artery-coronary artery anastomosis as method of treatment for angina pectoris. *J. Thorac. Cardiovasc. Surg.* **54,** 535–544.
17. The GUSTO Angiographic Investigators (1993) The effect of tissue plasminogen activator, streptokinase, or both on coronary patency, ventricular function and survival after acute myocardial infarction. *N. Engl. J. Med.* **329,** 1615–1622.
18. Spalteholz, W. (1907) Die Coronararterien des Herzens. *Verh. Anat. Ges.* **21,** 141–153.
19. Gregg, D. E., Thornton, J. J., and Mautz, F. R. (1939) The magnitude, adequacy and source of the collateral blood flow and pressure in chronicallyoccluded coronary arteries. *Am. J. Physiol.* **127,** 161–175.
20. Blumgart, H. L., Schlesinger, M. J., and Davis, D. (1940) Studies on the relation of the clinical manifestation of angina pectoris, coronary thrombosis, and myocardial infarction to the pathologic findings: with particular reference to the significance of the collateral circulation. *Am. Heart J.* **19,** 1–91.
21. Eckstein, R., Gregg, D., and Pritchard, H. (1941) *Am. J. Physiol.* **132,** 351–361.
22. Wiggers, C. J. (1952) The functional importance of coronary collaterals. *Circulation* **5,** 609–615.
23. Kattus, A. A. and Gregg, D. E. (1959) Some determinants of coronary collateral blood flow in the open-chest dog. *Circ. Res.* **7,** 628–642.
24. Paulin, S. (1967) Interarterial coronary anastomoses in relation to arterial obstruction demonstrated in coronary arteriography. *Invest. Radiol.* **2,** 147–159.
25. Habib, G. B., Heibig, J., Forman, S. A., Brown, G. G., Roberts, R., Terrin, M. L., and Bolli, R. (1991) Influence of coronary collateral vessels on myocardial infarct size in humans: results of phase I Thrombolysis In Myocardial Infarction (TIMI) trial. *Circulation* **83,** 739–746.

26. Hansen, J. F. (1989) Coronary collateral circulation: clinical significance and influence on survival in patients with coronary artery disease. *Am. Heart J.* **117,** 290–295.
27. Williams, D. O., Amsterdam, E. A., Miller, R. R., and Mason, D. T. (1976) Functional significance of coronary collateral vessels in patients with acute myocardial infarction. Relation to pump performance, cardiogenic shock and survival. *Am. J. Cardiol.* **37,** 345–351.
28. Sasayama, S. (1994) Effect of coronary collateral circulation on myocardial ischemia and ventricular dysfunction. *Cardiovasc. Drug Ther.* **8,** 327–334.
29. Bonetti, F., Margonato, A., Mailhac, A., Carandente, O., Cappelletti, A., Ballarotto, C., and Chierchia, S. L. (1992) Coronary collaterals reduce the duration of exercise-induced ischemia by allowing a faster recovery. *Am. Heart J.* **124,** 48–55.
30. Cohen, M. and Rentrop, K. P. (1986) Limitation of myocardial ischemia by collateral circulation during sudden controlled coronary artery occlusion in human subjects: a prospective study. *Circulation* **74,** 469–476.
31. Ramanathan, K. B., Wilson, J. L., Ingram, L. A., and Mirvis, D. M. (1995) Effects of immature recruitable collaterals on myocardial blood flow and infarct size after acute coronary occlusion. *J. Lab. Clin. Med.* **125,** 66–71.
32. Frank, M. W., Harris, K. R., Ahlin, K. A., and Klocke, F. J. (1996) Endothelium-derived relaxing factor (nitric oxide) has a tonic vasodilating action on coronary collateral vessels. *J. Am. Coll. Cardiol.* **27,** 658–663.
33. Eckstein, R. W. (1957) Effect of exercise and coronary artery narrowing on coronary collateral circulation. *Circ. Res.* **5,** 230–235.
34. Schaper, W. and Schaper, J. (1993) *Collateral Circulation: Heart, Brain, Kidney, Limbs.* Dordrecht, Kluwer Academic Publishers, Boston.
35. Litvak, J., Siderides, L. E., and Vineberg, A. M. (1957) Experimental production of coronary artery insufficiency and occlusion. *Am. Heart J.* **53,** 505–518.
36. Eng, C., Cho, S., Factor, S. M., Sonnenblick, E. H., and Kirk, E. S. (1984) Myocardial micronecrosis produced by microsphere embolization. Role of an a-adrenergic tonic influence on the coronary microcirculation. *Circ. Res.* **54,** 74–82.
37. Chilian, W. M., Mass, H. J., Williams, S. E., Layne, S. M., Smith, E. E., and Scheel, K. W. (1990) Microvascular occlusions promote coronary collateral growth. *Am. J. Physiol.* **258,** H1103–H1111.
38. Gwirtz, P. A. (1986) Construction and evaluation of a coronary catheter for chronic implantation in dogs. *J. Appl. Physiol.* **60,** 720–726.
39. Rugh, K. S., Garner, H. E., Hatfield, D. G., and Miramonti, J. R. (1987) Ischaemia induced development of functional coronary collateral circulation in ponies. *Cardiovasc. Res.* **21,** 730–736.
40. Cohen, M. V., Yipintsoi, T., and Scheuer, J. (1982) Coronary collateral stimulation by exercise in dogs with stenotic coronary arteries. *J. Appl. Physiol.* **52,** 664–671.
41. Bloor, C. M., White, F. C., and Sanders, T. M. (1984) Effect of exercise on collateral development in myocardial ischemia in pigs. *J. Appl. Physiol.* **56,** 656–665.
42. Roth, D. M., White, F. C., Nichols, M. L., Dobbs, S. L., Longhurst, J. C., and Bloor, C. M. (1990) Effect of long-term exercise on regional myocardial function and coronary collateral development after gradual coronary artery occlusion in pigs. *Circulation* **82,** 1778–1789.
43. Schaper, W., Sharma, H. S., Quinkler, W., Markert, T., Wünsch, M., and Schaper, J. (1990) Molecular biologic concepts of coronary anastomoses. *J. Am. Coll. Cardiol.* **15,** 513–518.
44. Schaper, W. (1995) Control of coronary angiogenesis. *Eur. Heart J.* **16(Suppl. C),** 66–68.
45. White, F. C., Carroll, S. M., Magnet, A., and Bloor, C. M. (1992) Coronary collateral development in swine after coronary artery occlusion. *Circ. Res.* **71,** 1490–1500.
46. Schaper, J. and Weihrauch, D. (1993) Collateral vessel development in the porcine and canine heart. Morphology revisited, in *Collateral Circulation: Heart, Brain, Kidney, Limbs* (Schaper, W. and Schaper, J., eds.), Kluwer Academic Publishers, Boston, pp. 65–102.
47. Dumont, D. J., Fong, G.-H., Puri, M. C., Gradwohl, G. J., Alitalo, D., and Breitman, M. L. (1995) Vascularization of the mouse embryo: a study of flk-1, tek, tie, and vascular endothelial growth factor expression during development. *Dev. Dyn.* **203,** 80–92.
48. Schaper, W. and Buschmann, I. (1999) Collateral circulation and diabetes (editorial). *Circulation* **99,** 2224–2226.
49. Kranz, A., Mayr, U., Frank, H., and Waltenberger, J. (1999) The coronary endothelium: a target for VEGF. Human coronary artery endothelial cells express functional receptors for VEGF *in vitro* and *in vivo*. *Lab. Invest.* **79,** 985–991.

50. Banai, S., Shweiki, D., Pinson, A., Chandra, M., Lazarovici, G., and Keshet, E. (1994) Upregulation of vascular endothelial growth factor expression induced by myocardial ischaemia: implications for coronary angiogenesis. *Cardiovasc. Res.* **28,** 1176–1179.

51. Kranz, A., Rau, C., Kochs, M., and Waltenberger, J. (2000) Elevation of vascular endothelial growth factor-A serum levels following acute myocardial infarction. Evidence for its origin and functional significance. *J. Mol. Cell. Cardiol.* **im Druck,**

52. Li, J., Brown, L. F., Hibberd, M. G., Grossman, J. D., Morgan, J. P., and Simons, M. (1996) VEGF, *flk-1*, and *flt-1* expression in a rat myocardial infarction model of angiogenesis. *Am. J. Physiol.* **270,** H1803–H1811.

53. Waltenberger, J., von Bonin, J., Scheunert, T., Gerber, J., Göller, V., Theiss, A., et al. (1998) Molecular mechanisms of collateral-formation in the ischemic myocardium. *Thorac. Cardiovasc. Surg.* **46(Suppl. 1),** 184.

54. Shweiki, D., Itin, A., Soffer, D., and Keshet, E. (1992) Vascular endothelial growth factor induced by hypoxia may mediate hypoxia-initiated angiogenesis. *Nature* **359,** 843–845.

55. Brogi, E., Schatteman, G., Wu, T., Kim, E. A., Varticovski, L., Keyt, B., and Isner, J.M. (1996) Hypoxia-induced paracrine regulation of vascular endothelial growth factor receptor expression. *J. Clin. Invest.* **97,** 469–476.

56. Waltenberger, J., Mayr, U., Pentz, S., and Hombach, V. (1996) Functional upregulation of the vascular endothelial growth factor receptor KDR by hypoxia. *Circulation* **94,** 1647–1654.

57. Sunderkötter, C., Steinbrink, K., Goebeler, M., Bhardwaj, R., and Sorg, C. (1994) Macrophages and angiogenesis. *J. Leukocyte Biol.* **55,** 410–422.

58. Brogi, E., Wu, T., Namiki, A., and Isner, J. M. (1994) Indirect angiogenic cytokines upregulate VEGF and bFGF gene expression in vascular smooth muscle cells, whereas hypoxia upregulates VEGF expression only. *Circulation* **90,** 649–652.

59. Cohen, T., Nahari, D., Cerem, C. W., Neufeld, G., and Levi, B.-Z. (1996) Interleukin 6 induces the expression of vascular endothelial growth factor. *J. Biol. Chem.* **271,** 736–741.

60. Clauss, M., Weich, H., Breier, G., Knies, U., Röckl, W., Waltenberger, J., and Risau, W. (1996) The vascular endothelial growth factor receptor FLT-1 mediates biological activities: Implications for a functional role of placenta growth factor in monocyte activation and chemotaxis. *J. Biol. Chem.* **271,** 17,629–17,634.

61. Arras, M., Ito, W. D., Scholz, D., Winkler, B., Schaper, J., and Schaper, W. (1998) Monocyte activation in angiogenesis and collateral growth in the rabbit hindlimb. *J. Clin. Invest.* **101,** 40–50.

62. Ito, W. D., Arras, M., Winkler, B., Scholz, D., Schaper, J., and Schaper, W. (1997) Monocyte chemotactic protein-1 increases collateral and peripheral conductance after femoral artery occlusion. *Circ. Res.* **80,** 829–837.

63. Waltenberger, J., Lange, J., and Kranz, A. (2000) Vascular endothelial growth factor-induced chemotaxis of monocytes is attenuated in patients with diabetes mellitus. A potential predictor for the individual capacity to develop collaterals. *Circulation* **101,** in press.

64. Abaci, A., Oguzhan, A., Kahraman, S., Eryol, N.K., Ünal, S., Arinc, H., and Ergin, A. (1999) Effect of diabetes mellitus on formation of coronary collateral vessels. *Circulation* **99,** 2239–2242.

65. Höckel, M. and Burke, F. J. (1989) Angiotropin treatment prevents flap necrosis and enhances dermal regeneration in rabbits. *Arch. Surg.* **124,** 693–698.

66. Takeshita, S., Zheng, L. P., Brogi, E., Kearney, M., Pu, L.-Q., Bunting, S., et al. (1994) Therapeutic angiogenesis. A single intraarterial bolus of vascular endothelial growth factor augments revascularization in a rabbit ischemic hind limb model. *J. Clin. Invest.* **93,** 662–670.

67. Waltenberger, J., Usuki, K., Fellström, B., Funa, K., and Heldin, C.-H. (1992) Platelet-derived endothelial cell growth factor: Pharmacokinetics, organ distribution and degradation after intravenous administration in rats. *FEBS Lett.* **313,** 129–132.

68. Yanagisawa-Miwa, A., Uchida, Y., Nakamura, F., Tomaru, T., Kido, H., Kamijo, T., et al. (1992) Salvage of infarcted myocardium by angiogenic action of basic fibroblast growth factor. *Science* **257,** 1401–1403.

69. Horrigan, M. C. G., MacIsaac, A. I., Nicolini, F. A., Vince, D. G., Lee, P., Ellis, S. G., and Topol, E. J. (1996) Reduction of myocardial infarct size by basic fibroblast growth factor after temporary coronary occlusion in a canine model. *Circulation* **94,** 1927–1933.

70. Lopez, J. J., Edelman, E. R., Stambler, A., Thomas, K. A., DiSalvo, J., Hibberd, M. G., et al. (1996) Perivascular delivery of prolonged half-life aFGF via EVAC results in angiographic collateral development, improvement in coronary flow and function in chronic myocardial ischemia. *J. Am. Coll. Cardiol.* **27,** 30A.

71. Giordano, F. J., Ping, P., McKirnan, M. D., Nozaki, S., DeMaria, A. N., Dillmann, W. H., et al. (1996) Intracoronary gene transfer of fibroblast growth factor-5 increases blood flow and contractile function in an ischemic region of the heart. *Nature Med.* **2,** 534–539.

72. Schumacher, B., Pecher, P., von Specht, B. U., and Stegmann, T. (1998) Induction of neoangiogenesis in ischemic myocardium by human growth factors. First clinical results of a new treatment of coronary heart disease. *Circulation* **97,** 645–650.

73. Ware, J. A. and Simons, M. (1997) Angiogenesis in ischemic heart disease. Inducing the formation of new blood vessels - a novel approach to treating myocardial ischemia. *Nature Med.* **3,** 158–164.

74. Laham, R. J., Sellke, F. W., Edelman, E. R., Pearlman, J. D., Ware, J. A., Brown, D. L., et al. (1999) Local perivascular delivery of basic fibroblast growth factor in patients undergoing coronary bypass surgery: results of a phase I randomized, double-blind, placebo-controlled trial. *Circulation* **100,** 1865–1871.

75. Henry, T. D., Annex, B. H., Azrin, M. A., McKendall, G., Willerson, J. T., Giordano, F. J., et al. (1999) Final results of the VIVA trial of rhVEGF for human therapeutic angiogenesis. *Circulation* **101,** I–476.

76. Rosengart, T. K., Lee, L. Y., Patel, S. R., Sanborn, T. A., Parikh, M., Bergman, G. W., et al. (1999) Angiogenesis gene therapy: phase I assessment of direct intramyocardial administration of an adenovirus vector expressing VEGF121 cDNA to individuals with clinically significant severe coronary artery disease. *Circulation* **100,** 468–474.

77. Losordo, D. W., Vale, P. R., Symes, J. F., Dunnington, C. H., Esakof, D. D., Maysky, M., et al. (1998) Gene therapy for myocardial angiogenesis: initial clinical results with direct myocardial injection of phVEGF(165) as sole therapy for myocardial ischemia. *Circulation* **98,** 2800–2804.

78. Beyer, M., Hoffer, H., Eggeling, T., Goertz, A., Mierdl, S., and Hannekum, A. (1992) Cardiomyoplasty to improve myocardial collateral blood supply as an alternative to transplantation in intractable angina. *J. Heart Lung Transpl.* **11,** 189–191.

79. Beyer, M., Hoffer, H., Eggeling, T., Matt, O., Beyer, U., and Hannekum, A. (1993) Free skeletal muscle transplantation to an infarction area: an experimental study in the dog. *Microsurg.* **14,** 125–129.

80. Beyer, M., Beyer, U., Mierdl, S., Sirch, J., von Behren, H., and Hannekum, A. (1994) Indirect myocardial revascularization: an experimental study in the dog. *Eur. J. Cardiothorac. Surg.* **8,** 557–562.

81. Beyer, M., Mierdl, S., Scheunert, T., Schleich, S., Oertel, F., and Hannekum, A. (1996) Erste klinische Erfahrungen mit indirekter Myokardrevaskularisation - freie Skelettmuskeltransplantation zur Induktion epi-myokardialer Gefäßeinsprosung. *Z. Kardiol.* **85(Suppl. 4),** 29–33.

82. Beyer, M., Hoffer, H., Matt, O., Hemmer, W., and Hannekum, A. (1993) Myocardial revascularization with a free skeletal muscle transplant: a functional analysis of angiogenesis. *Vasa* **22,** 113–119.

83. Mannion, J. D., Blood, V., Bailey, W., Bauer, T. L., Magno, M. G., DiMeo, F., et al. (1996) The effect of basic fibroblast growth factor on the blood flow and morphologic features of a latissimus dorsi cardiomyoplasty. *J. Thorac. Cardiovasc. Surg.* **111,** 19–28.

84. Vineberg, A. M. (1947) Development of an anastomosis between the coronary vessels and a transplanted internal mammary artery. *Can. Med. Assoc. J.* **56,** 609–614.

85. Shrager, J. B. (1994) The Vineberg procedure: the immediate forerunner of coronary artery bypass grafting. *Ann. Thorac. Surg.* **57,** 1354–1364.

86. Shrager, J. B. (1994) The Vineberg procedure: reply. *Ann. Thorac. Surg.* **57,** 1794.

87. Schofield, P. M., Sharples, L. D., Caine, N., Burns, S., Tait, S., Wistow, T., et al. (1999) Transmyocardial laser revascularisation in patients with refractory angina: a randomised controlled trial. *Lancet* **353,** 519–524.

88. Lauer, B., Junghans, U., Stahl, F., Kluge, R., Oesterle, S. N., and Schuler, G. (1999) Catheter-based percutaneous myocardial laser revascularization in patients with end-stage coronary artery disease. *J. Am. Coll. Cardiol.* **34,** 1663–1670.

89. Burkhoff, D., Schmidt, S., Schulman, S. P., Myers, J., Resar, J., Becker, L. C., et al. (1999) Transmyocardial laser revascularisation compared with continued medical therapy for treatment of refractory angina pectoris: a prospective randomised trial. *Lancet* **354,** 885–890.

90. Gassler, N., Rastar, F., and Hentz, M. W. (1999) Angiogenesis and expression of tenascin after transmural laser revascularization. *Histol. Histopathol.* **14,** 81–87.

91. Chu, V., Kuang, J., McGinn, A., Giaid, A., Korkola, S., and Chiu, R. C. (1999) Angiogenic response induced by mechanical transmyocardial revascularization. *J. Thorac. Cardiovasc. Surg.* **118,** 849–856.

92. Bauters, C., Asahara, T., Zheng, L. P., Takeshita, S., Bunting, S., Ferrara, N., et al. (1995) Site-specific therapeutic angiogenesis after systemic administration of vascular endothelial growth factor. *J. Vasc. Surg.* **21,** 314–325.

93. Waltenberger, J., Gürtler, R., Frank, H., Böhmer, F., and Hombach, V. (1996) Elevated glucose concentrations impair the endothelial response to vascular endothelial growth factor. A potential mechanism leading to endothelial dysfunction in diabetes mellitus. *Circulation* **94(Suppl.),** I–230.

94. Lindner, V. and Reidy, M. A. (1991) Proliferation of smooth muscle cells after vascular injury is inhibited by an antibody against basic fibroblast growth factor. *Proc. Natl. Acad. Sci. USA* **88,** 3739–3743.

95. Edelman, E. R., Nugent, M. A., Smith, L. T., and Karnovsky, M. J. (1992) Basic fibroblast growth factor enhances the coupling of intimal hyperplasia and proliferation of vasa vasorum in injured rat arteries. *J. Clin. Invest.* **89,** 465–473.

96. Lazarous, D. F., Shou, M., Scheinowitz, M., Hodge, E., Thirumurti, V., Kitsiou, A. N., et al. (1996) Comparative effects of basic fibroblast growth factor and vascular endothelial growth factor on coronary collateral development and the arterial response to injury. *Circulation* **94,** 1074–1082.

97. Battler, A., Scheinowitz, M., Bor, A., Hasdai, D., Vered, Z., DiSegni, E., et al. (1993) Intracoronary injection of basic fibroblast growth factor enhances angiogenesis in infarcted swine myocardium. *J. Am. Coll. Cardiol.* **22,** 2001–2006.

98. Harada, K., Grossman, W., Friedman, M., Edelman, E. R., Prasad, P. V., Keighley, C. S., et al. (1994) Basic fibroblast growth factor improves myocardial function in chronically ischemic porcine hearts. *J. Clin. Invest.* **94,** 623–630.

99. Uchida, Y., Yanagisawa-Miwa, A., Ikuta, M., Makamura, F., Tomaru, T., Fujimori, Y., and Morita, T. (1994) Angiogenic therapy of acute myocardial infarction (AMI) by intrapericardial injection of basic fibroblast growth factor (bFGF) and haparan sulfate (HS): an experimental study. *Circulation* **90,** I–296.

100. Unger, E. F., Banai, S., Shou, M., Lazarous, D. F., Jaklitsch, M. T., Scheinowitz, M., et al. (1994) Basic fibroblast growth factor enhances myocardial collateral flow in a canine model. *Am. J. Physiol.* **35,** H1588–H1595.

101. Lazarous, D. F., Scheinowitz, M., Shou, M., Hodge, E., Rajanayagam, M. A. S., Hunsberger, S., et al. (1995) Effects of chronic systemic administration of basic fibroblast growth factor on collateral development in the canine heart. *Circulation* **91,** 145–153.

102. Barrios, V., Cuevas, B., Carceller, F., Asin, E., Jiménez, J.J., Navarro, J., et al. (1995) Angiogenesis in the rat heart induced by local delivery of basic fibroblast growth factor. *Eur. Heart J.* **16(Abstract Suppl.),** 171.

103. Banai, S., Jaklitsch, M. T., Casscells, W., Shou, M., Shrivastav, S., Correa, R., et al. (1991) Effects of acidic fibroblast growth factor on normal and ischemic myocardium. *Circ. Res.* **69,** 76–85.

104. Sellke, F. W., Li, J., Stamler, A., Lopez, J. J., Thomas, K. A., and Simons, M. (1996) Angiogenesis induced by acidic fibroblast growth factor as an alternative method of revascularization for chronic myocardial ischemia. *Surgery* **120,** 182–188.

105. Banai, S., Jaklitsch, M. T., Shou, M., Lazarous, D. F., Scheinowitz, M., Biro, S., et al. (1994) Angiogenic-induced enhancement of collateral blood flow to ischemic myocardium by vascular endothelial growth factor in dogs. *Circulation* **89,** 2183–2189.

106. Pearlman, J. D., Hibberd, M. G., Chuang, M. L., Harada, K., Lopez, J. J., Gladstone, S. R., et al. (1995) Magnetic resonance mapping demonstrates benefits of VEGF-induced myocardial angiogenesis. *Nature Med.* **1,** 1085–1089.

107. Harada, K., Friedman, M., Lopez, J. J., Wang, S. Y., Li, J., Prasad, P. V., et al. (1996) Vascular endothelial growth factor administration in chronic myocardial ischemia. *Am. J. Physiol.* **270,** H1791–H1802.

17 Contact-Guided Angiogenesis and Tissue Engineering

Robert A. Brown, Giorgio Terenghi, and Clive D. McFarland

Contents

INTRODUCTION

It is clear that angiogenesis is a critical component in almost all forms of tissue repair aside from cartilage and some cartilage-like tissues. The most widely studied example is in dermal repair *(1,2)* but others include repair of bone, tendon, and peripheral nerve. New microvessels form as part of the early granulation tissue, through invasion of the initial fibrin-based clot. In dermal repair, the fine, apparently random network of vessels at this stage *(2)* is remodeled in the maturing scar tissue to give microvascular loops reaching from the deeper layers to the dermal-epidermal junction *(3)*.

Therapeutic control of angiogenesis is a concept described in many forms throughout this volume. It is almost always considered in terms of controlling its rate, i. e., to increase, decrease, or completely stop the process, depending on the application. Most approaches to this type of control focus on the use of soluble biochemical signals, such as FGF and VEGF *(4–7)*, affecting one or more components of the angiogenic cascade *(1)*. In the field of tissue and cellular engineering, it is argued that control of organizational architecture is at least as important as rate control *(8)*. Without effective control of organization and architecture, success in tissue repair or production of bioartificial tissues/grafts will be limited. This is an inescapable feature of tissue function because it is intimately linked with the presence of appropriate cell layers and cell orientation, the pattern of cell types, extracellular matrix, innervation, and of course microvessel distribution. This is particularly obvious in skin where injury sites are repaired by a poorly organized and functionally impaired scar tissue. The same functional dependence on orientation is even more critical in repair of tissues such as tendon, ligament, and nerve

From: *The New Angiotherapy*
Edited by: T.-P. D. Fan and E. C. Kohn © Humana Press Inc., Totowa, NJ

(9,10). Indeed, in many repair situations it is now suggested that more rapid formation of new tissue, such as that stimulated by transforming growth factor (TGF)-β1 and -β2, may in fact promote scarring and so be detrimental to function *(11)*.

Tissue engineering of clinically useful "implantable devices" is a relatively recent approach to the problem of how to acquire significant amounts of safe, graftable tissues. This involves growing isolated cells (autologous or allogeneic) on synthetic or bio-artificial substrates for such a time and under organizing cues that will eventually guide the formation of normal tissue structure and composition. A major aim in this field is the tissue engineering on small-diameter (< 6 mm) vessels. Some early success has been claimed using systems based on synthetic bioresorbable polymers *(12,13)* and on native collagen gels *(14)* and without any external support matrix *(15)*. Cells from venous tissue, adipose, and bone marrow have been proposed as potentially useful for seeding of such tissue-engineered small vessels *(16)*. Although these are narrow vessels, they clearly still aim to provide conventional implants to replace damaged or diseased segments of the vasculature. This scale of application is distinct from the aim of creating a capillary bed or microvascular network (or the precursor pattern for this) structures that can be implanted to specific (frequently repair) tissue sites.

This review examines a novel concept of angiogenic guidance tracks for control of three-dimensional organization of new microvascular networks (summarized in Fig. 1), using the well-known principles of cell/tissue orientation by contact guidance.

Control of Tissue Organization

Soluble chemical signals regulating growth rate may influence tissue organization over short distances. For example, it is likely that short, stable diffusion gradients can be maintained, such as the release of vascular endothelial growth factor (VEGF) by keratinocytes to penetrate a few millimeters into underlying granulation tissue *(6,17)*. Such a short-range VEGF gradient could be responsible for direction of capillary loops from the deep to superficial wound zones. However, over longer distances (laterally through large dermal wounds or between long gaps in injured peripheral nerves; *10*) chemical gradients will be disrupted by a range of factors. These factors include distortion of the extracellular matrix, in which the gradient exists, by tissue and muscle contraction, tissue compression, and interstitial tissue-fluid flow. In addition, any pre-existing anisotropic organization of the matrix (even excluding the complexity of tissue movements)— for example, in obviously aligned structures like muscle and orientated collagen fibers—diffusion gradients will tend to be deflected towards the parallel axis. This will mean that tissue structure will become more influential on diffusion gradients as the repair tissue matures, and becomes better organized. This instability of chemical gradients is known from work in peripheral-nerve repair, where diffusion gradients are important in promoting neuronal outgrowth *(10)*, and yet containment or protection of that gradient is necessary for regeneration across significant gaps. A further example of distortion or deflection of diffusion gradients by anisotropic tissue features is evident in repairs involving tendon-sheath or tendon fascia where new vessels must grow across or close to gliding interfaces (reviewed in ref. *18*).

Although descriptions of in vitro models of microvessel formation in three-dimensional collagen lattices *(19)* support the idea that it will be possible to develop artificial vascular plexi by tissue engineering, these models tell us little about spatial control because the matrix is too simple (i. e., static and homogeneous). Consequently, long-range control of orientation through heterogeneous and moving tissues (new or pre-

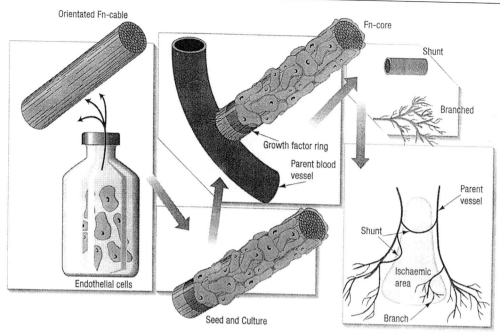

Fig. 1. Diagram showing a proposed scheme for the tissue engineering use of angiogenic tracks. In their simplest form angiogenic tracks of microvessel dimensions would be implanted directly with no requirement for cell-seeding. **(A)** Fn-cable support guides are prepared to a suitable diameter for the application and site and seeded onto the outer surface with suitable cultured endothelial cells. **(B)** These are then cultured to allow cell proliferation and distribution over the material, as required. The contact guidance surface means that a complete layer of cells is not necessary. A growth factor-rich zone at the end(s) to be attached to the existing vasculature (red-shaded ring), may be introduced to promote implant-vessel integration. The main point of probable variation of this scheme will be in stage **(C)**. Implantation techniques, including the means of attachment, site/vessel type, the type and density (if any) of cell-seeding, growth-factor additives to promote implant-vessel integration, will depend on the specific application involved. Induction of a lumen and so of flow at this stage will be either by physical clearance, for larger vessels or by activation of a latent protease in the Fn-cable. The two major formats in **(D)** are "branched" or unbranched or "shunt" forms would be suitable for different applications.

existing) is likely to be heavily dependent on solid-phase features of the intervening extracellular matrix. It may be better, for long range therapeutic guidance, to provide solid-phase cues within the matrix itself, rather than diffusion gradients. Such solid phase cues can be provided through cell-attachment sites using: (1) the chemical nature of the surface, (2) surface topography, and (3) mechanical forces, normally exerted through the substrate. In the case of (3), vascular endothelium is well-known to respond to mechanical stimuli, most notably the effects of fluid-flow shear, which produces dramatic alignment of cell-shape, cytoskeletal, and membrane components *(20–22)*. The most promising mechanisms at present seem to be based on examples (1) and (2).

Angiogenesis in Tissue Repair

Attempts to direct microvascular organization need to take account of the patterns and role of angiogenesis at particular repair sites and this has been examined most widely in association with dermal repair, although it is clearly critical in other tissues. The pattern of vessel invasion from the base of a full depth wound during healing around a skin graft indicated that there was little measurable new vessel formation before 3 d (23). Between days 3 and 5, immature lobular structures and sprouts appeared in the wound-base vasculature and by 5–10 d, discrete capillaries and microvascular plexi were evident. Revascularization of the graft was entirely by angiogenesis and new vessel formation (24), rather than insculation (new connections with existing capillaries in the graft). Recent work in the tissue engineering of skin equivalents (25) has also led to the identification of techniques to reconstruct "capillary-like" networks of endothelial cells (26). These have applications in clinical implantation and pharmaceutical testing and skin-permeability modeling (27,28). These networks represent nondirectional, random forms of substrate-based microvessel formation. Any their useful function in vivo would depend on ability to anastomose with surrounding vessels (insculation).

Wounding of large-vessel endothelium is followed by a change of endothelial cells from resting to migrating behavior. This transition to a "translocating cell" (29) is associated with a sequence of changes focused on actin microfilaments. These include a reduction of dense peripheral bands of microfilaments seen in the resting stage. This was followed by a reorientation of lamellipodia and associated microfilaments, and attachment plaques, to lie perpendicular to the wound margin as translocation begins. Comparable re-structuring of actin microfilament networks has been reported during hypoxia mediated changes in "in vitro angiogenesis" in collagen gels (30).

It is significant that these examples of endothelial-cell changes associated with movement, during injury-induced angiogenesis, are described in terms of sprouting, orientation, translocation, cytoskeletal reorganization, and so on. All forms of these activities that are not random must, by definition, include an element of direction. To be able to maintain an orientation (i.e., nonrandom direction), any cell requires cues (indicators of polarity and orientation) and predictable reference points. Whether these are available locally as endogenous cues or as external, "therapeutic" cues, it seems likely that the eventual orientation of a repaired vascular tissue will reflect the net influence on endothelial-cell guidance (8).

Repair of the meniscus is a particularly stark example of the importance to repair not only of a vascular network but also the orientation of vascular ingrowth. Meniscus has a rich vascular supply to its outer, peripheral edge, reaching in by 10–30% of the meniscal width (31), but is avascular in the central area. As in articular cartilage, damage to the avascular region that does not involve the vascular bed does not repair (32). However, damage frequently involves this avascular region and so attempts have been made to extend the peripheral vasculature towards the injury site (29). This has been attempted by creating full-depth access channels (33,34) or by trephining a discrete conduit, ~2 mm in diameter (35). Vessels from the peripheral vasculature migrate along these channels and initiate the formation of a fibrovascular scar tissue in the injury site. A simplified model form of this approach has been described, controlling short-range vessel polarity (directional angiogenesis) using shaped, biopolymer microspheres seeded with hepatocytes (36).

A tissue engineering approach would be to construct new tissues or tissue templates, based on appropriate cells growing in bioartificial materials, for use as implants. Interestingly, in this respect, there are indications that vascular smooth-muscle cells may prove useful in that they are able to function as pericytes during in vitro angiogenesis (37), suggesting a possible role in microvascular tissue engineering. However, angiogenesis in engineered tissues is currently considered as a process that will occur naturally in vivo, following implantation of the constructed tissue. Consequently, the present generation of bioartificial tissues is not designed to include a microvascular network that could be linked into the recipient tissue. Future tissue engineering research is likely to concentrate increasingly on the incorporation of more complex and subtle external guidance cues *(8)*. The remainder of this chapter will analyze: (1) why it may prove important to engineer this component of the tissue, and (2) how it could be achieved. Critical to each of these is the need to achieve particular three-dimensional organization or architecture and so to consider means of guiding microvascular architecture.

CONTACT GUIDANCE CUES
Cell Orientation by Topography and Surface Adhesion

The control of cell orientation and guidance of cell movement by surface shape or topography has been known for many years *(38,39)*. Early experimental studies, using smooth glass fibers as the topographical feature, indicated that diameters less than 100 μm are necessary to orientate cells parallel with a fiber axis *(40)*. More recently, cellular alignment has been characterized on micro-grooved or patterned silicone *(41,42)* titanium *(43,44)*, and silica *(45–47)*. The dimensions of topographical features in these substrates were between 2 and 10 μm for groove and ridge spacing. Groove dimensions of 5–10 μm in silica have been found to promote epithelial-cell, fibroblast, and neurone alignment. In addition, neurones migrated fourfold faster on grooved rather than on smooth surfaces *(47,48)*. In some instances, cell and substrate alignment have been related to orientation of cell-attachment plaques along the edge of the ridges *(49)*. In fibroblasts the first response is the alignment of microtubules, which precedes cell alignment itself *(49)*.

Guidance of cells has not been limited to synthetic surfaces and at least two forms of extracellular-matrix/cell-adhesion protein have been prepared in suitable forms. Fibroblast alignment on collagen fibrils in vitro has been described by a number of groups *(50–52)*. In addition, orientated forms of fibrillar fibronectin have been found to align fibroblasts *(54–56)*. Cell alignment, cytoskeletal re-organization, and increased rates of migration of fibroblasts, neurites, and macrophages have been reported on discrete fibers of fibronectin *(55)*. Hence the surface chemistry is at least as important to guidance as the substrate topography. Guidance through adhesion can operate independently of topography (i.e., through paths of adhesive protein on flat surfaces; *57*) as in Fig. 2A. However, topographic contact guidance must also include a cell adhesion component. Examples of adhesion-mediated guidance of cells includes neurite guidance on tracts of polylysine *(58)* and fibroblast orientation to linear tracts of fibronectin *(47)*. Surface adhesion properties also appear to be implicated in the rates at which cells migrate *(55,59)*.

Since cells interact with a substrate primarily through the protein layer which adsorbs to its surface *(60*; Fig. 2), controlling the nature of this protein film offers the potential for cell guidance. Adsorbed proteins modulate the cellular response to the substrate through cell membrane molecules such as the integrin family of receptors *(61)*. Although fibronectin can be considered the archetypal adhesion molecule for a wide range of cell types in vivo and in vitro *(62)*, vitronectin has been shown to be the key adhesive protein for many cultured cells, owing to its ability to adsorb to the substrate in the face of competition from other components of the serum used in the culture medium *(63)*. In this situation, fibronectin is unable to adsorb to the surface in sufficient amounts to support cell attachment *(64)*. Cell attachment can therefore be promoted by modifying the surface to enhance adsorption of adhesive proteins. In this way, oxygen- or nitrogen-rich surfaces have been shown to enhance the adsorption of vitronectin or fibronectin and hence

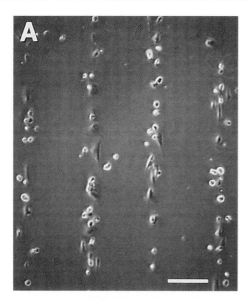
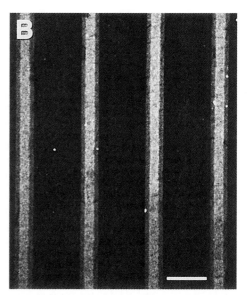

Fig. 2. Cell guidance by patterned surface chemistry. Flat quartz surfaces were patterned with N-(2-aminoethyl)-3-aminopropyl-trimethoxysilane and dimethyldichlorosilane (EDS/DMS)and examined for cell attachment and protein adsorption. Bone-cell attachment occurred preferentially on the aminosilane (EDS) regions (Panel **A**), and was dependent on the adsorption of Vn from serum. As visualized by immunofluorescent staining and confocal microscopy, Vn was preferentially adsorbed from serum onto the EDS regions (Panel **B**), thereby promoting cell attachment. When purified solutions of Vn or Fn were incubated with patterned surfaces, both proteins adsorbed preferentially to the EDS regions. In the presence of serum, however, only Vn was able to adsorb in the face of competition from other serum components. Removal of Vn from the serum virtually abolished attachment to the EDS regions, indicating the specificity of the effect of surface chemistry on protein-mediated cell attachment. Bars represent 100 µm.

encourage endothelial-cell attachment *(65)*. By generating adhesion-promoting chemistries in a patterned manner, cell guidance can be brought about *(66,67)*. Photolithographic techniques have been used to produce surfaces with chemistries that promote cell attachment in specific regions through the selective adsorption of vitronectin from culture serum *(68)*. In common with studies on cell shape *(69,70)*, the regulation of cell spatial distribution by patterned-surface chemistry can exert profound effects on the function, differentiation, and proliferation of anchorage-dependent cells *(66,71)*.

Because it has proved possible to guide the migration and to control the orientation of this range of cell types, it is tempting to suggest that a similar approach could be used to guide endothelial cells. However, there are here two aspects to the concept of endothelial-cell orientation. In mature vessels, the lining endothelial cells have a distinct polarity that is related to cues provided by the flow within that vessel *(20–22)*. Indeed this elongation and orientation of endothelial cells can be produced experimentally in vitro by culturing cells under fluid-flow conditions. Although this aspect of orientation is important to vascular function (and may indeed be possible to reproduce using contact guidance), the central aim in producing angiogenic guidance tracks is different. In this instance it is important to direct the orientation of endothelial-cell migration and, as a consequence, control the route taken by new capillary sprouts. Ideally, this should also hold cells in the three-dimensional configuration of a tube around the strand or guiding track (Fig. 1).

Contact Guidance: Fibronectin as a Base Material

The substrate material proposed here for production of angiogenic tracks is fibronectin, but other guidance substrates could also be used. For example, collagen substrates have been used to elicit contact guidance in vivo and in vitro *(50,51,72–74)*, in addition to a range of synthetic polymer surfaces *(48)*. Fibronectin appears to be a particularly promising substrate, however, for a number of reasons. In the first instance, implantation of significant amounts of this protein is unlikely to lead to resorption problems or abnormal cell responses because fibronectin is a normal matrix component involved in most stages of repair *(75,76)*. In addition, the aggregated fibronectin material (termed fibronectin- or Fn-mat) used most widely so far, releases significant amounts of weakly incorporated fibronectin over the first 48 h after rehydration *(77)*. Such a release of soluble protein or its fragments is, itself, likely to promote local recruitment of endothelial cells and new microvessels *(78,79)*.

The cell-adhesion function of Fn-mats is an additional benefit in achieving guidance, providing resident cells with directional attachment as well as topographical cues. The adherence of aortic endothelial cells under flow, for example, appears to be dependent on the presence and conformation of substrate fibronectin *(80)*. Recent studies have identified the combination of (1) substrate density of fibronectin (as one form of attachment ligand), and (2) cell-membrane density of appropriate integrins as the rate-limiting factor for cell migration *(59)*.

Endothelial cells at various times, express a wide array of integrins including $\alpha_1\beta_1$ *(81)*, $\alpha_2\beta_1$ *(82)*, $\alpha_3\beta_1$ *(83)*, $\alpha_5\beta_1$ *(84)*, $\alpha_v\beta_3$ *(85)*, four of which will bind fibronectin *(86)*. It is known from other systems that significant shifts in integrin expression are associated with the transitions that repair cells undergo as they are recruited from surrounding sites to migrate into the new provisional matrix *(87)*. In the case of endothelial cells, this is a transition from the differentiated lumenal cell to a migrating, matrix-invasive state, at the capillary sprout *(35)*. Loss of polarized attachment to basement-membrane components in the vessel wall and adoption of a migratory phenotype, with attachment to components, such as fibronectin and collagen types I and III, is comparable with a known switch in keratinocyte integrin expression. This switch in keratinocyte integrin expression parallels the loss of normal differentiated epithelial function and migration over wound granulation tissue *(87–89)*.

At least one such integrin switch is already known for endothelial cells. Endothelial cells in most mature vessels, such as uninjured dermis or unstimulated chick chorioallantoic membrane (CAM), are rich in integrins based on the $\beta 1$ subunit *(86,90; see* chapters 3 and 27, this volume). However, capillary sprouts, present in granulation tissue, tumors, and in stimulated regions of the CAM, express high levels of the unusual integrin, $\alpha_v\beta_3$ *(90)*. This integrin is not found in unstimulated vessels or after new vessels have become fully formed. There appears then to be a switch in expression to $\alpha_v\beta_3$, associated with migration during angiogenesis *(90–92)*. Indeed, expression of this integrin is stimulated by (FGF) *(93,94)* and its occupation by suitable ligands stimulates calcium-dependent signaling, leading to cell migration *(95)*. Inhibition of this integrin function with cyclic peptides *(91)* delayed granulation-tissue formation, apparently by inhibiting microvascular invasion. Consequently, this highly promiscuous integrin, reported to bind fibrin, fibronectin, vitronectin, thrombospondin, laminin, and von Willebrand factor (vWF) *(86,90,95)*, appears to be expressed to enable these cells to invade and attach to all components of the fibrin clot and provisional-repair matrix. Fibronectin-based materials, then, would be expected to be excellent adhesion substrates for promotion of this transient receptor pattern.

Physical and Chemical Forms of Fibronectin Guidance Substrates

The first forms of Fn-mat were prepared by aggregating fibers from purified solutions of fibronectin while concentrating under a fluid shear, in an ultrafiltration pressure cell *(54,77)*. Freeze-drying of these aggregates produced 1–2-mm thick, stable Fn-mats with a predominant fiber orientation (Fig. 3). Derivative forms of Fn-mat were described, incorporating heparin and basic fibroblast growth factor (bFGF) *(55,77)*. Either or both of these additives may enhance angiogenic responses to the fibronectin aggregates *(4,78,79)*. More recently, a modification of the aggregation process has been described to further stabilize the aggregate. This is based on the observation that Fn-mats have a high affinity for copper ions and that incorporation of traces of copper reduces the rate of protein loss in solution *(96)* and retards breakdown by trypsin. At the levels of copper required to produce a threefold increase in stability, growth of cells, even of sensitive cells such as Schwann cells, was not inhibited. Copper-stabilized Fn-mats would appear to have particular advantages for angiogenesis, not only for extending the survival of the guidance cue, but as a local source of copper as the mats degrade. Copper has been reported to promote angiogenesis *(97–100)*. Suggested mechanisms for this action have suggested that it acts together with a binding protein *(98)* or as an amine oxidase cofactor *(100)* potentially influencing collagen metabolism *(101)*. Evidence from other areas also indicates that local deficiencies of copper may indeed be important in retarding dermal repair following burn injury *(102)*.

Recent development of large-scale techniques for fibronectin aggregation have led to the production of cable forms, with diameters between 200 µm and 10 mm (Underwood, Ahmed et al., unpublished data). These cables can be pulled out to considerable lengths, with a view to implantation into nerve defects greater than 20 cm in length, but are equally suitable for construction of bioartificial blood vessels or implantation as long angiogenic tracks. Such new materials are effective substrates for a range of fibroblasts, endothelial-cell types, and nerve cells. In addition, they can, like Fn-mats, be stabilized by incorporation of traces of copper *(96)*.

Guidance In Vitro by Fibronectin Substrates

Although this is a new field, experimental work with fibronectin guidance materials in culture and in animal models (*see* below) suggests that guidance by angiogenic tracks is possible. The ability of endothelial cells to grow into and over fibronectin cables has been assessed in a two-dimensional system, where the guidance elements were attached to plastic culture dishes. Both human umbilical artery (HUACs) and bovine aortic endothelial cells (BAECs) were seeded onto such fibronectin cables and monitored over 7 d. Cells were either pre-labeled with a fluorescent tracking dye *(103)* or by staining for fibronectin receptor integrin, $\alpha_5\beta_1$, (Fig. 4). Both cell types clearly bound effectively to the fibronectin cables from an early stage (1 d). HUACs became closely bound to the surface of the cables but apparently did not penetrate into the body of the material. In this case, cell shape tended to be flattened and discoid rather than elongate. In contrast, there was evidence of extensive penetration into the fibronectin cable by BAECs with formation of a pronounced elongate morphology, relative to adjacent cells on plastic.

In addition, work in this lab (Harding, Ahmed, and Underwood, unpublished data) has led to the development of a simple model in which 200 µ*M* diameter fibronectin cables were embedded into three-dimensional collagen gels containing human umbilical vein

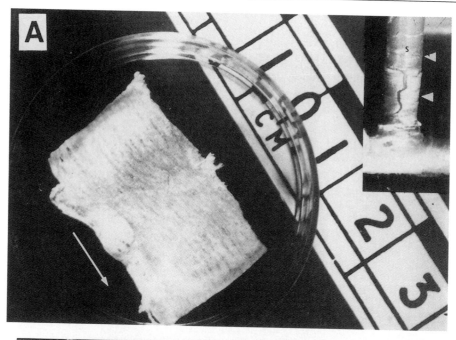

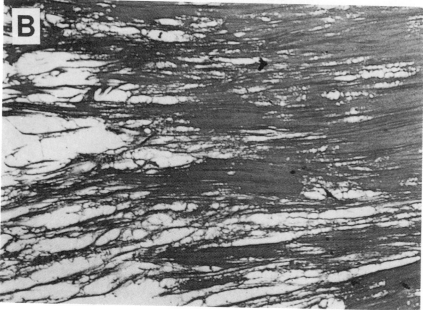

Fig. 3. (A) Gross view of a fibronectin-mat dried and flattened (cm scale to show dimensions). INSET shows a Fn-mat in the position which it aggregates (arrow heads), around the stirring shaft (S) of an ultrafiltration cell. Even at this level, the fibrous nature of the material and the fibrous orientation (arrow) are apparent. Adapted with permission from refs. *54* and *77*. **(B)** Light micrograph of a Fn-mat, cut parallel to the plane of fiber orientation (horizontal) showing the aggregation of fibers. Plastic-embedded specimen stained with Toluidine blue.

endothelial cells. This provided cells with the opportunity to interact with all surfaces of the Fn-guidance elements (i.e., in 3D). After 24 h, clear endothelial-cell attachment and

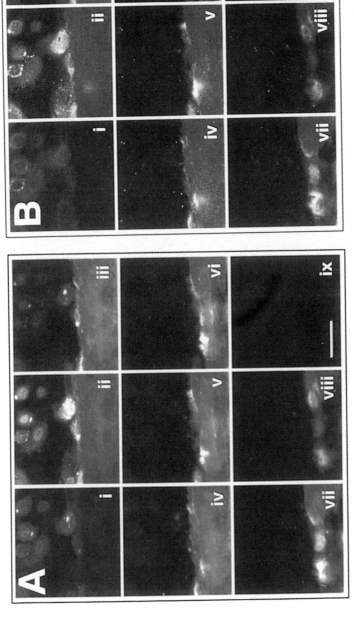

Fig. 4. Photomicrographs of directed cell migration using fibronectin cables in vitro. Endothelial-cells labeled with a fluorescent dye were incubated with glass coverslips bearing Fn-cables. After 1 d (Panels **A** and **B**) and 4 d (Panels **C** and **D**) in culture, samples were removed, fixed, and stained for the fibronectin integrin ($\alpha_5\beta_1$) receptor using polyclonal antisera. The dual-labeled samples were examined on a scanning-laser confocal microscope, enabling serial optical sections to be taken, starting at the surface of the coverslip (i) and ending at the top of the cable (ix). The cell distribution (left-hand panels, **A** and **C**) showed that although cells attached over the entire surface of the coverslip, there was preferential and rapid colonization of the Fn cables.

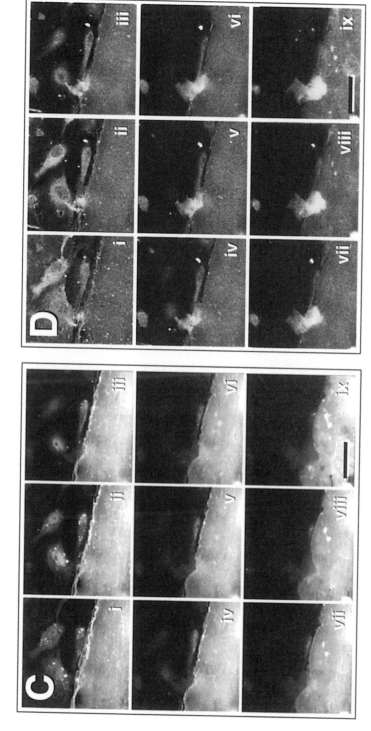

Fig. 4. (cont.) Although there was some expression of Fn receptors (right-hand panels, **B** and **D**), this was initially much lower on the glass substrate than on the Fn cables. This is expected in view of the different attachment mechanisms which will be operating on these two substrata. On glass, attachment will be primarily due to vitronectin, mediated via its $\alpha_v\beta_3$ integrin receptor, owing to the ability of this adhesive glycoprotein to adsorb to the surface in the face of competition from other serum components. On and within the cables, attachment was obviously primarily mediated by Fn and its $\alpha_5\beta_1$ receptor. As cells remained longer in culture, those adherent on the glass-surface synthesized fibronectin-rich matrix on their basal surface, and expression of the Fn receptor increased accordingly. Bars represent 50 µm.

aggregation to the cable was evident, as shown in Fig. 5. Under these conditions cells, attached principally to the outer surface of cables, producing a cellular tube, a number of cells thick, around the central fibronectin cable. Where Fn-materials are used in vivo, lumen formation would be expected to occur as a natural consequence of resorption of the fibronectin. Resorption in vivo involves neutrophils and macrophages in dermis and nerve (56). In a tissue-engineering context, lumen formation could be speeded up by incorporation of a latent protease, such as plasminogen, into the initial fibronectin cable, to be activated at an appropriate stage (Fig. 1). Results so far, then, suggest that fibronectin-guidance materials are effective as substrates for formation of endothelial-cell seeded implants. With suitable selection of the initial cable diameter, vessel templates could be engineered for a variety of sites and applications.

Guidance In Vivo by Fibronectin Substrates

Early experience of the effects of orientated Fn-mats on angiogenesis during in vivo tissue repair involve two models. Fn-mats, implanted into full-thickness porcine dermal wounds as 3–4 layers, were placed flat onto the wound bed with their fiber orientation parallel with the skin surface. Granulation-tissue alignment corresponded with orienta-tion of the implanted Fn-mat at the 14-d stage postinjury, by which time the Fn-mat had been largely resorbed (56). However, subsequent blood vessel ingrowth over the next 14 d took on a more normal orientation, running from the deep to surface layers of the dermis. Clearly, then, these vessels were perpendicular to the original Fn-mat contact-guidance cue. This deep to surface orientation of vessels is consistent with that expected from growth-factor gradients, such as VEGF, originating from the re-formed epidermal layer (6,17). This suggests that control of orientation was achievable but that contradictory directional cues were able to reorganize that structure once the Fn-mat guidance cue had disappeared (i.e., post-day 14).

In the second model, microvascular responses form part of the repair process follow-ing injury and regeneration of peripheral nerves. Changes in both angiogenesis (104) and microvascular permeability (105) have been reported, adjacent to sites of nerve regenera-tion. The importance of angiogenesis as part of this repair is evident because prevention of revascularization leads to necrosis and fibrosis (106). Re-innervation has been reported to follow slightly behind angiogenesis, following dermal injury (24). Attempts to improve revascularization clinically at the time of surgical nerve repair have proved equivocal (107). Studies using silicone-chamber implants (108) indicated that angiogenesis proceeded mainly in the proximal-distal direction, though it has remained uncertain whether ingrowth of microvessels preceded or followed that of Schwann cells and axons. Where nerve repair involves the use of bioartifical conduits, tubes, or other implants from silicone (109), bioresorbable polymer (110), fibronectin (111–115), or hyaluronan (116), revascularization is critical to repair.

Previous studies in which 1-cm defects were made in rat sciatic nerves and bridged by a guide or conduit of fibronectin mat have shown that a growth cone of axonal tissue extends progressively from the proximal to the distal ends of the implant (111–115). Guidance through fn mat conduits is particularly effective in promoting regeneration where growth factors NGF or NT-3 were incorporated (112,113,115). The pattern of angiogenesis associated with nerve regeneration in this model has identified a distinct linkage between the guidance of nerve elements and that of new capillaries (117). Dual immunolocalization of ingrowing endothelial cells and Schwann cells over the 30-d

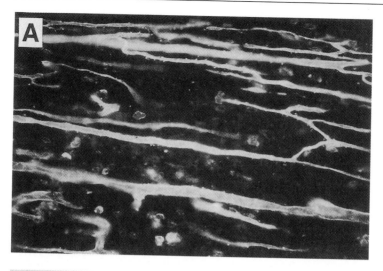

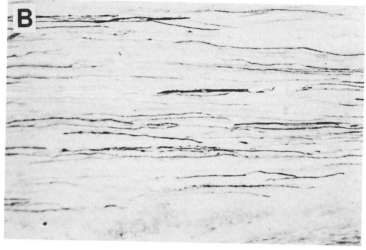

Fig. 5. (A) Endoneurial microvessels in a nerve that is regenerating through a fibronectin graft, immunostained with the endothelial cell marker RECA-1 (fluorescence labeling). Blood vessels are arranged parallel to the direction of the regenerating fibers (cf. Fig. 5B) with short anastomoses between vessels *(117)*. **(B)** Immunostaining for the neuronal marker CGRP on a section adjacent to that stained for RECA-1, showing a parallel orientation of the regenerating nerve fibers. The distribution is very similar to that of the blood vessels, although these are less numerous than the nerve fibers (ABC-peroxidase staining method).

period of nerve regeneration showed clearly that both cell types were orientated parallel with the Fn-mat fiber alignment (Fig. 5A). In small areas where microvessels were nonorientated, neural elements (axons and Schwann cells) had a similar random orientation and nerve regeneration was poor (Fig. 5B). In all implants, microvascular elements were the first to invade the Fn-mats, endothelial cells just preceding Schwann cell progression *(117)*. An earlier study found a similar pattern of microvascular invasion, relative to neural elements, in cutaneous wound healing *(3)*.

These studies suggest that the rate of angiogenesis could be rate limiting for the regeneration process *(117)* and use of Fn-mats can provide guidance for both invading microvessels and neural elements.

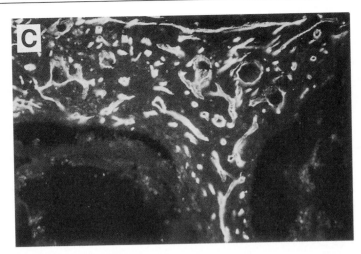

Fig. 5. (cont.) (C) RECA-1 immunofluorescent localization of blood vessels in a fibronectin graft. Here the vessels are more randomly orientated, and the level of penetration of regenerating nerve fibers is correspondingly very poor.

Future Applications for Angiogenic Tracks

Future strategies for the application of guidance tracks in angiogenesis will depend on the success of materials available at present but are likely to divide into three areas. In each case, use of the angiogenic tracks can be in vitro (i.e., for tissue engineering) or in vivo, normally to direct tissue repair. The three uses are: (1) to guide collateral vessel growth to improve local perfusion; (2) to deflect vessel growth away from a site, to reduce perfusion; and (3) to help organize a particular tissue architecture.

The most obvious and common application is (1) where collateral vessels are needed to supply an implant, repair site, or around an ishaemic area. Examples include neovascularization of poorly perfused skin flaps; to promote repair in chronic wounds and meniscal tears; perfusion of tissue-engineered glands *(118)* and cardiac infarct sites; or to promote calcification in nonunion fractures. The "diversion" application (2) is more likely to be effective in conjunction with an inhibitor of microvessel formation. Use of guidance tracks to direct architecture (3) is a potential solution to some applications of tissue engineering where tissue organization and function requires that certain areas are better-perfused than others (e.g., in the meniscus or the eye), or where the orientation of new vessels is critical to function and so needs to be specified (e.g., in and around nerves and tendons).

Recent work on the mechanisms of attachment and migration of endothelial cells *(90,91)* is particularly important in this area because it presents opportunities for modification of the substrates used in guidance. Such developments of basic guidance materials (immediate examples would be incorporation of nonadhesive layers containing hyaluronan or copper), representing cell-selective materials, would give more complex spatial control. Interestingly, cell-selective materials, using binding and non-binding substrates in conjunction with guidance tracks, tend to become mimics of natural-guidance mechanisms. The central part played by angiogenesis in many types of tissue repair makes further development of such guidance tracks and constructs an attractive general therapeutic goal.

ACKNOWLEDGMENTS

The authors are grateful to Sarah Harding for expert technical assistance and images of contact-guided endothelial cells and to the Engineering and Physical Sciences Research Council, together with the Augustus Newman and Welton Foundations (RAB) for financial support.

REFERENCES

1. Madri, J. A., Sankar, S., Romanic, A. M. (1996) Angiogenesis, in *The Molecular and Cellular Biology of Wound Repair*, 2nd ed., (Clark, R. A. F., ed.), Plenum, New York, pp. 355–371.
2. Arbiser, J. L. (1996) Angiogenesis and the skin: a primer. *J. Am. Acad. Dermatol.* **34**, 486–497.
3. Gu, X. H., Terenghi, G., Purkis, P. E., Leigh, I. M., and Polak, J. M. (1994) Morphological changes of neural and vascular peptides in human skin suction blister injury. *J. Pathol.* **172**, 61–72.
4. Schweigerer, L., Neufeld, G., Friedman, J., Abraham, J. A., Fiddes, J. C., and Gospodarowicz, D. (1987) Capillary endothelial cells express basic fibroblast growth factor, a mitogen that promotes their own growth. *Nature* **325**, 257–259.
5. Broadley, K. N., Aquino, A. M., Woodward, S. C., Buckley-Sturrock, A., Sato, Y., Rifkin, D. B., and Davidson, J. M. (1989) Monospecific antibodies implicate basic fibroblast growth factor in normal wound repair. *Lab. Invest.* **61**, 571–575.
6. Brown, L. F., Yeo, K.-T., Berse, B., Yeo, T-K., Senger, D. R., Dvorak, H. F., and van der Water, L. (1992) Expression of vascular permeability factor (vascular endothelial growth factor) by epidermal keratinocytes during wound healing. *J. Exp. Med.* **176**, 1375–1379.
7. Takeshita, S., Pu, L. Q., Stein, L. A., et al. (1994) Intramuscular administration of vascular endothelial growth factor induces dose-dependent collateral artery augmentation in a rabbit model of chronic limb ischemia. *Circulation* **90**, 228–234.
8. Brown, R. A., Smith, K. D., and McGrouther, D. A. (1997) Strategies for cell engineering in tissue repair. *Wound Repair. Regen.* **5**, 212–221.
9. Frank, C., Amiel, D., Woo, S. L.-Y., and Akeson, W. (1985) Normal ligament properties and ligament healing. *Clin. Orth. Rel. Res.* **196**, 15–25.
10. Lundborg, G. (1988) in *Nerve Injury and Repair*. Churchill Livingstone, Edinburgh, pp. 149–195.
11. Shah, M., Foreman, D. M., and Ferguson, M. W. (1995) Neutralisation of TGF–β1 and TGF–β2 or exogenous addition of TGF–β3 to cutaneous rat wounds reduces scarring. *J. Cell Sci.* **108**, 985–1002.
12. Shinoka, T., Shum-Tim, D., Ma, P. X., Tanel, R. E., Isoqai, N., Langer, R., et al. (1998) Creation of viable pulmonary artery autografts through tissue engineering. *J. Thorac. Cardiovasc. Surg.* **115**, 536–545.
13. Nikalson, L. E. and Langer, R. S. (1997) Advance in tissue engineering of blood vessels and other tissues. *Trans. Immunol.* **5**, 303–306
14. L'Heureux, N., Germain, L., Labbe, R., and Auger, F. A. (1993) In vitro construction of a human blood vessel from cultured vascular cells: a morphological study. *J. Vasc. Surg.* **17**, 499–509.
15. L'Heureux, N., Paquet, S., Labbe, R., Germain, L., and Auger, F. A. (1998) A completely biological tissue engineered blood vessel. *FASEB. J.* **12**, 47–56.
16. Noishiki, Y., Yamane, Y., Okashi, T., Tomizawa, Y., and Satoh, S. (1998) Choice, isolation and prepartion of cells for bioartificial vascular grafts. *Artif. Organs* **22**, 50–62.
17. Frank, S., Hubner, G., Breier, G., Longaker, M. T., Greenhalgh, D. G., and Werner, S. (1995) Regulation of vascular endothelial growth factor expression in cultured keratinocytes. *J. Biol. Chem.* **270**, 12,607–12,613.
18. Gelberman, R., Goldberg, V., An, K.-A., and Banes, A. (1988) Tendon, in *Injury and Repair of the Musculoskeletal Soft Tissues* (Woo, S. L.-Y. and Buckwalter, J. A., eds.), American Academy Orthopedic Surgeons, Park Ridge, IL, pp. 5–40.
19. Merwin, J. R., Anderson, J., Kocher, O., van Itallie, C., and Madri, J. A. (1990) Transforming growth factor beta 1 modulates extracellular matrix organization and cell-cell junctional complex formation during in vitro angiogenesis. *J. Cell Physiol.* **142**, 117–128.
20. Levesque, M. J. and Nerem, R. M. (1985) The elongation and orientation of cultured endothelial cells in response to shear stress. *J. Biomech. Eng.* **107**, 341–347.
21. Barbee, K. A., Mundel, T., Lal, R., and Davies, P. F. (1995) Subcellular distribution of shear stress at the surface of flow aligned and non-aligned endothelial monolayers. *Am. J. Physiol.* **268**, 1765–1772.

22. Davies, P. F. (1995) Flow-mediated endothelial mechanotransduction. *Physiol Rev.* **75,** 519–557.

23. Goretsky, M. J., Breeden, M., Pisarski, G., Harriger, D., Boyce, S. T., and Greenhalgh, D. G. (1995) Capillary morphogenesis during healing of full thickness skin grafts: an ultrastructural study. *Wound Rep. Reg.* **3,** 213–220.

24. Gu, X. H., Terenghi, G., Kangesu, T., et al. (1995) Regeneration pattern of blood vessels and nerves in cultured keratinocyte grafts assessed by laser confocal scanning microscopy. *Br. J. Dermatol.* **132,** 376–383.

25. Michel, M., L'hereux, N., Pouloit, R., Xu, W., Auger, F. A., and Germain, L. (1999) Characterization of a new tissue–engineered human skin equivalent with hair. *In Vitro Cell Dev Biol Anim.* **35,** 318–326.

26. Black, A. F., Berthod, F., L'heureux, N., Germain, L., and Auger, F. A. (1998) In vitro reconstruction of a human capillary-like network in a tissue-engineered skin equivalent. *FASEB J.* **12,** 1331–1340.

27. Li, H., Berthod, F., Xu, W., Damour, O., and Auger, F. A. (1997) Use of in vitro reconstructed skin To cover skin flap donor site. *Surg Res.* **73,** 143–148.

28. Auger, F. A., Rouabhia, M., Goulet, F., Berthod, F., Moulin, V., and Germain, L. (1998) Tissue-engineered human skin substitutes developed from collagen-populated hydrated gels: clinical and fundamental app. lications. *Med. Biol. Eng. Comput.* **36,** 801–812.

29. Lee, T. Y., Rosenthal, A., and Gotlieb, A. I. (1996) Transition of aortic endothelial cells from resting to migrating cells is associated with three sequential patterns of microfilament organization. *J. Vasc. Res.* **33,** 13–24.

30. Phillips, R. G., Birnby, L. M., and Narendran, A. (1995) Hypoxia induces capillary network formation in cultured bovine pulmonary microvessel endothelial cells. *Am. J. Physiol.* **268,** 789–800.

31. Arnoczky, S., Adams, M., DeHaven, K., et al. (1988) Meniscus, in *Injury and Repair of the Musculoskeletal Soft Tissues* (Woo, S. L.-Y. and Buckwalter, J. A., eds.), American Academy Orthopedic Surgeons, Park Ridge, IL, pp. 483–537.

32. Heatley, F. W. (1980) The meniscus: can it be repaired? An experimental investigation in rabbits. *J. Bone Joint Surg.* **62B,** 397–402.

33. Ghadially, F. N., Wedge, J. H., and Lalonde, J. M. A. (1986) Experimental methods of repairing injured menisci. *J. Bone Joint Surg.* **68B,** 106–110.

34. Vewth, R. P. H., den Heeten, G. J., Jansen, H. B. W., et al. (1983) Repair of the meniscus: an experimental investigation in rabbits. *Clin Orthop.* **175,** 258–262.

35. Gershuni, D. H., Skyhar, M. J., Danzig, L. A., et al. (1985) Healing of tears in the avascular segment of the canine lateral meniscus. *Trans. Orth. Res. Soc.* **10,** 294.

36. Wintermantel, E., Cima, L., Schloo, B., and Langer R. (1992) Angiopolarity of cell carriers: directional angiogenesis in resorbable liver cell transplantation devices. *EXS.* **61,** 331–334.

37. Nicosia, R. F. and Villaschi, S. (1995) Rat aortic smooth muscle cells become pericytes during angiogensis in vitro. *Lab. Invest.* **73,** 658–666.

38. Weiss, P. (1945) Experiments on cell and axon orientation in vitro: the role of colloidal exudates in tissue organization. *J. Exp. Zool.* **100,** 353–386.

39. Curtis, A. S. G. and Varde, M. (1964) Control of cell behaviour: topographical factors. *J. Natl. Can. Inst.* **33,** 15–26.

40. Dunn, G. A. and Heath, J. P. (1976) A new hypothesis of contact guidance in tissue cells. *Exp. Cell Res.* **101,** 1–14.

41. den Braber, E. T., de-Ruijter, J. E., Smits, H. T., Ginsel, L. A., von Recum, A. F., and Jansen, J. A. (1995) The effect of parallel surface microgrooves and surface energy on cell growth.

42. Green, A. M., Jansen, J. A., van der Waerden, J. P., and von Recum, A. F. (1994) Fibroblast response to microtextured silicone surfaces: texture orientation into or out of the surface. *J. Biomed. Mater. Res.* **28,** 647–653.

43. Lin, Y, Nishimura, R, Nozaki, K., Sasaki, N., Kadosawa, T., Goto, N., et al. (1992) Effects of pulsing electromagnetic fields on the ligament healing in rabbits. *J. Vet. Med. Sci.* **54,** 1017–1022.

44. Chehroudi, B., Gould, T. R., and Brunette, D. M. (1991) A light and electron microscopic study of the effects of surface topography on the behavior of cells attached to titanium–coated percutaneous implants. *J. Biomed. Mater. Res.* **25,** 387–405.

45. Clark, P., Connolly, P., Curtis, A. S., Dow, J. A., and Wilkinson, C. D. (1991) Cell guidance by ultrafine topography in vitro. *J. Cell Sci.* **99,** 73–77.

46. Wojciak-Stothard, B., Crossan, J., Curtis, A. S. G., and Wilkinson, C. D. (1995) Grooved substrata facilitate in vitro healing of completely divided flexor tendons. *J. Mater. Sci. Mater. Med.* **6,** 266–271.

47. Curtis, A. S. G. and Clark, P. (1990) The effects of topographic and mechanical properties of materials on cell behaviour. *Crit. Rev. Biocompat.* **5,** 343–362.

48. Curtis, A. S. G., Wilkinson, C. D., and Wojciak-Stothard, B. (1995) Cellular guidance, movement and growth: accelerating cell movement. *J. Cell. Eng.* **1,** 35–38.
49. Oakley, C. and Brunette, D. M. (1993) The sequence of alignment of microtubules, focal contacts and actin filaments in fibroblasts spreading on smooth and grooved titanium substrata. *J. Cell. Sci.* **106,** 343–354.
50. Dickinson, R. B., Guido, S., and Tranquillo, R. T. (1994) Biased cell migration of fibroblasts exhibiting contact guidance in oriented collagen gels. *Ann. Biomed. Eng.* **22,** 342–356.
51. Guido, S. and Tranquillo, R. T. (1993) A method for the systematic and quantitative study of cell contact guidance in orientated collagen gels. Correlation of fibroblast orientation and gel birefringence. *J. Cell Sci.* **105,** 317–331.
52. Dunn, G. A. and Ebendal, T. (1978) Contact guidance on orientated collagen gels. *Exp. Cell Res.* **111,** 475–479.
53. Elsdale, T. and Bard, J. (1972) Collagen substrata for studies on cell behaviour. *J. Cell Biol.* **54,** 626–637.
54. Ejim, O. S., Blunn, G. W., and Brown, R. A. (1993) Production of artificial-orientated mats and strands from plasma fibronectin: a morphological study. *Biomaterials* **14,** 743–748.
55. Wojciak-Stothard, B., Denyer, M., Mishra, M., and Brown, R. A. (1997) A study of the adhesion, orientation and movement of cells cultured on ultrathin fibronectin fibres. *In Vitro Cell Dev. Biol.* **33,** 110–117.
56. Ahmed, Z. A. and Brown, R. A. (1999) Adhesion and alignment of cultured Schwann cells on ultrathinn fibronectin fibres. *Cell Motil. Cytoskel.* **42,** 331–343.
57. Chiquet, M., Eppenberger, H. M., and Turner, D. C. (1981) Muscle morphogenesis: evidence for the organising function of exogenous fibronectin. *Dev. Biol.* **88,** 230–235.
58. Corey, J. M., Wheeler, B.C., and Brewer, G. J. (1991) Compliance of hipp. ocampal neurons to patterned substrate networks. *J. Neurosci. Res.* **30,** 300–307.
59. Palecek, S. P., Loftus, J. C., Ginsberg, M. H., Lauffenburger, D. A., and Horwitz, A. F. (1997) Integrin–ligand binding properties govern cell migration speed through cell-substratum adhesiveness. *Nature* **385,** 537–540.
60. Horbett, T. A. (1994) The role of adsorbed proteins in animal cell adhesion. *Coll. Surf. B: Biointerfaces* **2,** 225–240.
61. Hynes, R. (1992) Integrins: versatility, modulation, and signalling in cell adhesion. *Cell* **69,** 11–25.
62. Mohri, H. (1996) Fibronectin and integrins interactions. *J. Investig. Med.* **44,** 429–441.
63. Bale, M. D., Wohlfahrt, L. A., Mosher, D. F., Tomasini, B., and Sutton, R. C. (1989) Identification of vitronectin as a major plasma protein adsorbed on polymer surfaces of different copolymer composition. *Blood* **74,** 2698–2706.
64. Steele, J., Johnson, G., and Underwood, P. (1992) Role of serum vitronectin and fibronectin in adhesion of fibroblasts following seeding onto tissue culture polystyrene. *J. Biomed. Mater. Res.* **26,** 861–884.
65. Steele, J., Johnson, G., McFarland, C., Dalton, B., Gengenbach, T., Chatelier, R., et al. (1994) Roles of serum vitronectin and fibronectin in initial attachment of human vein endothelial cells and dermal fibroblasts on oxygen- and nitrogen-containing surfaces made by radiofrequency plasmas. *J. Biomater. Sci. Polym. Ed.* **6,** 511–532.
66. Healy, K. E., Thomas, C. H., Rezania, A., Kim, J. E., McKeown, P. J., Lom, B., and Hockberger, P. E. (1996) Kinetics of bone cell organization and mineralization on materials with patterned surface chemistry. *Biomaterials* **17,** 195–208.
67. Matsuda, T. and Sugawara, T. (1996) Control of cell adhesion, migration, and orientation on photo-chemically microprocessed surfaces. *J. Biomed. Mater. Res.* **32,** 165–173.
68. Thomas, C. H., McFarland, C. D., Jenkins, M. L., Rezania, A., Hockberger, P. E., Steele, J. G., and Healy, K. E. (1997) The role of vitronectin in the attachment and spatial distribution of bone-derived cells on materials with patterned chemistry. *J. Biomed. Mater. Res.* **37,** 81–93.
69. Singhvi, R., Kumar, A., Lopez, G. P., Stephanopoulos, G. N., Wang, D. I., Whitesides, G. M., and Ingber, D. E. (1994) Engineering cell shape and function. *Science* **264,** 696–698.
70. Folkman, J. and Moscona, A. (1978) Role of cell shape in growth control. *Nature* **273,** 345–349.
71. Opas, M. (1994) Substratum mechanics and cell differentiation. *Intl. Rev Cytol.* **150,** 119–137.
72. Yannas, I. V. (1988) Regeneration of skin and nerve by use of collagen templates in, *Collagen vol. III, Biotechnology*, (Nimni, M. E., ed.), CRC Press, FL, pp. 87–115.
73. Chang, A. S. and Yannas, I. V. (1992) Peripheral nerve regeneration, in *Neuroscience Year: suppl. 2* (Smith, B. and Adelman, G., eds.), Birkhauser, Boston, pp. 125–126.
74. Tranquillo, R. T. and Barocus, V. H. (1997) An anisotropic, biphasic theory of tissue equivalent mechanics. *J. Biomech. Eng.* **119,** 137–145.
75. Grinnell, F. (1984) Fibronectin and wound healing. *J. Cell Biochem.* **26,** 107–112.

76. Grinnell, F., Billingham, R. E., and Burgers, L. (1984) Distribution of fibronectin during wound healing in vivo. *J. Invest. Dermatol.* **76,** 181–189.

77. Brown, R. A., Blunn, G. W., and Ejim, O. S. (1994) Preparation of orientated fibrous mats from fibronectin: composition and stability. *Biomaterials* **15,** 475–464.

78. Bowersox, J. C. and Sorgente, N. (1982) Chemotaxis of aortic endothelial cells in response to fibronectin. *Cancer Res.* **42,** 2547–2551.

79. Ungari, S., Katari, R. S., Alessandri, G., and Gullino, P. M. (1985) Cooperation between fibronectin and heparin in the mobilisation of capillary endothelium. *Invasion Metastasis* **5,** 193–205.

80. Iuliano, D. J., Saavedra, S. S., and Truskey, G. A. (1993) Effect of the conformation and orientation of absorbed fibronectin on endothelial cell spreading and the strength of adhesion. *J. Biomed. Mater. Res.* **27,** 1103–1113.

81 Albelda, S. M. and Buck, C. A. (1990) Integrins and other cell adhesion molecules. *FASEB J.* **4,** 2868–2872.

82. Elices, M. J. and Hemler, M. E. (1989) The human integrin VLA-2 is a collagen receptor on some cells and a collagen/laminin receptor on others. *Proc. Natl. Acad. Sci. USA* **86,** 9906–9910.

83. Wayne, E. A. and Carter, W. G. (1987) Identification of multiple cell adhesion receptors for collagen and fibronectin in human fibrosarcoma cells possessing unique a and common b subunits. *J. Cell Biol.* **105,** 1873–1884.

84. Pytela, R., Pierschbacher, M. D., and Ruoslahti, E. (1985) Identification and isolation of a 140kd cell surface glycoprotein with properties expected of a fibronectin receptor. *Cell* **40,** 191–198.

85. Cheresh, D. (1987) Human endothelial cells synthesize and express an arg-gly-asp directed adhesion receptor involved in attachment to fibrinogen and von Willebrand factor. *Proc. Natl. Acad. Sci. USA* **84,** 6471–6475.

86. Dejana, E., Zanetti, A., Dominguez, C., and Conforti, G. (1992) Role of integrins in endothelial cell function, in *Angiogenesis in Health and Disease* (Maragoudakis, M. E., et. al., eds.), Plenum, New York, pp. 91–98.

87. Grinnell, F. (1992) Wound repair, keratinocyte activation and integrin modulation. *J. Cell Sci.* **101,** 1–5.

88. Adams, J. C. and Watt, F. M. (1991) Expression of β1/3/4 and 5 integrins by human epidermal keratinocytes and non–differentiating keratinocytes. *J. Cell. Biol.* **115,** 829–841.

89. Larjava, H., Salo, H., Haapasalmi, K., Kramer, R. H., and Heino, J. (1993) Expression of integrins and basement menbrane components by wound keratinocytes. *J. Clin. Invest.* **92,** 1425–1435

90. Brooks, P. C., Clark, R. A. F., and Cheresh D. A. (1994) Requirement of vascular integrin αvβ3 for angiogenesis. *Science* **264,** 569–571.

91. Clark, R. A. F., Tonnesen, M. G., Gailit, J., and Cheresh, D. A. (1996) Transient functional expression of αvβ3 on vascular cells during wound repair. *Am. J. Pathol.* **148,** 1407–1421.

92. Brooks, P. C., Montgomery, A. M. P., Rosenfeld, M., Reisfeld, R. A., Hu, T., Klier, G., and Cheresh, D. A. (1994) Integrin αvβ3 antagonists promote tumour regression by inducing apoptosis of angiogenic blood vessels. *Cell* **79,** 1157–1164.

93. Enenstein, J., Waleh, N, S., and Kramer, R. H. (1992) Basic FGF and TGF–β differentially modulate integrin expression of human microvascular endothelial cells. *Exp. Cell Res.* **203,** 499–503.

94. Swerlick, R. A., Brown, E. J., Xu, Y., Lee, K. H., Manos, S., and Lawley, T. J. (1993) Expression and modulation of the vitronectin receptor on human dermal microvascular endothelial cells. *J. Invest. Dermatol.* **99,** 715–722.

95. Leavesley, D. I., Schwartz, M. A., Rosenfeld, D., and Cheresh, D. A. (1993) Integrin β1 and β3-mediated endothelial cell migration is triggered through distinct signaling mechanisms. *J. Cell Biol.* **121,** 163–170.

96. Ahmed, Z., Idowu, B. D., and Brown, R. A. (1999) Stabilisation of fibronectin mats with micromolar concentrations of copper. *Biomaterials* **20,** 201–209.

97. Raju, K. S., Alessandri, G., Ziche, M., and Gullino, P. M. (1982) Ceruloplasmin, copper ions and angiogenesis. *J. Natl. Cancer Inst.* **69,** 1183–1188.

98. McAuslan, B. R. (1980) A new theory of neovascularisation based on identification of an angiogenic factor and its effect on cultured endothelial cells, in *Control Mechanisms in Animal Cells* (Jumemez, L., et. al., eds.), Raven Press, New York, pp. 285–292.

99. Brem, S. S., Zagzag, D., Tsanaclis, A. M. C., Gatley. S., Elkouby, M.-P., and Brien, S. E. (1990) Inhibition of angiogenesis and tumour growth in the brain. *Am. J. Pathol.* **137,** 1121–1142.

100. Ziche, M., Branchelli, G., Caderni, G., Raimondi, L., Dolara, P., and Buffoni, F. (1987) Copper–dependent amine oxidases in angiogenesis induced by prostaglandin E_1. *Microvascular Res.* **34,** 133–136.

101. Siegel, R. C. (1979) Lysyl oxidase. I*nt. Rev. Connect. Tissue Res.* **8,** 73–118.

IV ANTI-ANGIOGENESIS

18
Inhibitors of Matrix Metalloproteinases

Peter D. Brown
and William G. Stetler-Stevenson

CONTENTS

MATRIX METALLOPROTEINASES

Matrix metalloproteinases are a family of closely related enzymes that degrade extracellular-matrix proteins. All members of the family contain a zinc-binding catalytic domain and are active at neutral pH. A generic domain structure is shown in Fig. 1. Matrix metalloproteinase activity is thought to be responsible for much of the degradation of extracellular matrix that is necessary for normal development and is a central feature in the pathogenesis of diseases such as cancer and arthritis. The importance of degradative enzymes in the process of tissue remodeling was recognized long before the first matrix metalloproteinases were isolated and characterized. Writing in 1949, Gersch and Catchpole postulated that "during rapid growth of a tumor, perhaps even as a condition of tissue invasion by a neoplasm, the ground substance of neighboring connective tissue stroma, including the basement membrane of small blood vessels, may become more fluid as a result of the depolymerisation of the ground substance. This may be effected through the action of depolymerizing enzymes possibly secreted by fibroblasts" (1). In view of the now generally accepted role of fibroblasts in the secretion and/ or activation of matrix metalloproteinases in the process of tumor invasion this statement seems particularly far sighted.

It was another 18 years before the first mammalian matrix metalloproteinase, interstitial collagenase, was described (2). Shortly thereafter several groups showed that neoplastic transformation was accompanied by a marked increase in the expression of degradative enzymes, including collagenase (3,4). A second matrix metalloproteinase active in degrading the type IV collagen of basal laminae was isolated from metastatic sarcoma cells (5,6). The

From: *The New Angiotherapy*
Edited by: T.-P. D. F@an and E. C. Kohn © Humana Press Inc., Totowa, NJ

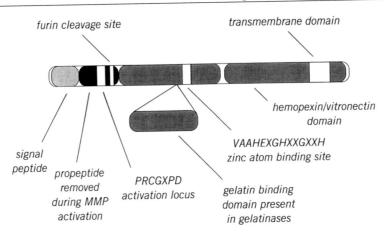

Fig. 1. Generic domain structure of matrix metalloproteinases. The hemopexin/vitronectin carboxy-terminal domain is severely truncated in the smallest matrix metalloproteinase, matrilysin. This domain also contains a transmembrane domain in the MT-MMP subfamily. The gelatin binding domain is unique to the two gelatinases and the furin cleavage site is only present in stromelysin-3 and the MT-MMPs. Latency is conferred through coordination of the zinc atom by the cysteine residue in the PRCGXPD activation locus in the amino-terminal propeptide.

human matrix metalloproteinase family is now known to include at least 15 enzymes, which collectively are capable of degrading all components of the extracellular matrix (Table 1). Many of these enzymes were originally identified because they were overexpressed in tumor cells or tumor tissue extracts. However, it is now known that matrix metalloproteinases are not tumor-specific but are expressed at low levels in a number of physiologic conditions, such as wound healing, placental development, and embryogenesis.

Three collagenases have been identified, interstitial collagenase (MMP-1), neutrophil collagenase (MMP-8), and collagenase 3 (MMP-13). These enzymes can degrade the generally proteolytic resistant fibrillar collagens making a characteristic 3/4 length break in the α-chain *(7,8)*. There are two type IV collagenases *(9,10)*, now termed gelatinase A (MMP-2) and gelatinase B (MMP-9), which, as described by Liotta and colleagues *(6)*, can degrade type IV collagen of basal laminae as well as other "nonhelical" collagen domains and proteins such as fibronectin and laminin. The gelatinases have also been shown to degrade native insoluble elastin *(11)*. Three enzymes have been classified as "stromelysins" although only stromelysin 1 (MMP-3) and stromelysin 2 (MMP-10) are closely related functionally, degrading various proteoglycan components of the extracellular matrix as well as fibronectin and laminin *(12,13)*. Stromelysin 3 (MMP-11) was identified relatively recently in the tissue surrounding invasive breast carcinoma *(14)*. Its preferred substrate remains a matter of debate. It does not appear to breakdown known extracellular matrix proteins but it is effective in degrading the serine proteinase inhibitor (serpin) α-1 antitrypsin and in doing so may potentiate the action of serine proteinases such as urokinase-type plasminogen activator (uPA) *(15)*. This serpinase activity is also displayed by other matrix metalloproteinases and supports the hypothesis that the metallo- and serine proteinase families act in an interdependent manner.

Two enzymes have been identified that, on the basis of sequence homology, do not belong in the three subgroups described earlier. These are matrilysin (MMP-7, formerly known as Pump) *(16)* and metalloelastase (MMP-12) *(17)*. Matrilysin is a short "truncated" proteinase that can degrade nonfibrillar collagen, fibronectin, and laminin.

Table 1
Human Matrix Metalloproteinase Family

Enzyme	Number	Principal substrates[a]
Interstitial collagenase	MMP-1	Fibrillar collagens, types I, II, III
Neutrophil collagenase	MMP-8	Fibrillar collagens, types I, II, III
Collagenase-3	MMP-13	Type I collagen
Gelatinase A	MMP-2	Nonfibrillar collagens, fibronectin, laminin
Gelatinase B	MMP-9	Nonfibrillar collagens, types IV and V
Stromelysin-1	MMP-3	Nonfibrillar collagens, proteoglycan, laminin
Stromelysin-2	MMP-10	Nonfibrillar collagens, proteoglycan, laminin
Stromelysin-3	MMP-11	Serine protease inhibitors (serpins)
Matrilysin	MMP-7	Nonfibrillar collagens, fibronectin, laminin
Metalloelastase	MMP-12	Elastin, nonfibrillar collagen
MT1-MMP[b]	MMP-14	Progelatinase A
MT2-MMP	MMP-15	Not defined
MT3-MMP	MMP-16	Progelatinase A
MT4-MMP	MMP-17	Not defined
— —	MMP-18	Not defined

[a]The principal substrates listed are only helpful as a guide; in practice, the substrate specificity shown in vitro is broad with considerable overlap between matrix metalloproteinases.
[b]MT stands for membrane-type.

Metalloelastase, as the name suggests, is capable of degrading elastin. In the past two years, the matrix metalloproteinase family has grown by the addition of a new subgroup, the membrane-type-, or MT-, MMPs. Currently four members have been identified (MMP-14 to MMP-17) *(18–21)*. These proteinases have a c-terminal transmembrane domain that allows them to be anchored in the cell membrane. The susbstrates for most of these enzymes have yet to be established, however, MT1-MMP and MT3-MMP (MMP-14, MMP-16) appear to be specific activators of latent gelatinase A *(20,22)*. More recently MMP-18, an enzyme with some homology to the stromelysins, has been added to the family *(23)* and it is likely that other members will be discovered in the next few years.

Another recent discovery is the finding that matrix metalloproteinases can hydrolyse the membrane-bound precursor form of tumor necrosis factor-α (TNF-α) as well as various other cytokines. Several members of the matrix metalloproteinase family show some activity in this form of cytokine processing but the identity of the enzyme or enzymes responsible in vivo remains to be determined, as does the physiological and pathological relevance of the activity *(24)*.

It is now generally accepted that matrix metalloproteinases play an important role in normal processes of tissue remodeling such as trophoblast implantation, embryogenesis, mammary involution, tissue growth, and wound repair. In these processes, the activity of these degradative enzymes can be kept in check at three levels. Firstly, gene expression is often tightly controlled with most, but not all, matrix metalloproteinases being expressed only when their activity is required. Secondly, matrix metalloproteinases are synthesized as latent proenzymes that require the proteolytic removal of a 10 kDa amino-terminal domain in order to become proteolytically active. For most of the matrix metalloproteinases, this occurs after secretion from the cell. The activation step is initiated by several possible mechanisms involving either an enzymatic activation cascade and/or cell-surface regulation. In the case of stromelysin-3 and MT1-MMP, the presence of a furin-processing motif (Arg-Xaa-Lys-Arg) suggests that these enzymes can be processed intracellularly in the Golgi vesicles. Thirdly, the activated matrix metalloproteinases can be inhibited by endogenous proteinase inhibitors such as α2-macroglobulin and more importantly the family of tissue inhibitors of metalloproteinases (TIMPs 1–4) *(25–28)*.

The secretion and activation of gelatinase A has been studied in some detail. This matrix metalloproteinase is secreted as the pro-enzyme with its native inhibitor TIMP-2 bound at a noninhibitory site. The pro-gelatinase-TIMP-2 complex is believed to be activated at the cell surface by MT1-MMP. TIMP-2 released from the complex is presumably in a good position to re-bind to activated gelatinase A, this time blocking the active site *(22)*. This abundance of negative regulatory mechanisms may explain how gelatinase A can be expressed constitutively in some tissues, such as arteriolar smooth muscle, without causing extensive degradation. Its activation in this tissue is likely to be tightly controlled and the active species short-lived.

Despite all of this negative regulation, there are several disease states in which matrix metalloproteinase activity is increased. In these pathogenic conditions it seems that rather than a complete uncoupling of inhibitory controls there is a "reprogramming" of enzymes and inhibitors involved in tissue remodeling. This allows the construction of new tissue, including new blood vessels. This is perhaps best illustrated by cancer, where simple tissue destruction would not be of advantage to the growing malignancy. In effect the tumor must remodel the local tissue to suit its own needs. The generation of a modified and increased vasculature is perhaps the most obvious feature of this remodeling, but associated with this must be the generation of supportive connective tissue.

Synthetic matrix metalloproteinase inhibitors were initially developed as agents to block tissue degradation in rheumatoid arthritis. As the role of matrix metalloproteinases in tissue remodeling and angiogenesis in different diseases has become better defined, the potential of these inhibitors as treatments for cancer and neurodegenerative diseases has also been explored. This chapter will review the experimental evidence for the role of matrix metalloproteinases in angiogenesis and describe the development of synthetic matrix metalloproteinase inhibitors, including results from the first clinical trials in cancer patients.

ROLE OF MATRIX METALLOPROTEINASES IN ANGIOGENESIS

Functional analysis clearly demonstrates the requirement for proteolytic activity in the process of angiogenesis. Less understood are the relative contributions of various classes of extracellular matrix degrading proteinases. This is almost certainly owing to the interdependence of the different proteinase systems, which must act in concert during the processes of endothelial-cell migration, invasion and vessel formation. Early studies with bovine corneal endothelial cells demonstrated that in vitro invasion through human amniotic membrane can be blocked by both serine protease inhibitors, such as aprotinin, and by the matrix metalloproteinase inhibitor, TIMP-1 *(29)*. Anti-gelatinase A antibodies also blocked invasion. In each case invasion was inhibited by 80–90% independently for each inhibitor, supporting the hypothesis that invasion may require the coordinate expression of both classes of proteinase. A role for the cysteine proteinase, cathepsin B, has also been suggested *(30,31)*.

Recent evidence for a role of matrix metalloproteinases in angiogenesis comes from studies with synthetic and endogenous matrix metalloproteinase inhibitors. The synthetic matrix metalloproteinase inhibitor, batimastat (British Biotech), was shown to reduce the angiogenic response in vivo to heparin-Matrigel implants to levels comparable to controls without added heparin *(32)*. In the same study it was shown that batimastat inhibited the invasion of human umbilical-vein endothelial cells through Matrigel in vitro, but did not significantly alter endothelial cell proliferation, haptotaxis, or chemotaxis. In this regard it appears that endogenous matrix metalloproteinase inhibitors may differ in their anti-angiogenic activity from synthetic inhibitors because TIMPs also appear to block endothelial-cell proliferation and/or migration. Studies with a cartilage-derived matrix metalloproteinase inhibitor have demonstrated the ability of this TIMP-related protein to block both capillary endothelial-cell proliferation and migration, as well as in vivo angiogenesis in the chick chorioallantoic membrane (CAM) assay *(33)*. Similarly TIMP-2 was shown to inhibit the proliferation of human microvascular endothelial cells in conditions where neither batimastat nor anti-gelatinase A antibodies were effective *(34)*. This suggests that TIMP-2 may modulate the proliferation of these human endothelial cells in a protease-independent fashion. TIMP-1 did not slow endothelial-cell proliferation in this study but did inhibit endothelial-cell chemotaxis and angiogenesis in more recent study *(35)*.

TIMPs, and synthetic inhibitors such as batimastat, are "broad spectrum" matrix metalloproteinase inhibitors and their anti-angiogenic activity reveals little about the contribution of individual matrix metalloproteinases to the process of angiogenesis. An immunohistochemical study of angiogenesis in skin during both fetal development and in adult cutaneous tumors has identified interstitial collagenase as being the principal matrix metalloproteinase expressed in developing microvessels. Expression of stromelysin, matrilysin, gelatinase A, and gelatinase B was not detected *(36)*. However, earlier studies have shown that anti-gelatinase A antibodies are able to inhibit endothelial-cell invasion in vitro *(29)*. Activation of gelatinase A has also been observed in tubule formation in vitro in cocultures of glial cells and central nervous system (CNS) microvascular endothelial cells *(37)*. As has been suggested by Pepper and others, the proteinase(s) used in the process of angiogenesis may change according to the type of tissue being vascularized. In analysing vascularization of tissue in uPA-deficient mice, they raised the possibility that uPA may only be necessary for vessel development when endothelial cells are invading fibrin *(38)*. The inhibition of cytokine-processing by matrix metalloproteinases may also modulate angiogenesis indirectly.

Synthetic matrix metalloproteinase inhibitors have been widely tested in animal models of cancer. These compounds have been shown to block both invasion and metastasis in both syngeneic and xenograft models and have improved survival *(39)*. Unfortunately, microvessel density has rarely been assessed in these models and much less is known about the effect of synthetic matrix metalloproteinase inhibitors on tumor angiogenesis. In one of the first studies with batimastat, Davies et al reported that treatment of nude mice bearing human ovarian cancer malignant ascites resulted in the formation of dense avascular nodules with small islands of tumor cells. However, this is a specialized setting in which vascularization is not a major factor *(40)*. More recently, Sledge and colleagues used antibodies to the endothelial-cell antigen CD31 to analyze blood-vessel density in MDA-MB-435 xenografts treated with batimastat. The tumors were grown in the mammary fat pads of nude mice and resected after 9 wk. The mice were then treated with batimastat or vehicle to investigate the ability of this inhibitor to inhibit regrowth. The rate of regrowth was significantly reduced in the batimastat-treated animals but the microvessel density appeared unchanged in the tumors that did develop *(41)*. In these sorts of studies, it may not be possible to resolve direct effects of matrix metalloproteinase inhibitors on tumor-cell invasion from effects on endothelial cell invasion and angiogenesis.

One interesting feature of certain experimental tumors treated with matrix metalloproteinase inhibitors is the development of an enlarged necrotic core. This was reported for C170HM$_2$ human colon tumors grown in the intraperitoneal cavity of nude mice *(42)*. These tumors grow rapidly by invading the liver. In addition to reducing the number and size of the liver tumors, batimastat treatment was associated with a marked increase in the size of necrotic core. An increase in the proportion of necrotic tumor was also observed in the treatment of Mat Ly Lu rat prostate tumors with the synthetic matrix metalloproteinase inhibitors, GI168 and GI173 (Glaxo Inc.) *(43)*. This increase in necrosis may be the result of anti-angiogenic activity. Alternatively, it is possible that in certain tumors constriction of invasive growth by matrix metalloproteinase inhibitors results in increased interstitial pressure. This in turn leads to compression of blood vessels in the center of the tumor causing ischaemia and subsequent necrosis *(44,45)*.

DEVELOPMENT OF MATRIX METALLOPROTEINASE INHIBITORS

Both endogenous and synthetic inhibitors have been considered as potential therapies for the treatment of arthritis and cancer. TIMP-1 and TIMP-2 were cloned and sequenced in 1985 and 1989, respectively *(25,26)*, and both have shown activity in models of tumor invasion, metastasis, and angiogenesis *(35,46–49)*. Unfortunately, the therapeutic use of these molecules has been limited by the fact that they are proteins (M_r 20,000–28,000), which makes long-term systemic administration particularly difficult. The possibility that TIMPs may have protease-independent inhibitory effects on endothelial-cell proliferation and motility *(34)* means that these proteins will remain of great interest in the development of "gene therapies."

The first synthetic matrix metalloproteinase inhibitors were developed in the early 1980s. These molecules were pseudopeptide derivatives based on the structure of the collagen molecule at the site of cleavage by interstitial collagenase. Compounds designed from the Ile-Ala-Gly and Leu-Leu-Ala sequences on the right-hand side of the cleavage site have emerged as the most promising drugs. The structure of one such compound, marimastat (BB-2516, British Biotech) is shown in Fig. 2. The inhibitor binds reversibly at the active site of the matrix metalloproteinase in a stereospecific manner. The zinc-binding group, in this case hydroxamic acid, is then positioned to chelate the active site zinc ion. Modification of the stereochemistry of the molecule results in loss of inhibitory activity. Several zinc-binding groups have been tested including carboxylates, aminocarboxylates, sulphydryls, and derivatives of phosphorus acids *(50)*, but hydroxamates have proved to be the most useful and the majority of inhibitors currently in clinical testing contain this group.

Highly potent compounds with K_i values in the low nanomolar range were developed early without the assistance of X-ray crystal structures. These compounds, typified by batimastat, showed broad specificity for members of the matrix metalloproteinase family but displayed little detectable activity against other classes of metalloproteinase such as angiotensin converting enzyme and enkephalinase *(39)*. Unfortunately, these early compounds showed poor oral bioavailability and long-term therapeutic use was problematic.

The design of synthetic matrix metalloproteinase inhibitors then proceeded with two goals, the development of compounds with good oral bioavailability and the development of compounds with selective inhibitory activity against individual matrix metalloproteinases. In both cases the design of new compounds was assisted by X-ray crystallography data on the three-dimensional structure of the collagenase active site *(51)*. Marimastat (M_r 333) was one of the first inhibitors to show good oral bioavailability

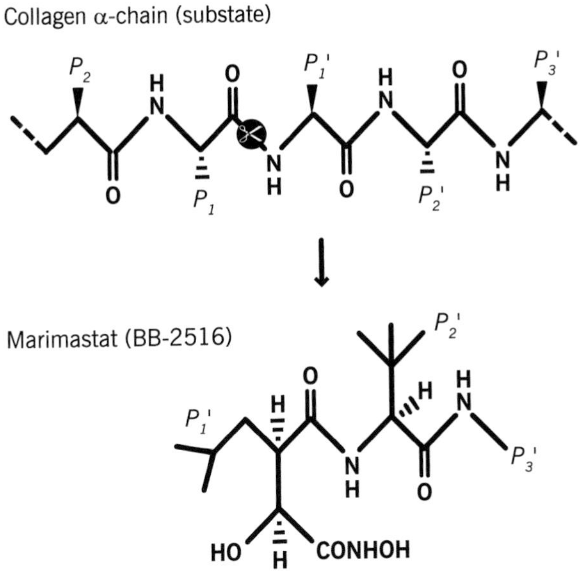

Collagen α-chain (substate)

Fig. 2. Structure of marimastat. Many of the inhibitors currently being studied are derived from the peptide structure of the α-chain of type I collagen at the point at which collagenase first cleaves the molecule. Marimastat is based on the right-hand side of this cleavage site, although the chemical groups at the P1', P2', and P3' positions are different from the original amino acid residues. The hydroxamate (-CONHOH) group binds the zinc atom in the active site of the MMP enzyme.

in both animals and humans, differing from its predecessor batimastat in the group adjacent to the hydroxamate and the group at the P2' position. In both positions a small substituent, -hyroxyl and -t-butyl, respectively, replaces a larger cyclic group.

More selective compounds have also been developed. In practice, these compounds are not selective for one particular matrix metalloproteinase but instead show a selective loss of activity against one or more of the enzymes. A series of compounds described by Morphy et al. take advantage of differences in the active site of gelatinase A and B which allow larger hydrophobic groups at the P1' position (52). These compounds show greater than 1000-fold selectivity for gelatinases over interstitial collagenase but are also quite potent inhibitors of stromelysin-1. Unfortunately, these early selective inhibitors have not shown good bioavailability when given orally and CDP-845 (Celltech), a potent selective gelatinase inhibitor, has recently been withdrawn from clinical development partly for this reason. Ro 32-3555 (Roche) is a hydroxamate-based inhibitor with relatively weak activity against gelatinase A and stromelysin-1, but good activity against interstitial collagenase. This compound shows good activity when given orally in animal models of arthritis and is currently in clinical development as a treatment for rheumatoid arthritis (53). It is expected that other orally bioavailable selective matrix metalloproteinase inhibitors will follow Ro 32-3555 into the clinic.

Low molecular-weight matrix metalloproteinase inhibitors have also been developed from natural products such as the tetracylines. Chemical modification of this group of molecules has led to the separation of antibiotic and protease-inhibitory activity (54). Interestingly, the more potent natural products such as BE16627B (55) and matlystatin (56) are structurally very similar to the right-hand side pseudopeptide inhibitors obtained by rational substrate-based design.

PRECLINICAL STUDIES

Studies of the effects of matrix metalloproteinase inhibitors in experimental models of disease are an important part of the preclinical development of potential drugs and provide some indication of what might be expected in the way of therapeutic effect in the subsequent clinical trials. Cancer models are a relevant example because the first clinical testing of matrix metalloproteinase inhibitors has been in cancer patients. Early studies with synthetic matrix metalloproteinase inhibitors, such as the hydroxamate SC44463 (G.D. Searle), and recombinant TIMPs demonstrated that these inhibitors could block tumor-cell invasion through matrix barriers in vitro and inhibit organ colonization by tumor cells (experimental metastasis) in vivo (46,57). At this time matrix metalloproteinase inhibitors were primarily thought of as anti-metastatic drugs; that is, drugs to block the passage of metastatic cells "into" and "out of" lymphatic and vascular channels. However, as further studies were carried out, it was realized that these inhibitors might have the potential to inhibit the growth of established tumors, either at their primary or secondary site.

Mechanistically it was proposed that matrix metalloproteinase inhibitors could inhibit tumor growth either by encouraging "stromal encapsulation" of the tumor, thereby preventing invasive growth, or by inhibiting angiogenesis. In a model of rat mammary carcinoma, batimastat was shown to reduce both the spread of metastatic cells and the growth of established metastases (58). Batimastat was also shown to inhibit loco-regional regrowth and metastasis of a human breast carcinoma, MDA-MB-435, following resection in athymic nude mice (41). In another series of experiments, increased expression of TIMP-2, in clones of rTIMP-2 transfected metastatic 4R cells, was associated with marked suppression of tumor growth and local invasion following subcutaneous implantation. Clones showing suppressed growth were surrounded by a capsule of dense connective tissue (49). Also, as mentioned previously, inhibition of the growth of some tumors by synthetic matrix metalloproteinase inhibitors is associated with an increase in the extent of the necrotic core (42,43). These changes in histological appearance offer one means of looking for anti-tumor activity in clinical studies and an example of this approach is described in the next section. Detection of a reduction in metastasis is not easily measured in the clinical setting. Metastases establish and grow rapidly in animal models and through various techniques can be counted when less than 1 mm in diameter. By contrast, metastasis in the clinic is a slow and unpredictable process. Metastases must grow to a size of approx 1 cm before being detectable by conventional imaging techniques. For these reasons, the effect of matrix metalloproteinase inhibitors on metastasis has not been analyzed in the first clinical trials.

Recent studies have also shown that matrix metalloproteinase inhibitors may be effectively combined with established cytoreductive cancer treatments. In a study of the synthetic inhibitor CT1746 (Celltech) and cyclophosphamide the two compounds combined were shown to be significantly more effective in inhibiting the growth and metastasis of the murine Lewis lung carcinoma than either agent used alone (59). Similarly, in a model of human ovarian carcinoma, batimastat and cisplatin were shown to be significantly more effective in prolonging survival than either single agent and, as in the study with CT1746, the additive therapeutic effects did not appear to be accompanied by additive toxicity (R. Giavazzi, personal communication). Although the mechanisms underlying these changes are not well-understood, these results have already led to clinical studies of the combined use of matrix metalloproteinase inhibitors and cytotoxic agents.

CLINICAL TRIALS WITH MATRIX METALLOPROTEINASE INHIBITORS

The first two matrix metalloproteinase inhibitors to be tested in patients were ilomastat (GM6001, Glycomed) (60) and batimastat (BB-94, British Biotech) (61). Neither compound showed good oral bioavailability and indications were sought that allowed alternative routes of administration. Ilomastat was administered as a topical agent in patients with corneal ulceration while batimastat was given as an intraperitoneal or intrapleural suspension in patients with malignant effusions. Currently, at least three matrix metalloproteinase inhibitors are believed to be in clinical trial in cancer patients as oral treatments; AG 3340 (Agouron), CGS-27023A (Novartis), and marimastat (BB-2516, British Biotech). A fourth compound developed by Bayer, but not named, is also understood to started clinic trials in cancer patients. Two compounds have also started clinical testing in patients with RA; Ro 32-3555 (Roche) and D5410 (Chiroscience). To date, results have only been presented for marimastat.

Marimastat displays limited oral bioavailability in rodents and systemic delivery by mini-pump is required for therapeutic blood concentrations of the drug to be maintained in these animals. However, preliminary results from healthy volunteer studies showed high blood concentrations of marimastat following oral administration with pharmacokinetic parameters indicating once or twice daily administration (50). Marimastat is currently being tested in a series of trials in cancer patients. Results from the first of these trials were presented at a recent European Society for Medical Oncology meeting and provide the first indications that the therapeutic potential seen in animal cancer models may be realized in the clinic. A series of studies in patients with advanced malignancy examined the effect of different doses of marimastat on the serum cancer antigens CA125, CEA, PSA, and CA19-9. Serum concentrations of these antigens are followed clinically as surrogate markers of disease progression (62–65). There was a dose-related reduction in the rate of rise of these markers, with a proportion of patients showing a fall in the absolute cancer antigen serum concentration over the 28-d study period (66–68).

In a separate study in patients with advanced gastric cancer, treatment with marimastat was associated with changes in the macroscopic and histological appearance of the tumors consistent with an increase in the quantity of fibrotic stromal tissue. The changes were very similar to those seen in various cancer models and several of the patients appeared to benefit from these alterations in tumor/stroma ratio (69).

Preliminary indications are that marimastat is generally well tolerated when given for periods of 3–6 mo. The nature of trials in patients with advanced malignancy complicates the analysis of potential side-effects and a clearer picture must await randomized placebo-controlled trials. Musculo-skeletal pain has emerged as the principal treatment related side effect with marimastat. The severity and rate of onset of symptoms were found to be dose-related and the effects were considered manageable at the dose range selected for future studies. The condition generally resolved rapidly on discontinuation of marimastat and several patients restarted treatment after an interruption of 2–4 wk (66–69). The mechanism responsible for the musculo-skeletal pain has not been established, but it seems likely that it is related to inhibition of metalloproteinase activity in the normal physiologic remodeling of tendons and joints.

PROMISE AND EXPECTATIONS

The therapeutic potential of matrix metalloproteinase inhibitors can now be studied in a range of diseases in which extracellular-matrix degradation or angiogenesis is part of the pathogenic mechanism. Trials in arthritis and cancer patients have already begun and trials in other diseases will follow. Studies in various models of neurodegenerative disease and cerebral hemorrhage indicate that both of these conditions may respond to matrix metalloproteinase inhibitor treatment (70,71). As more selective inhibitors become available for clinical testing, we might expect different inhibitors to be used in different diseases, possibly with an improved side-effect profile.

In the particular case of cancer, the use of matrix metalloproteinase inhibitors represents a fundamentally different approach from conventional treatments. A malignant tumor shows a remarkable ability to adapt to the various cytotoxic agents directed towards it, driven both by its genetic instability and high proliferative rate. Matrix metalloproteinase inhibitors, and other anti-angiogenic compounds, differ from cytoreductive treatments in that they are essentially targeting the other component of malignancy, the stroma. The tumor stroma, including the vasculature, plays a vital role in the growth, invasion, and spread of malignant disease. Perhaps this target will be less able than the tumor to evade treatment. In blocking the ability of the tumor to utilize the adjacent tissue for its own purposes, these new treatments may reveal an "Achilles heel" in the malignant phenotype; namely, its reliance on the "collaboration" of nonmalignant tissue.

If significant inhibition of tumor growth and spread can be achieved, it will alter the way both surgeons and oncologists view their respective means of intervention. Resection of more widespread disease might become worthwhile if it is known that the residual tumor can be held in check. Equally, the use of radiotherapy and chemotherapy in patients where the responses are short-lived should become more worthwhile if the time to relapse can be significantly extended. The next two years are likely to reveal whether matrix metalloproteinase inhibitors such as AG 3340, CGS-27023A, and marimastat will become part of a new generation of anti-neoplastic agents.

REFERENCES

1. Gersh, I. and Catchpole, H. R. (1949) The organization of ground substance and basement membrane and its significance in tissue injury, disease and growth. *Am. J. Anat.* **85,** 457–507.
2. Jeffrey, J. J. and Gross, J. (1967) Isolation and characterisation of a mammalian collagenolytic enzyme. *Fed. Proc.* **26,** 670.
3. Taylor, A. C., Levy, B. M., and Simpson, J. W. (1970) Collagenolytic activity of sarcoma tissues in culture. *Nature* **228,** 366–367.
4. Dresden, M. H., Heilman, S. A., and Schmidt, J. D. (1972) Collagenolytic enzymes in human neoplasms. *Cancer Res.* **32,** 993–996.
5. Liotta, L. A., Tryggvason, S., Garbisa, S., Hart, I., Foltz, C. M., and Shafie S. (1980) Metastatic potential correlates with enzymatic degradation of basement membrane collagen. *Nature* **284,** 67–68.
6. Liotta, L. A., Tryggvason, K., Garbisa, S., Robey, P. G., and Abe, S. (1981) Partial purification and characterisation of a neutral protease which cleaves type IV collagen. *Biochemistry* **20,** 100–104.
7. Wilhelm, S. C., Eisen, A. Z., Teter, M., Clark, S. D., Kronberger, A., and Goldberg, G. (1986) Human fibroblast collagenase: glycosylation and tissue-specific levels of enzyme synthesis. *Proc. Natl. Acad. Sci. USA* **83,** 3756–3760.
8. Hasty, K. A., Pourmotabbed, T. F., Goldberg, G. I., Thompson, J. P., Spinella, D. G., Stevens, R. M., and Mainardi, C. L. (1990) Human neutrophil collagenase; a distinct gene product with homology to other matrix metalloproteinases. *J. Biol. Chem.* **265,** 11,421–11,424.
9. Collier, I. E., Wilhelm, S. M., Eisen, A. Z., Marmer, B. L., Grant, G. A., Seltzer, J. L., et al. (1988) H-ras oncogene-transformed human bronchial epithelial cells (TBE-1) secrete a single metalloprotease capable of degrading basement membrane collagen. *J. Biol. Chem.* **263,** 6579–6587.
10. Wilhelm, S. M., Collier, I. E., Marmer, B. L., Eisen, A. Z., Grant, G. A., and Goldberg, G. I. (1989) SV40-transformed human lung fibroblasts secrete a 92-kDa Type IV collagenase which is identical to that secreted by normal human macrophages. *J. Biol. Chem.* **264,** 17,213–17,221.

11. Senior, R. M., Griffin, G. L., Fliszar, C. J., Shapiro, S. D., Goldberg, G. I., and Welgus, H. G. (1991) Human 92- and 72-kilodalton type IV collagenases are elastases. *J. Biol. Chem.* **266,** 7870–7875.

12. Wilhelm, S. M., Collier, I. E., Kronberger, A., Eisen, A. Z., Marmer, B. L., Grant, G. G., et al. (1987) Human skin fibroblast stromelysin: Structure, glycosylation, substrate specificity, and differential expression in normal and tumorigenic cells. *Proc. Natl. Acad. Sci. USA* **84,** 6725–6729.

13. Muller, D., Quantin, B., Gesnel, M. C., Millon-Collard, R., Abecassis, J., and Breathnach, R. (1988) The collagenase gene family in humans consists of at least four members. *Biochem. J.* **253,** 187–192.

14. Basset, P., Bellocq, J. P., Wolf, C., Stoll, I., Hutin, P., Limacher, J. M., et al. (1990) A novel metalloproteinase gene specifically expressed in stromal cell of breast carcinomas. *Nature* **348,** 699–704.

15. Pei, D., Majmudar, G., and Weiss, S. J. (1994) Hydrolytic inactivation of a breast carcinoma cell-derived serpin by human stromelysin-3. *J. Biol. Chem.* **269,** 25,849–25,855.

16. Quantin, B., Murphy, G., and Breathnach, R. (1989) Pump-1 cDNA codes for a protein with characteristics similar to those of classical collagenase family members. *Biochemistry* **28,** 5325–5334.

17. Shapiro, S. D., Kobayashi, D. K., and Ley, T. J. (1993) Cloning and characterisation of a unique elastolytic metalloproteinase produced by human alveolar macrophages. *J. Biol. Chem.* **268,** 23,824–23,829.

18. Sato, H., Takino, T., Okada, Y., Cao, J., Shinagawa, A., Yamamoto, E., and Seiki, M. (1994) A matrix metalloproteinase expressed on the surface of invasive tumor cells. *Nature* **370,** 61–65.

19. Will, H. and Hinzmann, B. (1995) cDNA sequence and mRNA tissue distribution of a novel human matrix metalloproteinase with a potential transmembrane segment. *Eur. J. Biochem.* **231,** 602–608.

20. Takino, T., Sato, H., Shinagawa, A., and Seiki, M. (1995) Identification of the second membrane-type matrix metalloproteinase (MT-MMP2) gene from a human placenta cDNA library. MT-MMPs form a unique membrane-type subclass in the MMP family. *J. Biol. Chem.* **270,** 23,013–23,020.

21. Puente, X. S., Pendas, A. M., Llano, E., Velasco, G., and López-Otin, C. (1996) Molecular cloning of a novel membrane-type matrix metalloproteinase from a human breast carcinoma. *Cancer Res.* **56,** 944–949.

22. Strongin, A., Collier, I., Bannikov, G., Marmer, B. L., Grant, G. A., and Goldberg G. I. (1995) Mechanism of cell surface activation of 72kDa type IV collagenase. *J. Biol. Chem.* **270,** 5331–5338.

23. Cossins, J., Dudgeon, T. J., Catlin, G., Gearing, A. J. H., and Clements, J. M. (1996) Identification of MMP-18, a putative novel human matrix metalloproteinase. *Biochem. Biophys. Res. Commun.* **228,** 494–498.

24. Gearing, A. J. H., Beckett, P., Christodoulou, M., Churchill, M., Clements, J., Davidson A. H., et al. (1994) Processing of tumor necrosis factor-α precursor by metalloproteinases. *Nature* **370,** 555–557.

25. Docherty, A. J. P., Lyons, A., Smith, B. J., Wright, E. M., Stephens, P. E., and Harris, T. J. R. (1985) Sequence of human tissue inhibitor of metalloproteinases and its identity to erythroid-potentiating activity. *Nature* **318,** 66–69.

26. Stetler-Stevenson, W. G., Krutzsch, H. C., and Liotta, L. A. (1989) Tissue inhibitor of metalloproteinase (TIMP-2). A new member of the metalloproteinase inhibitor family. *J. Biol. Chem.* **264,** 17,374–17,378.

27. Apte, S. S., Mattei, M. G., and Olsen, B. R. (1994) Cloning of the cDNA encoding human tissue inhibitor of metalloproteinases-3 (TIMP-3) and the mapping of the TIMP-3 gene to chromosome 22. *Genomics* **19,** 86–90.

28. Greene, J., Wang, M. S., Liu, Y. L. E., Raymond, L. A., Rosen, C., and Shi, Y. N. E. (1996) Molecular cloning and characterisation of human tissue inhibitor of metalloproteinase 4. *J. Biol. Chem.* **271,** 30,375–30,380.

29. Mignatti, P., Tsuboi, R., Robbins, E., and Rifkin, D. B. (1989) In vitro angiogenesis on the human amniotic membrane: Requirements for basic fibroblast growth factor-induced proteinases. *J. Cell Biol.* **108,** 671–682.

30. Mikkelsen, T., Yan, P. S., Ho, K. L., Sameni, M., Sloane, B. F., and Rosenblum, M. L. (1995) Immunolocalization of cathepsin B in human glioma: implications for tumor invasion and angiogenesis. *J. Neurosurg.* **83,** 285–290.

31. Sinha, A. A., Gleason, D. F., Staley, N. A., Wilson, M. J., Sameni, M., and Sloane, B. F. (1995) Cathepsin B in angiogenesis of human prostate: an immunohistochemical and immunoelectron microscopic analysis. *Anat. Record* **241,** 353–362.

32. Taraboletti, G., Garofalo, A., Belotti, D., Drudis, T., Borsotti, P., Scanziani, E., et al. (1995) Inhibition of angiogenesis and murine hemangioma growth by batimastat, a synthetic inhibitor of matrix metalloproteinases. *J. Natl. Cancer Inst.* **87,** 293–298.

33. Moses, M. A., Sudhalter, J., and Langer, R. (1990) Identification of an inhibitor of neovascularization from cartilage. *Science* **248,** 1408–1410.

34. Murphy, A. N., Unsworth, E. J., and Stetler-Stevenson, W. G. (1993) Tissue inhibitor of metalloproteinases-2 inhibits bFGF-induced human microvascular endothelial cell proliferation. *J. Cell. Physiol.* **157,** 351–358.

35. Johnson, M. D., Kim, H. R., Chesler, L., Tsao-Wu, G., Bouck, N., and Polverini, P. J. (1994) Inhibition of angiogenesis by tissue inhibitor of metalloproteinase. *J. Cell. Physiol.* **160,** 194–202.

36. Karelina, T. V., Goldberg, G. I., and Eisen, A. Z. (1995) Matrix metalloproteinases in blood vessel development in human fetal skin and in cutaneous tumors. *J. Invest. Dermatol.* **105,** 411–417.

37. Rao, J. S., Sawaya, R., Gokaslan, Z. L., Yung, W. K. A., Goldstein, G. W., and Laterra, J. (1996) Modulation of serine proteinases and metalloproteinases during morphogenic glial-endothelial interactions. *J. Neurochem.* **66,** 1657–1664.

38. Pepper, M. S., Montesano, R., Mandriota, S. J., Orci, L., and Vassalli, J. D. (1996) Angiogenesis- a paradigm for balanced extracellular proteolysis during cell migration and morphogenesis. *Enzyme Prot.* **49,** 138–162.

39. Brown, P. D. and Giavazzi, R. (1995) Matrix metalloproteinase inhibition: a review of anti-tumor activity. *Ann. Oncol.* **6,** 967–974.

40. Davies, B., Brown, P. D., East, N., Crimmin, M. J., and Balkwill, F. R. (1993) A synthetic matrix metalloproteinase inhibitor decreases tumor burden and prolongs survival of mice bearing human ovarian carcinoma xenografts. *Cancer Res.* **53,** 2087–2091.

41. Sledge, G. W., Qulali, M., Goulet, R., Bone, E. A., and Fife, R. (1995) Effect of matrix metalloproteinase inhibitor batimastat on breast cancer regrowth and metastasis in athymic mice. *J. Natl. Cancer Res.* **87,** 1546–1550.

42. Watson, S. A., Morris, T. M., Robinson, G., Crimmin, M., Brown, P. D., and Hardcastle, J. D. (1995) Inhibition of organ invasion by metalloproteinase inhibitor, BB-94 (batimastat) in two human colon metastasis models. *Cancer Res.* **55,** 3629–3633.

43. Conway, J. G., Trexler, S. J., Wakefield, J. A., Marron, B. E., Emerson, D. L., Bickett, D. M., et al. (1996) Effect of matrix metalloproteinase inhibitors on tumor growth and spontaneous metastasis. *Clin. Exp. Metastasis* **14,** 115–124.

44. Jain, R. K. (1994) Barriers to drug delivery in solid tumors. *Sci. Am.* **271,** 58–65.

45. Folkman, J. (1996) New perspectives in clinical oncology from angiogenesis research. *Eur. J. Cancer* **32A,** 2535–2539.

46. Schultz, R. M., Silberman, S., Persky, B., Bajkowski, A. S., and Carmichael, D. F. (1988) Inhibition by human recombinant tissue inhibitor of metalloproteinases of human amnion invasion and lung colonization by murine B16-F10 melanoma cells. *Cancer Res.* **48,** 5539–5545.

47. Albini, A., Melchiori, A., Santi, L., Liotta, L. A., Brown, P. D., and Stetler-Stevenson, W. G. (1991) Tumor cell invasion inhibited by TIMP-2. *J. Natl. Cancer Inst.* **83,** 775–779.

48. DeClerck, Y. A., Yean, T.-D., Chan, D., Shimada, H., and Langley, K. E. (1991) Inhibition of tumor invasion of smooth muscle cell layers by recombinant human metalloproteinase inhibitor. *Cancer Res.* **51,** 2151–2157.

49. DeClerck, Y. A., Perez, N., Shimada, H., Boone, T. C., Langley, K. E., and Taylor, S. M. (1992) Inhibition of invasion and metastasis in cells transfected with an inhibitor of metalloproteinases. *Cancer Res.* **52,** 701–708.

50. Beckett, R. P., Davidson, A. H., Drummond, A. H., Huxley, P., and Whittaker, M. (1996) Recent advances in matrix metalloproteinase inhibitor research. *Drug. Dev. Today* **1,** 16–26.

51. Grams, F., Crimmin, M., Hinnes, L., Huxley, P., Pieper, M., Tschesche, H., and Bode, W. (1995) Structure determination and analysis of human neutrophil collagenase complexed with a hydoxamate inhibitor. *Biochemistry* **34,** 14,012–14,020.

52. Morphy, J. R., Beeley, N. R. A., and Boyce, B. A. (1994) Potent and selective inhibitors of gelatinase A. 2. Carboxylic acids and phosphonic acid derivatives. *Bioorg. Med. Chem. Lett.* **4,** 2747–2752.

53. Beckett, R. P. (1996) Recent advances in the field of matrix metalloproteinase inhibitors (patent update). *Exp. Opin. Ther. Patents* **6,** 1305–1315.

54. Golub, L. M., McNamara, T. F., D'Angelo, G., Greenwald, R. A., and Ramamurthy, N. S. (1987) A nonantibacterial chemically-modified tetracycline inhibits mammalian collagenase activity. *J. Dental Res.* **66,** 1310–1314.

55. Naito, K., Nakajima, S., Kanbayashi, N., Okuyama, A., and Goto, M. (1993) Inhibition of metalloproteinase activity of rheumatoid arthritis synovial cells by a new inhibitor [BE16627B; L-N-(N-hydroxy-2-isobutylsuccinamoyl)-seryl-L-valine]. *Agents Actions* **39,** 182–186.

56. Tamaki, K., Tanzawa, K., Kurihara, S., Oikawa, T., Monma, S., Shimada, K., and Sugimura, Y. (1995) Synthesis and structure-activity relationships of gelatinase inhibitors derived from matlystatins. *Chem. Pharm. Bull.* **43,** 1883–1893.

57. Reich, R., Thompson, E. W., Iwamoto, Y., Martin, G. R., Deason, J. R., Fuller, G. C., and Miskin, R. (1988) Effects of inhibitors of plasminogen activator, serine proteinases, and collagenase IV on the invasion of basement membranes by metastatic cells. *Cancer Res.* **48,** 3307–3312.

58. Eccles, S. A., Box, G. M., Court, W. J., Bone, E. A., Thomas, W., and Brown, P. D. (1996) Control of lymphatic and hematogenous metastases of a rat mammary carcinoma by the matrix metalloproteinase inhibitor batimastat (BB-94). *Cancer Res.* **56,** 2815–2822.
59. Anderson, I. C., Shipp, M. A., Docherty, A. J. P., and Teicher, B. A. (1996) Combination therapy including a gelatinase inhibitor and cytotoxic agent reduces local invasion and metastasis of murine Lewis lung carcinoma. *Cancer Res.* **56,** 715–710.
60. Galardy, R. E., Cassabone, M. E., Giese, C., Gilbert, J. H., Lapierre, F., Lopez, H., et al. (1994) Low molecular weight inhibitors in corneal ulceration. *Ann. NY Acad. Sci.* **732,** 315–323.
61. Macaulay, V. M., O'Byrne, K. J., Saunders, M. P., Salisbury, A., Long, L., Gleeson, F., et al. (1995) Phase I study of matrix metalloproteinase (MMP) inhibitor batimastat (BB-94) in patients with malignant pleural effusions. *Br. J. Cancer* **71,** 11 (Abstract).
62. Rubin, S. C., Hoskins, W. J., and Hakes, T. B. (1989) CA 125 levels and surgical findings in patients undergoing secondary operations for epithelial ovarian cancer. *Am. J. Obstet. Gynecol.* **160,** 667–671.
63. Goldenberg, D. M., Neville, A., and Carter, A. (1981) CEA (carcinoembryonic antigen): Its role as a marker in the management of cancer. *J. Cancer Res. Clin. Oncol.* **101,** 239–242.
64. Stamey, T. A., Kabalin, J. W., and McNeal, J. E. (1989) Prostate-specific antigen in the diagnosis and treatment of adenocarcinoma of the prostate II radical prostatectomy treated patients. *J. Urol.* **141,** 1076–1083.
65. Steinberg, W., Gelfand, R., and Anderson, K. (1986) Comparison of the sensitivity and specificity of the CA 19-9 and CEA assays in detecting cancer of the pancreas. *Gastroenterology* **90,** 343–349.
66. Primrose, J., Bleiberg, H., Daniel, F., Johnson, P., Mansi, J., Neoptolemos, J., et al. (1996) A dose-finding study of marimastat, an oral matrix metalloproteinase inhibitor, in patients with advanced colorectal cancer. *Ann. Oncol.* **7,** 35 (Abstract).
67. Poole, C., Adams, M., Barley, V., Graham, J., Kerr, D., Louviaux, I., et al. (1996) A dose-finding study of marimastat, an oral matrix metalloproteinase inhibitor, in patients with advanced ovarian cancer. *Ann. Oncol.* **7,** 68 (Abstract).
68. Millar, A. and Brown, P. (1996) 360 patient meta-analysis of studies of marimastat, a novel matrix metalloproteinase inhibitor. *Ann. Oncol.* **7,** 123 (Abstract).
69. Parsons, S. L., Watson, S. A., Griffin, N. R., and Steele, R. J. C. (1996) An open phase I/II study of the oral matrix metalloproteinase inhibitor marimastat in patients with inoperable gastric cancer. *Ann. Oncol.* **7,** 47 (Abstract).
70. Gijbels, K., Masure, S., Carton, H., and Opdenakker, G. (1992) Gelatinase in cerebrospinal fluid of patients with multiple sclerosis and other inflammatory neurological disorders. *J. Neuroimmunol.* **41,** 29–34.
71. Rosenberg, G. A. (1995) Matrix metalloproteinases in brain injury. *J. Neurotrauma* **12,** 833–842.

19 Control of Angiogenesis by Microbial Products

Tsutomu Oikawa

CONTENTS

INTRODUCTION

Vascular formation is a dynamic morphogenic event essential for establishing the circulatory system during embryonic development. The establishment of a vascular network system requires both vasculogenesis and angiogenesis. Vasculogenesis is the formation of blood vessels from endothelial precursor cells, hemangioblasts, whereas angiogenesis is the growth of new vessels through the sprouting of pre-existing vasculature *(1–3)*. The mechanisms underlying vascular development have been an intriguing problem for biologists and medical scientists alike.

Recently, angiogenesis has also attracted the attention of investigators and clinicians engaged in research on and treatment of cancer. The reason for this is that the concept is now widely accepted that angiogenesis plays a fundamental role in the progressive growth and metastasis of tumors, and thus represents a novel target for cancer treatment.

For modern medical research, the important problem of how neoplasias can be overcome remains largely unresolved, though a variety of efforts have been made. Conventional therapeutic strategies, such as surgery, radiation therapy, and chemotherapy, have mainly involved strategies for directly killing tumor cells or reducing a tumor mass for a clinical effect. Unfortunately, it seems that the limits of such cytotoxic strategies have been reached *(4–7)*, and it is unlikely that remission or eradication, which is presently used as a clinical endpoint when assessing the efficacy of cancer treatment, is the best predicator of the long-term survival of patients. Against such a background a shift in the strategic approach for better cancer therapy has begun to occur *(4–7)*, while the traditional cytotoxic approaches remain in use.

From: *The New Angiotherapy*
Edited by: T.-P. D. Fan and E. C. Kohn © Humana Press Inc., Totowa, NJ

New strategies aim to regulate or control specific biological processes essential for the malignant phenotype of cancer cells. One such approach involves the inhibition of angiogenesis induced by tumors. Several anti-angiogenic agents are presently under clinical trial for patients with cancer and/or AIDS-associated Kaposi's sarcoma (KS), and a large number of inhibitors of neovascularization are being investigated in the laboratory.

Current medical research also faces the critical problem of how effective means of treatment for diseases difficult to cure, including rheumatoid arthritis and diabetic retinopathy, can be developed. A number of reports have revealed that angiogenesis plays an essential role in the induction and/or maintenance of such refractory diseases, clearly indicating that angioinhibitory therapy will become a new strategy for their treatment. These disorders, including cancer, are referred to as angiogenic diseases.

To develop such anti-angiogenic therapeutic strategies, it appears most important to find useful inhibitors of angiogenesis. From this viewpoint, a number of research groups have focused their efforts on the search for effective antagonists of neovascularization, as well as on elucidation of the mechanisms of action of angiogenesis with the aim of identifying promising targets.

Because all angiogenic diseases are chronic, and thus require long-term treatment, putative therapeutic agents should have sufficient bioavailability, half-lives, and safety, to allow oral dosing once or twice a day *(5)*. Considering the pharmacokinetic standpoint and application to clinical use, angiogenesis-antagonists with molecular weights smaller than 1,000 would be of greater therapeutic interest than large molecules such as neutralizing antibodies against certain angiogenic mitogens, as revealed by previous studies on drug development, even though such large molecules have been proven to exhibit effective therapeutic efficacy at the animal experimental level. In addition to these pharmaceutical properties, anti-angiogenic agents must preferably be nonpeptidyl organic compounds, as in the case of other therapeutic agents.

Studies on microbial products conducted so far have shown that micro-organisms produce numerous substances, like antibiotics, useful for maintaining human or other vegetable life. Thus it is rational to consider that they could produce useful inhibitors of angiogenesis as well. Indeed our group and others have found that a number of seemingly unrelated classes of small molecules derived from microorganisms interfere with angiogenesis. Several of these antagonists are currently under clinical trial for patients with solid tumors and/or AIDS-related KS, and many preclinical trials of microbial angiogenesis inhibitors for the treatment of angiogenic diseases such as solid tumors and rheumatoid arthritis are in progress.

This chapter will focus on potential control of angiogenesis by means of microbial products. The major part of this chapter will be based on information derived from in vivo rather than in vitro studies, because for the past 15 years our group has focused its efforts on the finding and development of angiogenesis-antagonists that elicit their effects in vivo and thus are efficacious against angiogenesis-dependent diseases, particularly solid tumors *(8)*. Thus the reader is referred to recent reviews for a broad coverage of the inhibitors, biology, and mechanism of neovascularization *(9–19)*.

OVERVIEW OF ANGIOGENESIS PROCESS

Because the concept of angiogenesis is thoroughly reviewed in other chapters, neovascularization will be briefly discussed to help the reader understand the contents of this chapter.

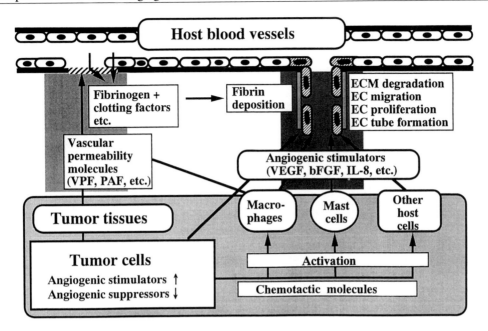

Fig. 1. Proposed scheme for the process of tumor angiogenesis.

Events Occurring During Angiogenesis

It has been recognized that angiogenesis is a cascade reaction. However, the exact biological mechanism of neovascular action has not yet been fully established, owing to the complexity of this phenomenon. Although there have been some advances in our understanding of the mechanism, an overall picture of angiogenesis is only just emerging. Because advances in our understanding of the process of angiogenesis have been largely owing to studies on tumor-related angiogenesis, the typical proposed scheme for the overall process of tumor angiogenesis is shown in Fig. 1. This scheme can be basically expanded, to varying extents, to other angiogenic responses that occur under non-neoplastic pathological conditions, including rheumatioid arthritis and proliferative diabetic retinopathy, and probably to physiological settings such as wound healing and corpus luteum formation, regardless of whether the key factor that triggers angiogenesis is the same or different in a certain situation. In the case of tumor angiogenesis, the functional cells are tumor cells, vascular endothelial cells (ECs), and/or other host cells recruited in the tumor site, including macrophages, mast cells, and fibroblast cells. The extent that these three types of host cells other than ECs contribute to the induction of angiogenesis seems to vary in the respective settings, and probably with the type of tumor. In contrast, there seems to be no convincing evidence that these three types of host cells play roles during embryonic angiogenesis.

An interesting point to emphasize here is that most, if not all, newly formed blood vessels are distinguishable from the pre-existing vasculature by their zigzagging character, although why new vessels display such a property remains largely unknown. Use of the mouse dorsal air-sac assay system involving a tumor cell-containing chamber might have revealed the possibility that such zigzagging vessels might be linked with changes in the tumor extracellular matrix (ECM), including fibrin deposition, ultimately induced by vascular hyperpermeability occurring in the early stage of angiogenesis. This problem will also be discussed in a later section of this chapter.

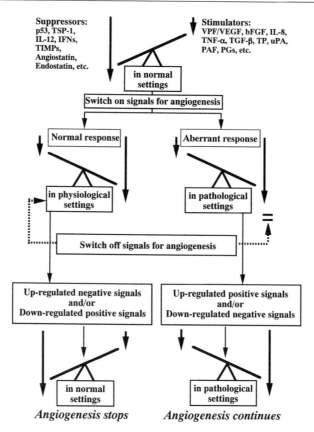

Fig. 2. Control of angiogenic responses by endogenous positive and negative regulators involved in the responses. Physiological neovascularization is self-controlled, and thus tightly regulated as to time and space. In contrast, angiogenic responses occurring in pathological settings are not self-controlled, and are in general endless. Note that angiogenesis is the result of a net balance between positive and negative regulators involved in angiogenesis; this phenomenon is induced by both upregulated angiogenesis-promoting signals and downregulated angiogenesis-suppressing signals. TP, thymidine phosphorylase; TIMPs, tissue inhibitors metalloproteinases.

An additional crucial aspect is that normal neovascularization is tightly regulated as to time and space; this response occurs under control of the homeostasis in the body. In contrast, angiogenic responses occurring in pathological settings are not self-controlled, and thus are in general endless. Also, one should note that angiogenesis is the result of a net balance between positive and negative regulators involved in angiogenesis; this phenomenon is induced through both upregulation of angiogenesis-promoting signals and downregulation of angiogenesis-suppressing signals (Fig. 2).

Function and States of Differentiation of Endothelial Cells During Angiogenesis

Normal vascular ECs are considered to be quiescent and in a well-differentiated state in vivo. During angiogenesis, differentiated ECs de-differentiate into cells with an undifferentiated phenotype, which exhibit both proliferative and migratory properties, as well as the ability to produce the proteolytic enzymes necessary for degrading extracellular matrix components, including urokinase-type plasminogen activator (uPA) and matrix metalloproteinases (MMPs). These cells subsequently differentiate into vessel-forming cells with a quiescent phenotype: eventually such upregulated activities have to be reduced to the basal level in differentiated cells, whereas capillary sprouts differentiate into mature capillaries with a new basement membrane.

Angiogenesis and Hyperpermeability

New blood vessels induced by tumors (and presumably those seen in other angiogenesis-dependent settings) exhibit a tortuous morphology, and this could be associated with increased vascular permeability. Vasopermeability-inducing factors include vascular permeability factor (VPF), also known as vascular endothelial growth factor (VEGF), platelet-activating factor (PAF), bradykinin, prostaglandins (PGs), histamine, and nitric oxide (NO or endothelium-derived relaxing factor), all of which induce an angiogenic response in in vivo model systems through their direct or indirect action on ECs (20–30). Interestingly, recent studies have suggested that the mechanism of vascular hyperpermeability induced by VPF/VEGF is different from those by the other factors, although VPF/VEGF and histamine may share a mechanism. VPF/VEGF acts on ECs to primarily increase the trans-endothelial permeability of plasma proteins through upregulation of the function of vesiculo-vacuolar organelles (31–33), whereas it is widely accepted that the increased vasopermeability induced by the other effectors is largely owing to the increased passage of plasma macromolecules through inter-EC junctions. Also, the mechanism of action of VPF/VEGF in causing vasopermeability does not require the activation of a transduction pathway involving PAF, bradykinin, or histamine (34). These vasopermeable molecules, including VPF/VEGF and PAF, are produced by different types of cells, such as tumor cells and activated macrophages (3,35,36–43). With respect to the effect of NO as a pro-angiogenic molecule, there is one contrary claim; sodium nitroprusside, which releases NO spontaneously, was reported to suppress angiogenesis in a model system involving chorioallantoic membranes (CAMs) of 9-d-old chick embryos (44).

HISTORY OF ANGIOGENESIS INHIBITOR RESEARCH

Before discussing inhibitors of angiogenesis derived from microorganisms, the history of the research on anti-angiogenic substances will be briefly reviewed.

Angioinhibitory activity was firstly detected in cartilage (45). This finding was based on the observation that this tissue is normally avascular, and is resistant to invasion or metastasis by most tumors, suggesting the presence of angiogenesis inhibitor(s). To date, several large molecules with anti-angiogenic activity have been found to present in this tissue, including a cartilage-derived inhibitor, a member of the tissue inhibitors of MMPs, and an unknown heat-resistant factor (46–48). A variety of endogenous suppressive factors of angiogenesis have been identified in other tissues, including factors transcriptionally regulated by the product of p53 tumor-suppressor gene, such as thrombospondin-1 (TSP-1) and a tentatively named glioma-derived angiogenesis-inhibitory factor, interferons (IFNs), angiostatin (a 38-kD fragment of plasminogen), interleukin 12 (IL-12) (8–16,49,50) and more recently identified endostatin (50a). Neutralizing antibodies directed against angiogenic peptides, such as basic fibroblast growth factor (bFGF), VPF/VEGF, and IL-8, as well as blocking antibodies to integrin $\alpha_v\beta_3$, have been shown to interfere with angiogenesis and/or to have anti-tumor effects (51–61). Several of these endogenous as well as exogenous inhibitors are currently under clinical trial for patients with cancer and/or AIDS-related KS, including IFNα-2a, platelet factor 4, carboxyaminotriazole, BB-94, BB-2516, and linomide.

MICROBIAL ANGIOGENESIS INHIBITORS

The information derived from studies on angiogenesis and/or ones previously unrelated to angiogenesis has just begun to uncover the mechanism of the angiogenic action, including signaling pathways, as well as cells and factors involved in the induction of neovascularization (Fig. 1). It seems impossible to say, however, that there is now an angiogenesis inhibitor whose mechanism of action has been entirely clarified. This might be owing to the fact that the mechanism of angiogenesis remains largely unknown, and that we still do not have sufficient information to determine how the in vitro effect(s) of a certain antagonist is related to its in vivo anti-angiogenic action. Thus, in this chapter most microbial angiogenesis inhibitors (Fig. 3) will be classified, based on findings seemingly unrelated to their previously reported in vitro effects. In particular, I shall focus on their effects on vascular ECs such as proliferation, migration, uPA production, and tube-formation.

Inhibitors with Modulatory Effects on Cellular Signaling Pathways

Studies in molecular and cellular biology have revealed that protein phosphorylation events mediated by a variety of protein kinases, including tyrosine kinases and protein kinase C (PKC), represent a key mechanism in triggering several cellular signaling pathways *(62–70)*. Also, other enzymes, such as phospholipases and phosphatidylinositol 3-kinase, have been shown to play roles in these signal-transduction pathway systems *(71–73)*. Thus, it is possible that agents that affect the functions of these enzymes deeply involved in these systems, could interfere with cellular events related to angiogenesis.

TYROSINE KINASE INHIBITORS

It has been found that a number of protein tyrosine kinases function as key factors in cellular signaling pathways. There is increasing evidence that this is also probably true in the case of endothelial responses to angiogenic signals.

Herbimycin A. Herbimycin A was originally identified as a benzoquinoid ansamycin antibiotic with herbicidal activity produced by a strain of *Streptomyces (74)*. The molecular formula and weight of herbimycin A are $C_{30}H_{42}N_2O_9$ and 574, respectively.

Subsequent studies demonstrated that this antibiotic is a potent inhibitor of protein tyrosine kinases such as p60[src] tyrosine kinase *(75,76)*. Acidic and basic FGFs, and closely related molecules were found to induce angiogenesis *(77–91)*. The membrane receptors for these angiogenic mitogens contain a functional tyrosine kinase domain, which transmits the biological signals of their ligands to intracellular transduction pathways *(92–94)*. These findings led to the working hypothesis that inhibitors of tyrosine kinase could affect angiogenic responses. As anticipated, topical treatment with herbimycin A inhibited angiogenesis in an in vivo assay system involving CAMs of developing 5-d-old chick embryos, the minimum effective dose and ID_{50} values being 100 and 150 ng (260 pmol) per egg, respectively *(95)*. This was the first evidence of a tyrosine kinase inhibitor exhibiting anti-angiogenic activity, but a direct cause-effect relationship has not yet been established. However, this finding indicated the following two possibilities.

First, microbial metabolites could provide an appealing treasury of useful angiogenesis inhibitors. Second, tyrosine kinase inhibitors could be angiogenesis-inhibitor candidates. This is supported by the studies on other microbial tyrosine kinase inhibitors described later, as well as the more recently synthesized inhibitors of the tyrosine-kinase activity of Flk-1/KDR, a receptor for VPF/VEGF *(96)*. It should be noted that the receptors of several other angiogenic mitogens (epidermal growth factor [EGF], hepatocyte growth factor) also exhibit functional tyrosine kinase activity *(3,65,97)*.

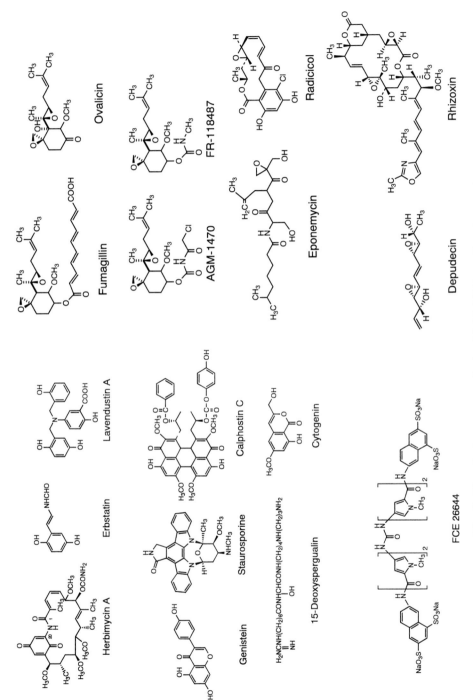

Fig. 3. Chemical structures of microbial inhibitors of angiogenesis.

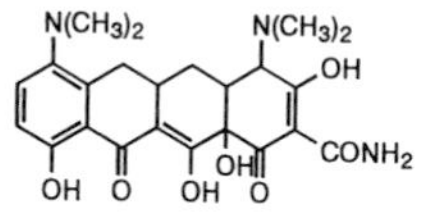

Fig. 3. (cont.) Chemical structures of microbial inhibitors of angiogenesis.

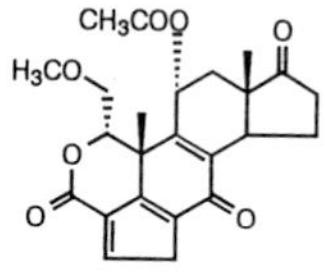

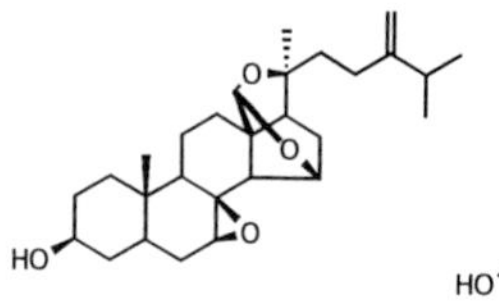

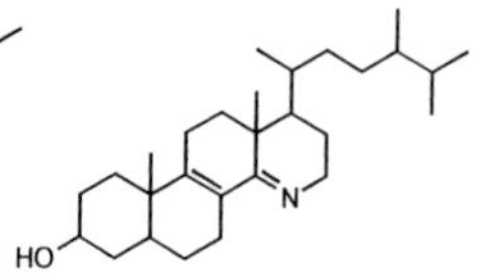

A recent study suggested that some functional groups in the herbimycin A molecule, including that at the C-19 position, the amino group between positions C-1 and C-20, and the carbamoyl group in C-7, might participate in its anti-angiogenic activity (98). Most surprisingly, the anti-angiogenic activity of herbimycin A was independently found by another group, who searched for inhibitors of angiogenesis using a random screening assay (99). The effect of systemic administration of herbimycin A on angiogenic responses has still not be mentioned in the literature. This is likely to be partly owing to the instability of herbimycin A when administered systemically, as observed for other tyrosine kinase inhibitors except lavendustin A.

Erbstatin. Erbstatin was isolated from *Streptomyces* MH435-hF3 (100,101). Its molecular formula and weight are $C_9H_9NO_3$ and 179, respectively.

Erbstatin inhibited angiogenesis in the 5-d-old CAM assay system, with an ID_{50} value of 450 pmol/egg (102). This activity appeared to be related to its inhibitory effect on EC proliferation ($IC_{50} = 3.6 \mu M$). In combination with foroxymithin, which prevents decomposition of the antibiotic through an iron-chelating action, erbstatin was found to inhibit tumor growth in vivo, although the mechanism underlying this anti-tumor activity remains unclear (103).

Lavendustin A. Lavendustin A is a tyrosine kinase inhibitor isolated from a culture filtrate of the fungus, *Streptomyces griseolavendus* (104). The molecular formula and weight of lavendustin A are $C_{12}H_{19}NO_6$ and 381, respectively.

Topical administration of lavendustin A alone inhibited VPF/VEGF-induced angiogenesis in a rat sponge-implant model (105). VPF/VEGF is a heparin-binding angiogenic mitogen that seems to selectively act on ECs through two distinct membrane-spanning tyrosine kinase receptors, Flt-1 and KDR/Flk-1 (3,33,106,107). The effect of lavendustin A on angiogenesis-dependent diseases like cancer has still not been reported. It would be very interesting to determine the effect of lavendustin A on angiogenic disorders, in which VPF/VEGF plays a predominant role.

Genistein. Genistein was originally identified as an isoflavone compound, which is an inhibitor of β-galactosidase produced by *Streptomyces xanthrophaeus* (108). Subsequently, the agent has been shown to have a tyrosine kinase-inhibitory effect, but to have little effect on the activities of other protein kinases such as cAMP-dependent kinase (109). Its molecular formula and weight are $C_{15}H_{10}O_5$ and 270, respectively.

At the dose of 100 ng/egg, genistein appeared to inhibit 5-d-old CAM angiogenesis, although the inhibition was not statistically significant *(110)*. A subsequent study revealed that genistein inhibited EC proliferation and in vitro angiogenesis at half maximal inhibition of 5 and 150 μM, respectively *(111)*. It is interesting to note that genistein was present at a high concentration in urine of individuals consuming a traditional soy-rich Japanese diet. These authors suggested that genistein may represent a member of a new class of dietary-derived anti-angiogenic compounds.

SERINE-THREONINE PROTEIN KINASE INHIBITORS

In addition to various angiogenic peptides, several chemicals like phorbol 12-myristate 13-acetate (PMA), a potent tumor promoter, have been shown to cause an angiogenic response *(112)*. PMA exhibits its tumor-promoting activity by binding to and activating PKC, a key enzyme involved in signal transduction and cell proliferation *(62)*. PMA also stimulates the proliferation of ECs and this stimulation is suppressed by staurosporine (*see* below), which is a very potent inhibitor of different types of protein kinases, including PKC *(113)*. These findings might partly form a basis for the examination of angioinhibitory activities of agents that inhibit PKC activity.

Staurosporine. Staurosporine was originally reported to be a microbial alkaloid produced by *Strepromyces* species *(114)*, and then found to be a potent protein kinase inhibitor *(115)*. The molecular formula and weight of staurosporine are $C_{28}H_{26}N_4O_3$ and 466, respectively.

Staurosporine dose-dependently inhibits angiogenesis, as evaluated in the 5-d-old CAM assay *(110)*. This inhibition started at a dose as low as 21 pmol/egg, the ID_{50} value being 71 pmol/egg. Staurosporine affected the proliferation of bovine carotid-artery ECs, with an IC_{50} value of 0.88 nM, suggesting that this inhibition might be responsible for its potent angio-inhibitory effect.

Fisetin, which is a plant flavonoid and has an inhibitory effect on PKC, also had a significant anti-angiogenic effect at the dose of 100 ng/egg under the same conditions as those used for staurosporine, although it was less potent than staurosporine *(110)*.

Calphostin C. Calphostin C is a potent and selective inhibitor of PKC isolated from the culture broth of a fungus, *Cladosporium caldosporioides (115,116)*. Its molecular formula and weight are $C_{44}H_{38}O_{14}$ and 790, respectively.

Topical administration of calphostin C (4 μg/d) significantly suppresses angiogenic responses induced by cytokines, such as tumor necrosis factor-α (TNF-α) and bFGF, and PMA in a rat sponge-implant model *(117)*. Based on these findings, the authors of this study proposed that a part of cytokine-induced neovascularization might occur through activation of PKC, and that selective inhibition of this enzyme could be efficacious against angiogenic diseases. In contrast, another group showed that in an in vivo assay system involving 10-d-old CAMs, topical treatment with calphostin C has only a small effect on angiogenesis in response to bFGF and TNF-α, but blocks the angiogenic responses induced by VEGF, tumor growth factor-α (TGF-α), and PMA *(118)*. Conceivably, the apparent discrepancy of these two studies might be related to the differences in the assay systems and/or the mode of administration of calphostin C. But, one should note that this explanation could not account for the fact that calphostin C was effective against PMA-mediated angiogenesis in these two different assay systems. It would be interesting to assess the effect of calphostin C on angiogenic diseases like cancer and rheumatoid arthritis, because it is likely that this agent will retain its angio-inhibitory action even when administered systemically.

Substances with Immunomodulatory Effects

Some immunomodulators of microbial origin, including 15-deoxyspergualin and cytogenin, have been shown to inhibit angiogenesis, although it is unclear whether their inhibitory activity is related to their immunomodulating effects. Interestingly, recent studies have suggested that the angiostatic fumagillin derivative, AGM-1470, has an immunomodulating effect *(119–122)*, and that VPF/VEGF prevents the functioning and maturation of dendritic cells. It should be noted that dendritic cells are the most effective antigen-presenting cells in the induction of primary immune responses, and are thought to be the best vehicle for the delivery of tumor-specific antigens for the immunotherapy of cancer *(123)*. As described earlier, blocking antibodies against VPF/VEGF have been found to exhibit efficacy in the treatment of solid tumors. Thus, the possibility exists that the previously observed anti-tumor effects of these two anti-angiogenic agents involve their immunomodulatory effects.

15-DEOXYSPERGUALIN

15-Deoxyspergualin exhibits the most potent biological activity among analogs of spergualin that show anti-tumor and immunomodulating activity *(124–127)*. The molecular formula and weight of this analog are $C_{17}H_{37}N_7O_3$ and 387.

15-Deoxyspergualin inhibits angiogenesis in the 5-d-old CAM assay, the ID_{50} value being 960 pmol/egg *(128)*. The agent has the distinct property that it inhibits angiogenesis in a relatively wide dose range, consistent with the results regarding its anti-tumor property *(125)*. Systemic administration of 15-deoxyspergualin significantly suppressed the angiogenic response induced by human glioma cells in the mouse dorsal air-sac assay *(129)*.

Experiments involving cultured bovine carotid-artery ECs showed that 10 μM 15-deoxyspergualin caused a 40% inhibition of cell proliferation in a three-dimensional collagen-gel assay, whereas the same concentration of 15-deoxyspergualin is ineffective in a two-dimensional culture assay *(130)*. This suggests that a three-dimensional culture assay, which more closely resembles EC proliferation in in vivo angiogenesis, would be useful for identifying novel compounds with a mechanism of action different from those of angiogenesis inhibitors found using a two-dimensional culture system. The greater usefulness of a three-dimensional culture system in angiogenesis research has been independently proposed *(131)*. There is an urgent need to develop a more complete angiogenesis assay system in order to avoid the possibility of overlooking potential angioinhibitory agents *(8,132)*.

CYCLOSPORIN A

Cyclosporin A is a nonpolar cyclic undecapeptide isolated from the fungus *Tolypocladium inflatum Grams*. Its molecular formula and weight are $C_{62}H_{111}N_{11}O_{12}$ and 1201, respectively.

In addition to its immunosuppresive property, there have been some reports that cyclosporin A causes improvement in patients with psoriasis, an angiogenic disease *(133–137)*, and suppresses tumor promotion induced by PMA *(138)*. Based on these findings, Norrby examined the anti-angiogenic activity of cyclosporin A *(139)*. At a s.c. dose of 4 mg/kg/d, cyclosporin A caused suppression of angiogenesis induced by endotoxins in a rat mesenteric-window assay system. Although the mechanism whereby cyclosporin A prevented angiogenesis remains unknown, in vitro experiments by other groups showed that at μM concentrations it affects the proliferation of ECs of different origins, including human umbilical vein ECs (HUVECs) *(140–143)*. In contrast to these results, D'Amato et al. reported that in the rabbit cornea micropocket assay, p.o. administration of cyclosporin A at a dose of 25 mg/kg had no ability to suppress bFGF-induced angiogenesis, whereas orally administered thalidomide at the dose of 200 mg/kg inhibited this angiogenic response *(144)*. Thus, it is likely that the effect of cyclosporin A on angiogenesis is dependent on the experimental conditions used, including the nature of the angiogenic stimulus. More recently, Butman et al. showed, however, that thalidomide has no effect on angiogenesis induced by and the growth of B16-melanoma or CT-26 colon carcinoma cells *(145)*. Taking this finding together with the previous observation that a neutralizing anti-bFGF antibody only has an effect in a specialized setting *(51)*, a bFGF-induced angiogenesis system may represent a model only for a limited numbers of different angiogenic responses in vivo, although a firm conclusion must await further investigation.

CYTOGENIN

Cytogenin is a small molecular agent, which was isolated from a culture filtrate of *Streproverticillium eurocidicum (146)*. Its molecular formula and weight are $C_{11}H_{10}O_5$ and 222. It exhibits anti-tumor activity in vivo, but only weak cytotoxicity toward murine and human tumor cells in vitro, even at concentrations higher than 0.2 mM *(146,147)*. It also has efficacy against arthritis induced by the injection of type II collagen in mice and adjuvant arthritis in rats, both of which are animal experimental models for human RA *(148)*. However, the mechanism by which cytogenin elicits these two activities has not yet been clarified, although there are some suggestive findings that its activities are host-mediated *(146,147,149,150)*.

Based on the fact that cytogenin exhibits efficacy against two different models of angiogenic disease, we proposed that this microbial metabolite could suppress angiogenesis and that this suppression might contribute to its therapeutic effects on these two diseases. To examine this possibility, the anti-angiogenic effects of cytogenin in the two in vivo assay systems were examined *(151)*.

Cytogenin at doses up to 100 μg/egg did not significantly affect embryonic angiogenesis when topically applied on the surface of 5-d-old CAM, suggesting that it has no effect on the normal angiogenic response. In contrast, the systemic administration of cytogenin (100 mg/kg p.o., for 5 consecutive days) significantly suppressed angiogenesis induced by S-180 sarcoma cells, one example of pathological neovascularization (Fig. 4). A pharmacokinetic study revealed that the maximal concentration of cytogenin in the plasma after a single oral injection of the compound was 32 μM. In vitro experiments showed that cytogenin at concentrations determined in the pharmacokinetic study had little effect on uPA secretion, or tube formation by or proliferation of HUVECs and/or bovine carotid-artery ECs. On the basis of these results, we proposed that cytogenin represents a novel oral anti-angiogenic agent. Its inhibitory action is probably responsible for its efficacy against both tumor growth and rheumatoid arthritis we previously found. Thus, cytogenin could be developed as a potential therapeutic agent for cancer, rheumatoid arthritis, and other angiogenesis-dependent disorders, such as diabetic retinopathy.

Although the mechanism underlying the angio-inhibitory action of cytogenin remains unclear, it might involve the following three effects: (1) an enhancing effect of cytogenin on the production of IL-1, which is induced by activated macrophages recruited in the lesion sites *(146,150)*. Indeed this cytokine inhibits bFGF-induced angiogenesis in a rabbit corneal implant model and suppresses HUVEC proliferation in vitro *(152)*; (2) the stimulatory effect of cytogenin on IFN-γ production by T lymphocytes *(150)*. Indeed IFN γ-inducible protein 10

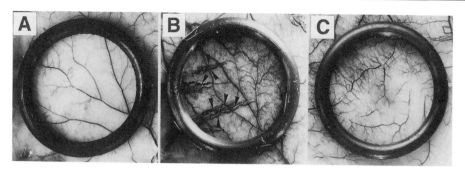

Fig. 4. Effect of cytogenin on angiogenesis induced by S-180 tumor cells. Groups A (panel **A**) and B (panel **B**) received chambers containing PBS and S-180 tumor cells, respectively, and each group was treated with the vehicle. Group C (panel **C**) received S-180 tumor cell-containing chambers, followed by the p.o. administration of cytogenin (100 mg/kg) for 5 consecutive days from the day of implantation of the chamber. Note that in panel **B**, the S-180 tumor cell-containing chamber produced zigzagging blood vessels characteristic of newly formed vasculature (arrowheads) and that the formation of such new vessels was suppressed on treatment with cytogenin (panel **C**) to roughly the extent of the angiogenesis index in group A (panel **A**). Magnification (× 3.8). (From: Oikawa, T., et al. (1997) *Anticancer Res.* **17**, 1881–1886; reproduced with permission.)

and/or monokine induced by IFN-γ have inhibitory effects on in vivo angiogenic responses induced by different angiogenic stimulators *(153–155)*, and the anti-angiogenic effect of IL-12 might be mediated through IFN-γ *(156)*. (3) The suppressive effect of cytogenin on the production of NO by activated macrophages *(149)* because, as described earlier, NO induces angiogenesis *(29,30)*. Collectively, it is likely that cytogenin inhibits tumor-induced angiogenesis via interference with multiple functions of host cells, including macrophages and/or T lymphocytes, related to angiogenesis.

Treatment involving an anti-angiogenic agent is anticipated to have to be relatively long-term. Hence it is desirable that an angioinhibitory agent be administered orally. In view of this, it should be noted that cytogenin inhibits tumor-induced angiogenesis even when given orally. Cytogenin is the first oral anti-angiogenic agent that exerts activity without affecting EC functions associated with angiogenesis: the oral administration of several compounds, including linomide *(157)* and carboxyamido-triazole *(158)*, caused the suppression of angiogenesis, probably through the inhibition of angiogenic EC functions such as the proliferation of and/or tube formation by ECs.

Sulfated Substances

Heparin is a highly sulfonated substance, which modulates an angiogenic response by binding to angiogenic molecules with affinity to heparin, but causes hemorrhage owing to its anticoagulant activity. This might be the basis for the development of sulfonated compounds that have angio-inhibitory but not anticoagulant activity. Examples are protamine sulfate, suramin and its derivative, pentosan polysulfate, platelet factor-4, and microbial-sulfonated substances, some of which are currently under clinical trial for patients with solid tumors and/or KS *(9–16,164)*.

TECOGALAN (DS-4152)

Tecogalan is a sulfated polysaccharide-peptidoglycan complex, which is derived from the bacterium, *Arthrobacter* species, with a D-gluco-D-galactan sulfate as the major component, and organic phosphates and peptidoglycan as minor ones *(159,160)*.

Tecogalan alone inhibits 5-d-old CAM angiogenesis, the ID_{50} value being 160–180 ng/egg *(161)*. This inhibition is enhanced in the presence of cortisone acetate, the ID_{50} value being 2–5 ng/egg. Tecogalan in combination with tetrahydro S, significantly suppressed M5076 tumor cell-induced angiogenesis, inhibited this tumor growth, and prolonged the survival time of animals bearing s.c. solid M5076 tumors *(161)*. Tecogalan also interfered with the in vitro proliferation of AIDS-associated KS derived spindle-shaped cells (AIDS-KS cells) at noncytotoxic concentrations, the IC_{50} value being 100 nM *(162)*. Furthermore, the compound not only suppressed angiogenesis induced by AIDS-KS cells in the 9-d-old CAM assay system, but also blocked the vascular hyperpermeability and neovascularization induced on s.c. inoculation of these cells into nude mice. Its anti-angiogenic action has been suggested to involve the prevention of bFGF binding to its receptor proteins resulting from the binding of tecogalan to bFGF *(163)*. Tecogalan is currently under clinical trial for patients with advanced malignancies and HIV-related KS. Disease stabilization, but not objective tumor regression, has been observed *(164)*.

SULFONATED DISTAMYCIN A DERIVATIVES

A series of sulfonated distamycin A derivatives have been synthesized, with the aim of identifying new agents that can form complexes with bFGF and other factor in tumor angiogenesis and thereby block the angiogenic process *(165,166)*.

Among eight derivatives, FCE 26644 was reported to be the most active, and to block entirely 5-d-old CAM neovascularization at the dose of 350 nmol/egg. This derivative at the dose of 200 mg/kg i.v. also prevented bFGF-induced angiogenesis in a mouse sponge model. Systemic administration of FCE 26644 produced anti-tumor activity against M5076 sarcomas, S180 sarcomas, or MXT fibrosarcomas.

Epoxide-Containing Substances

On the basis of the findings of our and other groups, we propose that an epoxide group is a useful indicator for finding new angiogenesis inhibitors. The results of studies performed so far seem to support the validity of this hypothesis, although not all epoxide-containing compounds are angioinhibitory.

FUMAGILLIN ANALOGS

AGM-1470 (TNP-470). AGM-1470 is an analog of fumagillin, an antibiotic produced by the fungus *Aspergillus fumigatus*. Its molecular formula is $C_{19}H_{28}NO_6Cl_2/5H_2O$ *(167)*. The analog has a potent anti-angiogenic effect, and is one of the most exhaustively studied agents.

Fumagillin suppresses the proliferation of HUVECs in vitro, the IC_{50} being 0.5 ng/mL, and prevents 6-d-old CAM angiogenesis at doses above 2 μg/egg *(168)*. Systemic administration of fumagillin (100 mg/kg s.c., for 3 d) affects the S-180 cell-induced angiogenic response in a mouse dorsal air sac assay system, but causes severe weight loss.

AGM-1470 is a less toxic and more potent inhibitor of angiogenesis than the parent compound *(167,168)*. In a monolayer culture, HUVECs appeared to be more susceptible to AGM-1470 than different human tumor-cell lines, like squamous-cell HSC-1, the IC_{50} value for HUVECs being around 10 pg/mL, yet no significant difference seemed to exist in the sensitivity to AGM-1470 between HUVECs and human embryonic lung fibroblast cells (or nonmalignant cells) *(168,169)*. Recent studies revealed that AGM-1470 directly inhibits the proliferation of human glioblastoma cells in vitro at concentrations similar to those that cause EC growth inhibition *(170)*. In addition, in a soft-agar culture, AGM-1470 inhibited the growth of hormone-independent-prostate cancer PC-3 cells, the IC_{50} value being 50 pg/mL, while it inhibited these cells in a monolayer culture with an IC_{50} value of about 5 µg/mL *(171)*. Overall, it is most likely that the cell sensitivity to AGM-1470 is largely dependent on the culture conditions used, and that the effect of AGM-1470 on EC growth is less specific than was previously claimed. Furthermore, as described earlier, recent studies have indicated that AGM-1470 also has an immunomodulatory effect *(119–122)*. Thus, it seems logical to consider that the in vivo anti-tumor activity of AGM-1470 observed so far might be the result of the combined direct effects of this agent on angiogenesis, tumor cell growth and the immune system. AGM-1470 also had efficacy against collagen-induced arthritis in a rat model of RA *(172,173)*. Clinical trials of AGM-1470 on cancer patients are currently in progress *(14,164)*.

FR-111142 and Its Derivative (FR-118487). Since FR-111142 and FR-118487 are extensively reviewed in another chapter *(see* Chapter 23, Terano et al.), only a brief comment will be made here.

FR-118487 is a semisynthetic derivative of FR-111142, which is an inhibitor of angiogenesis isolated from fermentation broth of the fungus, *Scolecobasidium arenarium*, and exhibits about 5–10 times stronger activities than the parent compound with respect to the inhibitory effects on HUVEC growth and 6-d-old CAM angiogenesis *(174,175)*. Also, this derivative inhibits neovascularization induced by a pellet containing an EC growth supplement and heparin in the rabbit corneal-implantation assay system, and has an anti-tumor effect in vivo.

(–)-Ovalicin. A method was established for the large-scale synthesis of (–)-ovalicin, a microbial product, which contains two epoxide groups, is structurally similar to fumagillin and exhibits almost as potent anti-angiogenic activity as AGM-1470 *(176)*. Ovalicin was reported to be advantageous over AGM-1470 in physico-chemical stability. However, there is no further information on this agent.

Eponemycin. Eponemycin is an antitumor antibiotic produced by *Streptomyces hygroscopicus (177)*. The molecular formula and molecular weight of eponemycin are $C_{20}H_{35}N_2O_6$ and 398, respectively.

This antibiotic induces significant prolongation of the survival time of mice transplanted with B16 melanoma cells, but exhibits no anti-tumor activity toward P388 leukemia cells. This suggested that the mechanism of its anti-tumor action involves an angioinhibitory effect. In fact, eponemycin inhibited angiogenesis on 5-d-old CAM *(178)*. This inhibition was detectable at the dose of 7.5 fmol/egg, the ID_{50} value being 250 fmol/egg, which might imply that eponemycin is one of the most potent anti-angiogenesis agents. It prevented the three-dimensional proliferation and migration of bovine carotid-artery ECs, the IC_{50} values being 77 and 740 nM, respectively.

Radicicol (Monorden). Radicicol, which was isolated from the mold, *Monosporium bonorden*, was originally identified as an antibiotic showing anti-fungal activity with relatively low toxicity *(179–181)*. Its molecular formula and weight are $C_{18}H_{17}ClO_6$ and 365, respectively.

Radicicol suppresses 5-d-old CAM angiogenesis, the ID_{50} value being 540 pmol/egg *(182)*. It seems most likely that the identification of radicicol as an angiogenesis inhibitor can be achieved by combining our hypothesis that cell-differentiation modulators, including natural and synthetic retinoids like TAC-101 (also named Am 555S), could affect angiogenesis *(8,183–186)*, and recent finding that radicicol exhibits differentiation-modulatory activity *(187,188)*. Radicicol inhibits the proliferation of and uPA secretion by bovine carotid-artery ECs at low nanomolar concentrations. Thus it is likely that radicicol affects angiogenesis by interfering with multiple EC functions related to neovascularization.

When administered systemically, radicicol prevented neither tumor cell-induced angiogenesis nor tumor growth, while its dipalmitoylated derivative totally blocked both neovascularization and tumor growth under the same experimental conditions (189). Thus, one can assume that even though agents identified as inhibitors of angiogenesis in the CAM assay fail to inhibit tumor-induced angiogenesis when given systemically, it might still be possible to develop effective derivatives.

Although circumstantial, the results of studies on the fumagillin analogs, eponemycin, and radicicol, have suggested that an epoxide group(s) is responsible for their anti-angiogenic activity, and thus will become a potential indicator for finding new inhibitors of angiogenesis. A study along these lines is beginning to yield exciting findings such as that depudecin, rhizoxin, other microbial products, and certain synthetic compounds are novel inhibitors of neovascularization.

Depudecin. Depudecin is a modulator of cell differentiation containing two epoxide groups, which was isolated from the fungus, *Alternaria brassiciola* (190,191). Its molecular formula and weight are $C_{11}H_{16}O_4$ and 212, respectively.

Depudecin inhibited 5-d-old CAM angiogenesis, the ID_{50} being 1.5 nmol/egg, and prevented HUVEC proliferation, the IC_{50} being 13 μM (192). The efficacy of depudecin against angiogenic diseases remains to be determined.

Rhizoxin. Rhizoxin is an epoxide-containing macrocyclic lactone produced by the plant pathogenic fungus, *Rhizopus chinensis* (193). Its molecular formula and weight are $C_{35}H_{47}NO_9$ and 625, respectively. Rhizoxin was found to inhibit tubulin polymerization (194,195). The anti-angiogenic effect of 2-methoxyestradiol has been suggested to involve its effect on tubulin polymerization in ECs (196). Based on these findings, rhizoxin was tested for its anti-angiogenic activity. As expected, the agent dose-dependently inhibited embryonic neovascular growth in 5-d-old CAMs, and suppressed tumor cell-induced neovascularization, suggesting that it is a novel inhibitor of angiogenesis, and has the potential as a new therapeutic agent for angiogenesis-dependent diseases like cancer (197). In fact, the previous study showed that this antibiotic has antitumor activity toward several murine tumors in vivo (198).

MMP Inhibitors

MINOCYCLINE

Minocycline is a semi-synthetic derivative of the antibiotic tetracycline. The molecular formula and weight of minocycline are $C_{23}H_{27}N_3O_7$ and 457, respectively.

Tamargo et al. showed that minocycline inhibits VX2 carcinoma-induced angiogenesis using the rabbit micropocket implantation assay (199). This inhibition was comparable to that elicited by the combination of heparin and cortisone. The authors suggested that the anti-MMP activity of minocycline could participate in the mechanism of its anti-angiogenic action. In contrast, Gilbertson-Beadling et al. suggested that minocycline exerts its angioinhibitory activity through an MMP-independent mechanism since, although this antibiotic is inhibitory in an in vitro model of angiogenesis (aortic sprouting in fibrin gels), BB-94, a synthetic agent that exhibits more potent anti-MMP activity and an anti-angiogenic effect, and is currently under clinical trial (200), has no such effect (201). Guerin et al. showed that several tetracycline derivatives including minocycline suppressed the proliferation of cultured bovine retinal ECs, but had little or no effect on the proliferation of other cells such as rat C6 glioma cells, suggesting the possible involvement of this effect of minocycline in the mechanism of its angio-inhibitory action (202). Combination therapy with minocycline and other anti-angiogenic compounds or chemotherapeutic agents exhibits greater therapeutic efficacy compared with single therapy (203–206).

Steroids

In 1985, Crum et al. reported that certain steroids devoid of glucocorticoid or mineralcorticoid effect, were able to prevent 6-d-old CAM angiogenesis in the presence of heparin. They named these compounds angiostatic steroids *(207)*. Subsequent studies have shown that some endogenous steroids are inhibitory in the standard angiogenesis assay *(8–10,12–16)*.

WORTMANNIN

Wortmannin is a fungal sterol originally identified as an antifungal agent *(72)*. Its molecular formula and weight are $C_{23}H_{24}O_8$ and 428, respectively. It blocks angiogenesis, as determined with the 5-d-old CAM assay *(208)*. This inhibition occurs at doses as low as 1 ng (2.3 pmol) per egg, the ID_{50} value being 30 ng/egg.

Previous findings have suggested the possibility that different cellular signaling systems are involved in the induction of in vivo angiogenesis, including those involving tyrosine phosphorylation and probably G-protein-coupled-receptor pathways *(3,7–19,209)*. It is known that the activation of phosphatidylinositol 3-kinase is a crucial step downstream of these signaling systems in various cellular responses *(72,73,210)*. Recently, wortmannin was shown to be a potent and selective inhibitor of phosphatidylinositol 3-kinase, the inhibition occurring at low nanomolar concentrations *(72)*. Thus it is likely that wortmannin interferes with embryonic angiogenesis by inhibiting phosphatidylinositol 3-kinase activity, suggesting that this enzyme is a novel target for the identification of new inhibitors of angiogenesis. An effort to learn how wortmannin blocks angiogenesis should lead to a better understanding of the mechanism of angiogenesis.

PAXISTEROL

Paxisterol was identified as an analgesic sterol containing an epoxide group without anti-inflammatory activity, and was isolated from the culture broth of a strain of *Penicillium (211)*. Its molecular formula and weight are $C_{28}H_{42}O_4$ and 442, respectively. This microbial sterol inhibits 5-d-old CAM angiogenesis, the ID_{50} value being 1.1 μmol/egg (T. Oikawa, et al., unpublished data). Thus, on a molar basis, paxisterol has fourfold weaker anti-angiogenic activity than medroxyprogesterone acetate (MPA), which is widely used as a therapeutic agent for breast and other cancers *(95)*. In this regard, we recently developed a 9α-fluorinated derivative of MPA (FMPA), which exhibits about two orders of magnitude stronger anti-angiogenic activity in the 5-d-old CAM assay than the parent compound *(212)*. The oral administration of FMPA leads to more potent inhibitory activity against both tumor-cell induced angiogenesis and growth of solid tumors *(213)*.

UCA1064-B

UCA1064-B is an azasterol produced by the fungus, *Wallemia sebi*. Its molecular formula and weight are $C_{28}H_{47}NO$ and 413, respectively. This microbial sterol suppresses 5-d-old CAM angiogenesis, the ID_{50} value being 73 nmol/egg (T. Oikawa, et al., unpublished data), and exhibits anti-tumor activity in vivo *(214)*.

Others

WF-16775 A₁ AND A₂

WF-16775A$_1$ and A$_2$ are inhibitors of angiogenesis produced by the fungus, *Chaetasbolisia erysiophoides (215)*. The molecular formulae and weights are $C_{15}H_{21}C_{12}NO_5$ and 366 for WF-16775 A$_1$, and $C_{15}H_{20}Cl_3NO_5$ and 400 for WF-16775 A$_2$, respectively.

WF-16775 A_1, at doses of 0.5–2.5 µg/egg, and WF-16775 A_2, at doses of 0.1–2.5 µg/egg, prevent 6-d-old CAM neovascularization. These two agents inhibit the proliferation of HUVECs, the IC_{50} values for WF-16775 A_1 and A_2 being 440 and 50 nM, respectively.

TAN-1120

TAN-1120 is one of the baumycin-group anthracyclines produced by a *Streptomyces* species *(216)*. Its molecular formula and weight are $C_{34}H_{41}NO_{13}$ and 671, respectively.

TAN-1120 inhibited 6-d-old CAM angiogenesis, the ID_{50} value being 69 pmol/egg, and suppressed bFGF-induced angiogenesis in the rat corneal micropocket assay. It also suppressed the proliferation of bovine fetal-heart ECs ($IC_{50} = 1$ pM), but not endothelial tube-formation on Matrigel at concentrations up to 10 µg/mL.

LACTACYSTIN

Lactacystin was originally identified as a microbial metabolite that induces neuritogenesis of neuroblastoma cells *(217)*. The molecular formula and weight of lactacystin are $C_{15}H_{24}N_2O_7$ S and 376, respectively.

Subsequent study involving tritium-labeled lactacystin identified the proteasome as its specific cellular target *(218)*. The proteasome is a recently identified intracellular protease whose catalytic active site is a threonine residue and has been shown to play critical roles in a variety of important intracellular events, including antigen-presenting pathway, cell-cycle progression, and apoptosis *(219–221)*. Cell growth largely depends on cell-cycle progression and is an important phase in the process of angiogenesis. Furthermore, there is increasing evidence suggesting a correlation between apoptosis and angiogenesis. These findings formed a basis for the examination of antiangiogenic activity of lactacystin.

Treatment with lactacystin inhibited 5-d-old CAM angiogenesis, the ID_{50} value being 9.6 nmol/egg *(222)*. It also suppressed vascular endothelial-tube formation on Matrigel, a model for in vitro angiogenesis, the IC_{50} value being 1.6 µM. This IC_{50} value is comparable to those for its inhibition in other experiments, such as on the inductions of neuritogenesis *(217)*, cell-cycle arrest *(223)* and apoptosis *(224)*. Moreover, lactacystin inhibited production of plasminogen activator, an important protease responsible for induction of angiogenesis, by ECs. These findings suggest that the proteasome operates in the process of angiogenesis.

NEOMYCIN B

Neomycin B is an aminoglycoside antibiotic, whose molecular formula and weight are $C_{23}H_{46}N_6O_{13}$ and 615, respectively.

Recent study has shown that neomycin B inhibits angiogenin-induced proliferation of sparsely cultured human ECs and suppresses angiogenin-induced angiogenesis in a bioassay system involving 10-d-old CAM *(225)*. It has been suggested that phospholipase C-inhibiting activity of neomycin B is involved in its inhibition of angiogenesis.

Special Note

TAC-101, a new synthetic retinoid, and NM-3, an analog of Cytogenin, are undergoing clinical trials in patients with cancer in the United States.

CONCLUSIONS AND PERSPECTIVES

It is obvious that a major goal of the study of angiogenesis is to develop a therapeutic strategy for controlling and treating aberrant angiogenic responses occurring in refractory diseases, including cancer, rheumatoid arthritis, and proliferative diabetic retinopathy.

Because anti-angiogenic therapy is cytostatic but not cytotoxic, when developing inhibitors of angiogenesis as therapeutic agents for angiogenic diseases we should always keep in mind the following points:

1. An ideal anti-angiogenic agent is one that has sufficient efficacy without unacceptable side effects even when given orally once or twice daily, all angiogenic diseases are most likely chronic, anti-angiotherapy has to be long-term.
2. Compounds, which exert their anti-angiogenic effects by making ECs unresponsive to any angiogenic signal, are most promising as therapeutic agents for angiogenic diseases because it is rational to consider that different angiogenic responses are all induced by the sum of the activities of multiple angiogenic signals rather than by only one angiogenic stimulus.
3. An angiogenesis inhibitor that upregulates the activity of endogenous angiogenesis suppressors would be useful, because it is most likely that in terms of side effects, such an agent has advantages over compounds that evoke anti-angiogenic activity though inhibition of the increased activities of angiogenesis inducers.
4. Angiostatic therapy, in combination with other treatments that can modulate the downregulated abilities of defense mechanisms like the immune system, will lead to a better outcome, because angiostatic therapy alone is in general unlikely to produce a complete cure, and because most, if not all, angiogenic diseases are also considered to be immunodeficient ones.

At present there seems to be no angio-inhibitory agents that satisfy all of these requirements, yet compounds that satisfy more than two of the criteria are likely to exist. Examples are carboxyamido-triazole, linomide, Irsogladin®, and probably tecogalan, which are currently under clinical trial in patients with cancer and/or diabetic retinopathy. At the preclinical level, there are also other promising candidates; some examples are cytogenin, newly synthesized FMPA and a new synthetic retinoid, TAC-101 (also named Am 555S). These three agents exhibit satisfactory therapeutic efficacy against certain angiogenic diseases without unacceptable side effects like weight loss even when administered orally once a day, and probably have no direct effect on EC proliferation. The point to emphasize here is that the three agents have all been found by using strategies different from the strategy widely used at present, which focuses on finding agents that specifically cause EC growth inhibition.

Finally, the establishment of new clinical-trial designs (Chapter 31) for optimally assessing the paradigm of angiostasis is critically important, because treatment with anti-angiogenic agents is cytostatic, but not cytotoxic (7,226). Indeed, a clinical study on carboxyamido-triazole was performed in patients with refractory cancers, including renal-cell carcinomas, pancreaticobiliary carcinomas, and melanomas, using disease stabilization as an end-point. This study showed that disease stabilization and improvement in performance status occurred in 49% of the patients who displayed disease progression before treatment with this agent (227).

ACKNOWLEDGMENTS

I wish to thank Dr. Tooru Sasaki for his assistance in the preparation of this review. I am also grateful to all the members of our laboratory and all coworkers in other laboratories for the helpful discussions on angiogenesis and its control, and to the Ministry of Education, Science, Sports and Culture of Japan for the funding of our laboratory work.

REFERENCES

1. Risau W., Sariola, H., Zerwes, H.-G., Sasse, J., Ekblom, P., Kemler, R., and Doetschman, T. (1988) Vasculogenesis and angiogenesis in embryonic-stem-cell-derived embryoid bodies. *Development* **102,** 471–478.
2. Risau, W. (1995) Differentiation of endothelium. *FASEB J.* **9,** 926–933.
3. Shibuya, M. (1995) Role of VEGF-Flt receptor system in normal and tumor angiogenesis. *Adv. Cancer Res.* **67,** 281–316.
4. Astrow, A. B. (1994) Rethinking cancer. *Lancet* **343,** 494–495.
5. Gibbs, J. B. and Oliff, A. (1994) Pharmaceutical research in molecular oncology. *Cell* **79,** 193–198.
6. Schipper, H., Goh, C. R., and Wang, T. L. (1995) Shifting the cancer paradigm: must we kill to cure? *J. Clin. Oncol.* **13,** 801–807.
7. Kohn, E. C. and Liotta, L. A. (1995) Molecular insights into cancer invasion: strategies for prevention and intervention. *Cancer Res.* **55,** 1856–1862.
8. Oikawa, T. (1995) Strategies to find novel angiogenesis inhibitors as potential therapeutic agents for cancer. *Curr. Med. Chem.* **1,** 406–417.
9. Herblin, W. F., Brem, S., Fan, T.-P., and Gross, J. L. (1994) Recent advances in angiogenesis inhibitors. *Exp. Opin. Ther. Patents* **4,** 641–654.
10. Auerbach, W. and Auerbach, R. (1994) Angiogenesis inhibition: a review. *Pharmacol. Ther.* **63,** 265–311.
11. Fidler, I. J. and Ellis, L. M. (1994) The implications of angiogenesis for the biology and therapy of cancer metastasis. *Cell* **79,** 185–188.
12. Hayes, D. F. (1994) Angiogenesis and breast cancer. *Hematol./Oncol. Clin. North Am.* **8,** 51–71.
13. Folkman, J. (1995) Angiogenesis in cancer, vascular, rheumatoid and other disease. *Nature Med.* **1,** 27–31.
14. Folkman, J. (1995) Clinical applications of research on angiogenesis. *N. Engl. J. Med.* **333,** 1757–1763.
15. Battegay, E. J. (1995) Angiogenesis: mechanistic insights, neovascular diseases, and therapeutic prospects. *J. Mol. Med.* **73,** 333–346.
16. Cockerill, G. W., Gamble, J. R., and Vadas, M. A. (1995) Angiogenesis: models and modulators. *Int. Rev. Cytol.* **159,** 113–160.
17. Polverini, P. J. (1996) Cellular adhesion molecules. Newly identified mediators of angiogenesis. *Am. J. Pathol.* **148,** 1023–1029.
18. Strömblad, S. and Cheresh, D. A. (1996) Cell adhesion and angiogenesis. *Trends Cell Biol.* **6,** 462–468.
19. Bouck, N., Stellmach, V., and Hsu, S. C. (1996) How tumors become angiogenic. *Adv. Cancer Res.* **69,** 135–174.
20. Connolly, D. T., Heuveiman, D. M., Nelson, R., Olander, J. V., Eppley, B. L., Delfino, J. J., et al. (1989) Tumor vascular permeability factor stimulates endothelial cell growth and angiogenesis. *J. Clin. Invest.* **84,** 1470–1478.
21. Leung, D. W., Cachianes, G., Kuang, W.-J., Goeddel, D. V., and Ferrara, N. (1989) Vascular endothelial growth factor is a secreted angiogenic mitogen. *Science* **246,** 1306–1309.
22. Wilting, J., Christ, B., and Weich, H. A. (1992) The effects of growth factors on the day 13 chorioallantoic membrane (CAM): a study of $VEGF_{165}$ and PDGF-BB. *Anat. Embryol.* **186,** 251–257.
23. Andrade, S. P., Vieira, L. B., Bakhle, Y. S., and Piper, P. J. (1994) Effect of platelet activating factor (PAF) on the formation of blood vessels in subcutaneous implants in mice. *J. Lipid Mediators Cell Signal.* **9,** 117–121.
24. Montrucchio, G., Lupia, E., Battaglia, E., Passerini, G., Bussolino, F., Emanuelli, G., and Camussi, G., (1994) Tumor necrosis factor α-induced angiogenesis depends on in situ platelet-activating factor biosynthesis. *J. Exp. Med.* **180,** 377–382.
25. Hu, D.-E. and Fan, T.-P. D. (1993) [Leu^8]des-Arg^9-bradykinin inhibits the angiogenic effects of bradykinin and interleukin-1 in rats. *Br. J. Pharmacol.* **109,** 14–17.
26. Ziche, M., Jones, J., and Gullino, P. M. (1982) Role of prostaglandin E1 and copper in angiogenesis. *J. Natl. Cancer Inst.* **69,** 475–482.
27. Form, D. M. and Auerbach, R. (1983) PGE_2 and angiogenesis. *Proc. Soc. Exp. Biol. Med.* **172,** 214–218.
28. Sorbo, J., Jakobsson, A., and Norrby, K. (1994) Mast-cell histamine is angiogenic through receptors for histamine 1 and histamine 2. *Int. J. Exp. Pathol.* **75,** 43–50.
29. Leibovich, S. J., Polverini, P. J., Fong, T. W., Harlow, L. A., and Koch, A. E. (1994) Production of angiogenic activity by human monocytes requires an L-arginine/nitric oxide-synthase-dependent effector mechanism. *Proc. Natl. Acad. Sci. USA* **91,** 4190–4194.

30. Ziche, M., Morbidelli, L., Masini, E., Amerini, S., Granger, H. J., Maggi, C. A., et al. (1994) Nitric oxide mediates angiogenesis in vivo and endothelial cell growth and migration in vitro promoted by substance P. *J. Clin. Invest.* **94,** 2036–2044.

31. Kohn, S., Nagy, J. A., Dvorak, H. F., and Dvorak, A. M. (1992) Pathways of macromolecular tracer transport across venules and small veins: structural basis for the hyperpermeability of tumor blood vessels. *Lab. Invest.* **67,** 596–607.

32. Qu-Hong, Nagy, J. A., Senger, D. R., Dvorak, H. F., and Dvorak, A. M. (1995) Ultrastructual localization of vascular permeability factor/vascular endothelial growth factor (VPF/VEGF) to the abluminal plasma membrane and vesiculovacuolar organelles of tumor microvascular endothelium. *J. Histochem. Cytochem.* **43,** 381–389.

33. Dvorak, H. F., Brown, L. F., Detmar, M., and Dvorak, A. M. (1995) Review: vascular permeability factor/vascular endothelial growth factor, microvascular hyperpermeability, and angiogenesis. *Am. J. Pathol.* **146,** 1029–1039.

34. Collins, P. D., Connolly, D. T., and Williams, T. L. (1993) Characterization of the increase in vascular permeability induced by vascular permeability factor in vivo. *Br. J. Pharmacol.* **109,** 195–199.

35. McManus, L. M., Woodard, D. S., Deavers, S. I., and Pinckard, R. N. (1993) Biology of disease: PAF molecular heterogeneity: pathobiological implications. *Lab. Invest.* **69,** 639–650.

36. Bussolino, F. and Camussi, G. (1995) Review: platelet-activating factor produced by endothelial cells: a molecule with autocrine and paracrine properties. *Eur. J. Biochem.* **229,** 327–337.

37. Sunderkötter, C., Steinbrink, K., Goebeler, M., Bhardwaj, R. and Sorg, C. (1994) Review: macrophages and angiogenesis. *J. Leukocyte Biol.* **55,** 410–422.

38. Colville-Nash, P. R. and Scott, D. L. (1992) Review: angiogenesis and rheumatoid arthritis: pathogenic and therapeutic implications. *Ann. Rheum. Dis.* **51,** 919–925.

39. Flier, J. S. and Underhill, L. H. (1993) New concepts about the mast cell. *N. Engl. J. Med.* **328,** 257–265.

40. Regoli, D. and Barabe, J. (1980) Pharmacology of bradykinin and related kinins. *Pharmacol. Rev.* **32,** 1–46.

41. Proud, D. and Kaplan, A. P. (1988) Kinin formation: mechanisms and role in inflammatory disorders. *Ann. Rev. Immunol.* **6,** 49–83.

42. Matsumura, Y., Kimura, M., Yamamoto, T., and Maeda, H. (1988) Involvement of the kinin-generating cascade in enhanced vascular permeability in tumor tissue. *Jpn. J. Cancer Res. (Gann)* **79,** 1327–1334.

43. Moncada, S., Palmer, R. M., and Higgs, E. A. (1988) The discovery of nitric oxide as the endogenous nitrovasodilator. *Hypertension* **12,** 365–372.

44. Pipili-Synetos, E., Sakkoula, E., Haralabopoulos, G., Andriopoulou, P., Peristeris, P. and Maragoudakis, M.E. (1994) Evidence that nitric oxide is an endogenous antiangiogenic mediator. *Br. J. Pharmacol.* **111,** 894–902.

45. Brem, H. and Folkman, J. (1975) Inhibition of tumor angiogenesis mediated by cartilage. *J. Exp. Med.* **141,** 427–439.

46. Moses, M. A., Sudhalter, J., and Langer, R. (1990) Identification of an inhibitor of neovascularization from cartilage. *Science* **248,** 1408–1410.

47. Dean, D. D. and Woessner, J. F., Jr. (1984) Extracts of human articular cartilage contain an inhibitor of tissue metalloproteinases. *Biochem. J.* **218,** 277–280.

48. Oikawa, T., Ashino-Fuse, H., Shimamura, M., Koide, U., and Iwaguchi, T. (1990) A novel angiogenic inhibitor derived from Japanese shark cartilage (I). Extraction and estimation of inhibitory activities toward tumor and embryonic angiogenesis. *Cancer Lett.* **51,** 181–186.

49. Van Meir, E. G., Polverini, P. J., Chazin, V. R., Huang, H.-J. S., de Tribolet, N., and Cavenee, W. K. (1994) Release of an inhibitor of angiogenesis upon induction of wild type *p53* expression in glioblastoma cells. *Nature Genet.* **8,** 171–176.

50. Bouck, N. (1996) P53 and angiogenesis. *Biochim. Biophys. Acta* **1287,** 63–66.

50a. O'Reilly, M. S., Boehm, T., Shing, Y., Fukai, N., Vasios, G., Lane, W. S., et al. (1997) Endostatin: an endogenous inhibitor of angiogenesis and tumor growth. *Cell* **88,** 277–285.

51. Hori, A., Sasada, R., Matsutani, E., Naito, K., Sakura, Y., Fujita, T., and Kozai, Y. (1991) Suppression of solid tumor growth by immunoneutralizing monoclonal antibody against human basic fibroblast growth factor. *Cancer Res.* **51,** 6180–6184.

52. Kim, K. J., Li, B., Winer, J., Armanini, M., Gillett, N., Phillips, H. S., and Ferrara, N. (1993) Inhibition of vascular endothelial cell growth factor-induced angiogenesis suppresses tumor growth *in vivo*. *Nature* **362,** 841–844.

53. Asano, M., Yukita, A., Matsumoto, T., Kondo, S., and Suzuki, H. (1995) Inhibition of tumor growth and metastasis by an immunoneutralizing monoclonal antibody to human vascular endothelial growth factor/vascular permeability factor$_{121}$. *Cancer Res.* **55,** 5296–5301.

54. Borgström, P., Hillan, K. J., Sriramarao, P., and Ferrara, N. (1996) Complete inhibition of angiogenesis and growth of microtumors by anti-vascular endothelial growth factor neutralizing antibody: novel concepts of angiostatic therapy from intravital videomicroscopy. *Cancer Res.* **56,** 4032–4039.

55. Smith, D. R., Polverini, P. J., Kunkel, S. L., Orringer, M. B., Whyte, R. I., Burdick, M. D., et al. (1994) Inhibition of interleukin 8 attenuates angiogenesis in bronchogenic carcinoma. *J. Exp. Med.* **179,** 1409–1415.

56. Arenberg, D. A., Kunkel, S. L., Polverini, P. J., Glass, M., Burdick, M. D., and Strieter, R. M. (1996) Inhibition of interleukin-8 reduces tumorigenesis of human non-small cell lung cancer in SCID mice. *J. Clin. Invest.* **97,** 2792–2802.

57. Fett, J. W., Olson, K. A., and Rybak, S. M. (1994) A monoclonal antibody to human angiogenin: inhibition of ribonucleolytic and angiogenic activities and localization of the antigenic epitope. *Biochemistry* **33,** 5421–5427.

58. Olson, K. A., Fett, J. W., French, T. C., Key, M. E., and Vallee, B. L. (1995) Angiogenin anatagonists prevent tumor growth in vivo. *Proc. Natl. Acad. Sci. USA* **92,** 442–446.

59. Brooks, P. C., Clark, R. A. F., and Cheresh, D. A. (1994) Requirement of vascular integrin $\alpha_v\beta_3$ for angiogenesis. *Science* **264,** 569–571.

60. Brooks, P. C., Montgomery, A. M. P., Rosenfeld, M., Reisfeld, R. A., Hu, T., Klier, G., and Cheresh, D. A. (1994) Integrin $\alpha_v\beta_3$ antagonists promote tumor regression by inducing apoptosis of angiogenic blood vessels. Cell 79, 1157–1164.

61. Brooks, P. C., Strömblad, S., Klemke, R., Visscher, D., Sarkar, F. H., and Cheresh, D. A. (1995) Antiintegrin $\alpha_v\beta_3$ blocks human breast cancer growth and angiogenesis in human skin. J. Clin. Invest. 96, 1815–1822.

62. Nishizuka, Y. (1984) The role of protein kinase C in cell surface signal transduction and tumor promotion. *Nature* **308,** 693–698.

63. Ullrich, A. and Schlessinger, J. (1990) Signal transduction by receptors with tyrosine kinase activity. *Cell* **61,** 203–212.

64. Hunter, T. (1991) Cooperation between oncogenes. *Cell* **64,** 249–270.

65. Cross, M. and Dexter, T. M. (1991) Growth factors in development, transformation, and tumorigenesis. *Cell* **64,** 271–280.

66. Carpenter, G. (1992) Receptor tyrosine kinase substrates: *src* homology domains and signal transduction. *FASEB J.* **6,** 3283–3289.

67. Sun, H. and Tonks, N. K. (1994) The coordinated action of protein tyrosine phosphatases and kinases in cell signaling. *Trends Biochem. Sci.* **19,** 480–485.

68. Marshall, C. J. (1995) Specificity of receptor tyrosine kinase signaling: transient versus sustained extracellular signal-regulated kinase activation. *Cell* **80,** 179–185.

69. Carter-Su, C., Schwartz, J., and Smit, L. S. (1996) Molecular mechanism of growth hormone action. *Ann. Rev. Physiol.* **58,** 187–207.

70. Argetsinger, L. S. and Carter-Su, C. (1996) Mechanism of signaling by growth hormone receptor. *Physiol. Rev.* **76,** 1089–1107.

71. Kapeller, R. and Cantley, L. C. (1994) Phosphatidylinositol 3-kinase. *Bioessays* **16,** 565–576.

72. Ui, M., Okada, T., Hazeki, K., and Hazeki, O. (1995) Wortmannin as a unique probe for an intracellular signalling protein, phosphoinositide 3-kinase. *Trends Biochem. Sci.* **20,** 303–307.

73. Shepherd, P. R., Reaves, B. J., and Davidson, H. W. (1996) Phosphoinositide 3-kinases and membrane traffic. *Trends Cell Biol.* **6,** 92–97.

74. Omura, S., Iwai, Y., Takahashi, Y., Sadakane, N., Nakagawa, A., Oiwa, H., et al. (1979) Herbimycin, a new antibiotic produced by a strain of Streptomyces. *J. Antibiot.* **32,** 255–261.

75. Uehara, Y., Hori, M., Takeuchi, T., and Umezawa, H. (1985) Screening of agents which convert 'transformed morphology' of Rous sarcoma virus-infected rat kidney cells to 'normal morphology': identification of an active agent as herbimycin and inhibition of intracellular *src* kinase. *Jpn. J. Cancer Res. (Gann)* **76,** 672–675.

76. Uehara, Y. and Fukazawa, H. (1991) Use and selectivity of herbimycin A as inhibitor of protein-tyrosine kinases. *Methods Enzymol.* **201,** 370–379.

77. Gospodarowicz, D., Blalecki, H., and Thakral, T. K. (1979) The angiogenic activity of the fibroblast and epidermal growth factor. *Exp. Eye Res.* **28,** 501–514.

78. Glaser, B. M., D'Amore, P. A., Michels, R. G., Patz, A., and Fenselau, A. (1980) Demonstration of vasoproliferative activity from mammalian retina. *J. Cell Biol.* **84,** 298–304.

79. Shing, Y., Folkman, J., Sullivan, R., Butterfield, C., Murray, J., and Klagsbrun, M. (1984) Heparin affinity: purification of a tumor-derived capillary endothelial cell growth factor. *Science* **223,** 1296–1299.

80. Lobb, R. R., Alderman, E. M., and Fett, J. W. (1985) Induction of angiogenesis by bovine brain derived class 1 heparin-binding growth factor. *Biochemistry* **24,** 4969–4973.
81. Thomas, K. A., Rios-Candelore, M., Gimenez-Gallego, G., DiSalvo, J., Bennett, C., Rodkey, J. and Fitzpatrick, S. (1985) Pure brain-derived acidic fibroblast growth factor is a potent angiogenic vascular endothelial cell mitogen with sequence homology to interleukin 1. *Proc. Natl. Acad. Sci. USA* **82,** 6409–6413.
82. Shing, Y., Folkman, J., Haudenschild, C., Lund, D., Crum, R., and Klagsbrun, M. (1985) Angiogenesis is stimulated by a tumor-derived endothelial cell growth factor. *J. Cell. Biochem.* **29,** 275–287.
83. Esch, F., Baird, A., Ling, N., Ueno, N., Hill, F., Denoroy, L., et al. (1985) Primary structure of bovine pituitary basic fibroblast growth factor (FGF) and comparison with the amino-terminal sequence of bovine brain acidic FGF. *Proc. Natl. Acad. Sci. USA* **82,** 6507–6511.
84. Gospodarowicz, D., Cheng, J., Lui, G. M., Baird, A., Esch, F., and Bohlen, P. (1985) Corpus luteum angiogenic factor is related to fibroblast growth factor. *Endocrinology* **117,** 2383–2391.
85. Davidson, J. M., Klagsbrun, M., Hill, K. E., Buckley, A., Sullivan, R., Brewer, P. S., and Woodward, S. C. (1985) Accelerated wound repair, cell proliferation, and collagen accumulation are produced by cartilage-derived growth factor. *J. Cell Biol.* **100,** 1219–1227.
86. Risau, W. and Ekblom, P. (1986) Production of a heparin-binding angiogenesis factor by the embryonic kidney. *J. Cell Biol.* **103,** 1101–1107.
87. Moscatelli, D., Presta, M., and Rifkin, D. B. (1986) Purification of a factor from human placenta that stimulates capillary endothelial cell protease production, DNA synthesis, and migration. *Proc. Natl. Acad. Sci. USA* **83,** 2091–2095.
88. Risau, W. (1986) Developing brain produces an angiogenesis factor. *Proc. Natl. Acad. Sci. USA* **83,** 3855–3859.
89. Hayek, A., Culler, F. L., Beattie, G. M., Lopez, A. D., Cuevas, P., and Baird, A. (1987) An in vivo model for study of the angiogenic effects of basic fibroblast growth factor. *Biochem. Biophys. Res. Commun.* **147,** 876–880.
90. Thompson, J., Anderson, K. D., DiPietro, J. M., Zwiebel, J. A., Zametta, M., Anderson, W. F., and Maciag, T. (1988) Site-directed neovessel formation in vivo. *Science* **241,** 1349–1352.
91. Thomas, K. A. and Gimenez-Gallego, G. (1986) Fibroblast growth factors: broad spectrum mitogens with potent angiogenic activity. *Trends Biochem. Sci.* **11,** 81–84.
92. Huang, S. S. and Huang, J. S. (1986) Association of bovine brain-derived growth factor receptor with protein tyrosine kinase activity. *J. Biol. Chem.* **261,** 9568–9571.
93. Coughlin, S. R., Barr, P. J., Cousens, L. S., Fretto, L. J., and Williams, L. T. (1988) Acidic and basic fibroblast growth factors stimulate tyrosine kinase activity in vivo. *J. Biol. Chem.* **263,** 988–993.
94. Lee, P. L., Johnson, D. E., Cousens, L. S., Fried, V. A., and Williams, L. T. (1989) Purification and complementary DNA cloning of a receptor for basic fibroblast growth factor. *Science* **245,** 57–60.
95. Oikawa, T., Hirotani, K., Shimamura, M., Ashino-Fuse, H., and Iwaguchi, T. (1989) Powerful antiangiogenic activity of herbimycin A (named angiostatic antibiotic). *J. Antibiot.* **42,** 1202–1204.
96. Strawn, L. M., McMahon, G., App, H., Schreck, R., Kuchler, W. R., Longhi, M. P., et al. (1996) Flk-1 as a target for tumor growth inhibition. *Cancer Res.* **56,** 3540–3545.
97. Rosen, E. M. and Goldberg, I. D. (1995) Scatter factor and angiogenesis. *Adv. Cancer Res.* **67,** 257–279.
98. Oikawa, T., Ogasawara, H., Sano, H., Shibata, K., and Omura, S. (1994) Possible functional groups responsible for inhibition of *in vivo* angiogenesis by herbimycin A. *Biol. Pharm. Bull.* **17,** 1430–1432.
99. Yamashita, T., Sakai, M., Kawai, Y., Aono, M., and Takahashi, K. (1989) A new activity of herbimycin A: inhibition of angiogenesis. *J. Antibiot.* **42,** 1015–1017.
100. Umezawa, H., Imoto, M., Sawa, T., Isshiki, K., Matsuda, N., Uchida, T., et al. (1986) Studies on a new epidermal growth factor-receptor kinase inhibitor, erbstatin, produced by MH435-hF3. *J. Antibiot.* **39,** 170–173.
101. Umezawa, K. and Imoto, M. (1991) Use of erbstatin as protein-tyrosine kinase inhibitor. *Methods Enzymol.* **201,** 379–385.
102. Oikawa, T., Ashino, H., Shimamura, M., Hasegawa, M., Morita, I., Murota, S., et al. (1993) Inhibition of angiogenesis by erbstatin, an inhibitor of tyrosine kinase. *J. Antibiot.* **46,** 785–790.
103. Toi, M., Mukaida, H., Wada, T., Hirabayashi, N., Toge, T., Hori, T., and Umezawa, K. (1990) Antineoplastic effect of erbstatin on human mammary and esophageal tumors in athymic nude mice. *Eur. J. Cancer* **26,** 722–724.
104. Onoda, T., Iinuma, H., Sasaki, Y., Hamada, M., Isshiki, K., Naganawa, H., et al. (1989) Isolation of a novel tyrosine kinase inhibitor, lavendustin A, from Streptomyces griseolavendus. *J. Natural Products* **52,** 1252–1257.

105. Hu, D. E. and Fan, T.-P. D. (1995) Suppression of VEGF-induced angiogenesis by the protein tyrosine kinase inhibitor, lavendustin A. *Br. J. Pharmacol.* **114,** 262–268.
106. Ferrara, N., Houck, K., Jakeman, L., and Leung, D.W. (1992) Molecular and biological properties of the vascular endothelial growth factor family of proteins. *Endocr. Rev.* **13,** 18–32.
107. Ferrara, N. (1993) Vascular endothelial growth factor. *Trends Cardiovasc. Med.* **3,** 244–250.
108. Hazato, T., Naganawa, H., Kumagai, M., Aoyagi, T., and Umezawa, H. (1979) β-Galactosidase-inhibiting new isoflavonoids produced by Actinomycetes. *J. Antibiot.* **32,** 217–222.
109. Akiyama, T. and Ogawara, H. (1991) Use and specificity of genistein as inhibitor of protein-tyrosine kinases. *Methods Enzymol.* **201,** 362–370.
110. Oikawa, T., Shimamura, M., Ashino, H., Nakamura, O., Kanayasu, T., Morita, I., and Murota, S. (1992) Inhibition of angiogenesis by staurosporine, a potent protein kinase inhibitor. *J. Antibiot.* **45,** 1155–1160.
111. Fotsis, T., Pepper, M., Adlercreutz, H., Fleischmann, G., Hase, T., Montesano, R., and Schweigerer, L. (1993) Genistein, a dietary-derived inhibitor of in vitro angiogenesis. *Proc. Natl. Acad. Sci. USA* **90,** 2690–2694.
112. Morris, P. B., Hida, T., Blackshear, P. J., Klintworth, G. K., and Swain, J. L. (1988) Tumor-promoting phorbol esters induce angiogenesis in vivo. *Am. J. Physiol.* **254(Cell Physiol. 23),** C318–C322.
113. Daviet, I., Herbert, J. M., and Maffrand, J. P. (1989) Tumor-promoting phorbol esters stimulate bovine cerebral cortex capillary endothelial cell growth in vitro. *Biochem. Biophys. Res. Commun.* **158,** 584–589.
114. Omura, S., Iwai, Y., Hirano, A., Nakagawa, A., Awaya, J., Tsuchiya, H., et al. (1977) A new alkaloid AM-2282 of Streptomyces origin: taxonomy, fermentation, isolation and preliminary characterization. *J. Antibiot.* **30,** 275–282.
115. Tamaoki, T. (1991) Use and specificity of staurosporine, UCN-01, and calphostin C as protein kinase inhibitors. *Methods Enzymol.* **201,** 340–347.
116. Kobayashi, E., Ando, K., Nakano, H., Iida, T., Ohno, H., Morimoto, M., and Tamaoki, T. (1989) Calphostins (UCN-1028), novel and specific inhibitors of protein kinase C. I. Fermentation, isolation, physico-chemical properties and biological activities. *J. Antibiot.* **42,** 1470–1474.
117. Hu, D. E. and Fan, T. P. (1995) Protein kinase C inhibitor calphostin C prevents cytokine-induced angiogenesis in the rat. *Inflammation* **19,** 39–54.
118. Friedlander, M., Brooks, P. C., Shaffer, R. W., Kincaid, C. M., Varner, J. A., and Cheresh, D. A. (1995) Definition of two angiogenic pathways by distinct α$_v$ integrins. *Science* **270,** 1500–1502.
119. Berger, A. E., Dortch, K. A., Staite, N. D., Mitchell, M. A., Evans, B. R., and Holm, M. S. (1993) Modulation of T lymphocyte function by the angiogenesis inhibitor AGM-1470. *Agents Actions* **39,** C86–C88.
120. Schoof, D. D., Obando, J. A., Cusack, J. C., Jr., Goedegebuure, P. S., Brem, H., and Eberlein, T. (1993) The influence of angiogenesis inhibitor AGM-1470 on immune system status and tumor growth *in vitro. Int. J. Cancer* **55,** 630–635.
121. Antoine, N., Bours, V., Heinen, E., Simar, L. J., and Castronovo, V. (1995) Stimulation of human B-lymphocyte proliferation by AGM-1470, a potent inhibitor of angiogenesis. *J. Natl. Cancer Inst.* **87,** 136–139.
122. Antoine, N., Daukandt, M., Heinen, E., Simar, L. J., and Castronovo, V. (1996) *In vitro* and *in vivo* stimulation of the murine immune system by AGM-1470, a potent angiogenesis inhibitor. *Am. J. Pathol.* **148,** 393–398.
123. Gabrilovich, D., Chen, H. L. Girgis, K. R., Cunningham, H. T., Meny, G. M., Nadaf, S., et al. (1996) Production of vascular endothelial growth factor by human tumors inhibits the functional maturation of dendritic cells. *Nature Med.* **2,** 1096–1103.
124. Takeuchi, T., Iinuma, H., Kunimoto, S., Masuda, T., Ishizuka, M., Takeuchi, M., et al. (1981) A new antitumor antibiotic, spergualin: isolation and antitumor activity. *J. Antibiot.* **34,** 1619–1621.
125. Umeda, Y., Moriguchi, M., Kuroda, H., Nakamura, T., Iinuma, H., Takeuchi, T., and Umezawa, H. (1985) Synthesis and antitumor activity of spergualin analogs. I. Chemical modification of 7-guanidino-3-hydroxyacyl moiety. *J. Antibiot.* **38,** 886–898.
126. Nishikawa, K., Shibasaki, C., Takahashi, K., Nakamura, T., Takeuchi, T., and Umezawa, T. (1986) Antitumor activity of spergualin, a novel antitumor antibiotic. *J. Antibiot.* **39,** 1461–1466.
127. Masuda, T., Mizutani, S., Iijima, M., Odai, H., Suda, H., Ishizuka, M., et al. (1987) Immunosuppressive activity of 15-deoxyspergualin and its effect on skin allografts in rats. *J. Antibiot.* **40,** 1612–1618.
128. Oikawa, T., Shimamura, M., Ashino-Fuse, H., Iwaguchi, T., Ishizuka, M., and Takeuchi, T. (1991) Inhibition of angiogenesis by 15-deoxyspergualin. *J. Antibiot.* **44,** 1033–1035.
129. Kiue, A., Abe, T., Morimoto, A., Okamura, K., Ono, M., Kohno, K., et al. (1992) Anti-angiogenic effect of 15-deoxyspergualin in angiogenesis model system involving human microvascular endothelial cells. *Cancer J.* **5,** 267–271.

130. Oikawa, T., Hasegawa, M., Morita, I., Murota, S., Ashino, H., Shimamura, M., et al. (1992) Effect of 15-deoxyspergualin, a microbial angiogenesis inhibitor, on the biological activities of bovine vascular endothelial cells. *Anti-Cancer Drugs* **3,** 293–299.

131. Williams, S. (1993) Angiogenesis in three-dimensional cultures. *Lab. Invest.* **69,** 491–493.

132. Kerbel, R. S. and Hawley, R. G. (1995) Interleukin 12: new member of the antiangiogenesis club. *J. Natl. Cancer Inst.* **87,** 557–559.

133. Müller, W. and Graf, U. (1981) The treatment of psoriais-arthritis with cyclosporin A, a new immunosuppressive agent. *Schweiz. Med. Wschr.* **111,** 408–413.

134. Harper, J. I., Keat, A. C., and Staughton, R. C. (1984) Cyclosporin for psoriasis. *Lancet* **2,** 981–982.

135. van Joost, T., Heule, F., Stolz, E., and Beukers, R. (1986) Short-term use of cyclosporin A in severe psoriasis. *Br. J. Dermatol.* **114,** 615–620.

136. Ellis, C. N., Gorsulowsky, D. C., Hamilton, T. A., Billings, J. K., Brown, M. D., Headington, J. T., et al. (1986) Cyclosporine improves psoriasis in a double-blind study. *JAMA* **256,** 3110–3116.

137. van Joost, T., Bos, J. D., Heule, F., and Meinardi, M. M. (1988) Low-dose cyclosporin A in severe psoriasis. A double-blind study. *Br. J. Dermatol.* **118,** 183–190.

138. Gschwendt, M., Kittstein, W., and Marks, F. (1987) Cyclosporin A inhibits phorbol ester-induced cellular proliferation and tumor promotion as well as phosphorylation of a 100-kd protein in mouse epidermis. *Carcinogenesis* **8,** 203–207.

139. Norrby, K. (1992) Cyclosporine is angiostatic. *Experientia* **48,** 1135–1138.

140. Sharpe, R. J., Arndt, K. A., Bauer, S. I., and Maione, T. E. (1989) Cyclosporine inhibits basic fibroblast growth factor-driven proliferation of human endothelial cells and keratinocytes. *Arch. Dermatol.* **125,** 1359–1362.

141. Lau, D. C. and Wong, K. L. (1987) Effect of cyclosporine on microvascular endothelial cell growth in culture. *Transpl. Proc.* **19,** 3496–3498.

142. Ferns, G., Reidy, M., and Ross, R. (1990) Vascular effects of cyclosporine A in vivo and in vitro. *Am. J. Pathol.* **137,** 403–413.

143. Zoja, C., Furci, L., Ghilardi, F., Zilio, P., Benigni, A., and Remuzzi, G. (1986) Cyclosporin-induced endothelial cell injury. *Lab. Invest.* **55,** 455–462.

144. D'Amato, R. J., Loughnan, M. S., Flynn, E., and Folkman, J. (1994) Thalidomide is an inhibitor of angiogenesis. *Proc. Natl. Acad. Sci. USA* **91,** 4082–4085.

145. Gutman, M., Szold, A., Ravid, A., Lazauskas, T., Merimsky, O., and Klausner, J. M. (1996) Failure of thalidomide to inhibit tumor growth and angiogenesis *in vivo. Anticancer Res.* **16,** 3673–3677.

146. Kumagai, H., Masuda, T., Ohsono, M., Hattori, S., Naganawa, H., Sawa, T., et al. (1990) Cytogenin, a novel antitumor substance. *J. Antibiot.* **43,** 1505–1507.

147. Kumagai, H., Masuda, T., Ishizuka, M., and Takeuchi, T. (1995) Antitumor activity of cytogenin. *J. Antibiot.* **48,** 175–178.

148. Hirano, S., Wakazono, K., Agata, N., Mase, T., Yamamoto, R., Matsufuji, M., et al. (1994) Effects of cytogenin, a novel anti-arthritic agent, on type II collagen-induced arthritis in DBA/1J mice and adjuvant arthritis in Lewis rat. *Int. J. Tissue Reac.* **16,** 155–162.

149. Kumagai, H., Masuda, T., Sakashita, M., Ishizuka, M., and Takeuchi, T. (1995) Modulation of macrophage activity in tumor bearing mice by cytogenin. *J. Antibiot.* **48,** 321–325.

150. Kumagai, H., Osono, M., Iijima, M., Sakashita, M., Ishizuka, M., and Takeuchi, T. (1995) Action of cytogenin on lymphoid cells and their cytokine production. *J. Antibiot.* **48,** 317–320.

151. Oikawa, T., Sasaki, M., Inose, M., Shimamura, M., Kuboki, H., Hirano, S., et al. (1997) Effects of cytogenin, a novel microbial product, on embryonic and tumor cell-induced angiogenic responses *in vivo. Anticancer Res.* **17,** 1881–1886.

152. Cozzolino, F., Torcia, M., Aldinucci, D., Ziche, M., Almerigogna, F., Bani, D., and Stern, D. M. (1990) Interleukin 1 is an autocrine regulator of human endothelial cell growth. *Proc. Natl. Acad. Sci. USA* **87,** 6487–6491.

153. Angiolillo, A. L., Sgadari, C., Taub, D. D., Liao, F., Farber, J. M., Maheshwari, S., et al. (1995) Human interferon-inducible protein 10 is a potent inhibitor of angiogenesis in vivo. *J. Exp. Med.* **182,** 155–162.

154. Strieter, R. M., Kunkel, L., Arenberg, D. A., Burdick, M. D., and Polverini, P. J. (1995) Interferon γ-inducible protein 10 (IP-10), a member of the C-X-C chemokine family, is an inhibitor of angiogenesis. *Biochem. Biophys. Res. Commun.* **210,** 51–57.

155. Strieter, R. M., Polverini, P. J., Kunkel, S. L., Arenberg, D. A., Burdick, M. D., Kasper, J., et al. (1995) The functional role of the ELR motif in CXC chemokine-mediated angiogenesis. *J. Biol. Chem.* **270,** 27,348–27,357.

156. Voest, E. E., Kenyon, B. M., O'Reilly, M. S., Truitt, G., D'Amato, R. J., and Folkman, J. (1995) Inhibition of angiogenesis in vivo by interleukin 12. *J. Natl. Cancer Inst.* **87,** 581–586.

157. Vukanovic, J., Passaniti, A., Hirata, T., Traystman, R. J., Hartley-Asp, B., and Isaacs, J. T. (1993) Antiangiogenic effects of the quinoline-3-carboxamide linomide. *Cancer Res.* **53**, 1833–1837.

158. Kohn, E., Alessandro, R., Spoonster, J., Wersto, R. P., and Liotta, L. A. (1995) Angiogenesis: role of calcium-mediated signal transduction. *Proc. Natl. Acad. Sci. USA* **92**, 1307–1311.

159. Inoue, K., Korenaga, H., and Kadoya, S. (1982) A sulfated polysaccharide produced by an *Arthrobactor* species. *J. Biochem.* **92**, 1775–1784.

160. Inoue, K., Korenaga, H., Tanaka, N. G., Sakamoto, N., and Kadoya, S. (1988) The sulfated polysac-charide-peptidoglycan complex potently inhibits embryonic angiogenesis and tumor growth in the presence of cortisone acetate. *Carbohydrate Res.* **181**, 135–142.

161. Tanaka, N. G., Sakamoto, N., Inoue, K., Korenaga, H., Kadoya, S., Ogawa, H., and Osada, Y. (1989) Antitumor effects of an antiangiogenic polysaccharide from an *Arthrobactor* species with or without a steroid. *Cancer Res.* **49**, 6727–6730.

162. Nakamura, S., Sakurada, S., Salahuddin, S. Z., Osada, Y., Tanaka, N. G., Sakamoto, N., et al. (1992) Inhibition of development of Kaposi's sarcoma–related lesions by a bacterial cell wall complex. *Science* **255**, 1437–1440.

163. Nakayama, Y., Iwahana, M., Sakamoto, N., Tanaka, N. G., and Osada, Y. (1993) Inhibitory effects of a bacteria-derived sulfated polysaccharide against basic fibroblast growth factor-induced endothe-lial cell growth and chemotaxis. *J. Cell. Physiol.* **154**, 1–6.

164. Hawkins, M. J. (1995) Clinical trials of antiangiogenic agents. *Curr. Opin. Oncol.* **7**, 90–93.

165. Sola, F., Biasoli, G., Pesenti, E., Farao, M., Della Torre, P., Mongelli, N., and Grandi, M. (1992) In vivo activity of novel sulphonic derivatives of distamycin A, in Angiogenesis: Key Principles–Science–Technology–Medicine (Steiner, R., Weisz, P. B., and Langer, R., ed.), Birkháuser Verlag, Basel, Switzerland, pp. 459–462.

166. Ciomei, M., Pastori, W., Mariani, M., Sola, F., Grandi, M., and Mongelli, N. (1994) New sulfonated distamycin A derivatives with bFGF complexing activity. *Biochem. Pharmacol.* **47**, 295–302.

167. Marui, S., Itoh, F., Kozai, Y., Sudo, K., and Kishimoto, S. (1992) Chemical modification of fumagillin. I. 6-*O*-Acyl, 6-*O*-sulfonyl, 6-*O*-alkyl, and 6-*O*-(*N*-substituted-carbamyl)fumagillols. *Chem. Pharm. Bull.* **40**, 96–101.

168. Ingber, D., Fujita, T., Kishimoto, S., Sudo, K., Kanamaru, T., Brem, H., and Folkman, J. (1990) Synthetic analogues of fumagillin that inhibit angiogenesis and suppress tumor growth. *Nature* **348**, 555–557.

169. Kusaka, M., Sudo, K., Matsutani, E., Kozai, Y., Marui, S., Fujita, T., et al. (1994) Cytostatic inhibition of endothelial cell growth by the angiogenesis inhibitor TNP-470 (AGM-1470). *Br. J. Cancer* **69**, 212–216.

170. Takamiya, Y., Brem, H., Ojeifo, J., Mineta, T. and Martuza, R. L. (1994) AGM-1470 inhibits the growth of human glioblastoma cells in vitro and in vivo. *Neurosurgery* **34**, 869–875.

171. Yamaoka, M., Yamamoto, T., Ikeyama, S., Sudo, K., and Fujita, T. (1993) Angiogenesis inhibitor TNP-470 (AGM-1470) potently inhibits the tumor growth of hormone-independent human breast and prostate carcinoma cell lines. *Cancer Res.* **53**, 5233–5236.

172. Peacock, D. J., Banquerigo, M. L., and Brahn, E. (1992) Angiogenesis inhibition suppresses collagen arthritis. *J. Exp. Med.* **175**, 1135–1138.

173. Oliver, S. J., Cheng, T. P., Banquerigo, M. L., and Brahn, E. (1995) Suppression of collagen-induced arthritis by an angiogenesis inhibitor, AGM-1470, in combination with cyclosporin: reduction of vascular endothelial cell growth factor (VEGF). *Cell. Immunol.* **166**, 196–206.

174. Otsuka, T., Shibata, T., Tsurumi, Y., Takase, S., Okuhara, M., Terano, H., et al. (1992) A new angiogenesis inhibitor, FR-111142. *J. Antibiot.* **45**, 348–354.

175. Otsuka, T., Ohkawa, T., Shibata, T., Oku, T., Okuhara, M., Terano, H., et al. (1991) A new potent angiogenesis inhibitor, FR-118487. *J. Microbiol. Biotechnol.* **1**, 163–168.

176. Corey, E. J., Guzman-Perez, A., and Noe, M. (1994) Short enantioselective synthesis of (–)-ovalicin, a potent inhibitor of angiogenesis, using substrate-enhanced catalytic asymmetric dihydroxylation. *J. Am. Chem. Soc.* **116**, 12,109–12,110.

177. Sugawara, K., Hatori, M., Nishiyama, Y., Tomita, K., Kamei, H., Konishi, M., and Oki, T. (1990) Eponemycin, a new antibiotic active against B16 melanoma. I. Production, isolation, structure and biological activity. *J. Antibiot.* **43**, 8–18.

178. Oikawa, T., Hasegawa, M., Shimamura, M., Ashino, H., Murota, S., and Morita, I. (1991) Eponemycin, a novel antibiotic, is a highly powerful angiogenesis inhibitor. *Biochem. Biophys. Res. Commun.* **181**, 1070–1076.

179. Delmotte, P. and Delmotte-Plaquee, J. (1953) A new antifungal substrate of fungal origin. *Nature* **171**, 344.

180. Mirrington, R. N., Richie, E., Shoppee, C. W., Taylor, W. C., and Sternhell, S. (1964) The constitution of radicicol. *Tetrahedron Lett.* **7**, 365–379.

181. McCapra, F., Scott, A. X., Delmotte, P., Delmotte-Plaquee, J., and Bhacca, N. S. (1964) The consti-
     tution of monorden, an antibiotic with tranquilizing action. *Tetrahedron Lett.* **15**, 869–875.
182. Oikawa, T., Ito, H., Ashino, H., Toi, M., Tominaga, T., Morita, I., and Mutota, S. (1993) Radicicol, a
     microbial cell differentiation modulator, inhibits in vivo angiogenesis. *Eur. J. Pharmacol.* **241**, 221–227.
183. Oikawa, T., Hirotani, K., Nakamura, O., Shudo, K., Hiragun, A., and Iwaguchi, T. (1989) A highly
     potent antiangiogenic activity of retinoids. *Cancer Lett.* **48**, 157–162.
184. Oikawa, T., Okayasu, I., Ashino, H., Morita, I., Murota, S., and Shudo, K. (1993) Three novel syn-
     thetic retinoids, Re 80, Am 580 and Am 80, all exhibit anti-angiogenic activity in vivo. *Eur. J.
     Pharmacol.* **249**, 113–116.
185. Oikawa, T., Shimamura, M., Shibata, J., Murakami, K., Wierzba, K., Yamada, Y., and Shudo, K.
     (1996) Effects of a novel synthetic retinoid Am 555S (TAC-101) on embryonic and tumor angiogen-
     esis. Proceedings of the 55th Annual Meeting of the Japanese Cancer Association. Yokohama, p. 463.
186. Oikawa, T., Hirotani, K., Ogasawara, H., Katayama, T., Nakamura, O., Iwaguchi, T., and Hiragun,
     A. (1990) Inhibition of angiogenesis by vitamin D_3 analogues. *Eur. J. Pharmacol.* **178**, 247–250.
187. Kwon, H. J., Yoshida, M., Fukui, Y., Horinouchi, S., and Beppu, T. (1992) Potent and specific
     inhibition of p60[v-src] protein kinase both *in vivo* and *in vitro* by radicicol. *Cancer Res.* **52**, 6926–6930.
188. Shimada, Y., Ogawa, T., Sato, A., Kaneko, I., and Tsujita, Y. (1995) Induction of differentiation of
     HL-60 cells by the anti-fungal antibiotic, radicicol. *J. Antibiot.* **48**, 824–830.
189. Oikawa, T., Ashino, H., Osada, H., Toi, M., Tominaga, T., Okayasu, I., et al. (1994) Inhibition of in
     vivo angiogenesis by radicicol, a microbial product showing cell differentiation-modulating activity.
     Proceedings of the 53rd Annual Meeting of the Japanese Cancer Association, p. 497.
190. Matsumoto, M., Matsutani, S., Sugita, K., Yoshida, H., Hayashi, F., Terui, Y., et al. (1992) Depudecin:
     a novel compound inducing the flat phenotype of NIH3T3 cells doubly transformed by *ras*- and *src*-
     oncogene, produced by *Alternaria brassiciola*. *J. Antibiot.* **45**, 879–885.
191. Sugita, K., Yoshida, H., Matsumoto, M., and Matsutani, S. (1992) A novel compound, depudecin,
     induces production of transformation to the flat phenotype of NIH3T3 cells transformed by *ras*-oncogene.
     Biochem. Biophys. Res. Commun. **182**, 379–387.
192. Oikawa, T., Onozawa, C., Inose, M., and Sasaki, M. (1995) Depudecin, a microbial metabolite contain-
     ing two epoxide groups, exhibits anti-angiogenic activity *in vivo*. *Biol. Pharm. Bull.* **18**, 1305–1307.
193. Iwasaki, S., Kobayashi, H., Furukawa, J., Namikoshi, M., Okuda, S., Sato, Z., et al. (1984) Studies on
     macrocyclic lactone antibiotics. VII. Structure of a phytotoxin "rhizoxin" produced by Rhizopus
     chinensis. *J. Antibiot.* **37**, 354–362.
194. Takahashi, M., Iwasaki, S., Kobayashi, H., Okuda, S., Murai, T., Sato Y., et al. (1987) Studies on
     macrocyclic lactone antibiotics. XI. Anti-mitotic and anti-tubulin activity of new antitumor antibiot-
     ics, rhizoxin and its homologues. *J. Antibiot.* **40**, 66–72.
195. Takahashi, M., Matsumoto, S., Iwasaki, S., and Yahara, I. (1990) Molecular basis for determining the
     sensitivity of eucaryotes to the antimitotic drug rhizoxin. *Mol. Gen. Genet.* **222**, 169–175.
196. Fotsis, T., Zhang, Y., Pepper, M. S., Adlercreutz, H., Montesano, R., Nawroth, P. P., and Schweigerer, L.
     (1994) The endogenous oestrogen metabolite 2-methoxyoestradiol inhibits angiogenesis and suppresses
     tumor growth. *Nature* **368**, 237–239.
197. Oikawa, T., Shimamura, M., and Iwasaki, S. (1995) Inhibitory effects of rhizoxin on embryonic and
     tumor angiogenesis. Proceedings of 54th Annual Meeting of Japanese Cancer Association, p. 483.
198. Tokui, T., Kuroiwa, C., Tokui, Y., Sasagawa, K., Kawai, K., Kobayashi, T., et al. (1994) Contribution
     of serum lipoproteins as carriers of anti-tumor agent RS-1541 (palmitoyl rhizoxin) in mice. *Biopharm.
     Drug Disposit.* **15**, 93–107.
199. Tamargo, R. J., Bok, R. A., and Brem, H. (1991) Angiogenesis inhibition by minocycline. *Cancer Res.*
     51, 672–675.
200. Brown, P. D. (1995) Matrix metalloproteinase inhibitors: a novel class of anticancer agents. *Adv.
     Enzyme Regul.* **35**, 293–301.
201. Gilbertson-Beadling, S., Powers, E. A., Stamp-Cole, M., Scott, P. S., Wallace, T. L., Copeland, J.,
     et al. (1995) The tetracycline analogs minocycline and doxycycline inhibit angiogenesis in vitro by
     a non-metalloproteinase-dependent mechanism. *Cancer Chemother. Pharmacol.* **36**, 418–424.
202. Guerin, C., Laterra, J., Masnyk, T., Golub, L. M., and Brem, H. (1992) Selective endothelial growth
     inhibition by tetracyclines that inhibit collagenase. *Biochem. Biophys. Res. Commun.* **188**, 740–745.
203. Teicher, B. A., Sotomayor, E. A., and Huang, Z. D. Antiangiogenic agents potentiate cytotoxic cancer
     therapies against primary and metastatic disease. *Cancer Res.* **52**, 6702–6704.
204. Teicher, B. A., Holden, S. A., Ara, G., and Northey, D. (1993) Response of the FSaII fibrosarcoma
     to antiangiogenic modulators plus cytotoxic agents. *Anticancer Res.* **13**, 2101–2106.

205. Sipos, E. P., Tamargom R. J., Weingart, J. D., and Brem, H. (1994) Inhibition of tumor angiogenesis. *Ann. NY Acad. Sci.* **732**, 263–272.

206. Parangi, S., O'Reilly, M., Christofori, G., Holmgren, L., Grosfeld, J., Folkman, J., and Hanahan, D. (1996) Antiangiogenic therapy of transgenic mice impairs de novo tumor growth. *Proc. Natl. Acad. Sci. USA* **93**, 2002–2007.

207. Crum, R., Szabo, S., and Folkman, J. (1985) A new class of steroids inhibits angiogenesis in the presence of heparin or a heparin fragment. *Science* **230**, 1375–1378.

208. Oikawa, T. and Shimamura, M. (1996) Potent inhibition of angiogenesis by wortmannin, a fungal metabolite. *Eur. J. Pharmacol.* **318**, 93–96.

209. Bauer, J., Margolis, M., Schreiner, C., Edgell, C.J., Azizkhan, J., Lazarowski, E., and Juliano, R. L. (1992) In vitro model of angiogenesis using a human endothelium-derived permanent cell line: contributions of induced gene expression, G-proteins, and integrins. *J. Cell. Physiol.* **153**, 437–449.

210. Stephens, L. R., Jackson, T. R., and Hawkins, P. T. (1993) Agonist-stimulated synthesis of phosphatidylinositol(3,4,5)-triphosphate: a new intracellular signalling system? *Biochim. Biophys. Acta* **1179**, 27–75.

211. Nakano, H., Nara, M., Yamashita, Y., Ando, K., and Shuto, K. (1988) Paxisterol, a new analgesic sterol without anti-inflammation activity from *Penicillium. J. Antibiot.* **41**, 409–410.

212. Sugino, E., Fujimori, S., Hibino, S., Choshi, T., Ichihara, Y., Sato, Y., et al. (1997) Synthesis of a new potent anti-angiogenic agent, 17α-acetoxy-9α-fluoro-6α-methylprogesterone (9α-fluoromedroxyprogesterone acetate [FMPA]). *Chem. Pharm. Bull.* **45**, 421–423.

213. Yamaji, T., Tsuboi, H., Murata, N., Fujimori, S., Ichihara, Y., Sato, Y., et al. (1997) Inhibitory effect of FMPA on angiogenesis and its antitumor effect on rat mammary carcinomas induced by 7,12-dimethylbenz[a]anthracene. Proceedings of the 117th Annual Meeting of the Pharmaceutical Society of Japan.

214. Takahashi, I., Matuta, R., Ando, K., Yoshida, M., Iwasaki, T., Kanazawa, J., et al. (1993) UCA1064-B, a new antitumor antibiotic isolated from Wallemia sebi: production, isolation and structural determination. *J. Antibiot.* **46**, 1312–1314.

215. Otsuka, T., Takase, S., Terano, H., and Okuhara, M. (1992) New angiogenesis inhibitors, WF-16775 A$_1$ and A$_2$. *J. Antibiot.* **45**, 1970–1973.

216. Nozaki, Y., Hida, T., Iinuma, S., Ishii, T., Sudo, K., Muroi, M., and Kanamaru, T. (1993) TAN-1120, a new anthracycline with potent angiostatic activity. *J. Antibiot.* **46**, 569–579.

217. Omura, S., Fujimoto, T., Otoguro, K., Matsuzaki, K., Moriguchi, R., Tanaka, H., and Sasaki, Y. (1991) Lactacystin, a novel microbial metabolite, induces neuritogenesis of neuroblastoma cells. *J. Antibiot.* **44**, 113–116.

218. Fenteany, G., Standaert, R. F., Lane, W. S., Choi, S., Corey, E. J., and Schreiber, S. L. (1995) Inhibition of proteasome activities and subunit-specific amino-terminal threonine modification by lactacystin. *Science* **268**, 726–731.

219. Hochstrasser, M. (1995) Ubiquitin, proteasomes, and the regulation of intracellular protein degradation. *Curr. Opin. Cell Biol.* **7**, 215–223.

220. Coux, O., Tanaka, K., and Goldberg, A. L. (1996) Structure and functions of the 20S and 26S proteasomes. *Ann. Rev. Biochem.* **65**, 801–847.

221. Hilt, W. and Wolf, D. H. (1996) Proteasomes: destruction as a programme. *Trends Biochem. Sci.* **21**, 96–102.

222. Oikawa, T., Sasaki, T., Nakamura, M., Shimamura, M., Tanahashi, N., Omura, S., and Tanaka, K. (1998) The proteasome is involved in angiogenesis. *Biochem. Biophys. Res. Commun.* **246**, 243–248.

223. Fenteany, G., Standaert, R. F., Reichard, G. A., Corey, E. J., and Schreiber, S. L. (1994) A b-lactone related to lactacystin induces neurite outgrowth in a neuroblastoma cell line and inhibits cell cycle progression in an osteosarcoma cell line. *Proc. Natl. Acad. Sci. USA* **91**, 3358–3362.

224. Imajoh-Ohmi, S., Kawaguchi, T., Sugiyama, S., Tanaka, K., Omura, S., and Kikuchi, H. (1995) Lactacystin, a specific inhibitor of the proteasome, induces apoptosis in human monoblast U937 cells. *Biochem. Biophys. Res. Commun.* **217**, 1070–1077.

225. Hu, G.-H. (1998) Neomycin inhibits angiogenin-induced angiogenesis. *Proc. Natl. Acad. Sci. USA* **95**, 9791–9795.

226. Marshall, J. L. and Hawkins, M. J. (1995) The clinical experience with antiangiogenic agents. *Breast Cancer Res. Treat.* **36**, 253–261.

227. Kohn, E. C., Reed, E., Sarosy, G., Christian, M., Link, C. J., Cole, K., et al. (1996) Clinical investigation of a cytostatic calcium influx inhibitor in patients with refractory cancers. *Cancer Res.* **56**, 569–573.

20

Interaction of Angiogenic Growth Factors with Endothelial Cell Heparan Sulfate Proteoglycans

Implications for the Development of Angiostatic Compounds

Marco Rusnati, Giovanni Tulipano, and Marco Presta

CONTENTS

INTRODUCTION

Glycosaminoglycans (GAGs) are negatively charged polysaccharides composed of repeating disaccharide units. GAGs are normally found as proteoglycans (PGs) composed of one or more polysaccharide chains attached to a core protein *(1)*.

PGs are present throughout all the animal kingdom, including organisms at very low levels of evolution *(2)*. Accordingly, PGs are present in almost all the cell types where they can be found in soluble forms, in the extracellular matrix (ECM), associated to plasma membrane, or segregated into intracellular granules *(1)*. The wide spectrum of distribution of PGs is the first prove of their biological relevance.

In the last few years the studies about GAGs and PGs have increased dramatically, leading to the comprehension of their biosynthesis and structure, together with the demonstration of the involvement of GAGs and PGs in various physiological processes. The biological functions of GAGs and PGs are highly diversified, ranging from relatively simple mechanical-support functions to more intricate effects on various cellular processes

From: *The New Angiotherapy*
Edited by: T.-P. D. Fan and E. C. Kohn © Humana Press Inc., Totowa, NJ

such as cell adhesion, proliferation, and differentiation. These effects are owing to the ability of PGs to act as "receptors" for adhesion molecules and free molecules such as growth factors, cytokines, and a variety of enzymes including proteases and coagulation enzymes.

A particular class of PGs, namely the heparan sulfate PGs (HSPGs), have been demonstrated to be involved in the modulation of the neovascularization that takes place in different physiological and pathological conditions. This modulation occurs through the interaction of HSPGs with angiogenic growth factors or with negative regulators of angiogenesis, suggesting that the study of the biochemical bases of protein-HSPG interaction may help to design synthetic GAG analogs endowed with angiostatic properties.

The purpose of this chapter is to provide an overview of the structure/function of HSPGs, to examine the biochemical bases and physiological significance of the interaction of angiogenic growth factors with heparin and HSPGs in endothelium, and to summarize the angiostatic properties of natural and synthetic heparin-like and heparin-binding molecules.

HEPARAN SULFATE PROTEOGLYCANS
Classification

The classification of GAGs is based on the structure of the repeating disaccharide units present in their chain and the species shown in Fig. 1 have been recognized. PGs can be classified on the basis of their localization, GAG-chain composition, and on the type of the core protein. As shown in Table 1, HSPGs are localized mainly in the basement membrane and on the cell surface (*see* below).

Synthesis

The biosynthesis of HSPGs is a process that leads to the production of molecules characterized by great structural heterogeneity with respect to the size of the polysaccharide chain, the ratio of iduronic (IdoA) to glucuronic acid (GlcA) units, and the amount and distribution of sulfate groups along the carbohydrate backbone. The biosynthesis of heparin/HS can be conveniently separated into three steps: 1) formation of the linkage region to the core protein; 2) chain elongation; 3) chain modifications (*see* ref. *1* for a detailed description of the process).

1. Polysaccharide formation is initiated by the transfer of a xylose (Xyl) unit from UDP-Xyl to a serine residue in the core protein. Then, two galactose units are transferred from corresponding UDP nucleotides to the xylosylated core protein. Amino acid sequences flanking the linking serine residue and/or 3D structures of the core protein seem to act as signals for directing the assembly of heparin/HS chains.
2. The nonreducing end of the neutral trisaccharide xylosyl-galactosyl-galactose becomes the primer for the elongation of the polysaccharide. In the case of HS and heparin, polymer formation occurs through an alternating transfer of GlcA units and N-acetylglucosamine (GlcNAc) units to the growing chain. The mechanisms that control the length of the fully growth polysaccharides are not fully elucidated. In general, the length of the final chain increases with the availability of the UDP-sugar precursor and decreases with the availability of the core protein.
3. Subsequent to polymer formation, the repeating GlcA-GlcNAc disaccharide chain undergoes a number of enzymatic modifications that occur in the following order:
    a. *N*-deacetylation of GlcNAc units that originates glucosamine (GlcN) residues.
    b. *N*-sulfation of newly formed GlcN residues.
    c. C5 epimerization of GlcA residues; this reaction leads to the formation of IdoA units.
    d. 2-*O*-sulfation of newly originated IdoA residues.

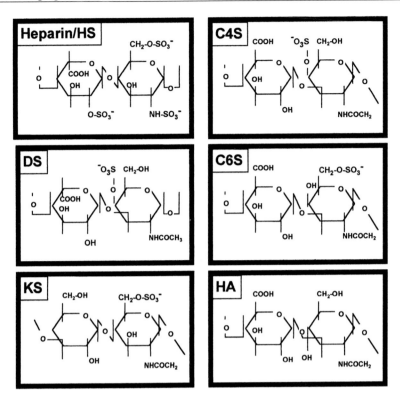

Fig. 1. Schematic structures of GAGs. Heparin/HS and hyaluronic acid (HA) are glycosaminoglycans; chondroitin-4-sulfate (C4S), chondroitin-6-sulfate (C6S), and dermatan sulfate (DS) are galactosaminoglycans; keratan sulfate (KS) is a sulfated polylactosamine. Because heparin/HS structures are highly heterogeneous, only their most abundant disaccharide unit IdoA(2-OSO_3)-GlcNSO$_3$(6-OSO_3) is shown here (*see* text for further details).

Table 1
Classification of Proteoglycans on the Basis of their Localization and Type of Core Protein

Localization	GAG-chain	M_r of the core protein (kD)	Principal members
ECM	HA, CS, KS	225–250	Aggrecan, versican
Collagen-associated	CS, DS, KS	40	Decorin, biglycan fibromodulin
Basement membrane	HS	120	Perlecan
Cell-surface	HS, CS	33^a-60^b-92^c	Syndecans[a], glypican[b], betaglycan[c], CD44E, cerebroglycan
Intracellular granules	Heparin, CS	17–19	Serglycin

CS, chondroitin sulfate; DS, dermatan sulfate; KS, keratan sulfate; HA, hyaluronic acid; HS, heparan sulfate.
[abc]: M_r of the corresponding HSPGs.

    e. 6-O-sulfation of GlcN residues.

    f. Sulfation can also occur at C3 of GlcN units and at C2 or C3 of GlcA units to a limited extent.

All these polymer modifications are incomplete in vivo. In other words, not all the sugar residues that are potential substrate for the various enzymes are transformed into their relative products. Because 2-O- and 6-O-sulfation occur only after C5 epimerization that, in turn, needs the preceding N-deacetylation/N-sulfation reaction, the distribution of 2-O- and 6-O-sulfate groups is restricted to N-sulfated regions. This partial modification process is the biosynthetic basis for the structural heterogeneity of heparin/HS, but its fine regulation remains unexplained. In this regard, it has been demonstrated that the product of the preceding biosynthetic step is the substrate for the next enzyme. This makes the first enzyme of the biosynthetic pathway, namely the deacetylase, the key molecule for regulating the whole process. This and the following enzymes may be regulated in their activity by cellular factors such as ions, pH, cofactors, and other metabolites, and by the epigenetic control of the expression of the corresponding genes. The regulation of the chain modification process leads to cell- or organ-specific HS structures that may allow a fine modulation of the biological functions of HSPGs.

Structure

As stated earlier, the final structure of heparin/HS depends upon the incompleteness of the reactions that occur during the biosynthetic process. The modification process is more complete in heparin where the final disaccharide IdoA(2-OSO_3)-GlcNSO$_3$(6-OSO_3) represents up to 70% of the chain, leading to a heavily O-sulfated polysaccharide with a high IdoA/GlcA ratio. In contrast, the modifications that occur during the biosynthesis of HS are less extensive, leading to HS molecules characterized by lower IdoA content and a lower overall degree of O-sulfation and resulting in high heterogeneity of distribution of the sulfate groups along the chain. Eventually, disaccharides containing GlcNAc or GlcNSO$_3$ may form clusters ranging from 2–20 adjacent GlcNAc-containing disaccharides and from 2 to 10 adjacent GlcNSO$_3$-containing disaccharides. However, about 20–30% of the chain contains alternate GlcNAc- and GlcNSO$_3$-disaccharide units (2).

Cell Association of HSPGs

Typical concentrations of HSPGs on the cell surface are in the range of 10^5–10^6 molecules/cell as measured in various cell-culture systems. HSPGs can link to plasma membrane through a hydrophobic transmembrane domain of their core protein or through a glycosyl-phosphatidylinositol (GPI) anchor covalently bound to the core protein (transmembrane HSPGs). Also, HSPGs can interact with the cell by noncovalent linkage to different cell-surface macromolecules (peripheral membrane HSPGs) (Fig. 2). Interestingly, interaction of free sulfated GAGs or soluble HSPGs with the cell surface can lead to intracellular signaling and modulation of gene expression (3,4).

Transmembrane HSPGs are glypican (5), cerebroglycan (6), betaglycan (7), CD44 (8), and the members of the syndecan family (9): syndecan 1, fibroglycan (syndecan 2), N-syndecan (syndecan 3), and ryudocan (syndecan 4). Glypican and cerebroglycan are typical GPI-anchored HSPGs. Syndecans and betaglycan are typical transmembrane HSPGs characterized by a core protein composed of an extracellular domain, a single membrane-spanning domain and a short cytoplasmic domain (28–34 amino acid residues) that can interact with the cytoskeleton. In the extracellular domain are present the consensus sequences for glycosylation and a conserved putative proteolytic cleavage site. Four tyrosine residues are highly conserved in the C-terminal of all the members of

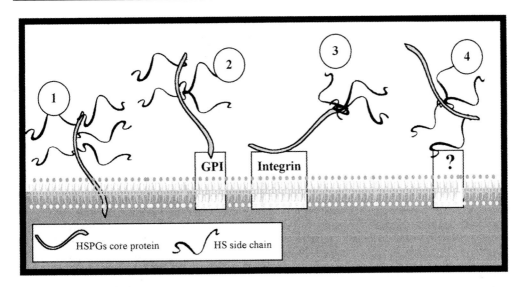

Fig. 2. Association of HSPGs with the cell surface. (**1**) HSPG linked to plasma membrane through a hydrophobic transmembrane domain of the core protein; (**2**) HSPG associated to plasma membrane through a glycosyl-phosphatidylinositol (GPI) anchor covalently bound to the core protein; (**3**) Noncovalent linkage between the core protein of HSPG and a cell-surface receptor (e.g., integrin receptor); (**4**) interaction of the saccharidic chain of HSPG with cell membrane (specific receptor ?).

the syndecan family and one of them fits a consensus sequence for tyrosine phosphorylation *(9)*. Recently, tyrosine phosphorylation of the intracellular domain of syndecan-1 by cytoplasmic tyrosine kinases has been described in intact cells *(10)*, thus supporting the hypothesis of HSPGs involvement in signal transduction.

Perlecan is a typical peripheral membrane HSPG that interacts with the cell surface through its core protein *(11)*. The cell-adhesion motif Arg-Gly-Asp within the core protein of perlecan binds integrins β_1 or β_3 present on endothelial cell surface *(12)*. However, HSPGs may associate to the cell surface and/or ECM also through their GAG-chain, as demonstrated by the observation that half of the total content of HSPGs in endothelial cells can be released after incubation with soluble heparin *(13)*.

HSPGs also exist in soluble form following their mobilization from the cell surface. Transmembrane HSPGs are released after proteolytic digestion of their core protein *(14)*. HSPGs bound to the cell surface via their GAG-chain can be mobilized by free GAGs by a simple law mass action *(13)* or by enzymatic digestion of their polysaccharidic backbone *(15)*. GPI-anchored HSPGs can be released by action of endogenous phospholipase *(16)*.

Finally, it is important to recall that cell-associated HSPGs can be internalized via endocytosis and metabolized in the lysosomal compartment *(1)*. In some cell types, oligosaccharides originated during intracellular degradation appears to be delivered specifically to the nucleus *(17)*.

Endothelium and HSPGs

HSPGs are necessary for the structural and functional integrity of the endothelium. HSPGs present at the basal site of blood vessels act as matrix receptors by interacting with a variety of basement-membrane proteins *(12)*. Moreover, basal HSPGs are responsible for the charge selectivity of filtration in endothelium *(18)* and inhibit smooth-muscle cell proliferation and migration *(19)*. HSPGs are also present at the luminal surface of endothelium *(20)*, where they are involved in the binding and internalization of lipoprotein lipase *(21)*. Moreover, luminal HSPGs play a major role in determining the anticoagulant properties of the vessel surface by binding to proteases of the intrinsic coagulation cascade, thrombin, and protease inhibitors, including antithrombin III *(22)*. Finally, endothelial cell-surface HSPGs act as co-receptors for a wide spectrum of angiogenic growth factors, being involved in the control of angiogenesis *(see* below).

Both macro- and microvascular endothelial cells synthesize HSPGs *(23–25)*. Different HSPGs have been identified in endothelial cells in culture *(26–28)*, where they account for the majority of extracellular sulfated GAGs *(23)*. Endothelial HSPGs may be found at intracellular level *(9)*, associated to plasma membrane and ECM, or in a soluble form *(13,29)*. Syndecan 1 is the most represented HSPG in microvascular endothelial cells *(27)*. It is mainly stored inside the cell, a small portion being present at the basal surface *(30)*. Syndecan 4 is also expressed on the surface of endothelial cells *(28)*, whereas perlecan is abundant in endothelial ECM *(31)*. Finally, a variety of poorly characterized soluble HSPGs with molecular weight spanning from 28–800 kD have been isolated from cultured media of endothelial cells *(14,32)*. The observation that the levels of HSPGs in endothelial cells derived from the microvasculature, where the angiogenic process takes place, are 10–15 times higher than those found in macrovascular endothelial cells *(33)* is in keeping with the role played by endothelial HSPGs in the modulation of angiogenesis. Indeed, depletion of HSPGs from endothelial-cell surface inhibits neovascularization *(34)*.

The HSPG-dependent regulation of angiogenesis is owing, at least in part, to their capacity to bind to and modulate the activity of angiogenic growth factors *(see* below), and contrasting effects can be obtained depending on the types of HSPGs and/or on the experimental conditions adopted. For instance, purified perlecan enhances angiogenesis induced by fibroblast growth factor-2 (FGF-2), whereas other purified HSPGs are ineffective *(31)*. Glypican augments the binding of FGF-1 (acidic FGF; aFGF) and FGF-2 to human tyrosine kinase FGF receptor-1 (FGFR-1) in a cell free-system and replaces heparin in supporting FGF-2-induced cellular proliferation of HS-negative cells expressing FGFR-1 *(35)*.

Overexpression of syndecan 1 on the surface of NIH 3T3 cells inhibits FGF-2-induced cell proliferation *(36)*. In contrast, syndecan 1 stimulates FGF-2-mediated cell growth when immobilized to matrix *(37)*. However, soluble syndecan, glypican, and fibroglycan block the restoration of FGF-2 receptor binding induced by heparin/HS in cell mutants deficient in cell-surface HSPGs *(38)* and soluble heparin/HS inhibit the binding of FGF-2 to FGFRs and HSPGs present on the surface of endothelial cells *(39)*. These data suggest that negative effects on angiogenesis may be exerted by the binding of angiogenic growth factors to soluble HSPGs or GAGs rather than to cell-associated HSPGs. Besides their capacity to modulate receptor binding, HSPGs may modulate angiogenesis also by protecting angiogenic growth factors from inactivation by heat *(40)* and proteolytic degradation *(14,41)* and by affecting their radius of diffusion *(42)*. Finally, HSPGs present in the ECM may act as a reservoir for angiogenic growth factors that will reach higher local concentrations and will sustain the long-term stimulation of endothelial cells *(15,43–45)*.

Given the aforementioned considerations, the expression of endothelial HSPGs during the angiogenic process must be tightly enforced. This kind of control may take place at different levels: 1) quantitative and qualitative differential expression of the various HSPG species; 2) modulation of the composition of GAG chains; 3) digestion of cell-associated GAGs by degrading enzymes; 4) induction of HSPG mobilization from cell surface. It is interesting to note that angiogenic growth factors and cytokines can effectively operate some of the controls described earlier. For instance, FGF-2 and transforming growth factor-β1 (TGF-β1) increase the expression of HSPGs, in particular of syndecan 1, in 3T3 fibroblasts (46,47). Moreover, heparan sulfate complexed with FGF-2 is protected from degradation by Chinese hamster-ovary (CHO) cell heparanase (48). A similar action may take place also in endothelial cells. On the other hand, the levels of endothelial HSPGs decrease significantly in growing microvessels of the rabbit eye (49) and of chick chorio-allantoic membrane (CAM) (50). Accordingly, total HSPG content decreases in sprouting endothelial cells in vitro (24). Concomitantly, a relative increase in soluble, low molecular-weight HSPGs occurs in endothelial cells during migration and sprouting, reflecting an enhanced HSPG turnover (24,32). Accordingly, FGF-2 increases the amount of soluble, FGF-2-binding HSPG species in the conditioned medium of cultured endothelial cells as the consequence of an increased proteolytic plasmin-dependent activity (29). Other authors have reported a decrease of HSPG content in migrating endothelial cells concomitant with an increase of chondroitin sulfate and dermatan sulfate PGs (32). Accumulation of chondroitin sulfate can be obtained also by stimulation of endothelial cells by different interleukins (ILs) (51). Finally, it has been demonstrated that FGF-2 modulates the expression and processing of biglycan in migrating endothelial cells (52). These observations point to the existence of an accurate, mutual control between growth factors and HSPGs in endothelium that may be of particular relevance during the angiogenic process (Fig. 3).

INTERACTION OF ANGIOGENIC GROWTH FACTORS WITH HEPARIN/HS
An Overview

The biological functions of HSPGs depend on their capacity to bind different molecules including extracellular matrix proteins, enzymes, and protease inhibitors (1,53). Of major interest for the aim of this chapter is the capacity of HSPGs to bind several growth factors, cytokines, and chemokines involved in the angiogenesis process (Table 2), thus affecting their biological activity.

HSPGs modulate the biological activity of heparin-binding growth factors and cytokines through different mechanisms.

1. The optional binding of the growth factor to soluble, ECM-associated or cell-surface HSPGs results in a fine control of the bioavailability of the protein. This is the case for TGF-β that binds betaglycan (7), a cell-associated PG, and decorin (54), which is present in the ECM, and for FGF-2 that binds basement membrane perlecan as well as cell-membrane syndecans (28,33).
2. The association with HSPGs stabilizes the growth factor and protects it from proteolytic degradation (14,41).
3. HSPGs modulate the access of growth factors to specific signaling receptors by different mechanisms (Fig. 4) (55).
4. HSPGs can control the intracellular fate of the growth factor (56).

Finally, the possibility exists that:

5. Transmembrane HSPGs themselves may transduce an intracellular signal (3,4).
6. HSPGs may activate an intracellular transduction signal by interacting directly with growth-factor receptors (57,58).

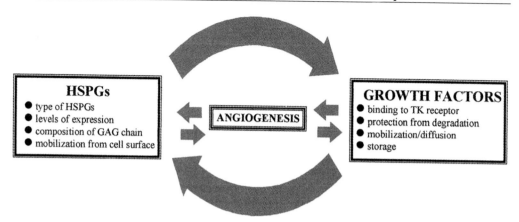

Fig. 3. Relationship between HSPGs and growth factors in angiogenesis.

Table 2
Angiogenesis-Related Heparin-Binding Growth Factors, Cytokines, and Chemokines

Fibroblast growth factors (FGFs)	Platelet-derived growth factor (PDGF)
Vascular endothelial growth factor (VEGF)	Pleiotrophin
Placenta growth factor (PlGF)	Midkine
Heparin-binding EGF-like growth factor	Platelet factor-4 (PF-4)
Hepatocyte growth factor (HGF)	Interleukin-8 (IL-8)
Angiogenin	Macrophage inflammatory protein-1 (MIP-1)
Transforming growth factor-β (TGF-β)	Interferon-γ-inducible protein-10 (IP-10)
Interferon-γ (IFN-γ)	HIV-Tat transactivating factor

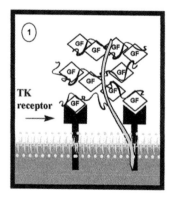
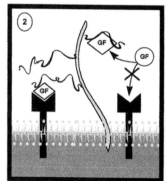
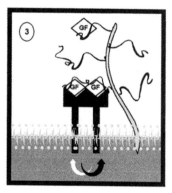

Fig. 4. Modulation of growth factor binding to tyrosine-kinase (TK) receptors by cell-surface HSPGs. (**1**) HSPGs increase local concentration of the growth factor (GF) in close vicinity to the TK receptor; (**2**) HSPGs induce a conformational change of the growth factor facilitating its interaction with TK receptor; (**3**) HSPGs induce growth-factor oligomerization leading to TK receptor dimerization and activation.

Whatever the mechanism(s) of regulation of growth factor activity by HSPGs, it is interesting to note that the binding of the same growth factor to different HSPGs may have different biological consequences. This is the case for syndecan *(49,59)*, betaglycan *(60)*, and perlecan *(31)*, all able to bind FGF-2 but with different effects. Indeed, syndecan inhibits the mitogenic activity of FGF-2 *(36)*, whereas perlecan promotes FGF-2-induced cell proliferation and angiogenesis *(31)*.

Conversely, modifications of HSPG composition can regulate the sensitivity of the cell to different growth factors. This may be of particular relevance when the spatial and temporal control of the activity of different growth factors must be tightly enforced. This possibility is exemplified by the shift in cell-surface HSPG properties from an FGF-2- to an FGF-1-binding phenotype in murine neuronal cells during embryonic development *(61)*.

The modality by which the various HSPGs "discriminate" among the several heparin-binding growth factors is based on their different core proteins, the high heterogeneity of GAG-chain composition, and on the possibility that both the protein moiety and GAG-chains may interact with different growth factors. For instance, betaglycan can exist as a "nude" core protein and the presence and composition of the GAG-chains of this HSPG can be regulated in response to FGF-2 *(11)*. FGF-2 itself binds the GAG-chain of betaglycan while the core protein can interact with TGF-β *(60)*. Also, the number and fine structure of HS chains in syndecan 1 vary in different tissues and in relation to cell differentiation *(62)*. Finally, different sulfated groups and distinct oligosaccharide sequences of the GAG-chain are responsible for the binding to different growth factors (*see* below).

In conclusion, HSPGs are characterized by a structural variability that appears to be highly regulated and that offers virtually unlimited possibilities for selective interactions with different growth factors, cytokines, and chemokines.

Molecular Basis of Growth Factor-Heparin/HS Interaction

Heparin consists largely of 2-*O*-sulfate IdoA → *N*,6-disulfate GlcN disaccharide units. Other disaccharides containing unsulfated IdoA or GlcA and *N*-sulfated or *N*-acetylated GlcN are also present as minor components. This heterogeneity is more pronounced in HS, where the low-sulfated disaccharides are the most abundant. As stated earlier, heparin/HS interacts with various angiogenic growth factors. These interactions depend on the size of the polysaccharide chain and on the degree and distribution of sulfate groups. Interestingly, distinct oligosaccharide sequences have been identified to retain angiogenic growth factor-binding capacity. For instance, the minimal FGF-2-binding sequence in HS has been identified as a pentasaccharide that contains the disaccharide units IdoA(2-OSO_3)-GlcNSO_3 or IdoA(2-OSO_3)-GlcNSO_3(6-OSO_3) *(63)*. Accordingly, binding studies involving chemically modified heparins or HS preparations have shown that 2-*O*- and *N*-sulfate groups are important for FGF-2 interaction (Fig. 5). However, FGF-1 and FGF-4 differ distinctly from each other and from FGF-2 in their interaction with selectively *O*-desulfated heparins, 6-*O*-sulfate groups being required in addition to 2-*O*-sulfate groups for GAG interaction *(64)*. Also, hepatocyte growth factor (HGF) interacts mainly with 6-*O*-sulfate groups of GlcNSO_3 residues while *N*-sulfates and IdoA(2-OSO_3) units play a limited role *(65)*. Both the HIV-Tat protein *(66)* and the longer spliced variant of platelet-derived growth factor A (PDGF-A$_L$) *(67)* require 2-*O*-, 6-*O*- and *N*-sulfate groups for optimal interaction with heparin, whereas *N*-sulfate groups are critically important for the interaction of the GAG with midkine *(68)*. Finally, heparin/HS subpopulations with chemokine-binding selectivity exist *(16)* and IL-8 has been dem-

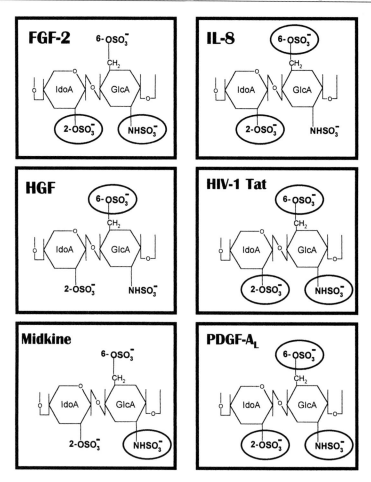

Fig. 5. Role of distinct sulfate groups of heparin/HS in growth-factor interaction. The sulfate groups mainly involved in high-affinity interaction with different angiogenic growth factors are circled.

onstrated to interact preferentially with the 6-O- and 2-O-sulfate groups of heparin (69). However, it should be pointed out that the binding of growth factors to heparin/HS does not depend only on their interaction with sulfate groups of the GAG chain. For instance, it has been shown that carboxyl groups of heparin contribute to FGF-2 interaction (70) and that small nonsulfated di- and tri-saccharides compete with radiolabeled heparin for the binding to FGF-2, albeit with a potency that is about 100 fold lower than that of unlabeled heparin (71).

Taken together, the data indicate that distinct structural requirements are necessary for the interaction of heparin/HS with different growth factors. Even though these specific binding sequences may be hidden in heparin owing to its high degree of sulfation, the high heterogeneity in HS structure allows a more refined tailoring of selective binding regions that may influence the biological activity and bioavailability of heparin/HS-binding growth factors.

Interestingly, also inhibitors of angiogenesis bind heparin/HS via specific sulfate groups. For instance, platelet factor 4 (PF-4), a chemokine able to inhibit angiogenesis in vivo (*see* below), binds to a HS sequence enriched in *N*-sulfated disaccharides and 2-*O*-sulfated iduronate residues, the latter being particularly important for the binding to the chemokine *(72)*. These observations rise the hypothesis that the structural composition and pattern of sulfation of endothelial-cell GAGs may affect the angiogenic balance by favoring the accumulation of angiogenic growth factors or of their inhibitors. Also, the possibility exists that some angiogenic inhibitors may act as growth-factor antagonists for cell-associated HSPG interaction when the two molecules share similar structural requirements for heparin interaction (*see* below).

The interaction of angiogenic growth factors and inhibitors with heparin depends also on distinctive biochemical features of the protein. For instance, heparin-binding domain(s) have been tentatively identified in the NH_2 terminus *(73)* and COOH terminus *(74,75)* of FGF-2 where basic amino acid residues may interact with sulfate groups of heparin. X-ray crystallography has identified a cluster of basic amino acids that form a "basic task" in the 3D structure of FGF-2 that is able to interact with 1–2 sulfate groups, thus representing a putative heparin-binding region *(76–78)*. A similar mechanism of interaction with heparin has been described for macrophage inflammatory protein-1α (MIP-1α), a chemokine able to modulate angiogenesis (*see* below). Folding of the protein originates a heparin-binding site formed by noncontiguous arginine residues in position 18, 46, and 48 and by the hystidine residue in position 45 *(79)*. Also, the resolution of the crystal structure of endostatin, a potent angiostatic heparin-binding peptide (*see* below), reveals that heparin interaction is mediated by a "basic task" originated by the clustering of 11 out of the 15 arginine residues of the protein *(80)*. Finally, heparin-binding regions have been tentatively identified in angiogenin *(81)* and midkine *(82)*. These observations implicate that an appropriate 3D structure of the protein is required for GAG interaction. Also, uncharged amino acids of FGF-2 have been shown to participate to heparin interaction, indicating that hydrogen bonds, van der Waals packing, and hydrophobic interactions, as well as ionic interactions, provide a significant contribution to the formation of the FGF-2-heparin complex *(71,83)*.

At variance with FGF-2, the heparin-binding capacity of different angiogenic factors may depend on linear stretches of contiguous basic amino acids. These basic regions are present in the heparin-binding isoforms of vascular endothelial growth factor (VEGF), placenta growth factor (PlGF), and PDGF-A_L *(84,85)*, and in the first exon of HIV-Tat protein *(86)*.

Interaction of Angiogenic Growth Factors with Extracellular Matrix

Heparin-binding angiogenic growth factors bind to HSPGs associated with ECM and endothelial cell surface with a Kd equal to approx 5–50 nM. Thus, ECM may act as a physiological reservoir for extracellular angiogenic factors. For instance, $VEGF_{145}$ *(87)* and HIV-Tat *(88)* accumulate in ECM by binding to HSPGs. Also, FGF-2 has been found in endothelial ECM in vitro *(45,89,90)* and basement membranes in vivo *(91–93)*. Newly synthesized FGF-2 is stored in ECM from where it can be released to induce long-term stimulation of target cells *(15,43–45)*. Mobilization of ECM-stored growth factors may occur through different enzymatic and nonenzymatic mechanisms. Plasmin, a serine protease, releases FGF-2-GAGs complexes by degrading the core protein of cell-associated HSPGs *(14)*. Because of its association with GAGs, released FGF-2 is protected from proteolytic inactivation and endowed with a larger radius of diffusion. Indeed, both heparin and solubilized GAGs of endothelial origin bind FGF-2 and protect it from heat and acidic inactivation *(40)* and from proteolytic degradation *(14,41)*. Moreover, soluble

GAGs may favor the delivery of FGF-2 to the blood supply to stimulate angiogenesis by increasing the radius of diffusion of FGF-2 *(42)*. This kind of releasing mechanism is strictly controlled by cytokines such as TGF-β and FGF-2 itself that affect the synthesis of plasminogen activators and their inhibitors in endothelial cells, thus modulating the activation of the proenzyme plasminogen to plasmin *(29)*. Heparitinase, heparinase, and heparanase, but not chondroitinase or hyaluronidase, also release biologically active FGF-2 from ECM by degrading the saccharidic backbone of immobilized HSPGs *(15)*. Phospholipase C releases FGF-2 as a biologically active complex with a GPI-anchored HSPG, suggesting that also endogenous phospholipase may be involved in the processes of mobilization of FGF-2 from cell-associated HSPGs *(16)*. Finally, free GAGs inhibit the binding of FGF-2 to cell-associated HSPGs with a potency that decreases in the following order: heparin > HS > dermatan sulfate. Hyaluronic acid, chondroitin-6-sulfate and chondroitin-4-sulfate are ineffective *(94)*. This suggests that soluble HSPGs generated by partial hydrolysis or by proteolysis of cell-associated HSPGs may mobilize heparin-binding angiogenic growth factors from ECM. A competitive effect on angiogenic growth factor binding to ECM HSPGs can be exerted also by the heparin-binding basic sequence of the PlGF-2 isoform *(95)*.

From these data, it appears that the balance between storage and release of angiogenic growth factors in ECM, as well as the integrity of the matrix, may regulate the biological effects of these molecules on endothelium *(96,97)*. For instance, the capacity of nitric oxide (NO) to mediate IL-1-induced degradation of ECM in cultured chondrocytes, with consequent release of extracellular FGF-2, has been implicated in the neovascularization of the inflamed synovia of arthritic patients *(98)*.

HSPGs Mediate the Binding of Angiogenic Growth Factors to Tyrosine-Kinase Receptors

Angiogenic growth factors induce response in target endothelial cells by binding to cognate cell-surface tyrosine kinase (TK) receptors *(99)*. The interaction of heparin-binding growth factors to TK receptors is modulated by HSPGs. For instance, the interaction of FGF-2 or of the heparin-binding $VEGF_{165}$ isoform to TK receptors is strongly reduced in cells made HSPG-deficient by treatment with heparinase or chlorate *(100,101)*. However, controversial results exist about the absolute requirement for HSPGs in FGF-2/receptor interaction. Yayon et al. *(102)* reported that HS-deficient CHO cells transfected with FGFR-1 do not bind FGF-2 unless heparin or HS are added to the cell culture medium. Accordingly, stable expression of perlecan antisense cDNA in mouse fibroblasts and human melanoma cells causes a dramatic reduction of the capacity of transfected cells to interact and to proliferate in response to FGF-2. FGF-2-binding capacity and responsiveness can be recovered by addition of soluble heparin to the cell culture *(103)*. In contrast, Roghani et al. *(104)* have shown that FGFRs expressed in CHO cell mutants or myeloid cells retain the capacity to bind FGF-2 also in absence of heparin. In these experimental conditions, heparin induces a three-fold increase in the affinity of the growth factor for its receptor. Controversial results were obtained also in cell-free systems. Ornitz et al. *(105)* showed that heparin represents an absolute requirement for cell-free binding of FGF-2 to a soluble form of the extracellular portion of FGFR-1, while Roghani et al. *(104)* reported that heparin is not necessary for the binding of FGF-2 to soluble FGFR. In agreement with these latter results, we have found that the formation of the FGF-2-FGFR complex in solution occurs also in the absence of heparin and it is enhanced by the GAG *(106)*. Similar results were obtained for the interaction of VEGF$_{165}$ with soluble KDR/flk-1 receptor (107). Interestingly, HSPGs are required also for receptor interaction of VEGF$_{121}$, a VEGF isoform lacking heparin binding ability (108). This latter observation, as well as the capacity of heparin to induce FGF-2-FGFR interaction in HS-deficient cells, can be interpreted on the basis of the capacity of GAGs to form ternary complexes by interacting with both ligand and receptor proteins $(64,106,109)$. Indeed, a heparin-binding domain has been identified in the NH$_2$-terminus of Ig-like domain II of FGFR-1 (110). The puzzling observation that heparin itself can activate FGFR in the absence of the growth factor (58) further increases the complexity of the ternary interaction among GAGs, growth factors, and TK receptors.

From the aforementioned considerations, it derives that: 1) heparin-related molecules can be used to modulate the biological activity of heparin-binding angiogenic growth factors and cognate TK receptors; 2) the structural requirements of heparin necessary to bind the growth factor and the TK receptor or to affect their mutual interaction may be different; 3) heparin-related molecules with different structures able to differently affect the biological activities of angiogenic growth factors can be designed. For instance, the identification of the structural requirements of heparin responsible for its interaction with FGF-2 and FGFR have been investigated by several laboratories with different experimental models. The results indicate that size $(111,112)$ and degree of sulfation $(38,64,113)$ are critical for the capacity of heparin to induce FGF-2-FGFR interaction. We have observed that heparin requires both 2-O- and 6-O-sulfate groups, as well as N-sulfate groups, to promote the binding of FGF-2 to soluble FGFR-1 (94). Thus, the binding of heparin/HS to FGF-2, which does not require 6-O-sulfate groups, is not sufficient to induce FGF-2 interaction with FGFR. Accordingly, unmodified heparin, but not 6-O-desulfated heparin, protects FGFR-1 from trypsin digestion (94). These data support the hypothesis that HSPGs modulate the binding of FGF-2 to FGFR through the formation of a ternary complex in which the GAG chain interacts with FGF-2 via 2-O- and N-sulfate groups while 6-O-sulfate groups are required for its interaction with FGFR (64).

A single molecule of heparin/HS may bind several molecules of FGF-2 (114) or of angiogenin (81), suggesting that GAGs induce oligomerization of angiogenic growth factors. Indeed, it has been demonstrated that heparin induces dimerization of FGF-2 in a cell-free system (105). A common theme among growth factors interacting with TK receptors is the involvement of ligand-induced receptor dimerization in receptor activation (115). It has been demonstrated that the dimerization and activation of FGFR catalyzed by heparin-dependent oligomerization of FGF-1 is required to induce a mitogenic response (116). Heparin has been hypothesized to play a similar role also for FGF-2 $(55,97,117)$ and HGF (118).

GROWTH FACTOR-HEPARIN/HS INTERACTION AS A TARGET FOR ANGIOGENESIS INHIBITORS

The capacity of various angiogenic factors to interact with heparin/HS raises the possibility that molecules able to interfere with this interaction may act as angiogenesis inhibitors. Two classes of compounds can be envisaged to have the capacity to exert angiostatic activity via this mechanism of action (Fig. 6): 1) heparin-binding, polycationic compounds able to compete with heparin-binding growth factors for HSPG interaction; 2) heparin-like, polyanionic compounds able to compete with HSPGs for heparin-binding growth factor interaction. In both cases, the binding of angiogenic factors to endothelial-cell surface would be hampered with consequent inhibition of their angiogenic capacity. Recent findings on the capacity of low molecular-weight heparin

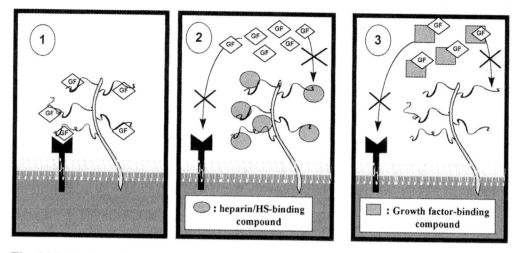

Fig. 6. Mechanisms of inhibition of the HSPG-dependent interaction between growth factors and TK receptors. HSPGs facilitate GF/TK receptor interaction (**1**). This can be prevented by polycationic compounds that bind to and mask HSPGs (**2**) or by polyanionic compounds that bind the GF hampering its interaction with HSPGs (**3**).

fragments administered systemically to reduce the angiogenic activity of FGF-2 and VEGF support this hypothesis *(119,120)*. Here it follows a brief description of natural and synthetic angiostatic compounds whose putative mechanism of action is based, at least in part, on their capacity to affect growth factor-heparin/HS interaction.

Natural Inhibitors of Angiogenesis

PROTAMINE

Protamine is a small sperm-derived, DNA-binding cationic protein (Mr = 4,300). It inhibits neovascularization in embryogenesis, inflammation, immune reaction, and tumor growth, even though its efficacy is limited by toxicity at high doses *(121)*. In vitro, protamine inhibits the mitogenic activity of FGF-2 *(122)* and hampers the capacity of heparin to prevent trypsin digestion of the growth factor *(114)*. This suggests that protamine may compete with heparin-binding growth factors for interaction with sulfated GAGs.

CHEMOKINES

Chemokines belong to a superfamily of low molecular-weight chemotactic proteins that are active on different leukocyte populations. They are divided into three structural subclasses depending on whether the first two of the four invariant cysteine residues are adjacent (C-C chemokines), separated by an intervening residue (C-X-C chemokines), or whether the first cysteine is missing (C chemokines) *(123–125)*. Moreover, C-X-C chemokines are subdivided further depending on the presence or the absence of the sequence Glu-Leu-Arg (the ELR motif) *(123)*. Chemokine receptors are members of the G protein-coupled 7 transmembrane family and they bind either C-C or C-X-C chemokines *(126)*. An exception to this ligand specificity is the promiscuous Duffy antigen/erythrocyte chemokine receptor (DARC), which can bind members of both the C-X-C and C-C class *(127)*. The expression of chemokine receptors CXCR4 and DARC has been demonstrated in human umbilical vein *(128)* and postcapillary venule *(129)* endothelial cells, respectively.

Besides a high-affinity receptor interaction, chemokines bind sulfated glycosaminogly-cans including heparin and HS *(130)* and thus can interact with HSPGs of the cell membrane and extracellular matrix. HSPGs on endothelial cells have been shown to present some chemokines to leukocytes in the multistep process of recruitment *(131)* and to facilitate chemokine oligomerization and receptor interaction *(132)*.

Recent work indicates that various chemokines may affect endothelial-cell function. In particular, PF-4 and other C-X-C chemokines lacking the ELR motif (ELR⁻ C-X-C chemokines) exert an angiostatic activity in vivo and inhibit FGF-2-induced proliferation and migration in cultured endothelial cells *(133,134)*. Recombinant human PF-4 has been tested in clinical trials that include Kaposi's sarcoma, colon and kidney carcinomas, and melanoma *(135)*. In particular, intralesional injection of PF-4 is effective in the treatment of Kaposi's sarcoma *(136)*. The role of HSPG interaction in mediating the anti-angiogenic activity of chemokines has not been clearly established and some contradictory findings have been reported. For instance, interferon-γ (IFN-γ)-inducible protein-10 (IP-10) and PF-4, that share a specific HSPG binding site in SV-40-transformed murine endothelial cells, cause inhibition of FGF-2-induced proliferation in human umbilical-vein endothelial cells, which is abrogated by soluble heparin *(137)*. Similarly, inhibition of FGF-2 activity by PF-4 is overcome by exogenous heparin in 3T3 fibroblasts *(138)*. Nevertheless, a PF-4 mutant called rPF-4-241, in which the heparin-binding site has been mutated such that the molecule no longer binds to heparin, retains a full anti-angiogenic activity *(139)*, thus suggesting that this chemokine may interact directly with the growth factor rather than with the GAG. Indeed, the capacity of PF-4 to complex to FGF-2 and to inhibit heparin-depen-dent FGF-2 dimerization has been demonstrated *(140)*. Also, the ELR⁺ C-X-C chemokines growth-related oncogene α (GROα) and GROβ, but not GROγ, have been shown to inhibit the mitogenic activity of FGF-2 in bovine capillary endothelial cells but their antagonist action is not reversed by heparin *(141)*. In the same study, GROβ reduced FGF-2-stimulated mouse corneal neovascularization and tumor growth. In contrast, a second study *(133)* has shown that GROα, GROβ, and GROγ can stimulate chemotaxis in bovine capillary endothelial cell and neovascularization of the rat cornea (limited to GROα). Others have failed to observe any activity of GROα on endothelial cells *(132)*.

Recent work in our laboratory underlines the complexity of the interaction among chemokines, angiogenic growth factors, and HSPGs. We have shown that IL-8 inhibits the mitogenic activity exerted by FGF-2 on some endothelial-cell types by a protein kinase C (PKC)-dependent, noncompetitive mechanism of action that causes FGFR downregulation. This activity is shared by several C-X-C and C-C chemokines and requires endothelial-cell surface HSPGs. Soluble heparin, 6-*O*-desulfated heparin, *N*-desulfated heparin, but not 2-*O*-desulfated heparin, abrogated IL-8 inhibitory activity, consistently with the presence of low-affinity, high-capacity HSPG-like chemokine bind-ing sites on endothelial cells. Finally, neovascularization induced by FGF-2 in murine subcutaneous sponge implants was reduced significantly by IL-8 *(142)*.

TECOGALAN SODIUM

D-gluco-D-galactan sulfate (DS-4152 or tecogalan) is a sulfated polysaccharide isolated from *Arthrobacter* species. It exerts a potent inhibitory activity against tumor-induced angiogenesis and the growth of solid tumors *(143)*. It also inhibits FGF-2-induced endot-helial-cell growth, chemotaxis, and morphogenesis by preventing the binding of the growth factor to HSPGs and high-affinity TK receptors *(144,145)*. In vivo, tecogalan inhibits neovascularization induced by FGF-2 in the CAM and in the rabbit cornea *(146,147)* and the development of Kaposi's sarcoma-like lesions in nude mice *(148)*. Eckhardt et al. *(149)* have found that the plasma levels of tecogalan sodium achieved in patients with advanced malignancies or HIV-related Kaposi's sarcoma are in the range of concentrations biologically active in experimental models and stabilization of the disease has been reported.

α_2-MACROGLOBULIN

α_2-Macroglobulin is a major serum protein originally characterized as a protease inhibitor. It binds several heparin-binding proteins, including FGF-2 and VEGF, thus neutralizing their receptor binding capacity and biological activity in cultured endothelial cells *(150,151)*. Heparin completely prevents the binding of VEGF and TGF-β to α_2-macroglobulin, but not that of FGF-2. Because α_2-macroglobulin does not interact with heparin, these results suggest that both molecules compete for the binding to the heparin-binding domain of the growth factor.

THROMBOSPONDIN

Platelet thrombospondin-1 (TSP), also secreted by several cell types including endothelial and inflammatory cells, belongs to a family of at least five related glycoproteins *(152,153)*. Multiple and sometimes opposite functions have been attributed to TSP. Indeed, TSP both promotes and inhibits cell adhesion, motility, proliferation, tumor growth, metastasis formation, and angiogenesis *(154)*. These pleiotropic functions possibly reflect the modular structure of TSP that enables it to affect cell functions through binding to specific cell receptors, HSPGs, and growth factors, such as FGF-2 *(155)*, HGF *(156)*, and TGF-β *(157)*.

TSP is thought to be an important modulator of angiogenesis, although its exact role in this process is still controversial *(154)*. In vitro, TSP prevents the motility and proliferative response of endothelial cells to FGF-2 *(158,159)*. In vivo, TSP inhibits the angiogenic activity of FGF-2 in the rabbit cornea *(158)*. We recently reported that TSP binds FGF-2 and that this interaction is fully prevented by heparin, a mechanism that might contribute to the described inhibition of FGF-2 angiogenic activity by TSP *(155)*. The capacity of TSP to bind to and inhibit the biological activity of HGF has been also described *(156)*, thus indicating that different angiogenic factors share the capacity to interact with TSP.

ENDOSTATIN

Recently, an angiogenesis inhibitor has been isolated from a murine hemangioendothelioma cell line and named endostatin *(160)*. Endostatin has been identified as a Mr 20,000 C-terminal fragment of collagen XVIII able to inhibit endothelial-cell proliferation, angiogenesis, and tumor growth. Interestingly, cycled therapy with recombinant endostatin caused tumor dormancy and did not induce resistance *(161)*. The mechanism of action of endostatin is still unclear, even though its high affinity for heparin, owing to the presence of a basic amino acid cluster on the surface of the molecule *(80)*, suggests the possibility that it may act by binding to HSPGs relevant for angiogenic growth-factor(s) activity.

Synthetic Inhibitors of Angiogenesis

SURAMIN DERIVATIVES

Suramin is a polysulfonated naphthylurea originally developed for the treatment of trypanosomiasis and onchocerciasis. Recent studies have shown that suramin possesses a variety of biological effects. The compound has been evaluated for antiviral therapy in the acquired immunodeficency syndrome (AIDS) because of its capacity to inhibit reverse transcriptase and to prevent HIV entry into the cell *(162)*. More recently, suramin has been used experimentally in the treatment of cancer *(163)*. In vitro, suramin blocks the activity of several growth factors by inhibiting their binding to cognate receptors *(164–166)*. Also, suramin is internalized into the cell *(167,168)* where it may affect the activity of various key enzymes involved in the intracellular transduction of mitogenic signals including PKC, DNA and RNA polymerases, topoisomerase II, phosphoinositol, and diacylglycerol kinases *(167,169–171)*. As observed for different heparin derivatives, suramin inhibits the activity of heparanase *(172)* and of urokinase-type plasminogen activator *(173)*, thus exerting an anti-invasive effect. The anti-proliferative and anti-invasive action of suramin, together with its inhibitory activity on cell adhesion and migration *(174)*, may explain, at least in part, the capacity of this molecule to inhibit tumor growth and metastasis in different experimental models *(175,176)*. On this basis, suramin has been employed in patients unresponsive to conventional chemotherapy and anti-tumor activity has been reported in the treatment of adrenocortical carcinoma and prostate carcinoma *(163)*. However, a limitation on the clinical use of suramin is represented by the serious toxic side-effects consequent to the administration of the high doses of the molecule required to achieve anti-tumor activity. For instance, in vivo administration of suramin, that shows a plasma half-life equal to 30–50 d *(177)*, dramatically increases tissue GAGs, leading to mucopolysaccharidosis-like pathologic conditions *(178)*, and elevates the concentration of circulating HS and dermatan sulfate, thus inducing coagulopathy *(163)*.

As an angiogenesis inhibitor, suramin has been demonstrated to inhibit the activity exerted by FGFs and VEGF on cultured endothelial cells by preventing their interaction with cell-surface HSPGs and TK receptors and to block their angiogenic activity in different animal models *(see* ref. *179* and references therein). This is owing, at least in part, to the capacity of suramin to bind to the heparin-binding region of the growth factor via one or more of its sulfonate groups *(180,181)*. Indeed, suramin is ineffective against angiogenesis elicited by nonheparin binding growth factors *(179)*. Accordingly, suramin is able to mimic heparin/HS for the capacity to protect FGF-2 from trypsin digestion. Interestingly, the same capacity is observed for the related polysulfonated compound trypan blue *(114)*. In order to improve the therapeutic ratio of this class of compounds, various polysulfonated naphthylureas structurally related to suramin have been investigated for the capacity to inhibit the activity exerted by FGF-2 on cultured endothelial cells and in a rat sponge angiogenesis assay *(165,182)*. Also, a series of sulfonated distamicyn A derivatives structurally related to suramin have been developed *(180,183)*. The results demonstrate that the number of sulfonate groups and modifications of the backbone of the molecule significantly affect the activity of these compounds. In particular, an extended multiple-ring structure with at least two aromatic groups intervening between the two terminal naphthyl rings confers to suramin derivatives a reduced toxicity without affecting, or even improving, their FGF-2 antagonist capacity. One of these compounds have been demonstrated to reduce the rate of growth and blood-vessel density of vascular lesions induced in immunodeficient mice by the injection of FGF-2-overexpressing murine endothelial cells *(184)*.

Interestingly, suramin and its derivatives have been shown to exert an anti-HIV activity *(185,186)*. Relevant to this observation is the capacity of polysulfonated compounds to interact with the heparin-binding domain of HIV-Tat and to inhibit several biological activities of extracellular Tat protein *(86)*, including its angiogenic activity (Corallini et al., manuscript in preparation).

PENTOSAN POLYSULFATE

Pentosan polysulfate is a polymer of xylose hydrogen sulfate (Mr = 3100) and contains two sulfate groups per carbohydrate monomer. It binds FGFs as well as other heparin-binding growth factors *(187,188)* and it has been shown to interact also with the heparin-binding site of FGFR-1 *(83)*. It inhibits the growth of SW13 adrenocortical cells transfected with FGF-4 *(189)* and of gastric cancer-cell lines overexpressing the angiogenic factor midkine *(190)* and suppresses tumorigenicity of MCF-7 breast carcinoma cells transfected with FGF-1 or FGF-4 *(191)*. Even though the contribution of a possible angiostatic effect of pentosan polysulfate was not investigated in these studies, independent observations have shown that cultured endothelium is sensitive to inhibition by pentosan polysulfate. Interestingly, microvascular endothelium appears to be more sensitive to inhibition by pentosan polysulfate and suramin derivatives than large-vessel endothelium *(165)*. Also, some observations have suggested that pentosan polysulfate may be more effective in inhibiting FGF-4-dependent than FGF-2-dependent cell proliferation. If confirmed, these findings support previous observations about different structural requirements in FGF-4-heparin interaction when compared to FGF-2-heparin interaction *(64)*. Pentosan polysulfate has been found to inhibit the growth of Kaposi's sarcoma-derived spindle cells in vitro *(148)*. As observed for suramin, pentosan polysulfate might be worth exploring as a potential agent for the treatment of Kaposi's sarcoma. A trial in patients with HIV-related Kaposi's sarcoma has shown that the maximally tolerated dose of pentosan polysulfate given by continuous venous infusion is 3 mg/kg per day. No patient had an objective clinical anti-tumor response to either systemic or intralesional pentosan polysulfate administration; however, three patients had stable Kaposi's sarcoma for 3–27 wk. Dose-limiting toxic effects were characterized by anticoagulation and thrombocytopenia and were reversible *(163,193,194)*.

MISCELLANEOUS

Besides the molecules described above, various polyanionic compounds have been described as potential angiostatic drugs. A non-comprehensive list includes: chemically sulfated malto-oligosaccharides (195); sulfated chitin derivatives *(196,197)*; β-cycodextrin tetradecasulfate in combination with angiostatic steroids *(198)*; heparin-steroid conjugates *(199,200)*; various sulfonic acid polymers *(201)*; the nonsulfated polyanionic compounds triphenylmethane derivative aurintricarboxylic acid (ATA) *(202,203)* and poly-4-hydroxyphenoxy acetic acid (RG-13577) *(204,205)*.

Malto-oligosaccharides, sulfated chitin derivatives, and sulfonic acid polymers exert they inhibitory activity, at least in part, by acting as antagonists for heparin-binding angiogenic growth factors. As observed for suramin derivatives and pentosan polysulfate, they inhibit cultured endothelial cell proliferation, chemotaxis, morphogenesis, and/or in vitro endothelial cell sprouting in rat aorta rings embedded in collagen gel. In vivo, they inhibit neovascularization in different assays and suppress tumor angiogenesis and growth. Similar biological activities have been demonstrated for ATA and RG-13577, thus indicating that also nonsulfated polyanionic compounds may act as angiostatic compounds.

In contrast, the rationale for the use of heparin-steroid conjugates or of β-cyclodextrin tetradecasulfate in combination with angiostatic steroids was based on pioneer observations on the capacity of defined batches of commercial heparin preparations to magnify the angiostatic capacity of corticosteroids devoid of glucocorticoid and mineralcorticoid activity *(206,207)*. The mechanism of action of these compounds is unclear, even though their primary action appears to be exerted on basement membrane integrity and synthesis *(208)*.

Recently, the capacity of phosphorothioate oligodeoxynucleotides to interact with heparin-binding growth factors, including FGF-2, FGF-1, FGF-4, and VEGF, has been demonstrated. This interaction is reversed by heparin or suramin *(209,210)*. Phosphorothioate oligodeoxynucleotides are isoelectronic congeners of phosphodiester oligodeoxynucleotides that contain internucleoside linkages in which one of the nonbridging oxygen atoms has been replaced by a sulfur atom. In analogy with other polyanions, they inhibit the binding of FGF-2 to HSPGs and TK receptors, thus preventing its mitogenic activity. Interestingly, the antagonist activity of phosphorothioate oligodeoxynucleotides depends only in part on their size and sequence and is independent of P-chirality *(211)*. In contrast, RNA ligands with defined consensus sequences and secondary structures have been described to interact specifically with FGF-2 or FGF-7 with nanomolar affinity *(212,213)*. Also in this case, interaction with the growth factor was prevented by heparin. At present, no data are available on the effect of phosphorothioate oligodeoxynucleotides and RNA ligands in angiogenesis-related assays in vitro and in vivo.

CONCLUDING REMARKS

The consequences of the interaction of angiogenic growth factors with heparin/HS in endothelium can result either in the inhibition or in the enhancement of their biological activity. Generally speaking, the binding of the growth factor to cell-associated HSPGs causes its storage in the ECM with consequent increase in local concentration, prolonged half-life, and decrease in the radius of diffusion. This will favor growth factor oligomerization, TK receptor interaction, and signaling. Conversely, the binding of the growth factor to soluble HSPGs may antagonize all or part of these effects, resulting in a potential angiostatic action. Exceptions can be represented by heparin/HS-derived oligosaccharides whose size and sequence allow a ternary interaction among soluble GAG, growth factor, and TK receptor. Thus, the biological activity of angiogenic growth factors on endothelial cells is controlled by a complex interplay among free and cell-associated heparin/HS. In this scenario, natural and synthetic heparin-related angiostatic compounds play their pharmacological action.

These considerations point to the importance of the accurate definition of the molecular bases of protein-heparin/HS interaction for the design of molecules endowed with angiogenic agonist or antagonist activity. As stated earlier, specific oligosaccharide sequences appear to be involved in the interaction with different growth factors and their receptors. In theory, this may allow the specific tailoring of molecules with selective action towards defined heparin-binding growth factors. To this respect, the synthetic angiostatic compounds described earlier are quite "nonselective," being able to affect the activity of a variety of growth factors. The lack of selectivity may be responsible, at least in part, for the side effects of these compounds, including their anticoagulant activity. On the other hand, because of the apparent redundancy of angiogenic growth factors possibly involved in different pathological conditions, the multiple-target action of the heparin/HS-related angiostatic molecules characterized so far may represent a therapeutical advantage. This may not be the case for synthetic GAG analogs aimed to potentiate the activity of a defined growth factor for which the selectivity of action appears to be of paramount importance. New methods are emerging for modeling carbohydrate interaction with protein combining site *(192)*. These strategies will help to optimize the chemical structure of saccharide species and pharmacological analogues in order to widen their therapeutic window and to increase their specificity of action.

ACKNOWLEDGMENTS

The work from our laboratory described in this chapter was supported in part by M.U.R.S.T. (Project "Inflammation: Biology and Clinics"), and by grants from C.N.R. (Progetto Finalizzato Biotecnologie, no. 97.01186.PF49), Centro per lo Studio del Trattamento dello Scompenso Cardiaco (University of Brescia, Italy), Associazione Italiana per la Ricerca sul Cancro (Special Project Angiogenesis), Istituto Superiore di Sanità (AIDS Project), and European Communities (Human Capital Mobility Project "Mechanisms for the Regulation of Angiogenesis") to M.P.

REFERENCES

1. Lindahl, U., Lidholt, K., Spillmann, D., and Kjellen, L. (1994) More to "heparin" than anticoagulation. *Thromb. Res.* **75**, 1–32.
2. Maccarana, M. (1994) *O*-sulfate groups in heparin and heparan sulfate. Formation and roles in protein binding. Ph. D. Dissertation Thesis. Acta Universitatis Upsaliensis, Uppsala, Sweden.
3. Wrenshall, L. E., Cerra, F. B., Singh, P. K., and Platt, J. L. (1995) Heparan sulfate initiates signals in murine macrophages leading to divergent biological outcomes. *J. Immunol.* **154**, 871–879.
4. Weiser, M. C. M., Grieshaber, N. A., Schwartz, E., and Majak, R. A. (1997) Perlecan regulates Oct-1 gene expression in vascular smooth muscle cells. *Mol. Biol. Cell* **8**, 999–1011.
5. Doolittle, R. F. (1992) Reconstructing history with amino acid sequences. *Protein Sci.* **1**, 191–200.
6. Stipp, C. S., Litwack, E. D., and Lander, A. D. (1994) Cerebroglycan: an integral membrane heparan sulfate proteoglycan that is unique to the developing nervous system and expressed specifically during neuronal differentiation. *J. Cell Biol.* **124**, 149–160.
7. Massaguè, J. (1992) Receptors for the TGF-beta family. *Cell* **69**, 1067–1070.
8. Brown, T. A., Bouchard, T., St John, T., Wayner, E., and Carter, W. G. (1991) Human keratinocytes express a new CD44 core protein (CD44E) as a heparan sulfate intrinsic membrane proteoglycan with additional exones. *J. Cell Biol.* **113**, 207–221.
9. Bernfield, M., Kokenyesi, R., Kato, M., Hinkes, M. T., Spring, J., Gallo, R. L., and Lose, E. J. (1992) Biology of the syndecans: a family of transmembrane heparan sulfate proteoglycans. *Annu. Rev. Cell Biol.* **8**, 165–193.
10. Reiland, J., Ott, V. L., Lebakken, C. S., Yeaman, C., McCarthy, J., And Rapraeger, A. C. (1996) Pervanadate activation of intracellular kinases leads to tyrosine phosphorylation and shedding of syndecan-1. *Biochem. J.* **319**, 39–47.
11. Lopez-Casillas, F., Cheifetz, S., Doody, J., Andres, J. L., Lane, W. S., and Massague, J. (1991) Structure and expression of the membrane proteoglycan betaglycan, a component of the TGF-β receptor system. *Cell* **67**, 785–795.
12. Hayashi, K., Madri, J. A., and Yurchenco, P. D. (1992) Endothelial cells interact with the core protein of basement membrane perlecan through β1 and β3 integrins: an adhesion modulated by glycosaminoglycans. *J. Cell Biol.* **119**, 945–959.
13. Lowe-Krentz, L. J., Thompson, K., and Patton II, W. A. (1992) Heparin releasable and nonreleasable forms of heparan sulfate proteoglycan are found on the surfaces of cultured porcine aortic endothelial cells. *Mol. Cell. Biochem.* **109**, 51–60.
14. Saksela, O., Moscatelli, D., Sommer, A., and Rifkin, D. B. (1988) Endothelial cell-derived heparan sulfate binds basic fibroblast growth factor and protects it from proteolytic degradation. *J. Cell Biol.* **107**, 743–751.
15. Bashkin, P., Doctrow, S., Klagsbrun, M., Svahn, C. M., Folkman, J., and Vlodavsky, I. (1989) Basic fibroblast growth factor binds to subendothelial extracellular matrix and is released by heparitinase and heparin-like molecules. *Biochemistry* **28**, 1737–1743.
16. Brunner, G., Gabrilove, J., Rifkin, D. B., and Wilson, E. L. (1991) Phospholipase C release of basic fibroblast growth factor from human bone marrow cultures as a biologically active complex with a phosphatidylinositol-anchored heparan sulfate proteoglycan. *J. Cell Biol.* **114**, 1275–1283.
17. Fedarko, N. S. and Conrad, E. (1986) A unique heparan sulfate in the nuclei of hepatocytes: structural changes with the growth state of the cells. *J. Cell Biol.* **102**, 587–599.
18. Kanwar Y. S. and Farquhar, M. G. (1979). Presence of heparan sulfate in the glomerular basement membrane. *Proc. Natl. Acad. Sci. USA* **76**, 1303–1307.

19. Castellot, J. J., Jr, Addonizio, M. L., Rosenberg, R., and Karnovsky, M. J. (1981) Cultured endothelial cells produce a heparinlike inhibitor of smooth muscle cell growth. *J. Cell Biol.* **90,** 372–379.

20. Marcum, J. A., McKenney, J. B., and Rosenberg, R. D. (1984) Acceleration of thrombin-antithrombin complex formation in rat hindquarters *via* heparin-like molecules bound to the endothelium. *J. Clin. Invest.* **74,** 341–350.

21. Williams, M. P., Steeter, H. B., Wusteman, F. S., and Cryer, A. (1983) Heparan sulfate and the binding of lipoprotein lipase to porcine thoracic aorta endothelium. *Biochem. Biophys. Res. Commun.* **756,** 83–91.

22. Danielsson, A., Raub, E., Lindahl, U., and Bjork, I. (1986) Role of ternary complexes, in which heparin binds both antithrombin and proteinase, in the acceleration of the reactions between antithrombin and thrombin or factor Xa. *J. Biol. Chem.* **261,** 15,467–15,473.

23. Kramer, R. H., Voegel, K. G., and Nicolson, G. L. (1982) Solubilization and degradation of subendothelial matrix glycoproteins and proteoglycans by metastatic tumor cells. *J. Biol. Chem.* **257,** 2678–2686.

24. Oohira, A., Wight, T. N., and Bornstein, P. (1983) Sulfated proteoglycans synthesized by vascular endothelial cells in culture. *J. Biol. Chem.* **258,** 2014–2021.

25. Busch, P. C. (1984) Sulfated glycosaminoglycans and vascular endothelial cells, in *Biology of Endothelial Cells* (Jaffe, E., ed.), Martinus Nijhoff Publisher, Boston, pp. 178–188.

26. Kojima, T., Leone, C. W., Marchildon, G. A., Marcum, J. A., and Rosenberg, R. D. (1992) Isolation and characterization of heparan sulfate proteoglycans produced by cloned rat microvascular endothelial cells. *J. Biol. Chem.* **267,** 4859–4869.

27. Kojima, T., Shworak, N. W., and Rosenberg, R. D. (1992) Molecular cloning and expression of two distinct cDNA-encoding heparan sulfate proteoglycan core proteins from a rat endothelial cell line. *J. Biol. Chem.* **267,** 4870–4877.

28. Kojima, T., Katsumi, A., Yamazaki, T., Muramatsu, T., Nagasaka, T., Ohsumi, K., and Saito, H. (1996) Human ryudocan from endothelium-like cells binds basic fibroblast growth factor, midkine, and tissue factor pathway inhibitor. *J. Biol. Chem.* **271,** 5914–5920.

29. Saksela, O. and Rifkin, D. B. (1990). Release of basic fibroblast growth factor-heparan sulfate complexes from endothelial cells by plasminogen activator-mediated proteolytic activity. *J. Cell Biol.* **110,** 767–775.

30. Lose, E. and Bernfield, M. (1991) Pulmonary artery endothelial cells produce syndecan, a cell surface proteoglycan and possible low-affinity bFGF receptor. *J. Cell Biol.* **115,** 417a.

31. Avezier, D., Hecht, D., Safran, M., Elsinger, M., David, G., and Yayon, A. (1994) Perlecan, basal lamina proteoglycan, promotes basic fibroblast growth factor-receptor binding, mitogenesis, and angiogenesis. *Cell* **79,** 1005–1013.

32. Kinsella, M. G. and Wight, T. N. (1988) Structural characterization of heparan sulfate proteoglycan subclasses isolated from bovine aortic endothelial cell cultures. *Biochemistry* **27,** 2136–2144.

33. Marcum, J. A. and Rosenberg, R. D. (1985) Heparin-like molecules with anticoagulant activity are synthesized by cultured endothelial cells. *Biochem. Biophys. Res. Commun.* **126,** 365–372.

34. Sasisekharan, R., Moses, M., Nugent, M. A., Cooney, C. L., and Langer, R. (1994) Heparinase inhibits neovascularization. *Proc. Natl. Acad. Sci. USA* **91,** 1524–1528.

35. Bonneh-Barkay, D., Shlissel, M., Berman, B., Shaoul, E., Admon, A., Vlodavsky, I., et al. (1997) Identification of glypican as a dual modulator of the biological activity of fibroblast growth factors. *J. Biol. Chem.* **272,** 12,415–12,421.

36. Mali, M., Elenius, K., Miettinen, H. M., and Jalkanen, M. (1993) Inhibition of basic fibroblast growth factor-induced growth promotion by overexpression of syndecan-1. *J. Biol. Chem.* **268,** 24,215–24,222.

37. Samivirta, M., Heino, J., and Jalkanen, M. (1992) Basic fibroblast growth factor-syndecan complex at cell surface or immobilized to matrix promotes cell growth. *J. Biol. Chem.* **267,** 17,606–17,610.

38. Avezier, D., Levy, E., Safran, M., Svahn, C., Buddeke, E., Shmidt, E., et al. (1994) Differential structural requirements of heparin and heparan sulfate proteoglycans that promote binding of basic fibroblast growth factor to its receptor. *J. Biol. Chem.* **269,** 114–121.

39. Coltrini, D., Rusnati, M., Zoppetti, G., Oreste, P., Grazioli, G., Naggi, A., and Presta, M. (1994) Different effects of mucosal, bovine lung and chemically modified heparin on selected biological properties of basic fibroblast growth factor. *Biochem. J.* **303,** 583–590.

40. Gospodarowicz, D. and Cheng, J. (1986) Heparin protects basic and acidic FGF from inactivation. *J. Cell. Physiol.* **128,** 175–184.

41. Sommer, A. and Rifkin, D. B. (1989) Interaction of heparin with human basic fibroblast growth factor: protection of the angiogenic protein from proteolytic degradation by a glycosaminoglycan. *J. Cell. Physiol.* **138,** 215–220.

42. Flaumenhaft, R., Moscatelli, D., and Rifkin, D. B. (1990) Heparin and heparan sulfate increase the radius of diffusion and action of basic fibroblast growth factor. *J. Cell Biol.* **111,** 1651–1659.

43. Flaumenhaft, R., Moscatelli, D., Saksela, O., and Rifkin, D. B. (1989) Role of extracellular matrix in the action of basic fibroblast growth factor: matrix as a source of growth factor for long-term stimulation of plasminogen activator production and DNA synthesis. *J. Cell. Physiol.* **140,** 75–81.

44. Presta, M., Maier, J. A. M., Rusnati, M., and Ragnotti, G. (1989) Basic fibroblast growth factor is released from endothelial extracellular matrix in a biologically active form. *J. Cell. Physiol.* **140,** 68–74.

45. Rogelj, S., Klagsbrun, M., Atzmon, R., Kurokawa, M., Haimovitz, A., Fuks, Z., and Vlodavsky, I. (1989) Basic fibroblast growth factor is an extracellular matrix component required for supporting the proliferation of vascular endothelial cells and the differentiation of PC12 cells. *J. Cell Biol.* **109,** 823–831.

46. Nugent, M. A. and Edelman, E. R. (1992) Transforming growth factor β1 stimulates the production of basic fibroblast growth factor binding proteoglycans in Balb/c3T3 cells. *J. Biol. Chem.* **267,** 21,256–21,264.

47. Elenius, K., Maata, A., Salmivirta, M., and Jalkanen, M. (1992) Growth factors induce 3T3 cells to express bFGF-binding syndecan. *J. Biol. Chem.* **267,** 6435–6441.

48. Tumova, S., and Bame, K. J. (1997) Interaction between basic fibroblast growth factor and heparan sulfate can prevent the in vitro degradation of the glycosaminoglycan by chinese hamster ovary cell heparanase. *J. Biol. Chem.* **272,** 9078–9085.

49. Ausprunk, D. H., Boudreau, C. L., and Nelson, D. A. (1981) Proteoglycans in the microvasculature. Histochemical localization in microvessel of the rabbit eye. *Am. J. Pathol.* **103,** 353–366.

50. Ausprunk, D. H. (1982) Synthesis of glycoproteins by endothelial cells in embryonic blood vessels. *Dev. Biol.* **90,** 79–90.

51. Montesano, R., Mossaz, A., Ryser, J.-E., Oril, L., and Vassalli, P. (1984) Leukocyte interleukines induce cultured endothelial cells to produce a highly organized, glycosaminoglycan-rich pericellular matrix. *J. Cell Biol.* **99,** 1706–1715.

52. Kinsella, M. G., Tsoi, C. K., Jarvelainen, H. T., and Wight T. N. (1997) Selective expression and processing of biglycan during migration of bovine endothelial cells. *J. Biol. Chem.* **272,** 318–325.

53. Spillmann, D. and Lindahl, U. (1994) Glycosaminoglycan-protein interactions. A question of specificity. *Curr. Opin. Struct. Biol.* **4,** 677–682.

54. Yamaguchi, Y., Mann, D. M., and Ruoslahti, E. (1990) Negative regulation of transforming growth factor-β by the proteoglycan decorin. *Nature (Lond.)* **346,** 281–284.

55. Ruoslahti, E. and Yamaguchi, Y. (1991) Proteoglycans as modulator of growth factor activities. *Cell* **64,** 867–869.

56. Rusnati, M., Urbinati, C., and Presta, M. (1993) Internalization of basic fibroblast growth factor (bFGF) in cultured endothelial cells: role of the low affinity heparin-like bFGF receptors. *J. Cell. Physiol.* **154,** 152–161.

57. Revis-Gupta, S., Abdel-Ghany, M., Koland, J., and Racker, E. (1991) Heparin stimulates epidermal growth factor receptor-mediated phosphorylation of tyrosine and threonine residues. *Proc. Natl. Acad. Sci. USA* **88,** 5954–5958.

58. Gao, G. and Goldfarb, M. (1995) Heparin can activate a receptor tyrosine kinase. *EMBO J.* **14,** 2183–2190.

59. Chernousov, M. A. and Carey, D. J. (1993) N-syndecan (syndecan-3) from neonatal rat brain binds basic fibroblast growth factor. *J. Biol. Chem.* **268,** 16,810–16,814.

60. Andres, J. L., DeFalcis, D., Noda, M., and Massague, J. (1992) Binding of two growth factor families to separate domains of the proteoglycan betaglycan. *J. Biol. Chem.* **267,** 5927–5930.

61. Nurcombe, V., Ford, M. D., Wildschut, J. A., and Bartlett, P. F. (1995) Developmental regulation of neuronal response to FGF-1 and FGF-2 by heparan sulfate proteoglycan. *Science* **260,** 103–106.

62. Bernfield, M. and Sanderson, R. D. (1990) Syndecan, a developmentally regulated cell surface proteoglycan that binds extracellular matrix and growth factors. *Phil. Trans. R. Soc. Lond.* **327,** 171–186.

63. Maccarana, M., Casu, B., and Lindahl, U. (1993) Minimal sequence in heparin/heparan sulfate required for binding of basic fibroblast growth factor. *J. Biol. Chem.* **268,** 23,898–23,905.

64. Guimond, S., Maccarana, M., Olwin, B. B., Lindahl, U., and Rapraeger, A. C. (1993) Activating and inhibitory heparin sequences for FGF-2 (basic FGF). Distinct requirements for FGF-1, FGF-2, and FGF-4. *J. Biol. Chem.* **268,** 23,906–23,914.

65. Lyon, M. and Gallagher, J. T. (1994) Hepatocyte growth factor/scatter factor: a heparan sulphate-binding pleiotropic growth factor. *Biochem. Soc. Trans.* **22,** 365–370.

66. Rusnati, M., Coltrini, D., Oreste, P., Zoppetti, G., Albini, A., Noonan, D., et al. (1997) Interaction of HIV-1 Tat protein with heparin. *J. Biol. Chem.* **272,** 11,313–11,320.

67. Feyzi, E., Lusting, F., Fager, G., Spillmann, D., Lindahl, U., and Salmivitra M. (1997) Characterization of heparin and heparan sulfate domains binding to the long splice variant of platelet-derived growth factor A chain. *J. Biol. Chem.* **28,** 5518–5524.

68. Kaneda, N., Talukder A. H., Ishihara M., Hara, S., Yoshida, K., and Muramatsu, T. (1996) Structural characteristics of heparin-line domain required for interaction of midkine with embryonic neurons. *Biochem. Biophys. Res. Comm.* **7,** 108–112.

69. Spillmann, D., Witt, D., and Lindahl, U. (1998) Defining the interleukin-8-binding domain of heparan sulfate. *J. Biol. Chem.* **273,** 15,487–15,493.

70. Ishihara, M., Shaklee, P. N., Yang, Z., Liang, W., Wei, Z., Stack, R. J., and Holme, K. (1994) Structural features in heparin which modulate specific biological activities mediated by basic fibroblast growth factor. *Glycobiology* **4,** 451–458.

71. Ornitz, D. M., Herr, A. B., Nilsson, M., Westman, J., Svahn, C. M., and Waksman, G. (1995) FGF binding and FGF receptor activation by synthetic heparan-derived di- and trisaccharides. *Science* **268,** 432–436.

72. Stringer S. E. and Gallagher J. T. (1997) Specific binding of the chemokine platelet factor 4 to heparan sulfate. *J. Biol. Chem.* **272,** 20,508–20,514.

73. Baird, A., Schubert, D., Ling, N., and Guillemin, R. (1988) Receptor- and heparin-binding domains of basic fibroblast growth factor *Proc. Natl. Acad. Sci. USA* **85,** 2324–2328.

74. Seno, M., Sasada, R., Kurokawa, T., and Igarashi, K. (1990) Carboxyl-terminal structure of basic fibroblast growth factor significantly contributes to its affinity for heparin. *Eur. J. Biochem.* **188,** 239–245.

75. Li, L., Safran, M., Aviezer, D., Bohlen, P., Seddon, A. P., and Yayon, A. (1994) Diminished heparin binding of a fibroblast growth factor mutant is associated with reduced receptor binding, mitogenesis, plasminogen activator induction, and in vitro angiogenesis. *Biochemistry* **33,** 10,999–11,007.

76. Zhang, J., Cousens, L. S., Barr, P. J., and Sprang, S. R. (1991) Three-dimensional structure of human basic fibroblast growth factor, a structural homologue of interleukin 1β. *Proc. Natl. Acad. Sci. USA* **88,** 3446–3450.

77. Zhu, X., Komiya, H., Chirino, A., Faham, S., Fox, G. M., Arakawa, T., et al. (1990). Three-dimensional structures of acidic and basic fibroblast growth factors. *Science* **251,** 90–93.

78. Eriksson, A. E., Cousens, L. S., Weaver, L. H., and Matthews, B. W. (1991) Three-dimensional structure of human basic fibroblast growth factor. *Proc. Natl. Acad. Sci. USA* **88,** 3441–3445.

79. Koopmann, W. And Krangel M. S. (1997) Identification of a glycosaminoglycan-binding site in chemokine macrophage inflammatory protein-1α. *J. Biol. Chem.* **272,** 10,103–10,109.

80. Hohenester, E., Sasaki, T., Olsen B. R., and Timpl, R. (1998) Crystal structure of the angiogenesis inhibitor endostatin at 1.5 Å resolution. *EMBO J.* **17,** 1656–1664.

81. Soncin, F., Strydom, D. J., and Shapiro, R. (1997) Interaction of heparin with human angiogenin. *J. Biol. Chem.* **272,** 9818–9824.

82. Asai, T., Watanabe, K., Ichihara-Tanaka, K., Kaneda, N., Kojima S., Iguchi, A., et al. (1997) Identification of the heparin-binding sites in midkine and their role in neurite-promotion. *Biochem. Biophys. Res. Comm.* **236,** 66–70.

83. Thompson, L. D., Pantoliano, M. W., and Springer, B. A. (1994) Energetic characterization of the basic fibroblast growth factor-heparin interaction: identification of the heparin binding domain. *Biochemistry* **33,** 3831–3840.

84. Kennet, A. T. (1996) Vascular endothelial growth factor, a potent and selective angiogenic agent. *J. Biol. Chem.* **271,** 603–606.

85. Andersson, M., Ostman, A., Westermark, B., and Heldin, C.-H. (1994) Characterization of the retention motif in the C-terminal part of the long splice form of platelet-derived growth factor A-chain. *J. Biol. Chem.* **269,** 926–930.

86. Rusnati, M., Tulipano, G., Urbinati, C., Tanghetti, E., Giuliani, R., Giacca, M., et al. (1998) The basic domain in HIV-1 Tat protein as a target for polysulfonated heparin-mimicking extracellular Tat antagonists. *J. Biol. Chem.* **273,** 16,027–16,037.

87. Polotrak, Z., Cohen, T., Sivan, R., Kandelis, Y., Spira, G., Vlodavsky, I., et al. (1997) VEGF$_{145}$, a secreted vascular endothelial growth factor isoform that binds to extracellular matrix. *J. Biol. Chem.* **272,** 7151–7158.

88. Chang, H. C., Samaniego, F., Nair, B. C., Buonaguro, L., and Ensoli, B. (1997) HIV-Tat protein exits from intact cells through a leaderness secretory pathway and binds to extracellular matrix-associated heparan sulfate proteoglycans. *AIDS* **11,** 1421–1431.

89. Baird, A. and Ling, N. (1987) Fibroblast growth factors are present in the extracellular matrix produced by endothelial cells in vitro: implications for a role of heparinase-like enzymes in the neovascular response. *Biochem. Biophys. Res. Comm.* **142,** 428–435.

90. Vlodavsky, I., Folkman, J., Sullivan, R., Fridman, R., Ishai-Michaeli, R., Sasse, J., and Klagsbrun, M. (1987) Endothelial cell-derived basic fibroblast growth factor: synthesis and deposition into subendothelial extracellular matrix. *Proc. Natl. Acad. Sci. USA* **84,** 2292–2296.

91. Folkman, J., Klagsbrun, M., Sasse, J., Wadzinsky, M., Ingber, D., and Vlodavsky, I. (1988) A heparin-binding angiogenic protein-basic fibroblast growth factor is stored within basement membrane. *Am. J. Pathol.* **130,** 393–400.

92. DiMario, J., Buffinger, N., Yamada, S., and Strohman, R. C. (1989) Fibroblast growth factor in the extracellular matrix of dystrophic (mdx) mouse muscle. *Science* **244,** 688–690.

93. Hageman, G. S., Kirchoff-Rempe, M. A., Lewis, G. P., Fisher, S. K., and Anderson, D. H. (1991) Sequestration of basic fibroblast growth factor in the primate retinal interphotoreceptor matrix. *Proc. Natl. Acad. Sci. USA* **88,** 6706–6710.

94. Rusnati, M. and Presta, M. (1996) Interaction of angiogenic basic fibroblast growth factor with endothelial cell heparan sulfate proteoglycans. *Int. J. Clin. Lab. Res.* **26,** 15–23.

95. Barillari, G., Albonici, L., Franzese, O., Modesti, A., Liberati, F., Barillari, P., et al. (1998) The basic residues of placenta growth factor type 2 retrieve sequestered angiogenic factors into a soluble form: implications for tumor angiogenesis. *Am. J. Pathol.* **152,** 1161–1166.

96. Ingber, D. E. and Folkman, J. (1989) Mechano-chemical switching between growth and differentiation during fibroblast growth factor-stimulated angiogenesis in vitro: role of extracellular matrix. *J. Cell Biol.* **109,** 317–330.

97. Vlodavsky, I., Bar-Shavit, R., Ishai-Michaeli, R., Bashkin, P., and Fuks Z. (1991) Extracellular sequestration and release of fibroblast growth factor: a regulatory mechanism? *Trends Biol. Sci.* **16,** 268–271.

98. Tamura, T., Nakanishi, T., Kimura, Y., Hattori, T., Sasaki, K., Norimatsu, H., et al. (1996) Nitric oxide mediates interleukin-1-induced matrix degradation and basic fibroblast growth factor release in cultured rabbit articular chondrocytes: a possible mechanism of pathological neovascularization in arthritis. *Endocrinology* **137,** 3729–3737.

99. Mustonen, T. and Alitalo, K. (1995) Endothelial receptor tyrosine kinases involved in angiogenesis. *J. Biol. Chem.* **129,** 895–898.

100. Rapraeger, A. C., Krufka, A., and Olwin, B. B. (1991) Requirement of heparan sulfate for bFGF-mediated fibroblast growth and myoblast differentiation. *Science* **252,** 1705–1708.

101. Gitay-Goren, H., Soker, S., Vlodavsky, I., and Neufeld, G. (1992) The binding of vascular endothelial growth factor to its receptor is dependent on cell surface-associated heparin-like molecules. *J. Biol. Chem.* **267,** 6093–6098.

102. Yayon, A., Klagsbrun, M., Esko, J. D., Leder, P., and Ornitz, D. M. (1991) Cell surface, heparin-like molecules are required for binding of basic fibroblast growth factor to its high affinity receptor. *Cell* **64,** 841–848.

103. Avezier, D., Iozzo, R. V., Noonan, D. M., and Yayon, A. (1997) Suppression of autocrine and paracrine functions of basic fibroblast growth factor by stable expression of perlecan antisense cDNA. *Mol. Cell. Biol.* **17,** 1938–1946.

104. Roghani, M., Mansukhani, A., Dell'Era, P., Bellosta, P., Basilico, C., Rifkin, D. B., and Moscatelli, D. (1994) Heparin increases the affinity of basic fibroblast growth factor for its receptor but is not required for binding. *J. Biol. Chem.* **269,** 3927–3984.

105. Ornitz, D. M., Yayon, A., Flanagan, J. G., Svahn, C. M., Levi, E., and Leder, P. (1992) Heparin is required for cell-free binding of basic fibroblast growth factor to a free receptor and for mitogenesis in whole cells. *Mol. Cell. Biol.* **12,** 240–247.

106. Rusnati, M., Coltrini, D., Caccia, P., Dell'Era, P., Zoppetti, G., Oreste, P., et al. (1994) Distinct role of 2-O-, N-, and 6-O-sulfate groups of heparin in the formation of the ternary complex with basic fibroblast growth factor and soluble FGF receptor-1. *Biochem. Biophys. Res. Commun.* **203,** 450–458.

107. Tessler, S., Rockwell, P., Hicklin, D., Cohen, T., Levi, B.-Z., Witte, L., et al. (1994) Heparin modulates the interaction of $VEGF_{165}$ with soluble and cell associated flk-1 receptors. *J. Biol. Chem.* **269,** 12,456–12,461.

108. Choen, T., Gitay-Goren, H., Sharon, R., Shibuya, M., Halaban, R., Levi, B.-Z., and Neufeld, G. (1995) $VEGF_{121}$, a vascular endothelial growth factor (VEGF) isoform lacking heparin binding ability, requires cell-surface heparan sulfates for efficient binding to the VEGF receptors of human melanoma cells. *J. Biol. Chem.* **270,** 11,322–11,326.

109. Turnbull, J. E. and Gallagher, J. T. (1993) Heparan sulfate: functional role as modulator of fibroblast growth factor activity. *Biochem. Soc. Transact.* **21,** 477–482.

110. Kan, M., Wang, F., Xu, J., Crabb, J. W., Hou, J., and McKeehan, L. W. (1993) An essential heparin-binding domain in the fibroblast growth factor receptor kinase. *Science* **259,** 1918–1921.

111. Ishihara, M., Tyrrell, D. J., Stauber, G. B., Brown, S., Cousens, L. S., and Stack, R. J. (1993) Preparation of affinity-fractionated, heparin-derived oligosaccharides and their effects on selected biological activities mediated by basic fibroblast growth factor. *J. Biol. Chem.* **268,** 4675–4683.

112. Tyrrell, D. J., Ishihara, M., Rao, N., Horne, A., Kiefer, M. C., Stauber, G. B., et al. (1993) Structure and biological activities of a heparin-derived hexasaccharides with high affinity for basic fibroblast growth factor. *J. Biol. Chem.* **268,** 4684–4689.

113. Walker, A., Turnbull, J. E., and Gallagher, J. T. (1994) Specific heparan sulfate saccharides mediate the activity of basic fibroblast growth factor. *J. Biol. Chem.* **269,** 931–935.

114. Coltrini, D., Rusnati, M., Zoppetti, G., Oreste, P., Isacchi, A., Caccia, P., Bergonzoni, L., and Presta, M. (1993) Biochemical bases of the interaction of human fibroblast growth factor with glycosaminoglycans. *Eur. J. Biochem.* **214,** 51–58.

115. Ullrich, A. and Schlessinger, J. (1990) Signal transduction by receptors with tyrosine-kinase activity. *Cell* **61,** 203–212.

116. Spivak-Krolzman, T., Lemmon, M. A., Dikic, I., Ladbury, J. E., Pinchasi, D., Huang, J., et al. (1994) Heparin-induced oligomerization of FGF molecules is responsible for FGF receptor dimerization, activation, and cell proliferation. *Cell* **79,** 1015–1024.

117. Klagsbrun, M. and Baird, A. (1991) A dual receptor system is required for basic fibroblast growth factor activity. *Cell* **67,** 229–231.

118. Sakata, H., Stahl, S. J., Taylor, W. G., Rosenberg, J. M., Sakaguchi, K., Wingfield, P. T., and Rubin, J. S. (1997) Heparin binding and oligomerization of hepatocyte growth factor/scatter factor isoforms. *J. Biol. Chem.* **272,** 9457–9463.

119. Norrby, K. and Ostergaard, P. (1996) Basic-fibroblast-growth-factor-mediated de novo angiogenesis is more effectively suppressed by low-molecular-weight than by high-molecular-weight heparin. *Int. J. Microcirc. Clin. Exp.* **16,** 8–15.

120. Norrby, K. and Ostergaard, P. (1997) A 5.0-kD heparin fraction systemically suppresses VEGF165-mediated angiogenesis. *Int. J. Microcirc. Clin. Exp.* **17,** 314–321.

121. Taylor, S. and Folkman, J. (1982) Protamine is an inhibitor of angiogenesis. *Nature* **297,** 307–312.

122. Neufeld, G. and Gospodarowicz, D. (1987) Protamine sulfate inhibits mitogenic activities of the extracellular matrix and fibroblast growth factor, but potentiates that of epidermal growth factor. *J. Cell. Physiol.* **132,** 287–294.

123. Baggiolini, M., Dewald, B., and Moser, B. (1994) Interleukin-8 and related chemotactic cytokines - CXC and CC chemokines. *Adv. Immunol.* **55,** 97–179.

124. Mantovani, A., Bussolino, F., and Introna, M. (1997) Cytokine regulation of endothelial cell function: from molecular level to the bed side. *Immunol. Today* **18,** 231–239.

125. Kelner, G. S., Kennedy, J., Bacon, K. B., Kleyensteuber, S., Largaespada, D. A., Jenkins, N. A., et al. (1994) Lymphotactin: a cytokine that represents a new class of chemokine. *Science* **266,** 1395–1399.

126. Murphy, P. M. (1996) Chemokine receptors: structure, function and role in microbial pathogenesis. *Cytokine Growth Factors Rev.* **1,** 47–64.

127. Horuk, R. (1994) The interleukin-8-receptor family: from chemokines to malaria. *Immunol. Today* **15,** 169–174.

128. Gupta, S. K., Lysko, P. G., Pillarisetti, K., Ohlstein, E., and Stadel, J. M. (1998) Chemokine receptors in human endothelial cells. Functional expression of CXCR4 and its transcriptional regulation by inflammatory cytokines. *J. Biol. Chem.* **273,** 4282–4287.

129. Hadley, T. J., Lu, Z. H., Wasniowska, K., Martin, A. W., Peiper, S. C., Hesselgesser, J., and Horuk, R. (1994) Postcapillary venule endothelial cells in kidney express a multispecific chemokine receptor that is structurally and functionally identical to the erythroid isoform, which is the Duffy blood group antigen. *J. Clin. Invest.* **94,** 985–991.

130. Witt, D. P. and Lander, A. D. (1994) Differential binding of chemokines to glycosaminoglycan subpopulations. *Curr. Biol.* **4,** 394–400.

131. Rot, A. (1992) Endothelial cell binding of NAP-1/IL-8 role in neutrophil emigration. *Immunol. Today* **13,** 291–294.

132. Hoogewerf, A. J., Kuschert, G. S., Proudfoot, A. E., Borlat, F., Clark-Lewis, I., Power, C. A., and Wells, T. N. (1997) Glycosaminoglycans mediate cell surface oligomerization of chemokines. *Biochemistry* **36,** 13,570–13,578.

133. Strieter, R. M., Polverini, P. J., Kunkel, S. L., Arenberg, D. A., Burdick, M. D., Kasper, J., et al. (1995) The functional role of the ELR motif in CXC chemokine-mediated angiogenesis. *J. Biol. Chem.* **270,** 27,348–27,357.

134. Maione, T. E., Gray, G. S., Petro, J., Hunt, A. J., Donner, A. L., Bauer, S. I., et al. (1990) Inhibition of angiogenesis by recombinant human platelet factor-4 and related peptides. *Science* **247**, 77–79.

135. Fan, T.-P. (1994) Angiosuppressive therapy for cancer. *Trends Pharmacol. Sci.* **15**, 33–36.

136. Staddon, A., Henry, D., and Bonnem, E. (1994) A randomized dose finding study of recombinant platelet factor 4 (rPF4) in cutaneous AIDS-related Kaposi's sarcoma. *Proc. Am. Soc. Clin. Oncol.* **13**, 50.

137. Luster, A. D., Greenberg, S. M., and Leder, P. (1995) The IP-10 chemokine binds to a specific cell surface heparan sulfate site shared with platelet factor 4 and inhibits endothelial cell proliferation. *J. Exp. Med.* **182**, 219–231.

138. Watson, J. B., Getzler, S. B., and Mosher, D. F. (1994) Platelet factor 4 modulates the mitogenic activity of basic fibroblast growth factor. *J. Clin. Invest.* **94**, 261–268.

139. Maione, T. E., Gray, C. S., Hunt, A. J., and Sharpe, R. J. (1991) Inhibition of tumor growth in mice by an analogue of platelet factor 4 that lacks affinity for heparin and retains potent angiostatic activity. *Cancer Res.* **51**, 2077–2083.

140. Perollet, C., Han, Z. C., Savona, C., Caen, J. P., and Bikfalvi, A. (1998) Platelet factor 4 modulates fibroblast growth factor 2 (FGF-2) activity and inhibits FGF-2 dimerization. *Blood* **91**, 3289–3299.

141. Cao, Y., Chen, C., Weatherbee, J. A., Tsang, M., and Folkman, J. (1995) Gro-γ, a -C-X-C- chemokine, is an angiogenesis inhibitor that suppresses the growth of Lewis lung carcinoma in mice. *J. Exp. Med.* **182**, 2069–2072.

142. Presta, M., Belleri, M., Vecchi, A., Hesselgesser, J., Mantovani, A., and Horuk, R. (1998) Non-competitive, chemokine-mediated inhibition of basic fibroblast growth factor-induced endothelial cell proliferation. *J. Biol. Chem.* **273**, 7911–7918.

143. Inoue, K., Korenaga, H., Tanaka, N. G., Sakamoto, N., and Kadoya, S. (1988) The sulfated polysac-charide-peptidoglycan complex potently inhibits embryonic angiogenesis and tumor growth in the presence of cortisone acetate. *Carbohydr. Res.* **181**, 135–142.

144. Nakayama, Y., Iwahana, M., Sakamoto, N., Tanaka, N. G., and Osada, Y. (1993) Inhibitory effects of a bacteria-derived sulfated polysaccharide against basic fibroblast growth factor-induced endothe-lial cell growth and chemotaxis. *J. Cell. Physiol.* **154**, 1–6.

145. Chleboun, J. O., Sellers, P., Muir, G., Chew, P., and Martins, R. N. (1994) The effect of tecogalan sodium on the development of the collateral circulation after acute arterial occlusion. *Biochem. Biophys. Res. Comm.* **202**, 1149–1155.

146. Murata, T., Ishibashi, T., Yoshikawa, H., Khalil, A., and Inomata, H. (1995) Tecogalan sodium inhibits corneal neovascularization induced by basic fibroblast growth factor. *Ophthalmol. Res.* **27**, 330–334.

147. Sakamoto, T., Ishibashi, T., Kimura, H., Yoshikawa, H., Spee, C., Haris, M. S., et al. (1995) Effect of tecogalan sodium on angiogenesis in vitro by choroidal endothelial cells. *Invest. Ophthalmol. Visual Sci.* **36**, 1076–1083.

148. Nakamura, S., Sakurada S., Salahuddin, S. Z., Osada, Y., Tanaka, N. G., Sakamoto, N., et al. (1992) Inhibition of development of Kaposi's sarcoma-related lesions by a bacterial cell wall complex. *Science* **255**, 1437–1440.

149. Eckhardt, S. G., Burris, H. A., Eckhardt, J. R., Weiss, G., Rodriguez, G., Rothenberg, M., et al. (1996) A phase I clinical and pharmacokinetic study of the angiogenesis inhibitor tecogalan sodium. *Ann. Oncol.* **7**, 265–311.

150. Dennis, P. A., Saksela, O., Harpel, P., and Rifkin, D. B. (1989) α2-Macroglobulin is a binding protein for basic fibroblast growth factor. *J. Biol. Chem.* **264**, 7210–7216.

151. Socker, S., Svahn, C. M., and Neufeld, G. (1993) Vascular endothelial growth factor is inactivated by binding to α2-macroglobulin and the binding is inhibited by heparin. *J. Biol. Chem.* **268**, 7685–7691.

152. Mosher, D. F. (1990) Physiology of thrombospondin. *Annu. Rev. Med.* **41**, 85–97.

153. Bornstein, P., and Sage, E. H. (1994) Thrombospondins. *Methods Enzymol.* **245**, 62–85.

154. Bornstein, P. (1995) Diversity of function is inherent in matricellular proteins: an appraisal of thrombospondin 1. *J. Cell Biol.* **130**, 503–506.

155. Taraboletti, G., Belotti, D., Borsotti, P., Vergani, V., Rusnati, M., Presta, M., and Giavazzi, R. (1997) The 140 kD, anti-angiogenic fragment of thrombospondin binds to basic fibroblast growth factor. *Cell Growth Differ.* **8**, 471–479.

156. Lamszus, K., Joseph, A., Jin, L., Yao, Y., Chowdhury, S., Fuchs, A., et al. (1996) Scatter factor binds to thrombospondin and other extracellular matrix components. *Am. J. Pathol.* **149**, 805–819.

157. Schultz-Cherry, S. and Murphy-Ullrich, J. E. (1993) Thrombospondin causes activation of latent transforming growth factor-beta secreted by endothelial cells by a novel mechanism. *J. Cell Biol.* **122**, 923–932.

158. Good, D. J., Polverini, P. J., Rastinejad, F., Le Beau, M. M., Lemons, R. S., Frazier, W. A., and Bouck, N. P. (1990) A tumor suppressor-dependent inhibitor of angiogenesis is immunologically

and functionally indistinguishable from a fragment of thrombospondin. *Proc. Natl. Acad. Sci. USA* **87,** 6624–6628.

159. Taraboletti, G., Roberts, D., Liotta, L. A., and Giavazzi, R. (1990) Platelet thrombospondin modulates endothelial cell adhesion, motility, and growth: a potential angiogenesis regulatory factor. *J. Cell Biol.* **111,** 765–772.

160. O'Reilly, M. S., Boehem, T., Shing, Y., Fukai, N., Vasios, G., Lane, W. S., et al. (1997) Endostatin: an endogenous inhibitor of angiogenesis and tumor growth. *Cell* **88,** 277–285.

161. Bohem, T., Folkman, J., Browder, T., and O'Reilly, M. S. (1997) Anti-angiogenic therapy of experimental cancer does not induce acquired drug resistance. *Nature* **390,** 404–407.

162. De Clerque, E. (1987) Suramin in the treatment of AIDS: mechanism of action. *Antiviral Res.* **7,** 1–10.

163. Hawkins, M. J. (1995) Clinical trials of antiangiogenic agents. *Curr. Opin. Oncol.* **7,** 90–93.

164. Coffey, R. J., Leof, E. B., Shipley, G., and Moses, H. L. (1987) Suramin inhibition of growth factor receptor binding and mitogenicity in AKR-2B cells. *J. Cell. Physiol.* **132,** 143–148.

165. Braddock, P. S., Hu, D. E., Fan, T. P., Stratford, I. J., Harris, A. L., and Bicknell, R. (1994) A structure-activity analysis of antagonism of the growth factor and angiogenic activity of basic fibroblast growth factor by suramin and related polyanions. *Br. J. Cancer* **69,** 890–898.

166. Rusnati, M., Dell'Era, P., Urbinati, C., Tanghetti, E., Massardi, M. L., Nagamine, Y., et al. (1996) A distinct basic fibroblast growth factor (FGF-2)/FGF receptor interaction distinguishes urokinase-type plasminogen activator induction from mitogenicity in endothelial cells. *Mol. Biol. Cell.* **7,** 369–381.

167. Bojanowski, K., Lelievre, S., Markovits, J., Couprie, J., Jacquemin-Sablon, A., and Larsen, A. K. (1992) Suramin is an inhibitor of DNA topoisomerase II in vitro and in Chinese hamster fibrosarcoma cells. *Proc. Natl. Acad. Sci. USA* **89,** 3025–3029.

168. Gagliardi, A. R., Taylor, M. F., and Collins, D. C. (1998) Uptake of suramin by human microvascular endothelial cells. *Cancer Lett.* **125,** 97–102.

169. Khaled, Z., Rideout, D., O'Driscoll, K. R., Petrylak, D., Cacace, A., Patel, R., et al. (1995) Effects of suramin-related and other clinically therapeutic polyanions on protein kinase C activity. *Clin. Cancer Res.* **1,** 113–122.

170. Kopp, R. and Pfeiffer, A. (1990) Suramin alters phosphoinositide synthesis and inhibits growth factor receptor binding in HT-29 cells. *Cancer Res.* **50,** 6490–6496.

171. Spigelman, Z., Dowers, A., Kennedy, S., DiSorbo, D., O'Brien, M., Barr, R., and McCaffrey, R. (1987) Anti-proliferative effects of suramin on lymphoid cells. *Cancer Res.* **47,** 4694–4698.

172. Nakajima, M., DeChavigny, A., Johnson, C. E., Hamada J., Stein, C. A., and Nicolson, G. L. (1991) Suramin. A potent inhibitor of melanoma heparanase and invasion. *J. Biol. Chem.* **266,** 9661–9666.

173. Behrendt, N., Ronne, E., and Dano, K. (1993) Binding of urokinase-type plasminogen activator to its cell surface receptors is inhibited by low doses of suramin. *J. Biol. Chem.* **268,** 5985–5989.

174. Zabrenetzky, V. S., Kohn, E. C., and Roberts, D. D. (1990) Suramin inhibits laminin- and thrombospondin-mediated melanoma cell adhesion and migration and binding to these adhesive proteins. *Cancer Res.* **50,** 5937–5942.

175. Sola F., Farao, M., Marsiglio, A., Mariani, M., and Grandi, M. (1993) Inhibition of lung and liver tumor colonies in mice pretreated with suramin. *Invasion Metastasis* **13,** 163–168.

176. Pesenti, E., Sola, F., Mongelli, N., Grandi, M., and Spreafico, F. (1992) Suramin prevents neovascularization and tumor growth through blocking of basic fibroblast growth factor activity. *Br. J. Cancer* **66,** 367–372.

177. Collins, J. M., Klecker, R. W., Yarchoan, R., Lane, H. C., Fauci, A. S., Redfield, R. R., et al. (1986) Clinical pharmaco-kinetics of suramin in patients with HTLV-III/LAV infection. *J. Clin. Pharmacol.* **26,** 22–26.

178. Constantopoulos, G., Ress, S., Cragg, B. G., Barranger, J. A., and Brady, R. O. (1983) Suramin-induced storage disease mucopolysaccharidosis. *Am. J. Pathol.* **113,** 266–268.

179. Fan, T.-P., Jaggar, R., and Bicknell, R. (1995) Controlling the vasculature: angiogenesis, anti-angiogenesis and vascular targeting of gene therapy. *Trends Pharmacol. Sci.* **16,** 57–66.

180. Ciomei, M., Pastori, W., Mariani, M., Sola, F., Grandi, M., and Mongelli, N. (1994) New sulfonated distamycin A derivatives with bFGF complexing activity. *Biochem. Pharmacol.* **47,** 295–302.

181. Middaugh, C. R., Mach, H., Burke, C. J., Volkin, D. B., Dabora, J. M., Tsai, P. K., et al. (1992) Nature of the interaction of growth factors with suramin. *Biochemistry* **31,** 9016–9024.

182. Takano, S., Gately, S., Neville, M. E., Herblin, W. F., Gross, J. L., Engelhard, H., et al. (1994) Suramin, an anticancer and angiosuppressive agent, inhibits endothelial cell binding of basic fibroblast growth factor, migration, proliferation, and induction of urokinase-type plasminogen activator. *Cancer Res.* **54,** 2654–2660.

183. Sola, F., Farao, M., Pesenti, E., Marsiglio, A., Mongelli, N., and Grandi, M. (1995) Antitumor activity of FCE 26644 a new growth-factor complexing molecule. *Cancer Chemother. Pharmacol.* **36,** 217–222.

184. Sola, F., Gualandris, A., Belleri, M., Giuliani, R., Coltrini, D., Bastaki, M., et al. (1997) Endothelial cells overexpressing basic fibroblast growth factor (FGF2) induce vascular tumors in immunodeficient mice. *Angiogenesis* **1,** 102–116.

185. Witvrouw, M., Desmyter, J., and De Clerq, E. (1994) Antiviral portrait series: 4. Polysulfonates as inhibitors of HIV and other enveloped viruses. *Antiviral Chem. Chemother.* **5,** 345–359.

186. Kreimeyer, A., Muller, G., Kassack, M., Nickel, P., and Gagliardi, A. R. (1998) Suramin analogues with a 2-phenylbenzimidazole moiety as partial structure; potential anti HIV- and angiostatic drugs, 2: sulfanilic acid-, benzenedisulfonic acid-, and naphthalenetrisulfonic acid analogues. *Arch. Pharm. (Weinheim)* **331,** 97–103.

187. Zugmaier, G., Lippman, M. E., and Wellstein, A. (1992) Inhibition by pentosan polysulfate (PPS) of heparin-binding growth factors released from tumor cells and blockage by PPS of tumor growth in animals. *J. Natl. Cancer Inst.* **84,** 1716–1724.

188. Belford, D. A., Hendry, I. A., and Parish, C. R. (1993) Investigation on the ability of several naturally occurring and synthetic polyanions to bind to and potentiate the biological activity of acidic fibroblast growth factor. *J. Cell. Physiol.* **157,** 184–189.

189. Wellstein, A., Zugmaier, G., Califano, J. A., Kern, F., Paik, S., and Lippman, M. E. (1991) Tumor growth dependent on Kaposi's sarcoma-derived fibroblast growth factor inhibited by pentosan polysulfate. *J. Natl. Cancer Inst.* **83,** 716–720.

190. Rha, S. Y., Noh, S. H., Kwak, H. J., Wellstein, A., Kim, J. H., Roh, J. K., et al. (1997) Comparison of biological phenotypes according to midkine expression in gastric cancer cells and their autocrine activities could be modulated by pentosane polysulfate. *Cancer Lett.* **118,** 37–46.

191. McLeskey, S. W., Zhang, L., Trock, B. J., Kharbanda, S., Liu, Y., Gottardis, M. M., et al. (1996) Effects of AGM-1470 and pentosan polysulphate on tumorigenicity and metastasis of FGF-transfected MCF-7 cells. *Br. J. Cancer* **73,** 1053–1062.

192. Baba, M., Nakajima, M., Schols, D., Pauwels, R., Balzarini, J., and De Clercq, E. (1988) Pentosan polysulfate, a sulfated oligosaccharide, is a potent and selective anti-HIV agent in vitro. *Antiviral Res.* **9,** 335–343.

193. Parker, B. W., Swain, S. M., Zugmaier, G., DeLap, R. L., Lippman, M. E., and Wellstein, A. (1993) Detectable inhibition of heparin-binding growth factor activity in sera from patients treated with pentosan polysulfate. *J. Natl. Cancer Inst.* **85,** 1068–1073.

194. Pluda, J. M., Shay, L. E., Foli, A., Tannenbaum, S., Cohen, P. J., Goldspiel, B. R., et al. (1993) Administration of pentosan polysulfate to patients with human immunodeficiency virus associated Kaposi's sarcoma. *J. Natl. Cancer Inst.* **85,** 1585–1592.

195. Foxall, C., Wei, Z., Schaefer, M. E., Casabonne, M., Fugedi, P., Peto, C., et al. (1996) Sulfated malto-oligosaccharides bind to basic FGF, inhibit endothelial cell proliferation, and disrupt endothelial cell tube formation. *J. Cell. Physiol.* **168,** 657–667.

196. Saiki, I., Murata, J., Nakajima, M., Tokura, S., and Azuma, I. (1990) Inhibition of by sulfated chitin derivatives of invasion through extracellular matrix and enzymatic degradation by metastatic melanoma cells. *Cancer Res.* **50,** 3631–3637.

197. Murata, J., Saiki, I., Makabe, T., Tsuta, Y., Tokura, S., and Azuma, I. (1991) Inhibition tumor-induced angiogenesis by sulfated chitin derivatives. *Cancer Res.* **51,** 22–26.

198. Li, W. W., Casey, R., Gonzalez, E. M. and Folman, J. (1991) Angiostatic steroids potentiated by sulfated cyclodextrins inhibit corneal neovascularization. *Invest. Ophthalmol. Visual Sci.* **32,** 2898–2905.

199. Thorpe, P. E., Derbyshire, E. J., Andreade, S. P., Press, N., Knowles, P. P., King, S., et al. (1993) Heparin-steroid conjugates: new angiogenesis inhibitors with antitumor activity in mice. *Cancer Res.* **53,** 3000–3007.

200. Derbyshire, E. J., Yang, Y. C., Li, S., Comin, G. A., Belloir, J., and Thorpe, P. E. (1996) Heparin-steroid conjugates lacking glucocorticoid or mineralcorticoid activities inhibit the proliferation of vascular endothelial cells. *Biochim. Biophys. Acta* **1310,** 86–96.

201. Liekens, S., Neyts, J., Degreve, B., and De Clerque, E. (1997) The sulphonic acid polymers PAMPS [poly(2-acrylamido-2-methyl-1-propanesulfonic acid)] and related analogues are highly potent inhibitors of angiogenesis. *Oncol. Res.* **9,** 173–181.

202. Gagliardi, A. R. and Collins, D. C. (1994) Inhibition of angiogenesis by aurintricarboxylic acid. *Anticancer Res.* **14,** 475–479.

203. Lozano, R. M., Rivas, G., and Gimenez-Gallego, G. (1997) Destabilization, oligomerization and inhibition of the mitogenic activity of acidic fibroblast growth factor by aurintricarboxylic acid. *Eur. J. Biochem.* **248,** 30–36.

204. Miao, H. Q., Ornitz, D. M., Aingorn, E., Ben-Sasson, S. A., and Vlodavsky, I. (1997) Modulation of fibroblast growth factor-2 receptor binding, dimerization, signaling, and angiogenic activity by a synthetic heparin-mimicking polyanionic compound. *J. Clin. Invest.* **99,** 1565–1575.

205. Medalion, B., Merin, G., Aingorn, H., Miao, H. Q., Elami, A., Ishai-Michaeli, R., and Vlodavsky, I. (1997) Endogenous basic fibroblast growth factor displaced by heparin from the lumenal surface of human blood vessels is preferentially sequestered by injured regions of the vessel wall. *Circulation* **95,** 1853–1862.

206. Folkman, J., Langer, R., Linhardt, R. J., Haudenschild, C., and Taylor, S. (1983) Angiogenesis inhibition and tumor regression caused by heparin or a heparin fragment in the presence of cortisone. *Science* **221,** 719–725.

207. Crum, R., Szabo, S., and Folkman, J. (1985) A new class of steroids inhibits angiogenesis in the presence of heparin or a heparin fragment. *Science* **230,** 1375–1378.

208. Ingber, D. E., Madri, J. A., and Folkman, J. (1986) A possible mechanism for inhibition of angiogenesis by angiostatic steroids: induction of capillary basement membrane dissolution. *Endocrinology* **119,** 1768–1775.

209. Guvakova, M. A., Yakubov, L. A., Vlodavsky, I., Tonkinson, J. L., and Stein C. A. (1995) Phosphortothioate oligodeoxynucleotides bind to basic fibroblast growth factor, inhibit its binding to cell surface receptors, and remove it from low affinity binding sites on extracellular matrix. *J. Biol. Chem.* **270,** 2620–2627.

210. Fennewald, S. M. and Rando, R. F. (1995) Inibition of high affinity basic fibroblast growth factor binding by oligonucleotides. *J. Biol. Chem.* **270,** 21,718–21,721.

211. Benimetskaya, L., Tonkinson, J. L., Koziolkiewicz, M., Karwowski, B., Guga, P., Zeltser, R., et al. (1995) Binding of phosphorothioate oligodeoxynucleotides to basic fibroblast growth factor, recombinant soluble CD4, laminin and fibronectin is P-chirality independent. *Nucleic Acids Res.* **23,** 4239–4245.

212. Jellinek, D., Lynott, C. K., Rifkin, D. B., and Janjic, N. (1993) High-affinity RNA ligands to basic fibroblast growth factor inhibit receptor binding. *Proc. Natl. Acad. Sci. USA* **90,** 11,227–11,231.

213. Pagratis, N. C., Bell, C., Chang, Y.-F., Jennings, S., Fitzwater, T., Jellinek, D., and Dang, C. (1997) Potent 2'-amino-, and 2'-fluoro-2'-deoxyribonucleotide RNA inhibitors of keratinocyte growth factor. *Nature Biotech.* **15,** 68–73.

214. Peters, T. and Pinto, B. M. (1996) Structure and dynamics of oligosaccharides: NMR and modeling studies. *Curr. Opin. Struct. Biol.* **6,** 710–720.

21

2-Methoxyestradiol

A Novel Endogenous Chemotherapeutic and Anti-Angiogenic Agent

Victor S. Pribluda, Theresa M. LaVallee, and Shawn J. Green

CONTENTS

INTRODUCTION
BIOSYNTHESIS AND METABOLIC FATE OF 2-METHOXYESTRADIOL
ANTIPROLIFERATIVE EFFECTS OF 2-METHOXYESTRADIOL
PATHOPHYSIOLOGICAL EFFECTS OF 2-METHOXYESTRADIOL
MECHANISM OF ACTION OF 2-METHOXYESTRADIOL
CONCLUSION: AN IDEAL ANTI-PROLIFERATIVE AGENT
ACKNOWLEDGMENTS
REFERENCES

INTRODUCTION

Once largely dismissed and viewed as an inert metabolic end-product of estrogen, 2-methoxyestradiol is now recognized as a potent endogenous antimitogen. Its ability to selectively inhibit the growth of rapidly proliferating endothelial cells and tumors has generated new interest in this long overlooked molecule. Its candidacy as a viable antimitotic drug is supported by experimental evidence demonstrating that 2-methoxyestradiol is orally-active, and at therapeutic doses exhibits minimal, if any, toxicity. Although much research is focused on this compound as a potential drug candidate for the treatment of cancer, preliminary data that will not be reviewed in detail here suggest that it may also impact on other diseases, including psoriasis, arthritis, and osteoporosis.

Rediscovery of 2-Methoxyestradiol

Over the past 50 years, the use of natural and synthetic estrogens, including antiestrogens, to regulate endocrine function and treat various disorders has been widespread and extensive. Estrogens have effectively been used as contraceptives, for the treatment of breast cancer, and to ameliorate cardiovascular disease and bone loss in post menopausal women. Unfortunately, chronic administration of estrogens unveiled the

From: *The New Angiotherapy*
Edited by: T.-P. D. Fan and E. C. Kohn © Humana Press Inc., Totowa, NJ

potential risk of cancer. It has often been argued that the metabolic conversion of estrogens to reactive metabolites is the culprit for initiating, if not promoting, cancers. Such arguments have prompted researchers to search for analogs of estrogens and alternative treatment strategies. As a result of many of these studies, it appeared that among all the metabolites of estrogens, only 2-methoxyestrogens, and in particular 2-methoxyestradiol, were devoid of any obvious physiological significance.

During this period, the vast majority of the scientific literature defined 2-methoxestrogens as the inactive byproducts of estrogen. The relatively high levels found in plasma during the third trimester of pregnancy further supported this conclusion, which did not show any physiological or pathological correlation with the outcome of pregnancy. In the late 1980s, the first reports of the cytotoxic and cytostatic activities of 2-methoxyestradiol emerged, and subsequent studies revealed its effectiveness in inhibiting angiogenesis and in repressing the growth of a variety of tumors. Such findings provoked others to begin the search for molecular target(s) of 2-methoxyestradiol. In this review, we highlight those observations that provide the basis of why 2-methoxyestradiol is an ideal drug candidate for the treatment of a wide variety of afflictions, including angiogenesis-based diseases, e.g., cancer, arthritis, and psoriasis.

BIOSYNTHESIS AND METABOLIC FATE OF 2-METHOXYESTRADIOL

2-methoxyestradiol ($2ME_2$) is synthesized in vivo by the sequential hydroxylation and O-methylation of estradiol at the 2-position. Estradiol is largely converted to estrone, which is further metabolized to 2-hydroxyderivatives, and to a far less extent to 4-hydroxyderivatives. Hydroxyderivatives, e.g., 2-hydroxyestrone and 2-hydroxyestradiol, are subsequently methylated by catechol-O-methyltransferase (COMT) to methoxyderivatives. The high level of COMT in erythrocytes favors the formation of 2-methylated derivatives in plasma. Estrone and estradiol, as well as the 2-hydroxyderivatives and their respective 2-methyl ethers, coexist in equilibrium as free molecules or conjugates with sulfate and glucuronic acid *(1–3)*.

The majority of the studies assessed the plasma concentration of total methoxyestrones, or 2-methoxyestrone alone *(1,4–7)*. The liver is the principal organ responsible for the biotransformation of estrogen, and incubation of rat-liver slices with 2-hydroxyestradiol resulted in a twofold higher concentration of 2-methoxyestrone than $2ME_2$ *(2)*. If plasma concentrations reflect the liver ratio, under normal physiological conditions $2ME_2$ will be in the picomolar range; however, during late pregnancy, these values may reach the tens of nanomolar *(7)*. Owing to the ubiquity of the enzymes responsible for its synthesis, the actual intracellular levels of $2ME_2$ in various tissues may be significantly higher than the circulating levels in plasma *(8–10)*. A high endogenous level might be related to the very low toxicity reported after prolonged treatment with therapeutically effective doses.

Because it is beyond the scope of this review to discuss the regulation of estrogen and its derivatives, we will briefly highlight the enzymatic activities involved in the conversion of these precursors to $2ME_2$ and relevant metabolites.

Hydroxylase

Hydroxylation of estrogens occurs in a wide variety of organs including placenta, prostate, adrenal, pituitary, brain, kidney, lung, heart, liver, testes, ovary, and uterus *(2,11,12)*. As mentioned previously, hydroxylation at the 4-position occurs as well, but to a lesser extent. Once estrogens undergo hydroxylation at either of these positions, there is no evidence of biotransformation from the 2-hydroxyderivatives to the 4-hydroxyderivatives. The relative amounts of 2- and 4-hydroxyestrogens are both tissue- and estrogen-dependent, and the 4-position is more favored in uterus, brain, and kidney *(13–16)*. 4-hydroxyestradiol has higher estrogenic activity than 2-hydroxyestradiol, and has been associated with kidney cancer in Syrian male hamsters *(17)*. Interestingly, $2ME_2$ has been shown to inhibit hydroxylase activity *(18)*, hence, it may exert additional antitumor activity indirectly by decreasing the formation of the carcinogenic 4-hydroxyestradiol derivative.

Catechol-O-Methyl Transferase

Catechol-O-methyl transferase (COMT) converts 2-hydroxyestradiol to $2ME_2$. This enzyme is ubiquitous: it is present in the liver, placenta, uterus, testis, adrenals, kidney, spleen, lung, intestine, pituitary, brain, and blood *(2,19)*. Of particular importance is the high activity found in erythrocytes *(20)*, which is responsible for the 10 to 100-fold lower level of 2-hydroxyestradiol found in plasma relative to estrogens and 2-methoxyestrogens *(7)*. Clearance rate studies strongly suggest that 2-hydroxyestradiol is methylated before leaving the blood compartment *(20)*.

COMT is also responsible for the metabolism and inactivation of catecholamines *(21)*. 2-Hydroxyestradiol is a better substrate of COMT than catecholamines, and a very potent inhibitor of their methylation *(22)*.

Conjugation

Conjugation may occur at different stages of estrogen biotransformation, and there is evidence that conjugates may act as substrates for hydroxylation and methylation reactions of estrogens and hydroxyestrogens, respectively *(3,23)*. Conjugation at the 17β-position of 2-hydroxyestradiol enhanced O-methylation at the 2-position and strongly inhibited methylation at position 3; this is in agreement with the levels observed in vivo, suggesting that conjugation occurs before methylation *(3)*. In addition, there is evidence for conjugation of $2ME_2$ after oral administration in mice, which could be partially responsible for the rapid clearance observed from plasma *(24)*.

Glucuronates and sulfates are the most prominent conjugates found in blood, urine, and feces *(23,25,26)*, though thioether conjugates with aminoacids and peptides have also been described *(25,27)*. Incubation of 2-hydroxyestradiol with rat liver slices resulted in the conjugation of the methyl ethers in addition to the estrogens; sulfates were predominantly intracellular, while glucuronates were only found in the incubation media *(26)*. This observation is consistent with the in vivo finding that glucuronates constitute the main fraction of excreted conjugates *(25)*.

Demethylases

Methylation by COMT is not a reversible reaction. However, there is ample evidence that free catechols are produced from the 2-methoxyderivatives in certain rat and human tissues. This is the result of the action of a distinct set of enzymes called demethylases *(12,28)*. Demethylation of 2-methoxyestrone and $2ME_2$ in rat liver proceeds through two different enzymes whose activity is regulated independently *(29)*. 2-methoxyestrone demethylase, but not $2ME_2$ demethylase, shows sexual dimorphism and is regulated by estrogens and thyroid hormones. Demethylases may also have a role in the toxicity of certain estrogen derivatives, because demethylation of 4-methoxyestradiol to 4-hydroxyestradiol has been associated with the carcinogenic potential of the former *(17)*.

Table 1
Anti-Proliferative Activity of 2ME$_2$ In Vitro

Cell Type	Inhibitory Concentration (μM)	Reference
Human Tumor		
Lung (HOP-62)	0.7[a]	(30)
Lung (H460)	5.0[b]	(31)
Lung (A549)	5.0[b]	(31)
Colon (HCT-116)	0.47[a]	(30)
CNS (SF-539)	0.32[a]	(30)
CNS (SH-SY5Y)	1.3[a,b]	(32)
Melanoma (UACC-62)	0.36[a]	(30)
Ovarian (OVCAR-3)	0.21[a]	(30)
Renal (SN12-C)	0.95[a]	(30)
Prostates (DU-145)	1.8[a]	(30)
Breast (MDA-MB-435)	0.08–0.61[a,b]	(33–34)
Breast (MDA231)	1.03[a]	(34)
Breast (MCF-7)	0.45[a,b]	(34)
Lymphoblast (Jurkat)	0.3	(35)
Lymphoblast (TK6)	1–2[b]	(36)
Lymphoblast (WTK1)	1–2[a]	(36)
Human Nontumor		
Skin Fibroblast (HFK2)	2.0[a]	(37)
Human Endothelial		
HUVEC	0.45[a,b]	(34)
Non-Human Tumor		
Lung (Lewis lung - Murine)	1.68[a,b]	(34)
Melanoma (B16 BL6 - Murine)	0.40[a,b]	(34)
Melanoma (B16 F10 - Murine)	0.30[a,b]	(34)
Endothelial (EOMA - Murine)	0.89[a,b]	(34)
Endothelial (H5V - Murine)	1.0	(38)
Nonhuman Nontumor		
Lung (V79-Hamster)	3.0	(39)
Ovarian (Granulosa - Porcine)	3.0	(40)
Smooth Muscle (Aorta - Rabbit)	1.0	(41)
Adipocytes (Murine)	1.7	(42)
Non-Human Endothelial		
Brain Capillary (Bovine)	0.19–0.49[a,b]	(33,3437)
Pulmonary artery (Bovine)	0.5[b]	(43)

[a]IC$_{50}$ measured by metabolic labeling or cell count.
[b]Cells assessed for apoptosis. In every instance, when evaluated, 2ME$_2$ inhibition was accompanied by apoptosis.

ANTIPROLIFERATIVE EFFECTS OF 2-METHOXYESTRADIOL

Over the past decade, a number of investigators have reported on the anti-mitotic properties of 2ME$_2$. Initially, its action was investigated on cell types associated with estrogen-responsive tissues, however subsequent studies clearly established that its anti-proliferative activity was not limited to estrogen-dependent cells. Table 1 lists different cell lines that are inhibited by 2ME$_2$. Two noteworthy features of this list are: 1) a wide diversity of cell types are sensitive to 2ME$_2$; and 2) the inhibitory concentrations are

Table 2
Biological Activities of 2ME$_2$

Biological activity	Target cells	Response inhibited	Reference
Anti-angiogenic	Endothelial	Proliferation Migration Tubule formation	(33,37,43)
Anti-tumor	Endothelial Tumor	Angiogenesis Tumor-cell proliferation	(33,37,50,52,54)
Anti-inflammatory	Endothelial	Angiogenesis NO production	(38)
Anti-estrogenic and anti-androgenic	Liver Prostate	Binding of sex hormones to sex hormone binding globulin	(58,59,63)
Stimulation of progesterone production	Ovary		(102,103)
Inhibition of prostaglandin synthesis	Endometrium		(104)
Enhancement of cathecolamine activity	Aorta	Catecholamine uptake	(105)
Hypocholesterolemic effect	Liver	reduced levels of serum cholesterol	(106)

limited to a relatively narrow range. This partial list includes both tumor and nontumor cell lines, and various primary cultures.

Inhibition of proliferation by 2ME$_2$ results mainly from induction of apoptosis (Table 1). Actually, it appears that 2ME$_2$ targets only actively proliferating cells, and it is not cytotoxic to quiescent cells; however, confluent endothelial cells become sensitive to the apoptotic effects of 2ME$_2$ after stimulating the cells with basic fibroblast growth factor (bFGF) (37). Moreover, human lymphoblasts and human skin fibroblast become more sensitive to 2ME$_2$ under conditions that favor an increased proliferation rate (36).

A number of reports showed that the cell count in cultures treated with 2ME$_2$ did not go below seeding density, regardless of whether apoptosis was detected (34,40,41). When 2ME$_2$ was removed and the cells were placed in media without drug, viable cells entered G$_1$ phase (35,40), or became apoptotic (36). The extent of cell-cycle arrest, and the conditions favoring it over apoptosis warrants further investigation.

Finally, a number of these studies compared the anti-proliferative action of 2ME$_2$ with estrogens, and other catechol and methoxyestrogens; in every instance 2ME$_2$ was the most effective inhibitor (37–40,43–45). Furthermore, inhibiting their conversion to 2ME$_2$ (45) eliminated the inhibitory effect of estradiol and 2-hydroxyestradiol.

The various biological activities described for 2ME$_2$ are summarized in Table 2. The following sections highlight the anti-angiogenic and anti-tumor activities, which are by far the most extensively studied.

Antiangiogenic

Although 2ME$_2$ has been coined as an anti-angiogenic, endothelial cells are not necessarily more sensitive to its anti-proliferative effect. In addition to its anti-proliferative effects, 2ME$_2$ also affects other steps in the angiogenesis cascade. Invasion through a collagen matrix, as

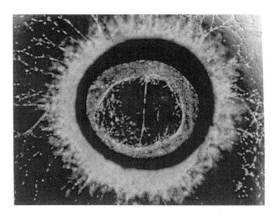
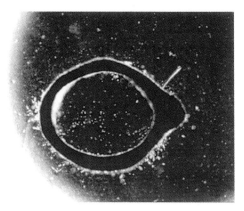

Fig. 1. Inhibition of microvessel growth from aorta sections by 2ME$_2$. Thoracic aortic rings from rats were incubated in medium in the absence (left) or the presence (right) of 2.5 μM 2ME$_2$. Microvessel growth was assessed after 5 d of incubation *(46,47)* (Dr. W.D. Figg, National Cancer Institute, NIH, Bethesda, MD, USA).

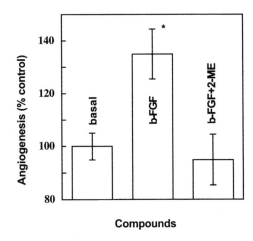

Fig. 2. Inhibition of bFGF-induced angiogenesis in chick choroallantoic membranes (CAM) by 2ME$_2$. CAM from 10-d-old chick embryos were treated with filter disks saturated with PBS buffer (basal) or 1 μg/mL bFGF. 2 μM 2ME$_2$ or vehicle was then added to the bFGF disks. This graph represents the quantitation of the number of vessels after 72-h treatment. Adapted with permission from ref. *(43)*.

well as tubule formation was blocked by 2ME$_2$ *(37)*. Similarly, in a rat-aorta ex-vivo model, 2ME$_2$ inhibited proliferation, migration, and tube formation (Fig. 1) *(46,47)*. In a study in which both matrix metalloproteinase/tissue inhibitor of metalloproteinase and urokinase/ plasminogen-activator inhibitor proteolytic balances were assessed in twelve human tumor cell lines, 2ME$_2$ did not produce a clear shift of the proteolytic balance. A clear increase in urokinase-type plasminogen-activator activity was observed only in a neuroblastoma cell line *(48)*. However, in endothelial cells 2ME$_2$ was shown to inhibit bFGF-mediated stimulation of urokinase-type plasminogen activator activity *(37)*.

The inhibitory effects of 2ME$_2$ on neovascularization has also been observed in the chick chorioallantoic membrane (CAM) *(43)* (Fig. 2) and the corneal micropocket vascularization

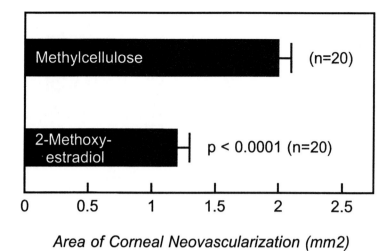

Fig. 3. Inhibition of bFGF-induced corneal neovascularization by $2ME_2$. This graph represents the quantitation of the area of neovascularization induced by a bFGF pellet 5 d after implantation. Mice were treated p.o. daily with methylcellulose or 150 mg/kg $2ME_2$. Adapted with permission from ref. *(33)*.

assays *(33)* (Fig. 3). In the former, $2ME_2$ at low micromolar concentrations, similar to those inhibiting migration and inducing apoptosis, inhibited angiogenesis induced by bFGF. In the corneal micropocket assay, oral administration of $2ME_2$ inhibited angiogenesis induced by either bFGF or vascular endothelial growth factor (VEGF).

These data support the notion that $2ME_2$ can effectively disrupt angiogenesis at different stages in the formation of new blood vessels. The antiangiogenic activity of $2ME_2$ in tumors will be described in the following section.

Anti-Tumor

Recent evidence provides encouraging results for the use of $2ME_2$ in cancer. Some of these studies suggest that $2ME_2$ targets both the tumor cell and the endothelial-cell compartment of a growing tumor.

Oral administration of $2ME_2$ was effective at reducing the rate of tumor growth in mice without signs of toxicity. After 2 wk of treatment, the primary tumor mass of Meth A sarcoma and B16 melanoma were reduced by 66 and 85%, respectively. A concomitant reduction in tumor vascularization was observed *(37)* (Fig. 4).

In a xenograft model, the estrogen receptor-negative human breast cell line, MDA-MB-435, was also sensitive to $2ME_2$ *(33)* (Fig. 5). The rate of growth was significantly reduced during this period: tumor volume of the treated animals was 40% of the controls. Immunohistochemical assessment of endothelial-cell markers in the tumor revealed a 60% reduction of the vascular density (Fig. 5). The number of proliferating cells in the tumor was reduced by a similar extent.

Preliminary results show that $2ME_2$ reduced the incidence and severity of brain lesions in an experimental hemangioma model, induced by infecting new born rats with murine polyoma virus, which results in transformation of the endothelial cells (Dr. J. Neyts, Katholieke Universiteit Leuven, Leuven, Belgium). In this same model, TNP-470, which is considered a pure antiangiogenic drug, was an effective inhibitor of hemangioma

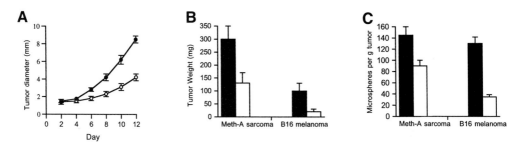

Fig. 4. Inhibition of growth and neovascularization of Meth-A sarcoma and B16 melanoma tumors in mice by oral administration of $2ME_2$. Tumor cells were inoculated s.c. in the dorsal skin of C3H mice. Mice received daily treatments with olive oil or 100 mg/kg $2ME_2$ p.o. from the day of inoculation. On day 12 the mice were killed and the tumor weighed. **(A)** Inhibition of Meth-A sarcoma tumor growth. Closed circles, control; open circles, $2ME_2$. **(B)** Tumor weight on day 12 after inoculation of Meth-A sarcoma or B16 melanoma cells. Closed bars, control; open bars, $2ME_2$. **(C)** Neovascularization of Meth-A sarcoma or B16 melanoma tumors. Vascularization was quantified by counting of microspheres injected 5 min before the mice were killed. Closed bars, control; open bars, $2ME_2$. Adapted with permission from ref. *(37)*.

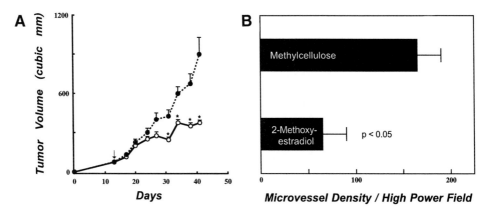

Fig. 5. Inhibition of tumor growth and associated vascularization in an estrogen receptor-negative human breast-cancer xenograft by $2ME_2$. SCID mice were inoculated with MDA-MB-435 on day 0. Mice were treated daily with either methylcellulose or 75 mg/kg $2ME_2$ p.o. was started on day 12 after the tumors became measurable (arrow). **(A)** Inhibition of tumor growth. Closed circles, control; open circles, $2ME_2$. **(B)** Quantitation of microvessel density. Animals were sacrificed 42 d after tumor inoculation. Tumor vascularization was analyzed by staining with polyclonal antibodies against von Willebrand factor. Adapted with permission from ref. *(33)*.

development *(49)*. In a human neuroblastoma xenograft model in mice, $2ME_2$ resulted in a significant reduction in tumor growth after 14 d of treatment of tumors that had reached a volume of at least 300 mm^3 (Fig. 6). In this study, $2ME_2$ was equally effective in male as in female mice, and there was a very clear antiangiogenic and apoptotic effect on the tumor (Table 3) *(50)*. Brain tumors are of particular interest, because of the absence of any effective treatment strategies. The hydrophobic nature of $2ME_2$, which allows passage through the blood-brain barrier, in conjunction with the relatively high content of 2-hydroxylase and COMT in brain, make $2ME_2$ particularly appealing for brain cancer treatment. The extent of growth inhibition of the neuroblastoma tumor by TNP-470 in rats

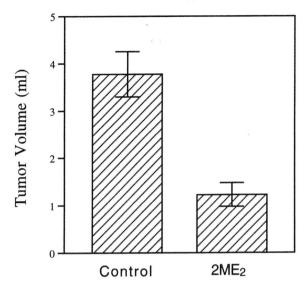

Fig. 6. Inhibition of tumor growth in a human neuroblastoma xenograft by 2ME$_2$. Nude mice, NMRI-nu, were inoculated with SH-SY5Y cells, and treated p.o with 100 mg/kg/d 2ME$_2$. Treatment was initiated when the tumors reached a volume of at least 0.3 mL. The volumes were reassessed after 14 d of treatment *(50)*.

Table 3
Effects of 2ME$_2$ on Neuroblastoma

Tumor parameters	2ME$_2$ (100 mg/kg/day)
Volume	↓ 63%
Angiogenesis[a]	↓ 40%
Proliferative cells	Unchanged
Apoptotic cells	↑ 208%

[a]Length of vessels per tumor volume.

was similar to the inhibition by 2ME$_2$ in mice *(51)*. Similarly, 2ME$_2$ inhibited the growth of angiosarcoma in mice, a model in which TNP-470 also was effective *(52)*. Further comparative studies between these two compounds will hopefully bring forth new information on the cellular target of 2ME$_2$.

In addition to primary tumors, 2ME$_2$ was recently found to be effective in controlling metastatic disease. Low doses (25 mg/kg/d) of 2ME$_2$ orally administrated commencing 3 days after mice were injected intravenously with B16BL6 melanoma resulted in a 70% reduction in the number of lung metastases. Higher doses cleared the lungs of surface metastases by more than 90%. Similar results were obtained with the Lewis Lung tumor cell line (Fig. 7). In the latter, 2ME$_2$ inhibits proliferation and induces apoptosis in the tumor-cell compartment, and also has antiangiogenic activity *(34)*. Consistent with these observations, a 60% inhibition in the number of lung colonies from an i.v. injected pancreatic cancer-cell line has been recently reported *(53)*. Similarly, orally administrated 2ME$_2$ also inhibited metastatic lung cancer cell colonies in the lung, and this effect was potentiated by simultaneous administration of adenoviral p53 *(54)*.

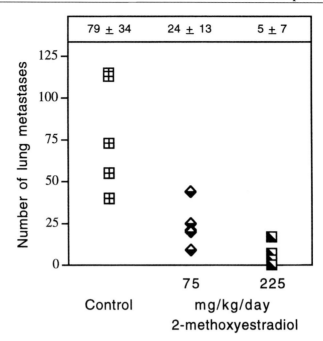

Fig. 7. Inhibition of melanoma lung colony formation by 2ME$_2$. B16-BL6 melanoma cells were i.v. injected into the tail vein of C57BL/6 mice. Three days later, mice were treated orally with 2ME$_2$ or vehicle (0.5% carboxymethyl cellulose). Fourteen days after tumor-cell inoculation, lungs were removed and surface pulmonary metastases were counted. The symbols correspond to counts from individual mice (n = 5 per group), and the values are the average ± standard deviation *(34)*.

To date, there are no data indicating that 2ME$_2$ treatment generates resistance although as more tumors are assessed resistance to 2ME$_2$ may surface. Transfection of the P-glycoprotein, which confers multidrug resistance *(55)*, did not affect the sensitivity of MDA-231 human breast cancer cell line to 2ME$_2$ *(34)*. We have examined the sensitivity to 2ME$_2$ of a variety of cell lines that have been made resistant to several chemotherapeutic agents including etoposide, adriamycin, methotrexate and taxol, and have found that none of these resistant cell lines is cross-resistant to 2ME$_2$ *(34;* Pribluda, V. S., et al., manuscript in preparation). Our efforts to directly generate resistance to 2ME$_2$ using a high-dose selection protocol have failed and we are currently evaluating the ability of cell lines to develop resistance to 2ME$_2$ using a step-wise selection protocol, a method that proved to be effective with other cell lines (Pribluda, V. S., et al., unpublished observations). In vivo, if 2ME$_2$ inhibits tumor growth by blocking angiogenesis, tumor resistance becomes less of a concern, because the development of resistance is not associated with anti-angiogenic therapy in humans and animal models *(56,57)*.

An additional level at which 2ME$_2$ may affect the proliferation of tumor growth in vivo is through interaction with the sex hormone binding globulin (SHBG). 2ME$_2$ enhances the expression of this protein *(58)*, to which it binds with higher affinity than testosterone and estradiol *(59)*. This interaction results in an inactive complex that blocks the activity of estrogens and androgens mediated through this protein *(60–62)*. In canine prostate tissue, in the presence of SHBG, 2ME$_2$ inhibited the production of the equivalent of the human prostate-specific antigen induced by estradiol and androgens *(63)*.

Recently, the allele coding for a low-activity variant of COMT was associated with the risk for breast cancer, and this risk was correlated with an increase in the concentration of catechol estrogens, in particular 4-hydroxyestradiol *(64)*. An additional factor, not considered in this report, is that low COMT activity could result in lower $2ME_2$ levels. The subsequent reduction in $2ME_2$ levels may contribute to the increased risk of breast cancer *(65)*.

PATHOPHYSIOLOGICAL EFFECTS OF 2-METHOXYESTRADIOL
Toxicity

Unlike the toxicity usually associated with conventional chemotherapy, therapeutic doses of $2ME_2$ did not result in hair loss, gastrointestinal disturbance, or leukocyte reduction in bone marrow and thymus *(33,37,38)*. A slight decrease in the number of B-cells in spleen was observed after 35 d of continuous exposure to subcutaneous implants containing 2–3 mg of $2ME_2$, although CD4+ and CD8+ cells were unaffected *(38)*. Subcutaneous treatment of pre-pubertal rats resulted in an increase in plasma levels of VLDL lipoproteins *(66)*, and in tumor-bearing mice minor weight loss was reported after oral doses of 150 mg/kg/d were administrated for 25 d. However, subsequent studies performed by the same lab, under the same conditions, showed no major weight loss after 42 d of continuous treatment *(33)*.

The plasma levels attained after administration of therapeutically effective doses are in the same range or slightly higher than the physiological levels found during the third trimester of pregnancy in women *(7,24)*. This is an important aspect, because there is no correlation between the methoxyestrogens levels found during pregnancy and pregnancy outcome.

Carcinogenicity

An obvious concern with the administration of $2ME_2$ is its conversion back to the parent estrogens and associated cancer-promoting potential, because administration of estrogens has been linked with tumorigenesis *(67)*. However, numerous studies suggest that this is not a concern with $2ME_2$ administration. In the male Syrian hamster model, where a large number of estrogen derivatives and estrogen preparations including 4-hydroxyestradiol were found to be carcinogenic, 2-hydroxyestradiol and $2ME_2$ did not induce renal carcinoma *(68)*. Consistent with these results, 4-hydroxyestradiol and related epoxide-intermediates were associated with transforming and mutagenic capacity to a much larger extent than 2-hydroxyestradiol and its derivatives *(69)*. The high ratio of $2ME_2$ to 2-hydroxyestradiol in plasma during late pregnancy shows that the equilibrium favors the methylated derivatives, rather than the estrogenic catechols *(7)*. Analysis of the plasma levels of $2ME_2$ and 2-hydroxyestradiol after intravenous administration of 2-hydroxyestradiol supports a similar conclusion: >90% of plasma 2-hydroxyestradiol undergoes biotransformation within 5 min *(70,71)*. The data suggest that 2-methoxyestrogens are favored metabolites of estrogens and the only ones that are not associated with tumor development.

Estrogenic Activity

Another concern with the chronic administration of $2ME_2$ is its ability to function as an estrogen agonist. The result summarized in Table 4, clearly indicates that administration of $2ME_2$ at doses and under conditions in which other estrogens had a distinct positive effect, failed to induce an estrogenic response.

$2ME_2$ was found to be completely ineffectual in sustaining uterine growth when administered continuously by means of osmotic pumps implanted in ovariectomized rats; whereas, in sharp contrast, 2-hydroxyestrone, 4-methoxyestrone and estradiol had strong

Table 4
Estrogenic Activity of 2ME$_2$

Assessed response	Estrogens[a]	2ME$_2$	Reference
E.R. Affinity[b,c]	High	Low (< 0.1%)	(72,77)
Uterotropic Activity[c]	+	–	(66,72)
Carcinogenesis[c]	+	–	(67–69)
Feminizing Activity[d]	+	–	(38)
Inhibition of leukopoiesis[d]	+	–	(38)

[a]+, activity present, – , activity absent.
[b]Measure the ability to displace estradiol from the uterine cytosol estrogen receptor (E.R.). Percentage (%) of estradiol binding. 2ME$_2$ exhibits 2,000-fold less affinity to the estrogen receptor in comparison to estradiol.
[c]2ME$_2$ and estradiol were compared with other natural and synthetic estrogens.
[d]Only 2ME$_2$ and estradiol were compared.

uterotropic activity (72). In a study with prepubertal rats, 2ME$_2$ induced a mild increase in uterus weight at the highest dose tested, which was only 15% of the effect observed with estradiol administered at one-tenth the dose (66). Furthermore, ovariectomized mice receiving microgram quantities of 2ME$_2$ twice a week remained at the diestrus stage, whereas a similar treatment with estradiol induced estrus phase within 6 d. As predicted, seminal vesicles in males were significantly reduced by estradiol treatment, but were unaffected with 2ME$_2$. Similarly, the inhibition of leukopoiesis induced by estrogens was not observed with 2ME$_2$ (38). In male hamsters, estradiol, 4-hydroxestradiol and 2-hydroxyestradiol, but not 2ME$_2$, sustained the tumor growth of H-301 cells, an estrogen-dependent hamster-kidney tumor cell line (68).

Consistent with these findings, proliferation of human umbilical endothelial cells (73,74) and MCF-7 cells, an estrogen-dependent human breast cancer cell line (44,45), were sustained by estradiol, but not by 2ME$_2$ (34,37). While estradiol sustained growth in media stripped of estrogens and rescued endothelial cells from apoptosis induced by tumor necrosis factor-α (TNF-α) (74), 2ME$_2$ inhibited cell growth and was a potent inducer of apoptosis (34,37).

The absence of functional estrogenic activity by the therapeutic doses of 2ME$_2$ is consistent with its weak binding activity to the uterine cytosol estrogen receptor: 2,000-fold lower affinity than estradiol for the estrogen receptor (72). Recently, a second estrogen receptor was identified (75,76). We find that the binding affinity for recombinant estrogen receptor β (ERβ) is even lower than for recombinant estrogen receptor α (ERα) (LaVallee, T. M., et al., manuscript in preparation). The estrogen receptor needs to be occupied for several hours for a full estrogenic response, a condition that is easily satisfied by a single administration of the high affinity binding estradiol. Conversely, 2-hydroxyestradiol with an estrogen receptor binding affinity of 20% of that of estradiol — and 400-fold higher than 2ME$_2$ — is ineffective when administrated by pulse injection and requires constant infusion to show estrogenic activity (77).

The likelihood that 2ME$_2$ mediates estrogenic activity via the estrogen receptor is further diminished because of rapid metabolic clearance from plasma and binding to plasma proteins. When 2ME$_2$ is administered orally or intravenously, peak plasma levels in the micromolar range are observed 15–30 min after administration, then rapidly decline and are not detectable after 1.5 h (24). Presumably, a large fraction of 2ME$_2$ becomes complexed with SHBG *(59)*. In addition, the formation of conjugates with sulfate and glucuronic acid *(23–26)* accelerates its clearance and reduce its ability to engage the target cell by preventing it from crossing the cell membrane.

Collectively, these findings suggest that $2ME_2$ is not able to engage estrogen receptors as an agonist.

Moreover, there is no correlation between estrogen-receptor expression and the antiproliferative and cytotoxic activity of $2ME_2$. $2ME_2$ has a similar antiproliferative activity on MCF7 cells (ER$\alpha^+\beta^+$), MDA-MB-435 cells (ER$\alpha^-\beta^+$) and MDA-231 cells (ER$\alpha^-\beta^-$) (Table 1). Blocking the estrogen receptor with antiestrogens does not obstruct the antiproliferative activity of $2ME_2$ (LaVallee, T. M., et al., manuscript in preparation). These data suggest that the estrogen receptor is not the molecular target for the antiproliferative activities of $2ME_2$.

MECHANISM OF ACTION OF 2-METHOXYESTRADIOL

The process by which $2ME_2$ affects cell growth remains unclear, however, a number of studies have implicated various mechanisms of action and cellular targets. Concentration and duration of exposure to $2ME_2$ may determine whether rapidly proliferating cells recover from G_2/M arrest *(35,40)* or become apoptotic *(36)*. As highlighted in Table 5, $2ME_2$ induced changes in the levels and activities of various proteins involved in the progression of the cell cycle. These include cofactors of DNA replication and repair, e.g., proliferating-cell nuclear antigen (PCNA) *(33,78)*; cell-division cycle kinases and regulators, e.g., p34^{cdc2} and cyclin B *(35,78,79)*; transcription factor modulators, e.g., SAPK/JNK *(43,80)*; and regulators of cell arrest and apoptosis, e.g., p21$^{WAF1/CIP1}$ *(31)*, bcl-2 and FAS *(43,80)*, and p53 *(31,36,54)*. These cellular targets are not necessarily mutually exclusive to the inhibitory effects of $2ME_2$ in actively dividing cells. The effects on the level of cAMP, calmodulin activity, and protein phosphorylation may also be related to each other *(35,45,78)*.

It is clear from Table 5 that all the observed effects are consistent with the ultimate cellular outcome, e.g., cell arrest or apoptosis. In every case, $2ME_2$ interferes with the cell-cycle machinery, not with housekeeping functions: the low toxicity in nonproliferating cells in culture and in vivo are consistent with a cellular target operating during a proliferative state.

Tubulin

In cells treated with $2ME_2$, histological staining and immunofluorescence with anti-tubulin antibodies clearly shows an increase in the percentage of mitotic figures, particularly during metaphase *(35,39,44,45)*. In endothelial cells, $2ME_2$ caused selective disruption of microtubules as opposed to other cytoskeletal structures *(37)*. Likewise, micromolar amounts caused disruption of the microtubular network in nonsynchronized Chinese hamster V79 cells *(39)*, and multipolar and irregular spindles in synchronized MCF-7 cells *(44)*. However, with Jurkat cells and other leukemia cell lines, the ability of $2ME_2$ to cause disruption of microtubules was challenged. Although cell arrest was observed at submicromolar concentrations of $2ME_2$, exposure of Jurkat cells to 20 μM for 24 h failed to show disassembly of microtubules *(35)*. $2ME_2$ has also been shown to inhibit aromatase activity; an activity observed with drugs that stabilize tubulin and not with agents that inhibit tubulin polymerization *(81)*.

Because microtubule poisons such as colchicine and taxol induce similar in vivo and in vitro changes *(33,82)*, the interaction of $2ME_2$ with tubulin was assessed *(83,84)*. $2ME_2$ inhibited the rate but not the degree of polymerization and depolymerization of tubulin induced by other agents. Morphological studies did not reveal major differences when tubulin was polymerized in the presence or absence of $2ME_2$.

Table 5
Mechanism of Action of 2ME$_2$; Potential Targets and Cellular Effects

Observed response	Probable targets or mediators of 2ME$_2$ action	Potential pathways affected by the observed response	Expected proliferative outcome	Reference
Damaged microtubular network / Abnormal mitotic spindle	Tubulin and/or microtubules / p53	p53 activation / bcl-2 phosphorylation	Arrest at G$_1$ phase / Arrest at G$_2$/M phase / Apoptosis	(35,37,39,44,45)
Increased levels of cAMP at S phase	Inhibition of calmodulin dependent phosphodiesterase	Reduced DNA synthesis by inhibition of ribonucleoside reductase	Apoptosis	(35,45)
Reduced levels and activity of the proliferating cell nuclear antigen	p53 and p21 [WAF1/CIP1]	Inhibition of DNA synthesis and repair	Cell arrest at G$_1$ phase / Apoptosis	(78)
Enhanced expression of p21[WAF1/CIP1]	p53		Cell arrest at G$_1$ phase	(31)
Enhanced expression and phosphorylation of p53	Activation of DNA-dependant kinase mdm2 phosphorylation		Cell arrest at G$_2$/M phase / Apoptosis	(31,36,54)
Unscheduled activation of p34[cdc2]	p53 / Microtubules	Premature exit of the S phase p34[cdc2]/Cyclin A and p34[cdc2]/Cyclin B activation	Cell arrest at G$_2$/M phase / Apoptosis	(35,78)
Enhanced expression of: SAPK/JNK FAS			Apoptosis	(42,80)
Enhanced expression and phosphorylation of bcl-2			Inhibition or stimulation of apoptosis	(42,80) 42, 80
Enhanced expression of DR5		Caspase cascade activation	Apoptosis	(97)

Owing to some structural similarities between $2ME_2$ and colchicine, the interaction of $2ME_2$ with the colchicine binding site was also assessed *(83)*. The inhibition of colchicine binding to tubulin by $2ME_2$ was competitive, but the K_i (22 µM) was 40 to 200-times higher than that observed with other competitive inhibitors of tubulin binding. In a panel of tumor cell lines, the IC_{50}'s for cell proliferation were one to two orders of magnitude lower than those for inhibition of tubulin polymerization and interaction with the colchicine binding site *(85)*. Hence, it is still not clear how $2ME_2$'s interaction with tubulin could account for inhibition of proliferation.

p53

By altering the progression of the cell cycle, apoptosis may also be triggered through the induction of p53 *(86–88)*. $2ME_2$ has been reported to increase the expression of functional or wild-type p53 in cancer cells resulting in programmed cell death *(31)*. If p53 was mutated, which often inactivates the tumor-suppressive activity of the p53 gene, $2ME_2$ was found to be ineffective at inhibiting proliferation. Along similar lines, if wild-type cells are treated with anti-sense p53 oligonucleotides, cells become refractory to the inhibitory effects of $2ME_2$. With an anti-p53 antibody, using nuclear extracts, super-shift analysis confirmed that an increase of p53-DNA complexes were present in $2ME_2$-treated cells compared to the control untreated extracts *(31)*.

After $2ME_2$ treatment, the enhanced phosphorylation of p53 may be responsible for its augmented expression, without an increase in the levels of mRNA. Post-transcriptional changes in the levels of p53 occur with different agents in other cellular systems *(89–93)*. Increased p53 expression by $2ME_2$ has also been associated with increased expression of cyclin-dependent kinase inhibitor p21[WAF1/CIP1], which results in G_1 phase arrest *(86)*. Although both p53 and p21[WAF1/CIP1] proteins increased in human lung cancer cells, cell-cycle analysis showed no evidence of G_1 phase arrest after $2ME_2$ treatment.

Interestingly, transformation of normal fibroblast with plasmids containing the gene for SV40 T antigen results in a dramatic increase in the number of cells undergoing apoptosis after treatment with $2ME_2$ *(36)*. Flow cytometry and immunofluorescence analyses showed that transformed cells had a higher content of p53 than the nontransformed cell line, and that p53 accumulated preferentially in $2ME_2$-treated cells arrested at G_2/M. The ability of the T antigen to bind both microtubules and p53 *(94–96)* suggest an intriguing mechanism of action, however, it does not address the action of $2ME_2$ in cells devoid of the T antigen.

Although these studies suggest that p53 plays a role in the mechanism of action of $2ME_2$ in these cell lines, a recent study reports apoptosis induced by $2ME_2$ to be independent of p53 *(53)*. Recently, we also have found that $2ME_2$-induced apoptosis does not require upregulation of p53 protein in all cell types. $2ME_2$ treatment of an endothelial-cell line, HUVEC, or two tumor-cell lines, ECV and HL60 cells, results in a similar antiproliferative and cytotoxic response; however, p53 protein is upregulated only in HUVEC. Using flow cytometric analysis we demonstrate that HUVEC and ECV cells have a similar response in terms of apoptosis and G_2/M arrest to $2ME_2$ treatment. These data suggest that although p53 may play a role in the mechanism of action of $2ME_2$, in some cell lines $2ME_2$ can induce apoptosis in a p53-independent manner *(97)*.

DR5

Apoptosis is an intracellular suicide program that is executed by the activation of caspases, a family of cytoplasmic proteases that have a cysteine residue at their active site

(98). The caspase-signaling cascade is induced by cellular stress that triggers a set of intracellular proteins or by the activation of cell-surface receptors. These receptors belong to the tumor necrosis factor receptor (TNFR) superfamily and include CD95 (Fas/Apo-1), TNFR-1, DR4, DR5 *(99)*. DR5 is a p53-regulated gene that is induced in response to genotoxic stress, cytokines, and exposure to chemotherapeutics by both a p53-dependent and p53-independent mechanism *(100,101)*. We have found that treatment of HUVEC, ECV, or HL60 cells to 2ME$_2$ results in upregulation of DR5 protein and activation of caspase 8 *(97)*. 2ME$_2$-induced apoptosis requires the activation of caspases because apoptosis is almost completely blocked by the caspase inhibitor zVAD-fmk. We are currently investigating whether 2ME$_2$ upregulates DR5 in other cell types and also if 2ME$_2$ induces other death receptors.

CONCLUSION: AN IDEAL ANTI-PROLIFERATIVE AGENT

As part of a new generation of anti-cancer agents, several of the properties described in this review make 2ME$_2$ distinctively attractive as a drug candidate.

- It is a naturally occurring metabolite in humans.
- It is orally active at inhibiting tumor growth.
- Experimental animal models had shown little or no toxicity at therapeutically effective doses.
- The plasma levels attained after administration of therapeutically effective doses are in the same range or slightly higher than the physiological levels found during the third trimester of pregnancy in women. This is an important aspect, because there is no correlation between the methoxyestrogens levels found during pregnancy and pregnancy outcome.
- Despite being an estrogen derivative, it does not display estrogenic activity in vitro or in vivo at efficacious doses.
- There is no apparent interrelation between 2ME$_2$ and carcinogenesis.
- 2ME$_2$ exhibits nonspecific, anti-proliferative action on a wide variety of tumor cells.
- 2ME$_2$ has anti-angiogenic properties beyond its anti-proliferative action on endothelial cells, e.g., blocks cell migration and tube formation.
- In contrast to conventional chemotherapeutics, 2ME$_2$ targets proliferating cells with relative high specificity and is not cytotoxic for quiescent cells.
- The plasma levels attained after administration of therapeutically effective doses are in the range of concentrations that inhibit proliferation of various tumor-cell lines in vitro.
- It does not readily induce resistance and does not show cross-resistance with other chemoterapeutic agents in vitro.
- Experimental models suggest that 2ME$_2$ may be effective in the treatment of other diseases, e.g., psoriasis, arthritis, atherosclerosis.

ACKNOWLEDGMENTS

We thank Dr. Adonia Papathanassiu and Dr. Anthony Treston for their careful reading of the manuscript.

REFERENCES

1. Martucci, C. P. (1983) Metabolic fate of catechol estrogens, in *Catechol Estrogens* (Merriam, G. R. and Lipsett, M. B., eds.), Raven Press, NY, pp. 115–122.
2. Ball, P., Haupt, M., and Knuppen, R. (1983) Biogenesis and metabolism of catechol estrogens *in vitro*, in *Catechol Estrogens* (Merriam, G. R. and Lipsett, M. B., eds.), Raven Press, NY, pp. 91–104.
3. Yoshizawa, I., Nakagawa, A., Kamiya, E., Itoh, S., and Ogiso, T. (1980) Evidence of the directive effect of 17β-conjugate group on the enzymatic o-methylation of catechol estrogen. *J. Pharm. Dyn.* **3,** 317–319.

4. Sagara, Y., Okatani, Y., and Takeda, Y. (1996) Studies of catecholestrogen metabolism during normal pregnancy: changes of plasma catecholestrogen levels after DHA-S or E1-S injection. *Nippon Sanka Fujinka Gakkai Zasshi* **38**, 89–94.

5. Emons, G., Ball, P., von Postel, G., and Knuppen, R. (1979) Radioimmunoassay for 2–methoxyestrone in human plasma. *Acta Endocrinol.* **91**, 158–166.

6. Longcope, C. (1983) Summary of discussion: Assay and metabolism of catechol estrogens, in *Catechol Estrogens* (Merriam, G. R. and Lipsett, M. B., eds.), Raven Press, NY, pp. 141–150.

6a. Berg, F. D. and Kuss, E. (1992) Serum concentration and urinary excretion of "classical" estrogens, cate cholestrogens and 2-methoxyestrogens in normal pregnancy. *Arch. Gynecol. Obstet.* **251**, 17–27.

7. Berg, F. D. and Kuss, E. (1991) Urinary excretion of catecholestrogens, 2-methoxyestrogens and "classical estrogens" throughout the normal menstrual cycle. *Arch. Gynecol. Obstet.* **249**, 201–207.

8. Ball, P., Haupt, M., and Knuppen, R. (1978) Comparative studies on the metabolism of oestradiol in the brain, the pituitary and the liver of the rat. *Acta Endocrinol.* **87**, 1–11.

9. Ball, P. and Knuppen, R. (1978) Formation of 2- and 4-hydroxyestrogens by brain, pituitary, and liver of the human fetus. *J. Clin. Endocrinol. Metab.* **47**, 732–737.

10. Dehennin, L., Blacker, C., Reiffsteck, A., and Scholler, R. (1984) Estrogen 2-, 4-, 6- or 16-hydroxylation by human follicles shown by gas chromatography-mass spectrometry associated with stable isotope dilution. *J. Steroid Biochem.* **20**, 465–471.

11. Fishman, J. (1983) Aromatic hydroxylation of estrogens. *A. Rev. Physiol.* **45**, 61–72.

12. Ball, P. and Knuppen, R. (1980) Catecholoestrogens (2-and 4-hydroxyestrogens). Chemistry, biogenesis, metabolism, occurrence and physiological significance, *Acta Endocrinol.* **232(Suppl)**, 1–127.

13. Liehr, J. G., Ricci, M. J., Jefcoate, C. R., Hannigan, E. V., Hokason, J. A., and Zhu, B. T. (1995) 4–Hydroxylation of estradiol by human uterine myometrium and myoma microsomes: implications for the mechanism of uterine tumorigenesis. *Proc. Natl. Acad. Sci. USA* **92**, 9220–9224.

14. Paria, B. C., Chakraborty, C., and Dey, S. K. (1990) Catechol estrogen formation in the mouse uterus and its role in implantation. *Mol. Cell. Endocrinol.* **69**, 25–32.

15. Bui, Q. D. and Weisz, J. (1989) Monooxygenase mediating catecholestrogen formation by rat anterior pituitary is an estrogen-4-hydroxylase. *Endocrinology* **124**, 1085–1087.

16. Weisz, J., Bui, Q. D., Roy, D., and Liehr, J. G. (1992) Elevated 4-hydroxylation of estradiol by hamster kidney microsomes: a potential pathway of metabolic activation of estrogens. *Endocrinology* **131**, 655–661.

17. Zhu, B. T., Evaristus, E. N., Antoniak, S. K., Sarabia, S. F., Ricci, M. J., and Liehr J. G. (1996) Metabolic deglucuronidation and demethylation of estrogen conjugates as a source of parent estrogens and catecholestrogen metabolites in syrian hamster kidney, a target organ of estrogen-induced tumorigenesis. *Toxicol. Appl. Pharmacol.* **136**, 186–193.

18. Brueggemeier, R. W. and Singh, U. (1989) Inhibition of rat liver microsomal estrogen 2-hydroxylase by 2-methoxyestrogens. *J. Steroid Biochem.* **33**, 589–593.

19. Bates, G. W., Edman, C. D., Porter, J. C., and MacDonald, P. C. (1997) Metabolism of catechol estrogen by human erythrocytes. *J. Clin. Endrocrinol. Metab.* **45**, 1120–1123.

20. Kono, S., Brandon, D. D., Merriam, G. R., Loriaux, D. L., and Lipsett, M. B. (1980) Low plasma levels of 2-hydroxyestrone are consistent with its rapid metabolic clearance. *Steriods* **36**, 463–472.

21. Ball, P., Knuppen, R., and Breuer, H. (1971) Purification and properties of a catechol O-methyltransferase of human liver. *Eur. J. Biochem.* **21**, 517–525.

22. Ball, P., Knuppen, R., Haupt, M., and Breuer, H. (1972) Interactions between estrogens and catecholamines III. Studies on the methylation of catecholestrogens, catecholamines, and other catechols by the catechol O-methyltransferase of human liver. *J. Clin. Endocrinol. Metab.* **34**, 736–746.

23. Diczfalnsy, E. and Levitz, M. (1970) Formation, metabolism, and transport of estrogen conjugates, in *Chemical and Biological Aspects of Steriod Conjugation* (Bernstein, S. and Solomon, S., eds.), Springler-Verlag, NY, pp. 291–367.

24. Squillace, D. P., Reid, J. M., Kuffel, M. J., and Ames, M. M. (1998) Bioavailability and *in vivo* metabolism of 2-methoxyestradiol in mice. *Proc. Am. Assoc. Cancer Res.* **39, a3560**, p. 523.

25. Ball, P., Farthmann, E., and Knuppen, R. (1976) Comparative studies on the metabolism of oestradiol-17β and 2-hydroxyestradiol-17β in man in vitro and in vivo. *J. Steroid Biochem.* **7**, 139–143.

26. Ball, P., Hoppen, H.-O., and Knuppen, R. (1974) Metabolism of oestradiol-17β and 2-hydorxyestradiol-17β in rat liver slices. *Hoppe Seylers Z. Physiol. Chem.* **355**, 1451–1462.

27. Riegel, I. L. and Mueller, G. C. (1954) Formation of a protein-bound metabolite of estrodiol-16-C^{14} by rat liver homogenates. *J. Biol. Chem.* **210**, 249–257.

28. Hoppen, H.-O., Ball, P., Hoogen, H., and Knuppen, R. (1973) Metabolism of 2-hydroxyestrogen methyl ethers in the rat liver in vitro. *Hoppe Seylers Z. Physiol. Chem.* **354**, 771–780.

29. Hoffman, A. R., Paul, S. M., and Axelrod, J. (1980) The enzymatic formation of catecholestrogens from 2-methoxyestrogens by rat liver microsomes. *Endocrinology* **107**, 1192–1197.
30. Cushman, M., He, H.-M., Katzenellenbogen, J. A., Lin, C. M., and Hamel, E. (1995) Synthesis, antitubulin and antimitotic activity, and cytotoxicity of analogs of 2-methoxyestradiol, an endogenous mammalian metabolite of estradiol that inhibits tubulin polymerization by binding to the colchicine binding site. *J. Med. Chem.* **38**, 2041–2049.
31. Mukhopadhyay, T. and Roth, J. A. (1997) Induction of apoptosis in human lung cancer cells after wild–type p53 activation by methoxyestradiol. *Oncogene* **14**, 379–384.
32. Nakagawa-Yagi, Y., Ogane, N., Inoki, Y., and Kitoh, N. (1996) The endogenous estrogen metabolite 2-methoxyestradiol induces apoptotic neuronal cell death in vitro. *Life Sci.* **58**, 1461–1467.
33. Klauber, N., Parangi, S., Flynn, E., Hamel, E., and D'Amato, R. J. (1997) Inhibition of angiogenesis and breast cancer in mice by the microtubule inhibitors 2–methoxyestradiol and Taxol. *Cancer Res.* **57**, 81–86.
34. Pribluda, V. S., LaVallee, T. M., Swartz, G., Johnson, M., Fogler, W., and Green S. J. (manuscript in preparation).
35. Attalla, H., Mäkelä, T. P., Adlercreutz, H., and Andersson, L. C. (1996) 2-methoxyestradiol arrests cells in mitosis without depolymerizing tubulin. *Biochem. Biophys. Res. Comm.* **228**, 467–473.
36. Seegers, J. C., Lottering, M.-L., Grobler C. J. S., van Papendorp, D. H., Habbersett, R. C., Shou, Y., and Lehnert B. E. (1997) The mammalian metabolite, 2–methoxyestradiol, affects p53 levels and apoptosis induction in transformed cells but not in normal cells. *J. Steroid Biochem. Mol. Biol.* **62**, 253–267.
37. Fotsis, T., Zhang, Y., Pepper M. S., Adlercreutz, H., Montesano, R., Nawroth P. P., and Schweigerer, L. (1994) The endogeneous oestrogen metabolite 2-methoxyestradiol inhibits angiogenesis and suppresses tumor growth. *Nature* **368**, 237–239.
38. Josefsson, E. and Tarkowski, A. (1997) Suppression of type II collagen-induced arthritis by the endogenous estrogen metabolite 2-methoxyestradiol. *Arth. Rheum.* **40**, 154–163.
39. Aizu-Yokota, E., Susaki, A., and Sato, Y. (1995) Natural estrogens induce modulation of microtubules in chinese hamster V79 cells in culture. *Cancer Res.* **55**, 1863–1868.
40. Spicer, L. J. and Hammond, J. M. (1989) Catecholestrogens inhibit proliferation and DNA synthesis of porcine granulosa cells in vitro: comparison with estradiol, 5α-dihydrotestosterone, gonadotropins and catecholamines. *Mol. Cell. Endocrinol.* **64**, 119–126.
41. Nishigaki, I., Sasaguri, Y., and Yagi, K. (1995) Anti-proliferative effect of 2–methoxyestradiol on cultured smooth muscle cells from rabbit aorta. *Atherosclerosis* **113**, 167–170.
42. Picó, C., Puigserver, P., Oliver, P., and Palou, A. (1998) 2-Methoxyestradiol, an endogenous metabolite of 17β-estradiol, inhibits adipocyte proliferation. *Mol. Cell. Biochem.* **189**, 1–7.
43. Yue, T.-L., Wang, X., Louden, C. S., Gupta, L. S., Pillarisetti, K., Gu, J.-L., et al. (1997) 2-methoxyestradiol, an endogenous estrogen metabolite induces apoptosis in endothelial cells and inhibits angiogenesis: possible role for stress–activated protein kinase signaling pathway and fas expression. *Mol. Pharmacol.* **51**, 951–962.
44. Seegers, J. C., Aveling, M.-L., van Aswegen, C. H., Cross, M., Koch, F., and Joubert, W. S. (1989) The cytotoxic effects of estradiol-17β, catecholestradiols and methoxyestradiols on dividing MCF-7 and HeLa cells. *J. Steroid Biochem.* **32**, 797–809.
45. Lotering, M.-L., Haag, M., and Seegers, J. C. (1992) Effects of 17β-estradiol metabolites on cell cycle events in MCF-7 cells. *Cancer Res.* **52**, 5926–5932.
46. Nicosia, F. R. and Ottinetti, A. (1990) Growth of microvessels in serum-free matrix cultures of rat aorta. *Lab. Invest.* **63**, 115–121.
47. Bauer, K. S., Dixon, S. C., and Figg, W. D. (1998) Inhibition of angiogenesis by thalidomide requires metabolic activation which is species-dependent. *Biochem. Pharmacol.* **55**, 1827–1834.
48. Fajardo, I., Quesada, A. R., Nuñez de Castro, I., Sánchez-Jiménez, F., and Medina, M. A. (1999) A comparative study of the effects of genistein and 2–methoxyestradiol on the proteolytic balance and tumor cell proliferation. *Br. J. Cancer* **80**, 17–24.
49. Liekens, S., Verbeken, E., Andrei, G., Vandeputte, M., De Clercq, E., and Neyts, J. Inhibition of hemangioma development in rats by TNP-470: A novel model for the study of therapeutic strategies for the treatment of hemangiomas. Submitted.
49a. Liekens, S., Verbeken, E., Vandebutte, M., DeClerq, E., and Neyts, J. (1999) A novel animal model for hemangiomas: inhibition of hemangioma development by the angiogenesis inhibitor TNP-470. *Cancer Res.* **59**, 2376–2383.
50. Wassberg, E., Sundelöf, J., Pribluda, V. S., Green, S. J., Hedborg, F., and Christofferson, R. The antiangiogenic and chemotherapeutic natural steroid 2–methoxyestradiol and its derivative 2-propynylestradiol are potent suppressors of neuroblastoma growth when administered orally. Submitted.

51. Wassberg, E., Påhlman, S., Westlin, J.-E., and Christofferson, R. (1997) *Pediatr. Res.* **41,** 327–333.
52. Arbiser, J. L., Panigrathy, D., Klauber, N., Rupnick, M., Flynn, E., Udagawa, T., and D'Amato R. (1999) The antiangiogenic agents TNP-470 and 2-methoxyestradiol inhibit the growth of angiosarcoma in mice. *J. Am. Acad. Dermatol.* **40,** 925–929.
53. Schumacher, G., Kataoka, M., Roth, J. A., and Mukhopadhyay, T. (1999) Potent antitumor activity of 2-methoxyestradiol in human pancreatic cancer cell lines. *Clin. Cancer Res.* **5,** 493–499.
54. Kataoka, M., Schumacher, G., Cristiano, R. J., Atkinson, E. N., Roth, J. A., and Mukhopadhyay, T. (1998) An agent that increases tumor suppressor transgene product coupled with systemic transgene delivery inhibits growth of metastatic lung cancer *in vivo. Cancer Res.* **58,** 4761–4765.
55. Shapiro, A. B. and Ling, V. (1995) Using purified P-glycoprotein to understand multidrug resistance. *J. Bioenerg. Biomembr.* **27,** 7–13.
56. Boehm, T., Folkman, J., Browder, T., and O'Reilly, M. S. (1997) Antiangiogenic therapy of experimental cancer does not induce acquired drug resistance. *Nature* **390,** 404–407.
57. Kerbel, R. S. (1997) A cancer therapy resistant to resistance. *Nature* **290,** 335–336.
58. Loukovaara, M., Carson, M., and Adlercreutz, H. (1995) Regulation of sex-hormone-binding globulin production by endogenous estrogens in vitro. *Biochem. Biophys. Res. Comm.* **206,** 895–901.
59. Dunn, J. F., Merraim, G. R., Eil, C., Kono, S., Loriaux, D. L., and Nisula, B. C. (1980) Testosterone-estradiol binding globulin binds to 2-methoxyestradiol with greater affinity than to testosterone. *J. Clin. Endocrino. Metab.* **51,** 404–406.
60. Nakhla, A. M., Khan, M. S., and Rosner, W. (1990) Biologically active steroids activate receptor-bound human sex hormone-binding globulin to cause LNCaP cells to accumulate adenosine 3', 5'-monophosphate. *J. Clin. Endocrinol. Metab.* **71,** 398–404.
61. Hryb, D. J., Khan M. S., Romas, N. A., and Rosner, W. (1990) The control of the interaction of sex hormone-binding globulin with its receptor by steroid hormones. *J. Biol. Chem.* **265,** 6048–6054.
62. Rosner, W., Hryb, D. J., Khan, M. S., Nakhla, A. M., and Romas, N. A. (1992) Sex hormone-binding globulin. Binding to cell membranes and generation of a second messenger. *J. Androl.* **13,** 101–106.
63. Ding, V. D., Moller, D. E., Feeney, W. P., Didolkar, V., Nakhla, A. M., Rhodes, L., et al. (1998) Sex hormone-binding globulin mediates prostate androgen receptor action via a novel signaling pathway. *Endocrinology* **139,** 213–218.
64. Lavigne, J. A., Helzlsouer, K. J., Huang, H.-Y, Strickland, P. T., Bell, D. A., Selmin, O., et al. (1997) An association between the allele coding for a low activity variant of catechol-O-methyltransferase and the risk for breast cancer. *Cancer Res.* **57,** 5493–5497.
65. Pribluda, V. S. and Green, S. J. (1998) A good estrogen. *Science* **280,** 987–988.
66. Rajan, R., Reddy, V. V. R., Reichle, F., David, J. S. K., and Daly, M. J. (1984) Effects of catechol estogen methyl ethers on lipid metabolism in prepubertal rats. *Steriods* **43,** 499–507.
67. Yager, J. D. and Liehr, J. G. (1996) Molecular mechanisms of estrogen carcinogenesis. *Annu. Rev. Pharmacol. Toxicol.* **36,** 203–232.
68. Liehr, J. G., Fang, W. F., Sirbasku, D. A., and Ari-Ulubelen (1986) Carcinogenesis of catechol estrogens in Syrian hamsters. *J. Steroid Biochem.* **24,** 353–356.
69. Purdy, R. H., Goldzieher, J. W., Le Quesne, P. W., Abdel-Baky, S., Durocher, C. K., Moore, P. H., Jr., and Rhim, J. S. (1983) Active intermediates and carcinogenesis, in *Catechol Estrogens* (Merriam, G. R. and Lipsett, M. B., eds.), Raven Press, NY, pp. 123–140.
70. Kono, S., Merriam, G. R., Brandon, D. D., Loraiux, D. L., and Lipsett, M. B. (1982) Radioimmunoassay and metabolism of the catechol estrogen 2-hydroxyestradiol. *J. Clin. Endocrinol. Metab.* **54,** 150–154.
71. Longcope, C., Femino, A., Flood, C., and Williams, K. I. H. (1982) Metabolic clearance rate and conversion ratios of [^{3}H]2-hydroxyestrone in normal men. *J. Clin. Endocrinol. Metab.* **54,** 374–380.
72. Martucci, C. P. and Fishman, J. (1979) Impact of continuously administrated catechol estrogens on uterine growth and luteinizing hormone secretion. *Endocronology* **105,** 1288–1292.
73. Morales, D. E., McGowan, K. A., Grant, D. S., Maheshwari, S., Bhartiya, D., Cid, M. C., et al. (1995) Estrogen promotes angiogenic activity in human umbilical vein endothelial cells in vitro and in a murine model. *Circulation* **91,** 755–763.
74. Spyridopoulos, I., Sullivan, A. B., Kearney, M., Isner, J. M., and Losordo, D. W. (1997) Estrogen-receptor-mediated inhibition of human endothelial cell apoptosis: estradiol as a survival factor. *Circulation* **95,** 1505–1514.
75. Mosselman, S., Polman, J., and Dijkema, R. (1996) ER beta: identification and characterization of a novel human estrogen receptor. *FEBS Lett* **392,** 49–53.
76. Kuiper, G. G. and Gustafsson, J. A. (1997) The novel estrogen receptor-beta subtype: potential role in the cell-and promoter-specific actions of estrogens and anti-estrogen. *FEBS Lett* **410,** 87–90.

77. MacLusky, N. J., Barnea, E. R., Clark, C. R., and Naftolin, F. (1983) Catechol estrogens and estrogen receptors, in *Catechol Estrogens* (Merriam, G. R. and Lipsett, M. B., eds.), Raven Press, NY, pp. 151–166.

78. Lottering, M.-L., de Kock, M., Viljoen, T. C., Grobler, C. J. S., and Seegers, J. C. (1996) 17β-estradiol metabolites affect some regulators of the MCF-7 cell cycle. *Cancer Lett.* **110**, 181–186.

79. Zoubine, M. N., Weston, A. P., Johnson, D. C., Campbell, D. R., and Banerjee, S. K. (1999) 2-Methoxyestradiol-induced growth suppression and lethality in estrogen- responsive MCF-7 cells may be mediated by down regulation of p34cdc2 and cyclin B1 expression. *Int. J. Oncol.* **15**, 639–646.

80. Attalla, H., Westberg, J. A., Andersson, L. C., Aldercreutz, H., and Makela, T. P. (1998) 2-Methoxyestradiol-induced phosphorylation of bcl–2: uncoupling from JNK/SAPK activation. *Biochem. Biophys. Res. Commun.* **247**, 616–619.

81. Purohit, A., Singh, A., Ghilchik, M. W., and Reed, M. J. (1999) Inhibition of Tumor Necrosis Factor α-stimulated aromatase activity by microtubule-stabilizing agents, paclitaxel and 2-methoxyestradiol. *Biochem. Biophys. Res. Comm.* **261**, 214–217.

82. Tishler, R. B., Lamppu, D. M., Park, S., and Price, B. D. (1995) Microtubule-active drugs taxol, vinblastine, and nocodazole increase the levels of transcriptionally active p53. *Cancer Res.* **55**, 6021–6025.

83. D'Amato, R. J., Lin, C. M., Flynn, E., Folkman, J., and Hamel, E. (1994) 2-Methoxyestradiol, and endogenous mammalian metabolite, inhibits tubulin polymerization by interacting at the colchicine site. *Proc. Natl. Acad. Sci. USA* **91**, 3964–3968.

84. Hamel, E., Lin, C. M., Flynn, E., and D'Amato, R. J. (1996) Interactions of 2-methoxyestradiol, and endogenous mammalian metabolite, with unploymerized tubulin and with tubulin polymers. *Biochemistry* **35**, 1304–1310.

85. Cushman, M., He, H.-M., Katzenellenbogen, J. A., Varma, R. K., Hamel, E., Lin, C. M., Ram, S., and Sachdeva, Y. P. (1997) Synthesis of analogs of 2-methoxyestradiol with enhanced inhibitory effects on tubulin polymerization and cancer cell growth. *J. Med. Chem.* **40**, 2323–2334.

86. Agarwal, M. L., Taylor, W. R., Chernov, M. V., Chernova, O. B., and Stark, G. R. (1998) The p53 network. *J. Biol. Chem.* **273**, 1–4.

87. Paulovich, A. G., Toczyski, D. P., and Hartwell, L. H. (1997) When checkpoints fail. *Cell* **88**, 315–321.

88. Nurse, P. (1997) Checkpoint pathways come of age. *Cell* **91**, 865–867.

89. Kubbutat, M. H., Jones, S. N., and Vousden, K. H. (1997) Regulation of p53 stability by mdm2. *Nature* **387**, 299–303.

90. Mayo, L. D., Turchi, J. J., and Berberich, S. J. (1997) Mdm-2 phosphorylation by DNA-dependent protein kinase prevents interaction with p53. *Cancer Res.* **57**, 5013–5016.

91. Shieh, S. Y., Ikeda, M., Taya, Y., and Prives, C. (1997) DNA damage-induced phosphorylation of p53 alleviates inhibition by MDM2. *Cell* **91**, 325–334.

92. Frattini, M. G., Hurst, S. D., Lim, H. B., Swaminathan, S., and Laimins, L. A. (1997) Abrogation of a mitotic checkpoint by E2 proteins from oncogenic human papillomaviruses correlates with increased turnover of the p53 tumor suppressor protein. *EMBO J.* **16**, 318–331.

93. Blagosklonny, M. V. (1997) Loss of function and p53 protein stabilization. *Oncogene* **15**, 1889–1893.

94. Maxwell, S. A., Ames, S. K., Sawai, E. T., Decker, G. L., Cook, R. G., and Butel, J. S. (1991) Simian virus 40 large T antigen and p53 are microtubules-associated proteins in transformed cells. *Cell Growth. Diff.* **2**, 115–127.

95. Kernohan, N. M., Hupp, T. R., and Lane D. P. (1996) Modification of an N-terminal regulatory domain of T antigen restores p53-T antigen complex formation in the absence of an essential metal ion cofactor. *J. Biol. Chem.* **271**, 4954–4960.

96. Carbone, M., Rizzo, P., Grimley, P. M., Procopio, A., Mew, D. J., Shridhar, V., et al. (1997) Simian virus-40 large-T antigen binds p53 in human mesotheliomas. *Nature Med.* **3**, 908–912.

97. LaVallee, T. M., Hembrough, W. A., Williams, M. S., Zhan, X. H., Pribluda, V. S., Papathanassiu, A., and Green, S. J. 2–Methoxyestradiol upregulates DR5 and induces apoptosis independently of p53. Submitted.

98. Earnshaw, W. C., Martins, L. M., and Kaufmann, S. H. (1999) Mammalian caspases: structure, activation, substrates, and functions during apoptosis. *Annu. Rev. Biochem.* **68**, 383–424.

99. Smith, C. A., Farrah, T., and Goodwin, R. G. (1994) The TNF receptor superfamily of cellular and viral proteins: activation, costimulation, and death. *Cell* **76**, 959–962.

100. Wu, G. S., Burns, T. F., McDonald, E. R., Jiang, W., Meng, R., Krantz, I. D., et al. (1997) KILLER/ DR5 is a DNA damage-inducible p53-regualted death receptor gene. *Nature Genet.* **17**, 141–143.

101. Sheikh, M. S., Burns, T. F., Huang, Y., Wu, G. S., Amundson, S., Brooks, K. S., et al. (1998) P53-dependent and –independent regulation of death receptor KILLER/DR5 gene expression in response to genotoxic stress and tumor necrosis factor α. *Cancer Res.* **58**, 1593–1598.

102. Spicer, L. J., Walega, M. A., and Hammond, J. M. (1987) Metabolism of [^{3}H]2-hydroxy-estradiol by cultured porcine granulosa cells: evidence for the presence of a catechol-O-methyl-transferase pathway and direct stimulatory effect of 2-methoxyestradiol on progesterone production. *Biol. Reprod.* **36,** 562–571.

103. Spicer, L. J. and Hammond, J. M. (1988) Comparative effects of androgens and catecholestrogens on progesterone production by porcine granulosa cells. *Mol. Cell. Endocrinol.* **56,** 211–217.

104. Zhang, Z. and Davis, D. L. (1992) Cell-type specific responses in prostaglandin secretion by glandular and stromal cells from pig endomerium treated with catecholestrogens, methoxyestrogens and progesterone. *Prostaglandins* **44,** 53–64.

105. Barone, S., Panek, D., Bennett, L., Stitzel, R. E., and Head, R. J. (1987) The influence of oestrogen and oestrogen metabolites on the sensitivity of the isolated rabbit aorta to catecholamines. *Naunyn-Schmiedeberg's Arch. Pharmacol.* **335,** 513–520.

106. Liu, D. and Bachmann, K. A. (1998) An investigation on the relationship between estrogen, estrogen metabolites and blood cholesterol levels in ovariectomized rats. *J. Pharmacol. Exp. Ther.* **286,** 561–568.

V   NOVEL TARGETS

22 Receptor Tyrosine Kinases in Angiogenesis

Laura K. Shawver, Kenneth E. Lipson, T. Annie T. Fong, Gerald McMahon, and Laurie M. Strawn

HISTORY AND REVIEW OF RECEPTOR TYROSINE KINASES

Cell to cell communication is imperative for physiological and pathological processes associated with multicellular organisms. This is demonstrated in the process of angiogenesis where the blood vessel endothelial cells require signals generated from cells in the hypoxic tissue in order to initiate the process of forming new capillaries. The transduction of signals from the extracellular milieu of the endothelial cell to the nucleus are receptor-mediated events. It is clear, from the body of research, that some of the receptors that mediate critical events in angiogenesis are receptor tyrosine kinases. Receptor tyrosine kinases (RTKs), also known as growth factor receptors, are a family of transmembrane proteins with a large extracellular ligand-binding domain, a transmembrane domain, and an intracellular domain with intrinsic tyrosine kinase activity (for review, *see* ref. *1*).

Tyrosine kinase research can be traced to the studies emanating from transforming viruses. In 1911, Peyton Rous discovered that sarcomas in chickens could be passed by filterable agents *(2)*. It was not until years later that viruses, later shown to be retroviruses, were discovered to cause mammary carcinomas and leukemias in mice*(3,4)*. In 1966, it was learned that *src* was the transforming gene of Rous sarcoma virus *(5)*. The gene product of *src* was characterized as a 60 kDa protein in 1978 *(6)* and shown to have kinase activity *(7,8)*. However, it was not until 1979–1980 that it was discovered that kinase activity associated with oncogenes such as *src* resulted in the transfer of phosphates to tyrosine

From: *The New Angiotherapy*
Edited by: T.-P. D. Fan and E. C. Kohn © Humana Press Inc., Totowa, NJ

residues in substrate proteins (*9*; for review, *see* ref. *10*). Also in 1980, the EGF receptor was shown to have tyrosine kinase activity *(11)*. Although it has been almost 30 yr since the discovery of protein tyrosine kinases and their roles in physiological and pathological processes, the vast research in the field has only recently led to a greater understanding of the molecular mechanisms underlying the signaling cascades in human diseases.

Historically, evidence that growth factors might be involved in malignant transformation emanated from the observation that chick embryo fibroblasts grew well in medium supplemented with serum. Plasma, however, was unable to support the growth of the chicken cells suggesting that a serum factor was required for cell growth. Rous sarcoma virus-infected fibroblasts, on the other hand, grew well in either plasma- or serum-supplemented media *(12,13)* indicating that the virus-infected cells could bypass the normal requirement for serum. The factor in serum required for growth of the chicken embryo fibroblasts was later shown to be released by platelets and subsequently became known as the platelet-derived growth factor (PDGF) *(14,15)*. At this time, it also became evident that cells stimulated by growth factors or transformed by viruses were very similar, exhibiting increases in amino acid, glucose, and ion transport as well as increases in DNA synthesis, loss of contact inhibition and continued cell division when compared to normal, unstimulated cells. In 1983, Waterfield et al. and Doolittle et al. *(16,17)* showed that the B chain of PDGF was >90% homologous to the v-*sis* oncogene product p28v^{sis}. This discovery marked the first observation that an oncogene product was related to a known growth factor. When it was discovered in 1984 that v-*erbB* was derived from the EGF receptor *(18)*, the theory of cancer cells being normal cells with aberrant signal transduction was confirmed. Since that time, numerous oncogenes have been shown to encode altered proteins that represent members of growth factor signaling cascades (for review *see* ref. *10*).

It is now understood that any one of many alterations in the growth factor signaling cascade can result in growth factor-independent proliferation. Although intracellular signaling pathways leading from RTKs to the nucleus are still being elucidated, they are likely to vary between RTKs as well as between target cells. Intracellular signaling has become quite complex as the individual components are unfolding. (For review, *see 10*.) A summary of the major second messenger signaling pathways utilized by RTKs is shown in Fig. 1.

Growth factor binding to its cognate RTK results in receptor dimerization with conformational changes that result in an intermolecular phosphorylation at tyrosine residues at multiple sites (for review, *see* ref. *19*). The exceptions to this are the insulin and insulin-like growth factor (IGF-1) receptor families, which exist as pre-formed dimers of α and β chains. However the induction of phosphorylation following receptor activation by ligand binding is similar. The phosphotyrosines on the receptor serve as attachment sites for substrates or adapter molecules. An example of a substrate is phosphotidylinositol 3-kinase (PI 3-kinase). The regulatory subunit of PI 3-kinase contains two SH2 (Src homology region 2) domains that are known to bind phosphotyrosine residues embedded in a unique consensus sequence that is present in the primary amino acid sequence of particular RTKs. The association of PI 3-kinase to the intracellular domain of the tyrosine phosphorylated RTK greatly enhances the activity of the enzyme through allosteric activation of the catalytic subunit. Activated PI 3-kinase catalyzes the transfer of phosphate from ATP to various positions of inositol resulting in phosphatidylinositol (PI), PI-4 monophosphate and PI-4, 5 bisphosphate. The PI 3-kinase pathway has been

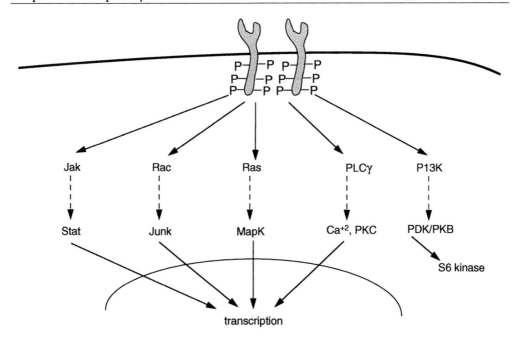

Fig. 1. Signaling pathways for receptor tyrosine kinases. Major pathways activated by RTKs include Jak, Rac, Ras, PLCγ, and PI3-kinase. These pathways are activated via binding of adaptor moleculesand/or substrates to phosphorylated receptors. The major pathways utilized by RTKs vary between RTKs, the cell types, and the type of second messenger expressed in a given cell. Activation of these signaling pathways leads to changes in gene transcription that affect growth, survival, motility, and metabolism.

shown to be important in diverse cellular responses by its action on multiple downstream effectors that include SH2 and pleckstrin homology domains of serine/threonine, tyrosine kinases, and various cytoskeletal proteins (for review, *see* ref. *20*). PI3 kinase-mediated cellular responses include cellular proliferation, GLUT 4 translocation, histamine release, calcium signaling, and respiratory bursts by neutrophils (for review, *see* ref. *21*).

Unlike PI3-kinase, adapter molecules contain no intrinsic catalytic activity. An example of an adapter molecule important in RTK signaling is Grb2. Grb2 functions by directly coupling activated RTKs to the Ras-activating nucleotide exchange factor SOS *(22,23)*. mediated through SH3 interactions with proline-rich consensus sequences. Grb2/SOS can bind to phosphorylated RTKs either directly or indirectly through SH2 interactions with RTKs or other adapter proteins such as Shc and Syp *(24,25)*. Activation of Ras or Ras-family members (e.g., Rho, Racl, etc.) through binding of Grb2/SOS to phosphotyrosine sites on RTKs leads to in activation of the raf/MAPKK/MAPK pathway. This has been implicated as a necessary component of intracellular signaling to elicit a range of cellular responses including mitogenesis, differentiation, and cell survival (for review, *see* ref. *10*). Thus, the cascade triggered by RTK activation leads to a variety of cellular events and in the case of angiogenesis might contribute to cell leakage, cellular motility, and cellular proliferation.

Although the role of aberrant RTK signaling was established with oncogenes and cancer, they have now been shown to be associated with many pathological conditions including psoriasis, cardiovascular disease, immunological dysfunctions, and metabolic disorders. In this context, a plethora of studies have emerged that implicate growth factors and RTK signaling in angiogenesis. This chapter will focus on a review of the RTKs implicated in angiogenesis and relevant data implicating each RTK type in therapeutic areas where angiogenesis is a critical component of the disease pathology. In this chapter, reference will be made to the RTK genes as well as their protein products. The gene, or in some cases mRNA will be denoted in italics where as standard format will be used when discussing the protein.

Receptor Tyrosine Kinases in Angiogenesis

A number of receptor tyrosine kinases are thought to be involved in angiogenesis, either directly or indirectly (Fig. 2). Of particular interest are Flt-1 and Flk-1, the receptors for VEGF, as well as Tie-1 and Tie-2/Tek. Flt-1 and Flk-1 are also known as VEGFR1 and VEGFR2, respectively, and the human homolog of Flk-1 is KDR. These receptors, as well as Tie-1 and Tie-2, are expressed primarily on endothelial cells and play a direct role in angiogenesis. Other RTKs of potential interest in angiogenesis include the epidermal growth factor (EGF) receptor, the platelet-derived growth factor (PDGF) receptor, the fibroblast growth factor (FGF) receptor family, insulin-like growth factor (IGF-1) receptor, Met and Eck. Although they have also been implicated in angiogenesis, they have broader expression patterns that encompass other cell types including endothelial cells and a broader range of physiological functions.

VEGF Receptor Family

Vascular endothelial growth factor (VEGF) is so named because it stimulates growth of endothelial cells during the process of angiogenesis *(26)*, but it was also independently isolated as vascular permeability factor (VPF) *(27)*. In its role as a permeability factor, it contributes to the hyperpermeability of tumor vasculature that may allow for deposition of proteins that form a substrate for growth of tumor and endothelial cells.

VEGF can be found as four different splice variants known as $VEGF_{121}$, $VEGF_{165}$, $VEGF_{189}$, and $VEGF_{206}$, where the number refers to the number of amino acids in the polypeptide. All four isoforms exist as disulfide-linked homodimers with some structural similarities to the PDGFs. There are differences in the secretion patterns of the isoforms from various cell types with $VEGF_{165}$ being the most common isoform observed. A fifth variant, $VEGF_{145}$, was recently found in three human carcinoma cell lines that originated from the female reproductive tract *(28)*. The five isoforms bind with high affinity to two receptors, Flt-1 and Flk-1/KDR (Fig. 3), but they differ in their binding affinity for heparin and extracellular matrix. The biological significance of multiple VEGF forms is not understood.

VEGF is induced by growth factors such as EGF and PDGF, as well as hypoxia. Many cell lines have been shown to have increased VEGF mRNA and protein levels when kept under hypoxic conditions for 24 h *(29)*. The 5'-promoter region of VEGF contains a site for hypoxia-inducible factor-1 (HIF-1) and mutation of this site eliminates VEGF induction in response to hypoxia. Furthermore, VEGF mRNA is stabilized under hypoxic conditions by the formation of an mRNA-protein complex in the 3'-untranslated region. It is also stabilized by inactivation of the von Hippel-Lindau tumor-suppressor gene in many tumor types. The induction of VEGF can lead to increased angiogenesis, and thus increased oxygen and nutrient supplies to hypoxic organs and tumors.

Placenta growth factor (PlGF) is similar to VEGF, but binds only to Flt-1 *(30)*. Three splice variants have been isolated *(30,31)*. Their biological roles are unknown, but they do not appear to be involved in angiogenesis because P1GFs are not expressed at concen-

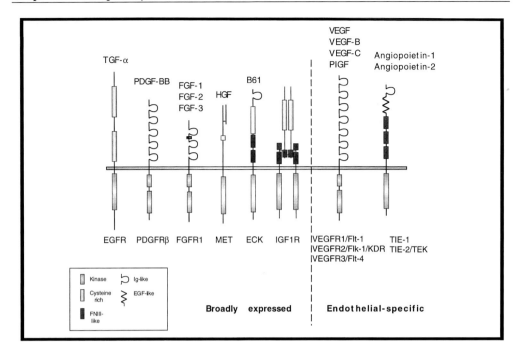

Fig. 2. Receptor tyrosine kinases (RTKs) in angiogenesis. Multiple sequence alignments of tyrosine kinase catalytic domains allow RTKs to be classified into distinct families. RTKs implicated in angiogenesis are shown. The horizontal line represents the plasma membrane with the extracellular domain above and the cytoplasmic domain below. FNIII, fibronectin type III repeat. Ig, Immunoglobulin.

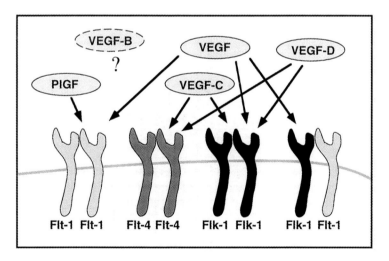

Fig. 3. The VEGF receptor family. This family consists of Flk-1, Flt-1, and Flt-4. In addition to existing as homodimers upon ligand binding, VEGF is thought to induce heterodimerization between Flk-1 and Flt-1.

trations required for Flt-1 activation. Recently, three new members of the VEGF family have been identified: VEGF-B, VEGF-C, and VEGF-D (Fig. 3). Two splice variants of VEGF-B have also been found *(32,33)*. It stimulates the growth of endothelial cells, but it is not yet clear what receptor or receptors it binds *(33)*. VEGF-C, also known as vascular endothelial growth factor-related protein, was identified as a ligand for Flt-4, which is primarily expressed on lymphatic endothelial cells *(34,35)*. The distribution of VEGF-C in mouse embryos suggest that it is involved in angiogenesis of lymphatic vasculature *(36)*. VEGF-C also binds to Flk-1/KDR; possibly its in vitro mitogenic *(35)* and migratory *(34)* effects on vascular endothelial cells are mediated through this receptor. VEGF-D is most closely related to VEGF-C structurally *(37,38)* and in the fact that it binds to and activates Flk-1/KDR and Flt-4 *(38)*. It is mitogenic for bovine aortic endothelial cells, but is significantly less potent that VEGF. There is some evidence that co-expression of two VEGF family members in the same cell type leads to the formation of heterodimers. The functions of such proteins remains to be elucidated.

The VEGF receptor family of tyrosine kinases (Figs. 2 and 3) is characterized by seven immunoglobin-like sequences in the extracellular domain and a split tyrosine kinase domain. The first member to be identified was Flt-1 (fms-like tyrosine kinase), which is also known as VEGFR1 *(39,40)*. The mouse receptor tyrosine kinase, Flk-1 (fetal liver kinase) *(41,42)*, and its human homolog, KDR (kinase insert domain -containing receptor) *(43)*, were shown to be a related but distinct VEGF receptor. Flt-4 is another member of the family that is expressed on lymphatic endothelium but not vascular endothelium *(44)*.

The receptor tyrosine kinases, Flk-1 and Flt-1, and their ligand, VEGF, are expressed in angiogenic tissues at a time when angiogenesis is known to occur. During development, transcripts for *flk-1* and *flt-1* were detected by *in situ* hybridization in mouse embryos, initially in the endothelial cell precursors and later in the endothelial cells of vessels throughout the embryos *(42,45,46)*. The distribution of *flt-1* and *flk-1* transcripts in human fetal tissues is comparable to that of the mouse and rat embryos as determined by Northern blotting *(47)*. Furthermore, protein expression of VEGF receptors was confirmed along the lumina of vessels in rat embryos by binding of [^{125}I]VEGF *(48)*. VEGF mRNA has been identified during the same stages of development as the receptors in mouse *(49)* and rat embryos *(48)*. The temporal and spatial patterns of expression of VEGF and its receptors support that they are involved in angiogenesis during development.

A number of techniques have been utilized to investigate the roles of Flk-1, Flt-1, and VEGF in angiogenesis. Measurement of mitogenesis in VEGF-stimulated endothelial cells is commonly used as an in vitro model. In such a system, addition of an anti-Flk-1 neutralizing antibody inhibited mitogenesis *(50)*, as did addition of a truncated soluble form of Flt-1, which competed for binding of VEGF to its receptors *(51)*. Similarly, ribozymes that cleave *flk-1* or *flt-1* mRNAs reduced the growth of human microvascular endothelial cells, presumably by decreasing the amount of receptors on the cells *(52)*. Despite these results with Flt-1, the role of Flt-1 in endothelial-cell growth is not clear. Engineered mutant forms of VEGF were found to bind differentially to Flk-1 and Flt-1 *(53)*. Mutant VEGFs that had reduced binding to Flt-1 but normal binding to Flk-1-stimulated endothelial cells similar to wild-type VEGF. These studies suggested that Flk-1 and not Flt-1 may be involved in the growth of endothelial cells.

In vivo models have also indicated that VEGF and its receptors are involved in angiogenesis. The genes for all three proteins have been disrupted through targeted mutagenesis in mice. Embryos that were homozygous for mutant forms of *flk-1*, *flt-1*, or *VEGF* forms were resorbed by days 10–12 of development. In the case of the *flk-1* disruption, only markers of immature endothelial cells were found and no vessels formed in the embryo or yolk sac *(54)*. This indicated that Flk-1 was required for development of mature endothelial cells. In contrast, embryos lacking Flt-1 had mature endothelial cells but the vessels were large and disorganized *(55)*. This suggested that Flt-1 was probably involved in the adhesion process between endothelial cells or between endothelial cells and matrix that is required for normal vessel assembly. In two studies following disruption of the VEGF gene, heterozygous as well as homozygous embryos were resorbed *(56,57)*, strongly suggesting that the amount of VEGF expressed during embryonic development is critical. Also, mature endothelial cells were detected, but the vessels in the embryos and yolks were abnormal, as in the case of the *flt-1*-deficient embryos. It has been suggested that the newly identified ligand for Flt-4, VEGF-C *(34)* or VRP *(35)*, may substitute for VEGF, allowing maturation of endothelial cells in the embryos with the disrupted VEGF genes. Currently, there is no evidence for a direct role of Flt-4 in angiogenesis.

A specific receptor for VEGF$_{165}$, neuropilin-1, was recently identified *(58)*. Neuropilin-1 had previously been described for its role in neuronal-cell guidance in developing embryos, but has now been shown to bind VEGF$_{165}$ as well as collapsin/semaphorin. The VEGF isoform specificity occurs because the binding sequence for neuropilin-1 is coded within exon 7 of VEGF, which is lacking in VEGF$_{121}$. Unlike Flk-1/KDR, neuropilin-1 is expressed in many cell types in adult tissue, including heart, placenta, lung, liver, skeletal muscle, kidney, and pancreas. It has also been found in endothelial cells and a number of tumor-derived cell lines. Neuropilin-1 does not have enzymatic activity but, when co-expressed with Flk-1/KDR, it enhanced binding of VEGF$_{165}$ to cells fourfold. It also increased chemotaxis in response to VEGF$_{165}$ when coexpressed with Flk-1/KDR, but did not mediate chemotaxis when expressed alone. Neuropilin-1 most likely contributes to angiogenesis by enhancing the effects of VEGF$_{165}$ on cells. Placenta growth factor-2 (PlGF-2) is also a ligand for neuropilin-1, although PlGF-2 does not stimulate mitogenesis of HUVECs and neuropilin-1 does not appear to mediate migration induced by PlGF-2 *(59)*. The role of neuropilin-1 in angiogenesis is supported by the results of studies with transgenic mice *(60)*. Overexpression of neuropilin-1 in embryos caused increased formation of capillaries and blood vessels, dilation of vessels, and hemorrhage, as well as nervous system abnormalities.

Angiopoietin Receptor Family

Angiopoietin-1 has been described as a ligand for Tie-2/Tek, a receptor tyrosine kinase expressed primarily on endothelial cells *(61)*. It has a structure unlike other known angiogenic factor, consisting of a coiled-coil domain, which may be involved in formation of multimers, and a fibrinogen-like domain. In embryos, angiopoietin-1 is expressed near the developing vasculature in proximity to its receptor. Addition of angiopoietin-1 to endothelial cells does not have a mitogenic effect, despite the finding that it binds and stimulates autophosphorylation of Tie-2/Tek. Disruption of the angiopoietin-1 gene in mice suggests that it is involved in the interaction of endothelium with the surrounding matrix and cells, which are necessary for structural integrity of newly formed vessels *(62)*. Transgenic mice in which the angiopoietin gene was expressed in skin under the control of the keratin 14 promoter had a red appearance owing to increased vascularization *(63)*. The vessels were larger and had a greater degree of branching than those of wild-type mice. Angiopoietin-1 appears to play a role in vasculature remodeling and maturation in the later stages of development. Recently, angiopoietin-2 was identified as another ligand for Tie-2/Tek and is related to angiopoietin-1 *(64)*. However, angiopoietin-2 was found to inhibit the function of angiopoietin-1 and Tie-2/Tek. Angiopoietin-2 was found to be expressed in adult mice and humans at sites of vascular remodeling. Overexpression of angiopoietin-2 in transgenic mice was found to disrupt blood vessel formation in the developing embryo.

The Tie family of receptors has a unique structure: the extracellular domain consists of three epidermal growth factor homology motifs, two immunoglobulin-like sequences, and three fibronectin type III repeats. The known family members (Fig. 4) are Tie-1 (originally known as Tie: tyrosine kinase with immunoglobin and EGF homology domains [65]) and Tie-2/TEK (tunica interna endothelial cell kinase) (66–68).

Tie-1 and Tie-2 are receptor kinases whose expression is most prevalent in the vascular endothelium during embryonic development (66,69,70). In adults, the Tie receptors are weakly expressed, but are induced during active angiogenesis. For example, Tie-1 expression is upregulated in skin capillaries during wound healing (71) and in angiogenesis associated with metastatic melanomas (72). Transgenic mouse embryos expressing a dominant-negative form of the Tie-2 receptor were developmentally delayed, had compromised heart development, and exhibited signs of hemorrhage (73). Embryos lacking Tie-2 died earlier in gestation and had retarded growth of the head and heart (73,74). The vasculature of *Tie-2* null mice was found to be abnormal, suggesting that Tie-2 is important for vasculogenesis. Mouse embryos lacking Tie-1 (74,75) exhibited somewhat different embryonic phenotypes: embryos died in mid- to late-gestation or shortly after birth owing to breathing problems. In addition, embryos or mice lacking Tie-1 exhibited peripheral and abdominal hemorrhage or edema. Because the vasculature appeared to be properly developed, these observations suggest that Tie-1 may be important for maintaining vascular integrity. Thus, the expression patterns of Tie receptors in developing embryos and adults, the effect of expressed dominant-negative receptors in transgenic mice, and the embryonic phenotypes following deletion of Tie receptor or angiopoietin genes strongly implicate the Tie receptors as important mediators of angiogenesis and vasculogenesis.

EGF Receptors

Ligands for the EGF receptor encompass a number of structurally homologous mitogens (76,77), which include EGF, transforming growth factor-α (TGF-α), amphiregulin (AR), heparin-binding EGF-like growth factor (HB-EGF), betacellulin (78), and epiregulin (79) (Fig. 5). EGF is a 6 kDa protein that was first purified in 1962 as a substance that produced tooth eruption in newborn mice (80). AR is a larger (18–35 kDa), glycosylated, heparin-binding protein. TGF-α exists in several forms, including a secreted 6 kDa protein. AR, HB-EGF, TGF-α, and EGF all have a conserved cysteine-rich consensus that, in the case of EGF, results in formation of three disulfide bonds.

The EGF receptor was cloned in 1984 by Ullrich and coworkers (81). The receptor contains two cysteine-rich regions in the extracellular domain and a single intracellular kinase domain. There are three other members of the EGF receptor family (Fig. 5), known as Her-2, Her-3 and Her-4 (homologous to the EGF receptor) also known as erbB2, erbB3, and erbB4. Coexpression of these family members resulted in heterodimer formation following ligand addition. Ligands that have been identified for Her-2, Her-3, and HER-4 include NRG-1 (neuregulin, also known as heregulin [HRG], glial growth factor [GGF], acetylcholine-receptor inducing factor [ARIA], new differentiation factor [NDF]) and NRG-2 (82). The EGF receptor family of ligands result in complex patterns of receptor activation; some of the peptides activate signaling by more than one EGF receptor family member. Her-2, Her-3, Her-4, and the ligands NRG-1 and NRG-2 have not been implicated in angiogenesis.

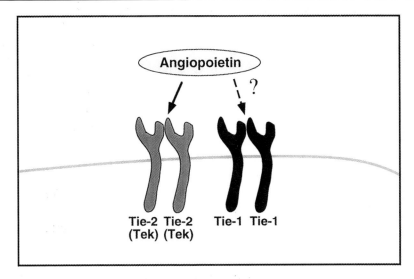

Fig. 4. Tie/Tek RTK family. Both family members of this RTK family have been implicated in vasculogenesis and angiogenesis. Although angiopoietin was only recently identified, there are likely to be other ligands.

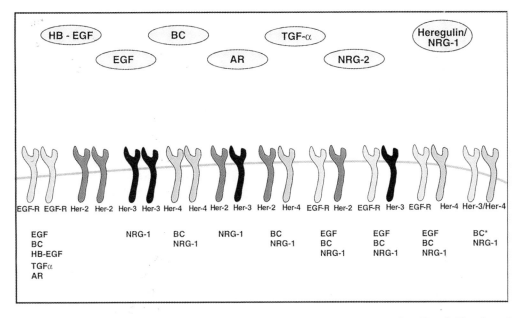

Fig. 5. EGF receptor family. This family consists of the EGF receptor as well as Her-2, Her-3, and Her-4. Receptors in this family not only undergo homodimerization but actively form heterodimers when stimulated by the appropriate ligand. Her-2, Her-3, and Her-4 have not been directly implicated in angiogenesis. For a review of the interactions of the EGF family ligands and EGF receptor family members, *see* ref. *(355)*. BC, Betacellulin; AR, amphiregulin. *Phosphorylation of Her-4 only.

EGF and TGF-α bind to EGF receptors with comparable affinity but TGF-α has been shown to be a more potent mediator of angiogenesis in the hamster cheek pouch assay *(83)*. TGF-α has been shown to be secreted from some tumor cells *(84)* and has been seen in psoriatic epidermis *(85)*. Thus, signaling through EGF receptors has been implicated as angiogenic. In support of this, inhibitors of EGF or TGF-α binding have been used in experimental models to validate the receptor in angiogenesis. For example, a fragment of EGF has been shown to inhibit EGF-induced angiogenesis in a vitelline membrane assay *(86)*. Furthermore, anti-TGF-α neutralizing antibodies prevented TGF-α-induced tube formation by human omentum microvascular endothelial cells in collagen gels *(87)*. Although these observations appear to confirm EGF-dependent angiogenesis, studies have not shown EGF receptors as critical for the angiogenesis process. For instance, gross abnormalities of the vasculature have not been reported in mouse embryos lacking EGF *(88)*, TGF-α*(89)*, or EGF receptors *(90–92)*, or with an EGF receptor mutation that attenuates signaling *(93)*. However, the observation that activation of EGF receptors can induce the expression of VEGF *(94)* have suggested that EGF and TGF-α may contribute indirectly to the angiogenic process. HB-EGF may also participate indirectly. It is not mitogenic to endothelial cells, but was found to induce the migration of bovine endothelial cells and the release of endothelial-cell motogenic activity from bovine vascular smooth-muscle cells *(95)*. This activity was specifically blocked by neutralizing anti-VEGF antibodies. EGF or TGF-α had no effect on release of endothelial-cell motogenic activity from smooth muscle cells.

FGF Receptor Family

FGF was originally identified as a soluble factor that promoted fibroblast proliferation in vitro *(96,97)*. Since then, the FGF gene family has shown to become quite large (Fig. 6). Thus, although originally given different names, a standardized naming system has recently been employed. Where possible, the alternative names will be mentioned. A FGF2/bFGF was partially purified from bovine pituitary *(98)*, whereas an FGF1/aFGF was partially purified from bovine brain *(99)*. These studies led to the eventual cloning of *FGF1/aFGF* *(100)* and *FGF2/bFGF (101,102)*. FGF3/int2 *(103,104)*, FGF4/hst/kFGF *(105–107)*, and FGF5 *(108–110)*, were also identified as oncogene products. *FGF6* was cloned by low-stringency hybridization with a *FGF4* probe *(111)*. FGF7/KGF was identified and subsequently cloned by its ability to stimulate keratinocyte proliferation *(112)*. The mouse homolog of human FGF8 *(113)* was originally identified and cloned as an androgen-induced autocrine growth factor for a mouse mammary carcinoma cell *(114)*. FGF9/GAF was identified in the supernatant of a human glioma cell line as a novel factor that stimulated the growth of glial cells *(115)*. The DNA sequence for *FGF10* corresponds to myocyte activating factor (GenBank accession no. U76381) but has not as yet been published. Also, DNA sequences for *FGF11* and *FGF12* were identified through database searching *(116)*. In addition, four FGF-homologous factors, designated FHF1-FHF4, have been implicated in nervous system development *(117)*. Thus, at the present time, there appear to be 16 members of the FGF family (Fig. 6). The receptor binding characteristics of the first 9 members of the family have been characterized *(118)*. FGF1 binds to all known splice isoforms for each of the signaling FGF receptors, whereas the other family members bind to more limited subsets of receptors and their splice variants *(118)*.

Currently, there are four related genes encoding human FGF receptors (Fig. 6) containing cytoplasmic tyrosine kinase domains *(119–123)* and one gene encoding an unrelated cysteine-rich FGF receptor that lacks a tyrosine kinase domain *(124)*. The latter receptor may function as the E-selectin ligand *(125)*. *FGF-R1/flg* (fms-like gene) was originally cloned by low stringency hybridization with a probe derived from v-*fms*, and subse-

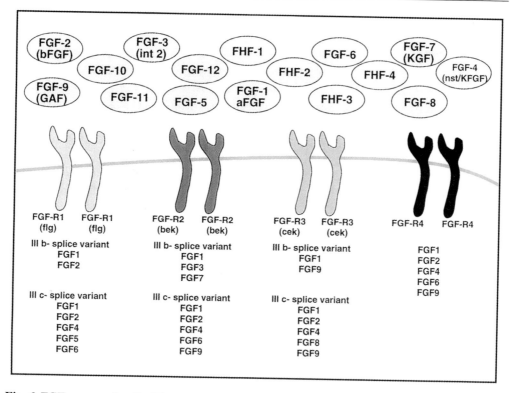

Fig. 6. FGF receptor family. The extracellular domain of the FGF receptors contains three immunoglobulin-like domains (*see* Fig. 2). Messenger RNA splice variants result in FGF receptors that differ in these Ig-domains. One splicing event gives rise to a short, two Ig-domain form owing to skipping of the amino-terminal Ig-like domain. The ligand binding properties of the short and long forms are similar although the affinities for some FGFs may differ. Another splicing event gives rise to three alternative versions of the third Ig-like domain (referred to as IIIa, IIIb, and IIIc). The IIIa form yields a secreted extracellular FGF-binding protein with no known signaling capabilities. FGFs containing alternatively spliced "b" and "c" forms bind FGFs in a differing fashion as shown. FHF, FGF-homologus factors.

quently shown to be a receptor for FGF1 *(126)*. A partial cDNA for *FGF-R2/bek* (<u>b</u>acterially <u>e</u>xpressed <u>k</u>inase) was originally identified by expression cloning using anti-phosphotyrosine detection *(127)*. Its homology with *FGF-R1/flg* suggested it might be an FGF receptor, which was confirmed upon cloning of the human *FGF-R2 (120)*. *FGF-R3/cek2* (<u>c</u>hicken <u>e</u>mbryo <u>k</u>inase 2) was also identified by expression cloning and probing with antiphosphotyrosine antibodies *(128)*. Human *FGF-R3* was subsequently cloned from K562 cells *(121,123)*. *FGF-R4* was also identified in K562 cells *(121,123)* and lung *(129)* by polymerase chain reaction (PCR) using DNA sequences derived from kinase domains. The four human FGF receptors have a variety of alternative splice variants (Fig. 6), including some that are not membrane localized or that do not contain the kinase domains *(97,130–132)*. Splice variant receptor forms have been shown to bind a restricted set of FGFs and transduce mitogenic signaling with different efficacies *(118)*.

A secreted form of FGF-1 (aFGF) was expressed in porcine arteries by in vivo gene transfer and found to induce neointimal hyperplasia and angiogenesis within the neointima *(133)*. Neointimal hyperplasia was not observed in ePTFE vascular grafts coated with

FGF-1 *(134)* but significant enhancement of endothelialization was induced by the FGF-1 coating. Blocking FGF-2 (bFGF) interactions with its receptor by antibodies to FGF-2 *(135,136)*, addition of platelet factor 4 *(136)*, or mutations in *FGF-2* in the heparin binding site *(137)* resulted in inhibition of various steps involved in in vitro angiogenesis. These included induction of endothelial cell protease expression *(135,137)*, cellular invasion *(135)*, and formation of capillary-like tubes *(136,137)*. There are also correlative observations relating the expression of FGF-2 and FGF-R1 to cardiac development *(138,139)* and endothelium re-establishment after vessel injury *(140)*. Dominant-negative FGF receptors have been targeted to the eye lens *(141,142)*, epidermis *(143)*, and lung *(144)*, but not endothelium. Mouse embryos homozygous for deletion of the *FGF-R1* gene died early in development (prior to E10.5) and exhibited gross abnormalities in mesodermal patterning *(145,146)*, however, effects of the gene disruption on vasculogenesis has not been reported. Although FGFs have been implicated in angiogenesis, direct validation of a role for the known human FGF receptors or known FGFs is still lacking.

HGF/SF Receptor (Met)

Hepatocyte growth factor (HGF) or scatter factor (SF), was originally described by its biological activities. HGF/SF was first observed in the serum of partially hepatectomized rats and which stimulated the growth of hepatocytes *(147)*. Molecular cloning of the cDNA for human HGF was reported 5 years later *(148,149)*. Scatter factor (SF) was identified as a protein expressed by fibroblasts and other cells of mesenchymal origin that induced the motility of epithelial cells *(150)*. SF was subsequently demonstrated to be identical to HGF *(151,152)*. Tumor cytotoxic factor (TCF) is related to HGF by physico-chemical properties *(153)*. It was identified as a protein secreted by human lung fibroblasts that when added to Sarcoma 180 cells was found to be cytotoxic, and when added to KB cells, was found to be cytostatic to KB cells. Molecular cloning of TCF confirmed that it was identical to HGF *(154)*. A fibroblast-derived epithelial growth factor was also demonstrated to be identical to HGF *(155)*. HGF/SF also has two splice variants, NK1 and NK2 *(156)*. Both consist of the N-terminal domain and first kringle domain and NK2 also has the second kringle domain. Depending on the cell line and the heparin concentration, these variants may have agonistic or antagonistic properties.

The HGF/SF receptor, Met was originally identified as an oncogene in human osteosarcoma cells derived by chemical treatment with N-methyl-N'-nitro-N-nitrosoguanidine *(157)*. The oncogene transformed NIH 3T3 cells and was subsequently demonstrated to be a fusion protein resulting from the DNA translocation of the *tpr* (translocated promoter region) gene and the Met protooncogene *(158)*. Molecular cloning of the Met proto-oncogene cDNA identified it as a receptor tyrosine kinase *(159)*. Crosslinking studies using [135]I-labeled HGF demonstrated that Met was the receptor for HGF *(160)*. A receptor gene structurally related to Met has been designated Ron, although ligands have not been identified nor has its role in angiogenesis been established.

Hepatocyte growth factor/scatter factor (HGF/SF) and its receptor Met have many important roles in embryogenesis *(161)*. However, regulation of vasculogenesis does not appear to be one. Embryos homozygous for deletions of HGF/SF *(161,163)* or Met *(164)* developed a normal vascular system, but died between E13.5 and E16.5 from abnormal development of the placenta and liver. In Matrigel plug and cornea models, HGF/SF induced angiogenesis, which was inhibited with anti-HGF/SF antibodies *(165,166)*. Reverse transcription (RT)-PCR analysis of cells infiltrating a Matrigel plug containing HGF/SF revealed the expression of several angiogenic factors and chemokines, including VEGF *(167)*. However, anti-VEGF antibodies were effective to only partial attenuate HGF/SF-induced angiogenesis *(167)*. In other studies platelet-activating factor (PAF) was subsequently demonstrated to be a potent mediator of HGF-induced angiogenesis *(168)*. The addition of PAF receptor antagonist, WEB2170, or inhibition of macrophage infiltration with antibodies were very effective means to inhibit HGF-induced angiogenesis in using Matrigel plugs *(168)*. Thus, it appears that the role of HGF/SF in angiogenesis may occur though indirect effects, including those mediated by PAF and VEGF.

B61 Receptor

The Eck/Eph subfamily represents the largest group of RTKs (Fig. 7) although their biological roles are not well understood. The receptors in this subclass are largely orphan receptors without known ligands. B61 (LERK-1) was identified by receptor affinity chromatography as a ligand for Eck (epithelial cell kinase) *(169)*. B61 had been previously identified as the protein product of a response gene induced by TNF-α. In addition to being a secreted protein, it was found that B61 can exist as a cell-surface glycosylphosphatidylinositol-linked protein, which is capable of activating Eck *(170)*. *Eck* was cloned from a cDNA human keratinocyte library using a partial clone isolated from a HeLa library that had been screened with degenerate oligonucleotides to conserved regions of tyrosine kinase domains *(171)*. The protein product of the Eck gene encodes a 130 kDa protein that was found to be expressed in rat organs (skin, intestine, lung, and ovary) that contain high proportions of epithelial cells *(171)*.

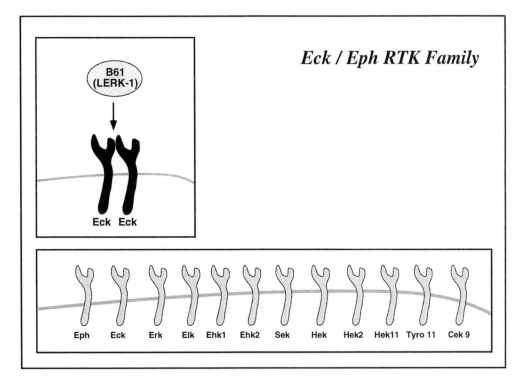

Fig. 7. Eck/Eph RTK family. This family is the largest family of RTKs although their biological roles are not well-understood. Most are orphan receptors without known ligands. One identified ligand for Eck is B61. Other ligands for this receptor as well as other family members most likely exist but have not yet been discovered.

During embryogenesis, Eck has been implicated as having a role in pattern formation in gastrulation, hindbrain segmentation, and limb development (172). In this study, expression of Eck in the developing vascular system was not reported. In contrast, B61 was found to be expressed in endothelial cells of the developing vascular system, in the endocardium of the developing heart, and has been postulated to have a role in vasculogenesis and angiogenesis (173). The expression of Eck was demonstrated in human umbilical-vein endothelial cells, and B61 was shown to induce angiogenesis in an angiogenic cornea model (174). Because B61 can be induced by TNF-α (175), which has been reported to be an angiogenic factor (176), Pandey et al. (174) investigated the putative role of B61 in TNF-α-mediated angiogenesis. In this study, ant-B61 antibodies inhibited TNF-α-induced angiogenesis in the angiogenic cornea model (174). It has yet to be determined if B61 induction of Eck represents a direct or indirect mechanism in the angiogenic process.

PDGF Receptors

As described earlier, Ross et al. (14), Kohher and Lipton (15), and Westermark and Wasteson (177) found direct evidence for the presence of a potent growth factor derived from platelets. Since then, many studies have shown unequivocally that PDGF is made by a number of cell types under normal or pathologic conditions including atherosclerosis, fibrotic disease, and cancer. PDGF consists of two related polypeptide chains (A and B), which are assembled as biologically active hetero- and homodimers. The three isoforms of PDGF (AA, AB, and BB; Fig. 8) have molecular weights of approx 28 kDa daltons and bind with different affinities to the two different receptor types, α and β (for review, see ref. 178). PDGF A chain binds to the α-receptor whereas the B chain binds both α- and β-receptors.

Characterization of the PDGF receptors was begun in the early 1980s when PDGF was found to induce tyrosine phosphorylation of a 185 kDa protein in plasma membranes from human and mouse cells (179,180). The initial receptor was purified from porcine uterus (181) and mouse fibroblasts (182), but subsequent findings about the different biological effects of the PDGF isoforms indicated that there may be more than one PDGF receptor (183,184). Binding studies produced further evidence for this hypothesis, leading to the designation of α- and β- receptors (Fig. 8). This was confirmed by cloning the receptors and conducting binding studies using expressed recombinant proteins (for review, see ref. 185).

Spatial and temporal expression of PDGF-BB and the PDGF β-receptors suggested that they may play a role in angiogenesis. Both are expressed in vessels in human placenta (186), healing wounds, adenocarcinoma (187), and glioblastoma (188). There is some discrepancy as to what cell types express the receptor and whether growth factor activation acts by an autocrine or paracrine mechanism, though this may be tissue-dependent. There are also conflicting reports on the expression patterns of the PDGF receptor in in vitro tube-formation assays (189–191). It is likely that PDGF is involved in angiogenesis, but has been suggested to play an indirect role by inducing VEGF (192,193). In addition, it may also exert growth-stimulatory effects on pericytes (187) and fibroblast-like cells (191,194) that surround the endothelial cells. Recently, more direct evidence has been found linking PDGF and PDGF receptors to vasculogenesis. Lindahl et al. found that mouse embryos deficient in PDGF-B lacked microvascular pericytes, which normally form part of the capillary wall and contribute to its stability (264). Endothelial cells of the sprouting capillaries in the mutant mice appeared unable to attract PDGF-β receptor-positive pericyte progenitor cells. Thus, the PDGF-B deficient mice developed numerous capillary microaneurysms that ruptured at late gestation.

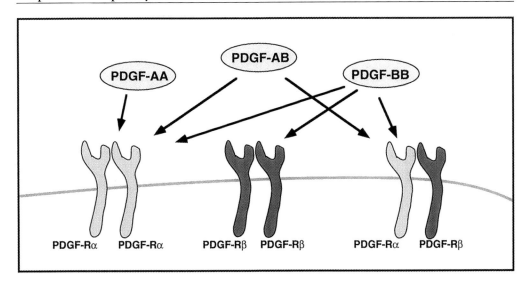

Fig. 8. PDGF receptors. PDGF exists as a homo- or heterodimer of A and B chains and the receptors, when activated by their appropriate ligand, can homo- or heterodimerize. PDGF-AA binds only to the PDGF-α receptor homodimer, whereas PDGF-BB can bind all three receptors although with differing affinities.

IGF-1 Receptor

The IGF are comprised of two ligands (IGF-1, IGF-2) that bind to three or four different receptors; insulin receptor, IGF receptor type-1 (IGF-1R), IGF receptor type-2 (IGF-2R; also known as the mannose-6-phosphate receptor), and an insulin/IGF-1 receptor hybrid (Fig. 9) *(195)*. IGF-1, IGF-2 and insulin are synthesized as prohormones, but after proteolytic processing, IGF-1 and IGF-2 still contain domain C, which is removed from insulin. The resulting IGF-1 peptide has a molecular weight of 7.5 kDa. One of the main roles of IGF-1 in the developing embryo appears to be to stimulate linear skeletal growth by increasing cartilage synthesis by chondrocytes.

The IGF-1 receptor is similar to the insulin receptor because it is translated as a single-chain that is later cleaved into α and β subunits. The two subunits exist as dimers linked through disulfide bonds. The β subunit spans the membrane and contains an intracellular tyrosine kinase domain. The α subunit is extracellular and contains the ligand binding domain.

IGF-1 binds with high affinity to the IGF-1 receptor and with lower affinity to the insulin receptor (Fig. 9). IGF-2 also binds with high affinity to the IGF-1 receptor, but also binds to its own receptor that is unrelated to the IGF-1 and insulin receptors. Insulin binds with low affinity to the IGF-1 receptor as well. It is thought that the IGF-1 receptor may mediate mitogenic effects of all three factors, where the insulin receptor mediates the metabolic effects of insulin. The insulin/IGF-1 hybrid receptor appears to function as a signaling molecule for IGF-1 but not insulin. IGF-1 is further regulated by six binding proteins. Some inhibit IGF-1 action by preventing it from binding to the receptor. Others appear to enhance the effects of IGF-1 binding.

As with PDGF, IGF-1 has been observed in angiogenic tissues and is released by monocytes *(196,197)*. IGF-1 also induces in vitro tube formation by endothelial cells

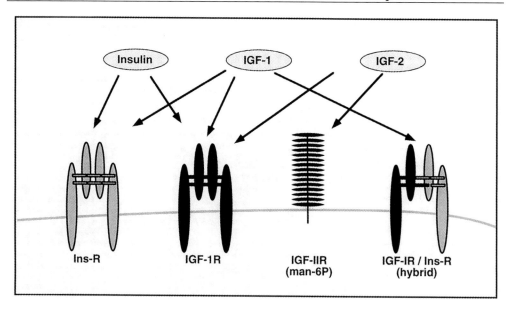

Fig. 9. IGF receptors. The IGF receptors, unlike the other receptor tyrosine kinases, exist as pre-formed heterotetramers of α and β subunits. Insulin, IGF-1, and IGF-2 bind with differing affinities to the various receptors. The IGF-2 receptor (also known as the mannose-6-phosphate receptor) is very different structurally and its short cytoplasmic domain lacks catalytic activity. Signal transduction through the IGF-2 receptor is unclear.

(198) and stimulates the growth of fibroblast-like cells in vascular explants *(194)*. IGF-1 has been implicated in the angiogenesis that occurs in diabetic retinopathy because its expression is increased in the vitreous of patients and can stimulate the growth of human retinal endothelial cells *(199)*. Furthermore, IGF-1 induces angiogenesis in rabbit corneas *(200)*. So far, it is not clear whether IGF-1 and its receptor play a direct or indirect role in angiogenesis.

ANGIOGENIC DISEASES AND RECEPTOR TYROSINE KINASES
Cancer and Metastasis

The link between angiogenesis and cancer is well-established. Neovascularization is an important step in the transition from hyperplasia to neoplasia and it must occur for tumors to grow beyond 1–2 mm *(201,202)*. A correlation between microvessel density and severity of disease and prognosis has been observed in a number of different tumor types including brain *(203,204)*, breast *(205)*, bladder *(206)*, colon *(207)*, cervical *(208)*, and endometrial cancer *(209–211)*.

Many activators of tumor angiogenesis are growth factors that stimulate proliferation of endothelial cells. The roles of VEGF and its cognate receptor Flk-1/KDR are well-established in this role. VEGF is secreted by a number of human tumor cell lines in culture including glioma *(193)*, melanoma *(212)*, Kaposi's sarcoma *(213)*, and epidermoid carcinoma cells *(214)*. More importantly, VEGF transcripts or protein has been identified by *in situ* hybridization or immunohistochemistry in primary gliomas *(215,216)*, hemangioblastomas *(217)*, and breast *(218–220)*, colon *(221,207)* and renal cell tumors *(222)*.

In glioblastoma, the message for VEGF is found in cells adjacent to necrotic regions, which is consistent with upregulation by hypoxia *(215,223)*. For some tumors, VEGF expression has been correlated with more aggresive disease and a poorer prognosis *(204,218,224)*. Furthermore, patients with cancer have significant higher serum VEGF levels than normal volunteers *(225)*. The highest VEGF concentrations were observed in patients with untreated metastatic cancers.

A number of animal models have been developed to investigate the function of VEGF in tumor angiogenesis. Rat C6 glioma and human U87MG glioblastoma cells secrete VEGF and grow subcutaneously in athymic mice *(226,227)*. The introduction of antisense constructs against VEGF mRNA into these cell lines reduces their in vivo growth, as well as the degree of neovascularization. Monoclonal antibodies (MAbs) against VEGF have been utilized to inhibit the subcutaneous growth of human rhabdomyosarcoma, glioblastoma, leiomyosarcoma *(228)*, and fibrosarcoma *(229)* in athymic mice. Metastasis of fibrosarcoma *(230)* and colon cancer tumors *(231)* was also shown to be blocked by anti-VEGF antibodies. The presence of VEGF in primary tumors and tumor cell lines, as well as the inhibitory activity of VEGF using antisense and neutralizing antibodies, indicated that VEGF is a significant player in tumor angiogenesis.

The contribution of the VEGF receptors, Flk-1/KDR and Flt-1, to tumor growth has also been studied extensively. Like VEGF, their mRNA has been detected in tumors such as gliomas *(215,216)*, hemangioblastomas *(217)*, colon cancer207 and adenocarcinomas *(221)*. In these cases, the receptors were detected on the endothelial cells of the vessels and not the tumor cells. This supports a paracrine mechanism in which VEGF secreted from tumor cells stimulates proliferation of endothelial cells. In contrast, KS cell lines and primary tissue express Flt-1 and KDR as well as VEGF *(213)*. This finding coupled with the observation that growth of KS cell lines is inhibited by VEGF antisense oligonucleotides, suggests that an autocrine loop may be present in KS leading to enhanced cell growth and vasculature. The capacity of Flk-1 to act as a modulator of tumor growth has also been studied in animal tumor models. Athymic mice were co-implanted with tumor cells and virus-producing cells that produced viral DNA encoding a truncated *flk-1* gene *(231,232)*. The co-implantation allowed the introduction of mutant receptor into endothelial cells, where it acted in a dominant-negative fashion to block activation of Flk-1 and effect the growth of the tumor. By this method, the subcutaneous growth of a variety of human, rat, and mouse tumor cells was shown to be inhibited. In addition the microvessel density was shown to be reduced in the small tumors that did form confirming the connection between Flk-1, angiogenesis, and tumor growth.

Flk-1/KDR has been proposed as a target for the development of novel anticancer agents. Because of its restricted role in angiogenesis, specific inhibitors of Flk-1/KDR would be expected to have fewer side effects than cytotoxic chemotherapy drugs. This is owing to the consideration that angiogenesis is thought to rarely occur in healthy adults (with the exception of angiogenesis that occurs following wound injury or during cyclical changes in the endometrium and ovary). In this regard, several modes of action are possible to inhibit VEGF signaling. For example, MAbs specific for VEGF *(228)* and Flk-1 *(233)* have been shown to inhibit tumor growth in animals by disrupting binding of VEGF to the receptor. Also, synthetic small molecule inhibitors of Flk-1 tyrosine kinase activity have been shown to block the effects of VEGF in several in vitro and in vivo systems *(234)*.

Like Flk-1/KDR, expression of Tie-1 and Tie-2 is primarily limited to endothelial cells. In one study, Tie-1 mRNA was shown to be highly expressed in capillaries and vessels of primary and metastatic melanoma, but only low levels were observed in normal tissue surrounding the tumors *(72)*. Tie-1 was also highly expressed on vessels of gliomas, meningiomas *(235)*, and hemangioblastomas *(217)*, although expression in vessels of breast tumors is comparable to normal tissue *(236)*. In a recent study of breast tissue, the strongest expression of Tie-2 was seen in vascular "hot spots" within the inflammatory infiltrate at the periphery of invasive tumors *(237)*. Also in this study it was found that the proportion of Tie-2 positive vessels was significantly higher in breast tumors compared to either normal breast tissue or benign lesions. Because Tie-1 and Tie-2 were only recently identified, their biologic roles in tumor angiogenesis are only now being elucidated. However, Tie-2/Tek and its ligand, angiopoietin-1 *(61)*, appear to be required for recruitment of pericytes and smooth muscle cells *(238)*. Thus, disruption of signaling through Tie-2 may prevent the formation of stable vessels leading to tumor growth inhibition.

Acidic and basic fibroblast growth factors (FGF1/aFGF and FGF2/bFGF) and their receptors, FGFR-1 and FGFR-2, have been identified in a variety of tumor types. Although FGFs have been implicated in a paracrine fashion for stimulation of angiogenesis, it is difficult to dissect their role in tumor growth given that autocrine stimulation of tumor cells is also playing a role. The distribution pattern of FGFs and their receptors implicate FGFs in tumor angiogenesis but clearly their expression is not limited to the endothelium. A human renal cell carcinoma cell line has been shown to secrete FGF2/bFGF *(239)* and two human prostate-tumor cell lines were found to make and respond to FGF2/bFGF *(240)*. Analysis of mRNA from various grades of astrocytomas revealed that the expression of different FGF receptors changes as the tumors progress to higher grades of malignancy *(241)*. Excised skin from melanoma patients was found to have high FGFR-1 expression in the invading melanoma cells and stroma, but not in the endothelial cells *(72)*. However, in a study of 45 cases of invasive breast cancer using immunhistochemistry, FGF2/bFGF expression showed a positive correlation with microvessel density *(242)*. Neutralizing antibodies specific for FGF2/bFGF have been used to investigate the role of FGF2/bFGF in cancer. FGF-induced mitogenesis of SC115 mouse mammary carcinoma cells was shown to be inhibited by anti-FGF antibodies *(243)*. Similarly, an anti-FGF2/bFGF MAb blocked the growth of U-87MG and T98G human glioblastoma cells in culture and as xenografts in nude mice *(244)*. In the latter case, it is unclear whether the anti-tumor effects of the antibody treatment are related to inhibition of tumor growth, tumor vasculature, or both.

Compounds that inhibit FGF signaling are currently under development as anti-cancer agents. Tecogalan sodium, an inhibitor of FGF2/bFGF binding to its receptor, is currently in clinical trials for the treatment of solid tumors and KS *(245)*. The polyanionic compound, suramin, is also under investigation as an FGF inhibitor *(246)*, although it blocks the binding of a number of growth factors to their receptors. Many other agents block FGF2/bFGF-induced angiogenesis, but it is not known that they work directly on signaling through the FGF receptor. This includes the synthetic compound, thalidomide *(247)*, and the protein-based angiogenesis inhibitors, angiostatin and endostatin *(248,249)*, all of which are being pursued as potential anti-angiogenic agents.

PDGF and its receptors have been detected in cancers such as gliomas *(188,250–252)*, ovarian carcinomas *(253)*, lung carcinomas *(254)*, melanoma *(254,255)*, colorectal carcinomas *(256)*, prostate carcinomas *(257)*, gastric carcinomas *(258)*, breast carcinomas *(259)*, choriocarcinoma *(260)*, esophageal carcinomas *(261)*, soft tissue tumors *(262)*, and AIDS-related KS *(263)*. Many reports have cited the co-expression of PDGF and its receptors by the tumor cells, suggesting that the tumor cells may stimulate their own proliferation through an autocrine mechanism *(250,252–256,258,260,261,263)*. Although the direct role of PDGF to influence tumor growth is well-established, PDGF is thought to be important for tumor angiogenesis. It has been shown that PDGF receptors are expressed on tumor neovasculature and are upregulated during tumor progression *(188)*. Furthermore, the β-receptor appears to play a role in angiogenesis by regulating the pericytes that surround the microvessels *(264)*. In addition, PDGF receptor expression on tumor stroma fibroblasts may support tumor cell growth *(256,265–268)*.

Scatter factor/hepatocyte growth factor (SF/HGF) is overexpressed in many human cancers including nonsmall cell lung tumors *(269)*, melanoma *(270)*, endothelial carcinoma *(211)*, leiomyosarcoma *(271)*, thyroid carcinoma *(272)*, and multiple myeloma *(273)*. It has been shown to play a role in tumor invasion as well as being an independent prognostic indicator *(211)*. In some cases it appears to be secreted from stromal fibroblasts and macrophages, and not from the tumor cells *(274)*, though SF/HGF has been identified in five myeloma cell lines *(275)*. Furthermore, overexpression of SF/HGF in transgenic mice resulted in formation of hepatocellular adenoma by the time the mice were 1.5 yr old *(276)*. Met is expressed on tumor endothelial cells and may contribute to tumor angiogenesis by induction of endothelial cell motility. In addition, SF/HGF has been shown to induce chemotactic migration of endothelial cells in vitro. However, the primary angiogenic contribution of MET may be induction of PAF from macrophages *(168)*. Thus, HGF signaling through MET may have a more indirect role in angiogensis.

Although EGF has been associated predominantly with autocrine growth of tumor cells, several studies have implicated a role for EGF receptor signaling in angiogensis associated with tumors. For example, in a study of 45 cases of invasive breast cancer *(242)*, expression of TGF-α and the EGF correlated positively with microvascular density. Co-expression of TGF-α/EGFR showed a stronger correlation with the microvascular density than either one alone *(242,277)*.

IGF-1 and its receptor clearly plays a role in cancer *(278)*, but as in the case of the FGF family, the effects of IGF-1 on tumor cells may also be as important as the effect on tumor vasculature. In this regard, IGF-1 has been shown to be required for transformation of fibroblasts *(278)* and protection of tumor cells from apoptosis *(279)*. As discussed earlier, it probably acts as an angiogenic factor by inducing other growth factors such as VEGF, so inhibition of its action may block tumor growth by acting directly on tumor cells and by inhibition of angiogenesis. Other growth factors and their receptors that play a supporting role in angiogenesis are probably involved in tumor growth. PDGF, EGF, and IGF-1 receptors have all been identified in various tumors and tumor cell lines and contribute to transformation of cells. As with the FGF receptors and Met, they may contribute to the growth of tumors by promoting angiogenesis and tumor-cell proliferation and survival.

Rheumatoid Arthritis

Rheumatoid arthritis (RA) is an inflammatory joint disease that is characterized by cellular infiltration of synovial fluid by neutrophils, and of the synovial membrane by T lymphocytes and macrophages, hyperproliferation of cells of the synovial membrane — which results in formation of a pannus — and destruction of cartilage and bone *(280,281)*. More than a decade ago, it was observed that synovial fluid from arthritis patients contained angiogenic factors *(282,283)*. Angiogenesis is currently thought to have an important role in the pathogenesis of RA *(284)*, and it has been demonstrated that inhibition of angiogenesis with the fumagillin analog AGM-1470 suppresses RA in experimental models of RA *(285,286)*. Many growth factors and cytokines have been implicated as having a role in RA *(280)*, some of which have also been implicated as angiogenic factors *(284,287)*. Putative angiogenic factors that have been reported to be expressed in RA synovial fluid or tissue include VEGF *(288–291)*, FGF2/bFGF *(292,293)*, FGF1/aFGF *(294)*, IL-8 *(295)*, TNF-α *(296)*, PAF *(296)*, and HGF/SF *(297)*. Of these, the strongest evidence for a role as a direct angiogenic factor exists for VEGF.

VEGF expression is significantly higher in synovial fluid and tissue from RA patients than from patients with other types of arthritis *(288,289)*. The source of this VEGF appears to be elevated expression in synovial lining cells, subsynovial macrophages, fibroblasts surrounding microvessels, and vascular smooth-muscle cells *(288–290)*. In addition, it has been reported that inflammatory mediators such as PGE_2 and IL-1 induce VEGF expression in synovial fibroblasts *(291)*. These observations indicate that tissue VEGF levels are elevated by expression in the infiltrating macrophages as well as in endogenous cells bathed in inflammatory mediators.

TNF-α is considered to be a central regulator of RA pathogenesis through direct and indirect induction of other cytokines and proteases *(280)*. Although TNF-α has been reported to be an angiogenic factor *(176,298)*, it appears to act via an indirect mechanism by induction of the expression of the Eck ligand, B61 *(174)*, and of platelet activating factor (PAF) *(296,299)*. PAF produced by macrophages has also been reported to be the active angiogenic agent mediating HGF-induced angiogenesis *(168)*. In an angiogenesis assay, PAF has been demonstrated to induce the expression of many cytokines, including VEGF *(300)*. Thus, TNF-α, HGF, and PAF all appear to induce angiogenesis by indirectly inducing signal transduction of VEGF (and perhaps other) receptors.

Synovial lining cells, macrophages, endothelial cells, and vascular smooth-muscle cells of rheumatoid joints *(301)* as well as mast cells in rheumatoid synovium *(302)* have been reported to express FGF2/bFGF. Its synthesis and release are enhanced by cytokines such as IL-1 or IFN-α and IL-2 *(292,293)* that are associated with RA *(280)*. However, FGF2/bFGF does not appear to be elevated in RA synovial fluid *(301)*. In addition, FGF1/aFGF is abundantly expressed in synovial tissues from RA patients *(294)*, and expression of FGF-R1, the receptor for FGF1 and FGF2 *(118)*, is enhanced on CD4+ T cells *(294)*. Because FGF1/aFGF is costimulatory for CD4+ T cells *(303)*, these observations suggest a mechanism for enhancing cytokine release that may contribute to RA pathogenesis, and to angiogenic responses via indirect mechanisms.

Psoriasis

Psoriasis is a chronic skin disorder that is characterized by hyperproliferation of the epidermis, inflammation, and angiogenesis. Angiogenesis appears to be crucial in the pathogenesis of psoriasis and microvascular changes are one of the earliest detectable events in developing psoriatic lesions *(304)*. Several reports have implicated the epidermis as the origin of angiogenic factors *(305–308)*. However, it has long been recognized that the inflammatory component of the disease complicates dissection of the angiogenic factors involved in the disease *(309)*, since cytokines secreted by lymphocytes, macrophages, mast cells, and neutrophils can also contribute to angiogenesis *(295,302,310,311)*.

Of the many angiogenic factors identified in skin *(312)*, VEGF has been the best characterized as a direct inducer of angiogenesis. VEGF is overexpressed in keratinocytes of psoriatic skin, but only minimally expressed in normal epidermis *(313)*. VEGF is also overexpressed in other skin diseases such as bullous pemphigoid, dermatitis herpetiformis, erythema multiforme *(314)*, delayed skin hypersensitivity reactions *(315)*, and probably after sun exposure, as suggested by the induction of VEGF expression in cultured keratinocytes following exposure to ultraviolet light *(316)*.

TGF-α has also been reported to be overexpressed in psoriatic epidermis *(85)*, and may signal the hyperproliferation of keratinocytes through the EGF receptor in an autocrine manner. TGF-α also induces the dose-dependent expression of VEGF in cultured keratinocytes *(313)*, suggesting that a TGF-α autocrine loop in psoriatic skin may induce a primary angiogenic stimulus. TGF-α expressed by cultured keratinocytes has been shown to stimulate tubule formation in human omental microvascular endothelial cells in collagen gels *(317)*. Thus, in addition to inducing the expression of VEGF, TGF-α may contribute to psoriatic angiogenesis by enhancing tubular morphogenesis.

FGF2/bFGF is expressed in keratinocytes and endothelial cells and stimulates the proliferation of both through autocrine and paracrine mechanisms *(318,319)*. Mast cells have also been reported to be a major source of FGF2/bFGF in chronic inflammatory diseases *(302)*, which may contribute to the link between inflammation and angiogenesis. The immunosuppressant, cyclosporin-A, improves psoriatic symptoms *(320)*. It has also been shown to inhibit keratinocyte proliferation induced by TGF-α or FGF2 *(321–323)*. Thus it is unclear if cyclosporin-A is effective in treating psoriasis by inhibiting inflammation or keratinocyte hyperproliferation. HGF/SF has been reported to be angiogenic, and to be present at sites of blood vessel formation in psoriatic skin *(166)*. The source of HGF/SF in psoriatic skin may be leukocytes associated with the inflammatory component of the disease. Although HGF/SF may induce angiogenesis in vivo, it appears to do so via an indirect mechanism that is mediated by PAF *(168)* and VEGF *(300)*.

Ocular Diseases

The release of angiogenic factors from the ischemic retina has been hypothesized to be the central stimulus for retinal neovascularization. Glaucoma, vitreous hemorrhage, and retinal detachment secondary to intraocular neovascularization accounts for the resultant vision loss in several ocular disorders such as retinopathy of prematurity, age-related macular degeneration, and diabetic retinopathy. The release of angiogenic factors by the ischemic retina to induce new blood-vessel growth and increase the oxygen supply to the area turns out to be harmful as the new vessels do not grow with normal architecture. Edema, hemorrhage, vessel tortuosity, and pathological neovascularization subsequently result in retinal detachment and lead to blindness.

The consideration of angiogenic factors in ocular diseases relies upon the presence in the eyes of patients or animals with retinopathy. Ideally, factor production would be triggered by oxygen-poor conditions and it should be able to induce ocular or retinal neovascularization *(324)*. Evidence in the literature indicates that both stimulatory and inhibitory activities on proliferation and migration of endothelial cells are present in retinal and vitreous extracts *(325–327)*. Some angiogenic factors such as IGF-1, FGF, and VEGF have elevated expression in vitreous and neovascular membranes from patients with retinal disorders *(326–332)*. Therefore, these growth factors are candidates for the angiogenic factors that modulate or initiate intraocular neovascularization in retinal disorders.

VEGF is constitutively expressed in the vascularized tissues of the normal eye *(333)*. Intraocular VEGF gene expression is increased in disease states like diabetic retinopathy *(330–332,334)*. Using neutralizing antibodies specific for VEGF and soluble VEGF-receptor proteins, it has been shown that VEGF is sufficient to induce neovascularization *(333,335–337)*. In animal models, intraocular injections of VEGF into normal eyes caused retinal edema, microaneurysms, hemorrhage, and intraretinal neovascularization *(336,338,339)*. Decreased levels of VEGF paralleled the regression of proliferative retinopathy. Stimuli associated with oxygen deprivation such as hypoxia *(215,223,338,339)*, generation of oxygen intermediates *(340)*, and accumulation of advanced glycation endproducts *(341)* in diabetics, increased endogenous VEGF expression in vivo. Inhibitors of VEGF signaling including antisense VEGF reagents *(342)*, soluble VEGF receptor proteins *(335)*, ribozymes targeting VEGF receptor subtype mRNAs *(56,343)*, and selective PKC inhibitors *(344)*, resulted in significant inhibition of corneal and retinal neovascularization, VEGF-stimulated cell growth in vitro and VEGF-induced retinal permeability in vivo. All of these data provide strong support for a direct role of VEGF in ocular angiogenesis.

IGF-1 is expressed in rapidly proliferating endothelium, suggesting that it may play a role in its growth *(196)*. In vitro studies support a role of IGF-1 in the pathogenesis of retinal neovascularization by demonstrating that IGF-1 acts at all the stages required for new vessel formation including endothelial cell proliferation *(345)*, migration *(346)*, and production of proteases relevant to basement membrane degradation *(347–349)*. In vivo, IGF-1 induces angiogenesis in the rabbit corneal model as well as retinal fibrovascular proliferation when injected into the vitreous cavity *(200)*. Recently, IGF-1 has been found to induce the expression of VEGF by increasing its rate of transcription in several colon carcinoma cell lines but it did not stimulate proliferation *(350)*. This suggests that the proliferative response induced by IGF-1 and its ability to induce VEGF expression may occur through different mechanisms. It is not known whether the effect of IGF-1 on VEGF induction is unique to cancer cells and whether its effects on retinal neovascularization is direct or indirect.

FGF2/bFGF also appears to play a role in diabetic retinopathy *(329,351)*. In addition to being present in vitrectomy samples from retinal disorders *(329)*, FGF2/bFGF induces endothelial-cell proliferation *(352,353)*, migration *(354)*, and the release of collagenase and plasminogen activators *(355)*. In vivo, FGF2/bFGF induces corneal neovascularization *(356,357)* as well as retinal fibrovascular proliferation with an enhanced fibrotic component when injected into the vitreous cavity *(200)*. The developed retinal capillary basement membrane thickening and subsequent retinal traction and detachment is similar to those occurring in humans and animals with diabetes.

Arterial Thickening and Restenosis

Arterial injury as part of the atherosclerotic process or as a consequence of balloon-mediated injury to treat coronary occlusions is known to be accompanied by thickening of the arterial wall. This response is also observed in cases of organ rejection where chronic vascular injury is associated with thickening of the arteries at the site of the organ transplant. RTKs have been implicated as important players within the disease process associated with the injury response. As in the case of atherosclerosis, both PDGF and FGFs are associated with the hyperproliferation of the arterial smooth-muscle cell. These cell layers, when they become ischemic, require new blood-vessel formation in order to support their hyperproliferation. In the case of smooth-muscle cell migration, the activation of mitogen-activated protein (MAP) kinase has been shown to be associated with PDGF-dependent cell movement *(358)*. A synthetic compound that blocks binding of PDGF to its receptor has been shown to inhibit chemotaxis of smooth muscle cells and inhibit neo-intimal formation in restenotic lesions following balloon-injury of carotid arteries in rats *(359)*. In addition, PDGF mRNA levels have been shown to be increased in human cardiac allografts *(360)*. In animal models, PDGF and FGF have been shown to be expressed in the injury response following cardiac *(360,361)* and renal *(362,363)* transplantation. However, the role of PDGF and FGF in directly stimulating angiogenesis into the newly forming smooth-muscle layer, beyond their chemotactic and proliferative properties, is less clear at this time.

Atherosclerosis

Atherosclerosis is a disease associated with the formation of arterial lesions or atheromas consisting of an endothelium-covered fibro-fatty plaques. Beneath the endothelial layer exists smooth-muscle cells and extracellular matrix components containing variable amounts of serum proteins. This overlies an area characterized by collections of lipid-laden macrophages. Significant numbers of lymphocytes, particularly T cells, are also present and may contribute to lymphocyte-mediated angiogenesis *(364)*. Both macrophages and lymphocytes traverse the endothelium in order to enter the atheroma lesion. The lesion is characterized by a flux of blood cells including platelets that enter or exit the endothelium. Similar to the restenotic lesion, the build-up of smooth-muscle cells is supported by angiogenesis and is likely to be stimulated by factors released from the smooth-muscle cells when they become hypoxic. In contrast to atheromas, thrombi of arteries and veins are characterized by structures containing a fibrin mesh in which blood cells are entrapped.

The presence of platelets and other cells in the lesion have led to a number of studies that implicate growth factors and their cognate receptor tyrosine kinases as players in the disease *(365)*. The most prominent player in this regard is PDGF. PDGF has been detected in atherosclerotic lesions of rat *(366)*, rabbit *(367)*, and human *(368,369)* origin. The release of PDGF from platelets and other lymphocytes is thought to elicit a pleiotrophy of paracrine effects on blood cells and smooth-muscle cells in the vicinity of the lesion. The chemoattractant, cell survival, migratory, and mitogenic properties of PDGF receptor function in cells may contribute directly or indirectly to different activities on different cell types. PDGF RNA expression has been shown to be associated with the presence of circulating mononuclear cells in hypercholesterolemic patients *(368)*. The presence of mononuclear and other blood cells in the atherosclerotic lesion has been shown to also elaborate the expression of VEGF and FGF growth factors. In smooth-muscle cells, PDGF has been shown to exert a number of effects that may directly or indirectly effect the angiogenic process *(370)*. For instance, it has been suggested that PDGF signaling may upregulate the expression of VEGF in smooth-muscle cells *(371)*. In addition, it is clear that PDGF is a player in myointimal proliferation associated with formation of atherosclerotic plaques. The proliferative *(372)*, migratory *(358,373,374)*, and cell survival *(375)* aspects of PDGF function in smooth-muscle cells may be a major determinant of the formation of the atherosclerotic lesion.

In addition, increased expression of PDGF *(365,371,376)*, VEGF *(371,377,378)*, and FGF *(375)* has been shown to occur in smooth muscle cells under conditions of hypoxia. It has been well-established that endothelial-cell growth and angiogenesis is triggered by conditions of low oxygen tension. The inducibility of these factors is consistent with previous association of these factors and Flk-1/KDR, Flt-1, PDGF receptors, and FGF receptors as participants in this process. In the case of a fibrotic thrombus, the fibrin gel itself is viewed as a provisional matrix into which vascularized connective tissue invades, similar to wound healing. FGF has been considered to be an important player in hyperproliferative and angiogenic aspects of this lesion. FGF1/aFGF and FGF2/bFGF or receptor expression has been shown to be increased rat aortic smooth-muscle cells *(379)*, human cardiac allografts *(360,361)*, CD4+ T cells *(303)*, and atherosclerotic human arteries *(380)*.

Because PDGF, VEGF, and FGF play a role in the formation of atheromas and fibrotic lesions, RTK-mediated signaling events may be important in the development and maintenance of the lesion. It has been suggested that interruption of these signaling systems may enable a means to inhibit the formation or disrupt the remodeling or integrity of the lesion. The angiogenic aspect of this process may be related to local hypoxic conditions that lead to paracrine effects of growth factors on endothelial cells, smooth-muscle cells, or infiltrating leukocytes. In all of these cases, intervention at the level of PDGF, VEGF, and FGF receptors may serve to block the chemotaxis, migratory, survival, and hyperproliferative aspects of cells involved in the disease. In the fibrotic thrombus, targeting of these receptors may be advantageous to reduce the number of connective tissues cells involved in fibrin deposition and development of the clot.

Tissue Ischemia

The formation of new blood vessels is tightly regulated by receptor tyrosine kinases and their cognate ligands. This has been best substantiated for the VEGF, FGF, and PDGF receptor systems where these receptors effect the growth and survival of endothelial cells, pericytes, and arterial smooth-muscle cells. In the case of tissue ischemia, the induction of new blood-vessel growth may be advantageous for the treatment of specific human diseases where oxygen and nutrient limitation is linked to the disease pathology. Because the expression of PDGF *(366,362,376)*, VEGF *(371,377,378)*, and FGF *(376)* have been shown to be expressed in cells under conditions hypoxic conditions, growth factor therapy leading to the induction of new blood vessels has been suggested as a mechanism to overcome myocardial ischemia *(381)*. This rationale suggests that treatment for diseased hearts may relieve symptoms by restoration of myocardial oxygen or restoration of blood flow and thereby prevent disease progression or in the case of treatments using angioplasty or coronary-bypass surgery. In this regard, animal experiments exhibiting acute ischemia models in dogs *(382,388)* and pigs *(383,385,386)* have suggested that intracoronary injection of FGF or perivascular delivery of FGF in a polymer may be beneficial. It is unclear, however, whether this benefit is owing to the generation of new collateral vessels or other aspects of FGF treatment leading to increased cell viability following myocardial injury. In additional studies, chronic administration of FGF2/bFGF to dogs with chronic coronary occlusion showed a fast improvement in function and increased number of vessels *(387,388)*. Moreover, chronic intracoronary infusion of VEGF resulted in substantial improvement of coronary flow of the diseased heart *(389,390)*. Peripheral ischemia has been shown to have improved collateral circulation upon injection of FGF2/bFGF *(391)*, VEGF *(392)*, and SF/HGF *(393)*. More recently, VEGF gene-therapy trials have been initiated to measure improved vascular function *(394,395)*. The encouraging initial findings with FGF and VEGF to improve circulation in coronary and peripheral circulation would provide a rationale to develop therapies to increase Flk-1/KDR or FGF receptor signaling.

Another use of the positive angiogenic activity of VEGF and FGF that has recently been studied is to improve graft survival, which is dependent on the rate and amount of vascular ingrowth. In studies examining revascularization of orthotopic canine autografts *(396)*, topical administration of FGF2/bFGF showed better graft viability than control.

FGF was also found to increase survival of a vascular pedicle implanted subcutaneously in rabbits *(397)* and to increase survival of a prefabricated myocutaneous flap placed subcutaneously in rats *(398)*. In addition to coronary and peripheral ischemia, FGF may be a useful treatment for graft survival.

SUMMARY AND FUTURE OUTLOOK

There is evidence for the role of several receptor tyrosine kinases in vasculogenesis and angiogenesis associated with pathological conditions. The predominant evidence, at this time, is associated with the VEGF receptor family and the angiopoietin receptor family. The expression of both of these receptor classes appears to be restricted to endothelial cells. Certainly, overwhelming evidence was obtained following targeted mutagenesis. *Flk-1, flt-1, VEGF, Tie-1*, and *Tie-2* knock-out mice all showed deficiencies in vascular endothelium. It appears that Flk-1 is important early in vasculogenesis as mature endothelial cells were not formed in the –/– embryos. Mature endothelial cells were formed in *Flt-1*-deficient embryos but the organization was disrupted. *Tie-1* and *Tie-2,* on the other hand, most likely play a role later in the process as mature endothelium can be found but it was disorganized. In the case of the *Tie-1* knock-out, embryos died much later, some not until after birth. Therefore *Tie-1* was postulated to be involved in vascular integrity. In angiogenesis associated with disease, there are many reports implicating a role for VEGF including solid tumors, rheumatoid arthritis, psoriasis, diabetic retinopathy, retinopathy of prematurity, and vascular disease. The number of studies examining a role for the angiopoietin receptors in disease is significantly fewer and more limited to detection of mRNA or protein rather than effects on disease by interfering with the activity of the receptors or altering expression via genetic manipulation. This is probably owing to the later cloning of the receptors and their cograte ligands. Future studies will likely shed additional light on the role for this class of RTKs.

Even though the VEGF and angiopoietin receptors have been clearly implicated in angiogenesis, it is unlikely, given the redundancies frequently found in signal transduction by growth factors, that these are the only important RTK families involved in angiogenesis. The FGF receptor family should also be considered a major contributor. Although FGF knock-out mice have not been reported to have deficiencies in the vasculature, FGFs are clearly angiogenic factors and blocking FGF activity has been found to inhibit various steps of angiogenesis. Studies examining the role of FGF inhibitors in disease are often confounded owing to the fact that nonendothelial cells express FGF receptors and direct effects on nonvasculature needs to be considered. For example tumor cells frequently show increased expression of FGF ligands as well as receptors, so activity by anti-FGF agents could be owing to direct action on the tumor cells. It is difficult to dissect the contributions of autocrine vs paracrine pathways.

Although it has not been given the same level of attention in angiogenic studies, the PDGF and PDGF-receptor family should also be considered an important player, particularly in light of the recent knock-out mice showing a role for PDGF-B chain in pericytes. This growth factor receptor family is an example of a role for nonendothelial cells in the vasculature and in the angiogenic process. PDGF has been known for some time to be the most potent mitogen for cells of mesenchymal origin. Kidney glomerular mesangial cells were the targets of disrupted PDGF-B or PDGF-β receptor *(399,400)* genes in mice and were found to lead to the development of lethal hemorrhage and edema in late embryogenesis. Mesangial cells are related to microvascular pericytes, another target of the disrupted PDGF-B gene. Pericytes encircle the microvessels in many different tissues. They are contractile cells and therefore may contribute to the mechanical stability of the capillary wall. Pericytes express PDGF receptors and respond to PDGF in vitro. Pericytes may also regulate endothelial-cell function. Thus, it appears clear that the importance of RTKs in angiogenesis and pathologies where angiogenesis plays a role is complex and extends beyond the direct focus of endothelial cells.

It is less clear what role other RTKs, EGF, IGF-1, HGF, and B61 receptors play in angiogenesis. Many of the ligands have been classified as angiogenic agents and indeed, have been found to induce angiogenesis in some model systems. Most evidence, however, supports a more indirect role. Nevertheless, it is important to consider that even though they have not been shown to play a direct role in normal angiogenesis, their influence could be considerable under pathological conditions. This is especially true for some of the factors that, in pathological conditions, may regulate the more direct-acting angiogenic factors.

It is likely that future work will bring to light the role of other growth factors and RTKs in angiogenesis. Many RTK families have been studied only in a limited fashion owing both to the inavailability of reagents and the lack of identity of specific ligands. Finally, this review has not touched on the potential for negative regulation of angiogenesis by growth factors and their RTKs. An example is the recently identified angiopoietin-2 *(64)*, which appears to be an antagonist for Tie-2. As recent and perhaps future work points to a role for growth factors in negative regulation, survival, or as apoptotic-inducing factors, the role of growth factors and RTKs may become more complex.

In addition to advances in understanding the biology of receptor tyrosine kinases and their roles in angiogenesis, clinical studies using inhibitors of RTK signaling will likely shed light on the therapeutic potential of blocking these biochemical events. Several approaches can be taken to inhibit growth factor signaling such as blocking the ligand, preventing ligand binding to the receptor, blocking the catalytic activity of the kinase enzyme, and inhibiting downstream signaling. Over the past 10 years, considerable research has been conducted in these areas and several molecules have made it through the preclinical challenges to enter clinical development. Indeed, Herceptin™ (Genentech), a MAb against HER-2 (erbβ-2) was recently approved by the United States Food and Drug Administration (FDA) for use in advanced breast cancer. Although this molecule represents a direct attack on tumor cells rather than tumor vasculature, it establishes an important "proof-of-concept" that blocking receptor tyrosine kinase pathways can have therapeutic benefit. Genentech is also developing a MAb against VEGF that is currently in Phase II trials. Imclone is developing an antibody against the extracellular domain of Flk-1/KDR (currently in preclinical development), which is also designed to prevent binding of VEGF to its receptor. A number of clinical trials are ongoing with small molecule inhibitors of receptor tyrosine kinases (for review, *see* ref. *401*). Zeneca (ZD-1839), Pfizer (CP-358774) and Novartis (CGP-57148) are in Phase II studies with EGF receptor inhibitors (for review, *see* ref. *401*). SUGEN has an ongoing Phase III study in recurrent glioblastoma multiforme for its PDGF receptor inhibitor (SU101) and Phase II studies in other types of cancer. Because of the interest in VEGF receptors, a number of companies have small molecule Flk-1/KDR inhibitors in preclinical or clinical development including SUGEN, Novartis, Zeneca, Parke-Davis, and Pfizer. SUGEN (SU5416) and Novartis (CGP79787) have begun Phase I and Phase I/II testing. In addition to targeting growth factor binding and enzymatic activity, a number of compounds that target downstream signaling molecules are under development. Although these may not specifically be developed as anti-angiogenesis agents, they may be useful in this regard. The next three to five years will likely see many additional compounds entering clinical trials and the emergence of some of these compounds into the mainstream of cancer treatment.

ACKNOWLEDGMENTS

The authors would like to thank Dr. Tai-Ping Fan for helpful discussions and Dr. Sara Courtneidge for her historical perspective on tyrosine kinases. The authors also gratefully acknowledge Tonia Muñoz and Kathy Burch for word processing and administrative help and Martha Velarde for her help with the figures.

REFERENCES

1. Plowman, G., Ullrich, A., and Shawver, L. K. (1994) Receptor tyrosine kinases as targets for drug intervention. *DNP* **7**, 334–339.
2. Rous, P. (1911) A sarcoma of the fowl transmissible by an agent separable from the tumor cells. *J. Exp. Med.* **13**, 397.
3. Bittner, J. J. (1936) Some possible effects of nursing on the mammary gland tumor incidence in mice. *Science* **84**, 162.
4. Gross, L. (1951) "Spontaneous" leukemia developing in C3H mice following inoculation, in infancy, with AK-leukemic extracts or AK-embryos. *Proc. Soc. Exp. Biol. Med.* **76**, 27–32.
5. Hanafusa, H. and Hanafusa, T. (1966) Determining factor in the capacity of Rous sarcoma virus to induce tumors in mammals. *Proc. Natl. Acad. Sci. USA* **55**, 532–538.
6. Brugge, J. S., Steinbaugh, P. J., and Erikson, R. L. (1978) Characterization of the avian sarcoma virus protein p60src. *Virology* **91**, 130–140.
7. Collett, M. S. and Erickson, R. L. (1992) Protein kinase activity associated with the avian sarcoma virus *src* gene product. *Proc. Natl. Acad. Sci. USA* **75**, 2021–2024.
8. Levinson, A. D., Oppermann, H., Varmus, H. E., and Bishop, J. M. (1980) The purified product of the transforming gene of avian sarcoma virus phosphorylates tyrosine. *J. Biol. Chem.* **255**, 11,973–11,980.
9. Sefton, B. M., Hunter, T., Beemon, K., and Eckhart, W. (1980) Evidence that the phosphorylation of tyrosine is essential for cellular transformation by Rous sarcoma virus. *Cell* **20**, 807–816.
10. Hunter, T. (1997) Oncoprotein Networks. *Cell* **88**, 333–346.
11. Cohen, S., Carpenter, G., and King, L. (1980) Epidermal growth factor-receptor-protein kinase interactions. *J. Biol. Chem.* **255**, 4834–4842.
12. Balk, S. D. (1971) Stimulation of the proliferation of chicken fibroblasts by folic acid or a serum factor(s) in a plasma-containing medium. *Proc. Natl. Acad Sci. USA* **68**, 1689–1692.
13. Balk, S. D., Whitfield, J. F., Youdale, T., and Braun, A. C. (1973) Roles of calcium, serum, plasma, and folic acid in the control of proliferation of normal and Rous sarcoma virus–infected chicken fibroblasts. *Proc. Natl. Acad. Sci. USA* **70**, 675–679.
14. Ross, R., Glomset, J., Kariya, B., and Harker, L. (1974) A platelet-dependent serum factor that stimulates the proliferation of arterial smooth muscle cells in vitro. *Proc. Natl. Acad. Sci. USA* **71**, 1207–1210.
15. Kohler, N. and Lipton, A. (1974) Platelets as a source of fibroblast growth-promoting activity. *Exp. Cell. Res.* **87**, 297–301.
16. Waterfield, M. D., Scrace, G. T., Whittle, N., Stroobant, P., Johnsson, A., Wasteson, A., et al. (1983) Platelet-derived growth factor in structurally related to putative transforming protein p28sis of simian sarcoma virus. *Nature* **304**, 35–39.
17. Doolittle, R. F., Hunkapiller, M. V., Hood, L. E., Devare, S. G., Robbins, K. C., Aaronson, S. A., and Antoniades, H. N. (1983) Simian sarcoma virus *onc* gene, v-*sis*, is derived from the gene (or genes) encoding a platelet-derived growth factor. *Science* **221**, 275–277.
18. Downward, J., Yarden, Y., Mayes, E., Scarce, G., Totty, N., Stockwell, P., et al. (1984) Close similarity of epidermal growth factor and v-*erb*B oncogene protein sequences. *Nature* **307**, 521–527.
19. Ullrich, A. and Schlessinger, J. (1990) Signal transduction by receptors with tyrosine kinase activity. *Cell* **61**, 203–212.
20. Carpenter, C. L. and Cantley, L. C. (1996) Phosphoinositide kinases. *Curr. Opin. Cell Biol.* **8**, 153–158.
21. Nakanishi, S., Yano, H., and Matsuda, Y. (1995) Novel functions of phosphatidylinositol 3-kinase in terminally differentiated cells. *Cell Sig.* **7**, 545–557.
22. Lowenstein, E. J., Daly, R. J., Batzer, A. G., Li, W., Margolis, B., Lammers, R., Ullrich, A., et al. (1992) The SH2 and SH3 domain-containing protein GRB2 links receptor tyrosine kinases to ras signaling. *Cell* **70**, 431–442.

23. Clark, S. G., Stern, M. J., and Horvitz, H. R. (1992) C. elegans cell-signalling gene sem-5 encodes a protein with SH2 and SH3 domains. *Nature (Lond.)* **356**, 340–344.
24. Puil, L., Liu, J., Gish, G., Mbamalu, G., Bowtell, D., Pelicci, P. G., Aet al. (1994) Bcr-Abl oncoproteins bind directly to activators of the Ras signalling pathway. *EMBO J.* **13**, 764–773.
25. Tauchi, T., Feng, G.-S., Shen, R., Song, H. Y., Donner, D., Pawson, T., and Broxmeyer, H. E. (1994) SH2-containing phosphotyrosine phosphatase syp is a target of p210bcr-abl tyrosine kinase. *J. Biol. Chem.* **269**,15,381–15,387.
26. Ferrara N. (1993) Vascular endothelial growth factor. *Trends Cardiovasc. Med.* **3**, 244–250.
27. Connolly, D. T., Olander, J. V., Heuvelman, D., Nelson, R., Monsell, R., Siegel, N., et al. (1989) Human vascular permeability factor. Isolation from U937 Cells. *J. Biol. Chem.* **264**, 20,017–20,024.
28. Poltorak, Z., Cohen, T., Sivan, R., Kandelis, Y., Spira, G., Vlodaushy, I., et al. (1997) VEGF145, a secreted vascular endothelial growth factor isoform that binds to extracellular matrix. *J. Biol. Chem.* **272**, 7157–7158.
29. Levy, A. P., Levy, N. S., Iliopoulos, O., Jiang, C., Kaelin, Jr., W. G., and Goldberg, M. A. (1997) Regulation of vascular endothelial growth factor by hypoxia and its modulation by the von Hippel-Lindau tumor suppressor gene. *Kidney Intl.* **51**, 575–578.
30. Park, M., Chen, H. H., Winer, J., Houck, K. A., and Ferrara, N. (1994) Placenta growth factor potentiation of vascular endothelial growth factor bioactivity, *in vitro* and *in vivo*, and high affinity binding to Flt–1 but not to Flk-1/KDR. *J. Biol. Chem.* **296**, 25,646–25,654.
31. Cao, Y., Ji, W. R., Qi, P., Rosin, A., and Cao, Y. (1997) Placenta growth factor: identification and characterization of a novel isoform generated by RNA alternative splicing. *Biochem. Biophys. Res. Comm.* **235**, 493–498.
32. Olofsson, B., Pajusola, K., von Euler, G., Chilov, D., Alitalo, K., and Eriksson, U. (1996) Genomic organization of the mouse and human genes for vascular endothelial growth factor B (VEGF-B) and characterization of a second splice isoform. *J. Biol. Chem.* **271**, 19,310–19,317.
33. Olofsson, B., Pajusola, K., Kaipainen, A., von Euler, G., Joukov, V., Saksela, O., et al. (1996) Vascular endothelial growth factor B, a novel growth factor for endothelial cells. *Proc. Natl. Acad. Sci. USA* **93**, 2576–2581.
34. Joukov, V., Pajusola, K., Kaipainen, A., Chilov, D., Lahtinen, I., Kukk, E., et al. (1996) A novel vascular endothelial growth factor, VEGF-C, is a ligand for the Flt4 (VEGFR-3) and KDR (VEGFR-2) receptor tyrosine kinases. *EMBO J.* **15**, 290–298.
35. Lee, J., Gray, A., Yuan, J., Luoh, H. M., Avraham, H., and Wood, W. I. (1996) Vascular endothelial growth factor-related protein: A ligand and specific activator of the tyrosine kinase receptor Flt4. *Proc. Natl. Acad. Sci. USA* **93**, 1988–1992.
36. Kukk, E., Lymboussaki, A., Taira, S., Kaipainen, A., Jeltsch, M., Joukov, V., and Alitalo, K. (1996) VEGF-C receptor binding and pattern of expression with VEGFR-3 suggests a role in lymphatic vascular development. *Development* **122**, 3829–3837.
37. Yamada, Y., Nezu, J.-I., Shimane, M., and Hirata, Y. (1997) Molecular Cloning of a Novel Vascular Endothelial Growth Factor, VEGF-D. *Genomics* **42**, 483–488.
38. Achen, M. G., Jeltsch, M., Kukk, E., Mäkinen, T., Vitali, A., Wilks, A. F., et al. (1998) Vascular endothelial growth factor D (VEGF-D) is a ligand for the tyrosine kinases VEGF receptor 2 (Flk1) and VEGF receptor 3 (Flt4). *Proc. Natl. Acad. Sci. USA* **95**, 548–553.
39. Shibuya, M., Yamaguchi, S., Yamane, A., Ikeda, T., Tojo, A., Matsushime, H., and Sato, M. (1990) Nucleotide sequence and expression of a novel human receptor-type tyrosine kinase gene (flt) closely related to the fms family. *Oncogene* **5**, 519–524.
40. De Vries, C., Escobedo, J. A., Ueno, H., Houck, K., Ferrara, N., and Williams, L. T. (1992) The *fms*-like tyrosine kinase, a receptor for vascular endothelial growth factor. *Science* **255**, 989–991.
41. Quinn, T. P., Peters, K. G., De Vries, C., Ferrara, N., and Williams, L. T. (1993) Fetal liver kinase 1 is a receptor for vascular endothelial growth factor and is selectively expressed in vascular endothelium. *Proc. Natl. Acad. Sci. USA* **90**, 7533–7537.
42. Millauer, B., Wizigmann-Voos, S., Schnürch, H., Martinez, R., Møller, N. P. H., Risau, W., and Ullrich, A. (1993) High affinity VEGF binding and developmental expression suggest Flk-1 as a major regulator of vasculogenesis and angiogenesis. *Cell* **72**, 835–846.
43. Terman, B. I., Dougher-Vermazen, M., Carrion, M. E., Dimitrov, D., Armellino, D. C., Gospodarowicz, D., and Böhlen, P. (1992). Identification of the KDR tyrosine kinase as a receptor for vascular endothelial cell growth factor. *Biochem. Biophys. Res. Comm.* **187**, 1579–1586.

44. Pajusola, K., Aprelikova, O., Korhonen, J., Kaipainen, A., Pertovaara, L., Alitalo, R., and Alitalo, K. (1992) FLT4 receptor tyrosine kinase contains seven immunoglobulin-like loops and is expressed in multiple human tissues and cell lines. *Cancer Res.* **52,** 5738–5743.

45. Yamaguchi, T. P., Dumont, D. J., Conlon, R. A., and Breitman, M. L. (1993) Flk–1, an flt–related receptor tyrosine kinase is an early marker for endothelial cell precursors. *Development* **118,** 489–98.

46. Breier, G., Clauss, M., and Risau, W. (1995) Coordinate expression of vascular endothelial growth factor receptor-1 (flt-1) and its ligand suggests a paracrine regulation of murine vascular development. *Dev. Dyn.* **204,** 228–239.

47. Kaipainen, A., Korhonen, J., Pajusola, K., Aprelikova, O., Persico, M. G., Terman, B. I., and Alitalo, K. (1993) The related FLT4, FLT1, and KDR receptor tyrosine kinases show distinct expression patterns in human fetal endothelial cells. *J. Exp. Med.* **178,** 2077–2088.

48. Jakeman, L. B., Armanini, M., Phillips, H. S., and Ferrara, N. (1993) Developmental expression of binding sites and messenger ribonucleic acid for vascular endothelial growth factor suggests a role for this protein in vasculogenesis and angiogenesis. *Endocrinology* **133,** 848–859.

49. Breier, G., Albrecht, U., Sterrer, S., and Risau, W. (1992) Expression of vascular endothelial growth factor during embryonic angiogenesis and endothelial cell differentiation. *Development* **114,** 521–532.

50. Rockwell, P., Neufeld, G., Glassman, A., Caron, D., and Goldstein, N. (1995) In vitro neutralization of vascular endothelial growth factor activation of Flk-1 by a monoclonal antibody. *Mol. Cell. Diff.* **3,** 91–109.

51. Kendall, R. L. and Thomas, K. A. (1993) Inhibition of vascular endothelial cell growth factor activity by an endogenously encoded soluble receptor. *Proc. Natl. Acad. Sci. USA* **90,** 10,705–10,709.

52. Cushman, C., Escobedo, J., Parry, T. J., Kisich, K. O., Richardson, M. L., Speirer, K. S., et al. (1996) Ribozyme inhibition of VEGF-mediated endothelial cell proliferation in cell culture and VEGF-induced angiogenesis in a rat corneal model. Abstract from Angiogenesis Inhibitors and Other Novel Therapeutic Strategies for Ocular Diseases of Neovascularization.

53. Keyt, B. A., Nguyen, H. V., Berleau, L. T., Duarte, C. M., Park, J., Chen, H., and Ferrara, N. (1996) Identification of vascular endothelial growth factor determinants for binding KDR and FLT-1 receptors. *J. Biol. Chem.* **271,** 5638–5646.

54. Shalaby, F., Rossant, J., Yamaguchi, T. P., Gertsenstein, M., Wu, X. F., Breitman, M. L., and A. C. Schuh, A. C. (1995) Failure of blood-island formation and vasculogenesis in Flk-1-deficient mice. *Nature* **376,** 62–66.

55. Fong, G. H., Rossant, J., and Gertsenstein, M. (1995) Role of the Flt-1 receptor tyrosine kinase in regulating the assembly of vascular endothelium. *Nature* **376,** 66–70.

56. Carmeliet, P., Ferreira, V., Breier, G., Pollefeyt, S., Kieckens, L., Gertsenstein, M., et al. (1996) Abnormal blood vessel development and lethality in embryos lacking a single VEGF allele. *Nature* **380,** 435–439.

57. Ferrara, N., Carver-Moore, K., Chen, H., Dowd, M., Lu, L., O'Shea, K. S., et al. (1996) Heterozygous embryonic lethality induced by targeted inactivation of the VEGF gene. *Nature* **80,** 439–442.

58. Soker, S., Takashima, S., Miao, H. Q., Neufeld, G., and Klagsbrun, M. (1998) Neuropilin-1 is expressed by endothelial and tumor cells as an isoform-specific receptor for vascular endothelial growth factor. *Cell* **92,** 735–745.

59. Migdal, M., Huppertz, B., Tessler, S., Comforti, A., Shibuya, M., Reich, R., et al. (1998) Neuropilin-1 is a placenta growth factor-2 recpeter. *J. Biol. Chem.* **273,** 22,272–22,278.

60. Kitsukawa, T., Shimono, A., Kawakami, A., Kondoh, H., and Fujisawa, H. (1995) Overexpression of a membrane protein, neuropilin, in chimeric mice causes anomalies in the cadiovascular system, nervous system and limbs. *Development* **121,** 4309–4318.

61. Davis, S., Aldrich, T. H., Jones, P. F., Acheson, A., Compton, D. L., Jain, V., et al. (1996) Isolation of angiopoietin-1, a ligand for the TIE2 receptor, by secretion-trap expression cloning. *Cell* **87,** 1161–1169.

62. Suri, C., Jones, P. F., Patan, S., Bartunkova, S., Maisonpierre, P. C., Davis, S., et al. (1996) Requisite role of angiopoietin-1, a ligand for the TIE2 receptor, during embryonic angiogenesis. *Cell* **87,** 1171–1180.

63. Suri, C., McClain, J., Thurston, G., McDonald, D. M., Zhou, H., Oldmixon, E. H., et al. (1998) Increased vascularization in mice overexpressing angiopoietin-1. *Science* **282,** 468–471.

64. Maisonpierre, P. C., Suri, C., Jones, P. F., Bartunkova, S., Wiegand, S. J., Radziejewski, C., et al. (1997) Angiopoietin-2, a natural antagonist for Tie2 that disrupts in vivo angiogenesis. *Science* **277,** 55–60.

65. Partanen, J., Armstrong, E., Makela, T. P., Korhonen, J., Sandberg, M., Renkonen, R., et al. (1992) A novel endothelial cell surface receptor tyrosine kinase with extracellular epidermal growth factor homology domains. *Mol. Cell. Biol.* **12,** 1698–1707.

66. Dumont, D. J., Yamaguchi, T. P., Conlon, R. A., Rossant, J., and Breitman, M. L. (1992) *Tek*, a novel tyrosine kinase gene located on mouse chromosome 4, is expressed in endothelial cells and their presumptive precursors. *Oncogene* **7,** 1471–1480.

67. Schnürch, H. and Risau, W. (1993) Expression of tie-2, a member of a novel family of receptor tyrosine kinase, in the endothelial cell lineage. *Development* **119,** 957–968.

68. Ziegler, S. F., Bird, T. A., Schneringer, J. A., Schooley, L. A., and Baum, P. R. (1993) Molecular cloning and characterization of a novel receptor protein tyrosine kinase from human placenta. *Oncogene* **8,** 663–670.

69. Sato, T. N., Qin, Y., Kozak, C. A., and Audus, K. L. (1993). *tie-1* and *tie-2* define another class of putative receptor tyrosine kinase genes expressed in early embryonic vascular system. *Proc. Natl. Acad. Sci. USA* **90,** 9355–9358.

70. Korhonen, J., Polvi, A., Partanen, J., and Alitalo, K. (1994) The mouse *tie* receptor tyrosine kinase gene: expression during embryonic angiogenesis. *Oncogene* **9,** 395–403.

71. Korhonen, J., Partanen, J., Armstrong, E., Vaahtokari, A., Elenius, K., Jalkanen, M., and Alitalo, K. (1992) Enhanced expression of the tie receptor tyrosine kinase in endothelial cells during neovascularization. *Blood* **80,** 2548–2555.

72. Kaipainen, A., Vlaykova, T., Hatva, E., Boehling, T., Jekunen, A., Pyrhoenen, S., and Alitalo, K. (1994) Enhanced expression of the Tie receptor tyrosine kinase mRNA in the vascular endothelium of metastatic melanomas. *Cancer Res.* **54,** 6571–6577.

73. Dumont, D. J., Gradwohl, G., Fong, G.-H., Puri, M. C., Gertsenstein, M., Auerbach, A., and Breitman, M. L. (1994) Dominant-negative and targeted null mutations in the endothelial receptor tyrosine kinase, *tek*, reveal a critical role in vasculogenesis of the embryo. *Genes Dev.* **8,** 1897–1909.

74. Sato, T. N., Tozawa, Y., Deutsch, U., Wolburg-Buchholz, K., Fujiwara, Y., Gendron-Maguire, M., et al. (1995) Distinct roles of the receptor tyrosine kinases Tie-1 and Tie-2 in blood vessel formation. *Nature* **376,** 70–74.

75. Puri, M. C., Rossant, J., Alitalo, K., Bernstein, A., and Partanen, J. (1995) The receptor tyrosine kinase TIE is required for integrity and survival of vascular endothelial cells. *EMBO J.* **14,** 5884–5891.

76. Carpenter, G., and Wahl, M. I. (1990) The epidermal growth factor family, in *Peptide Growth Factors and Their Receptors*, vol. 1. (Sporn, M. B. and Roberts, A. B., eds.), Springer-Verlag, New York, pp. 69–171.

77. Purchio, A. F. and Plowman, G. D. (1993) Transforming growth factors, in *The Molecular Basis of Human Cancer* (Neel, B. and Kumar, R., eds.), Futura Publishing, Mount Kisco, NY.

78. Riese, D. J., 2nd, Bermingham, Y., van Raaij, T. M., Buckley, S., Plowman, G. D., and Stern, D. F. (1996) Betacellulin activates the epidermal growth factor receptor and erbB-4, and induces cellular response patterns distinct from those stimulated by epidermal growth factor or neuregulin-beta. *Oncogene* **12,** 345–353.

79. Shelly, M., Pinkas-Kramarski, R., Cuarino, B. C., Waterman, H., Wang, L.-M., Lyass, L., et al. (1998) Epiregulin is a potent pan-ErbB ligand that preferentially activates heterodimeric receptor complexes. *J. Biol. Chem.* **273,** 10,496–10,4505

80. Cohen, S. (1962) Isolation of a mouse submaxillary gland protein accelerating incisor eruption and eyelid opening in the newborn animal. *J. Biol. Chem.* **237,** 1562–1568.

81. Ullrich, A., Coussens, L., Hayflick, J. S., Dull, T. J., Gray, A., Tam, A. W., et al. (1984) Human epidermal growth factor receptor cDNA sequence and aberrant expression of the amplified gene in A431 epidermoid carcinoma cells. *Nature* **309,** 418–425.

82. Carraway, K. L., 3rd, Weber, J. L., Unger, M. J., Ledesma, J., Yu, N., Gassmann, M., and Lai, C. (1997) Neuregulin-2, a new ligand of ErbB3/ErbB4-receptor tyrosine kinases. *Nature* **387,** 512–516.

83. Schreiber, A. B., Winkler, M. E., and Derynck, R. (1986) Transforming growth factor-α: A more potent angiogenic mediator than epidermal growth factor. *Science* **232,** 1250–1253.

84. Yeh, J. and Yeh, Y. C. (1989) Transforming growth factor alpha and human cancer. *Biomed. Pharmacother.* **43,** 651–659.

85. Elder, J. T., Fisher, G., Lindquist, P. B., Bennett, G. L., Pittelkow, M. R., Coffey, Jr., R. J., et al. (1989) Overexpression of transforming growth factor a in psoriatic epidermis. *Science* **243,** 811–814.

86. Nelson, J., Allen, W. E., Scott, W. N., Bailie, J. R., Walker, B., McFerran, N. V., and Wilson, D. J. (1995) Murine epidermal growth factor (EGF) fragment (33-42) inhibits both EGF- and Laminin-dependent endothelial cell motility and angiogenesis. *Cancer Res.* **55,** 3772–3776.

87. Okamura, K., Morimoto, A., Hamanaka, R., Ono, M., Kohno, K., Uchida, Y., and Kuwano, M. (1992) A model system for tumor angiogenesis: Involvement of transforming growth factor-α in tube formation of human microvascular endothelial cells induced by esophageal cancer cells. *Biochem. Biophys. Res. Comm.* **186,** 1471–1479.

88. Mann, G. B., Fowler, K. J., Gabriel, A., Nice, E. C., Williams, L., and Dunn, A. R. (1993) Mice with a null mutation of the TGFα gene have abnormal skin architecture, wavy hair, and curly wiskers and often develop corneal inflammation. *Cell* **73,** 249–261.

89. Luetteke, N. C., Qiu, T. H., Peiffer, R. L., Oliver, P., Smithies, O., and Lee, D. C. (1993) TGFα deficiency results in hair follicle and eye abnormalities in targeted and Waved–1 mice. *Cell* **7,** 263–278.

90. Threadgill, D. W., Dlugosz, A. A., Hansen L. A., Tennenbaum, T., Lichti, U., Yee, D., et al. (1995) Targeted disruption of mouse EGF receptor: Effect of genetic back ground on mutant phenotype. *Science* **269,** 230–234.

91. Sibilia, M. and Wagner, E. F. (1995) Strain-dependent epithelial defects in mice lacking EGF receptor. *Science* **26,** 234–238.

92. Miettinen, P. J., Berger, J. E., Meneses, J., Phung, Y., Pedersen, R. A., Werb, Z., and Derynck, R. (1995) Epithelial immaturity and multiorgan failure in mice lacking epidermal growth factor receptor. *Nature* **376,** 337–341.

93. Luetteke, N. C., Phillips, H. K., Qiu, T. H., Copeland, N. G., Earl, H. S., Jenkins, N. A., and Lee, D. C. (1994) The mouse Waved-2 phenotype results from a point mutation in the EGF receptor tyrosine kinase. *Genes Dev.* **8,** 399–413.

94. Goldman, C. K., Kim, J., Wong, W.-L., King, V., Brock, T., and Gillespie, G. Y. (1993) Epidermal growth factor stimulates vascular endothelial growth factor production by human malignant glioma cells: a model of glioblastoma multiforme pathophysiology. *Mol. Biol. Cell.* **4,** 121–133.

95. Abramovitch, R, Neeman, M., Reich R., Stein I., Keshet E., Abraham, J., et al. (1998) Intercellular communication between vascular smooth muscle and endothelial cells mediated by heparin-binding epidermal growth factor-like growth factor and vascular endothelial growth factor. *FEBS Lett.* **425,** 441–471.

96. Burgess, W. H. and Maciag, T. (1989) The heparin-binding (fibroblast) growth factor family of proteins. *Ann. Rev. Biochem.* **58,** 575–606.

97. Jaye, M., Schlessinger, J., and Dionne, C. A. (1992) Fibroblast growth factor receptor tyrosine kinases: molecular analysis and signal transduction. *Biochim. Biophys. Acta.* **1135,** 185–99.

98. Gospodarowicz, D. (1975) Purification of a fibroblast growth factor from bovine pituitary. *J. Biol. Chem.* **250,** 2515–2520.

99. Thomas, K. A., Riley, M. C., Lemmon, S. K., Baglan, N. C., and Bradshaw, R. A. (1980) Brain fibroblast growth factor: nonidentity with myelin basic protein fragments. *J. Biol. Chem.* **255,** 5517–5520.

100. Jaye, M., Howk, R., Burgess, W., Ricca, G. A., Chiu, I. M., Ravera, M. W., et al. (1986) Human endothelial cell growth factor: cloning, nucleotide sequence, and chromosome localization. *Science* **233,** 541–545.

101. Abraham, J. A., Whang, J. L., Tumolo, A., Mergia, A., Friedman, J., Gospodarowicz, D., and Fiddes, J. C. (1986) Human fibroblast growth factor: nucleotide sequence and genomic organization. *EMBO J.* **5,** 2523–2528.

102. Kurokawa, T., Sasada, R., Iwane, M., and Igarashi, K. (1987) Cloning and expression of cDNA encoding human basic fibroblast growth factor. *FEBS Lett.* **213,** 189–194.

103. Smith, R., Peters, G., and Dickson, C. (1988) Multiple RNAs expressed from the int-2 gene in mouse embryonal carcinoma cell lines encode a protein with homology to fibroblast growth factors. *EMBO J.* **7,** 1013–1022.

104. Brookes, S., Smith, R., Casey, G., Dickson, C., and Peters, G. (1989) Sequence organization of the human int-2 gene and its expression in teratocarcinoma cells. *Oncogene* **4,** 429–436.

105. Delli-Bovi, P., Curatola, A. M., Kern, F. G., Greco, A., Ittmann, M., and Basilico, C. (1987) An oncogene isolated by transfection of Kaposi's sarcoma DNA encodes a growth factor that is a member of the FGF family. *Cell* **50,** 729–737.

106. Taira, M., Yoshida, T., Miyagawa, K., Sakamoto, H., Terada, M., and Sugimura, T. (1987) cDNA sequence of human transforming gene hst and identification of the coding sequence required for transforming activity. *Proc. Natl. Acad. Sci. USA* **84,** 2980–2984.

107. Yoshida, T., Miyagawa, K., Odagiri, H., Sakamoto, H., Little, P. F., Terada, M., and Sugimura, T. (1987) Genomic sequence of hst, a transforming gene encoding a protein homologous to fibroblast growth factors and the int-2-encoded protein. *Proc. Natl. Acad. Sci. USA* **84,** 7305–7309.

108. Zhan, X., Bates, B., Hu, X. G., and Goldfarb, M. (1988) The human FGF-5 oncogene encodes a novel protein related to fibroblast growth factors. *Mol. Cell. Biol.* **8,** 3487–3495.

109. Haub, O., Drucker , B., and Goldfarb, M. (1990) Expression of the murine fibroblast growth factor 5 gene in the adult central nervous system. *Proc. Natl. Acad. Sci. USA* **87,** 8022–8026.

110. Bates, B., Hardin, J., Zhan, X., Drickamer, K., and Goldfarb, M. (1991) Biosynthesis of human fibroblast growth factor-5. *Mol. Cell. Biol.* **11,** 1840–1845.
111. Marics, I., Adelaide, J., Raybaud, F., Mattei, M. G., Coulier, F., Planche, J., et al. (1989) Characterization of the HST-related FGF. 6 gene, a new member of the fibroblast growth factor gene family.
Oncogene **4,** 335–340.
112. Finch, P. W., Rubin, J. S., Miki, T., Ron, D., and Aaronson, S. A. (1989) Human KGF is FGF-related
with properties of a paracrine effector of epithelial cell growth. *Science* **245,** 752–755.
113. Payson, R. A., Wu, J., Liu, Y., and Chiu, I. M. (1996) The human FGF-8 gene localizes on chromosome
10q24 and is subjected to induction by androgen in breast cancer cells. *Oncogene* **13,** 47–53.
114. Tanaka, A., Miyamoto, K., Minamino, N., Takeda, M., Sato, B., Matsuo, H., and Matsumoto, K. (1992)
Cloning and characterization of an androgen-induced growth factor essential for the androgen-depen-
dent growth of mouse mammary carcinoma cells. *Proc. Natl. Acad. Sci. USA* **89,** 8928–8932.
115. Miyamoto, M., Naruo, K.-I., Seko, C., Matsumoto, S., Kondo, T., and Kurokawa, T. (1993) Molecular
cloning of a novel cytokine cDNA encoding the ninth member of the fibroblast growth factor family,
which has a unique secretion property. *Mol. Cell. Biol.* **13,** 4251–4259.
116. Coulier, F., Pontarotti, P., Roubin, R., Hartung, H., Goldfarb, M., and Birnbaum, D. (1997) Of worms
and men: an evolutionary perspective on the fibroblast growth factor (FGF) and FGF receptor families.
J. Mol. Evol. **44,** 43–56.
117. Smallwood, P. M., Munoz-Sanjuan, I., Tong, P., Macke, J. P., Hendry, S. H. C., Gilbert, D. J., et al.
(1996) Fibroblast growth factor (FGF) homologous factors: new members of the FGF family implicated in nervous system development. *Proc. Natl. Acad. Sci. USA* **93,** 9850–9857.
118. Ornitz, D. M., Xu, J., Colvin, J. S., McEwen, D. G., MacArthur, C. A., Coulier, F., et al. (1996) Receptor
specificity of the fibroblast growth factor family. *J. Biol. Chem.* **271,** 15,292–15,297.
119. Isacchi, A., Bergonzoni, L., and Sarmientos, P. (1990) Complete sequence of a human receptor for
acidic and basic fibroblast growth factors. *Nucleic Acids Res.* **18,** 1906.
120. Dionne, C. A., Crumley, G., Bellot, F., Kaplow, J. M., Searfoss, G., Ruta, M., et al. (1990) Cloning and
expression of two distinct high-affinity receptors cross-reacting with acidic and basic fibroblast growth
factors. *EMBO J.* **9,** 2685–2692.
121. Keegan, K., Johnson, D. E., Williams, L. T., and Hayman, M. J. (1991) Isolation of an additional member
of the fibroblast growth factor receptor family, FGFR–3. *Proc. Natl. Acad. Sci. USA* **88,** 1095–1099.
122. Partanen, J., Makela, T. P., Alitalo, R., Lehvaslaiho, H., and Alitalo, K. (1990) Putative tyrosine kinases
expressed in K562 human leukemia cells. *Proc. Natl. Acad. Sci. USA* **87,** 8913–8917.
123. Partanen, J., Makela, T. P., Eerola, E., Korhonen, J., Hirvonen, H., Claesson-Welsh, L., and Alitalo,
K. (1991) FGFR-4, a novel acidic fibroblast growth factor receptor with a distinct expression pattern.
EMBO J. **10,** 1347–1354.
124. Burrus, L. W., Zuber, M. E., Lueddecke, B. A., and Olwin, B. B. (1992) Identification of a cysteine-
rich receptor for fibroblast growth factor. *Mol. Cell. Biol.* **12,** 5600–5609.
125. Steegmaier, M., Levinovitz, A., Isenmann, S., Borges, E., Lenter, M., Kocher, H. P., et al. (1995) The
E-selectin-ligand ESL-1 is a variant of a receptor for fibroblast growth factor. *Nature* **373,** 615–620.
126. Ruta, M., Burgess, W., Givol, D., Epstein, J., Neiger, N., Kaplow, J., et al. (1989) Receptor for acidic
fibroblast growth factor is related to the tyrosine kinase encoded by the fms-like gene (FLG). *Proc.
Natl. Acad. Sci. USA* **86,** 8722–8726.
127. Kornbluth, S., Paulson, K. E., and H., Hanafusa, H. (1988) Novel tyrosine kinase identified by
phosphotyrosine antibody screening of cDNA libraries. *Mol. Cell. Biol.* **8,** 5541–5544.
128. Pasquale, E. B. and Singer, S. J. (1989) Identification of a developmentally regulated protein-tyrosine
kinase by using anti-phosphotyrosine antibodies to screen a cDNA expression library. *Proc. Natl.
Acad. Sci. USA* **86,** 5449–5453.
129. Holtrich, U., Brauninger, A., Strebhardt, K., and Rubsamen-Waigmann, H. (1991) Two additional protein-tyrosine kinases expressed in human lung: fourth member of the fibroblast growth factor receptor family and an intracellular protein–tyrosine kinase. *Proc. Natl. Acad. Sci. USA* **88,** 10,411–10,415.
130. Givol, D. and Yayon, A. (1992) Complexity of FGF receptors: genetic basis for structural diversity and
functional specificity. *FASEB J.* **6,** 3362–3369.
131. Johnson, D. E. and Williams, L. T. (1993) Structural and functional diversity in the FGF receptor
multigene family. *Adv. Cancer Res.* **60,** 1–41.
132. Green, P. J., Walsh, F. S., and Doherty, P. (1996) Promiscuity of fibroblast growth factor receptors.
BioEssays **18,** 639–646.

133. Nabel, E. G., Yang, Z.-Y., Plautz, G., Forough, R., Zhan, X., Haudenschild, C. C., et al. (1993) Recombinant fibroblast growth factor-1 promotes intimal hyperplasia and angiogenesis in arteries in vivo. *Nature* **362,** 844–846.

134. Gray, J. L., Kang, S. S., Zenni, G. C., Kim, D. U., Burgess, W. H., Drohan,W., et al. (1994) FGF-1 affixation stimulates ePTFE endothelialization without intimal hyperplasia. *J. Surg. Res.* **57,** 596–612.

135. Mignatti, P., Tsuboi, R., Robbins, E., and Rifkin, D. B. (1989) In Vitro angiogenesis on the human amniotic membrane: requirement for basic fibroblast growth factor-induced proteinase. *J. Cell Biol.* **108,** 671–682.

136. Sato, Y., Shimada, T., and Takaki, R. (1991) Autocrinological role of basic fibroblast growth factor on tube formation of vascular endothelial cells in vitro. *Biochem. Biophys. Res. Comm.* **180,** 1098–11,102.

137. Li, L.-Y., Safran, M., Aviezer, D., Boehlen, P., Seddon, A. P., and Yayon, A. (1994) Diminished heparin binding of a basic fibroblast growth factor mutant is associated with reduced receptor binding, mitogenesis, plasminogen activator induction, and in vitro angiogenesis. *Biochem.* **33,** 10,999–1007.

138. Parlow, M. H., Bolender, D. L., Kokan-Moore, N. P., and Lough, J. (1991) Localization of bFGF-like proteins as punctate inclusions in the preseptation myocardium of the chicken embryo. *Dev. Biol.* **146,** 139–147.

139. Sugi, Y., Sasse, J., Barron, M., and Lough, J. (1995) Developmental expression of fibroblast growth factor receptor-1 (cek; flg) during heart development. *Dev. Dyn.* **202,** 115–125.

140. Lindner, V. and Reidy, M. A. (1993) Expression of basic fibroblast growth factor and its receptor by smooth muscle cells and endothelium in injured rat arteries. An en face study. *Circ. Res.* **73,** 589–595.

141. Robinson, M. L., MacMillan-Crow, L. A., Thompson, J. A., and Overbeek, P. A. (1995) Expression of a truncated FGF receptor results in defective lens development in transgenic mice. *Development* **121,** 3959–3967.

142. Chow, R. L., Roux, G. D., Roghani, M., Palmer, M. A., Rifkin, D. B., Moscatelli, D. A., and Lang, R. A. (1995) FGF suppresses apoptosis and induces differentiation of fibre cells in the mouse lens. *Development* **121,** 4383–4393.

143. Werner, S., Weinberg, W., Liao, X., Peters, K. G., Blessing, M., Yuspa, S. H., et al. (1993) Targeted expression of a dominant-negative FGF receptor mutant in the epidermis of transgenic mice reveals a role of FGF in keratinocyte organization and differentiation. *EMBO J.* **12,** 2635–2643.

144. Peters, K., Werner, S., Liao, X., Wert, S., Whitsett, J., and Williams, L. (1994) Targeted expression of a dominant negative FGF receptor blocks branching morphogenesis and epithelial differentiation of the mouse lung. *EMBO J.* **13,** 3296–3301.

145. Yamaguchi, T. P., Harpal, K., Henkemeyer, M., and Rossant, J. (1994) *fgfr1* is required for embryonic growth and mesodermal patterning during mouse gastrulation. *Genes Dev.* **8,** 3032–3044.

146. Deng, C.-X., Wynshaw-Boris, A., Shen, M. M., Daugherty, C., Ornitz, D. M., and Leder, P. (1994) Murine FGFR-1 is required for early postimplantation growth and axial organization. *Genes Dev.* **8,** 3045–3057.

147. Nakamura, T., Nawa, K., and Ichihara, A. (1984) Partial purification and characterization of hepatocyte growth factor from serum of hepatectomized rats. *Biochem. Biophys. Res. Commun.* **122,** 1450–1459.

148. Nakamura, T., Nishizawa, T., Hagiya, M., Seki, T., Shimonishi, M., Sugimura, A., et al. (1989) Molecular cloning and expression of human hepatocyte growth factor. *Nature* **342,** 440–443.

149. Miyazawa, K., Tsubouchi, H., Naka, D., Takahashi, K., Okigaki, M., Arakaki, N., et al. (1989) Molecular cloning and sequence analysis of cDNA for human hepatocyte growth factor. *Biochem. Biophys. Res. Comm.* **163,** 967–973.

150. Stoker, M., Gherardi, E., Perryman, M., and Gray, J. (1987) Scatter factor is a fibroblast derived modulator of epithelial cell mobility. *Nature* **327,** 239–242.

151. Gherardi, E. and Stoker, M. (1990) Hepatocytes and scatter factor. *Nature* **346,** 228.

152. Weidner, K. M., Arakaki, N., Hartmann, G., Vandekerckhove, J., Weingart, S., Rieder, H., et al. (1991) Evidence for the identity of human scatter factor and human hepatocyte growth factor. *Proc. Natl. Acad. Sci. USA* **88,** 7001–7005.

153. Higashio, K., Shima, N., Goto, M., Itagaki, Y., Nagao, M., Yasuda, H., and Morinaga , T. (1990) Identity of a tumor cytotoxic factor from human fibroblasts and hepatocyte growth factor. *Biochem. Biophys. Res. Comm.* **170,** 397–404.

154. Shima, N., Nagao, M., Ogaki, F., Tsuda, E., Murakami, A., and Higashio, K. (1991) Tumor cytotoxic factor/hepatocyte growth factor from human fibroblasts: cloning of its cDNA, purification and characterization of recombinant protein. *Biochem. Biophys. Res. Comm.* **180,** 1151–1158.

155. Rubin, J. S., Chan, A. M.-L., Bottaro, D. P., Burgess, W. H., Taylor, W. G., Cech, A. C., et al. (1991) A broad-spectrum human lung fibroblast-derived mitogen is a variant of hepatocyte growth factor. *Proc. Natl. Acad. Sci. USA* **88,** 415–419.

156. Chirgadze, D. Y., Hepple, J., Byrd, R. A., Sowdhamini, R., Blundell, T. L., and Gherardi, E. (1998) Insights into the structure of hepatocyted growth factor/scatter factor (HGF/SJ) and implications for receptor activation. *FEBS Lett.* **430,** 126–129.

157. Cooper, C. S., Park, M., Blair, D. G., Tainsky, M. A., Huebner, K., Croce, C. M., and Vande Woude, G. F. (1984) Molecular cloning of a new transforming gene from a chemically transformed human cell line. *Nature* **311,** 29–33.

158. Park, M., Dean, M., Cooper, C. S., Schmidt, M., O'Brien, S. J., Blair, D. G., and Vande Woude, G. F. (1986) Mechanism of *met* oncogene activation. *Cell* **45,** 895–904.

159. Park, M., Dean, M., Kaul, K., Braun, M. J., Gonda, M. A., and Vande Woude, G. (1987) Sequence of *MET* protooncogene cDNA has features characteristic of the tyrosine kinase family of growth-factor receptors. *Proc. Natl. Acad. Sci. USA* **84,** 6379–6383.

160. Bottaro, D. P., Rubin, J. S., Faletto, D. L., Chan, A. M.-L., Kmiecik, T. E., Vande Woude, G. F., and Aaronson, S. A. (1991) Identification of the hepatocyte growth factor receptor as the *c-met* proto-oncogene product. *Science* **251,** 802–804.

161. Matsumoto, K. and Nakamura, T. (1996) Emerging multipotent aspects of hepatocyte growth factor. *J. Biochem.* **119,** 591–600.

162. Schmidt, C., Bladt, F., Goedecke, S., Brinkmann, V., Zschiesche, W., Sharpe, M., et al. (1995) Scatter factor/hepatocyte growth factor is essential for liver development. *Nature* **373,** 699–702.

163. Uehara, Y., Minowa, O., Mori, C., Shiota, K., Kuno, J., Noda, T., and Kitamura, N. (1995) Placental defect and embryonic lethality in mice lacking hepatocyte growth factor/scatter factor. *Nature* **373,** 702–705.

164. Bladt, F., Riethmacher, D., Isenmann, S., Aguzzi, A., and Birchmeier, C. (1995) Essential role for the c-*met* receptor in the migration of myogenic precursor cells into the limb bud. *Nature* **376,** 768–771.

165. Bussolino, F., DiRenzo, M. F., Ziche, M., Bocchietto, E., Olivero, M., Naldini, L., et al. (1992) Hepatocyte growth factor is a potent angiogenic factor which stimulates endothelial cell motility and growth. *J. Cell Biol.* **119,** 629–641.

166. Grant, D. S., Kleinman, H. K., Goldberg, I. D., Bhargava, M. M., Nickoloff, B. J., Kinsella, J. L., et al. (1993) Scatter factor induces blood vessel formation in vivo. *Proc. Natl. Acad. Sci.* **90,** 1937–1941.

167. Silvagno, F., Follenzi, A., Arese, M., Prat, M., Giraudo, E., Gaudino, G., et al. (1995) In vivo activation of *met* tyrosine kinase by heterodimeric hepatocyte growth factor molecule promotes angiogenesis. *Athero. Throm. Vasc. Biol.* **15,** 1857–1865.

168. Camussi, G., Montrucchio, G., Lupia, E., Soldi, R., Comoglio, P. M., and Bussolino, F. (1997) Angiogenesis induced *in vivo* by hepatocyte growth factor is mediated by platelet-activating factor synthesis from macrophages. *J. Immunol.* **158,** 1302–1309.

169. Bartley, T. D., Hunt, R. W., Welcher, A. A., Boyle, W. J., Parker, V. P., Lindberg, R. A., et al. (1994) B61 is a ligand for the ECK receptor protein-tyrosine kinase. *Nature* **368,** 558–560.

170. Shao, H., Pandey, A., O'Shea, K. D., Seldin, M., and Dixit, V. M. (1995) Characterization of B61, the ligand for the Eck receptor protein-tyrosine kinase. *J. Biol. Chem.* **270,** 5636–5641.

171. Lindberg, R. A. and Hunter, T. (1997) cDNA cloning and characterization of eck, and epithelial cell receptor protein-tyrosine kinase in the eph/elk family or protein kinases. *Mol. Cell. Biol.* **10,** 6316–6324.

172. Ganju, P., Shigemoto, K., Brennan, J., Entwistle, A., and Reith, A. D. (1994) The Eck receptor tyrosine kinase is implicated in pattern formation during gastrulation, hindbrain segmentation and limb development. *Oncogene* **9,** 1613–1624.

173. Takahashi, H. and Ikeda, T. (1995) Molecular cloning and expression of rat and mouse B61 gene: implications on organogenesis. *Oncogene* **11,** 879–883.

174. Pandey, A., Shao, H., Marks, R. M., Polverini, P. J., and Dixit, V. M. (1995) Role of B61, the ligand for the Eck receptor tyrosine kinase, in TNF-α-induced angiogenesis. *Science* **268,** 567–569.

175. Holzman, L. B., Marks, R. M., and Dixit, V. M. (1990) A novel immediate-early response gene of enothelium is induced by cytokines and encodes a secreted protein. *Mol. Cell. Biol.* **10,** 5830–5888.

176. Leibovich, S. J., Polverini, P. J., Shepard, H. M., Wisemann, D. M., Shively, V., and Nuseir, N. (1987) Macrophage-induced angiogenesis is mediated by tumor necrosis factor-α. *Nature* **329,** 630–632.

177. Westermark, B. and Wasteson, A. (1976) A platelet factor stimulating human normal glial cells. *Exp. Cell. Res.* **98,** 170–174.

178. Ross, R., Raines, E. W., and Bowen-Pope, D. F. (1986) The biology of platelet-derived growth factor. *Cell* **46,** 155–169.

179. Nishimura, J., Huang, J. S., and Deuel, T. F. (1982) Platelet-derived growth factor stimulates tyrosine-specific protein kinase activity in Swiss mouse 3T3 cell membranes. *Proc. Natl. . Acad. Sci. USA* **79,** 4303–4307.

180. Cooper, J. A., Bowen-Pope, D. F., Raines, E., Ross, R., and Hunter, T. (1982) Similar effects of of platelet-derived growth factor and epidermal growth factor on the phosphorylation of tyrosine in cellular proteins. *Cell* **31,** 263–273.

181. Röhnstrand, L., Beckmann, M. P., Faulders, B., Östman, A., Ek, B., and Heldin, C. H. (1987) Structure of the receptor for platelet-derived growth factor from porcine uterus. *J. Biol. Chem.* **262,** 2929–2932.

182. Yarden, Y., Escobedo, J. A., Kuang, W.-J., Yang-Feng, T. L., Daniel, T. O., Tremble, P. M., et al. (1986) Structure of the receptor for platelet-derived growth factor helps define a family of closely related growth factor receptors. *Nature* **323,** 226–232.

183. Hart, C. E., Forstrom, J. W., Kelly, J. D., Seifert, R. A., Smith, R. A., Ross, R., et al. (1988) Two classes of PDGF receptor recognize different isoforms of PDGF. *Science* **240,** 1529–1531.

184. Heldin, C. H., Hammacher, A., Nister, M., and Westermark, B. (1988) Structural and functional aspects of platelet-derived growth factor. *Br. J. Cancer* **57,** 591–593.

185. Claessen-Welsh, L. (1993) PDGF receptors: Cytokines, structure and mechanism of action in *Biology of Platelet-Derived Growth Factor*, vol. 5(Westermark, B., and Sorg, C. ed.), Basel, Karfger, pp. 31–43.

186. Holmgren, L., Glaser, A., Pfeifer-Ohlsson, S., and Ohlsson, R. (1991) Angiogenesis during human extraembryonic development involves the spatiotemporal control of PDGF ligand and receptor gene expression. *Dev.* **113,** 749–754.

187. Sundberg, C., Ljungström, C., Lindmark, G., Gerdin, B., and Rubin, K. (1993) Microvascular pericytes express platelet-derived growth factor-β receptors in human healing wounds and colorectal adenocarcinoma. *Am. J. Pathol.* **143,** 1377–1388.

188. Plate, K. H., Breier, G., Farrell, C. L., and Risau, W. (1992) Platelet-derived growth factor receptor-beta is induced during tumor development and upregulated during tumor progression in endothelial cells in human gliomas. *Lab Invest.* **67,** 529–534.

189. Battegay, E. J., Rupp, J., Iruela-Arispe, L., Sage, E. H., and Pech, M. (1994) PDGF-BB modulates endothelial proliferation and angiogenesis in vitro via PDGF β-receptors. *J. Cell Biol.* **125,** 917–928.

190. Marx, M., Perlmutter, R. A., and Madri, J. A. (1994) Modulation of platelet-derived growth factor receptor expression in microvascular endothelial cells during in vitro angiogenesis. *J. Clin. Invest.* **93,** 131–139.

191. Sato, N., Beitz, J. G., Kato, J., Yamamoto, M., Clark, J. W., Calabresi, P., and Frackelton, Jr., A. (1993) Platelet-derived growth factor indirectly stimulates angiogenesis in vitro. *Amer. J. Pathol.* **142,** 1119–1130.

192. Brogi, E., Wu, T., Namiki, A., and Isner, J. M. (1994) Indirect angiogenic cytokines upregulate VEGF and bFGF gene expression in vascular smooth muscle cells, whereas hypoxia upregulates VEGF expression only. *Circulation* **90,** 649–652.

193. Tsai, J.-C., Goldman, C. K., and Gillespie, G. Y. (1995) Vascular endothelial growth factor in human glioma cell lines: induced secretion by EGF, PDGF-BB, and bFGF. *J. Neurosurg.* **82,** 864–873.

194. Nicosia, R. F., Nicosia, S. V., and Smith, M. (1994) Vascular endothelial growth factor, platelet-derived growth factor, and insulin-like growth factor-1 promote rat aortic angiogenesis in vitro. *Am. J. Pathol.* **145,** 1023–1029.

195. Krywicki, R. F. and Yee, D. (1992) The insulin-like growth factor family of ligands, receptors, and binding proteins. *Breast Cancer Res. Treat.* **22,** 7–19.

196. Hansson, H. A., Brandsten, C., Lossing, C., and Petruson, K. (1989) Transient expression of insulin-like growth factor: immunoreactivity by vascular cells during angiogenesis. *Exp. Mol. Path.* **50,** 125–138.

197. Kluge, A., Zimmermann, R., Munkel, B., Mohri, M., Sack, S., Schaper, J., and Schaper, W. (1995) Insulin-like growth factor I is involved in inflammation linked angiogenic processes after microembolisation in porcine heart. *Cardiovasc. Res.* **29,** 407–415.

198. Nakao-Hayashi, J., Ito, H., Kanayasu, T., Morita, I., and Murota, S. (1992) Stimulatory effects of insulin and insulin-like growth factor I on migration and tube formation by vascular endothelial cells. *Atherosclerosis* **92,** 141–149.

199. Grant, M. B., Caballero, S., and Millard, W. J. (1993) Inhibition of IGF-1 and b-FGF stimulated growth of human retinal endothelial cells by the somatostatin analogue, octreotide: a potential treatment for ocular neovascularization. *Reg. Peptides* **48,** 267–278.

200. Grant, M. B., Mames, R. N., Fitzgerald, C., Ellis, E. A., Aboufriekha, M., and Guy, J. (1993) Insulin-like growth factor I acts as an angiogenic agent in rabbit cornea and retina: comparative studies with basic fibroblast growth factor. *Diabetologia* **36,** 282–291.

201. Folkman, J. (1990) What is the evidence that tumors are angiogenesis dependent? *J. Natl. Cancer Inst.* **82,** 4–6.

202. Folkman, J., Watson, K., Ingber, D., and Hanahan, D. (1989) Induction of angiogenesis during the transition from hyperplasia to neoplasia. *Nature* **339,** 58–61.
203. Plate, K. H. and Risau, W. (1995) Angiogenesis in malignant gliomas. *GLIA* **15,** 339–347.
204. Abdulrauf, S., Edvardsen, K., Ho, K. L., Yang, X. Y., Rock J. P., and Rosenblum, M. L. (1998) Vascular endothelial growth factor expression and vascular density as prognostic markers of survival in patients with low-grade astrocytoma. *J. Neurosur.* **88,** 513–520.
205. Horak, E. R., Leek, R., Klenk, N., LeJeune, S., Smith, K., Stuart, N., et al. (1992) Angiogenesis, assessed by platelet/endothelial cell adhesion molecule antibodies, as indicator of node metastases and survival in breast cancer. *Lancet* **340,** 1120–1124.
206. Dickinson, A. J., Fox, S. B., Persad, R. A., Hollyer, J., Sibley, G. N. A., and Harris, A. L. (1994) Quantification of anigiogenesis as an independent predictor of prognosis in invasive bladder carcinomas. *Br. J. Urol.* **74,** 762–766.
207. Takahashi, Y., Kitadai, Y., Bucana, C. D., Cleary, K. R., and Ellis, L. M. (1995) Expression of vascular endothelial growth factor and its receptor, KDR, correlates with vascularity, metastasis, and proliferation of human colon cancer. *Cancer Res.* **55,** 3964–3968.
208. Obermair, A., Wanner, C., Bilgi, S., Speiser, P., Kaider, A., Reinthaller, A., et al. (1998) Tumor angiogenesis in stage IB cervical cancer: correlation of microvessel density with survival. *Am. J. Obstet. Gynecol.* **178,** 314–319.
209. Kirschner, C. V., Alanis-Amezcua, J. M., Martin, V. G., Luna, N., Morgan, E., Yang, J. J., and Yordan, E. L. (1996) Angiogenesis factor in endometrial carcinoma: a new prognostic indicator? *Am. J. Obstet. Gynecol.* **174,** 1879–1882.
210. Salvesen, H. B., Iversen, O. E., and Akslen, L. A. (1998) Independent prognostic importance of microvessel density in endometrial carcinoma. *Br. J. Cancer* **77,** 1140–1141.
211. Wagastuma, S., Konno, R., Sato, S., and Yajima, A. (1998) Tumor angiogenesis, hepatocyte growth factor, and c-Met expression in endometrial carcinoma. *Cancer* **82,** 520–530.
212. Claffey, K. P., Brown, L. F., del Aguila, L. F., Tognazzi, K., Yeo, K. T., Manseau, E. J., and Dvorak, H. F. (1996) Expression of vascular permeability factor/vascular endothelial growth factor by melanoma cells increases tumor growth, angiogenesis, and experimental metastasis. *Cancer Res.* **56,** 172–181.
213. Masood, R., Cai, J., Zheng, T., Smith, D. L., Naidu, Y., and Gill, P. S. (1997) Vascular endothelial growth factor/vascular permeability factor is an autocrine growth factor for AIDS-Kaposi sarcoma. *Proc. Natl. Acad. Sci. USA* **94,** 979–984.
214. Myoken, Y., Kayada, Y., Okamoto, T., Kan, M., Sato, G. H., and Sato, J. D. (1991) Vascular endothelial cell growth factor (VEGF) produced by A-431 human epidermoid carcinoma cells and identification of VEGF membrane binding sites. *Proc. Natl. Acad. Sci. USA* **88,** 5819–5823.
215. Plate, K. H., Breier, G., Weich, H. A., and Risau, W. (1992) Vascular endothelial growth factor is a potential tumour angiogenesis factor in human gliomas in vivo. *Nature* **359,** 845–848.
216. Plate, K. H., Breier, G., Weich, H. A., Mennel, H. D., and Risau, W. (1994) Vascular endothelial growth factor and glioma angiogenesis: coordinate induction of VEGF receptors, distribution of VEGF protein and possible in vivo regulatory mechanisms. *Int. J. Cancer* **59,** 520–529.
217. Hatva, E., Böhling, T., Jääskeläinen, J., Persico, G., Haltia, M., and Alitalo, K. (1996) Vascular growth factors and receptors in capillary hemangioblastomas and hemangiopericytomas. *Am. J. Pathol.* **148,** 763–775.
218. Toi, M., Hoshina, S., Takayanagi, T., and Tominaga, T. (1994) Association of vascular endothelial growth factor expression with tumor angiogenesis and with early relapse in primary breast cancer. *Jpn. J. Cancer Res.* **85,** 1045–1049.
219. Anan, K., Morisaki, T., Katano, M., Ikubo, A., Kitsuki, H., Uchiyama, A., et al. (1996) Vascular endothelial growth factor and platelet-derived growth factor are potential angiogenic and metastatic factors in human breast cancer. *Surgery* **119,** 333–339.
220. Yoshiji, H., Gomez, D. E., Shibuya, M., and Thorgeirsson, U. P. (1996) Expression of vascular endothelial growth factor, its receptor, and other angiogenic factors in human breast cancer. *Cancer Res.* **56,** 2013–2016.
221. Brown, L. F., Berse, B., Jackman, R. W., Tognazzi, K., Manseau, E. J., Senger, D. R., and Dvorak, H. F. (1993) Expression of vascular permeability factor (vascular endothelial growth factor) and its receptors in adenocarcinomas of the gastrointestinal tract. *Cancer Res.* **53,** 4727–4735.
222. Takahashi, A., Sasaki, H., Kim, S. J., Tobisu, K., Kakizoe, T., Tsukamoto, T., et al. (1994) Markedly increased amounts of messenger RNAs for vascular endothelial growth factor and placenta growth factor in renal cell carcinoma associated with angiogenesis. *Cancer Res.* **54,** 4233–4237.

223. Shweiki, D., Itin, A., Soffer, D., and Keshet, E. (1992) Vascular endothelial growth factor induced by hypoxia may mediate hypoxia-initiated angiogenesis. *Nature* **359**, 843–845.
224. Tokunaga, T., Oshika, Y., Abe Y., Ozeki, Y., Sadahiro, S., Kijima, H., et al. (1998) Vascular endothelial growth factor (VEGF) mRNA isoform expression pattern is correlated with liver metastasis and poor prognosis in colon cancer. *Br. J. Cancer* **77**, 998–1002.
225. Salven, P., Mäenpää, H., Orpana, A., Alitalo, K., and Joensuu, H. (1997) Serum vascular endothelial growth factor is often elevated in disseminated cancer. *Clin. Cancer Res.* **3**, 647–651.
226. Saleh, M., Stacker, S. A., and Wilks, A. F. (1996) Inhibition of growth of C6 glioma cells in vivo by expression of antisense vascular endothelial growth factor sequence. *Cancer Res.* **56**, 393–401.
227. Cheng, S.-Y., Huang, H.-J. S., Nagane, M., Ji, X.-D., Wang, D., Shih, C. C.-Y., et al. (1996) Suppression of Glioblastoma Angiogenicity and Tumorigenicity by Inhibition of Endogenous Expression of Vascular Endothelial Growth Factor. *Proc. Natl. Acad. Sci. USA* **93**, 8502–8507.
228. Kim, K. J., Li, B., Winer, J., Armanini, M., Gillett, N., Phillips, H. S., and Ferrara, N. (1993) Inhibition of vascular endothelial growth factor-induced angiogenesis suppresses tumour growth in vivo. *Nature* **362**, 841–844.
229. Asano, M., Yukita, A., Matsumoto, T., Kondo, S., and Suzuki, H. (1995) Inhibition of tumor growth and metastasis by an immunoneutralizing monoclonal antibody to human vascular endothelial growth factor/vascular permeability factor 121. *Cancer Res.* **55**, 5296–5301.
230. Warren, R. S., Yuan, H., Matli, M. R., Gillett, N. A., and Ferrara, N. (1995) Regulation by vascular endothelial growth factor of human colon cancer tumorigenesis in a mouse model of experimental liver metastasis. *J. Clin. Invest.* **95**, 1789–1797.
231. Millauer, B., Shawver, L. K., Plate, K. H., Risau, W., and Ullrich, A. (1994) Glioblastoma growth inhibited in vivo by a dominant-negative Flk-1 mutant. *Nature* **367**, 576–579.
232. Millauer, B., Longhi, M. P., Plate, K. H., Shawver, L. K., Risau, W., Ullrich, A., and Strawn, L. M. (1996) Dominant-negative inhibition of Flk-1 suppresses the growth of many tumor types in vivo. *Cancer Res.* **56**, 1615–1620.
233. Rockwell, P., Witte, L., Hicklin, D., Pytowski, B., and Goldstein, N. I. (1997) Antitumor activity of anti-flk-1 monoclonal antibodies. *Proc. Am. Assoc. Cancer Res.* **38**, 266.
234. Strawn, L. M., McMahon, G., App, H., Schreck, R., Kuchler, W. R., Longhi, M. P., et al. (1996) Flk-1 as a target for tumor growth inhibition. *Cancer Res.* **56**, 3540–3545.
235. Hatva, E., Kaipainen, A., Mentula, P., Jaaskelainen, J., Paetau, A., Haltia, M., and Alitalo, K. (1995) Expression of endothelial cell-specific receptor tyrosine kinases and growth factors in human brain tumors. *Am. J. Pathol.* **146**, 368–378.
236. Salven, P., Joensuu, H., Heikkila, P., Matikainen, M. T., Wasenius, V. M., Alanko, A., and Alitalo, K. (1996) Endothelial tie growth factor receptor provides antigenic marker for assessment of breast cancer angiogenesis. *Br. J. Cancer* **74**, 69–72.
237. Peters, K. G., Coogan, A., Berry D., Marks, J., Iglehart, J. D., Kontos, C. D., et al. Expression of Tie2/Tek in breast tumour vasculature provides a new marker for evaluation of tumour angiogenesis. *Br J. Cancer* **77**, 51–61.
238. Vikkula, M., Boon, L. M., Carraway, K. L. 3rd, Calvert, J. T., Diamonti, A. J., Goumnerov, B., et al. (1996) Vascular dysmorphogenesis caused by an activating mutation in the receptor tyrosine kinase TIE2. *Cell* **87**, 1181–1190.
239. Singh, R. K., Llansa, N., Bucana, C. D., Sanchez, R., Koura, A., and Fidler, I. J. (1996) Cell density-dependent regulation of basic fibroblast growth factor expression in human renal cell carcinoma cells. *Cell Growth Diff.* **7**, 397–404.
240. Nakamoto, T., Chang, C. S., Li, A. K., and Chodak, G. W. (1992) Basic fibroblast growth factor in human prostate cancer cells. *Cancer Res.* **52**, 571–577.
241. Yamaguchi, F., Saya, H., Bruner, J. M., and Morrison, R. S. (1994) Differential expression of two fibroblast growth factor-receptor genes is associated with malignant progression in human astrocytomas. *Proc. Natl. Acad. Sci. USA* **91**, 484–488.
242. de Jong, J. S., van Diest, P. J., van der Valk, P., and Baak, J. P. (1998) Expression of growth factors, growth-inhibiting factors, and their receptors in invasive breast cancer. II: correlations with proliferation and angiogenesis. *J. Pathol.* **184**, 53–71.
243. Lu, J., Nishizawa, Y., Tanaka, A., Nonomura, N., Yamanishi, H., Uchida, N., et al. (1989) Inhibitory effect of antibody against basic fibroblast growth factor on androgen- or glucocorticoid-induced growth of shionogi carcinoma 115 cells in serum-free culture. *Cancer Res.* **49**, 4963–4967.

244. Takahashi, J. A., Fukumoto, M., Kozai, Y., Ito, N., Oda, Y., Kikuchi, H., and Hatanaka, M. (1991) Inhibition of cell growth and tumorigenesis of human glioblastoma cells by a neutralizing antibody against human basic fibroblast growth factor. *FEBS Lett.* **288,** 65–71.

245. Eckhardt, S. G., Burris, H. A., Eckardt, J. R., Weiss, G., Rodriguez, G., Rothenberg, M., et al. (1996) A phase I clinical and pharmacokinetic study of the angiogenesis inhibitor, tecogalan sodium. *Ann. Oncol.* **7,** 491–496.

246. Takano, S., Gately, S., Neville, M. E., Herblin, W. F., Gross, J. L., Engelhard, H., et al. (1994) Suramin, an anticancer and angiosuppressive agent, inhibits endothelial cell binding of basic fibroblast growth factor, migration, proliferation, and induction of urokinase-type plasminogen activator. *Cancer Res.* **54,** 2654–2660.

247. D'Amato, R. J., Loughnan, M. S., Flynn, E., and Folkman, J. (1994) Thalidomide is an Inhibitor of Angiogenesis. *Proc. Natl. Acad. Sci. USA* **91,** 4082–4085.

248. O'Reilly, M. S., Holmgren, L., Shing, Y., Chen, C., Rosenthal, R. A., Moses, M., et al. (1994) Angiostatin: a novel angiogenesis inhibitor that mediates the suppression of metastases by a Lewis lung carcinoma. *Cell* **79,** 315–328.

249. O'Reilly, M. S., Boehm, T., Shing, Y., Fukai, N., Vasios, G., Lane, W. S., et al. (1997) Endostatin: an endogenous inhibitor of angiogenesis and tumor growth. *Cell* **88,** 277–285.

250. Hermanson, M., Funa, K., Hartman, M., Claesson-Welsh, L., Heldin, C. H., Westermark, B., and Nister, M. (1992) Platelet-derived growth factor and its receptors in human glioma tissue: expression of messenger RNA and protein suggests the presence of autocrine and paracrine loops. *Cancer Res.* **52,** 3213–3219.

251. Nister, M., Claesson-Welsh, L., Eriksson, A., Heldin, C. H., and Westermark, B. (1991) Differential expression of platelet-derived growth factor receptors in human malignant glioma cell lines. *J. Biol. Chem.* **266,** 16,755–16,7563.

252. Nister, M., Libermann, T. A., Betsholtz, C., Pettersson, M., Claesson-Welsh, L., Heldin, C. H., et al. (1988) Expression of messenger RNAs for platelet-derived growth factor and transforming growth factor-alpha and their receptors in human malignant glioma cell lines. *Cancer Res.* **48,** 3910–3918.

253. Henriksen, R., Funa, K., Wilander, E., Backstrom, T., Ridderheim, M., and Oberg, K. (1993) Expression and prognostic significance of platelet-derived growth factor and its receptors in epithelial ovarian neoplasms. *Cancer Res.* **53,** 4550–4554.

254. Antoniades., H. N., Galanopoulos, T., Neville-Golden, J., and O'Hara, C. J (1992) Malignant epithelial cells in primary human lung carcinomas coexpress in vivo platelet-derived growth factor (PDGF) and PDGF receptor mRNAs and their protein products. *Proc. Natl. Acad. Sci. USA* **89,** 3942–3946.

255. Krasagakis, K., Garbe, C., and Orfanos, C. E. (1993) Cytokines in human melanoma cells: synthesis, autocrine stimulation and regulatory functions - an overview. *Melanoma Res.* **3,** 425–433.

256. Lindmark, G., Sundberg, C., Glimelius, B., L., P., Rubin, K., and Gerdin, B. (1993) Stromal expression of platelet-derived growth factor beta-receptor and platelet-derived growth factor B-chain in colorectal cancer. *Lab. Invest.* **69,** 682–689.

257. Story, M. T. (1991) Polypeptide modulators of prostatic growth and development. *Cancer Surv.* **11,** 123–146.

258. Chung, C. K. and Antoniades, H. N. (1992) Expression of c-sis/platelet-derived growth factor B, insulin-like growth factor I, and transforming growth factor alpha messenger RNAs and their respective receptor messenger RNAs in primary human gastric carcinomas: in vivo studies with *in situ* hybridization and immunohistochemistry. *Cancer Res.* **52,** 3453–3459.

259. Seymour, L., Dajee, D., and Bezwoda, W. R. (1993) Tissue platelet derived-growth factor (PDGF) predicts for shortened survival and treatment failure in advanced breast cancer. *Breast Cancer Res. Treat.* **26,** 247–252.

260. Holmgren, L., Flan, F., Larsson, E., and Ohlsson, R. (1993) Successive activation of the platelet-derived growth factor beta receptor and platelet-derived growth factor B genes correlates with genesis of human choriocarcinoma. *Cancer Res.* **53,** 2927–2941.

261. Yoshida, K., Kuniyasu, H., Yasui, W., Kitadai, Y., Toge, T., and Tahara, E. (1993) Expression of growth factors and their receptors in human esophageal carcinomas: regulation of expression by epidermal growth factor and transforming growth factor alpha. *Cancer Res. Clin. Oncol.* **199,** 401–407.

262. Wang, J., Coltrera, D., and Gown, A. M. (1994) Cell proliferation in human soft tissue tumors correlates with platelet-derived growth factor B chain expression: an immunohistochemical and in situ hybridization study. *Cancer Res.* **54,** 560–564.

263. Sturzl, M., Roth, W. K., Brockmeyer, N. H., Zietz, C., Speiser, B., and Hofschneider, P. H. (1992) Expression of platelet-derived growth factor and its receptor in AIDS-related Kaposi sarcoma in

vivo suggests paracrine and autocrine mechanisms of tumor maintenance. *Proc. Natl. Acad. Sci. USA* **89,** 7046–7050.

264. Lindahl, P., Johansson, B. R., Levéen, P., and Betsholtz, C. (1997) Pericyte loss and microaneurysm formation in PDGF-B-deficient mice. *Science* **227,** 242–245.

265. Brouty-Boye, D. and Magnien, V. (1994) Myofibroblast and concurrent ED-b fibronectin phenotype in human stromal cells cultured from non-malignant and malignant breast tissue. *Eur. J. Cancer* **30A,** 66–73.

266. Forsberg, K., Valyi-Nagy, I., Heldin, C. H., Herlyn, M., and Westermark, B. (1993) Platelet-derived growth factor (PDGF) in oncogenesis: development of a vascular connective tissue stroma in xenotransplanted human melanoma producing PDGF-BB. *Proc. Natl. Acad. Sci. USA* **90,** 393–397.

267. Ponten, F., Ren, Z., Nister, M., Westermark, B., and Ponten, J. (1994) Epithelial-stromal interactions in basal cell cancer: the PDGF system. *Invest. Dermatol.* **102,** 304–309.

268. Westermark, B. and Heldin, C. H. (1993) Platelet-derived growth factor. Structure, function and implications in normal and malignant cell growth. *Acta. Oncol.* **32,** 101–105.

269. Siegfried, J. M., Weissfeld, L. A., Singh-Kaw, P., Weyant, R. J., Testa, J. R., and Landreneau, R. J. (1997) Association of immunoreactive hepatocyte growth factor with poor survival in resectable non-small cell lung cancer. *Cancer Res.* **57,** 433–439.

270. Hendrix, M. J., Seftor, E. A., Seftor, R. E., Kirschmann, D. A., Gardner, L. M., Boldt, H. C., et al. (1998) Regulation of uveal melanoma interconverted phenotype by hepatocyte growth factors/scatter factor (HGF/SF). *Am. J. Pathol* **152,** 855–863.

271. Jeffers, M., Rong, S., and Vande Woude, G. F. (1996) Enhanced tumorigenicity and invasion-metastasis by hepatocyte growth factor/scatter factor-met signalling in human cells concomitant with induction of the urokinase proteolysis network. *Mol. Cell. Biol.* **16,** 1115–1125.

272. Di Renzo, M. F., Narsimhan, R. P., Olivero, M., Bretti, S., Giordano, S., Medico, E., et al. (1991) Expression of the Met/HGF receptor in normal and neoplastic human tissues. *Oncogene* **6,** 1997–2003.

273. Börset, M., Hjorth-Hansen, H., Seidel, C., Sundan, A., and Waage, A. (1996) Hepatocyte growth factor and its receptor c-Met in multiple myeloma. *Blood* **88,** 3998–4004.

274. Rosen, E. M. and Goldberg, I. D. (1995) Scatter factor and angiogenesis. *Adv. Cancer Res.* **67,** 257–279.

275. Börset, M., Lien, E., Espevik, T., Helseth, E., Waage, A., and Sundan, A. (1996) Concomitant expression of hepatocyte growth factor/scatter factor and the receptor c-MET in human myeloma cell lines. *J. Biol. Chem.* **271,** 24,655–24,661.

276. Sakata, H., Takayama, H., Sharp, R., Rubin, J. S., Merlino, G., and LaRochelle, W. J. (1996) Hepatocyte growth factor/scatter factor overexpression induces growth, abnormal development, and tumor formation in transgenic mouse livers. *Cell Growth Diff.* **7,** 1513–1523.

277. de Jong, J. S., van Diest, P. J., van der Valk, P., and Baak, J. P. (1998) Expression of growth factors, growth inhibiting factors, and their receptors in invasive breast cancer. I: an inventrory in search of autocrine and paracrine loops. *J. Pathol.* **184,** 44–52.

278. Baserga, R. (1995) The insulin-like growth factor I receptor: a key to tumor growth? *Cancer Res.* **55,** 249–252.

279. Resnicoff, M., Abraham, D., Yutanawiboonchai, W., Rotman, H. L., Kajstura, J., Rubin, R., et al. (1995) The insulin-like growth factor I receptor protects tumor cells form apoptosis in vivo. *Cancer Res.* **55,** 2463–2469.

280. Feldman, M., Brennan, F. M., and Maini, R. N. (1996) Role of cytokines in rheumatoid arthritis. *Ann. Rev. Immunol.* **14,** 397–440.

281. Paleolog, E. M. (1996) Angiogenesis: a critical process in the pathogenesis of RA - a role for VEGF? *Br. J. Rheumatol.* **35,** 917–920.

282. Brown, R. A., Weiss, J. B., Tomlinson, I. W., Phillips, P., and Kumar, S. (1980) Angiogenic factor from synovial fluid resembling that from tumours. *Lancet.* **29,** 682–685.

283. Semble, E. L., Turner, R. A., and McCrickard, E. L. (1985) Rheumatoid arthritis and osteoarthritis synovial fluid effects on primary human endothelial cell cultures. *J. Rheumatol.* **12,** 237–241.

284. Colville-Nash, P. R. and Scott, D. L. (1992) Angiogenesis and rheumatic arthritis: pathogenic and therapeutic implications. *Annals. Rheumatic Dis.* **51,** 919–925.

285. Peacock, D. J., Banquerigo, M. L., and Brahn, E. (1992) Angiogenesis inhibition suppresses collagen arthritis. *J. Exp. Med.* **175,** 1135–1138.

286. Peacock, D. J., Banquerigo, M. L., and Brahn, E. (1995) A novel angiogenesis inhibitor suppresses rat adjuvant arthritis. *Cell. Immunol.* **160,** 178–184.

287. Shawver, L. K., Lipson, K. E., Fong, T. A. T., McMahon, G., Plowman, G. D., and Strawn, L. M. (1997) Receptor tyrosine kinases as targets for inhibition of angiogenesis. *Drug Discovery Today* **2,** 50–63.

288. Fava, R. A., Olsen, N. J., Spencer-Green, G., Yeo, K.-T., Yeo T.-K, Berse B., et al. (1994) Vascular permeability factor/endothelial growth factor (VPF/VEGF): accumulation and expression in human synovial fluids and rheumatoid synovial tissues. *J. Exp. Med.* **180**, 341–346.

289. Koch, A. E., Harlow, L. A., Haines, G. K., Amento, E. P., Unemori, E. N., Wong, W. L., et al. (1994) Vascular endothelial growth factor, a cytokine modulating endothelial function in rheumatoid arthritis. *J. Immunol.* **152**, 4149–4156.

290. Nagashima, M., Yoshino, S., Ishiwata, T., and Asano, G. (1995) Role of vascular endothelial growth factor in angiogenesis of rheumatoid arthritis. *J. Rheumatol.* **22**, 1624–1630.

291. Ben-Av, P., Crofford, L. J., Wilder, R. L., and Hla, T. (1995) Induction of vascular endothelial growth factor expression in synovial fibroblasts by prostaglandin E and interleukin–1: a potential mechanism for inflammatory angiogenesis. *FEBS Lett.* **372**, 83–87.

292. Cozzolino, F., Torcia, M., Lucibello, M., Morbidelli, L., Ziche, M., Platt, J., et al. (1993) Interferon-α and interleukin 2 synergistically enhance basic fibroblast growth factor synthesis and induce release, promoting endothelial cell growth. *J. Clin. Invest.* **91**, 2504–2512.

293. Tamura, T., Nakanishi, T., Kimura, Y., Hattori, T., Sasaki, K., Norimatsu, H., et al. (1996) Nitric oxide mediates interleukin-1-induced matrix degradation and basic fibroblast growth factor release in cultured rabbit articular chondrocytes: a possible mechanism of pathological neovascularization in arthritis. *Endocrinol.* **137**, 3729–3737.

294. Byrd, V., Zhao, X.-M., McKeehan, W. L., Miller, G. G., and Thomas, J. W. (1996) Expression and functional expansion of fibroblast growth factor receptor T cells in rheumatoid synovium and peripheral blood of patients with rheumatoid arthritis. *Arthritis Rheumatism* **39**, 914–922.

295. Koch, A. E., Polverini, P. J., Kunkel, S. L., Harlow, L. A., DiPietro, L. A., Elner, V. M., et al. (1992) Interleukin-8 as a macrophage-derived mediator of angiogenesis. *Science* **258**, 1798–1801.

296. Lupia, E., Montrucchio, G., Battaglia, E., Modena, V., and Camussi, G. (1996) Role of tumor necrosis factor-α and platelet-activating factor in neoangiogenesis induced by synovial fluids of patients with rheumatoid arthritis. *Eur. J. Immunol.* **26**, 1690–1694.

297. Koch, A. E., Halloran, M. M., Hosaka, S., Shah, M. R., Haskell, C. J., Baker, S. K., et al. (1996) Hepatocyte growth factor: a cytokine mediating endothelial migration in inflammatory arthritis. *Arthritis Rheumatism* **39**, 1566–1575.

298. Frater-Schroder, M., Risau, W., Hallaman, R., Gautschi, P., and Bohlen, P. (1987) Tumor-necrosis factor type α, a potent inhibitor of endothelial cell growth *in vitro*, is angiogenic *in vivo*. *Proc. Natl. Acad. Sci. USA* **84**, 5277–5281.

299. Montrucchio, G., Lupia, E., Battaglia, E., Passerini, G., Bussolino, F., Emanuelli, G., and Camussi, G. (1994) Tumor necrosis factor alpha-induced angiogenesis depends on in situ platelet-activating factor biosynthesis. *J. Exp. Med.* **180**, 377–382.

300. Bussolino, F., Arese, M., Montrucchio, G., Barra, L., Primo, L., Benelli, R., et al. (1995) Platelet activating factor produced in vitro by Kaposi's sarcoma cells induces and sustains *in vivo* angiogenesis. *J. Clin. Invest.* **96**, 940–952.

301. Hosaka, S., Shah, M. R., Barquin, N., Haines, G. K., and Koch, A. E. (1995) Expression of basic fibroblast growth factor and angiogenin in arthritis. *Pathobiology* **63**, 249–256.

302. Qu, Z., Liebler, J. M., Powers, M. R., Galey, T., Ahmadi, P., Huang, X.-N., et al. (1995) Mast cells are a major source of basic fibroblast growth factor in chronic inflammation and cutaneous hemangioma. *Am. J. Pathol.* **147**, 564–573.

303. Zhao, X. M., Byrd, V. M., McKeehan, W. L., Reich, M. B., Miller, G. G., and Thomas, J. W. (1995) Costimulation of CD4+ T cells by fibroblast growth factor-1 (acidic fibroblast growth factor) *J. Immunol.* **155**, 3904–3911.

304. Creamer, J. D. and Barker, J. N. W. N. (1995) Vascular proliferation and angiogenic factors in psoriasis. *Clin. Exp. Dermatol.* **20**, 6–9.

305. Nishioka, K. and Ryan, T. J. (1972) The influence of the epidermis and other tissues on blood vessel growth in the hamster cheek pouch. *J. Invest. Dermatol.* **58**, 33–45.

306. Wolf, J. E., Jr. and Harrison, R. G. (1973) Demonstration and characterization of an epidermal angiogenic factor. *J. Invest. Dermatol.* **59**, 40–43.

307. Barnhill, R. L., Parkinson, E. K., and Ryan, T. J. (1984) Supernatants from cultured human epidermal keratinocytes stimulate angiogenesis. *Br. J. Dermatol.* **110**, 273–281.

308. Malhotra, R., Stenn, K. S., Fernandez, L. A., and Braverman, I. M. (1989) The angiogenic properties of normal and psoriatic skin associate with the epidermis-not the dermis. *Lab. Invest.* **61**, 162–165.

309. Wolf, J. E., Jr. (1989) Angiogenesis in normal and psoriatic skin. *Lab. Invest.* **61**, 139–142.

310. Majewski, S., Kaminski, M., Jablonska, S., Szmurlo, A., and Pawinska, M. (1985) Angiogenic capability of peripheral blood mononuclear cells in psoriasis. *Arch. Dermatol.* **121**, 1018–1021.

311. Majewski, S., Tigalonowa, M., Jablonska, S., Polakowski, I., and Janczura, E. (1987) Serum samples from patients with active psoriasis enhance lymphocyte-induced angiogenesis and modulate endothelial cell proliferation. *Arch. Dermatol.* **123,** 221–225.

312. Arbiser, J. L. (1996) Angiogenesis and the skin: a primer. *J. Am. Acad. Derm.* **34,** 486–497.

313. Detmar, M., Brown, L. F., Claffey, K. P., Yeo, K.-T., Kocher, O., Jackman, R. W., et al. (1994) Overexpression of vascular permeability factor/vascular endothelial growth factor and its receptors in psoriasis. *J. Exp. Med.* **180,** 1141–1146.

314. Brown, L. F., Harrist, T. J., Yeo, K.-T., Stahle-Backdahl, M., Jackman, R. W., Berse, B., et al. (1995) Increased expression of vascular permeability factor (vascular endothelial growth factor) in bullous pemphigoid, dermatitis herpetiformis and erythema multiforme. *J. Invest. Dermatol.* **104,** 744–749.

315. Brown, L. F., Olbricht, S. M., Berse, B., Jackman, R. W., Matsueda, G., Tognazzi, K. A., et al. (1995) Overexpression of vascular permeability factor (VPF/VEGF) and its endothelial cell receptors in delayed hypersensitivity skin reactions. *J. Immunol.* **154,** 2801–2807.

316. Brauchle, M., Funk, J. O., Kind, P., and Werner, S. (1996) Ultraviolet B and H2O2 are potent inducers of vascular endothelial growth factor expression in cultured keratinocytes. *J. Biol. Chem.* **271,** 21,793–21,797.

317. Ono, M., Okamura, K., Nakayama, Y., Tomita, M., Sato, Y., Komatsu, Y., and Kuwano, M. (1992) Induction of human microvascular endothelial tubular morphogenesis by human keratinocytes: Involvement of transforming growth factor-α. *Biochem. Biophys. Res. Comm.* **189,** 601–609.

318. Schweigerer, L., Neufeld, G., Friedman, J., Abraham, J. A., Fiddes, J. C., and Gospodarowicz , D. (1987) Capillary endothelial cells express basic fibroblast growth factor, a mitogen that promotes their own growth. *Nature* **325,** 257–259.

319. O'Keefe, E. J., Dhiu, M. L., and Payne, R. E., Jr. (1988) Stimulation of growth of keratinocytes by basic fibroblast growth factor. *J. Invest. Dermatol.* **90,** 767–769.

320. Ellis, C. N., Gorsulowsky, D. C., Hamilton, T. A., Billings, J. K., Brown, M. D., Headington, J. T., et al. (1986) Cyclosporin improves psoriasis in a double-blind study. *JAMA* **256,** 3110–3116.

321. Furue, M., Gaspari, A. A., and Katz, S. I. (1988) The effects of cyclosporin on epidermal cells: II. Cyclosporin A inhibits proliferation of normal and transformed keratinocytes. *J. Invest. Dermatol.* **90,** 796–800.

322. Nickoloff, B. J., Fisher, G. J., Mitra, R. S., and Voorhees, J. J. (1988) Additive and synergistic antiproliferative effects of cyclosporin A and gamma interferon on cultured human keratinocytes. *Am. J. Pathol.* **131,** 12–18.

323. Sharpe, R. J., Arndt, K. A., Bauer, S. I., and Malone, T. E. (1989) Cyclosporin inhibits basic fibroblast growth factor-driven proliferation of human endothelial cells and keratinocytes. *Arch. Dermatol.* **125,** 1359–1362.

324. Barinaga, M. (1995) Shedding light on blindness. *Science* **267,** 452–454.

325. Chen, C. H. and Chen S. C. (1980) Angiogenic activity of vitreous and retinal extract. *Invest. Ophthalmol. Vis. Sci.* **6,** 596–592.

326. Felton, S., Brown, G., Felberg, N., and Federman, J. (1979) Vitreous inhibition of tumor neovascularization. *Arch. Ophthalmol.* **97,** 1710–1713.

327. Brem, S., Preis, I., Langer, R., Brem, H., Folkman, J., and Patz, A. (1977) Inhibition of neovascularization by an extract derived from vitreous. *Am. J. Ophthalmol.* **84,** 323–328.

328. Grant, M. B., Russel, B., Fitzgerald, C., and Merimee, T. J. (1986) Insulin-like growth factors in vitreous: studies in controls and diabetics with neovascularization. *Diabetes* **35,** 416–420.

329. Sivalingam, A., Kennery, J., Brown, G. C., Benson, W. E., and Donoso, L. (1990) Basic fibroblast growth factor levels in the vitreous of patients with proliferative diabetic retinopathy. *Arch Ophehalmol.* **108,** 869–872.

330. Aiello, L. P. and King G. L. (1994) Vascular endothelial growth factor in ocular fluid of patients with diabetic retinopathy and other retinal disorders. *New Engl. J. Med.* **331,** 1480–1487.

331. Malecaze, F., Clamens, S., Simorre-Pinatel, V., Mathis, A., Chollet, P., Favard, C., et al. (1994) Detection of vascular endothelial growth factor messenger RNA and vascular endothelial growth factor-like activity in proliferative diabetic retinopathy. *Arch. Ophthalmol.* **112,** 1476–1482.

332. Adamis, A. P., Miller, J. W., Bernal, M.-T., D'Amico, D. J., Folkman, J., Yeo, T.-K., and Yeo, K.-T. (1994) Increased vascular endothelial growth factor levels in the vitreous of eyes with proliferative diabetic retinopathy. *Am. J. Ophthalmology.* **118,** 445–450.

333. Adamis, A. P., Shima, D. T., Tolentino, M. J., Gragoudas, E. S., Ferrara, N., Folkman, J., et al. (1996) Inhibition of vascular endothelial growth factor prevents retinal ischemia-associated iris neovascularization in a nonhuman primate. *Arch. Ophthalmol.* **114,** 66–71.

334. Pe'er, J., Shweiki, D., Itin, A., Gnessin, H., and Keshtet, E. (1995) Hypoxia-induced expression of vascular endothelial growth factor by retinal cells is a common factor in neovascularizing ocular diseases. *Lab. Invest.* **72,** 638–645.

335. Aiello, L. P., Pierce, E. A., Foley, E. D., Takagi, H., Chen, H., Riddle, L., et al. (1995) Suppression of retinal neovascularization in vivo by inhibition of vascular endothelial growth factor (VEGF) using soluble VEGF-receptor chimeric proteins. *Proc. Natl. Acad. Sci. USA* **92,** 10,457–10,461.

336. Tolentino, M. J., Miller, J. W., Gragoudas, E. S., Jakobiec, F. A., Flynn, E., Chatzistefanou, K., et al. (1996) Intravitreal injections of vascular endothelial growth factor produce retinal ischemia and microangiopathy in an adult primate. *Ophthalmology* **103,** 1820–1888.

337. Tolentino, M. J., Miller, J. W., Gragoudas, E. S., Chatzistefanou, K., Ferrara, N., and Adamis, A. P. (1996) Vascular endothelial growth factor is sufficient to produce iris neovascularization and neovascular glaucoma in a non–human primate. *Arch. Ophthalmol.* **114,** 964–970.

338. Pierce, A. E., Avery, R. L., Foley, E. D., Aiello, L. P., and Smith, L. E. H. (1995) Vascular endothelial growth factor/vascular permeability factor expression in a mouse model of retinal neovascularization. *Proc. Natl. Acad. Sci. USA* **92,** 905–909.

339. Miller, J. W., Adamis, A. P., Shima, D. T., D'Armore, P. A., Moulton, R. S., O'Reilly, M. S., et al. (1994) Vascular endothelial growth factor/vascular permeability factor is temporally and spatially correlated with ocular angiogenesis in a primate model. *Am. J. Pathol.* **145,** 574–584.

340. Kuroki, M., Voest, E. E., Amano, S., Beerepoot, L. V., Takemura, T., Tolentino, M. J., et al. (1996) Reactive oxygen intermediates increase vascular endothelial growth factor expression in vitro and in vivo. *J. Clin. Invest.* **98,** 1667–1675.

341. Adamis, A. P. (1997) Regulation of vascular endothelial growth factor in the eye. *Angiogenesis Novel Therapeutic Development Conference.* Unpublished communication.

342. Smith, L. (1996) IBC Conference on Angiogenesis Inhibitors and Other Novel Therapeutic Strategies for Ocular Diseases of Neovascularization.

343. Pavco, P. (1997) Ribozyme inhibition of VEGF–mediated endothelial cell proliferation and neovascularization in a rat corneal model. IBC Conference on Novel Anti–angiogenic Therapy for Diabetic Retinopathy, Macular Degeneration and Other Ocular Diseases of Neovascularization.

344. Xia, P., Aiello, L. P., Ishii, H., Jiang, Z. Y., Park, D. J., Robinson, G. S., et al. (1996) Characterization of vascular endothelial growth factor's effect on the activation of protein kinase C, its isoforms, and endothelial cell growth. *J. Clin. Invest.* **98,** 2018–2026.

345. King, G. L., Goodman, A. D., Buzney, S., Moses, A., and Kahn, C. R. (1985) Receptors and growth promoting effect of insulin and insulin-like growth factors on cells from bovine retinal capillaries and aorta. *J. Clin. Invest.* **75,** 1028–1036.

346. Grant, M. B., Jerdan, J., and Merimee, T. J. (1987) Insulin-like growth factor I modulates endothelial cell chemotaxis. *J. Clin. Endocrinol. Metab.* **65,** 370–371.

347. Grant, M. B. and Guay, C. (1991) Plasminogen activator production by human retinal endothelial cells of non-diabetic and diabetic origin. *Invest. Ophthalmol. Vis. Sci.* **32,** 53–64.

348. Bauer, P. I., Machoric, R., Bokikg, C., Sanka, E., Koch, S. A., and Horvath, I. (1984) Interaction of plasmin with endothelial cells. *Biochem. J.* **218,** 119–124.

349. Moscatelli, D., Jaffe, E., and Rifkin, D. B. (1980) Tetradecanoyl phorbol acetate stimulates latent collagenase production by cultured human-endothelial cells. *Cell* **20,** 343–351.

350. Warren, R. S., Yuan, H., Matli, M. R., Ferrara, N., and Donner, D. B. (1996) Induction of vascular endothelial growth factor by insulin-like growth factor 1 in colorectal carcinoma. *J. Biol. Chem.* **271,** 29,483–29,488.

351. Hanneken, A., deJuan, E., Hutty, G. A., Fox, G. M., Schiffer, S., and Hjelmeland, H. L. (1991) Altered distribution of basic fibroblast growth factor in diabetic retinopathy. *Arch. Ophthalmol.* **109,** 1005–1011.

352. Gospodarowitz, D. (1976) Humoral control of cell proliferation: the role of fibroblast growth factor in regeneration, angiogenesis, wound healing and neoplastic growth. *Prog. Clin. Biol. Res.* **9,** 1–19.

353. D'Armore, P. and Klagsbrun, M. (1984) Endothelial cell mitogens derived from retina and hypothalamus: biochemical and biological similarities. *J. Cell Biol.* **99,** 1545–1549.

354. Herman, I. M. and D'Armore, P. (1984) Capillary endothelial cell migration: loss of stress fibers in response to retinal-derived growth factor. *J. Muscle Res. Cell Motil.* **5,** 697–709.

355. Presta, M., Moscatelli, D., Joseph-Silverstein, J., and Rifkin, D. B. (1986) Purification from a human hepatoma cell line of a basic fibroblast growth factor-like molecule that stimulates capillary endothelial cell plasminogen activator production, DNA synthesis, and migration. *Mol. Cell. Biol.* **6,** 4060–4066.

356. Gospodarowitz, D., Bialecki, H., and Thakral, T. K. (1979) The angiogenic activity of the fibroblast and epidermal growth factor. *Exp. Eye Res.* **28,** 501–514.

357. Risau, W. (1986) Developing brain produces an angiogenic factor. *Proc. Natl. Acad Sci. USA* **83,** 3855–3859.
358. Graf, K., Xi, X. P., Yang, D., Fleck, E., Hsueh, W. A., and Law, R. E. (1997) Mitogen-activated protein kinase activation is involved in platelet-derived growth factor-directed migration by vascular smooth muscle cells. *Hypertension* **29,** 334–339.
359. Mullins, D. E., Hamud, F., Reim, R., and Davis, H. R. (1994) Inhibition of PDGF receptor binding and PDGF-stimulated biological activity in vitro and of intimal lesion formation in vivo by 2-bromomethyl-5-chlorobenzene sulfonylphthalimide. *Arterioscler Thromb* . **14,** 1047–1055.
360. Zhao, X. M., Frist, W. H., Yeoh, T. K., and Miller, G. G. (1994) Modification of alternative messenger RNA splicing of fibroblast growth factor receptors in human cardiac allografts during rejection. *J. Clin. Invest.* **94,** 992–1003.
361. Zhao, X. M., Yeoh, T. K., Frist, W. H., Porterfield, D. L., and Miller G. G. (1994) Induction of acidic fibroblast growth factor and full-length platelet-derived growth factor expression in human cardiac allografts. Analysis by PCR, in situ hybridization, and immunohistochemistry. *Circulation* **90,** 677–685.
362. Alpers, C. E., Davis, C. L., Barr, D., Marsh, C. L., and Hudkins, K. L. (1996) Identification of platelet-derived growth factor A and B chains in human renal vascular rejection. *Am. J. Pathol.* **148,** 439–451.
363. Abboud, H. E. (1995) Role of platelet-derived growth factor in renal injury. *Annu. Rev. Physiol.* **57,** 297–309.
364. Kaminski, M. and Auerbach, R. (1988) Angiogenesis induction by CD-4 positive lymphocytes. *Proc. Soc. Exp. Biol. Med.* **188,** 440–443.
365. Chabrier, P. E. (1996) Growth factors and the vascular wall. *Int. Angiol.* **15,** 100–103.
366. Waltenberger, J., Akyurek, M. L., Aurivillius, M., Wanders, A., Larsson, E., Fellstrom, B., and Funa, K. (1996) Ischemia-induced transplant arteriosclerosis in the rat. Induction of peptide growth factor expression. *Arterioscler Thromb. Vasc. Biol.* **16,** 1516–1523.
367. Agapitos, E., Karayannacos, P., Donta, I., Kotsarelis, D., Iliopoulos, D., Davaris, P., et al. (1996) Immunohistochemical detection of platelet-derived growth factor (PDGF) in the aortic wall of atherosclerotic rabbits. *Int. Angiol.* **15,** 249–251.
368. Billett, M. A., Adbeish, I. S., Alrokayan, S. A., Bennet, A. J., Marenah, C. B., and White, D. A. (1996) Increased expression of genes for platelet-derived growth factor in circulating mononuclear cells of hypercholesterolemic patients. *Arterioscler. Thromb. Vasc. Biol.* **16,** 399–406.
369. Ito, M., Yamada, K., Masuda, J., Kinoshita, A., Otsuki, H., and Hayakawa, T. (1995) Expression of PDGF in relation to cell division in atherosclerotic intima of human carotid arteries. *Neurol. Res.* **17,** 345–348.
370. Newby, A. C. and George, S. J. (1996) Proliferation, migration, matrix turnover, and death of smooth muscle cells in native coronary and vein graft atherosclerosis. *Curr. Opin. Cardiol.* **11,** 574–582.
371. Stavri, G. T., Hong, Y., Zachary, I. C., Breier, G., Baskerville, P. A., Yla-Herttuala, S., et al. (1995) Hypoxia and platelet-derived growth factor-BB synergistically upregulate the expression of vascular endothelial growth factor in vascular smooth muscle cells. *FEBS Lett.* **358,** 311–315.
372. Randone, B., Sterpetti, A. V., Stipa, F., Proietti, P., Aromatario, C., Guglielmi, M. B., et al. (1997) Growth factors and myointimal hyperplasia in experimental aortic allografts. *Eur. J. Vasc. Endovasc. Surg.* **13,** 66–71.
373. Abedi, H. and Zachary, I. (1995) Signalling mechanisms in the regulation of vascular cell migration. *Cardiovasc. Res.* **30,** 544–556.
374. Koster, R., Windstetter, U., Uberfuhr, P., Baumann, G., Nicol, S., and Hofling, B. (1995) Enhanced migratory activity of vascular smooth muscle cells with high expression of platelet-derived growth factor A and B. *Angiology* **46,** 99–106.
375. Bennet, M. R., Evan, G. I., and Schwartz, S. M. (1995) Apoptosis of human vascular smooth muscle cells derived from normal vessels and coronary atherosclerotic plaques. *J. Clin. Invest.* **95,** 2266–2274.
376. Michiels, C., De Leener, F., Arnould, T., Dieu, M., and Remacle, J. (1994) Hypoxia stimulated human endothelial cells to release smooth muscle cell mitogens: role of prostaglandins and bFGF. *Exp. Cell. Res.* **213,** 43–54.
377. Knighton, D. R., Hunt, T. K., Scheusenluthl, H., Halliday, B. J., Werb, Z., and Banda, M. J. (1983) Oxygen tension regulates the expression of angiogenesis factor by macrophages. *Science* **221,** 1283–1285.
378. Li, J., Brown, L. F., Hibberd, M. G., Grossman, J. D., Morgan, J. P., and Simons, M. (1996) VEGF, flk-1, and flt-1 expression in rat myocardial infarction model of angiogenesis. *Am. J. Physiol.* **270,** 1803–1811.

379. van Neck, J. W., Medina, J. J., Onnekink, C., Schwartz, S. M., and Bloemers, H. P. (1995) Expression of basic fibroblast growth factor and fibroblast growth factor receptor genes in cultured rat aortic smooth muscles cells *Biochim. Biophys. Acta.* **1261,** 210–214.

380. Hughes, S. E. (1996) Localisation and differential expression of the fibroblast growth factor receptor (FGFR) multigene family in normal and atherosclerotic human arteries. *Cardiovasc. Res.* **32,** 557–569.

381. Ware, J. A. and Simons, M. (1997) Angiogenesis in disease. *Nature Med.* **3,** 158–164.

382. Yanigisawa-Miwa, A., Uchida, Y., Nakamura, F., Tomaru, T., Kido, H., Hamiho, T., et al. (1992) Salvage of infarcted myocardium by angiogenic action of basic fibroblast growth factor. *Science* **257,** 1401–1403.

383. Battler, A., Scheinowitz, M., Bor, A., Hasdai, D., Vered, Z., Di Segni, E., et al. (1995) Intracoronary injection of basic fibroblast growth factor enhances angiogenesis in infarcted swine myocardium. *J. Am. Coll. Cardio.* **22,** 2001–2006.

384. Padua, R. R., Sethi, R., Dhalla, N. S., and Kardami, E. (1995) Basic fibroblast growth factor is a cardioprotective in ischemia-reperfusion injury. *Mol. Cell. Biochem.* **143,** 129–135.

385. Watanabe, E., Smith, D. M., Sun, J., Smart, F. W., Delcaprio, J. B., Roberts T. B., et al. (1998) Effect of basic fibroblast growth factor on angiogenesis in the infarcted porcine heart. *Basic Red Cardiol.* **93,** 30–71.

386. Lopez, J. J., Edelman E. R., Stamler, A., Hibbard M. G., Prasad, P., Thomas, K. A., et al. (1998) Angiogenic potential of perivascularly delivered aFGF in a porcine model of chronic myocadial ischemia. *Am. J. Physiol.* **274,** 930–936.

387. Giordano, F. J., Ping, P., McKirnan, M. D., Nozaki, S., DeMaria, A. N., Dillmann, W. H., et al. (1996) Intracoronary transfer of fibroblast growth factor-5 increases blood flow and contractile function in an ischmic region of the heart. *Nature Med.* **2,** 534–539.

388. Lazarous, D. F., Scheinowitz, M., Shou, M., Hodge, E., Rajanayagam, S., Hunsberger, S., et al. (1995) Effects of chronic systemic administration of basic fibroblast growth factor on collateral development in the canine heart. *Circulation* **91,** 145–153.

389. Pearlman, J. D., Hibberd, M. G., Chuang, M. L., Harada, K., Lopez, J. J., Gladstone, S. R., et al. (1995) Magnetic resonance mapping demonstrates benefits of VEGF-induced myocardial angiogenesis. *Nature Med.* **1,** 1085–1089.

390. Harada, K., Friedman, M., Lopez, J. J., Wang, S. Y., Li, S., Prasad, Y., et al. (1996) Vascular endothelial growth factor in chronic myocardial ischemia. *Am. J. Physiol.* **270,** 1792–1802.

391. Baffour, R., Berman, J., Garb, J. L., Sang, M. S., Rhee, W., Kaufman, J., and Friedmann, P. (1992) Enhanced angiogenesis and growth of collaterals by in vivo adminsitration of recomibant basic fibroblast growth factor in a rabbit model of acute lower limb ischemia: Dose-response effect of basic fibroblast growth factor. *J. Vasc. Surg.* **16,** 181–191.

392. Takeshita, S., Zheng, L. P., Brohi, E., Kearney, M., Pu, L.-Q., Bunting, S., et al. (1994) Therapeutic angiogenesis. A single intra-arterial bolus of vascular endothelial growth factor augments revascularization in a rabbit ischemic hind limb model. *J. Clin. Invest.* **93,** 662–670.

393. Van Belle, E., Witzenbichler, B., Chen D., Silver, M., Chang, L., Schwall, R., and Isner, J. M. (1998) Potentiated angiogenic effect of scatter factor/hepatocyte growth factor via induction of vascular endothelial growth factor: the case for paracrine amplification of angiogenesis. *Circulation* **97,** 381–390.

394. Isner, J. M. (1996) Clinical evidence of angiogenesis after arterial gene transfer of phVEGF165 in patient with ischaemic limb. *Lancet* **348,** 370–374.

395. MacCarthy M. J., Crowther, M., Bell, P. R., and Brindle, N. P. (1998) The endothelial receptor tyrosine kinase tie-1 is upregulated by hypoxia and vascular endothelial growth factor. *FEBS Lett* **423,** 334–338.

396. Nakanishi, R., Hashimoto, M., and Yasumoto, K. (1998) Improved airway healing using basic fibroblast growth factor in a canine tracheal autotransplantation model. *Ann. Surg.* **227,** 446–454.

397. Hickey, M. J., Wilson, Y., Hurley, J. V., and Morrison, W. A. (1998) Mode of vascularization of control and basic fibroblast growth factor-stimulated prefabricated skin flaps. *Plast Reconstr Surg* **101,** 1296–1304.

398. Bayati, S., Russell, R. C., and Roth A. C. (1998) Stimulation of angiogenesis to improve the viability of prefabricated flaps. *Plast. Reconstr. Surg.* **101,** 1290–1295.

399. Levéen, P., Pekny, M., Gebre-Medhin, S., Swolin, B., Larsson, E., and Betsholtz, C. (1994) Mice deficient for PDGF B show renal, cardiovascular, and hematological abnormalities. *Genes Dev.* **8,** 1875–1887.

400. Soriano, P. (1994) Abnormal kidney development and hematological disorders in PDGF β-receptor mutant mice. *Genes Dev.* **8,** 1888–1896.

401. Strawn, L. M. and Shawver, L. K. (1998) Tyrosine kinases in disease: overview of kinase inhibitors as therapeutic agents and current drugs in clinical trials. *Exp. Opin. Invest Drugs* **7,** 553–573.

23 Targeting Gene Therapy to the Tumor Vasculature

Kelvin K. W. Lau and Roy Bicknell

"...to render the enemy's armies helpless is best..." The Art of War, Sun Tzu.

CONTENTS

INTRODUCTION

Targeting therapy to tumor blood supply has been established as a valid adjuvant to cancer therapy. Proof-of-concept experiments have shown that both antiangiogenic and antivascular approaches can cause dramatic tumor regression in animal models. Several groups are now attempting "gene therapy" using the tumor endothelium as a target. In this chapter, the concept of gene transfer to the tumor endothelium will be discussed. The available vectors will be reviewed for their use in gene delivery to the tumor vasculature, followed by a discussion on methods for targeting transgene expression specifically to this tissue. Finally, the problem of target definition in the tumor endothelium will be described.

Advances in our understanding of tumor biology in the past decade suggest that tumor growth, like development, depends on tightly regulated homeostatic mechanisms ranging from hormonal interactions to oxygen regulation. For instance, tumor growth is strongly dependent on a supporting vasculature for the supply of nutrients *(1)*. Because of the intimate physiological interdependency between the tumor and its blood supply, modification of the

From: *The New Angiotherapy*
Edited by: T.-P. D. Fan and E. C. Kohn © Humana Press Inc., Totowa, NJ

tumor vasculature is a valid way to interfere with tumor growth and physiology. First, simple interruption of this blood supply can lead to ischaemia and consequently cell death (2,3). In gene therapy, this can be accomplished using a suicide gene. Second, if the tumor vasculature could be made to express tumor modifying molecules basolaterally, such as toxins or chemotherapeutic agent carriers, the problem of tumor penetration presented by current therapeutics can be circumvented. Third, because of the genetic stability of endothelium, this tissue can be relied on as a faithful therapy target for histologically different types of tumors, and is furthermore not susceptible to the drug resistance that is encountered with all other anti-cancer therapy (4). Now that human gene therapy is a reality, genetic modification of the tumor endothelium is being explored as a possible adjuvant to the therapy of cancer.

Targeting gene therapy to the tumor endothelium can be achieved by manipulation at two levels: firstly by limiting gene delivery to the target tissue, and secondly by restricting gene expression to the target tissue. Targeted gene delivery and expression is very important, especially if the gene product is toxic (such as a toxigene or a pro-drug activator) as would be the case for destructive vascular targeting. Furthermore, gene delivery is most likely to be via the intravenous route to maximize bioavailability, taking advantage of the direct contact of the endothelium with the bloodstream. The expression system itself needs to be very specific to reduce the danger of transducing endothelium outside of the tumor. Thus the use of vascular targeting in cancer therapy requires that four issues be resolved: to achieve (1) targeting of the gene-carrying vector; (2) targeted expression of the transgene to the tumor endothelium and away from other tissues; (3) selection of an optimal transgene for delivery; and (4) achieving an understanding of the physiological responses associated with the delivery and expression of such a transgene. However, because the ultimate aim of genetic modification of the tumor vasculature is tumor regression, many other principal concerns of gene therapy such as persistence of expression or vector capacity become relatively unimportant.

METHODS OF GENE DELIVERY

Strategies of gene delivery have generally been of two kinds: nonviral and viral. In general, transduction by viral methods is more efficient than by nonviral methods, owing in part to natural selection of viral mechanisms for their ability to infect their host cells. Nonviral methods of delivery are extensions of pre-existing methods of cell transfection in tissue culture; naked DNA has been used, as well as DNA packaged into liposomes and condensation agents. More effective gene transduction efficiencies have been observed with viral vectors. The first human gene therapy trial in 1989 utilizsed retroviruses for the ex-vivo transduction of tumor-infiltrating lymphocytes (5). Since then, many vector systems have become available (such as adenoviruses and adeno-associated viruses [AAV]) and many more are being developed, exploiting the many subtle facets of viral behaviour for different gene therapeutic aims. An example of this is herpesvirus: its latent infection in neurones is being exploited for neurone-directed gene therapy. In the following sections, the currently available vector systems will be reviewed and their use in targeting genes to tumor endothelium assessed.

NON-VIRAL METHODS

The simplest form of gene delivery is by injection of naked DNA. Injected DNA is believed to be taken up nonspecifically through endocytic vesicles, where it undergoes purely diffusive movement into the cytosol and then on into the nucleus. Most of the DNA that gets taken up in this fashion will be trafficked to the lysosome for rapid degradation (teleologically, this mechanism would have evolved to protect the genotype of cells from exogenous DNA in the environment), thus the dose of DNA given needs to be very high (in the order of g/m^2) to achieve physiologically meaningful transduction. Naked DNA transduction of endothelium has been reported both in animals and in humans. In an ischaemic model, Isner and colleagues transduced the internal iliac artery of rabbits percutaneously with a plasmid-encoding human vascular endothelial growth factor (VEGF) using a hydrogel-covered angioplasty balloon inflated at 4 atmospheres *(6)*. Transgene expression was detected not only in the endothelium but also in the tunica media (probably as a direct result of the high pressure exerted on the vessel wall), with expression lasting for 2 wk postoperatively. β-galactosidase staining showed a transfection efficiency of about 1%. Despite the low level of transduction, VEGF was expressed at physiological levels and enhanced collaterals were clearly visible at day 30 postoperative. Thus naked DNA appears to transduce endothelial cells inefficiently and with a short time-course of transgene expression. However, physiologically meaningful levels of transgene expression are possible. This was further confirmed in a 70-yr old patient suffering from lower-limb ischaemia *(7)*. She received 2000 µg of plasmid DNA transferred to the distal popliteal artery under a similar protocol, resulting in marked collateral vessel formation, thus confirming the ability of naked DNA to transduce endothelium in humans to produce physiological quantities of a protein. More recently, a phase I clinical study showed that direct injection of naked DNA encoding VEGF into the ventricular wall of patients with refractory angina was able to substantially alleviate both haemodynamic and subjective parameters *(8)*.

To enhance gene delivery, DNA can be wrapped up in lipids as a liposome. Cationic liposomes are positively charged, allowing DNA to condense within them, and thus greatly increasing the size of the DNA that can be carried relative to conventional liposomes. Furthermore, most biological surfaces are negatively charged, and will interact spontaneously with the liposomes, leading to fusion. After fusing directly with the cell membrane, the DNA is delivered to the cytosol where some translocates to the nucleus, bypassing degradation in the lysosomes. Indeed, transfection efficiencies with cationic liposomes are considerably higher than with naked DNA. In a porcine arterial model, the liposome formulation GAP-DLRIE/ DOPE has been shown to offer high transduction efficiencies nearing those achieved by viral vectors *(9)*. Reporter gene expression was confined mostly to the endothelium. Under optimized conditions, the transduction efficiency was only 20-fold lower than a high-titer adenoviral vector (10^{10} pfu/injection) carrying the same gene. Another advantage to using nonviral vectors is the stability of liposomes in serum, a property shared by few viral vectors. As a recent report has shown, delivery using these vectors intravenously can achieve physiologically effective levels of gene product expression *(10)*. Systemic delivery of liposomes is showing promise, and they are the first vectors that can achieve a meaningful level of gene transduction in vivo using this route. Rapid developments in the field will, however, lead to liposomes capable of delivering genes at even higher efficiency. Nonviral based vectors are promising and avoids many of the problems that plague viral vectors such as reversions to wild-type or vector-associated immune responses.

Nonviral methods appear to offer acceptable levels of transduction and transgene expression. So far as expressing a tumor-toxin or endothelial killing is concerned, a low efficiency of transduction is not as important as high-level expression of the gene product. Gene expression can be targeted by manipulation of the transgene promoter to suppress expression outside the target tissue. However, in the ideal situation, the transduction of such toxic products is further complemented by a specific targeting vehicle. The vectors described above deliver genes irrespective of cell type; tissue transduction is limited only by the mechanical procedure of administration and diffusion barriers such as the internal elastic lamina. More specificity in delivery can be achieved by conjugating the delivery vehicle to a "magic bullet" such as monoclonal antibodies (MAbs) or peptide ligands. Naked DNA can be condensed onto polylysine or protamine (both strongly cationic proteins) and linked to moieties that recognize tumor endothelium. In one study, DNA was targeted to integrins using RGD-peptides linked to polylysine, and showed targeted delivery to integrin-expressing cells *(11)*, delivery can further be enhanced when the peptide-DNA complex was complexed to lipofectin (DOTMA/DOPE) and showed very high specificity for endothelial cells in an organ culture assay *(12)*. We have recently shown that certain integrins are upregulated on proliferating endothelium *(13)*, integrin-targeting peptides could show efficacy for targeted delivery to tumor endothelium.

Antibodies can be incorporated into liposomes to form immunoliposomes which have increased tissue-specificity for gene delivery. The ability of such modified liposomes to target has been demonstrated in several studies *(14)*. The targeting mechanisms in turn depend on the existence of tumor endothelium markers for which antibodies could be raised. Further increases in transduction efficiency are now being explored through the attachment of proteins with nuclear localization signals to the plasmid DNA in order to reduce loss of DNA while in the cytosol. These signals are gradually being elucidated *(15)*.

RETROVIRUSES: BIOLOGY

Retroviruses received considerable attention as a viral vector for gene delivery for several reasons. Firstly, their biology is relatively well-understood and they have been used for many years in the study of oncogenes and oncogenesis. The initial observation that transforming retroviruses act as delivery vehicles for oncogenes led to the first considerations of therapeutic gene transfer *(16)*. Furthermore, although nonviral methods of gene delivery may nonetheless lead to expression of genes, episomal DNA is unstable and is gradually degraded within the cell, especially those undergoing cell division. Transgene expression is therefore transient. The ability of retroviruses to integrate into host chromosomal DNA made them a good candidate for long-term stable gene delivery in gene augmentation therapy.

Retroviruses contain two single-stranded RNA molecules that replicate through a double-stranded DNA intermediate before integrating into the genome. The RNA is packaged with essential proteins necessary in *trans*, inside a protein viral capsid, which is in turn surrounded by a lipid bilayer envelope containing retroviral glycoproteins (*see* Fig. 1). All these functions are encoded within the three genes in the retroviral genome: *gag* encodes the structural proteins of the capsid, *pol* encodes the enzymes necessary for replicative and integrative functions, and *env* encodes the glycoprotein on the envelope. These genes are located in that order between two flanking long-terminal repeats (LTRs, which contain many of the viral regulatory sequences), which also function as a strong viral promoter. There is in addition a packaging signal ψ, which is necessary for the genome to be packaged. Without this signal, empty virions are produced. The gene order LTR-gag-pol-env-LTR is faithfully maintained between virus budding and viral integration. Thus retroviral vectors have the advantage of low frequency of gene rearrangement and efficient yet low-copy number gene transfers (mostly single-copy transfers), features not found in other vectors such as AAV.

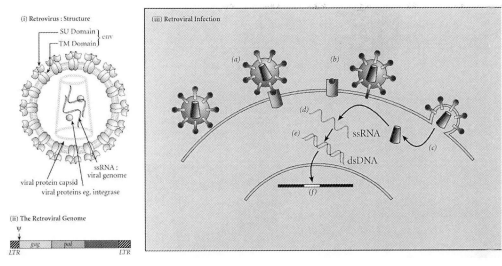

Fig. 1. (*See* color plate 2 appearing after page 490). (i) Structure of Retrovirus; (ii) Structure of the Retroviral Genome; (iii) Infection by a Retrovirus. (**A**) The retrovirus envelope SU domain binds to its cellular receptor and is followed by membrane fusion. (**B**) The SU domain is shed and the TM domain mediates fusion of the envelope with the membrane. (**C**) The protein capsid is released into the cytoplasm where it dismantles, releasing the RNA genome. (**D,E**) Reverse Transcriptase and DNA polymerase reverse transcribes this into the dsDNA provirus. (**F**) This enters the nucleus and integrates randomly into the host chromosomes.

Retroviral infection starts with the binding of the retroviral envelope protein to its cellular receptor on the cell surface. The identity of these receptors for the type C mammalian retroviruses is now clear and they appear to belong to a group of permeases. For example, the ecotropic MuLV (murine leukaemia virus), which infects rodent cells but not others, uses the cationic amino acid transporter MCAT-1 as the cellular receptor *(17)*, whereas the amphotropic MuLV, which infects not only rodent cells but also cells from other species including humans, uses a phosphate transporter Pit-2 as its cellular receptor *(18)*. This suggests that a common determinant or function of the permeases exists and is required for retroviral cell entry. Many viruses including the orthomyxoviruses and togaviruses require low pH for activation of the fusion machinery. The amphotropic MuLV, on the other hand, is able to cause syncytia formation at neutral pH, thus the binding of the retrovirus to its cellular receptor is believed to be followed directly by pH-independent fusion at the cell surface *(19)*. It is noted, however, that certain cell lines can only be infected at low pH with the ecotropic retrovirus, therefore it remains a possibility that there exist auxiliary mechanisms of entry *(20)*.

After viral-cell fusion, the virus enters the cytosol and undergoes uncoating into a nucleoprotein complex. Reverse transcriptase reverse-transcribes the RNA genome into DNA. The integrase then inserts the viral DNA into the host chromosome, where it remains latent as a provirus. It appears that for efficient integration, the cell must be actively dividing *(21)*. This has become a safety concern in the use of retroviruses as a gene delivery vector owing to the apparently random site of integration of the viral genome; fear that insertion mutagenesis may activate oncogenes or inactivate tumor suppression became a pertinent issue in the review process of retroviral gene-therapy protocols. Despite numerous studies, such vector-related tumor generation has yet to be observed, and furthermore, current protocols in cancer therapy utilize highly mutagenic agents such as radiation and chemotherapy, so that the relatively small elevated risk is considered acceptable and relatively low-risk in the context of anti-cancer therapies.

RETROVIRUSES AS A VECTOR

In the generation of a retroviral vector, the ability of the retrovirus to replicate must be eliminated to prevent infection of the host and uncontrollable gene transduction. Such replication-incompetent retroviruses are formed by deletion of the structural and replicative genes necessary for productive infection. This is necessary also to provide space for the transgene, as the retroviruses have a packaging limit for a transgene of about 7–8 kb. Thus, retroviral vectors are designed to incorporate the transgene and any other *cis* elements necessary for infection such as LTRs and packaging signals. The structural and replicative functions needs to be provided in *trans*. Packaging cell lines have been developed to provide these elements. The first packaging cell lines created in the early 1980s consisted of cells stably transfected with the entire provirus lacking a packaging signal ψ *(22)*. However, wild-type viruses were frequently produced. A single recombination event between the packaging and vector constructs can introduce the packaging signal back, rescuing the provirus. The risk of such rescuing events can be further reduced by modifying other aspects of the packaging cell lines. The second generation packaging construct has deletions at the 5' end of both the LTRs *(23)*. In this case, 2 recombination events are necessary for rescue. Further modifications include the introduction of packaging functions as two separate construct, encoding *gag-pol* and *env* separately *(24)*, and removal from the vector construct of the residual γαγ start codon located within ψ *(25)*.

Upon transfection of the packaging cell line with the vector construct, a retroviral vector is produced. The tropism of this new virus is identical to the retrovirus from which the packaging construct is derived. The broad host range of the amphotropic retrovirus has led this retrovirus to be used in in vivo attempts to transduce vascular endothelial cells in various animal models. Many studies have shown transduction of reporter genes to be inefficient, with efficiencies ranging from 0.1–5% *(26,27)*, mainly owing to poor efficiency of successful gene delivery *(28)*. This may be owing in part to the dependency of retroviral gene transduction on cell proliferation. If the transduction efficiency is significantly higher in proliferating cells in vivo, then the differential between quiescent endothelium in most tissues and proliferating endothelium in the tumor may mean that retroviral vectors would naturally target tumor endothelium. However, experimental evidence of such preferential transduction of tumor endothelium in vivo is lacking. Existing data on the transduction of proliferating endothelium have all been gathered in vitro, and it is becoming clear that, phenotypically, tumor endothelium and proliferating endothelium in culture behave very differently *(29)*.

Experience from using retroviral vectors for in vivo gene delivery have revealed many other obstacles. This is owing to a number of reasons. First, existing retroviral vectors cannot achieve the high titers that are necessary for systemic administration, especially in the face of rapid clearance from the circulation. Second, retroviruses are very labile in vivo, as they are inactivated and lysed by serum complement *(30)*, and third, whereas retroviruses has the advantage of integrating into the host genome, this requires that the target cells be actively dividing. In tumor endothelium, endothelial cells proliferate more than quiescent cells, but the level of proliferation may still be low compared to other rapidly proliferating cells such as lymphocytes. Most research into vector design now focuses on nonretroviral vectors.

THE TARGETABLE RETROVIRUS

As described earlier, endothelium can be transduced with low efficiency by simple retroviral vectors: further modification to build in a "homing" mechanism is needed to enhance infection of the tumor endothelium and reduce background infection of the rest of the vasculature. In vivo gene therapy will be possible when we can deliver a recombinant retrovirus systemically but be assured that the gene is delivered and expressed only in a predetermined population of cells. There are two ways in which targeting can be achieved: one is by host-range expansion, where a virus normally noninfective to a cell type is made infective—for example, an ecotropic retrovirus rendered infective to human cells; the other by host-range restriction, where a virus is rendered noninfective to its natural host—for example, an amphotropic retrovirus that will only infect human tumor endothelium. As described earlier, monoclonal antibodies (MAbs) can be used to confer specificity on the gene vehicle. Direct modification of the surface of the virus with the antibody can produce such targetable vectors. The host-range of a retrovirus appears to be determined by the distribution of its receptors and the env glycoprotein: more specifically the surface domain (SU) of the heterodimer. For example, MCAT-1 is not expressed in murine hepatocytes, a cell type that is resistant to infection by the ecotropic retrovirus *(31)*, and human cells can be made susceptible to infection by the ecotropic retrovirus by transfection with the MCAT-1 gene *(32)*. The converse is also true, thus pseudotyped viruses (where one virus is coated in the envelope of another virus) assume the host-range of the new envelope *(33–35)*, although it becomes more difficult to pseudotype viruses that are less closely related. Furthermore, although this confers upon the retroviral vector a new host-range that may be more appropriate for delivery of certain genes, there is no known virus that has a natural tropism for proliferating or tumor endothelium whose envelope we can use to target a retrovirus to the tumor endothelium, thus limiting this approach as a targeting mechanism for retroviral vectors.

Modification of retroviruses by pseudotyping allows us to redirect a virus's tropism, however, the new virus is still limited by the host range of the new env. The first attempts at direct engineering of novel tropisms to the retroviral envelope for targeting purposes involved the coupling of targeting moieties to the env glycoprotein. If the host-range determinant were simply a function of the binding activity of env to its receptor, then it should theoretically be possible to expand the host range by adding moieties that bind to, for example, human cells. Indeed, this approach met with some success. Using antibodies bridged with strepavidin, antibodies against molecules such as MHC and EGFR as well as ligands such as EGF can be linked to the env-glycoprotein, allowing viruses to bind to cells expressing these molecules *(36,37)*. Whereas binding to the new receptor occurred faithfully along with internalization of the vector, gene-transduction efficiency was very poor. Part of the explanation lies in inactivation owing to chemical manipulation of the viruses, and partly owing to the lack of translocation of the vector into the cytosol. Most of the internalized vectors were thought to have undergone degradation in the lysosome. The ecotropic receptor MCAT-1 does not differ significantly from its human homolog HCAT in its binding affinity to env, however, infection can be effected in the presence in the medium of adenovirus *(38)*. This suggests that binding is necessary but not sufficient for infection, and that another function such as endosomal escape or translocation is needed, a function that was provided by the adenoviral capsid. Recently, the structure of the retroviral env transmembrane domain (TM) was crystallized and elucidated *(39)*. Analogous to influenza haemagglutinin HA_1 and HA_2, it was suggested that on binding the cellular receptor, SU is shed leading to a conformational change similar to a loaded spring, where the fusogenic peptide forms an extended coil that inserts into the plasma membrane initiating fusion events. Therefore retargeting by coupling molecules to env with such a large bispecific antibody can disrupt the intra-molecular transmission of receptor binding to the fusion peptide at a different part of env.

An alternative method of retargeting is through direct modification of env. The receptor binding sites of env have been localized to two variable regions within the N-terminal parts of SU, thus host-range modification could conceivably be achieved through modification of these regions. Kasahara et al. *(40)* replaced this region of the ecotropic env with erythropoietin (EPO) and demonstrated an extended tropism for several human cell lines expressing EPO-receptors, although efficiency of infection were very low (50 cfu/mL). Furthermore, modified env needs to be coexpressed with wild-type env because modified env is not efficiently incorporated into virions. The same group subsequently inserted the heregulins α and β1, ligands for the EGF-receptor, into the same region of env. These modified retroviruses were able to infect human cell lines overexpressing EGF-R at a higher titer of 8×10^3 cfu/mL *(41)*, but the titer is still too low to be physiologically effective for systemic administration in animal models. In addition to receptor ligands, single-chain antibodies (scFvs) have been used to target retroviral infection to selected cell types. The first successful report of such a modification came from Russell et al. *(42)*. They produced a chimæric fusion protein with a scFv inserted between amino acids 6 and 7 at the N-terminal end of SU. Again, both wild-type and modified env were expressed for efficient incorporation into virions. The antibody was against the hapten NIP (4-hydroxy-5-iodo-3-nitrophenacetyl caproate), however, on treatment with NIP, nonpermissive human cells became permissive for the ecotropic retrovirus, thus host-range extension through the new fusion protein could not be shown. Since then, many attempts at inserting a scFv into the ecotropic retroviral env have failed to extend infection to the new target at anything but very low titers. The genetic modification of env appears to be a major obstacle in targeting retroviral infections, arising from the lack of detailed structural model of the envelope that would allow rational modification. The recent elucidation of the structure of the SU domain *(43)* indeed revealed the existence of two discrete structural domains within SU that are responsible for binding and transmission to TM respectively. These two domains are linked by a proline-rich hypervariable linker. Insertion of a single chain fragment into this region results in correct folding and virion maturation *(44)*. The titer of the viruses appear to be similar to the wild-type viruses, although the absolute titer achieved was not measured in the study.

ADENOVIRUSES

One of the main obstacles to using retroviruses in human gene therapy is the technical difficulty in obtaining an adequate titer for systemic administration. Furthermore, the size limit of 8kb limits the size of the input genome, which needs to comprise of at least a structural gene and a tightly regulated promoter (*see* Fig. 2). Thus many investigators have focused on other vectors that are easier to manipulate and have a higher capacity. Adenoviruses satisfy these requirements: they are more stable than retroviruses and can be prepared to titers of up to 10^{12} pfu/mL, they have a genome of 36kb in length allowing it to carry genes of substantial size, and, unlike retroviruses, they are able to infect

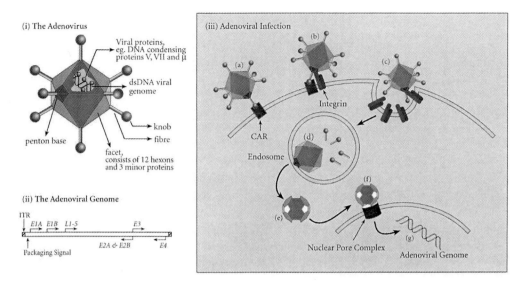

Fig. 2. (*See* color plate 3 appearing after page 490). (i) Structure of a Adenovirus; (ii) Structure of the Adenoviral Genome; (iii) Infection by an Adenovirus. (**A**) Adenovirus binds to its cellular receptor CAR. (**B**) This allows the penton base to bind to the α_v subunit of the integrins. (**C**) The adenovirus enters the endocytic pathway with the integrins. (**D,E**) In the endosome, the fibers dissociate and the penton base and other capsid components mediate endosomal escape of the capsid. (**F**) This complex targets to the nuclear pore complex where it docks. (**G**) Here it releases the viral genome through the pore into the nucleus.

nondividing cells, allowing the transduction of terminally differentiated tissues such as respiratory epithelia and neurones.

Adenoviruses infections are common and involve clinical symptoms such as acute febrile pharyngitis and pneumonia. Despite being a pathogen, most cases of infections are mild and self-limiting. Furthermore, the use of live adenovirus vaccines in the US military *(45)* further attest to the safety of adenovirus administration for gene delivery. Of the 47 serotypes known, serotypes Ad2 and Ad5 belonging to the nononcogenic subgenus C *(46)*. These two are the most intensively studied candidate vectors for gene delivery. Adenoviruses, however, do not integrate into the host chromosome. This could be seen as a benefit against insertional mutagenesis, although the episomal form of the input genome may be lost in dividing cells. In the context of gene delivery to tumor endothelium, the strength of adenoviruses lies in the high titer possible, in the light of dilution through intravenous administration.

Adenoviruses, like retroviruses, have a broad host-range. They can infect a large number of tissues although the infection efficiency differs for different cell types. In general, differentiated endothelial cells in vivo are relatively resistant to infection *(47)* requiring a high multiplicity of infection (MOI) and prolonged duration of exposure. Part of this phenomenon is likely to be mediated by charge interactions at the glycocalyx *(48)*, which can be neutralized in tissue culture with polycations such as polybrene or protamine and partly in the low level expression of the viral receptors. Future developments in adenoviral vectors will address this problem, which is important for in vivo delivery of the vector.

ADENOVIRUSES AS VECTORS

Adenoviruses consist of a linear double-stranded DNA genome of approx 36 kb packaged within a nonenveloped protein capsid. The protein capsid is icosahedral with 12 vertices and 20 facets. The facets are occupied by the hexon proteins whereas the vertices are occupied by the penton base protein. To the penton base are attached the trimeric fiber protein, which is globular distally, a region known as the "knob." This knob domain mediates the first binding step of the adenovirus to its target cell, in the case of serotypes 2 and 5, either through the coxsackievirus and adenovirus receptor (CAR) *(49)* or the α2 domain of the MHC class I molecules *(50)*. Binding of the knob domain to either of these primary receptors is followed by internalization mediated by the penton base and the $α_v$ integrins. The viral particle is subsequently trafficked to the endosomal compartment where the penton base is believed to mediate endosomal escape *(51)*. The release of the capsid into the cytosol is followed by dismantling of the virus. The viral genome is subsequently translocated into the nucleus: although the nuclear targeting signals and their mechanism of action are not clear, they appear to involve nuclear localization signals in the hexon protein as well as the cellular chaperone protein hsp70 *(52)*.

The adenoviral genome is flanked by two inverted terminal repeats (ITRs) and contains coding sequences for some 30 RNA species. The expression of these genes are organised into the early and late genes. The early genes are subdivided into 4 regions, E1-4. E1 encodes immediate early genes whose functions include *trans*-activation of the rest of the early regions. E2 encodes proteins necessary for replicative functions such as DNA polymerases. E3 encodes immunosuppressive peptides that block MHC Class 1 peptide presentation, and E4 encodes for functions that cause host-gene expression shut-down, accumulation of viral transcripts and onset of late gene expression. The 5 major late regions L1-5 encode the structural proteins that make up the virion capsid.

Most of the current adenoviral vectors are derived from adenovirus serotype 5 (Ad5) where E1 is deleted and replaced by foreign DNA. The effect of the E1 deletion (ΔE1) is to reduce viral-gene expression and prevents viral propagation. Furthermore, deletion of E1A removes a highly antigenic region dominantly displayed by MHC Class I molecules. These vectors have been used to deliver genes efficiently to the endothelium in animal experiments. The efficiency of delivery and expression can be seen in Zoldhelyi and colleagues' porcine model *(53)*. 10^{10} pfu/mL adenovirus vectors carrying the cyclooxygenase-1 *(COX-1)* gene was instilled into the carotid artery for 30 min after angioplasty injury. The subsequent levels of expression of COX-1 and a concomitant rise in prostacyclin synthesis is so high as to completely inhibit thrombus formation or any cyclic blood-flow changes. However, these results cannot be extrapolated directly to gene delivery to intact endothelium, such as found in tumors. More relevant are experiments performed on uninjured endothelium *(54,55)*. In a gene-augmentation experiment, Welling and colleagues *(55)* attempted to express systemically the interleukin-1 (IL-1) receptor antagonist IL-1ra by transducing the rat hindlimb vasculature with this gene. They injected 0.7 mL of the ΔE1 adenovirus at 10^{12} particles/mL into the isolated hindlimb vasculature and allowed it to incubate for 30 min. Highly efficient gene transfer was obtained, with 70% of the gastrocnemius endothelium transduced for the reporter gene 5 d post-operative. The high transduction efficiency is a result of the high titer of virus administered. When the experiment was performed at a titer of 10^9, transduction efficiency reduced to 2%. It is also important to note that the administration of adenoviral vectors with prolonged incubation to an isolated vasculature is not practical in in vivo human gene with therapy, where systemic intravenous administration will be required. However, intravenous delivery of present adenoviral vectors results in delivery of more than 90% of vector to the liver *(56)*, as a result of the high-affinity specific binding of the knob to the liver *(57)*. In fact, the estimated capacity of the murine liver for adenoviral knobs is near to the equivalent of more than the achievable titer of 10^{12} pfu *(57)*. Therefore the effective titer that is available to transduce endothelial cells becomes impracticably low.

Furthermore, systemic administration of adenoviruses in Welling's experiment led to lung and liver toxicity characterized by infiltrating lymphocytes and zones of necrosis. The risk of such toxicity is considerable if a titer of at least 10^{12} pfu/mL is needed locally before efficient gene transduction can take place, and furthermore the delivery of such high levels of toxic genes to the liver is likely to be lethal. A solution to this problem is to modify the tropism of the adenoviral vector in such a way to restrict the host range to the target-cell population similar to the attempts at modifying env in retroviral targeting *(58)*.

Another salient feature in Welling's experiment concerns the immune response induced by gene delivery. When transducd with Ad-IL-1ra, serum levels of the recombinant protein again reached a high level at day 5, but were undetectable at day 21. When repeated in athymic rats, this loss of expression was not observed, and the protein was still detectable at 98 d after transduction. This suggests that an immune mechanism against the transducted cells may be at leat responsible for the loss of expression of the transgene. Similar results have been obtained where murine and human erythropoietin alleles were delivered by an adenoviral vector to immunocompetent mice. Mice receiving the former continued to express the transgene and showed persistent elevation of haematocrit, whereas those receiving the latter induced an immune response that led to transient expression of the transgene with no persistent elevation haematocrit, *(59)*. Besides immune responses against the transgene, it is known that ΔE1 vectors continue to express viral genes at low levels thus allowing the development of Class (I) restricted CTL responses against transduced cells *(60)*, contributing to the small window of transgene expression. Despite the relative importance of responses against the transgene and viral antigens being contested by Michou et al. *(61)*, who suggests that the cellular response against viral antigens play only a small role in extinction of transgene expression, vectors have been developed that further suppress leaky viral-gene expression. One such vector is the ΔE1/ΔE4 vector *(62)*. Because E4 regulates the early-to-late phase transition, ΔE4 vectors will not be able to express late stage viral structural genes which are believed to be antigenic. Indeed, direct comparison between this vector and ΔE1 vector shows a considerably prolonged expression of reporter gene at greater levels than the latter. There is also a reduction in cytopathic effects in the liver that is believed to be mediated through L3 *(63)*.

The immune features of an immunogenic vector system can enhance destructive gene therapy, whereas with gene therapy aimed at modifying endothelial function, a less immunogenic vector system would be more appropriate. The one feature that will deny routine use of adenoviral vector is an effective neutralizing humoral response directed against the vector that develops after the first administration, indeed, the presence of immunity against many different serotypes have been found frequently in the population, and this may impinge on attempts to readminister the vector. One ingenious solution to this problem is to incorporate the apoptosis signaling molecule *fas* ligand into the vector, such that transduction is followed by expression of the transgene as well as *fas* ligand *(64)*, the latter inducing apoptosis in CTLs that recognize the transduced cell. These vectors have efficacy in immunologically primed animals as well as naive animals, and are therefore capable of overriding pre-existing immunity against the vector. One potential problem lies the resistance of transduced cell to CTL killing, which could lead to cells being more susceptible to oncogenic development, and loss of protection from intracellular pathogens such as viruses. Other methods of decreasing the immunogenicity of the vector is by deletion of endogenous viral sequences, many such gutless vectors have been produced, and most of them lead to persistent transgene expression in vivo. However, such vectors have a particularly high dependence on helper viruses, and the high level of wild-type virus contamination within these preparations preclude them from being used clinically (65).

The fiber protein knob domain is analogous to the SU domain of retroviral envelope proteins, because they are both involved in receptor recognition and binding. Many investigators have begun to explore the effect of modification of this domain to alter adenoviral tropism. In a recent report, Curiel's group (58) replaced the Ad5 fiber knob domain with the equivalent domain from Ad3. Viruses carrying this modified fiber adopted the receptor binding profile of Ad3. Unlike retroviruses, there is a structural model for the adenoviral fiber protein (66) allowing rational modification of the tropism. So far, targeting adenoviruses by modification of the capsid proteins have been considerably more successful than modification of env, this is in part owing to the segregation of functions to disparate proteins: the knob does not have a role in internalization, which is the function of the penton base. Both the knob domain and the penton base has been successfully modified to retarget the vector to a expanded host range (58,67). However, specific insertion of novel targeting ligands into the HI loop of the knob have accomplished only extended tropism, native tropism for the CAR/MHC Class I receptors has not been ablated, and therefore the modified vectors are still plagued with unwanted tropism for the liver (68). The precise location of the native receptor binding site within the knob is still unknown, but targeted mutations in this site will allow the production of adenoviruses of altered tropism.

ADENO-ASSOCIATED VIRUSES

Adeno-associated viruses (AAV) were discovered initially as cryptic infections in preparations of adenovirus from various isolates, including humans (69). They were subsequently found as co-infecting agents in adenoviral epidemics (70). However, further studies revealed no pathology or other adverse effects associated with AAV infection. Furthermore, AAVs are naturally replication-deficient, thus attention has turned to them as a safe but efficient vector for gene therapy. Most studies on AAV as a gene-therapy vector have been performed on AAV serotype 2 (AAV2).

AAV is a member of the *Parvoviridae* family of viruses, characterized by a nonenveloped icosahedral capsid containing the genome in the form of a single stranded DNA molecule. The virus is inherently replication defective. After infection, the integrated provirus remains latent in the host genome until infection by a helper virus such as adenovirus or herpesvirus rescues the provirus, leading to a productive infection. Like adenoviruses, AAV utilizes a primary receptor for attachment, and internalizes via secondary receptors. AAV first binds avidly to membrane-associated heparan sulfate proteoglycans on the target cells (71), followed by attachment to either fibroblast growth factor (FGF) receptor 1 (72) or the $\alpha_v\beta_5$ integrins (73), both of which promotes entry of AAV following binding to heparan sulfate. However, it is of interest to note that cells that do not express either of these molecules can still be readily transduced by AAV (74). Thus unlike adenoviruses, internalization with the secondary receptors does not appear to be rate-limiting. The virus has a broad host-range and infects most human, rodent, and simian cell lines. Upon infection, AAV integrates into the host chromosome very specifically at a single site on the long arm of chromosome 19 (19q13.3-qter) (75).

This integration site is upstream of an open reading frame that is transcribed at low levels in several tissues *(76)*, thus insertion is not associated with oncogenesis. This feature of site-specific integration makes AAV a superior vector to retroviruses where fear of insertional mutagenesis have limited its use in humans.

AAV AS A VECTOR

AAV is a very small virus and it is therefore not surprising that as a vector, it has limited capacity. The AAV genome is 4.68 kb in size consisting of two open reading frames *rep* and *cap* flanked by two 145 bp inverted terminal repeats (ITRs). The *rep* genes encode replicative and regulatory functions such as excision and accumulation of ssDNA, and the *cap* genes code for the 3 structural genes that form the viral capsid. The only *cis*-element necessary for packaging and infection are the 145 bp ITRs *(77)*. The upper limit for packaging AAV genomes is about 4.9 kb, thus the maximum size of the transgene in the minimal vector is about 4.4 kb including promoter and poly-adenylation sites, a severely limiting factor for the choice of genes that could be delivered. On the other hand, unlike, retroviruses, AAV can be purified to titers of 10^{12} infection units/mL, which approaches the levels necessary for efficient transduction of tissue in vivo, and transduction occurs in both dividing and nondividing cells *(78)*.

The gutless AAV vectors described earlier have been used to transduce cultured mammalian cells as well as to deliver genes in animal models of in vivo gene therapy. However, results regarding the preservation of integration-site specificity in the vectors have been disappointing both in in vitro *(78,79)* and in in vivo experiments *(80)*. The viral genome appears to remain in episomal form in most transduced cells; when integration events do occur, they do not do so in a site-specific manner and occur very infrequently (6% integrated). Recent elucidation of the recombination signals within the viral genome and the target sequence *(81)* suggest that rep68/78, two proteins encoded in the *rep* region are necessary for site-specific integration. These two proteins recognise homologous sequences present in both the viral ITR and the target-integration site and are absolutely needed in *trans* for the integration process. Thus the next generation of vectors need to incorporate rep-function to preserve the site-specificity of integration where required.

The first in vivo studies were carried out to deliver genes to respiratory epithelium in models of cystic fibrosis in rat, rabbits, and macaques *(82–84)*. In all cases, gene transduction was achieved with high efficiency (about 50%) for prolonged periods (transgene still detectable after 6 mo). Furthermore, there was no evidence of toxicity or inflammation associated with the procedure. These results suggest that immune responses against the transduced cell are considerably less severe than that observed with adenoviruses. In the case of gene delivery to macaques *(84)*, their sero-positivity to AAV antigens suggest that immune responses against viral vector antigens may not necessarily attenuate efficient delivery. Whereas AAV has been shown to infect microvascular endothelial cells in vitro efficiently *(85)*, it is only recently that in vivo gene delivery to endothelium was demonstrated *(86)*. In striking contrast to adenoviral vectors, AAV failed to transduce arterial vascular cells, including the endothelium in both injured and uninjured arteries. However, of great interest was the observation that gene transduction occurred only in the microvascular endothelium of the tunica adventitia vasa vasorum. Thus it remains to be determined whether AAV has a natural tropism for adventitial microvascular endothelium, or microvascular endothelium. It is perhaps of interest that labeled proliferating cells co-localized with the expression of reporter gene, suggesting that this vector may be used to target gene expression to tumor endothelium.

Just as retroviruses and adenoviruses have a broad host range, infecting most of the tissues, systemic AAV delivery results in infection of a large variety of cells and tissues including the haematopoietic cells and the lungs. Therefore retargeting AAV tropism is important to increase specificity to the target tissue, and also to increase the effective titer of viruses reaching the target tissue. Recently a first attempt has been made to develop one such vectors. Using bispecific antibodies against the megakaryocyte-specific integrin αIIbβ3 and the AAV capsid, Bartlett et al. have successfully transduced several AAV resistant megakaryocyte cell lines using AAV complexed to the bispecific antibodies *(87)*. Further structural studies of the binding domains of the AAV capsid will allow us to generate AAV with recombinant capsids and altered tropism.

ANTIANGIOGENIC GENE THERAPY

Currently vectors are modified to enhance specificity in transgene delivery to a desired cell type, another approach to target gene transduction involves manipulation of gene expression pattern itself. This is achieved by selecting promoters that limit transgene expression to the target cell, assuming that such tissue-specific promoters are available. Specific promoters which are uniquely activated in the tumor endothelium have not been identified. This is in part due to the arbitrary definition of tumor vasculature. Because tumor endothelium are themselves derived from the rest of the rest of the endothelium, attempts to restrict gene expression to it through endothelial-specific promoters such as the tie promoter *(88)* and vWF promoter *(89)* are inadequate. Instead differences in gene expression patterns between these cells and the endothelium of nontumorous tissues have to be exploited. These differences stem from interaction between the endothelium and the tumor. Such interactions include angiogenic signals emanating from hypoxic regions of the tumor, and cytokines secreted by the large number of inflammatory and immune cells within the tumor. Two such promoters have been described in vitro that can target gene expression to proliferating endothelium and tumor endothelium *(90)*. Promoter activity for the VEGF-receptor (KDR) and E-selectin was enhanced 5–10 fold in endothelial cell lines when compared to fibroblasts, however, gene expression in quiescent vs proliferating/stimulated endothelium were not described. Addition of other regulatory sequences may improve endothelial specificity, which would be necessary before systemic administration can be carried out. Because both KDR and E-selectin are upregulated in the tumor endothelium, these promoters can conceivably be used to restrict gene expression to this tissue. In the future, this approach as well as enhanced specificity of targeted gene delivery will allow high-level tissue-specific gene expression to be achieved. When vectors with a natural tropism for proliferating or tumor endothelium become available, they will provide more latitude in terms of the promoter specificity required. Then concerns for expression outside of the endothelium will be less, and an endothelial specific promoter such as vWF *(89)* may be adequate.

Many investigators over the past few years have taken a different approach. To avoid the problems of generalized toxicity associated with the use of cytotoxic genes, many have chosen to use antiangiogenic genes. The past few years have seen the identification of several potent endogenous angiogenesis inhibitors such as thrombospondin-1, a fragment of platelet factor-4, angiostatin and endostatin, as well as recombinant inhibitors of angiogenesis, such as sFLT-1 *(91)* and ExTek *(92)*. The group of molecules selectively inhibit angiogenesis without affecting other cell types, and some further induce apoptosis in proliferating endothelium (93,94). Therefore, gene therapy with these has an added level of in-built specifity. Furthermore, the cost of production of recombinant proteins is high, and the frequent administration required to maintain therapeutic concentrations over long periods makes it economically unviable. Gene-therapy delivery of angiogenic inhibitors is more cost-effective, and can theoretically result in steady-state levels of inhibitors after a single administration. Furthermore, when combined with specific promoters as discussed earlier, expression can be localized to specific areas of tumor growth. Indeed, tumor-suppressive effects have been observed after gene delivery of these inhibitors (95–98). However, efficient transduction and tumor regression awaits the development of highly efficient and specific vectors.

IN SEARCH OF TARGETS ON TUMOR ENDOTHELIUM

Solid tumors depend on a blood supply for survival and growth, thus attacking the tumor vasculature, like Achille's heel, could be crippling for the tumor. It has been more than a decade since this idea was first proposed (2). It is therefore surprising that progress in the area has been slow. The first demonstration of in vivo vascular targeting came only in 1993 (91) in a model where tumor endothelium was stimulated to express MHC Class II in response to a interferon-γ secreting tumor. Targeting and destruction was achieved using an immunotoxin against the MHC molecule. In a report published recently (3), tumor targeting was still carried out through an artificially induced marker. The lack of definitive targets that are characteristic of tumor endothelium has therefore hindered developments in this field. Two features of tumor endothelium can be exploited for target definition, the first is the proliferation phenotype. Endothelial cells in adult tissue proliferate at a very low rate, whereas those in the tumor proliferate at a faster rate in response to tumor growth and demand. Indeed, attempts at producing antibody specific for proliferating endothelium went back to 1986 when Hagemeier et al. (100) described an antibody EN7/44 that was reactive with proliferating endothelium including those in tumors. However, his results have not been reproduced. Other putative tumor endothelial markers have been described such as endoglin (101), however, their tissue distribution are too broad for vascular-targeting purposes. Another property of a tumor is the often high levels of cytokines produced by resident macrophages activating endothelium into the inflammatory phenotype (102). One of the consequence of the exposure of endothelium to cytokines is the expression of cell-surface adhesion molecules such as ICAMs, VCAMs, and selectins. These molecules can serve as potential markers for vector targeting.

With the advent of phage-display technology, true target definition becomes a reality for tumor endothelium. This technology allows a library of peptides or proteins to be selected for binding affinities (103). The M13 phage pili protein is engineered to carry the peptide or protein to be assayed, whereas the phage contains a copy of the gene. The library of phages is added to an antigen followed by several increasingly stringent washes, in the hope that low-affinity binders will be washed off. Phages that remain bound can be rescued subsequently and the gene recovered. Recent studies have shown that phenotypically endothelium cultured in vitro differ considerably from tumor endothelium in vivo and the true relationship between the former and latter are dubious (29,104,105). Panning should therefore be carried out in vivo to ensure all relevant antigens are present and irrelevant ones absent. Indeed, Pasqualini et al. (106) have injected phage libraries into mice followed by recovery from different tissues. Because the time frame of the experiment meant that the phage only has time to contact the endothelium, rescued phages would express true endothelium "addresses labels" for the tissue from which it is recovered. It should be feasible to extend this technique to identify molecular targets on tumor endothelium.

On the other hand, selection of targeting receptors is important, but the distribution of the receptor is not sufficient for it being used as a target for gene therapy: a rapidly internalized receptor can significantly decrease the titer by trafficking the virus to degradation within the lysosomal compartments *(107)*, leading to rapid degradation, whereas other receptors that are not internalized will not allow delivery into the cells.

SUMMARY

Human gene therapy is now a reality. Since the first retroviral-mediated gene transfer protocol commenced in May 1989 *(5)*, the number of clinical trials in gene therapy has grown exponentially. With a better understanding of vector biology and development of better vector systems, in vivo gene delivery to the endothelium became possible and advanced greatly in the past 5 yr. For the purpose of destroying or modifying tumor endothelium, gene therapy needs to be targeted specifically to the tissue. Retroviruses, adenoviruses, and adeno-associated viruses have all been shown to transduce endothelium in vivo, albeit with low efficiency. Retrovirus were the first viruses used for gene delivery. They preferentially infect dividing cells, thus making it an ideal candidate for selectively infecting tumor endothelium. Practical issues concerning the preparation of high-titer virus unfortunately prohibit the use of this vector in systemic gene delivery. Another factor that makes systemic delivery in humans unsuitable is that retroviruses are relatively promiscuous viruses. Further engineering the virus to restrict the host range to the target tissue is required to prevent unwanted transduction of other dividing cells. Adenoviruses have also been intensely studied as an alternative vector system based on their ability to transduce nondividing cells as well as having a substantially larger capacity for transgene insertion. Like retroviruses, the adenoviruses are relatively promiscuous, being able to transduce most human cell lines. However, re-engineering of tropism has met with fewer problems than found with retroviruses, thus this virus may become the first targetable vector used in the clinical setting. A problem that plagues adenoviral vectors is their high antigenicity and the development of strong immune response against transduced cell and transgene products. About 50–70% of the population have neutralizing antibodies to adenoviruses in their serum. Also, gene transduction using this vector is transient, lasting 2–3 wk, a phenomenon that appears to be immune-mediated. Nonetheless, this virus can be purified to considerably higher titers than retroviruses and has therefore been used in systemic intravenous administration, although toxicity in the lungs and liver have been noted using this route. Adeno-associated viruses, on the other hand, appears to be able to infect nondividing cells, can be produced at high titers, and can lead to long-term expression of transgene without eliciting strong immune responses. The presence of serum antibodies against AAV does not markedly reduce gene-delivery efficiency in an animal model, a factor with direct relevance to its use in humans. Reports of endothelial transduction with this vector are scarce, but results suggest that AAV may have a natural tropism for proliferating microvascular endothelium in vivo. Reengineering of AAV tropism is currently underway in several laboratories, and with the eventual identification of the AAV cellular receptor, targeted AAV delivery may soon be possible.

Targeting gene delivery to a specific tissue can be complemented with targeted expression of transgene. The problems with identification of a suitable promoter that is activated to high levels in tumor endothelium is the same as identification of targeting moieties to target gene delivery: there are no true cell markers for tumor endothelium to define the target for the vector or transgene. Recent advances in target definition technology may help us to identify genes that are activated in tumor endothelium in vivo using a Darwinian strategy rather than the laborious MAb screening procedure that have been used in the past, which was available only in vitro.

In summary, targeted gene therapy for tumor endothelial destruction or modification is conceptually simple. Existing vectors are able to transduce endothelium, and transgenes are available to express different functions in these cells, including cell death. However, the lack of markers for tumor endothelium has meant that targeted gene therapy is not yet possible. New methods of identifying cell markers have recently been developed, hence the next few years will prove to be very exciting as the few missing components of a vascular-targeting gene-therapy vehicle become available.

REFERENCES

1. Folkman, J. (1990)What is the evidence that tumors are angiogenesis dependent? *J. Natl. Cancer Inst.* **82(1),** 4–6.
2. Denekamp, J. (1984) Vascular endothelium as the vulnerable element in tumors. *Acta Radiol. Oncol.* **23(4),** 217–225.
3. Huang, X., Molema, S., King, L., Watkins, T., Edgington, S., and Thorpe, E. (1997)Tumor infarction in mice by antibody-directed targeting of tissue factor to tumor vasculature. *Science* **275,** 547–549.
4. Boehm, T., Folkman, J., Browder, T., and O'Reilly, M. S. (1997) Antiangiogenic therapy of experimental cancer does not induce acquired drug resistance. *Nature* **390(6658),** 404–407.
5. Rosenberg, S. A., Aebersold, P., Cornetta, K., Kasid, A., Morgan, R. A., Moen, R., et al. (1990) Gene transfer into humans: immunotherapy of patients with advanced melanoma, using tumor-infiltrating lymphocytes modified by retroviral gene transduction. *N. Engl. J. Med.* **323(9),** 570–578.
6. Takeshita, S., Tsurumi, Y., Couffinahl, T., Asahara, T., Bauters, C., Symes, J., et al. (1996) Gene transfer of naked DNA encoding for three isoforms of vascular endothelial growth factor stimulates collateral development in vivo. *Lab. Invest.* **75(4),** 487–501.
7. Isner, J. M., Pieczek, A., Schainfeld, R., Blair, R., Haley, L., Asahara, T, et al. (1996) Clinical evidence of angiogenesis after arterial gene transfer of phVEGF165 in patient with ischaemic limb. *Lancet* **348(9024),** 370–374.
8. Losordo, D. W., Vale, R., Symes, J. F., Dunnington, C. H., Esakof, D. D., Maysky, M. (1998) Gene therapy for myocardial angiogenesis: initial clinical results with. *Circulation* **98(25),** 2800–2804.
9. Stephan, D. J., Yang, Z. Y., San, H., Simari, R. D., Wheeler, C. J., Felgner, L., et al. (1996) Nabel, A new cationic liposome DNA complex enhances the efficiency of arterial gene transfer in vivo. *Hum. Gene Ther.* **7(15),** 1803–1812.
10. Liu, Y., Thor, A., Shtivelman, E., Cao, Y., Tu, G., Heath, T. D., and Debs, R. J. (1999) Systemic gene delivery expands the repertoire of effective antiangiogenic agents. *J. Biol. Chem.* **274(19),** 13,338–13,344.
11. Hart, S. L., Harbottle, R. P., Cooper, R., Miller, A., Williamson, R., and Coutelle, C. (1995) Gene delivery and expression mediated by an integrin-binding peptide. *Gene Ther.* **2(8),** 552–554.
12. Hart, S. L., Arancibia-Carcamo, C. V., Wolfert, M. A., Mailhos, C., O'Reilly, N. J., Ali, R. R., et al. (1998) Thrasher, and C. Kinnon, Lipid-mediated enhancement of transfection by a nonviral integrin-targeting vector. *Hum. Gene Ther.* **9(4),** 575–585.
13. Zhang, H. T., Smith, K., Graham, A. P., Lau, K. K. W., and Bicknell, R. Transcription Profiling of Humna Microvascular Endothelial Cells in the Proliferative and Quiescent State using cDNA Arrays, In press.
14. Khaw, B. A., Torchilin, V. P., Vural, I., and Narula, J. (1995) Plug and seal: prevention of hypoxic cardiocyte death by sealing membrane lesions with antimyosin-liposomes. *Nature Med.* **1(11),** 1195–1198.
15. Greber, U. F. and Kasamatsu, H. (1996) Nuclear targeting of SV40 and adenovirus. *Trends Cell Biol.* **6(5),** 189–195.
16. Friedmann, T. and Roblin, R. (1972) Gene therapy for human genetic disease? *Science* **175(25),** 949–955.

17. Albritton, L. M., Tseng, L., Scadden, D., and Cunningham, J. M. (1989) A putative murine ecotropic retrovirus receptor gene encodes a multiple membrane-spanning protein and confers susceptibility to virus infection. *Cell* **57(4)**, 659–666.

18. Kavanaugh, M. P., Miller, D. G., Zhang, W., Law, W., Kozak, S. L., Kabat, D., and Miller, A. D. (1994) Cell-surface receptors for gibbon ape leukemia virus and amphotropic murine retrovirus are inducible sodium-dependent phosphate symporters. *Proc. Natl. Acad. Sci. USA* **91(15)**, 7071–7075.

19. McClure, M. O., Sommerfelt, M. A., Marsh, M., and Weiss, R. A. (1990) The pH independence of mammalian retrovirus infection. *J. Gen. Virol.* **71(Pt 4)**, 767–773.

20. Wilson, C. A., Marsh, J. W., and Eiden, M. V. (1992) The requirements for viral entry differ from those for virally induced syncytium formation in NIH 3T3/DTras cells exposed to Moloney murine leukemia virus. *J. Virol.* **66(12)**, 7262–7269.

21. Miller, D. G., Adam, M. A., and Miller, A. D. (1990) Gene transfer by retrovirus vectors occurs only in cells that are actively replicating at the time of infection. *Mol. Cell. Biol.* **10(8)**, 4239–4242.

22. Mann, R., Mulligan, R. C., and Baltimore, D. (1983) Construction of a retrovirus packaging mutant and its use to produce helper. free defective retrovirus. *Cell* **33(1)**, 153–159.

23. Miller, A. D. and Buttimore, C. (1986) Redesign of retrovirus packaging cell lines to avoid recombination leading to helper virus production. *Mol. Cell. Biol.* **6(8)**, 2895–2902.

24. Markowitz, D., Goff, S., and Bank, A. (1988) A safe packaging line for gene transfer: separating viral genes on two different plasmids. *J. Virol.* **62(4)**, 1120–1124.

25. Bender, M. A., Palmer, T. D., Gelinas, R. E., and Miller, A. D. (1987) Evidence that the packaging signal of Moloney murine leukemia virus extends into the gag region. *J. Virol.* **61(5)**, 1639–1646.

26. Nabel, E. G., Plautz, G., and Nabel, G. J. (1990) Site-specific gene expression in vivo by direct gene transfer into the arterial wall. *Science* **249(4974)**, 1285–1288.

27. Flugelman, M. Y., Jaklitsch, M. T., Newman, K. D., Casscells, W., Bratthauer, G. L., and Dichek, D. A. (1992) Low level in vivo gene transfer into the arterial wall through a perforated balloon catheter. *Circulation* **85(3)**, 1110–1117.

28. Flugelman, M. Y. (1995) Inhibition of intravascular thrombosis and vascular smooth muscle cell proliferation by gene therapy. *Thromb. Haemost.* **74(1)**, 406–410.

29. Schnitzer, J. E., McIntosh, D. P., Dvorak, A. M., Liu, J., and Oh, P. (1995) Separation of caveolae from associated microdomains of GPI. anchored proteins. *Science* **269(5229)**, 1435–1439.

30. Welsh, R. M., Jr., Cooper, N. R., Jensen, F. C., and Oldstone, M. B. (1975) Human serum lyses RNA tumor viruses. *Nature* **257(5527)**, 612–614.

31. Closs, E. I., Rinkes, I. H., Bader, A., Yarmush, M. L., and Cunningham, J. M. (1993) Retroviral infection and expression of cationic amino acid transporters in rodent hepatocytes. *J. Virol.* **67(4)**, 2097–2102.

32. Albritton, L. M., Kim, J. W., Tseng, L., and Cunningham, J. M. (1993) Envelope. binding domain in the cationic amino acid transporter determines the host range of ecotropic murine retroviruses. *J. Virol.* **67(4)**, 2091–2096.

33. Takeuchi, Y., Simpson, G., Vile, R. G., Weiss, R. A., and Collins, M. K. L. (1992) Retroviral pseudotypes produced by rescue of a Moloney murine leukemia virus vector by C-type, but not D-type, retroviruses. *Virology* **186(2)**, 792–794.

34. Burns, J. C., Friedmann, T., Driever, W., Burrascano, M., and Yee, J. K. (1993) Vesicular stomatitis virus G glycoprotein pseudotyped retroviral vectors: concentration to very high titer and efficient gene transfer into mammalian and nonmammalian cells. *Proc. Natl. Acad. Sci. USA* **90(17)**, 8033–8037.

35. Dong, J., Roth, M. G., and Hunter, E. (1992) A chimeric avian retrovirus containing the influenza virus hemagglutinin gene has an expanded host range. *J. Virol.* **66(12)**, 7374–7382.

36. Roux, P., Jeanteur, P., and Piechaczyk, M. (1989) A versatile and potentially general approach to the targeting of specific cell types by retroviruses: application to the infection of human cells by means of major histocompatibility complex class I and class II antigens by mouse ecotropic murine leukemia virus-derived viruses. *Proc. Natl. Acad. Sci. USA* **86(23)**, 9079–9083.

37. Etienne-Julan, M., Roux, P., Carillo, S., Jeanteur, P., and Piechaczyk, M. (1992) The efficiency of cell targeting by recombinant retroviruses depends on the nature of the receptor and the composition of the artificial cell-virus linker. *J. Gen. Virol.* **73(Pt 12)**, 3251–3255.

38. Adams, R. M., Wang, M., Steffen, D., and Ledley, F. D. (1995) Infection by retroviral vectors outside of their host range in the presence of replication. defective adenovirus. *J. Virol.* **69(3)**, 1887–1894.

39. Fass, D., Harrison, S. C., and Kim, P. S. (1996) Retrovirus envelope domain at 1. 7 angstrom resolution. *Nat. Struct. Biol.* **3(5)**, 465–469.

40. Kasahara, N., Dozy, A. M., and Kan, Y. W. (1994) Tissue-specific targeting of retroviral vectors through ligand-receptor interactions. *Science* **266(5189)**, 1373–1376.
41. Han, X., Kasahara, N., and Kan, Y. W. (1995) Ligand-directed retroviral targeting of human breast cancer cells. *Proc. Natl. Acad. Sci. USA* **92(21)**, 9747–9751.
42. Russell, S. J., Hawkins, R. E., and Winter, G. (1993) Retroviral vectors displaying functional antibody fragments. *Nucleic. Acids. Res.* **21(5)**, 1081–1085.
43. Fass, D., Davey, R. A., Hamson, C. A., Kim, P. S., Cunningham, J. M., and Berger, J. M. (1997) Structure of a murine leukemia virus receptor. binding glycoprotein at 2.0 angstrom resolution. *Science* **277(5332)**, 1662–1666.
44. Kayman, S. C., Park, H., Saxon, M., and Pinter, A. (1999) The hypervariable domain of the murine leukemia virus surface protein tolerates large insertions and deletions, enabling development of a retroviral particle display system. *J. Virol.* **73(3)**, 1802–1808.
45. Rubin, B. A. and Rouke, L. B. (1988) Adenovirus vaccines, in *Vaccines*, (Plotkin S. A. and Mortimer, E. A., ed.), W. B. Saunders, Philadephia, PA, pp. 492–512.
46. Williams, J., Williams, M., Liu, C., and Telling, G. (1995) Assessing the role of E1A in the differential oncogenicity of group A and group C human adenoviruses. *Curr. Top. Microbiol. Immunol.* **199(Pt 3)**, 149–175.
47. Schachtner, S. K., Rome, J. J., Hoyt, R. F., Jr., Newman, K. D., Virmani, R., and Dichek, D. A. (1995) In vivo adenovirus-mediated gene transfer via the pulmonary artery of rats. *Circ. Res.* **76(5)**, 701–709.
48. Arcasoy, S. M., Latoche, J. D., Gondor, M., Pitt, B. R., and Pilewski, J. M. (1997) Polycations increase the efficiency of adenovirus. mediated gene transfer to epithelial and endothelial cells in vitro. *Gene Therapy* **4(1)**, 32–38.
49. Bergelson, J. M., Cunningham, J. A., Droguett, G., Kurt Jones, E. A., Krithivas, A., Hong, J. S., et al. (1997) Finberg, Isolation of a common receptor for Coxsackie B viruses and adenoviruses 2 and 5. *Science* **275(5304)**, 1320–1323.
50. Hong, S. S., Karayan, L., Tournier, J., Curiel, D. T., and Boulanger, P. A. (1997) Adenovirus type 5 fiber knob binds to MHC class I alpha2 domain at the surface of human epithelial and B lymphoblastoid cells. *EMBO J.* **16(9)**, 2294–2306.
51. Blumenthal, R., Seth, P., Willingham, M. C., and Pastan, I. (1986) pH-dependent lysis of liposomes by adenovirus. *Biochemistry* **25(8)**, 2231–2237.
52. Niewiarowska, J., D'Halluin, J. C., and Belin, M. T. (1992) Adenovirus capsid proteins interact with HSP70 proteins after penetration in human or rodent cells. *Exp. Cell. Res.* **201(2)**, 408–416.
53. Zoldhelyi, P., McNatt, J., Xu, X. M., Loose Mitchell, D., Meidell, R. S., Clubb, F. J., Jr., et al. (1996) Prevention of arterial thrombosis by adenovirus. mediated transfer of cyclooxygenase gene. *Circulation* **93(1)**, 10–17.
54. Lemarchand, P., Jones, M., Yamada, I., and Crystal, R. G. (1993) In vivo gene transfer and expression in normal uninjured blood vessels using replication-deficient recombinant adenovirus vectors. *Circ. Res.* **72(5)**, 1132–1138.
55. Welling, T. H., Davidson, B. L., Zelenock, J. A., Stanley, J. C., Gordon, D., Roessler, B. J., and Messina, L. M. (1996) Systemic delivery of the interleukin-1 receptor antagonist protein using a new strategy of direct adenoviral-mediated gene transfer to skeletal muscle capillary endothelium in the isolated rat hindlimb. *Hum. Gene. Ther.* **7(15)**, 1795–1802.
56. Kass-Eisler, A., Falck-Pedersen, E., Elfenbein, D. H., Alvira, M., Buttrick, P. M., and Leinwand, L. A. (1994) The impact of developmental stage, route of administration and the immune system on adenovirus. mediated gene transfer. *Gene Ther.* **1(6)**, 395–402.
57. Zinn, K. R., Douglas, J. T., Smyth, C. A., Liu, H. G., Wu, Q., Krasnykh, V. N., et al. (1998) Mountz, Imaging and tissue biodistribution of 99mTc-labeled adenovirus knob (serotype 5). *Gene Ther.* **5(6)**, 798–808.
58. Krasnykh, V. N., Mikheeva, G. V., Douglas, J. T., and Curiel, D. T. (1996) Generation of recombinant adenovirus vectors with modified fibers for altering viral tropism. *J. Virol.* **70(10)**, 6839–6846.
59. Tripathy, S. K., Black, H. B., Goldwasser, E., and Leiden, J. M. (1996) Immune responses to transgene-encoded proteins limit the stability of gene expression after injection of replication-defective adenovirus vectors. *Nature Med.* **2(5)**, 545–550.
60. Yang, Y., Ertl, H. C., and Wilson, J. M. (1994) MHC class I-restricted cytotoxic T lymphocytes to viral antigens destroy hepatocytes in mice infected with E1-deleted recombinant adenoviruses. *Immunity* **1(5)**, 433–442.

61. Michou, A. I., Santoro, L., Christ, M., Julliard, V., Pavirani, A., and Mentali, M. (1997) Adenovirus. mediated gene transfer: influence of transgene, mouse strain and type of immune response on persistence of transgene expression. *Gene Ther.* **4(5),** 473–482.

62. Wang, Q., Greenburg, G., Bunch, D., Farson, D., and Finer, M. H. (1997) Persistent transgene expression in mouse liver following in vivo gene transfer with ΔE1/ΔE4 adenovirus vector. *Gene Therapy* **4(5),** 393–400.

63. Chen, P. H., Ornelles, D. A., and Shenk, T. (1993) The adenovirus L3 23-kilodalton proteinase cleaves the amino. terminal head domain from cytokeratin 18 and disrupts the cytokeratin network of HeLa cells. *J. Virol.* **67(6),** 3507–3514.

64. Luo, Z., Sata, M., Nguyen, T., Kaplan, J. M., Akita, G. Y., and Walsh, K. (1999) Adenovirus. mediated delivery of fas ligand inhibits intimal hyperplasia after balloon injury in immunologically primed animals. *Circulation* **99(14),** 1776–1779.

65. Morsy, M. A. and Caskey, C. T. (1999) Expanded-capacity adenoviral vectors: the helper-dependent vectors. *Mol. Med. Today* **5(1),** 18–24.

66. Xia, D., Henry, L. J., Gerard, R. D., and Deisenhofer, J. (1994) Crystal structure of the receptor-binding domain of adenovirus type 5 fiber protein at 1. 7 A resolution. *Structure* **2(12),** 1259–1270.

67. Wickham, T. J., Segal, D. M., Roelvink, P. W., Carrion, M. E., Lizonova, A., Lee, G. M., and Kovesdi, I. (1996) Targeted adenovirus gene transfer to endothelial and smooth muscle cells by using bispecific antibodies. *J. Virol.* **70(10),** 6831–6838.

68. Douglas, J. T., Miller, C. R., Kim, M., Dmitriev, I., Mikheeva, G., Krasnykh, V., and Curiel, D. T. (1999) A system for the propagation of adenoviral vectors with genetically modified receptor specificities. *Nat. Biotechnol.* **17(5),** 470–475.

69. Blacklow, N. R., (1988) Adeno-associated viruses of humans, in *Parvoviruses and Human Diseases*, (Pattison, J., ed., CRC Press, Boca Raton, FL, pp. 165–174.

70. Blacklow, N. R., Hoggan, M. D., Sereno, M. S., Brandt, C. D., Kim, H. W., Parrott, R. H., and Chanock, R. M. (1971) A seroepidemiologic study of adenovirus-associated virus infection in infants and children. *Am. J. Epidemiol.* **94(4),** 359–366.

71. Summerford, C. and Samulski, R. J. (1998) Membrane. associated heparan sulfate proteoglycan is a receptor for adeno-associated virus type 2 virions. *J. Virol.* **72(2),** 1438–1445.

72. Qing, K., Mah, C., Hansen, J., Zhou, S., Dwarki, V., and Srivastava, A. (1999) Human fibroblast growth factor receptor 1 is a co-receptor for infection by adeno-associated virus 2. *Nature Med.* **5(1),** 71–77.

73. Summerford, C., Bartlett, J. S., and Samulski, R. J. (1999) AlphaVbeta5 integrin: a co-receptor for adeno-associated virus type 2 infection. *Nature Med.* **5(1),** 78–82.

74. Qiu, J., Mizukami, H., and Brown, K. E. (1999) Adeno-associated virus 2 co-receptors? *Nature Med.* **5(5),** 467–468.

75. Samulski, R. J., Zhu, X., Xiao, X., Brook, J. D., Housman, D. E., Epstein, N., and Hunter, L. A. (1991) Targeted integration of adeno. associated virus (AAV) into human chromosome 19. *EMBO J.* **10(12),** 3941–3950.

76. Kotin, R. M., Linden, R. M., and Berns, K. I. (1992) Characterization of a preferred site on human chromosome 19q for integration of adeno-associated virus DNA by non-homologous recombination. *EMBO J.* **11(13),** 5071–5078.

77. Srivastava, A., Lusby, E. W., and Berns, K. I. (1983) Nucleotide sequence and organization of the adeno. associated virus 2 genome. *J. Virol.* **45(2),** 555–564.

78. Flotte, T. R., Afione, S. A., and Zeitlin, P. L. (1994) Adeno-associated virus vector gene expression occurs in nondividing cells in the absence of vector DNA integration. *Am. J. Respir. Cell. Mol. Biol.* **11(5),** 517–521.

79. Kearns, W. G., Afione, S. A., Fulmer, S. B., Pang, M. C., Erikson, D., Egan, M., et al. (1996) Cutting, Recombinant adeno. associated virus (AAV-CFTR) vectors do not integrate in a site-specific fashion in an immortalized epithelial cell line. *Gene Ther.* **3(9),** 748–755.

80. Clark, K. R., Sferra, T. J., and Johnson, P. R. (1997) Recombinant adeno-associated viral vectors mediate long term transgene expression in muscle. *Hum. Gene. Ther.* **8,** 659–669.

81. Linden, R. M., Winocour, E., and Berns, K. I. (1996) The recombination signals for adeno-associated virus site-specific integration. *Proc. Natl. Acad. Sci. USA* **93(15),** 7966–7972.

82. Flotte, T. R., Afione, S. A., Conrad, C., McGrath, S. A., Solow, R., Oka, H., et al. (1993a) Stable in vivo expression of the cystic fibrosis transmembrane conductance regulator with an adeno. associated virus vector. *Proc. Natl. Acad. Sci. USA* **90(22),** 10,613–10,617.

83. Flotte, T. R. (1993b) Prospects for virus. based gene therapy for cystic fibrosis. *J. Bioenerg. Biomembr.* **25(1),** 37–42.

84. Conrad, C. K., Allen, S. S., Afione, S. A., Reynolds, T. C., Beck, S. E., Fee Maki, M., et al. (1996) Flotte, Safety of single-dose administration of an adeno-associated virus (AAV)-CFTR vector in the primate lung. *Gene Therapy* **3(8)**, 658–668.

85. Brookens, M., Calmiels, T., Samulski, R. J., Meyrick, B., Gao, X., Huang, L., and Pitt, B. R. (1992) Adeno-associated virus vector for gene transfer to cultured ovine pulmonary microvascular endothelial cells. *Am. Rev. Resp. Dis.* p.A834.

86. Lynch, C. M., Hara, P. S., Leonard, J. C., Williams, J. K., Dean, R. H., and Geary, R. L. (1997) Adeno-associated virus vectors for vascular gene delivery. *Circ. Res.* **80(4)**, 497–505.

87. Bartlett, J. S., Kleinschmidt, J., Boucher, R. C., and Samulski, R. J. (1999) Targeted adeno-associated virus vector transduction of nonpermissive cells mediated by a bispecific F (ab'gamma) 2 antibody. *Nat. Biotechnol.* **17(2)**, 181–186.

88. Korhonen, J., Lahtinen, I., Halmekyto, M., Alhonen, L., Janne, J., Dumont, D., and Alitalo, K. (1995) Endothelial. specific gene expression directed by the tie gene promoter in vivo. *Blood* **86(5)**, 1828–1835.

89. Ozaki, K., Yoshida, T., Ide, H., Saito, I., Ikeda, Y., Sugimura, T., and Terada, M. (1996) Use of von Willebrand factor promoter to transduce suicidal gene to human endothelial cells, HUVEC. *Hum. Gene Ther.* **7(13)**, 1483–1490.

90. Jaggar, R. T., Chan, H. Y., Harris, A. L., and Bicknell, R. (1997) Endothelial cell-specific expression of tumor necrosis factor-alpha from the KDR or E. selectin promoters following retroviral delivery. *Hum. Gene Ther.* **8(18)**, 2239–2247.

91. Goldman, C. K., Kendall, R. L., Cabrera, G., Soroceanu, L., Heike, Y., Gillespie, G. Y., et al. (1998) Paracrine expression of a native soluble vascular endothelial growth factor receptor inhibits tumor growth, metastasis, and mortality rate. *Proc. Natl. Acad. Sci. USA* **95(15)**, 8795–8800.

92. Lin, P., Buxton, J. A., Acheson, A., Radziejewski, C., Maisonpierre, P. C., Yancopoulos, G. D. (1998) Antiangiogenic gene therapy targeting the endothelium-specific receptor tyrosine kinase Tie2. *Proc. Natl. Acad. Sci. USA* **95(15)**, 8829–8834.

93. Guo, N., Krutzsch, H. C., Inman, J. K., and Roberts, D. D. (1997) Thrombospondin 1 type I repeat peptides of thrombospondin 1 specifically induce apoptosis of endothelial cells. *Cancer Res.* **57(9)**, 1735–1742.

94. Dhanabal, M., Ramchandran, R., Waterman, M. J, Lu, H., Knebelmann, B., Segal, M., and Sukhatme, V. P. (1999) Endostatin induces endothelial cell apoptosis. *J. Biol. Chem.* **274(17)**, 11,721–11,726.

95. Liu, Y., Thor, A., Shtivelman, E., Cao, Y., Tu, G., Heath, T. D., and Debs, R. J. (1999) Systemic gene delivery expands the repertoire of effective antiangiogenic agents. *J. Biol. Chem.* **274(19)**, 13,338–13,344.

96. Tanaka, T., Manome, Y., Wen, P., Kufe, D. W., and Fine, H. A. (1997) Fine, viral vector-mediated transduction of a modified platelet factor 4 cDNA inhibits angiogenesis and tumor growth. *Nature Med.* *3(4)*, 437–442.

97. Tanaka, T., Cao, Y., Folkman, J., and Fine, H. A. (1998) Viral vector-targeted antiangiogenic gene therapy utilizing an angiostatin complementary DNA. Cancer Res. 58(15), 3362–3369.

98. Blezinger, P., Wang, J., Gondo, M., Quezada, A., Mehrens, D., French, M., et al. (1999) Systemic inhibition of tumor growth and tumor metastases by intramuscular administration of the endostatin gene [In Process Citation]. *Nature Biotechnol.* **17(4)**, 343–348.

99. Burrows, F. J. and Thorpe, P. E. (1993) Eradication of large solid tumors in mice with an immunotoxin directed against tumor vasculature. *Proc. Natl. Acad. Sci. USA* **90(19)**, 8996–9000.

100. Hagemeier, H. H., Vollmer, E., Goerdt, S., Schulze, Osthoff, K., and Sorg, C. (1986) A monoclonal antibody reacting with endothelial cells of budding vessels in tumors and inflammatory tissues, and non-reactive with normal adult tissues. *Int. J. Cancer* **38(4)**, 481–488.

101. Thorpe, P. E. and Burrows, F. J. (1995) Antibody-directed targeting of the vasculature of solid tumors. *Breast Cancer Res. Treat.* **36(2)**, 237–251.

102. Ruco, L. P., Pomponi, D., Pigott, R., Stoppacciaro, A., Monardo, F., Uccini, S. et al. (1990) Cytokine production (IL-1) alpha, IL-1 beta, and TNF alpha) and endothelial cell activation (ELAM-1 and HLA-DR) in reactive lymphadenitis, Hodgkin's disease, and in non-Hodgkin's lymphomas. An immunocytochemical study. *Am. J. Pathol.* **137(5)**, 1163–1171.

103. Winter, G., Griffiths, A. D., Hawkins, R. E., and Hoogenboom, H. R. (1994) Making antibodies by phage display technology. *Annu. Rev. Immunol.* **12**, 433–455.

104. Modzelewski, R., Auerbach, R., Chang, M. J., and Johnson, C. S. (1992) Isolation of tumor endothelial cells using MoAb to angiotensin-converting enzyme. *Proc. Am. Assoc. Can. Res.* **33**, 100, Ab 598.

105. Wernert, N., Raes, M. B., Lassalle, P., Dehouck, M. P., Gosselin, B. Vandenbunder, B., and Stehelin, D. (1992) C-ets1 Proto-oncogene is a transcription factor expressed in endothelial cells during tumor vascularization and other forms of angiogenesis in humans. *Am. J. Pathol.* **140(1)**, 119–127.

24

Antibody Targeting of Tumor Vasculature

J. Wilson, David C. West, and Philip E. Thorpe

CONTENTS

INTRODUCTION: WHY TARGET THE ENDOTHELIUM?
THE TUMOR VASCULATURE AND PHENOTYPIC DIFFERENCES
ANTIGENS WITH POTENTIAL FOR VASCULAR TARGETING
SUMMARY AND CONCLUSIONS
ACKNOWLEDGMENTS
REFERENCES

INTRODUCTION: WHY TARGET THE ENDOTHELIUM?

For many years the idea of the "magic bullet" approach to target cells in the treatment of cancer and other pathological conditions has been a tempting scenario. One such approach is to develop monoclonal antibodies (MAbs) against defined cell-surface markers and use these antibodies to direct cytotoxic agents to specific cells. However, the use of such therapies to target the actual tumor cells within solid tumors has proved to be inefficient, with usually less than 0.01% of the injected dose of an antibody localising per gram of tumor in humans. Furthermore, owing to the density of the packed tumor cells and high interstitial pressure in the tumor core, this localization is uneven and the antibody tends to become adsorbed in the perivascular regions of the peripheral tumor cells, with none reaching the tumor cells at more distant sites.

It is well-established that most solid tumors require a blood supply to sustain their growth, invasion, and metastasis, and so are inescapably dependent on their ability to continuously elicit new blood-vessel formation *(1,2)*. Over the last 25 yr most research on tumor angiogenesis has been aimed at inhibiting the process of tumor-induced vessel formation. To date, many hundreds of compounds have been reported to possess "anti-angiogenic" activity (reviewed in refs. *3,4*). These fall into the following broad groups: antagonists of angiogenic growth factors and cytokines; metalloproteinase inhibitors; inhibitors of endothelial migration and capillary formation; inhibitors of basement-membrane synthesis; and endothelial-selective cytotoxic drugs. It is still uncertain as to whether neutralization of angiogenic factors, or disruption of their receptor interactions, is an effective approach to anti-angiogenesis therapy, especially on established tumors. Anti-

From: *The New Angiotherapy*
Edited by: T.-P. D. Fan and E. C. Kohn © Humana Press Inc., Totowa, NJ

angiogenic therapy is at present essentially a stasis approach, slowing or delaying tumor growth, rather than causing significant regression of established tumors. Additionally, few of the compounds in clinical trials are amenable to long-term oral administration, which will be a necessary feature of such treatments. In contrast, initial reports on other compounds, such as angiostatin and endostatin, which appear to be cytotoxic to tumor endothelium rather than cytostatic, suggest that apoptosis induction may be a practicable approach to solid tumor therapy, especially in combination with other chemotherapeutic agents (reviewed in ref. 5).

Denekamp (6) originally hypothesized that the local disruption of the tumor vasculature would result in the death of many thousands of tumor cells, and that only a few endothelial cells within the vessels need to be killed to completely occlude the vessels. This alternative approach, called "vascular targeting," aims to target the tumor endothelium with toxins or coagulants and disrupt the tumor's blood supply directly. Vascular endothelial cells within the tumor are in direct contact with the bloodstream and are readily accessible to intravenously injected macromolecules, such as immunoconjugates, thus overcoming the problem of poor penetration into solid tumors (7). It is also very likely that the targeting of the vasculature of solid tumors may be applicable to many tumor types, as they all must induce new capillary growth in order to form and maintain a mass larger than 1 mm^3.

Vascular targeting is not only a powerful approach to the treatment of solid tumors. Endothelial cells play a central role in other pathological conditions, especially inflammatory diseases such as psoriasis and rheumatoid arthritis (RA), and are an obvious target for novel therapies. For such strategies to be successful in humans, antigens that are preferentially expressed in tumor or activated vessels have to be identified. Ideally, such antigens would not be expressed on endothelial cells, or other cells in normal tissues and would be expressed on many tumor endothelial cells in diverse solid tumors or widely expressed in chronic inflammation. Much research is currently ongoing to identify such antigens and generate targeting antibodies, and the latest findings are described later.

THE TUMOR VASCULATURE AND PHENOTYPIC DIFFERENCES

In tumors, capillary formation follows the same sequence of events as in other tissues, but results in giant capillaries, blind vessels, arteriovenous shunts, capillaries connecting two venules, and compressed or damaged vessels in close proximity to each other (8,9). This produces a chaotic tumor vasculature with irregular inter-capillary spacing that is insufficient to meet the local nutrient requirements. This, together with local vascular collapse, results in areas of hypoxia, reduced pH, and necrosis (10). Also, the newly formed capillaries do not mature properly and lack some of the elements necessary for local homeostatic regulation. Tumor-derived soluble factors such as vascular endothelial growth factor (VEGF) and interleukin-1 (IL-1) induce procoagulative changes on endothelium, leading to hypercoagulability and the generation of microthrombi. These factors combine to produce a unique environment in which we might expect the endothelium to express proteins not found on the normal quiescent endothelium.

Increasing numbers of reports of organ and site-specific differences in protein synthesis, surface glycoproteins, lectin-binding specificity, tumor cell and lymphocyte adhesion, suggest that molecules specific for tumor endothelium may exist (11). In our own studies, two-dimensional electrophoretic analysis of total endothelial-cell protein synthesis and cell-surface glycoproteins has shown that treatment of cultured human large vessel and capillary endothelial cells with mitogens induces general, and also

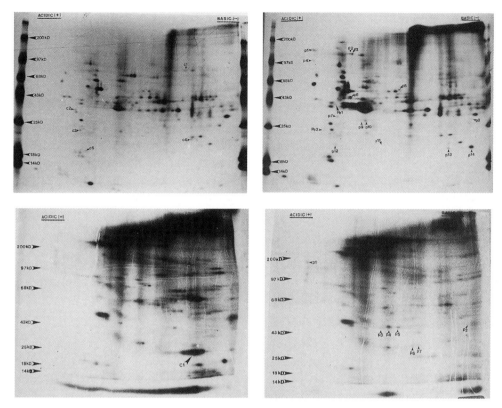

Fig. 1. 2-D PAGE gels of (^{35}S)-labeled (top) and (^{125}I) – surface-labeled (bottom) human umbilical-vein endothelial cells. (Left) confluent cultures and (Right) stimulated with tumor-conditioned medium. Arrows denote unique proteins. (*See* refs. *13,14* for details.)

mitogen-specific, surface glycoproteins *(12–14)*. Treatment of endothelial cells with tumor-conditioned medium induces proliferation and migration-related and new tumor vessel-associated proteins. Some of these proteins appear to be induced in several types of endothelial cells by different tumor-conditioned media *(14)*, Fig. 1, suggesting universal targets for tumor endothelium may exist. MAbs against four such tumor endothelial surface antigens stained the vasculature of several types of tumors but not that of normal tissues, including those containing proliferating endothelium, i.e., placenta and colon. Each MAb reacted with vessels in a different series of tumors but a combination of two MAbs stained vessels in 70% of the tumors screened. It is possible that these antigens are new tumor-induced endothelial cell-surface "activation" antigens.

VEGF and platelet-derived growth factor (PDGF) receptors, Tie receptor kinase, HSP70, endoglin and the endothelial adhesion molecules, P-selectin, E-selectin and VCAM-1 are upregulated on both wound and tumor vasculature. Data indicate that the angiogenic phenotype is, in part, similar to that induced by various forms of mechanical and environmental stresses or injury, as well as by biochemical/immunological stimuli. These stimuli induce a wide, but overlapping, spectrum of "activated" endothelial-cell responses that require altered gene expression and the acquisition of an "activated" phenotype. This is characterized by: increased proteolytic activity; enhanced, or de novo, expression of chemoattractants, MHC-I/MHC-II and adhesion molecules for inflammatory cells; altered vasoactive properties and growth factor production; and increased turnover rate. Many of these "injuries" also stimulate angiogenesis and endothelial cells in growing capillaries appear express many of the properties and molecules associated with the "activated" phenotype, which offers the prospect of new targets for therapy *(15)*.

ANTIGENS WITH POTENTIAL FOR VASCULAR TARGETING

Most of the MAbs described below were raised using cultured human endothelial cells, usually human umbilical vein, stimulated with either single angiogenic factors, tumor-conditioned medium, or by direct co-culture with tumor cells. Several were produced by injection of tumor tissue or tumor capillary fractions. The perfect antibody for solid tumor targeting would: (1) bind an epitope expressed by a high proportion of the tumor vasculature in diverse types of tumor, and (2) not bind to endothelial cells, or any other cells, in normal tissues.

Signal Transduction Pathways

Endothelial receptor tyrosine kinases appear to have a role in pathological vascular growth, particularly in tumors. Several receptors identified so far appear to be upregulated on vessels in solid tumors and are candidates for targeting (reviewed in ref. *16*).

TIE RECEPTOR TYROSINE KINASE

Partanen et al. *(17)* first described Tie-1, the protein product of a receptor tyrosine kinase cDNA. The expression of Tie-1 and the closely related Tie-2 (TEK) is most prevalent in the vascular endothelium during embryonic development. The Tie receptors, which are only weakly expressed in adults, are upregulated during angiogenesis. Using transgenic mice, the Tie2/Tie2 ligand pathway has been shown to play important roles during development of the embryonic vasculature. Its role in adult angiogenesis has been examined using a soluble form of mouse Tie-2 (ExTEK.6His) as a Tie-2 inhibitor. Soluble Tie-2 was found to reduce the growth of a mammary tumor inside a rat cutaneous window chamber, and the tumor vascular length density was also significantly reduced. In the rat cornea, this inhibitor protein also blocked angiogenesis stimulated by tumor-conditioned medium *(18)*. Tie-2 expression has been detected in the endothelium of normal breast tissue, benign breast lesions, and breast tumors. However, strongest expression was seen in vascular hotspots, and the proportion of Tie-2-positive vessels was significantly higher in breast tumors than in nonmalignant breast tissues *(19)*. Recently it has been demonstrated that angiopoietin-1 and angiopoietin-2 regulate angiogenesis as an agonist and antagonist, respectively, by triggering the Tie-2 receptor *(20,21)*.

THE EPH FAMILY RECEPTORS AND LIGANDS

The Eph family of receptors is a large subfamily of receptor tyrosine kinases (recently reviewed in ref. *22*). At least 14 Eph family members and 8 ephrin ligands for these receptors have been described. On the basis of sequence homology and binding specificities, the Eph receptors can be broadly divided into two groups, EphA and EphB. The ephrin ligands cannot act as soluble mediators, and must be membrane-bound in order to activate their receptors *(23)*. To date, most of the studies surrounding the Eph receptors and their ligands have been in the nervous system, where they have a role in guiding axons to their targets, and maintaining borders between distinct neuronal compartments by preventing cell mixing *(24,25)*.

More recently, a role for the Eph family has been suggested in the vasculature (reviewed by Yancopoulos et al. *[26]*). In the corneal assay, ephrin-A1 is highly angiogenic and anti-ephrin-A1 antibody significantly reduces the angiogenic effect of tumor necrosis factor (TNF)-α *(27)*. Ephrin-A1 is a chemoattractant for endothelial cells and so its effect on angiogenesis is as a result of promoting cell migration. The effect of this ligand is possibly mediated via the Eph receptor, EphA2, which is reportedly expressed on endothelial cells *(27)*.

Studies have demonstrated that EphB1 and EphA2 can direct vascular network assembly, affecting endothelial migration, capillary morphogenesis, and angiogenesis *(28)*. In addition, at the earliest stages of capillary-plexus formation, members of the Eph family distinctly mark arteries and veins. Wang et al. *(29)* demonstrated that the ligand ephrin-B2 marks future arterial but not venous endothelial cells, whereas the receptor Eph-B4 (one of the ephrin-B2 receptors) reciprocally marks the venous endothelium.

The Eph family receptors and their ligands are thought to participate in the morphogenesis of kidney microvascular structures *(30)*. The ephrin-B1 ligand induces the formation of capillary-like structures in human renal microvascular endothelial cells in vitro, and this effect is mediated by the receptor EphB1. Interestingly, in similar experiments, ephrin-B1 has no effect on human umbilical-vein endothelial cells, whereas ephrin-A1 induces the formation of capillary-like structures but has no effect on renal endothelial cells. This indicates that different ligands have specificity for different types of endothelial cells, suggesting they express different Eph receptors. It is possible that future work in this young field might identify Eph family members that are novel markers of neovascularization.

VEGF AND VEGF RECEPTORS

It has long been established that VEGF has a leading role in the regulation of angiogenesis, particularly as a mediator of tumor angiogenesis. Many human tumors exhibit a high level of expression of VEGF, and anti-VEGF MAbs can inhibit human tumor growth in nude mice *(31)*. VEGF conjugates with a mutated form of diphtheria toxin induces vascular-mediated injury in tumors in mice *(32)* and clinical studies are now in progress *(33)*.

Two endothelial-cell surface receptors, VEGFR-1 (flt-1) and VEGFR-2 (flk-1/KDR) have been established as the mediators of the angiogenic responses of VEGF. Blocking antibodies against VEGFR-2, which inactivate this receptor, disrupt ongoing angiogenesis and prevent malignant human keratinocyte invasion *(34)*. Also, a soluble VEGF receptor constructed by fusing the entire extracellular domain of murine flk-1 to a six-histidine tag at the C-terminus (ExFlk.6His) was found to inhibit VEGF action by a dominant-negative mechanism. This suggests that a soluble receptor may have potential in anti-angiogenic therapy for cancer and other angiogenesis-dependent conditions *(35)*. Novel MAbs, 2-10-1 and 2-7-9, have been generated against the extracellular domain of human VEGFR-II *(36)* that have potential for drug targeting in angiogenic diseases.

Within the tumor microenvironment, hypoxia and the local increase in the concentration of VEGF, results in the upregulation of VEGF receptor expression on tumor endothelial cells. The high concentration of both VEGF and its receptor leads to a high concentration of receptor-bound VEGF on the tumor endothelium. The production of MAbs against VEGF bound to the Flk-1 receptor, which bind with high affinity to frozen sections of human and rodent tumors and, selectively localize to the tumor endothelium following intravenous administration into mice bearing human tumor xenografts *(37)*. The upregulation of VEGF and the VEGF receptor, and the subsequent binding of VEGF to its receptor, is a feature of blood vessels supplying many types of solid tumors, suggesting that this type of immunoconjugate can be used to treat many different types of cancer. A similar antibody has been conjugated to ricin, and successfully used to target tumors in mice and guinea pigs *(38)*.

Cell Adhesion Molecules

INTEGRINS

The integrin $\alpha_v\beta_3$ is absent or expressed at low levels on normal, or resting blood vessels, but it is significantly upregulated in the vasculature of tumors (39–41). Furthermore, β_3 integrin expression in melanoma (42) and α_{v-3} expression in breast cancer (41) predicts subsequent metastases. Increased expression is also associated with the angiogenesis seen during wound healing (43,44), suggesting that α_{v-3} has a physiological role in the angiogenic process (43,45). In vivo studies have demonstrated that MAbs against $\alpha_v\beta_3$ interfere with adhesion-dependent signals, causing apoptosis of angiogenic endothelial cells in the chick chorioallantoic membrane (CAM) assay (46). Additionally, in a mouse model of human breast cancer, treatment with anti-$\alpha_v\beta_3$ MAb resulted in tumors having not only significantly fewer human blood vessels, but also in tumors that appeared to be considerably less invasive than in control animals (47). A further indication that $\alpha_v\beta_3$ is an excellent target for gene therapy comes from the report that the disintegrin, triflavin, which is more inhibitory than anti-$\alpha_v\beta_3$ MAbs on angiogenesis (48), disrupts only newly forming blood vessels without affecting the pre-existing vasculature.

CD44

Flow cytometry and immunohistochemical studies have demonstrated that endothelial cells from human solid tumors display enhanced expression of CD44, as compared to endothelial cells from normal tissue. The angiogenic stimuli, bFGF and VEGF, upregulated CD44 on cultured human endothelial cells, suggesting that CD44 is an activation antigen on human vasculature. Additionally, in vitro experiments showed the endothelial cells are efficiently killed by an immunotoxin directed against CD44, suggesting that CD44 may prove to be a useful endothelial target for therapy (49,50).

Inflammatory Adhesion Molecules

VASCULAR CELL ADHESION MOLECULE-1 (VCAM-1)

During inflammation, cytokines induce the expression of vascular cell adhesion molecule-1, or VCAM-1, on the endothelium, leading to the recruitment of leukocytes at these sites (reviewed by Granger and Kubes [51]). VCAM-1 is largely absent from normal vasculature. It is present, however, on the endothelium in many malignant tumors, such as renal carcinoma (52) and Hodgkin's disease (53), as well as in begnign tumors, such as hemangioma (54). However, in humans it is constitutively expressed on some vessels in the kidney, thymus, and thyroid (54,55). Recently it has been reported that a MAb to mouse VCAM-1 covalently linked to human tissue factor localized selectively to VCAM-1 expressing vessels in immunodeficient mice bearing human Hodgkin's tumors, following intravenous injection (56). Thrombosis of these vessels occurred and resulted in a slowing of tumor growth.

SIALYL LEWIS(X) AND SELECTINS

The inducible endothelial-adhesion molecules E- and P-selectin and their tetrasaccharide ligands, sialyl Lewis X (SLeX), and sialyl Lewis a (SLea), have mostly been studied in the context of leukocyte and tumor-cell adhesion to activated endothelial cells (57,58). However, endothelial E-selectin expression is upregulated by proliferative and migratory stimuli (50,59). Also, Nguyen et al. (60) have shown that E/P-selectin-SleX/a interactions are important mediators of endothelial-endothelial adhesion during lumen formation in vitro. The recent finding that soluble E-selectin can induce angiogenesis in vivo and stimulate endothelial-cell migration in vitro, suggests that E-selectin-SLeX interactions may play a role in endothelial-endothelial signaling during capillary formation (61). Furthermore, several workers, including ourselves, have found that in most solid tumors E-selectin is expressed by the intratumoral and peritumoral microvessels, and some small venules (54,62–64). In addition, increased circulating levels of soluble E-selectin have been reported for several solid tumors, especially metastatic tumors (63,65; West et al., unpublished results). In breast carcinoma, endothelia in primary breast lesions express more SLeX than in normal tissue and metastatic lesions express even higher amounts of SLeX compared with primary lesions. The expression of P- and E-selectin was also greatly enhanced in tumor-bearing tissue compared with normal (66). Given the endothelial specificity of E-selectin expression, and the correlation between tumor vessel density and metastasis in many tumors, increased circulating E-selectin probably reflects the level of tumor angiogenesis (67). Interestingly, it appears that the anti-angiogenic agents AGM-1470 and angiostatin also upregulate endothelial E-selectin expression (68,69).

Recently, anti-E-selectin conjugated liposomes and oligonucleotides have been shown to be phagocytosed by activated endothelial cells in vitro, suggesting that anti-E-selectin antibodies may be a useful targeting agent for toxin-mediated killing of tumor endothelium (70,71). Furthermore, ^{111}In-labeled anti-E-selectin antibodies have already been used to image rheumatoid joints (72,73).

Other Molecules Expressed on Endothelial Cell Surface

ENDOGLIN (CD105)

Endoglin or CD105 is a dimmeric glycoprotein consisting of two 95 kDa disulphide-linked subunits, which is part of the TGF- complex on human endothelial cells and binds TGF-1 and TGF-4 β243. It is expressed at low levels on most normal endothelium (74,75), but is strongly expressed on the vasculature of a wide range of solid tumors, and on proliferating endothelial cells in culture (76). It is also upregulated at other angiogenic locations, such as dermal endothelium in chronic inflammatory skin lesions (75). However, it is also expressed on some other cell types, including fetal syncytiotrophoblasts (77) and some leukemic and hemopoietic cell lines.

The MAb TEC-11, raised by immunizing BALB/c mice with human umbilical-vein cells (HUVEC) stimulated by culturing them with conditioned medium from a human colorectal carcinoma cell line, HT29 (76), has been successfully used to target the vasculature of tumors. Flow-cytometry studies of mouse L-cells transfected with human endoglin have demonstrated that the TEC-11 antibody recognizes endoglin (76). Early studies with a immunotoxin prepared by conjugating TEC-11 with deglycosylated ricin A chain demonstrated the therapeutic potential of this antibody, because in vitro this immunotoxin was much more potent at inhibiting protein synthesis in proliferating HUVEC cultures than to confluent cultures (76).

The E-9 MAb, raised against cultured HUVEC, also recognizes endoglin. However the epitope recognized appears to be different from that recognized by TEC-11, as E-9 stains all tumors, fetal organs, and inflamed tissues examined so far. E-9 exhibited weak staining of normal endothelium, with the exception of strong staining of tonsil. Placenta was reported to be negative (78).

ONCOFETAL FIBRONECTIN

Oncofetal fibronectin (B-FN) isoform is present in vessels of neoplastic tissues but, in normal adult tissues, expression is limited to sites of angiogenesis. Human antibody fragments with pan-species recognition of this isoform have been isolated from a phage-display library. These fragments were chemically coupled to a fluorophore and used to image in real time an aggressive tumor (F9 murine teratocarcinoma) in nude mice *(79)*.

Similar in vivo studies used a different MAb (BC-1) labeled with ^{125}I to examine the distribution of human oncofetal fibronectin in nude mice bearing subcutaneous human tumor implants of U87MG high-grade astrocytoma and SKMel28 melanoma. Following injection, ^{125}I-BC-1 was preferentially taken up in the human tumor implants; however, there was some nonspecific uptake in the bone marrow and skeletal muscle, but this was at much lower levels than in tumors *(80)*.

CD40 LIGAND

CD40 ligand is expressed by human vascular endothelial cells, smooth-muscle cells, and human macrophages in vitro and is co-expressed with its receptor CD40 on all three cell types in human atherosclerotic lesions *in situ (81)*. In neovascularized areas of renal-cell carcinoma, the endothelial cells have been reported to express CD40, and the presence of tumor cells is necessary for this expression, as substantiated by in vitro experiments *(82)*.

PROSTATE-SPECIFIC MEMBRANE ANTIGEN (PSMA)

As the name suggests, the expression of PSMA was originally thought to be exclusively restricted to the epithelial-cell membrane of the prostate *(83,84)*. It is an ideal candidate for prostate-specific targeting therapies, because PSMA is expressed in a high proportion of prostate cancers *(85)*, and this expression is increased in metastatic disease. However, it now appears that antibodies to PSMA also strongly react with the vascular endothelium in a wide range of carcinomas, including lung, colon, and breast *(86,87)*, but do not react with the normal endothelium. Thus, antibodies recently described *(86,88)* should prove useful for targeting not only prostate cancer, but also the vascular compartment of a wide variety of carcinomas.

EN 7/44 ANTIGEN

EN 7/44 was the first MAb reported to bind specifically to human tumor vasculature. It binds a 30.5 kDa antigen in endothelial cells of miscellaneous tumors, placenta, and sites of acute inflammation *(89)*. In most tumors, the strongest reaction is seen with capillary buds, but staining of large vessels, venules, veins, and some small arteries in normal and tumor tissues was observed. The antigen is largely a cytoplasmic antigen and, as such, of limited value as a target molecule.

ENDOSIALIN

Raised against cultured human fetal fibroblasts, the FB5 MAb detects a novel 165 kDa cell-surface highly-sialylated protein whose gene is located on chromosome 11q13-qtr *(90)*. Although normal blood vessels and adult tissues do not express endosialin, FB5 stains the endothelium of 67% of tumors. However, much of the staining is in the stroma adjacent to the vasculature and there is a large variability in the number of vessels stained in different tumors. This can range from a few capillaries to the entire tumor vasculature. FB5 is rapidly internalized by cultured HUVEC and may be a useful targeting agent for conjugated toxins.

TP-1/ TP-3 ANTIGEN

The MAbs TP-1 and TP-3, raised against cells from a human osteosarcoma xenograft, appear to recognize different epitopes on the same 80 kDa osteosarcoma-associated protein *(91)*. Both antibodies stained the vasculature of placenta and budding capillaries in tumors, but staining of normal tissues was limited to a few cells in the adrenal medulla and proximal-kidney tubules.

Potential Agents to Target

So far we have discussed only one component of vascular-targeting agents, the antibody that binds to antigens on the surface of blood vessels that supply tumors. The second key component is the drug molecule that kills the endothelial cells and occludes the vessels. A compelling feature of such treatments is that even tumor cells at the core are killed, and these are usually the most resistant to traditional anti-cancer drugs owing to their inaccessibility. However, cells in the periphery of the tumor can sometimes survive by obtaining necessary nutrients from the surrounding tissue, but these can be eradicated using orthodox anti-cancer agents.

COAGULANTS

Coagulants such as the human coagulation-initiating protein, tissue factor, can also be conjugated to the targeting antibody to bring about infarction of tumor vessels. Once the antibody is bound to the vessel wall, the tissue factor is brought into proximity with the endothelial-cell surface, takes part in its native function, and locally initiates thrombosis, leading to occlusion of the vessel.

The normal function of tissue factor is to induce coagulation at sites of injury. Tissue factor on cells outside the bloodstream comes into contact with factor VII/VIIa in the blood, and initiates the cascade of events leading to the production of the protein, fibrin, which is a major component of clots. Tissue factor has to be modified to prevent it from causing coagulation in the bloodstream, while it is on route to the tumor endothelium. Studies have centered on a soluble recombinant tissue factor (tTF) lacking the cytosolic and transmembrane domains. Truncated TF is virtually devoid of clotting ability because it lacks a phospholipid surface upon which to function *(92)*. Tissue factor needs to be associated with negatively charged phospholipids in order to activate the next stages of the clotting process. Once the antibody targets the tTF to the tumor vessels, it is brought back into proximity to a lipid surface and clotting activity is regained.

A mouse model was set up where the tumor endothelium expresses major histocompatibility complex class II antigens. These antigens are absent from normal endothelium in the mouse and so constitute a tumor endothelial cell-specific marker *(93)*. Immunoconjugates containing truncated tissue factor (tTF) linked to an antibody specific for class II antigens have been targeted to the tumor endothelium in this model *(94)*. Within 30 min, tumor vessels are coagulated and by 4 h there are signs of tumor-cell injury. This is followed by tumor collapse over the next few days and finally results in a fibrous scar visible at the location of the tumor mass *(94)*.

As already discussed, the main criteria for a targeting therapy to be successful in the clinic, is that the target molecule is expressed selectively on the tumor endothelium and is largely absent from the normal endothelium. In order to examine the feasibility of targeting tTF to human tumor vasculature, a "coaguligand" was constructed by covalently linking tTF to a MAb against VCAM-1. This was able to selectively induce thrombosis of tumor vessels and tumor infarction in human Hodgkin's lymphoma, grown as a xenograft in SCID mice *(56)*.

One of the main advantages of using tissue factor in vascular targeting is that it is a human protein, and so should have low immunogenicity in human subjects. Additionally, it is highly potent because one molecule is capable of activating a cascade of clotting proteins, thus greatly amplifying the effect. Even a small dose causes extensive coagulation in the tumor vessels. Additionally, in murine studies the binding of the coaguligand to VCAM-1 on normal vessels constitutively expressing VCAM-1, such as heart and lung, did not induce thrombosis *(56)*. It appears that an additional factor, phosphatidyl serine (PS) has to be present on the luminal side of vessels, to provide a procoagulant surface upon which the proteins of the clotting cascade can assemble *(95)*. Immunohistochemical studies showed that PS is positioned on the luminal surface of vessels in small tumors, but not in normal tissues *(56)*. This explains the lack of thrombotic activity in the normal tissues. The finding that the initiation of coagulation by anti-VCAM-1:tTF treatment requires expression of both the target molecule and PS should contribute to the selectivity of thrombosis induction and thus to the safety of coaguligands in clinical applications.

Toxins

Toxins commonly used in producing immunotoxins are derived from either bacteria (e.g., diphtheria toxin), or plants (e.g., ricin or abrin), and kill cells by inhibiting protein synthesis (reviewed by Thrush et al. *[96]*). Toxins, or their cytotoxic A-chains, can be conjugated to the targeting antibody and, once delivered to the tumor endothelial cells, the toxin enters the cells and kills them. As the cells in the vessel wall die, platelet activation and clot formation are triggered and the vessels supplying the tumor become occluded, leaving vessels in normal tissues unaffected. Using the mouse model expressing MHC class II antigens on the tumor endothelium *(93)*, a single intravenous injection of anti-class II ricin A-chain immunotoxin into mice bearing large solid tumors resulted in major tumor regressions *(7)*.

SUMMARY AND CONCLUSIONS

The antibody-directed targeting of toxins, coagulating agents, antisense and "suicide" genes to the tumor endothelium is an attractive therapeutic strategy. There are two major advantages of this approach over targeting the tumor cells themselves, namely: the endothelium is freely accessible to the antibody-drug conjugates, and the phenotype of tumor endothelium is reasonably uniform and stable. Thus a single agent may reasonably be expected to be applicable to many different tumors.

Much of this review has been directed towards the use of conjugated antibodies, where the antibodies are merely a delivery vehicle. The complex polysaccharide exotoxin CM101, which has been shown to target tumor endothelium, directly induces complement-dependent endothelial cytotoxicity *(97)*, as do many anti-endothelial IgM autoantibodies *(98)*. Tumor regression has been observed in the early clinical studies with CM101, an unusually high anti-tumor activity compared with other anti-angiogenesis drugs *(99)*. Many anti-tumor antibodies mediate considerable antibody-dependent cellular cytotoxicity (ADCC), especially high-affinity antibodies against high density epitopes *(100)*, although conjugation of toxins to the Fc region would greatly reduce this effect. These data suggest that more antibodies could be manufactured that produce anti-vascular effects directly through complement activation, ADCC or direct induction of endothelial cell apoptosis, as is the case with the anti- $\alpha_v\beta_3$ antibody LM609 *(see above)*.

As with CM101, targeting toxins and coagulating agents to the tumor endothelium appears to cause rapid and almost complete tumor regression. This is a definite advance over the present generation of anti-angiogenesis agents, but the residual tumor cells will need to be eliminated or controlled using chemotherapy or anti-angiogenesis therapy.

ACKNOWLEDGMENTS

DCW acknowledges the support of the NorthWest Cancer Research Fund.

REFERENCES

1. Folkman, J. (1990) What is the evidence that tumors are angiogenesis-dependent? *J. Natl. Cancer Inst.* **82,** 4–6.
2. Paweletz, N. and Knierim, M. (1989) Tumor-related angiogenesis. *Crit. Rev. Oncol. Hematol.* **9,** 197–242.
3. Holmgren, L. and Bicknell, R. (1997) Inhibition of tumor angiogenesis and the induction of tumor dormancy, in *Tumor Angiogenesis* (Bicknell, R., et al., eds.), Oxford University Press, Oxford, UK, pp. 301–307.
4. Fan, T. P., Jagger, R., and Bicknell, R. (1995) Controlling the vasculature: angiogenesis, anti-angiogenesis and vascular targeting of gene therapy. *Trends Pharmacol. Sci.* **16,** 57–66.
5. Sim, K. L. (1998) Angiostatin™ and Endostatin™: endothelial cell-specific endogenous inhibitors of angiogenesis and tumor growth. *Angiogenesis* **2,** 37–48.
6. Denekamp, J. (1982) Endothelial cell proliferation as a novel approach to targeting tumor therapy. *Br. J. Cancer* **45,** 136–139.
7. Burrows, F. J. and Thorpe, P. E. (1993) Eradication of large solid tumors in mice with an immunotoxin directed against tumor vasculature. *Proc. Natl. Acad. Sci. USA* **90,** 8996–9600.
8. Jain, R. K. (1988) Determination of tumour blood flow: a review. *Cancer Res.* **48,** 2641–2658.
9. Konerding, M. A., Fait, E., Dimitropoulou, C., Malkusch, W., Ferri, C., Giavazzi, R., et al. (1998) Impact of fibroblast growth factor-2 on tumor microvascular architecture. A tridimensional morphometric study. *Am. J. Path.* **152,** 1607–1616.
10. Chaplin, D. J., Trotter, M. J., and Dougherty, G. J. (1997) Microregional tumor blood flow: heterogeneity and therapeutic significance, in *Tumor Angiogenesis* (Bicknell, R., et al. , eds.), Oxford University Press, Oxford, UK, pp. 61–70.
11. Belloni, P. N. and Nicolson, G. L. (1988) Differential expression of cell surface glycoproteins on various organ-derived microvascular endothelia and endothelial cell cultures. *J. Cell Physiol.* **136,** 398–410.
12. Kumar, S., West, D. C., and Ager, A. (1987) Heterogeneity in endothelial cells from large vessels and microvessels. *Differentiation* **36,** 57–70.
13. Clarke, M. S., Kiff, R. S., Kumar, S., Kumar, P., and West, D. C. (1991) The identification of proliferation-related proteins in human endothelial cells as a possible target in tumor therapy. *Int. J. Radiat. Biol.* **60,** 17–23.
14. Clarke, M. S. and West, D. C. (1991) The identification of proliferation and tumour-induced proteins in human endothelial cells: a possible target for tumor therapy. *Electrophoresis* **12,** 500–508.
15. Griffioen, A. W. (1997) Phenotype of the tumor vasculature; cell adhesion as a target for tumor therapy. *Cancer J.* **10,** 249–254.
16. Shawver, L. K., Lipson, K. E., Fong, T. A. T., McMahon, G., Plowman, G. D., and Strawn, L. M. (1997) Receptor tyrosine kinases as targets for inhibition of angiogenesis. *Drug Discovery Today* **2,** 50–63.
17. Partanen, J., Armstrong, E., Makela, T. P., Korhonen, J., Sanberg, M., Renkonen, R., et al. (1992) A novel endothelial cell surface receptor tyrosine kinase with extracellular epidermal growth factor homology domains. *Mol. Cell Biol.* **12,** 1698–1707.
18. Lin, P., Polverini, P., Dewhirst, M., Shan, S., Rao, P. S., and Peters, K. (1997) Inhibition of tumor angiogenesis using a soluble receptor establishes a role for Tie2 in pathologic vascular growth. *J. Clin. Invest.* **100,** 72–78.
19. Peters, K. G., Coogan, A., Berry, D., Marks, J., Iglehart, J. D., Kontos, C. D., et al. (1998) Expression of Tie2/TEK in breast tumor vasculature provides a new marker for evaluation of tumor angiogenesis. *Br. J. Cancer* **77(1),** 51–56.
20. Davis, S., Aldrich, T. H., Jones, P. F., Acheson, A., Compton, D. L., Jain, V., et al. (1996) Isolation of angiopoietin-1, a ligand for the TIE2 receptor, by secretion-trap expression cloning. *Cell* **87,** 1161–1169.
21. Maisonpierre, P. C., Suri, C., Jones, P. F., Bartunkova, S., Wiegang, S. J., Radziejewski, C., et al. (1997) Angiopoietin-2, a natural antagonist for Tie2 that disrupts in vivo angiogenesis. *Science* **277,** 55–60.
22. Zhou, R. (1998) The Eph family receptors and ligands. *Pharmacol. Ther.* **77,** 151–181.
23. Davis, S., Gale, N. W., Aldrich, T. H., Maisonpierre, P. C., Lhotak, V., Pawson, T, et al. (1994) Ligands for EPH-related receptor tyrosine kinases that require membrane attachment or clustering for activity. *Science* **266,** 816–819.

24. Drescher, U. (1997) The Eph family in the patterning of neural development. *Curr. Biol.* **7**, R799–R780.
25. Flanagan, J. G. and Vanderhaeghen, P. (1998) The ephrins and Eph receptors in neural development. *Annu. Rev. Neurosci.* **21**, 309–345.
26. Yancopoulos, G. D., Klagsburn, M., and Folkman, J. (1998) Vasculogenesis, Angiogenesis, and growth factors: Ephrins enter the fray at the border. *Cell.* **92**, 661–664.
27. Pandey, A., Shao, H., Marks, R. M., Polverini, P. J., and Dixit, V. M. (1995) Role of B61, the ligand for the Eck receptor tyrosine kinase, in TNF-α induced angiogenesis. *Science* **268**, 567–569.
28. Stein, E., Lane, A. A., Cerretti, D. P., Schoecklmann, H. O., Schroff, A. D., Van Etten, R. L., and Daniel, T. O. (1998) Eph receptors discriminate specific ligand oligomers to determine alternative signaling complexes, attachment, and assembly responses. *Genes Dev.* **12**, 667–678.
29. Wang, H. U., Chen, Z. F., and Anderson, D. J. (1998) Molecular distinction and angiogenic interaction between embryonic arteries and veins revealed by ephrin-B2 and its receptor Eph-B4. *Cell* **93**, 741–753.
30. Daniel, T. O., Stein, E., Cerretti, D. P., St. John, P. L., Robert, B., and Abrahamson, D. R. (1996) Elk and Lerk-2 in developing kidney and microvascular endothelial assembly. *Kidney Int.* **50(Suppl. 57)**, S73–S81.
31. Kim, K. J., Li, B., Winer, J., Armanini, M., Gillet, N., Phillips, H. S., and Ferrara, N. (1993) Inhibition of vascular endothelial growth factor-induced angiogenesis suppresses tumor growth in vivo. *Nature.* **362**, 841–844.
32. Olson, T. A., Mohanraj, D., Roy, S., and Ramakrishnan, S. (1997) Targeting the tumor vasculature: inhibition of tumor growth by a vascular endothelial growth factor-toxin conjugate. *Int. J. Cancer* **10**, 865–870.
33. Molema, G. and Griffioen, A. W. (1998) Rocking the foundations of solid tumor growth by attacking the tumor's blood supply. *Immunol Today* **19**, 392–394.
34. Skobe, M., Rockwell, P., Goldstein, N., Vosseler, S., and Fusenig, N. E. (1997) Halting angiogenesis suppresses carcinoma cell invasion. *Nature Med.* 1222–1227.
35. Lin, P., Sankar, S., Shan, S., Dewhirst, M. W., Polverini, P.J., Quinn, T. Q., and Peters, K. G. (1998) Inhibition of tumor growth by targeting tumor endothelium using a soluble vascular endothelial growth factor receptor. *Cell Growth Differ.* **9**, 49–58.
36. Menrad, A., Thierauch, K. H., Martiny-Baron, G., Siemeister, G., Schirner, M., and Schneider, M. R. (1997) Novel antibodies directed against the extracellular domain of the human VEGF-receptor type II. *Hybridoma* **16**, 465–471.
37. Brekken, R. A., Huang, X., King, S. W., and Thorpe, P. E. (1998) Vascular endothelial growth factor as a marker of tumor endothelium. *Cancer Res.* **58**, 1952–1959.
38. Report. (1996) *New Scientist* 19 Oct, 25.
39. Gladson, C. L. (1996) Expression of integrin alpha v beta 3 in small blood vessels of glioblastoma tumors. *J. Neuropathol. Exp. Neurol.* **55**, 1143–1149.
40. Max, R., Gerritsen, R. R., Nooijen, P. T., Goodman, S. L., Sutter, A., Keilholz, U., et al. (1997) Immunohistochemical analysis of integrin alpha v beta 3 expression on tumor-associated vessels of human carcinomas. *Int. J. Cancer* **71**, 3–4.
41. Gasparini, G., Brooks, P. C., Biganzoli, E., Vermeulen, P. B., Bonoldi, E., Dirix, L. Y., et al. (1998) Vascular integrin alpha(v)beta3: a new prognostic indicator in breast cancer. *Clin. Cancer Res.* **4**, 2625–2634.
42. Hieken, T. J., Farolan, M., Ronan, S. G., Shilkaitis, A., Wild, L., and Das Gupta, T. K. (1996) Beta3 integrin expression in melanoma predicts subsequent metastasis. *J. Surg. Res.* **63**, 169–173.
43. Brooks, P. C., Clark, R. A. F., and Cheresh, D. A. (1994) Requirement of vascular integrin $\alpha_v\beta_3$ for angiogenesis. *Science* **264**, 569–571.
44. Clarke, R. A., Tonnesen, M. G., Gailit, J., and Cheresh, D. A. (1996) Transient functional expression of alphaVbeta 3 on vascular cells during wound repair. *Am. J. Pathol.* **148**, 1407–1421.
45. Varner, J. A. and Cheresh, D. A. (1996) Integrins and cancer. *Curr. Opin. Cell Biol.* **8**, 724–730.
46. Brooks, P. C., Montgomery, A. M., Rosenfeld, M., Reisfeld, R. A., Hu, T., Klier, G., and Cheresh, D. A. (1994) Integrin alpha v beta 3 antagonists promote tumor regression by inducing apoptosis of angiogenic blood vessels. *Cell* **79**, 1157–1164.
47. Brooks, P. C., Stromblad, S., Klemke, R., Visscher, D., Sarkar, F. H., and Cheresh, D. A. (1995) Antiintegrin alpha v beta 3 blocks human breast cancer growth and angiogenesis in human skin. *J. Clin Invest.* **96**, 1815–1822.
48. Sheu, J. R., Yen, M. H., Kan, Y. C., Hung, W. C., Chang, P. T., and Luk, H. N. (1997) Inhibition of angiogenesis in vitro and in vivo: comparison of the relative activities of triflavin, an Arg-Gly-Asp-containing peptide and anti-alpha(v)beta3 integrin monoclonal antibody. *Biochim. Biophys. Acta.* **1336**, 445–454.

49. Griffioen, A. W., Coenen, M.J., Damen, C. A., Hellwig, S. M., van Weering, D. H., Vooys, W., et al. (1997) CD44 is involved in tumor angiogenesis; an activation antigen on human endothelial cells. *Blood* **90,** 1150–1159.

50. West, D. C., Wilson, J., Lagoumintzis, G., and Joyce, M. (1999) Angiogenic hyaluronan oligosaccharides interact with endothelial cell CD44 to upregulate expression of adhesion molecules, vegf receptors and IL-8, in *Vascular endothelium: Mechanisms of Cell Signalling* (Catravas, J., ed.), Plenum Press, New York, pp. 233–241.

51. Granger, D. N. and Kubes, P. (1994) The microcirculation and inflammation: modulation of leukocyte-endothelial cell adhesion. *J. Leukocyte Biol.* **55,** 662–675.

52. Droz, D., Patey, N., Paraf, F., Chretien, Y., and Gogusev, J. (1994) Composition of extracellular matrix and distribution of cell adhesion molecules in renal cell tumours. *Lab Invest.* **71,** 710–718.

53. Patay, N., Vazeux, R., Canioni, D., Potter, T., Gallatin, W. M., and Brousse, N. (1996) Intercellular adhesion molecule-3 on endothelial cells: expression in tumors but not in inflammatory responses. *Am. J. Pathol.* **148,** 465–472.

54. Kuzu, I., Bicknell, R., Fletcher, C. D. M., and Gatter, K. C. (1993) Expression of adhesion molecules on the endothelium of normal tissue vessels and vascular tumors. *Lab. Invest.* **69,** 322–328.

55. Bruijn, J. A. and Dinklo, N. J. C. M. (1993) Distinct patterns of expression of intercellular adhesion molecule-1, vascular cell adhesion molecule-1 and endothelial-leukocyte adhesion molecule-1 in renal disease. *Lab Invest.* **69,** 329–335.

56. Ran, S., Gao, B., Duffy, S., Watkins, L., Rote, N., and Thorpe, P. E. (1998) Infarction of solid Hodgkin's tumors in mice by antibody-directed targeting of tissue factor to tumor vasculature. *Cancer Res.* **58,** 4646–4653.

57. Lasky, L. A. (1995) Selectin-carbohydrate interactions and the initiation of the inflammatory response. *Ann. Rev. Biochem.* **64,** 113–139.

58. Takada, A., Ohmori, K., Yoneda, T., Tsuyuoka, K., Hasegawa, A., Kiso, M., and Kannagi, R. (1993) Contribution of carbohydrate antigens sialyl Lewis-a and sialyl Lewis-x to adhesion of human cancer-cells to vascular endothelium. *Cancer Res.* **53,** 354–361.

59. Bischoff, J., Brasel. C., Kraling, B., and Vranovska, K. (1997) E-selectin is upregulated in proliferating endothelial cells In vitro. *Microcirculation* **4,** 279–287.

60. Nguyen, M., Strubel, N. A., and Bischoff, J. (1993) A role for sialyl Lewis-X/A glycoconjugates in capillary morphogenesis. *Nature* **365,** 149–152.

61. Koch, A. E., Halloran, M. M., Haskell, C. J., Shah, M. R., and Polverini, P. J. (1995) Angiogenesis mediated by soluble forms of E-selectin and vascular cell-adhesion molecule-1. *Nature* **376,** 517–519.

62. Zocchi, M. R. and Poggi, A. (1993) Lymphocyte endothelial-cell adhesion molecules at the primary tumor site in human lung and renal-cell carcinomas. *J. Natl. Cancer Inst.* **85,** 246–247.

63. Ye, C. L., Kiriyama, K., Mistuoka, C., Kannagi, R., Ito, K., Watanabe, T., et al. (1995) Expression of E-selectin on endothelial-cells of small veins in human colorectal-cancer. *Int. J. Cancer* **61,** 455–460.

64. Salmi, M. and Jalkanen, S. (1995) Different forms of human vascular adhesion protein-1 (VAP-1) in blood-vessels in-vivo and in cultured endothelial-cells implications for lymphocyte-endothelial cell-adhesion models. *Eur. J. Immunol.* **25,** 2803–2812.

65. Banks, R. E., Gearing, A. J. H., Hemingway, I. K., Norfolk, D. R., Perren, T. J., and Selby, P. J. (1993) Circulating intercellular-adhesion molecule-1 (ICAM-1), E-selectin and vascular cell-adhesion molecule-1 (VCAM-1) in human malignancies. *Br. J. Cancer* **68,** 122–124.

66. Renkonen, J., Paavonen, T., and Renkonen, R. (1997) Endothelial and epithelial expression of sialyl Lewis (x) and sialyl Lewis (a) in lesions of breast carcinoma. *Int. J. Cancer* **74,** 296–300.

67. Gasparini, G. and Harris, A. L. (1995) Clinical importance of the determination of tumor angiogenesis in breast-carcinoma - much more than a new prognostic tool. *J. Clin. Oncol.* **13,** 765–782.

68. Budson, A. E., Ko, L., Brasel, C., and Bischoff, J. (1996) The angiogenesis inhibitor AGM-1470 selectively increases E-selectin. *Biochem Biophys Res Comm.* **225,** 141–145.

69. Luo, J. Y., Lin, J., Paranya, G., and Bischoff, J. (1998) Angiostatin upregulates E-selectin in proliferating endothelial cells. *Biochem Biophys Res Comm.* **245,** 906–911.

70. Spragg, D. D., Alford, D. R., Greferath, R., Larsen, C. E., Lee, K. D., Gurtner G. C., et al. (1997) Immunotargeting of liposomes to activated vascular endothelial cells: a strategy for site-selective delivery in the cardiovascular system. *Proc. Natl. Acad. Sci. USA* **94,** 8795–8800.

71. Wickham, T. J., Haskard, D., Segal, D., and Kovesdi, I. (1997) Targeting endothelium for gene therapy via receptors up-regulated during angiogenesis and inflammation. *Cancer Immunol. Immunother.* **45,** 149–151.

72. Jamar, F., Chapman, P. T., Manicourt, D. H., Glass, D. M., Haskard, D. O., and Peters, A. M. (1997) A comparison between In-111-anti-E-selectin mAb and Tc-99(m)-labelled human non-specific immunoglobulin in radionuclide imaging of rheumatoid arthritis. *Br. J. Radiol.* **70,** 473–481.

73. Chapman, P. T., Jamar, F., Keelan. E. T. M., Peters. A. M., and Haskard, D. O. (1996) Use of a radiolabeled monoclonal antibody against E-selectin for imaging of endothelial activation in rheumatoid arthritis. *Arth. Rheum.* **39,** 1371–1375.

74. Gougos, A. and Letarte, M. (1988) Identification of a human endothelial cell antigen with monoclonal antibody 44G4 produced against a pre-B leukemic cell line. *J. Immunol.* **141,** 1925–1933.

75. Westphal, J. R., Willems, H. W., Schalkwijk, C. J., Ruiter, D. J., and deWaal, R. M. (1993) A new 180-kDa dermal endothelial cell activation antigen: in vitro and in situ characteristics. *J. Invest. Dermatol.* **100,** 27–34.

76. Burrows, F. J., Derbyshire, E. J., Tazzari, P. L., Amlot, P., Gazdar, A. F., King, S. W., et al. (1995) Up-regulation of Endoglin on vascular endothelial cells in human solid tumors: Implications for diagnosis and therapy. *Clin Cancer Res.* **1,** 1623–1634.

77. Gougos, A., St. Jacques, S., Greaves, A., O'Connell, P. J., d'Apice, A. J., Buhring, H. J., et al. (1992) Identification of distinct epipotes of endoglin, an RGD-containing glycoprotein of endothelial cells, leukemic cells and syncytiotrophoblasts. *Int. Immunol.* **4,** 83–92.

78. Wang, J. M., Kumar, S., Pye, D., Vanagthoven, A. J., Krupinski, J., and Hunter, R. D. (1993) A monoclonal antibody detecting heterogeneity in vascular endothelium of tumors and normal tissues. *Int. J. Cancer* **54,** 363–370.

79. Neri, D., Carnemolla, B., Nissim, A., Leprini, A., Querze, G., Balza, E., et al. (1997) Targeting by affinity-matured recombinant antibody fragments of an angiogenesis associated fibronectin isoform. *Nat. Biotechnol.* **15,** 1271–1275.

80. Mariani, G., Lasku, A., and Balza, E. (1997) Tumor targeting potential of the monoclonal antibody BC-1 against oncofetal fibronectin in nude mice bearing human tumor implants. *Cancer* **80,** 2378–2384.

81. Mach, F., Schonbeck, U., Sukhova, G. K., Bourcier, T., Bonnefoy, J. Y., Pober, J. S., and Libby, P. (1997) Functional CD40 ligand is expressed on human vascular endothelial cells, smooth muscle cells, and macrophages: implications for CD40-CD40 ligand signaling in atherosclerosis. *Proc. Natl. Acad. Sci. USA* **94,** 1931–1936.

82. Kluth, B., Hess, S., Engelmann, H., Schafnitzel, S., Riethmuller, G., and Feucht, H. E. (1997) Endothelial expression of CD40 in renal cell carcinoma. *Cancer Res.* **57,** 891–899.

83. Horoszewicz, J. S., Kawinski, E., and Murphy, G. P. (1987) Monoclonal antibodies to a new antigenic marker in epithelial cells and serum of prostatic cancer patients. *Anticancer Res.* **7,** 927–936.

84. Israeli, R. S., Powell, C. T., Fair, W. R., and Heston, W. D. W. (1993) Molecular cloning of a complementary DNA encoding a prostate-specific membrane antigen. *Cancer Res.* **53,** 227–230.

85. Wright, G. L., Jr., Haley, C., Beckett, M. L., and Schelhammer, P. F. (1995) Expression of prostate-specific antigen in normal, benign, and malignant prostate tissues. *Urol Oncol.* **1,** 18–28.

86. Liu, H., Moy, P., Kim, S., Xia, Y., Rajasekaran, A., Navarro, V., et al. (1997) Monoclonal antibodies to the extracellular domain of prostate-specific membrane antigen also reacts with tumor vascular endothelium. *Cancer Res.* **57,** 3629–3634.

87. Silver, D. A., Pellicer, I., Fair, W. R., Heston, W. D. W., and Cordon-Cardo, C. (1997) Prostate-specific membrane antigen expression in normal and malignant human tissues. *Clin. Cancer Res.* **3,** 81–85.

88. Murphy, G. P., Greene, T. G., Tino, W. T., Boynton, A. L., and Holmes, E. H. (1998) Isolation and characterization of monoclonal antibodies specific for the extracellular domain of prostate specific membrane antigen. *J. Urol.* **160,** 2396–2401.

89. Hagemeier, H. H., Vollmer, E., Goerdt, S., Schulze-Osthoff, K., and Sorg, C. (1986) A monoclonal antibody reacting with endothelial cells of budding vessels in tumors and inflammatory tissues, and non-reactive with normal adult tissues. *Int. J. Cancer* **38,** 481–488.

90. Rettig, W. J., Garinchesa, P., Healey, J. H., Su, S. L., Jaffe, E. A., and Sorg, C. (1992) Identification of endosialin, a cell surface glycoprotein of vascular endothelial cells in human cancer. *Proc. Natl. Acad. Sci. USA* **89,** 10,832–10,836.

91. Bruland, O. S., Fodstad, O., Stenwig, A. E., and Pihl, A. (1988) Expression and characteristics of a novel human osteosarcoma-associated cell surface antigen. *Cancer Res.* **48,** 5302–5309.

92. Stone, M. J., Ruf, W., Miles, D. J., Edgington, T. S., and Wright, P. E. (1995) Recombinant soluble human tissue factor secreted by Saccharomyces cerevisiae and refolded from E. coli inclusion bodies: glycosylation of mutants, activity and physical characterization. *Biochem. J.* **310,** 605–614.

93. Burrows, F. J., Watanabe, Y., and Thorpe, P. E. (1992) A murine model for antibody-directed targeting of vascular endothelial cells in solid tumors. *Cancer Res.* **52,** 5954–5962.

94. Huang, X., Molema, G., King, S., Watkins, L., Edgington, T. S., and Thorpe, P. E. (1997) Tumor infarction in mice by antibody-directed targeting of tissue factor to tumor vasculature. *Science* **275,** 547–550.

95. Williamson, P. and Schlegel, R. A. (1994) Back and forth: the regulation and function of transbilayer phospholipid movement in eukaryotic cells. *Mol. Membr. Biol.* 11, 199–216.

96. Thrush, G. R., Lark, L. R., Clinchy, B. C., and Vitetta. E. S. (1996) Immunotoxins: an update. *Ann. Rev. Immunol.* **14,** 49–71.

97. Yan, H. P., Carter, C. E., Wang, E. Z., Page, D. L., Washington, K., Wamil, B. D., et al. (1998) Functional studies on the anti-pathoangiogenic properties of CM101. *Angiogenesis* **2,** 219–233.

98. Fujieda, M., Oishi, N., and Kurashige, T. (1997) Antibodies to endothelial cells in Kawasaki disease lyse endothelial cells without cytokine pretreatment. *Clin. Exp. Immunol.* **107,** 120–126.

99. Harris, A. L. (1997) Clinical trials of anti-vascular agent group B Streptococcus toxin (CM101). *Angiogenesis* **1,** 36–37.

100. Velders, M. P., vanRhijn, C. M., Oskam, E., Fleuren, G. J., Warnaar, S. O., and Litvinov, S. V. (1998) The impact of antigen density and antibody affinity on antibody-dependent cellular cytotoxicity: relevance for immunotherapy of carcinomas. *Br. J. Cancer* **78,** 478–483.

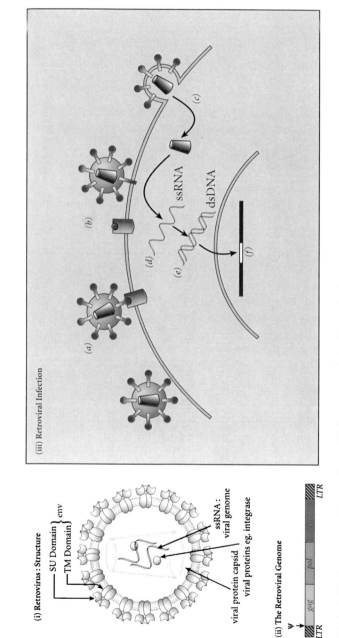

(iii) Retroviral Infection

(a)

(b)

(c)

(d)

ssRNA

(e)

dsDNA

(f)

(i) Retrovirus : Structure

SU Domain ⎫
          ⎬ env
TM Domain ⎭

ssRNA :
viral genome

viral protein capsid

viral proteins eg. integrase

(ii) The Retroviral Genome

ψ

LTR | gag | pol | env | LTR

Plate 2. (i) Structure of Retrovirus, (ii) Structure of the Retroviral Genome, (iii) Infection by a Retrovirus (*see* figure and full caption on page 457).

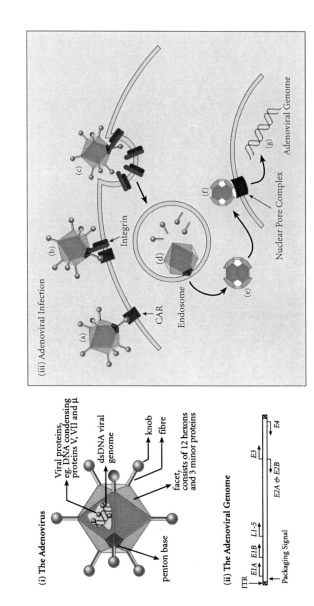

Plate 3. (i) Structure of Adenovirus, (ii) Structure of the Adenoviral Genome, (iii) Infection by an Adenovirus (*see* figure and full caption on page 461).

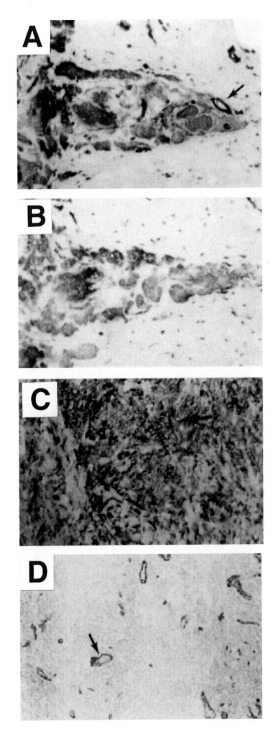

Plate 4. Reactivity of a crossreactive anti-CD105 MAb SN6f with vascular endothelium of malignant tissues of breast, lung, and lymph node (*see* figure and full caption on page 506).

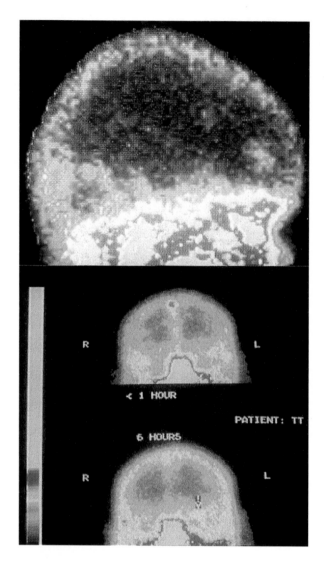

Plate 5. Immun oscintigraphs of two patients with tumors (*see* figure and full caption on page 512).

25

Endothelial Monocyte-Activating Polypeptide II

A Novel Injury Signal?

Cliff Murray and Maarten Tas

CONTENTS

INTRODUCTION

Tumor necrosis factor-α (TNF-α) has been shown to induce hemorrhagic necrosis and regression in experimental murine solid tumors *(1)*. When infused into mice bearing methylcholanthrene-A-induced (MethA) fibrosarcomas, there is rapid induction of intravascular coagulation at the tumor site resulting in a major drop in tumor blood flow *(2)*. In this model, intravascular coagulation is initiated by enhanced expression of tissue factor (or thromboplastin) on the luminal surface of the tumor-associated endothelial cells, ultimately leading to the deposition of insoluble fibrin on the endothelial surface *(2,3)*. It has been hypothesized that this excessive thrombus formation leads to vascular occlusion, precipitating tumor cell death and regression of the tumor.

Why does TNF-α have such profound effects upon the tumor vasculature while having relatively little effect on that of the normal tissues? During the late 1980s, the observations just described led to speculation that factors produced by tumor cells might specifically prime tumor-associated endothelial cells to respond to TNF-α. At about this time, Noguchi et al. *(4)* described a soluble factor in supernatants of a human bladder carcinoma cell line (BCDC), which induces tissue factor activity on the surface of human umbilical vein endothelial cells (HUVEC), and hypothesized that such a factor might contribute to the

From: *The New Angiotherapy*
Edited by: T.-P. D. Fan and E. C. Kohn © Humana Press Inc., Totowa, NJ

coagulopathies often associated with malignancy (for review, *see* ref. *5*). Subsequently, using bioassays based upon coagulant-inducing activity, several similar proteins that potentiate TNF-α-induced coagulation were isolated from a variety of tumor cell lines. One such factor, isolated from MethA cell conditioned medium, turned out to be the murine homolog of the potent angiogenic factor vascular endothelial cell growth factor (VEGF; *6*). Two more proteins with similar activities were isolated from MethA cells; the 44 kDa endothelial monocyte-activating polypeptide 1 (EMAP-1; *7*) and 22 kDa EMAP-II *(8)*. Unlike VEGF, these factors are not mitogenic for endothelial cells. Based on its apparent molecular weight and biological activities, MethA-derived EMAP-II is likely to be the mouse homolog of BCDC *(4)* and two other partially characterized proteins, FO-1 *(9)* and HS-1 *(10)*, derived from the FO-1 and BLM human melanoma cell lines, respectively.

STRUCTURE, SYNTHESIS, AND PROCESSING

Difficulties in obtaining sufficient material to carry out biological studies persuaded various groups of the need to clone the EMAP-II gene and generate recombinant material. In 1994, Stern's group at Columbia University isolated full-length cDNAs encoding murine and human EMAP-II from the MethA fibrosarcoma and U937 monocytic cell lines, respectively *(11)*. The deduced amino acid sequences appeared to be 86% identical between the two species. MethA cDNA libraries, primed with either oligo(dT)$_{17}$ or a sequence complementary to the putative 5' region (based on amino acid analysis), were used to generate overlapping clones, which were then sequenced. Based on these results, the full-length cDNA for mouse EMAP-II was estimated to be 1086 bp. This estimate was corroborated by Northern analysis of RNA from MethA cells, which indicated a single transcript of ~1070 bases. Analysis of this sequence suggested that the open reading frame encodes a protein of 310 amino acids (the human sequence appears to contain an extra 2 amino acids) with a predicted molecular weight of 34 kDa. Furthermore, what was thought to be the N-terminus appeared to be an internal sequence.

The discrepancy in size between the predicted 34 kDa molecule and the 22 kDa molecule detected in tumor-cell supernatants, led Kao et al. *(11)* to speculate that EMAP-II is synthesized as a leaderless precursor (which we will henceforth refer to as proEMAP-II), which is cleaved to an active 22 kDa mature form at a critical aspartate residue (Asp^{144} in mouse, Asp^{146} in human). This overall picture is reminiscent of the inflammatory cytokine interleukin-1β (IL-1β), which is synthesized as a leaderless 31 kDa precursor proIL-1β, and undergoes processing to the 17 kDa mature form during translocation through the plasma membrane *(12)*. Furthermore the amino acid sequence in the vicinity of the cleavage sight of proEMAP-II suggests the potential involvement of a caspase enzyme, as in the processing of proIL-1β by the caspase IL-1-converting enzyme (ICE).

The relationship between the mature form of EMAP-II and the putative precursor as described by Kao et al. *(11)* has recently been thrown into doubt by the work of Quevillon et al. *(13)*, who have cloned and characterized an apparently unrelated protein with a high degree of amino acid identity to EMAP-II. The mammalian multisynthetase complex is a high molecular-weight structure composed of nine aminoacyl-tRNA synthetases and three auxiliary proteins with molecular weights of 18, 38, and 43 kDa. The hamster p43 component is composed of 359 amino acids with a predicted molecular weight of 40 kDa. This protein shares 86 and 85% amino acid identity with human and murine proEMAP-II, respectively.

The cDNAs encoding human and mouse proEMAP-II are significantly shorter than that of hamster p43 (1070 bp vs 1254 bp), which has led Quevillon et al. *(13)* to suggest that those cDNAs originally isolated by Kao et al. *(11)* are incomplete. Kao et al. *(11)* identified three ATG start codons within the first 200 nucleotides of their proEMAP-II cDNA. However, they pointed out that only one, at position 64, meets the criteria of Kozak for initiation of translation, giving rise to a 310 amino acid protein in mouse and 312 amino acid protein in human. Furthermore, only the 1070 nucleotide transcript is evident on Northern blots of RNA isolated from MethA cells, while a 1254 nucleotide species is absent. Using Western blotting with polyclonal and monoclonal antibodies (PAbs/MAbs) against the mature form of EMAP-II, we have detected a 34 kDa species in a wide range of cultured cells and tissue extracts *(14,25,26)*, which tends to support the model proposed by Kao and colleagues.

Whether mature EMAP-II arises from the p43 component of the multi-synthetase complex, or from a precursor such as that described by Kao et al. *(11)*, it is almost certainly the product of some form of processing. While accepting the possibility that a caspase may be involved in cleavage at the critical Asp^{144} residue, Quevillon et al. *(13)* have suggested that the presence of a "KEKE" motif immediately upstream (between residues 110 and 147) of the putative cleavage site, may target the precursor molecule for processing by the multicatalytic protease, or 20S proteosome *(15)*.

Although nothing is known about subsequent processing of EMAP-II, the mature form appears to be relatively resistant to proteolytic degradation (Jakobsen et al., submitted). Mature recombinant EMAP-II is, however, sensitive to thrombin in vitro, being cleaved at a single site to yield two unequal fragments of approx 5 and 15 kDa (Tas et al., unpublished observations). It has yet to be determined whether this has implications for degradation or further functional processing of the polypeptide.

Knies et al. *(24)* have recently provided indirect evidence for the involvement of a previously unidentified caspase-like enzyme in the cleavage of proEMAP-II. We have investigated the processing of recombinant human proEMAP-II using Western blotting and proEMAP-II radio labeled with $[^{35}S]$-methionine by in vitro transcription/translation (Jakobsen et al., submitted). Our data suggest that the 34 kDa precursor form of EMAP-II is not susceptible to the major caspase enzymes, caspase I (ICE) and caspase 3 (CPP32/apopain). Furthermore, conversion of the precursor by membrane extracts of U937 monocytic cells, which constitutively process this molecule *(14)*, is not inhibited by the standard repertoire of caspase inhibitors. Indeed our data with U937 membrane extracts tend to support the contention of Quevillon et al. *(13)* that the processing may be mediated by a group of proteolytic activities, such as those associated with the proteosome, rather than a single enzyme.

DISTRIBUTION IN NORMAL TISSUES

As demonstrated by reverse transcription-polymerase chain reaction (RT-PCR), mRNA for EMAP-II is found in a wide range of human tissues, as well as in many normal and tumor cell lines (Tas et al., unpublished observations; Knies et al., personal communication). Schluesener et al. *(16)* published the first, somewhat selective, immunohistochemical study of EMAP-II expression using MAbs raised against recombinant EMAP-II and synthetic polypeptides based on the N-terminal region of mature EMAP-II. They reported on the expression of EMAP-II immuno-reactivity in certain normal tissues of the rat, including the spleen, lymph nodes, and liver, in which there was selective staining of a subpopulation of monocytes. In the normal brain they found positive staining in cells of the perivascular microglia.

We recently raised PAbs and MAbs against recombinant human EMAP-II produced as a fusion product with invertebrate glutathione-S-transferase (GST) *(14)*. After adsorbing out activity against GST, the EMAP-II-staining PAbs were used to survey the expression of the protein in formalin-fixed, paraffin-embedded sections of normal human tissues. EMAP-II expression was highly restricted; apart from strong staining of monocyte/macrophages, positive staining was seen in a number of secretory epithelial cells associated with endocrine organs and in neurons, suggesting that EMAP-II protein expression may be restricted essentially to cells of neuro-endocrine origin *(25)*.

DISTRIBUTION IN PATHOLOGICAL TISSUES

We have assessed a range of human tumors for EMAP-II expression by immunohistochemistry and observed strong expression, in carcinoma of the prostate *(26)*, in lung tumors showing neuro-endocrine differentiation, and in ductal carcinoma in situ (DCIS) and invasive carcinoma of the breast (Tas et al., in preparation).

Schluesener et al. *(16)* reported on the expression of EMAP-II in experimental models of auto-immune diseases of the central nervous system (CNS), including experimental encephalomyelitis, neuritis, and uveitis. Macrophages of inflammatory lesions were prominently stained. EMAP-II is also strongly expressed in microglial cells of the diseased brain, not only locally in inflammatory lesions but throughout the parenchyma. In inflammatory bowel disease (Jenkins et al., in preparation), including active ulcerative colitis and Crohn's disease, EMAP-II expression is enhanced in cells of the macrophage lineage, although significant staining was also observed in endothelial cells of granulation tissue (Jenkins et al., in preparation).

EFFECTS OF EMAP-II IN VITRO

Growth medium conditioned by a variety of tumor cell lines is found to induce tissue-factor synthesis in cultured HUVEC *(17)*. As mentioned earlier, EMAP-II appears to be one of a number of factors that mediate this effect, and that can be blocked by pre-incubation of the conditioned medium with antibodies against tissue factor. Co-incubation of endothelial cells with suboptimal concentrations of TNF-α and EMAP-II produces a supra-additive effect on coagulation. Similar effects are seen when endothelial cells are co-incubated with the melanoma-derived FO-1 factor *(9)*, previously described as identical to EMAP-II, and flavone acetic acid, a novel chemotherapeutic agent that causes hemorrhagic necrosis in murine solid tumors in vivo. The basis of this potentiating activity is not understood, although increases in EC procoagulant activity correlate with enhanced levels of mRNA for tissue factor *(9,11)*.

EMAP-II has a variety of biological effects on endothelial cells, monocytes, and neutrophils. Common to these three cell types in terms of their response to EMAP-II is a rapid rise in cytosolic free calcium *(11)*. Crosslinking studies have demonstrated binding of ^{125}I-labeled EMAP-II-derived peptides to a ~73 kDa protein associated with the monocyte cell surface *(18)*, suggesting the existence of a distinct receptor. Binding of EMAP-II to EC leads, in addition to tissue-factor expression, to release of von Willebrand Factor (vWF), and enhanced expression of the adhesion molecules E- and P-selectins. Monocytes synthesize TNF-α, IL-8, and tissue factor in response to EMAP-II, whereas neutrophils release myeloperoxidase activity. EMAP-II is chemotactic for both monocytes and neutrophils *(11)*.

EFFECTS OF EMAP-II IN VIVO

Local injection of EMAP-II into the mouse footpad evokes an acute inflammatory response. In one study *(8)*, systemic infusion of 10 µg of EMAP-II into C3H/HeJ or Balb/c mice was associated with systemic toxicity, pulmonary congestion, and the appearance of TNF-α, IL-1β, and IL-6 in the plasma. In the same study, C3H/He mice bearing MethA tumors received a single intra-tumor injection of EMAP-II. Hemorrhage and inflammatory infiltrates were observed, followed by decreases in tumor volume. In another study *(18)*, local injection of EMAP-II into immuno-compromised mice bearing B16 melanomas or HT-1080 human fibrosarcomas (tumors considered resistant to TNF-α treatment), followed ~15 h later by intravenous TNF-α, resulted in thrombo-hemorrhagic and acute inflammatory changes, and partial regression of the tumors. These findings support the notion that EMAP-II has the properties of a pro-inflammatory mediator and the capacity to prime the tumor vasculature for a locally destructive process.

Recently, Schwarz et al. *(19)* demonstrated that EMAP-II induces apoptosis in proliferating endothelial cells, and inhibits neovascularization of matrix gels implanted in mice. They suggested that EMAP-II suppresses the growth of Lewis lung carcinomas by inducing perivascular apoptosis, and concluded that EMAP-II is primarily an anti-angiogenic cytokine-targeting growing endothelium, with the potential to destroy the vasculature of solid tumors.

The reported effects of EMAP-II in vivo and in vitro are summarized in Table 1. As indicated earlier, mRNA for EMAP-II is found in several tumor cell lines by RT-PCR. However, many other cell lines and normal tissues are also positive for EMAP-II mRNA. It is not known how the presence of mRNA relates to protein expression, or whether proEMAP-II is always present within the cytoplasm, awaiting cleavage and secretion.

CONCLUSIONS AND FUTURE DIRECTIONS

Many of the fundamental questions surrounding the expression and function of EMAP-II remain unresolved. Perhaps the most important question concerns the normal function of EMAP-II. Current thinking would suggest that the protein probably exists for the most part in an inactive "precursor" form, awaiting an appropriate stimulus to be processed and released into the extracellular environment where it can perform its function. Our data indicate that a number of stresses may induce release and processing.

From the perspective of tumor biology, it is certainly unclear what benefit the production of active EMAP-II might confer on a tumor. Much of the evidence suggests that release of EMAP-II should, by one of several potential mechanisms, impede the growth of tumors. We should reflect on the fact that the protein was originally detected at extremely low levels in tumor-cell supernatants. Furthermore it has been suggested, but not proven, that caspases, enzymes closely associated with apoptosis, may be involved in the processing and release of mature EMAP-II. This argues in favor of a scenario in which the molecule is not constitutively released but may be released by dying or injured cells, at which point its function might be to attract, in particular, phagocytic cells into the area of damage/injury. Of course, recruitment of inflammatory cells per se is not a feature of apoptosis. However, this pre-supposes that apoptosis is indeed the trigger for the release of EMAP-II. Our data do not support this contention, but rather suggest that cell injury in general may lead to EMAP-II processing and release.

Table 1
Effects of EMAP-2 In Vitro and In Vivo

Target	Action
In vitro	
Endothelial cells	Potentiates TNF-induced tissue factor expression (8)
	Potentiates TF-induction by novel agent flavone acetic acid (9)
	Upregulates E- and P-selectin (11)
	Increases cytosolic Ca^{2+} (11)
	Induction of apoptosis (19)
Monocytes	Upregulation of tissue factor (8)
	Enhanced TNF expression (8)
	Enhanced IL-8 expression (11)
	Increased cytosolic Ca^{2+} (11)
	Chemotaxis (8)
Neutrophils	Release of myeloperoxidase (11)
	Increased cytosolic Ca^{2+} (11)
	Chemotaxis (8)
In Vivo	
Mouse	Induction of acute inflammatory response (8)
	Partial tumor regression (11)
	Sensitization of tumors to TNF (8,18)

Having been released, what is the function of processed EMAP-II in the extracellular environment? The best-characterized function of EMAP-II appears to be to upregulate the expression of tissue factor on endothelial cells. Although it is supposed that this inevitably leads to occlusion of blood vessels and necrosis, tissue factor clearly has a more complex role in vascular biology. Carmeliet et al. (20) have shown using "knock-out" technology that inactivation of the tissue-factor gene results in abnormal circulation and ultimately embryonic lethality at E10.5. Furthermore we know that coagulation, and in particular the deposition of fibrin within the extravascular compartment, probably plays a positive role in normal and pathological angiogenesis (21). Contrino et al. (22) have shown that active tissue factor is present within neovasculature of invasive breast carcinomas but not that of benign tumors, suggesting a role in tumor progression.

One in vitro study has suggested that EMAP-II induces apoptosis in cultured endothelial cells (19). It is interesting to note that a relationship between tissue-factor expression and apoptosis of endothelial cells has been demonstrated. Bombeli et al. (23) have shown that tissue-factor expression is enhanced at an early phase of staurosporine-induced apoptosis in cultured endothelial cells. This provides a potential link between the earlier observations of tissue factor upregulation, and more recent reports of apoptosis in endothelial cells. What then is the significance of EMAP-II as an inducer of endothelial cell-death: could its role be to eliminate unwanted endothelial cells during vascular remodeling, as in highly angiogenic situations? The answers to these and other questions await the development of EMAP-II knockout mice and further information about the processing of the molecule.

ACKNOWLEDGMENTS

The work of the authors is supported by the Cancer Research Campaign of the UK.

REFERENCES

1. Old, L. (1986) Tumor necrosis factor. *Science* **230,** 630–632.
2. Nawroth, P., Handley, D. A., Matsueda, G., de Waal, R., Gerlach, H., Blohm, D., and Stern, D. (1988) Tumor necrosis factor/cachectin-induced intravascular fibrin formation in MethA fibrosarcomas. *J. Exp. Med.* **168,** 637–647.
3. Zhang, Y., Deng, Y., Wendt, T., Liliensiek, B., Bierhaus, A., Greten, J., et al. (1996) Intravenous somatic gene transfer with antisense tissue factor restores blood flow by reducing tumor necrosis factor-induced tissue factor expression and fibrin deposition in mouse Meth-A sarcomas. *J. Clin. Invest.* **97,** 2213–2224.
4. Noguchi, M., Sakai, T., and Kisiel, W. (1989) Identification and partial purification of a novel tumor-derived protein that induces tissue factor on cultured human endothelial cells. *Biochem. Biophys. Res. Comm.* **160,** 222–227.
5. Murray, J. C. (1991) Coagulation and Cancer. *Br. J. Cancer* **64,** 422–424.
6. Clauss, M., Gerlach, M., Gerlach, H., Brett, J., Wang, F., Familletti, P. C., et al. (1990a) Vascular permeability factor: a tumor-derived polypeptide that induces endothelial cell and monocyte procoagulant activity, and promotes monocyte migration. *J. Exp. Med.* **172,** 1535–1545.
7. Clauss, M., Murray, J. C., Vianna, M., de Waal, R., Thurston, G., Nawroth, P., et al. (1990b) A polypeptide factor produced by fibrosarcoma cells that induces endothelial tissue factor and enhances the procoagulant response to tumor necrosis factor/cachectin. *J. Biol. Chem.* **265,** 7078–7083.
8. Kao, J., Ryan, J., Brett, J., Chen, J., Shen, H., Fan, Y.-G, et al. (1992) Endothelial monocyte-activating polypeptide II. A novel tumor-derived polypeptide that activates host-response mechanisms. *J. Biol. Chem.* **267,** 20,239–20,247.
9. Murray, J. C., Clauss, M., Denekamp, J., and Stern, D. (1991) Selective induction of endothelial cell tissue factor in the presence of a tumor-derived mediator: a potential mechanism of flavone acetic acid action in tumor vasculature. *Int. J. Cancer* **49,** 254–259.
10. Pötgens, A. J. G., Lubsen, N. H., van Altena, G., Schoenmakers, J. G. G., Ruiter, D. J., and de Waal, R. (1994) Measurement of tissue factor messenger RNA levels in human endothelial cells by a quantitative RT-PCR assay. *Thromb. Haemostasis* **71,** 208–213.
11. Kao, J., Houck, K., Fan, Y., Haehnel, I., Libutti, S. K., Kayton, M. L., et al. (1994) Characterization of a novel tumor-derived cytokine. Endothelial-monocyte activating polypeptide II. *J. Biol. Chem.* **269,** 25,106–25,119.
12. Singer, L. L., Scott, S., Chin, J., Bayne, E. K., Limjuco, G., Weidner, J., et al. (1995) The interleukin-1ϑ-converting enzyme (ICE) is localized on the external cell surface membranes and in the cytoplasmic ground substance of human monocytes by immuno-electron microscopy. *J. Exp. Med.* **182,** 1447–1459.
13. Quevillon, S., Agou, F., Robinson, J.-C., and Mirande, M. (1997) The p43 component of the mammalian multi-synthetase complex is likely to be the precursor of the endothelial monocyte-activating polypeptide II cytokine. *J. Biol. Chem.* **272,** 32,573–32,579.
14. Tas, M. P. R., Houghton, J., Jakobsen, A. M., Tolmachova, T., Carmichael, J., and Murray J. C. (1997) Cloning and expression of human endothelial monocyte-activating polypeptide 2 (EMAP-II) and identification of its putative precursor. *Cytokine* **9,** 535–539.
15. Realini, C., Rogers, S. W., and Rechsteiner, M. (1994) KEKE motifs: proposed roles in protein-protein association and presentation of peptides by MHC Class I receptors. *FEBS Lett.* **348,** 109–113.
16. Schluesener, H. J., Seid, K., Zhao, Y., and Meyerman, R. (1997) Localization of endothelial-monocyte-activating polypeptide II (EMAP II), a novel proinflammatory cytokine, to lesions of experimental autoimmune encephalomyelitis, neuritis and uveitis. *Glia* **20,** 365–372.
17. Hewett, P. W. and Murray, J. C. (1996) Modulation of human endothelial procoagulant activity in tumor models *in vitro*. *Int. J. Cancer* **66,** 784–789.
18. Marvin, M. R., Libutti, S. K., Kayton, M., Kao, J., Hayward, J., Grikscheit, T., et al. (1996) A novel tumor-derived mediator that sensitizes cytokine-resistant tumors to tumor necrosis factor. *J. Surg. Res.* **63,** 248–255.
19. Schwarz, M., Brett, J., Li, J., Hayward, J., Schwarz, R., Kao, J., et al. (1995) Endothelial-monocyte activating polypeptide (EMAP) II, a novel antiangiogenic protein, suppresses tumor growth and induces apoptosis in endothelial cells. *Circulation* **92(Sup.)** I–7.
20. Carmeliet, P., Mackman, N., Moons, L., Luther, T., Gressens, P., VanViaenderen, I., et al. (1996) Role of tissue factor in embryonic blood vessel development. *Nature* **383,** 73–75.
21. Dvorak, H. F. (1987) Abnormalities of hemostasis in malignancy, in *Hemostasis and Thrombosis: Basic Principles and Practice* (Colman, R. W., et al., eds.), J. B. Lippincott, Philadelphia.

22. Contrino, J., Hair, G., Kreutzer, D. L., and Rickles, F. R. (1996) *In situ* detection of tissue factor in vascular endothelial cells: correlation with the malignant phenotype of human breast disease. *Nature Med.* **2,** 209–215.
23. Bombeli, T., Karsan, A., Tait, J. F., and Harlan, J. M. (1997) Apoptotic vascular endothelial cells become procoagulant. *Blood* **89,** 2429–2442.
24. Knies, U., Behrensdorf, H. A., Mitchell, C. A., Deutsch, U., Risau, W., Drexler, H. C. A., and Clauss, M. (1998) Regulation of endothelial monocyte-activating polypeptide II release by apoptosis. *Proc. Natl. Acad. Sci. USA* **95,** 12,322–12,327.
25. Murray, J. C., Barnett, G., Tas, M. P. R., Jakdosen, A. M., Brown, J., Powe, D., and Clelland, C. (2000) Immunohistochemical analysis of endothelial-monocyte activating polypeptide-II (EMAP-II) expression in vivo. *Am. J. Pathol.* **157,** 2045–2053.
26. Barnett, G., Tas, M., Jakobsen, A. M., Rice, K., Carmichael, J., and Murray, J. C. (2000) Prostate adenocarcinoma cells release the novel pro-inflammatory protein EMAP-II in response to stress. *Cancer Res.* **60,** 2850–2857.

26

CD105 Antibody for Targeting of Tumor Vascular Endothelial Cells

Ben K. Seon and Shant Kumar

CONTENTS

INTRODUCTION

At present most treatments for cancers are designed to eliminate cancer cells directly. In a landmark publication nearly 30 years ago, Folkman *(1)* proposed antiangiogenesis as a potential target in cancer therapy. Numerous investigators have since attempted to exploit this concept (for recent reviews *see* refs. *2,3*). In particular, the development of monoclonal antibodies (MAbs) directed against tumor endothelium has attracted the greatest attention. The progressive growth of solid tumors beyond a few mm^3 requires the continuous formation of new blood vessels, a process known as tumor angiogenesis *(1,4)*. Tumor growth and metastasis are angiogenesis-dependent. Therefore, either prevention of tumor angiogenesis (antiangiogenic therapy)* or selective destruction of tumor's existing blood vessels (vascular targeting therapy)* may be a potentially effective strategy for the treatment of solid tumors and control of tumor metastasis *(1,5–8)*.

Antiangiogenic therapy has several advantages over conventional treatments for solid tumors. First, this approach may circumvent the problem of acquired drug resistance *(9,10)*. The rationale is that drug-resistant mutants are easily generated from tumor cells because of their inherent genetic instability, whereas genetically stable normal cells, such as vascu-

---

*In this review the term antiangiogenic targeting has been often used to cover both antiangiogenic therapy and vascular targeting.

From: *The New Angiotherapy*
Edited by: T.-P. D. Fan and E. C. Kohn © Humana Press Inc., Totowa, NJ

lar endothelial cells, would be far less adept at generating such mutants. Indeed, drug resistance has not been a significant problem in antiangiogenic therapy in animals *(10)* and patients *(11)*. Second, antiangiogenic vascular targeting therapy may be able to overcome the problem of tumor heterogeneity, a major problem with tumor cell targeting therapy. Thirdly, the physiologic barriers to penetration into solid tumors by high molecular-weight reagents (such as antibodies and immunoconjugates) *(12,13)* will be circumvented by targeting tumor vasculature rather than tumor cells. Unlike the cells in a tumor mass, vascular endothelial cells are directly accessible to circulating high molecular-weight drugs. Fourth, many thousands of dependent tumor cells will die of nutrient and oxygen deprivation if a capillary or a sector of the capillary bed fails *(6)*. Therefore, killing of only a minority of tumor vascular endothelial cells may be sufficient to eradicate vast numbers of malignant cells in tumors. Last, a single agent developed for antiangiogenic targeting could be applied to most or all types of solid tumor and angiogenesis-associated disease.

In order to apply effectively antiangiogenic therapy to cancer, it is imperative to develop appropriate reagents that selectively destroy tumor-associated vasculature without severely damaging the vasculature and other vital components of normal tissues. As MAbs are highly specific, MAb-based reagents may be appropriate candidates for such selective targeting. Endothelium in normal adults is quiescent and the turnover of these cells is very low (i.e., thousands of days) *(4,14,15)*. However, the same endothelial cells can undergo rapid proliferation during spurts of angiogenesis. Thus, a certain antigen may be expressed more strongly on tumor than on normal endothelium. This is the case for several endothelial cell markers defined by MAbs which are summarized in the next section. However, none of these markers is absolutely specific for tumor vascular endothelial cells. Therefore, targeting efficacy and potential side effects of these MAbs need to be evaluated in animals before their clinical potential can be ascertained in man. Until now, such evaluation has been carried out with only a few MAbs (*see* below). This chapter describes mainly our in vitro and in vivo experimental approaches to evaluate the usefulness of MAbs to CD105 (endoglin), initially reported as a leukemia-associated cell surface glycoprotein by Haruta and Seon *(16)*.

CELL SURFACE MARKERS ON ENDOTHELIAL CELLS OF TUMOR VASCULATURE

Only those that are integral cell-membrane antigens have been considered here. Some antigens such as vascular endothelial growth factor (VEGF) are attached to endothelial cells by virtue of binding to their receptors. Targeting of these nonintegral membrane antigens will be complicated because an administration of MAb to such a factor will bind free (noncell-bound) circulating factor as well as cell-bound factor in vivo. Antitumor efficacy of such a MAb would be the combined effects of the two different phenomenona, i.e., a direct and an indirect effect on the vasculature.

Integrin $\alpha_v\beta_3$

Intergrins are a widely expressed family of cell-surface adhesion receptors. They function both as cell-substratum and cell-cell adhesion receptors *(17,18)*. All integrins are heterodimers of α and β chains, which noncovalently associate to form the receptor. The α subunits vary in size between 120 and 180 kDa and are each noncovalently associated with a β subunit of 90–110 kDa. Integrin $\alpha_v\beta_3$ (vitronectin receptor) allows endothelial cells to interact with a wide variety of extracellular matrix components *(18,19)*. It is expressed on blood vessels in human wound granulation tissue and there is a fourfold increase in its expression during angiogenesis on the chick chorioallantoic membrane (CAM). An anti-$\alpha_v\beta_3$ MAb and $\alpha_v\beta_3$ antagonists have been used to suppress tumors transplanted onto the chicken CAM (*see* Mouse Model Studies and Chick Chorioallantoic Membrane sections).

TP Antigen

Two MAbs, TP-1 and TP-3, recognize two different epitopes of this antigen, which is a monomeric 80 kDa polypeptide *(20)*. Immunohistochemical studies using the MAbs showed that endothelial cells were stained in proliferating microvessels in placenta and in most tumors. The TP antigen was absent in resting, but present in actively proliferating osteoblastic cells. It was observed in all osteogenic sarcomas tested, and in most cases of malignant fibrous histiocytoma but not in the other main groups of sarcoma or nonsarcomatous malignancy. In normal tissues, the antigen was detected in clusters of cells in the adrenal medulla and in proximal kidney tubules.

Endosialin

A novel cell-surface antigen, termed endosialin, was defined by MAb FB5 raised against cultured fetal fibroblasts *(21)*. The antigen is a 165 kDa glycoprotein, comprised of a 95 kDa core polypeptide and highly sialylated O-linked oligosaccharides. The antigen was not detected on either normal or cytokine-activated human umbilical vein endothelial cells (HUVEC). Immunohistochemical analysis showed that endosialin was selectively expressed in vascular endothelial cells of malignant tumors but not in normal blood vessels or other normal adult tissues tested.

Platelet-Derived Growth Factor Receptor-β (PDGFR-β)

Plate et al. *(22)* performed *in situ* hybridization and immunocytochemical analyses of PDGFR-β in normal human brain, astrocytoma, anaplastic oligo-astrocytoma, and glioblastoma. The authors found that there was an upregulation of PDGFR-β on vascular endothelial cells of these tumors. The levels of PDGFR-β on endothelial cells of other types of tumor remains to be determined.

Endothelial Cell-Surface Receptor Tyrosine Kinase Tie

The receptor tyrosine kinase, Tie, is the protein product of a recently cloned cDNA *(23)*. Tie is a glycosylated polypeptide of 117 kDa. Preliminary studies have shown that the expression of the Tie gene appears to be restricted to endothelial and some myeloid leukemia cell lines.

VEGF Receptors

VEGF is a key regulator of angiogenesis and vasculogenesis. The receptors for VEGF are the tyrosine kinases *(24–26)*, expressed primarily in the endothelium, and thus are attractive targets for antiangiogenic targeting (*see* Mouse Model for Targeting VEGF Receptors section).

Cationic Heme-Protein Eosinophil Peroxidase (EPO)

Normally, EPO is exclusively confined to the intracellular granules within intact eosinophils. In a variety of pathological conditions, eosinophils release their granule contents, which then bind to the anionic surfaces of adjacent cells. Samoszuk et al. *(27)*

found that EPO was localized by *in situ* immunohistochemistry on the vascular endothelial cells and connective tissue stroma of human endometrial carcinoma and ovarian carcinoma. EPO was not detected in normal endometrial tissues or ovaries from healthy subjects, in adjacent uninvolved tissues from tumor-bearing subjects, or in any of the other normal organs examined. The results suggest that EPO is a marker for tumor blood vessels of human ovarian and endometrial cancers.

CD44 Antigen

CD44 is a broadly distributed family of glycoproteins of 80–95 kDa. It is expressed on red blood cells and several different leukocytes including T cells, granulocytes, and pre-B cells. Griffioen et al. *(28)* reported that endothelial cells from the vasculature of human solid tumors displayed an enhanced expression of CD44 as compared to those from normal tissues. Because of the wide distribution of this antigen in many different tissues, safe and effective targeting of this marker in antiangiogenic therapy will be unrealistic.

Prostate-Specific Membrane Antigen (PSMA)

PMSA is a type 2 integral membrane glycoprotein strongly expressed on prostate epithelial cells. Liu et al. *(29)* reported that anti-PMSA MAbs defining extracellular epitopes of PMSA strongly reacted with vascular endothelium within a wide variety of carcinomas but not with normal vascular endothelium. These MAbs also reacted with some normal tissues including prostate, duodenum, and some tubules in kidney. PSMA MAbs are likely to have limited potential for antiangiogenic therapy.

IN VIVO STUDIES

Mouse Model Studies Using Artificially-Induced Marker on Endothelial Cells

Burrows and Thorpe *(8)* inoculated nude mice with a mouse neuroblastoma cell line transfected with the mouse interferon-γ (IFN-γ) gene. IFN-γ secreted by the tumor induced the expression of MHC II antigens on the tumor vascular endothelium. They used these artificially induced MHC II antigens as the marker for vascular targeting using a rat anti-murine MHC II immunotoxin *(8)*. The immunotoxin caused occlusion of the tumor vasculature and regression of large solid tumors, although the anti-tumor effects were transient and the tumors regrew 7–10 d later. A conventional anti-tumor cell immunotoxin of equivalent in vitro potency produced only minor, transient anti-tumor effects. When the two immunotoxins were combined, they induced long-lasting complete remissions in over half of the animals. Thorpe and his colleagues *(30)* in a later study used a truncated form of human tissue factor bound to a bispecific MAb, directed to the murine MHC II antigen and human tissue factor, to target the artificially induced MHC II antigens on vascular endothelium of tumors in mice. Intravenous administration of the antibody-tissue factor complex into mice with large neuroblastomas resulted in complete tumor regressions in 38% of the mice.

CAM Model for Targeting Integrin $\alpha_v\beta_3$

Brooks et al. *(31)* reported that a MAb or cyclic peptide antagonist of integrin $\alpha_v\beta_3$ disrupted ongoing angiogenesis on the CAM. This led to the regression of human tumors transplanted onto the CAM. Antagonists of the integrin-induced apoptosis of proliferative angiogenic vascular cells did not affect the pre-existing quiescent blood vessels. It will be interesting to determine the antiangiogenic activity and side effects of this anti-$\alpha_v\beta_3$ MAb in animals.

Mouse Model for Targeting α_v Integrins and Undefined Marker(s)

Arap et al. *(32)* used in vivo selection of phage-display libraries to isolate peptides that home specifically to tumor blood vessels. When coupled to doxorubicin, two of these peptides, one containing an integrin-binding Arg-Gly-Asp motif and the other an Asn-Gly-Arg motif, enhanced the efficacy of the drug against human breast-cancer xenografts in nude mice and also reduced its toxicity.

Mouse Model for Targeting VEGF Receptors

Ramakrishnan and associates *(33)* used VEGF-toxin conjugate to target VEGF receptors on the tumor vasculature in nude mice inoculated subcutaneously (s.c.) with a human ovarian cancer cell line. Daily intraperitoneal (i.p.) injections of the conjugate showed a significant inhibition of tumor growth.

Mouse Model for Targeting CD105 on Endothelial Cells

Details of the studies are found in the next section.

CD105 TARGETING FOR ANTIANGIOGENIC AND VASCULAR TARGETING THERAPY

CD105

In 1986, a novel human leukemia associated homodimer, GP160, was identified using a MAb SN6 *(16)*. MAb SN6 exhibited a highly restricted reactivity to immature B-lineage ALL and myeloid/monocytic leukemia cells but not with various other normal human peripheral blood and bone marrow cells (*see* below). Subsequently, the expression of GP160 on leukemia cells was observed to be strongly upregulated by transformation with 12-O-tetradecanoylphorbol-13-acetate *(34)*. It was therefore concluded that GP160 is a transformation/proliferation-associated antigen. Two years later, Gougos and Letarte *(35)* reported a leukemia-associated glycoprotein of 170 kDa with an identical cell distribution to GP160. They also found that the 170 kDa homodimer was present on endothelial cells, determined the nucleotide sequence of the cDNA coding for it, and named it endoglin *(36)*. GP160 and endoglin are identical *(37)* and have since been assigned to cluster CD105. CD105 specifically binds transforming growth factor-β (TGF-β) and its deduced amino acid sequence possesses a strong homology to betaglycan, a TGF-β receptor type III (*38*; Fig. 1). The role of CD105 in TGF-β induced signal transduction is poorly understood.

In recent years, several MAbs that bind to distinct regions of the extracellular domains of CD105 have become available *(39–41)*. Letarte and her colleagues *(40)* have utilized many of these antibodies to map their respective epitopes. Figure 2 shows the position of exons and epitopes recognized by different MAbs to CD105. It is becoming apparent that these MAbs differ markedly in their tissue reactivity. For instance, MAb E9 shows considerable specificity for endothelial cells of blood vessels in tissues undergoing angiogenesis *(42,43)*. In contrast, another MAb CLE4 has no such selective reactivity for endothelial cells (*42*; Wang et al., unpublished data). Furthermore, unlike some other anti-CD105 antibodies, MAb E9 does not stain villus endothelium in placenta.

Although CD105 is highly expressed on tumor-associated blood vessels in human cancers *(42,44,45)* and thus is an attractive target for antiangiogenic targeting, this potential has not been fully explored. The main reason is that newly formed blood vessels in xenografts originate from the host's tissues and conventional anti-CD105 MAbs do not

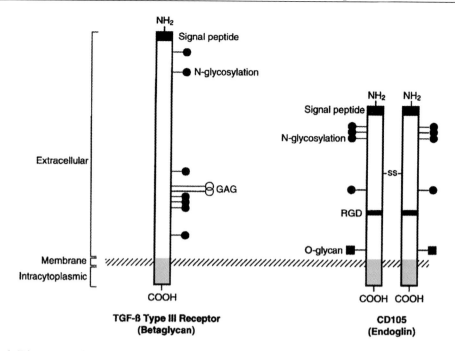

Fig. 1. Diagrammatic representation of CD105 and TGF-β III receptor (betaglycan). CD105 is a specialized type 111 TGF-β receptor whose tissue distribution is limited principally to EC. CD105 has significant homology (71%) to betaglycan in the transmembrane domain and cytoplasmic tail, whereas the homology of the extracellular domain is low. Betaglycan can bind all three TGF-β isoforms whereas CD105 binds with high affinity only to TGF-β1 and TGF-β3. The number and location of TGF-β binding regions is unknown, one is predicted to be within the N-terminal betaglycan related domain. CD105 forms heteromeric complexes with type 1 and type 11 receptors and is believed to function as an auxiliary receptor which contibutes to the regulation of TGF-β responses. CD105 has an extracellular cleavage site. CD105 is upregulated on EC at sites of neovascularization and loss of function mutaions in the CD105 gene on chromosome 9q34 result in the formation of vascular lesions. These findings implicate CD105 as a key mediator of EC activity in development, tissue repair, and disease.

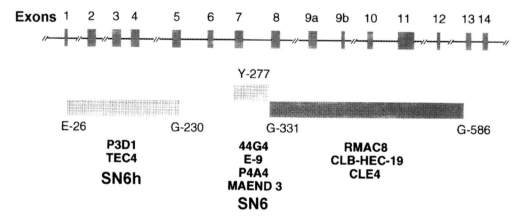

Fig. 2. Epitope mapping of CD105 using a panel of MAbs: position of exons and corresponding epitopes can be seen in this figure (for further details, *see* ref. *40*; we are most grateful to Prof. M. Letarte for use of some of her unpublished data).

react with endothelial cells of animal origin *(44)*. To overcome this problem, we have screened a panel of 12 anti-CD105 MAbs for their crossreactivity with mouse CD105. Four of the 12 MAbs crossreacted with mouse endothelial cells and have been used for antiangiogenic therapy in mice transplanted with human tumors. Details of the experimental procedures are given elsewhere *(46)*.

Reactivity of Anti-CD105 MAbs with Normal and Malignant Cells and Tissues

NORMAL CELLS AND TISSUES

Reactivity of various anti-CD105 MAbs with normal human tissues is variable but when present it is mainly restricted to vascular endothelium. Anti-CD105 MAbs react strongly with vascular endothelial cells of certain tissues such as inflammatory tonsil and appendix *(42)*. CD105 is expressed on syncytiotrophoblast of term placenta *(41,42)*. Anti-CD105 MAb, SN6, does not react with various normal human peripheral blood cells such as B cells, T cells, granulocytes, and erythrocytes, or monocytes, but it reacts with activated monocytes (macrophages) *(16)*. Lastres et al. *(47)* obtained similar results using two different anti-CD105 MAbs 44G4 and 8E11. Approximately 1% of normal human bone marrow cells reacted with MAb SN6 *(16)*. Studies using colony-forming unit (CFU) assays showed that the majority of CFU-GEMM pluripotent progenitor cells and CFU-GM myeloid progenitor cells in normal human bone marrow were viable after incubation with MAb SN6-immunotoxin. Under these conditions, over 99% of the colonies formed by CD105-expressing NALM-6 leukemia cells were suppressed. Bühring et al. *(48)* and Rokhlin et al. *(49)* reported that anti-CD105 MAbs reacted with a subpopulation of immature erythroid cells in normal human bone marrow and also with stromal cells derived from fetal bone marrow.

MALIGNANT CELLS AND TISSUES

In immunohistochemical analysis, our anti-CD105 MAbs belonging to series SN (e.g., MAb SN6) reacted strongly with the vascular endothelium in over 90% of the acetone-fixed cryostat sections of a large panel of human tumors. A different MAb (SN6f) was reactive with vascular endothelial cells of both mouse and human tissues (Fig. 3 and ref. *46*). It should be noted that such species crossreactive anti-CD105 MAb had not been reported previously.

Another anti-CD105 MAb SN6h reacted strongly with the majority of formalin-fixed and paraffin-embedded solid tumors *(46)*. Reactivity of MAb SN6f with various human malignant solid tumors was restricted to vascular endothelium *(45)*. However, some cultured epithelial malignant cell lines also reacted with MAb SN6f. For instance, three breast-cancer cell lines (MDA-231, SK-BR3 and T47D) were positive whereas the fourth (MCF-7) was negative. All anti-CD105 MAbs also stained immature B-lineage acute lymphoblastic and myeloid/monocytic leukemia cells *(16,35,49)*.

Detection of Anti-CD105 MAbs That Crossreact with Mouse Endothelial Cells

The initial screening of anti-human CD105 MAbs for their crossreactivity with mouse endothelial cells was carried out using a cellular radioimmunoassay (RIA), and the crossreactivity was confirmed by flow-cytometry analysis with mouse endothelial cells and by immunohistochemical staining of xenografts of human tumors in SCID mice *(46)*.

CELLULAR RADIOIMMUNOASSAY

Four of the 12 SN6 series MAbs reacted with SVEC4-10 mouse endothelial cells in RIA *(50)*. Binding of MAb SN6f to SVEC4-10 cells was weak but statistically significant compared to the isotype-matched control IgG. The rate of binding of this MAb to

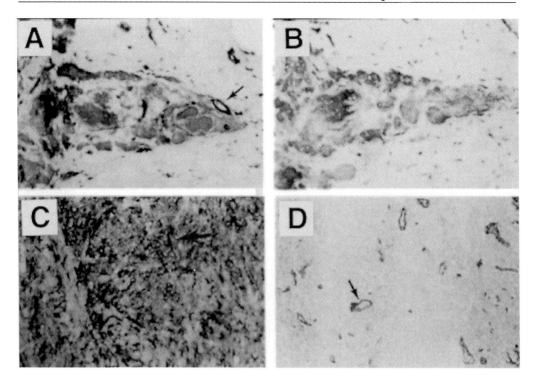

Fig. 3. (*See* color plate 4 appearing after page 490). Reactivity of a crossreactive anti-CD105 MAb SN6f with vascular endothelium of malignant tissues of breast, lung, and lymph node. Tissues of breast ductal carcinoma (**A** and **B**), lung adenocarcinoma (**C**), and B-cell lymphoma (**D**) were allowed to react with a 10,000-fold dilution of MAb SN6f ascites (A, C, and D) or the same dilution of isotype-matched control IgG ascites (B) and stained with DAKO staining kits. Counterstaining was performed with hematoxylin (× 50). An example of the stained blood vessels is indicated by an arrow in each of panels A, C, and D. Control IgG did not show any staining in each of the tested tissues and an example is presented in panel B.

SVEC4-10 cells was slow; maximum binding was obtained after a 24 h incubation. The MAb, SN6f, reacted much more strongly with HUVEC but no significant binding to MCF-7 breast-cancer cells was detected.

FLOW CYTOMETRY

The crossreactivity of anti-CD105 MAbs with mouse endothelial cells was confirmed by flow cytometry (Fig. 4). MAb SN6f showed significant binding to SVEC4-10 cells from subconfluent (i.e., proliferating) (Fig. 4A) but less well to (quiescent) cultures (Fig. 4B). Under the same conditions, MAb SN6f did not show any significant binding to control cells, e.g., BALL-1 leukemia cells that do not express CD105 *(46)*.

REACTIVITY WITH TUMOR VASCULATURE IN THE MOUSE AS DETERMINED BY IMMUNOHISTOCHEMISTRY

MAb SN6f showed substantial reactivity with the vasculature in xenografts of human tumors in SCID mice, but the vasculature in control skin tissues of tumor-free SCID mice was negative. An isotype-matched control MAb SN1 showed no significant staining *(46)*.

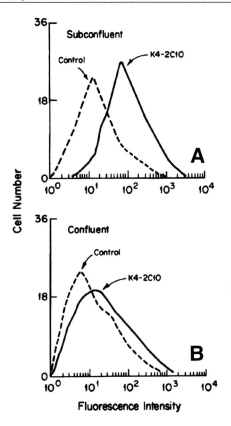

Fig. 4. Flow-cytometry analysis of binding of MAb SN6f to SVEC4-10 mouse endothelial cells. Direct binding of FITC-labeled MAb SN6f and an isotype-matched control IgG to target cells was measured using Becton Dickinson FACScan. The mean fluorescence intensity (MFI) of MAb SN6f was 182.5 and 64.1, respectively, for the subconfluent (proliferating; panel **A**) and confluent (quiescent) cells (panel **B**) while the MFI of the control IgG was 32.7 and 27.2, respectively, for the two cultures.

Immunoconjugates of the Crossreactive Anti-CD105 MAbs

Toxins, drugs and radioisotopes are most widely used for conjugation with a MAb to prepare an immunoconjugate *(51)*. Among the various toxins and toxin subunits available, the A-chain subunit of ricin, a plant toxin from castor beans, and truncated forms of *Pseudomonas* exotoxin (PE) have been used most widely in preparing immunotoxins for in vivo investigations. Previously, we have used ricin A chain (RA) and/or deglycosylated RA (dgRA; *52*) in preparing anti-human tumor immunotoxins (e.g., *53–56*). In the present studies, RA and dgRA were used to prepare immunotoxins of the crossreactive anti-CD105 MAbs.

IN VITRO CYTOTOXIC ACTIVITY OF THE CROSSREACTIVE ANTI-CD105 IMMUNOTOXINS (ITs)

RA and dgRA conjugates of the crossreactive MAbs and a control IgG (MOPC 195 variant) were tested against SVEC4-10 mouse endothelial cells in vitro. The conjugates of all these MAbs showed significant cytotoxicity against mouse endothelial cells compared with the control conjugate (Fig. 5).

Both RA and dgRA conjugates of MAb SN6f possessed weak, but significant, cytotoxicity against mouse endothelial cells; the 50% inhibitory concentrations (IC_{50})

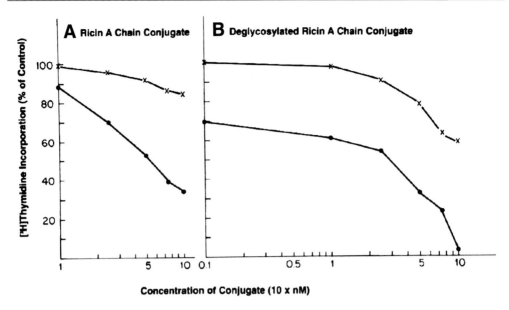

Fig. 5. Cytotoxic activity of RA and dgRA conjugates of MAb SN6f (•-•) and an isotype-matched control IgG (×-×) against murine endothelial cells. The IC$_{50}$ values of MAb SN6f and MAb SN6f-dgRA are 52 and 29 nM, respectively.

of these conjugates were 54 and 29 nM, respectively. Control RA and dgRA conjugates showed weak cytotoxic effects at concentrations higher than 25 nM (2.5×10^{-8} M). Such nonspecific cytotoxic effects of control RA and dgRA conjugates against various target cells in vitro have often been observed at concentrations higher than 25 nM *(44,57)*. MAb SN6f dgRA and control IgG-dgRA were further tested against MCF-7 human breast cancer cells, both showed very weak cytotoxic effects at concentrations higher than 50 nM.

IN VIVO ASSAY OF ANTIANGIOGENIC ACTIVITY OF THE CROSSREACTIVE ANTI-CD105 IMMUNOTOXIN IN MICE

Tumor-associated angiogenesis was induced in the dorsal air sac of mice by using HT1080, a human fibrosarcoma cell line, which is known to produce marked amounts of angiogenesis factors *(46)*. In this assay, HT1080 cells are potent inducers of angiogenesis. Treatment with MAb SN6f immunotoxin was strongly antiangiogenic, inhibiting both vasodilation and the formation of the tortuous microvessels *(46)*.

Antiangiogenic and Vascular Targeting Therapy of Human Tumors in SCID Mice by Intravenous Administration of MAb and Immunotoxin (IT)

SCID MOUSE MODEL OF HUMAN SUBCUTANEOUS TUMORS

We have established a highly reliable animal model that requires s.c. injection of 8×10^6 MCF-7 cells in SCID mice and results in 100% of animals developing tumor *(46)*.

ANTIANGIOGENIC THERAPY AND A NOVEL MODALITY

Therapeutic experiments were carried out using a crossreactive anti-CD105 MAb and dgRA conjugate of the MAb *(46)*. In addition, a novel modality of antiangiogenic therapy

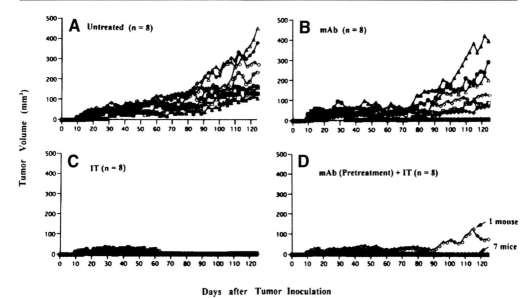

Days after Tumor Inoculation

Fig. 6. Lasting complete inhibition of the growth of human solid tumors in SCID mice. Mice were inoculated s.c. with MCF-7 human breast-cancer cells and divided into four groups (8 mice/group) and were: untreated (**A**), treated with MAb SN6f (**B**), or MAb SN6f-dgRA (**C**). The last group (**D**) was first pretreated with unconjugated MAb SN6f and subsequently treated with the SN6f-dgRA. The therapeutic MAb and IT were given on days 3, 5, and 7 post-tumor inoculation (day 0) via the tail vein of the mice. The pretreatment MAb was given i.v. 2 h post-tumor inoculation.

was also designed *(46)*. An example of the results in which MAb SN6f and SN6f-dgRA were used is shown in Fig. 6.

SCID mice that had been inoculated s.c. with MCF-7 tumor cells were divided into four groups (8 mice/group) comprising: untreated (A); treated with 17 µg unconjugated MAb (B), treated with 20 µg immunotoxin (IT) (C), or treatment with 75 µg MAb (over a four-molar excess) followed by 20 µg IT (D). The therapeutic MAb (group B) and IT (group C) were administered via the tail vein on day 3, 5 and 7 post-tumor-cell inoculation (day 0) while the pretreatment MAb (group D) was given 2 h post-tumor cell inoculation. The total dose (60 µg) of IT corresponded to 22% of the LD_{50} dose.

Palpable tumors began to appear 1–2 wk post-tumor inoculation in all groups of mice and grew beyond the size of the avascular phase, i.e., more than a few mm^3. However, there were remarkable differences in tumor growth between the IT-treated and untreated groups. Tumors in all eight untreated mice (group A) continued to grow, whereas tumors in 8/8 IT-treated mice (group C) regressed completely and remained so for as long as the mice were followed, i.e., 125 d (Fig. 6). Unconjugated MAb SN6f (IgG1-κ) was not effective in inhibiting tumor growth (group B). 7/8 in group D mice, which had been pretreated with an excess of MAb and subsequently treated with IT, regressed completely. No overt toxicity was detected in any of the treated mice. Thus, MAb SN6f IT is capable of exerting a complete and lasting inhibition of tumors without showing any undesirable side effects. Statistical analysis of the data was carried out using both Fisher's exact test and Student's *t*-test. In each test, the differences between the IT-treated groups (C and D) and the control group (A) were statistically highly significant ($p < 0.001$).

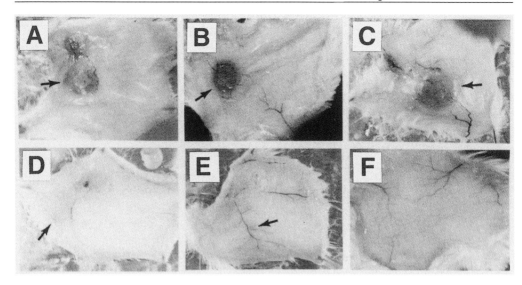

Fig. 7. Representative examples of anatomical examination of the mouse skin transplanted with human breast cancer cells. Tissues **(A)** and **(B)** were derived from the control untreated mice, while tissue **(C)** was from a MAb-treated mouse, tissue **(D)** from an IT-treated mouse and tissue **(E)** was from a mouse that was pretreated with unconjugated MAb followed by treatment with IT. Skin F was from a control SCID mouse that had not been inoculated with tumor cells and untreated. The size of the tumors was 8.2×8.1 mm (length $\times$ width), 7.1×6.4 mm and 9.0×8.6 mm, respectively, for tissues A, B, and C. Tumors in tissues (D) and (E) were undetectable. The distinct tumors (A, B, and C) and scars of individual regressed tumors (D and E) are indicated by arrows.

In an additional set of experiments, the effects of the dgRA conjugate of an isotype-matched control IgG (MOPC 195 variant) on tumor growth was investigated under the same conditions as described earlier. Unlike the crossreactive anti-CD105 IT, the control IT did not prevent tumor growth in any of the eight treated mice, although some inhibitory effect was observed in 5/8 mice *(46)*.

The therapeutic efficacy of the MAb and control IT was further evaluated by morphological examination of the tissues of the sacrificed mice. Representative examples of skin with tumors or where the tumors had regressed are illustrated in Fig. 7. Untreated control mice (groups A and B) as well as mice treated with unconjugated MAb (C) showed distinct tumors with multiple microvessels. In contrast, only a scar without microvessels was detected both in tissues of mice treated with IT (D) and with IT following pretreatment with MAb (E). Normal control skin from an untreated mouse is shown in panel F. Thus the gross tissue morphology agrees well with measurements on tumors *in situ*.

The strong anti-tumor efficacy of the MAb SN6f IT is remarkable in view of the facts that MAb SN6f and its IT showed only weak reactivity with mouse endothelial cells (less than one-tenth of the binding to human endothelial cells) and that a relatively small amount of IT was administered i.v. to treat s.c. tumors. It is anticipated that the MAb SN6f IT will show a much stronger anti-tumor efficacy and antiangiogenic activity in patients with solid tumors and other angiogenesis-associated diseases. The present results demonstrate for the first time that an anti-CD105 MAb or its immunoconjugate can effectively target tumor-associated vasculature in vivo.

A major concern in the antibody targeting of endothelial cell markers in antiangiogenic therapy and vascular-targeting therapy is undesirable side effects, because none of the known endothelial-cell markers is specific for tumor vasculature. To minimize this problem, a pretreatment protocol was devised as described in Fig. 6. It was hypothesized that pretreatment of tumor-bearing host with an unconjugated anti-CD105 MAb or its fragments (e.g., F[ab']$_2$) may reduce the undesirable side effects and further enhance the tumor-vasculature selectivity of an IT containing the same or a homologous MAb defining the same epitope on the CD105 molecule *(46)*. The rationale for this hypothesis is that endothelial-cell turnover in normal quiescent vasculature is very slow, whereas the turnover in the tumor-associated neovasculature is rapid. Therefore, pretreatment of tumor-bearing hosts with a free MAb (or its fragments) may be able to mask the weak binding sites on the quiescent endothelial cells in normal tissues while newly-generated binding sites on the proliferating endothelial cells in tumor tissues may be available for a subsequently administered IT. Thus, the pretreatment may reduce undesirable potential side effects of the administered IT. In addition, the pretreatment may enhance the anti-tumor efficacy of the IT because of the more efficient delivery of the systemically administered IT to tumor sites. Using this hypothesis, we carried out a pretreatment experiment, with unconjugated MAb SN6f followed by treatment with MAb SN6f-dgRA conjugate. The results of initial pretreatment experiments appear to support this hypothesis, although the optimal timing for the subsequent administration of an IT after pretreatment with an unconjugated MAb (or fragments) and the optimal molar ratio of unconjugated MAb to IT need to be determined. The optimal timing is influenced by several factors, such as the pharmacokinetics of the administered MAb (or fragments) and the rate of endocytosis/shedding of the MAb (or fragments) bound to CD105 on the endothelial-cell surface.

VASCULAR TARGETING THERAPY OF DISTINCT, PALPABLE TUMORS

In this assay, SCID mice were inoculated s.c. with MCF-7 cells and left untreated until palpable tumors of distinct size (4–6 mm^2 in diameter) appeared in the inoculated mice. Mice with tumors were selected, and groups of mice were either untreated (control), treated with a control IT, or treated with a crossreactive anti-CD105 IT. The anti-CD105 IT showed remarkable anti-tumor efficacy *(58)*.

Studies in Dogs with Spontaneous Ductal Breast Tumors

In an unpublished study, Jekunen et al. (personal communication) examined the uptake of radiolabeled anti-CD105 MAb MAEND3, in two dogs with spontaneous ductal breast carcinoma. They observed fast uptake, with tumor to background ratios of 6.2:1 and 9.3:1 in two dogs and during the follow up period of 3 mo, no side effects were noticed.

Studies in Cancer Patients

Tumors of the central nervous system (CNS) are among the most vascular tumors in humans and we have observed that CD105 is highly expressed in their vascular endothelium. In contrast, EC of normal brain contains only negligible amounts of CD105 or none at all. The overall survival for patients of many of these intracranial tumors has shown little signs of improvement over many years. In an unpublished study, we have examined the suitability of our anti-CD105 MAb E9, for targeted therapy in human CNS tumors. The antibody was labeled with ^{131}I, filtered, tested for pyrogenicity, and injected i.v. into 3 patients with highly malignant brain tumors. The biodistribution and pharma-

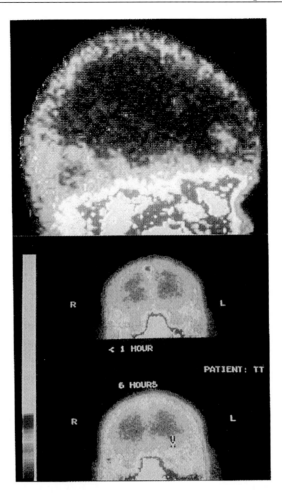

Fig. 8. (*See* color plate 5 appearing after page 490). Immunoscintigraphs of two patients with tumors. Iodinated anti-endothelial MAb failed to localize in a patient with a glioma-biodistribution and pharmacokokinetics of the conjugate was examined for up to 7 d. In a separate series of experiments a tumor was clearly localized (indicated by arrow) within 6 h following injection of radiolabeled antibody. (We are grateful to the Isotope Department of Christie Hospital for providing these figures.)

cokinetics of the conjugate was examined for up to 7 d following injection. Immunoscintigraphy showed no significant localization of radiolabeled antibody in or around the tumor mass (Fig. 8). The validity of the method was confirmed in a separate series of patients where specific localization of radiolabeled anti-tumor MAb can be seen. Whether the use of a different anti-CD105 antibody, e.g., SN6f or the preparation of radiolabeled MAb E9 F(ab) or F(ab)$_2$ fragments would further improve the immunocalization of CD105 remains to be determined.

ACKNOWLEDGMENTS

The authors wish to thanks Dr. Y. Haruta, Dr. F. Matsuno, Dr. M. Barcos, and Mrs. H. Tsai for their contributions to the work presented and Mrs. S. Sabadasz for help in the preparation of the manuscript. This work was supported in part by a US Army Breast Cancer

Research Grant # DAMD17-97-1-7197, American Cancer Society Grant # IM-741/ RPG-91-005-05-IM, and Roswell Park Alliance Grant (all to BKS). SK is in receipt of support from the Wellcome Trust.

REFERENCES

1. Folkman, J. (1972) Anti-angiogenesis: new concept for therapy of solid tumors. *Ann. Surg.* **175,** 409–416.
2. Brem, S. (1998) Angiogenesis antagonists: current clinical trials. *Angiogenesis* **2,** 9–20.
3. Sim, B. K. L. (1998) Angiostatin™ and Endostatin™: endothelial cell-specific endogenous inhibitors of angiogenesis and tumor growth. *Angiogenesis* **2,** 37–48.
4. Folkman, J. and Shing, Y. (1992) Angiogenesis. *J. Biol. Chem.* **267,** 10,931–10,934.
5. Bicknell, R. and Harris, A. L. (1992) Anticancer strategies involving the vasculature: Vascular targeting and the inhibition of angiogenesis. *Semin. Cancer Biol.* **3,** 399–407.
6. Denekamp, J. (1993) Angiogenesis, neovascular proliferation and vascular pathophysiology as targets for cancer therapy. *Br. J. Radiol.* **66,** 181–196.
7. Auerbach, W. and Auerbach, R. (1994) Angiogenesis inhibition: a review. *Pharmacol. Ther.* **63,** 265–311.
8. Burrows, F. J. and Thorpe, P. E. (1993) Eradication of large solid tumors in mice with an immunotoxin directed against tumor vasculature. *Proc. Natl. Acad. Sci. USA* **90,** 8996–9000.
9. Kerbel, R. S. (1991) Inhibition of tumor angiogenesis as a strategy to circumvent acquired resistance to anti-cancer therapeutic agents. *Bioessays* **13,** 31–36.
10. Boehm, T., Folkman, J., Browder, T., and O'Reilly, M. S. (1997) Antiangiogenic therapy of experimental cancer does not induce acquired drug resistance. *Nature* **390,** 404–407.
11. Folkman, J. (1995) Angiogenesis in cancer, vascular, rheumatoid and other disease. *Nature Med.* **1,** 27–31.
12. Jain, R. K. (1994) Barriers to drug delivery in solid tumors. *Sci. Am.* **271,** 58–65.
13. Dvorak, H. F., Nagy, J. A., and Dvorak, A. M. (1991) Structure of solid tumors and their vasculature: Implications for therapy with monoclonal antibodies. *Cancer Cells* **3,** 77–85.
14. Engerman, R. L., Pfaffenbach, D., and Davis, M. D. (1967) Cell turnover of capillaries. *Lab. Invest.* **17,** 738–743.
15. Risau, W. (1995) Differentiation of endothelium. *FASEB J.* **9,** 926–933.
16. Haruta, Y. and Seon, B. K. (1986.) Distinct human leukemia-associated cell surface glycoprotein GP160 defined by monoclonal antibody SN6. *Proc. Natl. Acad. Sci. USA* **83,** 7898–7902.
17. Albelda, S. M. and Buck, C. A. (1990) Integrins and other cell adhesion molecules. *FASEB J.* **4,** 2868–2880.
18. Hynes, R. O. (1992) Integrins: Versatility, modulation, and signaling in cell adhesion. *Cell* **69,** 11–25.
19. Cheresh, D. A. (1991) Structure, function and biological properties at integrin $\alpha v \beta_3$ on human melanoma cells. *Cancer Metastasis Rev.* **10,** 3–10.
20. Bruland, Ø. S., Fodstad, Ø., Stenwig, A. E., and Pihl, A. (1988) Expression and characteristics of a novel human osteosarcoma-associated cell surface antigen. *Cancer Res.* **48,** 5302–5309.
21. Rettig, W. J., Garin-Chesa, P., Healey, J. H., Su, S. L., Jaffe, E. A., and Old, L. J. (1992) Identification of endosialin, a cell surface glycoprotein of vascular endothelial cells in human cancer. *Proc. Natl. Acad. Sci. USA.* **89,** 10,832–10,836.
22. Plate, K. H., Breier, G., Farrell, C. L., and Risau, W. (1992) Platelet-derived growth factor receptor–β is induced during tumor development and upregulated during tumor progression in endothelial cells in human gliomas. *Lab. Inv.* **67,** 529–534.
23. Partanen, J., Armstrong, E., Mäkelä, T. P., Korhonen, J., Sandberg, M., Renkonen, R., et al. (1992) A novel endothelial cell surface receptor tyrosine kinase with extracellular epidermal growth factor homology domains. *Mol. Cell. Biol.* **12,** 1698–1707.
24. Beck, Jr., L. and D'Amore, P. A. (1997) Vascular development: cellular and molecular regulation. *FASEB J.* **11,** 365–373.
25. Ferrara, N., Houck, K., Jakeman, L., and Leung, D. W. (1992) Molecular and biological properties of the vascular endothelial growth factor family of proteins. *Endocrine Rev.* **13,** 18–32.
26. Senger, D. R., VanDeWater, L., Brown, L. F., Nagy, J. A., Yeo, K.-T., Yeo, T.-K.,, et al. (1993) Vascular permeability factor (VPF, VEGF) in tumor biology. *Cancer Metastasis Rev.* **12,** 303–324.
27. Samoszuk, M., Lin, F., Rim, P., and Strathearn, G. (1996) New marker for blood vessels in human ovarian and endometrial cancers. *Clin. Cancer Res.* **2,** 1867–1871.
28. Griffioen, A. W., Coenen, M. J. H., Damen, C. A., Hellwig, S. M. M., van Weering, D. H. J., Vooys, W., et al. (1997) CD44 is involved in tumor angiogenesis: an activation antigen on human endothelial cells. *Blood* **90,** 1150–1159.

29. Liu, H., Moy, P., Kim, S., Xia, Y., Rajasekaran, A., Navarro, V., et al. (1997) Monoclonal antibodies to the extracellular domain of prostate-specific membrane antigen also react with tumor vascular endothelium. *Cancer Res.* **57,** 3629–3634.

30. Huang, X., Molema, G., King, S., Watkins, L., Edgington, T. S., and Thorpe, P. E. (1997) Tumor infarction in mice by antibody-directed targeting of tissue factor to tumor vasculature. *Science* **275,** 547–550.

31. Brooks, P. C., Montgomery, A. M. P., Rosenfeld, M., Reisfeld, R. A., Hu, T., Klier, G., and Cheresh, D. A. (1994) Integrin $\alpha_v\beta_3$ Antagonists promote tumor regression by inducing apoptosis of angiogenic blood vessels. *Cell* **79,** 1157–1164.

32. Arap, W., Pasqualini, R., and Ruoslahti, E. (1998) Cancer treatment by targeted drug delivery to tumor vasculature in a mouse model. *Science* **279,** 377–380.

33. Olson, T. A., Mohanraj, D., Roy, S., and Ramakrishnan, S. (1997) Targeting the tumor vasculature: inhibition of tumor growth by a vascular endothelial growth factor-toxin conjugate. *Int. J. Cancer* **73,** 865–870.

34. Matsuzaki, H., Haruta, Y., and Seon, B. K. (1987) Effect of induced transformation of human leukemia cells on the expression of GP160, a novel human leukemia-associated cell surface glycoprotein. *Fed. Proc.* (Abstract) **46,** 1056.

35. Gougos, A. and Letarte, M. (1988) Identification of a human endothelial cell antigen with monoclonal antibody 44G4 produced against a pre-B leukemic cell line. *J. Immunol.* **141,** 1925–1933.

36. Gougos, A. and Letarte, M. (1990) Primary structure of endoglin, an RGD-containing glycoprotein of human endothelial cells. *J. Biol. Chem.* **265,** 8361–8364.

37. Bellón, T., Corbí, A., Lastres, P., Calés, C., Cebrián, M., Vera, S., et al. (1993) Identification and expression of two forms of the human transforming growth factor-β-binding protein endoglin with distinct cytoplasmic regions. *Eur. J. Immunol.* **23,** 2340–2345.

38. Cheifetz, S., Bellón, T., Calés, C., Vera, S., Bernabeu, C., Massagué, J., and Letarte, M. (1992) Endoglin is a component of the transforming growth factor-β receptor system in human endothelial cells. *J. Biol. Chem.* **267,** 19,027–19,030.

39. Seon, B. K., Haruta, Y., and Matsuno, F. (1996) Epitope mapping of endoglin, a TGF-β receptor, by use of twelve SN6 series monoclonal antibodies. *Proc. Am. Assoc. Cancer Res.* **37,** 59.

40. Pichuantes, S., Vera, S., Bourdeau, A., Pece, N., Kumar, S., Wayner, E. A., and Letarte, M. (1997) Mapping epitopes to distinct regions of the extracellular domain of endoglin using bacterially expressed recombinant fragments. *Tissue Antigens* **50,** 265–276.

41. Gougos, A., St. Jacques, S., Greaves, A., O'Connell, P. J., d'Apice, A. J. F., Buhring, H.-J., et al. (1992) Identification of distinct epitopes of endoglin, an RGD-containing glycoprotein of endothelial cells, leukemic cells and syncytiotrophoblasts. *Int. Immunol.* **4,** 83–92.

42. Wang, J. M., Kumar, S., Pye, D., van Agthoven, A. J., Krupinski, J., and Hunter, R. D. (1993) A monoclonal antibody detects heterogeneity in vascular endothelium of tumors and normal tissues. *Int. J. Cancer,* **54,** 363–370.

43. Krupinski, J., Kaluza, J., Kumar, P., Kumar, S., and Wang, J. M. (1994) The role of angiogenesis in cerebral ischaemia (stroke). *Stroke* **25,** 1794–1798.

44. Burrows, F. J., Derbyshire, E. J., Tazzari, P. L., Amlot, P., Gazdar, A. F., King, S. W., et al. (1995) Up-regulation of endoglin on vascular endothelial cells in human solid tumors: Implications for diagnosis and therapy. *Clin. Cancer Res.* **1,** 1623–1634.

45. Seon, B. K., Matsuno, F., Haruta, Y., Barcos, M., and Spaulding, B. (1998) CD105 Workshop: Immunohistochemical detection of CD105 in the vascular endothelium of human malignant and non-malignant tissues, in *Leukocyte Typing VI: White Cell Differentiation Antigens.*(Kishimoto, T., et al., eds.), Garland Publishing, New York, pp. 709–710.

46. Seon, B. K., Matsuno, F., Haruta, Y., Kondo, M., and Barcos, M. (1997) Long-lasting complete inhibition of human solid tumors in SCID mice by targeting endothelial cells of tumor vasculature with antihuman endoglin immunotoxin. *Clin. Cancer Res.* **3,** 1031–1044.

47. Lastres, P., Bellon, T., Cabañas, C., Sanchez-Madrid, F., Acevedo, A., Gougos, A., et al. (1992) Regulated expression on human macrophages of endoglin, an Arg-Gly-Asp-containing surface antigen. *Eur. J. Immunol.* **22,** 393–397.

48. Bühring, H.-J., Müller, C. A., Letarte, M., Gougos, A., Saalmüller, A., van Agthoven, A. J., and Busch, F.W. (1991) Endoglin is expressed on a subpopulation of immature erythroid cells of normal human bone marrow. *Leukemia* **5,** 841–847.

49. Rokhlin, O. W., Cohen, M. B., Kubagawa, H., Letarte, M., and Cooper, M. D. (1995) Differential expression of endoglin on fetal and adult hematopoietic cells in human bone marrow. *J. Immunol.* **154,** 4456–4465.

50. O'Connell K. A. and Edidin, M. (1990) A mouse lymphoid endothelial cell line immortalized by simian virus 40 binds lymphocytes and retains functional characteristics of normal endothelial cells. *J. Immunol.* **144,** 521–525.

51. Pietersz, G. A. and McKenzie, I. F. C. (1992) Antibody conjugates for the treatment of cancer. *Immunol. Rev.* **129,** 57–80.

52. Blakey, D. C., Watson, G. J., Knowles, P. P., and Thorpe, P. E. (1987) Effect of chemical deglycosylation of ricin A chain on the in vivo fate and cytotoxic activity of an immunotoxin composed of ricin A chain and anti-Thy 1.1 antibody. *Cancer Res.* **47,** 947–952.

53. Hara, H. and Seon, B. K. (1987) Complete suppression of in vivo growth of human leukemia cells by specific immunotoxins: Nude mouse models. *Proc. Natl. Acad. Sci. USA* **84,** 3390–3394.

54. Yokota, S., Hara, H., Luo, Y., and Seon, B. K. (1990) Synergistic potentiation of in vivo antitumor activity of anti-human T leukemia immunotoxins by recombinant α-interferon and daunorubicin. *Cancer Res.* **50,** 32–37.

55. Kawata, A., Yoshida, M., Okazaki, M., Yokota, S., Barcos, M., and Seon, B. K. (1994) Establishment of new SCID and nude mouse models of human B leukemia/lymphoma and effective therapy of the tumors with immunotoxin and monoclonal antibody: marked difference between the SCID and nude mouse models in the antitumor efficacy of monoclonal antibody. *Cancer Res.* **54,** 2688–2694.

56. Yoshida, M., Rybak, R. J., Choi, Y., Greenberg, S. J., Barcos, M., Kawata, A., et al. (1997) Development of a severe combined immunodeficiency (SCID) mouse model consisting of highly disseminated human B-cell leukemia/lymphoma, cure of the tumors by systemic administration of immunotoxin, and development/application of a clonotype-specific polymerase chain reaction-based assay. *Cancer Res.* **57,** 678–685.

57. Seon, B. K. (1984) Specific killing of human T leukemia cells by immunotoxins prepared with ricin A chain and monoclonal anti-human T-cell leukemia antibodies. *Cancer Res.* **44,** 259–264.

58. Matsuno, F., Haruta, Y. Kondo, M., Tsai, H., Barcos, M., and Seon, B. K. (1998) Induction of lasting complete regression of preformed distinct solid tumors by targeting the tumor vasculature using two new anti-endoglin monoclonal antibodies. *Clin. Cancer Res.* **5,** 371–382.

VI ANGIOTHERAPY IN THE CLINIC

27 Design of Pharmacological and Diagnostic Strategies for Angiogenesis-Dependent Diseases

Lucia Morbidelli and Marina Ziche

Contents

INTRODUCTION

Thanks to the advancement of knowledge in the field of angiogenesis, i.e., angiogenic/angiostatic factors and their receptors as well as the molecular mechanisms activated, it has been possible to design diagnostic tools for new therapeutic strategies for angiogenesis-dependent diseases and for assessing the angiogenic potential and malignancy of tumors. It is known that fibroblast growth factor-2 (FGF-2) and vascular endothelial growth factor (VEGF) play a critical role in the acquisition of an angiogenic phenotype. However, the blocking of these specific molecules might not be sufficient to suppress endothelial cell activation. Strategies targeting signal transduction cascades or the invasive phenotype acquired by the endothelium rather than individual factors and/or their receptors may be also proposed. Following this approach, we have targeted the nitric oxide synthase (NOS) pathway, the mitogen activated protein kinase (MAPK) cascade, and the urokinase-type plasminogen activator (uPA)-receptor, with encouraging results. The quantitation of the angiogenic output in tumor specimens or biopsies provides important information for the prognosis and the definition of biological endpoints to direct therapeutic decisions. Here we describe the development of quantitative methodologies for measuring the expression of angiogenic factors and modulators in tumor specimens. Assay methods, with good performance in practicability and analytical quality, when used to measure individual angiogenic factors in tumor specimens, are able to characterize tumor angiogenesis as a prognostic parameter and to select and monitor the efficacy of specific antiangiogenic drugs.

From: *The New Angiotherapy*
Edited by: T.-P. D. Fan and E. C. Kohn © Humana Press Inc., Totowa, NJ

NEW ANTIANGIOGENIC STRATEGIES

Angiogenesis is a tightly controlled process depending on the balance between stimulatory and inhibitory factors. When this balance is disrupted, angiogenesis acquires a pathological meaning *(1–3)*. The list of angiogenic molecules clearly illustrates the immense heterogeneity in chemical characteristics and biological properties. A large amount of literature has shown that fibroblast growth factor-2 (FGF-2) *(4)* and vascular endothelial growth factor (VEGF) *(5)* play important role in the acquisition of an angiogenic phenotype. High levels of VEGF and FGF-2 in body fluids and in tumor samples have been shown to correlate with poor prognosis *(6–10)*.

Several antiangiogenic drugs specifically targeting VEGF and its receptor on endothelial cells are now undergoing clinical testing. Examples are humanized anti-VEGF monoclonal antibody (MAb) by Genetech *(11)* and the VEGF receptor antagonist SU5416 by Sugen *(12)*. However, targeting VEGF may result in development of tumor-cell variants that may be able to stimulate neovascularization by secreting alternative growth factors and therefore, develop acquired resistance to VEGF-targeting agents. Thus, the impairment of these specific molecules might not be sufficient for turning off endothelial-cell activation. Thus it is important to consider the development of alternative strategies as:

1. Use of multiple therapies, i.e., antiangiogenic drugs targeting different pathways.
2. Combination of antiangiogenic drugs with low doses of conventional chemotherapy *(13,14)*.
3. Strategies targeting signal transduction cascades or the invasive phenotype acquired by the endothelium rather than individual factors and or their receptors.

Recently, a new concept has emerged suggesting that activated endothelial cells use the same pathways that are operative in tumor cells during their growth and dissemination. Different functional similarities can be found between tumor-cell invasion and angiogenesis: increased cell migration, increased cell proliferation, and increased activity of degradative enzymes (Fig. 1). Thus, novel therapeutic strategies have been developed aiming to hinder both tumor and endothelial-cell activation.

Antisense Oligonucleotides Targeting u-PA Receptor

The biochemical pathways involved in endothelial-cell as well as tumor cell migration and invasion are well-characterized. Key enzymes involved in the degradation of extracellular matrix are metalloproteinases (MMPs) and the urokinase-type plasminogen activator (u-PA)/u-PA receptor (u-PAR) system *(15)*. We have demonstrated that soluble u-PA induces neovascular growth in the avascular rabbit cornea and dose-dependently promotes growth, chemotaxis, and matrix invasion of cultured endothelial cells. Interaction of u-PA with its receptor appears to be mandatory for the angiogenic effect of u-PA since anti-u-PA and anti-u-PAR MAbs blocked the proangiogenic effects of u-PA at the endothelial-cell level. Impairment of u-PAR availability by monoclonal antibodies and by antisense oligonucleotides (aODN) against u-PAR mRNA inhibited endothelial cell proliferation, chemotaxis, and chemoinvasion *(16)*. These data suggest that u-PAR activation consequent to binding of u-PA can be regarded as an "angiogenic switch" and lead to the possibility that anti u-PAR aODN strategy could efficiently target endothelial-cell function in order to control angiogenesis in vivo. The use of an ODN against u-PAR as an anti-tumor strategy seems very promising because tumor-cell invasiveness will also be targeted (Fig. 1).

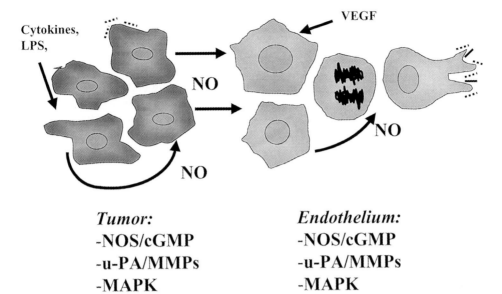

Cytokines,
LPS,

VEGF

NO

NO

NO

Tumor:
-NOS/cGMP
-u-PA/MMPs
-MAPK

Endothelium:
-NOS/cGMP
-u-PA/MMPs
-MAPK

Fig. 1. Common pathways in tumor and activated endothelial cells to be targeted by antiangiogenic strategies. i) Cytokines and endotoxins (e.g., *E. coli* lipopolysaccharide) induce nitric oxide synthase (NOS) expression and activity in tumour cells. NO, directly or indirectly through the production of growth factors, induces angiogenesis. The same endothelial cell is able to produce NO and cGMP in response to vasoactive substances and VEGF. The end result is the induction of angiogenesis. ii) Key enzymes involved in the degradation of extracellular matrix accompanying migration of both tumor and endothelial cells are metalloproteinases (MMPs) and the urokinase type plasminogen activator (u-PA)/u-PA receptor (u-PAR) system. iii) Finally, both proliferating tumor cells and activated endothelial cells use the mitogen-activated protein kinase (MAPK) pathway during cell cycle.

The current unresolved problems related to the use of ODN are their potential toxicity in vivo, often linked to the choice of the vehicle, and the difficulty in entering the cells in appropriate concentration.

Targeting of Nitric Oxide Synthase Pathway

The knowledge of the intracellular signaling pathways activated by angiogenic factors in endothelial cells allows for the development of highly selective inhibitors of these pathways. A pivotal role of the nitric oxide (NO) pathway in response to VEGF receptor activation has been extensively demonstrated by our group and others *(17–21)*. Because the tumor-derived NO synthase (NOS) pathway finely regulates angiogenesis and tumor spreading *(22)* (Fig. 1), we propose the measurement of NOS activity/expression as a diagnostic parameter and the use of NOS inhibitors to block tumor growth and dissemination. However, at present no specific tumor-selective NOS inhibitor is available for clinical use. Problems to be resolved are the presence of systemic side effects and the specific targeting to the tumor mass.

Gene Targeting of Endothelial Activation by Dominant Negatives for Signaling Cascade

We have recently reported that in microvascular endothelial cells, the mitogen-activated protein kinase (MAPK) ERK1/2 is a downstream signal of endothelial-NOS (e-NOS) activation *(23)*. In order to understand the temporal and spatial intracellular events linked to kimase domain region (KDR) activation, dominant negatives for raf and MEKK have been used. Preliminary results indicate that these experimental tools are specific for endothelial-cell response to VEGF or exogenous NO.

Because tumor cells widely use the MAPK pathway during cell cycle *(24,25)*, the use of dominant-negatives against the specific components of the MAPK cascade as anti-tumor agents is doubly justified because they block both proliferating tumor cells and activated endothelial cells (Fig. 1). As seen for ODN, the disadvantages related to this strategy are the lack of selective targeting and the presence of toxicity related to transfection reagents.

MEASUREMENT OF THE ANGIOGENIC OUTPUT

Tumor growth and spreading have been demonstrated extensively as being angiogenesis-dependent *(1,26–28)*. As documented in both clinical and experimental studies, the ability of tumors to induce a neovascular growth is a critical factor in determining their size as well as their distant dissemination *(1)*. At the clinical level, the angiogenic profile of a neoplasm represents an important prognostic and diagnostic parameter *(29)*, potentially yielding information on the clinical outcome following therapy.

Current Methods for Assessing Tumor Angiogenesis

Immunohistochemical and morphological studies have indicated that the number of microvessels in different types of tumors (breast, lung, and prostate) correlates with the metastatic potential and prognosis *(26)*. Moreover, the amount of angiogenic factors or their expression in pathological tissue is higher than in normal tissue. At present, the methods currently in use to delineate the angiogenic potential of a solid tumor are:

1. Microvessel density (MVD) in tumor specimens: capillaries are labeled with anti-CD31 and anti-factor VIII antibodies *(22,29,30)*.
2. Immunohistochemical assays on tumor sections *(6,7,31,32)* or Western blot on tumor lysates *(33)* for detecting VEGF, FGF, and their receptor protein expression.
3. Immunoassays for VEGF or FGF-2 in tumor samples or in body fluids as serum *(9,10,34–36)*.
4. Northern blot, RNase protection assay, and reverse transcription-polymerase chain reaction (RT-PCR) methods on RNA extracted from tumor fragments for evaluating the expression of VEGF, FGF, and their receptors *(33,37–40)*.

However, there are some disadvantages related to these methodologies:

1. They are not quantitative, i.e., for RT-PCR the quantitation is made in relation to reference genes as β-actin or GAPDH, or by the use of internal competitors.
2. They do not allow a comparison with healthy tissue.
3. They do not provide information on the relative contribution of the multiple factors involved in the angiogenic process.
4. They are not be feasible to be applied on fragments as small as biopsies.
5. They possess limitations in analytical standardization.
6. The clinical significance of angiogenic factor levels in serum of cancer patients, determined by immunochemical methods, is often controversial.

At present, microvessel density (MVD) counting is the gold standard in evaluating tumor angiogenesis. However, as different angiogenic factors can induce angiogenesis, MVD does not seem suitable for revealing which biochemical pathway is involved in inducing angiogenic activity. Different methodologies do not allow direct comparison between different laboratories and show poor practicability for routine clinical use, because some of them are expensive, difficult, and cumbersome. It has recently been reported that serum VEGF concentrations appear to reflect mainly platelet counts rather than tumor burden (35,36). Thus, VEGF in cancer patient serum cannot be indicative of tumor neovascularization and prognosis.

Quantitative Measurement of Tumor Angiogenesis

A prerequisite to achieve specific antiangiogenic therapeutic strategies is the availability of quantitative, inexpensive, rapid, and routine angiogenesis assays. The questions to be answered are: 1) which are the significant biological parameters to be measured? and 2) how can we measure them in patients affected by neoplasia, in order to direct and monitor the efficacy of antiangiogenic treatment? In fact, when patients are selected for clinical trials, surrogate markers for angiogenesis should be found in order to identify patients more likely to respond to specific antiangiogenic compounds, based on the angiogenic characterization of the tumor (41).

The efficacy of an antiangiogenic drug could be demonstrated by monitoring of circulating factors or MVD of metastases at recurrence. As discussed earlier, quantitation of circulating angiogenic factors is not reliable and MVD does not assess the functional angiogenic activity or give information about the biochemical pathways involved in tumor angiogenesis. Thus, these assays cannot readily be used for selection and monitoring of therapeutic effects. Likewise, they do not give an overall assessment of angiogenesis in the body or in metastasis.

It is now established that the measurement of a single angiogenic factor does not provide sufficient information on tumor progression. Moreover, different angiogenic factors are important for the progression of different tumors (41). A new technology, DNA microarray is now approaching clinical use. However, only a qualitative evaluation of the expression of multiple factors can be provided. On this basis we have contributed to the development of quantitative methodologies for the measurement of angiogenic/angiostatic factor expression in human tissues for clinical application. In particular, we have developed two quantitative methods for measuring the angiogenic profile of tumor samples: the TaqMan technology and the multiple competitive RT-PCR. By using these methods, quantitation of gene expression may be performed on tissue microbiopsies, circulating tumor cells, and blood.

TAQMAN TECHNOLOGY

We have developed a quantitative RT-PCR assay that measures the expression of specific factors in real time (42,43). With this technique, the measurement of the expression of angiogenic factors and inhibitors is also possible in specimens as small as biopsies. The quantitative RT-PCR method for measuring angiogenic factor (i.e., VEGF) mRNA expression based on the TaqMan technology presents the following characteristics: 1) results as absolute quantitative measurements (i.e., molecules of VEGF mRNA/μg of total RNA); 2) use of an external calibrator; 3) choice of a set of primers suitable for any of the VEGF isoforms expressed by the tumor or by normal tissue; 4) correlation between VEGF expression levels and angiogenesis in various experimental models using the in vivo rabbit cornea test and VEGF overexpressing cell lines.

This methodology, known as real time quantitative RT-PCR, is based on the use of a fluorogenic probe designed to hybridize within the target sequence and generates a signal that accumulates during PCR cycling proportionally to the amplification products *(42,43)*. Following this principle, the measurement of fluorescence in each sample provides a homogeneous signal, which is specifically associated with the amplified target and quantitatively related to the amount of PCR products. By using real-time quantitative RT-PCR, the specific RNA in the sample can eventually be reverse-transcribed, amplified, and quantitated without any further downstream processing, thus minimizing the risk of contamination. Native RNA, purified from cell lines overexpressing the gene under investigation, can be used as the standard preparation for the calibration curves.

The proposed methodological approach for a quantitative VEGF mRNA expression shows a good correlation with angiogenesis in vivo tested in the rabbit cornea and good performance of reproducibility and practicability suitable for routine use in large-scale clinical studies *(43)*. The preliminary results obtained in tumor specimens support the finding that VEGF mRNA is increased only in a subset of tumors. A significant increase in VEGF has been observed in renal tumors (mean 9.2×10^7 VEGF mRNA molecules/µg total RNA) compared to nonadjacent, nonneoplastic tissue (mean value 1.6×10^5 VEGF mRNA molecules/µg total RNA, $n = 6$, $p < 0.05$) with a ratio ranging from 181–2222. The pathophysiological meaning, as well as the clinical utility of these results, is under investigation using a larger number of patients and correlation studies with additional diagnostic and clinical parameters.

MULTIPLE COMPETITIVE RT-PCR

This assay is based on the construction of plasmids containing competitors for different angiogenic genes *(42,44)*. Competitors are characterized by:

1. Sequence homology with gene to be assayed,
2. Identical primer recognition sites with the gene of interest, and
3. Spacers or deletions enabling differentiation from authentic genes.

To obtain quantitative measurement of the expression of angiogenic factors/modulators within the same tumor with high accuracy, we have constructed a single synthetic RNA competitor for FGF-2, VEGF, TGF-β genes, and for the reference genes β-actin and GAPDH (Italian patent n. FI/A/000086). This competitor was constructed with the overlap-extension method, in a single-step recombinant PCR procedure and inserted as a 251 bp sequence in a plasmid. The order of primer insertion was designed to obtain competitors of comparable sizes to those of the respective genomic targets, but still easily recognizable from the latter ones by gel electrophoresis. Assays were performed in a single tube containing a known amount of the competitor and the mRNA to be quantified (Fig. 2). The cloned competitor was tested to evaluate the linearity range for each assay and validated for the measurements of the expression of the considered angiogenic factors in tumor cell lines stably transfected for the overexpression of the angiogenic factors FGF-2 and VEGF. Preliminary results indicate the applicability of the multiple competitor for the quantification of angiogenic factors/modulators in human tumor specimens. In Fig. 3, it is reported the quantitation of FGF-2, VEGF, and TGF-β mRNA expression in breast-cancer samples.

The present application of quantitative RT-PCR based on a multiple competitor represents a useful approach for the achievement of a single reagent for the evaluation of a panel of genes potentially overexpressed in human tumors. The plasmid represents a promising reagent for the sensitive and reproducible routine detection of angiogenic gene expression in the clinical laboratory.

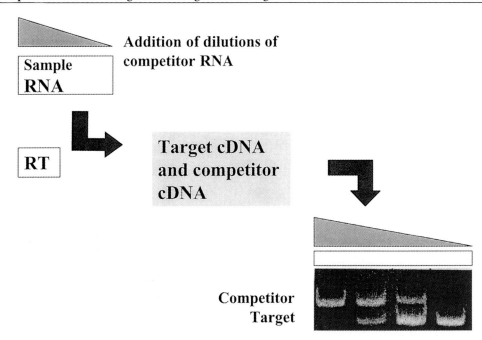

Fig. 2. Principle of competitive RT-PCR. Serial dilutions of the constructed competitor are added to fixed amount of RNA extracted from tumor or normal tissue samples in the same tube. After reverse-transcription (RT), the target cDNA and the competitor cDNA are amplified. Separation of the amplification products of the competitor and the genes of interest is performed by means of gel electrophoresis. Through densitometric analysis of the bands, it is possible to quantitate the concentration of target RNAm present in the samples. When the molar ratio is 1:1, [target] = [competitor].

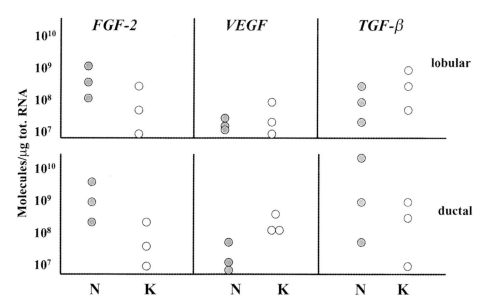

Fig. 3. Quantitation of angiogenic factor and modulator expression in breast cancer samples by multiple competitive RT-PCR. Total RNA extracted form tumor samples (K) and normal tissue (N) of human breast has been analyzed by the use of competitive RT-PCR (C-MZ Italian patent n. FI/A/000086). Data are reported considering lobular and ductal histotypes.

CONCLUSIONS

Antiangiogenic therapy has been proposed as an adjuvant therapy in combination with conventional anticancer therapies (surgery, chemotherapy, radiotherapy) for the treatment of neoplastic patients. An emerging concept is that direct targeting of specific angiogenic molecules might not be sufficient to hamper endothelial-cell activation. Thus, new strategies should be considered, as recently suggested by Kerbel *(13,14)*:

1. Combination of multiple antiangiogenic drugs,
2. Sequential administration of antiangiogenic drugs, and
3. Drugs targeting signal transduction cascades or the invasive phenotype acquired by activated endothelium.

By blocking different targets on activated endothelial cells and/or on proliferating tumor cells, we can increase the possibility of "killing" the tumor or reducing its burden. To obtain clear information about the efficacy of the aforementioned treatments, accurate but not invasive biological tests are necessary to document the patient response. Availability of quantitative, inexpensive, rapid, and routine angiogenesis assays, to be applied on small specimens as biopsies, is mandatory. The use of quantitative assays (TaqMan and multiple competitive RT-PCR) to measure the expression of all-important angiogenesis regulators (positive and negative) is promising for providing a measure of primary or metastatic tumor aggressiveness and monitoring the efficacy of antiangiogenic therapy. These assays can be performed on tissue microbiopsies, circulating tumor cells, and blood and results seem very promising.

ACKNOWLEDGMENTS

This work was supported by funds from the Azienda Ospedaliera Careggi, Florence, Italy (Project n. 94a), the National Research Council (Progetto Finalizzato Biotecnologie), the Italian Ministry of University and Scientific and Technological Research (MURST) and the Italian Association for Cancer Research (AIRC).

REFERENCES

1. Folkman, J. (1995) Angiogenesis in cancer, vascular rheumatoid and other diseases. *Nature Med.* **1**, 27–31.
2. Ziche, M., Morbidelli, L., and Donnini, S. (1996) Angiogenesis. *Exp. Nephrology* **4**, 1–14.
3. Keshet, E. and Ben-Sasson, A. B. (1999) Anticancer drug targets: approaching angiogenesis. *J. Clin. Invest.* **104**, 1497–1501.
4. Bikfalvi, A., Klein, S., Pintucci, G., and Rifkin, D.B. (1997) Biological roles of fibroblast growth factor-2. *Endocr. Rev.* **18**, 26–45.
5. Ferrara, N. (1999) Role of vascular endothelial growth factor in the regulation of angiogenesis. *Kidney Int.* **56**, 794–814.
6. Brown, L. F., Berse, B., Jackman, R. W., Tognazzi, K., Manseau, E. J., Dvorak, H. F., et al. (1993) Increased expression of vascular permeability factor (vascular endothelial growth factor) and its receptors in kidney and bladder carcinomas. *Am. J. Pathol.* **143**, 1255–1262.
7. Gasparini, G., Toi, M., Gion, M., Verderio, P., Dittami, R., Hanatani, M., et al. (1997) Prognostic significance of vascular endothelial growth factor protein in node negative breast carcinoma. *J. Natl. Cancer Inst.* **89**, 139–147.
8. Li, W. V., Folkerth, R. D., Watanabe, H., Yu, C., Rupnick, M., Barnes, P., et al. (1994) Microvessel count and cerebrospinal fluid fibroblast growth factor in children with brain tumours. *Lancet* **344**, 82–86.
9. Toi, M., Kondo, S., Suzuki, H., Yamamoto, Y., Inada, K., Imazawa, T., et al. (1996) Quantitative analysis of vascular endothelial growth factor in primary breast cancer. *Cancer Res.* **77**, 1101–1105.
10. Dirix, L. Y., Vermeulen, P. B., Pawinski, A., Prove, A., Benoi, I., De Pooter, C., et al. (1997) Elevated levels of the angiogenic cytokines basic fibroblast growth factor and vascular endothelial growth factor in sera of cancer patients. *Br. J. Cancer* **76**, 238–243.

11. Gordon, M. S., Talpaz, M., Margolin, K., et al. (1998) Phase I trial of recombinant humanized mono-clonal antivascular endothelial growth factor (anti VEGF MAB) in patients with metastatic cancer (abstract no 809). *Proc. Am. Soc. Clin. Oncol.* **17,** 210.

12. Strawn, L. M. and Shawver L. K. (1998) Tyrosine kinases in diseases: overview of kinase inhibitors as therapeutic agents and current drugs in clinical trials. *Exp. Opin. Invest. Drugs* **7,** 553–573.

13. Klement, G., Baruchel, S., Rak, J., Man, S., Clark, K., Hicklin, D. J., et al. (2000) Continuous low-dose therapy with vinblastine and VEGF receptor-2 antibody induces sustained tumor regression without overt toxicity. *J. Clin.Invest.* **105,** R15–R24.

14. Kerbel, R. S., Viloria-Petit, A., Klement, G., and Rak, J. (2000) 'Accidental' anti-angiogenic drugs, anti-oncogene directed signal transduction inhibitors and conventional chemoterapeutic agents as examples. *Eur. J. Cancer* **36,** 1248–1257.

15. Mazar, A. P., Henkin, J., and Goldfarb, R. H. (1999) The urokinase plasminogen activator system in cancer: implications for tumor angiogenesis and metastasis. *Angiogenesis* **3,** 15–32.

16. Fibbi, G., Caldini, R., Chevanne, M., Pucci, M., Schiavone, N., Morbidelli, L., et al. (1998) Urokinase-dependent angiogenesis in vitro and diacylglycerol production are blocked by antisense oligonucle-otides against the urokinase receptor. *Lab. Invest.* **78(9),** 1109–1119.

17. Morbidelli, L., Chang, C.-H., Douglas, J. G., Granger, H. J., Ledda, F., and Ziche, M. (1996) Nitric oxide mediates the mitogenic effect of VEGF on coronary venular endothelium. *Am. J. Physiol.* **39(1),** H411–H415.

18. Ziche, M., Parenti, A., Ledda, F., Dell'Era, P., Granger, H. J., Maggi, C. A., et al. (1997) Nitric oxide promotes proliferation and plasminogen activator production by coronary venular endothelium through endogenous bFGF. *Circ. Res.* **80,** 845–852.

19. Ziche, M., Morbidelli, L., Choudhuri, R., Zhang, H.-T., Donnini, S., Granger, H. J., et al. (1997) Nitric oxide-synthase lies downstream of vascular endothelial growth factor but not basic fibroblast growth factor induced angiogenesis. *J. Clin. Invest.* **99,** 2625–2634.

20. Kroll, J. and Waltenberger, J. (1998) VEGF-A induces expression of eNOS and iNOS in endothelial cells via receptor-2 (KDR). *Biochem. Biophys. Res. Commun.* **252,** 743–746.

21. Hood, J. D., Ziche, M., and Granger, H. J. (1998) VEGF upregulates ecNOS message, protein, and NO production. *Am. J. Physiol.* **274(3 Pt 2),** H1054–H1058.

22. Gallo, O., Masini, E., Morbidelli, L., Franchi, A., Fini-Storchi, I., Vergari, W. A., et al. (1998) Role of nitric oxide in angiogenesis and tumor progression in head and neck cancer. *J. Natl. Cancer Inst.* **90(8),** 587–595.

23. Parenti, A., Morbidelli, L., Cui, X. L., Douglas, J. G., Hood, J., Granger, H. J., et al. (1998) Nitric oxide is an upstream signal for vascular endothelial growth factor-induced extracellular signal-regulated kinases$_{1/2}$ activation in postcapillary endothelium. *J. Biol. Chem.* **273,** 4220–4226.

24. Robinson M. J. and Cobb, M. H. (1997) Mitogen-activated protein kinase pathways. *Curr. Opin. Cell Biol.* **9,** 180–186.

25. Schmidt C. M., McKillop I. H., Cahill P. A., and Sitzmann, J. V. (1997) Increased MAPK expression and activity in primary human hepatocellular carcinoma. *Biochem. Biophys. Res. Commun.* **236,** 54–58.

26. Folkman, J. (1990) What is the evidence that tumors are angiogenesis dependent? *J. Natl. Cancer Inst.* **82,** 4–6.

27. Folkman, J. (1982) Angiogenesis: initiation and control. *Ann. NY Acad. Sci.* **401,** 212–227.

28. Weidner, N., Semple, J., Welch, W. R., and Folkman, J. (1991) Tumor angiogenesis and metastasis: correlation in invasive breast carcinoma. *N. Engl. J. Med.* **324,** 1–8.

29. Weidner, N., Folkman, J., Pozza, F., Benilecqua, P., Allard, E. N., Moore, D. H., et al. (1992) Tumor angiogenesis: a new significant and independent prognostic indicator in early stage breast carcinoma. *J. Natl. Cancer Inst.* **84,** 1875–1887.

30. Bochner B. H., Cote, R. J., Weidner, N., Groshen, S., Chen, S.-C., Skinner D. G., et al. (1995) Angio-genesis in bladder cancer: relationship between microvessel density and tumor prognosis. *J. Natl. Cancer Inst.* **87,** 1603–1012.

31. Obermair, A., Bancher-Tedesca, D., Bilgi, S., Kaider, A., Kohlberger, P., Mullauer-Ertl, S., et al. (1997) Correlation of vascular endothelial growth factor expression and microvessel density in cervical intraepithelial neoplasia. *J. Natl. Cancer Inst.* **89,** 1212–1217.

32. Blanckaert, V. D., Hebbar, M., Louchez, M.-M., Vilain, M.-O., Schelling, M. E., and Peyrat, J.-P. (1998) Basic fibroblast growth factor receptors and their prognostic value in human breast cancer. *Clin. Cancer Res.* **2,** 2939–2947.

33. Nicol, D., Hii, S. I., Walsh, M., The, B., Thompson, L., Kennett, C., et al. (1997) Vascular endothelial growth factor expression is increased in renal cell carcinoma. *J. Urol.* **157,** 1482–1486.

34. Heer, K., Kumar, H., Speirs, V., Greenman, J., Drew, P. J., Fox J. N., et al. (1998) Vascular endothelial growth factor in premenopausal women: indicator of the best time for breast cancer surgery? *Br. J. Cancer* **78,** 1203–1207.

35. Verehul, H. M., Hoekman, K., Luykx-de Bakker, S., Eekman, C. A., Folman, C. C., Broxterman H. J., et al. (1997) Platelet: transporter of vascular endothelial growth factor. *Clin. Cancer Res.* **3,** 2187–2190.
36. Homer, J. J., Anyanwu, K., Ell, S. R., Greenman, J., and Stafford, N. D. (1999) Serum vascular endothelial growth factor in patients with head and neck squamous cell carcinoma. *Clin. Otolaryngol.* **24,** 426–430.
37. Inoue, K., Ozeki, Y., Saganuma, T., Sugiura, Y., and Tanaka, S. (1997) Vascular endothelial growth factor expression in primary esophageal squamous cell carcinoma. Association with angiogenesis and tumor progression. *Cancer* **79,** 206–213.
38. Yiangou, C., Gomm, J. J., Coope, R. C., Law, M., Luqmani, Y. A., Shousha, S., et al. (1997) Fibroblast growth factor 2 in breast cancer: occurrence and prognostic significance. *Br. J. Cancer* **75,** 28–33.
39. O'Brien, T., Cranston, D., Fuggle, S., Bicknell, R., and Harris, A. L. (1995) Different angiogenic pathways characterize superficial and invasive bladder cancer. *Cancer Res.* **55,** 510–513.
40. Relf, M., LeJeune, S., Scott, P. A., Fox, S., Smith, K., Leek, R., et al. (1997) Expression of the angiogenic factors vascular endothelial cell growth factor, acidic and basic fibroblast growth factor, tumor growth factor beta-1, platelet-derived endothelial cell growth factor, placenta growth factor, and pleiotrophin in human primary breast cancer and its relation to angiogenesis. *Cancer Res.* **57,** 963–969.
41. Ziche, M., Sorriso, C., Parenti, A., Brogelli, L., Tricarico, C., Villari, D., and Pazzagli, M.(1999) Biological parameters for the choice of antiangiogenic therapy and efficacy monitoring. *Int. J. Biol. Markers* **14,** 214–216.
42. Orlando, C., Pimzani, P., and Pazzagli, M. (1998) Developments in quantitative PCR. *Clin. Chem. Lab. Med.* **36,** 255–270.
43. Tricarico. C., Salvadori, B., Villari, D., Nicita, G., Della Melina, A., Pinzani, P., et al. (1999) Quantitative RT-PCR assay for VEGF mRNA in human tumors of the kidney. *Int. J. Biol. Markers.* **14,** 247–250.
44. Sestini, R., Orlando, C., Peri, A., Tricarico, C., Pazzagli, M., Serio, M., et al. (1996) Quantitation of somatostatin receptor type 2 gene expression in neuroblastoma cell lines and primary tumors using competitive reverse transcription-polymerase chain reaction. *Clin. Cancer Res.* **2,** 1757–1765.

28 Design of Clinical Trials for Anti-Angiogenics

Elise C. Kohn

INTRODUCTION

The development of new treatment programs is fraught frequently with similar conundrums. The backbone of the Hippocratic Oath, "First do no harm," counsels the clinical investigator to discover the safest mode, schedule, and dose for treatment administration. The requirement to treat the disease drives identification of the optimal schedule, trial endpoints, and analytic approaches. These same questions must be satisfied in order to bring new clinical interventions to the general community whether the pathology is systemic, such as in diabetes and cancer, or focal, as seen in epilepsy and appendicitis. These are the questions with which the new discipline of angiotherapy is now faced. The following issues will be discussed in the context of the development of anti-angiogenic agents for cancer treatment as the paradigm.

What is the physiologic target for angiotherapy?
How should angiotherapy be used?
When should angiotherapy be used?
Is there value in combination treatment approaches?
What surrogate markers or intermediate endpoints should be tested?
What are the expected toxicities of angiotherapy?
What are the testable clinical hypotheses, objectives, and endpoints for angiotherapy?

From: *The New Angiotherapy*
Edited by: T.-P. D. Fan and E. C. Kohn © Humana Press Inc., Totowa, NJ

Conventional Cancer Therapy Development Phases

The classical clinical paradigm for development of therapeutic interventions uses a graded clinical trial system, Phases I–III (Table 1) *(1,2)*. The objective of Phase I studies is to find an acceptable dose and schedule using toxicity as the primary endpoint. Safety is a paramount goal in any clinical setting. However, the definition of acceptable may vary with the clinical scenario. For example, myelosuppression may be an acceptable endpoint in the treatment of cancer patients, but it may be a dangerous side effect in patients who are immunocompromised and are at risk for infection, such as patients with inflammatory diseases, HIV, and vasculitides. A response to treatment, such as improvement in the disease state or reduction in tumor size, is not a prerequisite for Phase I analysis in this classical approach. Response criteria or use of validated surrogate markers may be incorporated into treatment design to provide supportive evidence for the further development of the agent or technique under investigation. Phase I cancer clinical trials focus on the use of new agents or new combinations and generally accrue patients for whom standard treatment options have been exhausted or for whom the likelihood of cure with conventional treatment is minimal. Patients who participate in Phase I clinical trials may be doing so for altruistic reasons, in the hope that there may be a benefit of this otherwise untested approach, or in response to family or physician guidance. Patients are not necessarily of a homogenous background and may have a variety of different tumors, prior treatment histories, underlying diseases, and pre-existent toxic injury. Frequent associated objectives of Phase I clinical trials may be pharmacokinetic and pharmacodynamic analyses, or clinico-laboratory correlates that may be related to the purported mechanism of action of the agents in question, the treatment targets, or the disease.

New treatments enter Phase II, or efficacy-oriented clinical trials upon clarification of a safe dose and administration schedule in Phase I. The primary objective of these trials is to identify beneficial effects of the tested treatment. Here, parameters for response such as tumor mass reduction, reduction in tumor-related symptoms and signs, or specifric regulation of validated markers of treatment activity are defined prospectively as the endpoints of the clinical trial *(1–3)*. In order to meet these objectives, this patient cohort must be more homogenous. Phase II trials are generally directed to a single cancer type and frequently include limits on the prior treatment exposure to minimize underlying end organ injury. Patients entering Phase II trials also may have failed prior regimens of anticipated benefit, and thus may not be the optimal test cohort as their likelihood of response may be poor. This may bias negatively the response rate seen for the given investigational agent and underestimate its potential benefits. The patient selection biases seen in Phase II studies may be minimized by randomization between two efficacy-oriented treatment arms. The clinical goal of randomized Phase II trials is still response outcome. These randomized trials generally need greater numbers of patients than single-arm Phase II studies, are more costly, and take a longer time to accomplish the clinical objectives than traditional Phase II trials.

Promising new regimens are then tested against the defined standards of care in Phase III trials to determine if the new approach is better than, equivalent to, or less effective than the given treatment standard. The defined outcome of these Phase III clinical trials in cancer treatment is response, time-to-progression or duration of disease response, and overall survival. Quality of life is becoming an important new endpoint for consideration. These Phase III trials are large, usually multi-institutional, and have defined control populations. They often have stratification for patient inclusion to optimize balance between the treatment populations.

Table 1
Phases of Clinical Investigation

Phase	Primary clinical objective	Ancillary objectives
I	Definition of a safe formulation, dose, and schedule for subsequent use	Pharmacokinetics, pharmacodynamics, Clinicolaboratory investigations, molecular markers, Quality of life measurements
II	Evaluation of clinical efficacy, e.g., tumor mass reduction	Pharmacokinetics, pharmacodynamics, Clinicolaboratory investigations, molecular markers, Quality of life measurements
III	Randomized evaluation against the defined treatment standards, response, time to disease progression, survival	Pharmacokinetics, pharmacodynamics, Clinicolaboratory investigations, molecular markers, Quality of life measurements

Cytotoxic or Cytostatic?

The primary tumor-response criteria used in oncologic clinical trials is tumor-mass reduction. It is a measured variable based upon the sum of the products of the bidirectional diameters of the defined index lesions as determined on physical examination and/or noninvasive tests such as radiographs and computed tomography (CT) scans (2). Tumor reduction as an endpoint would be expected based on the cytotoxic activity of most chemotherapeutic agents used in cancer treatment, those that cause cancer cell death. Diminished tumor mass would be anticipated in situations where the anti-neoplastic agent inhibits tumor cell replication sufficiently. The molecular targets of these varied chemotherapeutic agents are very central to cell function, at the level of nucleic acid synthesis, transcription, translation, and enzyme function (4). They are ubiquitous events, occurring both in tumor cells and normal cells. For example, the platinums, cisplatin, carboplatin, oxaliplatinum, and tetraplatinum, form adduct crosslinks with DNA and cause DNA strand-breaks in any cell type (5,6). Nucleotide excision repair pathways are required to repair the platinum damage, but may neither be quick enough nor successful enough to prevent a cytotoxic insult to the tumor cell or normal cell, thereby causing collateral damage to normal tissues (7).

The effect of cytotoxic agents may be beneficial against the disease for which they are administered as in the reduction of tumor volume, release of compromised normal tissues, and the reversal of paraneoplastic side effects in cancer patients. However, due to their promiscuity, cytotoxic agents may also injure normal tissues as is seen with mucosal damage, bone marrow suppression, and hair loss (4,8). These toxic effects are owing to injury to dividing cells that depend on the targeted molecular synthetic machinery. Inhibition of normal cell function or number by cytotoxic intervention may help in reducing tumor burden wherein the normal cells are facilitating tumor proliferation and progression. A secondary anti-angiogenic effect caused by the toxic effect of cytotoxic agents against activated, proliferating endothelial cells at the proliferative margin of a tumor is an example of this activity (9).

Cytostatic therapy is a newly emerging paradigm for the treatment of cancer (10,11). Cytostatic agents do not kill or irrevocably inhibit cell function leading to loss of cell viability after one or several cell cycles, as is seen with cytotoxic treatments and radiotherapy (12). They inhibit proliferation, activation, or other functions of the tumor or normal cells usually in a reversible manner. The molecular targets of cytostatic agents may be more selective and specific than the replication-targeted cytotoxic agents, wherein they may be directed to selected biochemical signaling pathways, growth factors or their receptors, endocrine functions, or specific cell types (Table 2). Thus, cytostatic agents may be focused at selected physiologic events during cancer or other disease progression.

Angiogenesis is an excellent target for cytostatic intervention. First, angiogenesis is a selective and focused physiologic event under normal circumstances, occurring during placentation, development, and wound repair *(13–15)*. Under normal differentiated and adult conditions, endothelial cells are generally functional but quiescent and terminally differentiated. Endothelial cells in differentiated adults appear to be a stable, minimally proliferative population *(16,17)*. The very small normal frequency of endothelial-cell proliferation is offset by an equally small and balanced cell attrition, attributed experimentally to apoptotic cell death *(18)*. It has been demonstrated that this balance can be upset by either induction of proliferation or reduction in the apoptotic index. Upon stimulation by inflammatory, neoplastic, or other injurious events, endothelial cells may proliferate and invade into local stroma for the initiation of new vessels *(11,15)*. Agents that directly target these activated endothelial cells may fall into the cytostatic category as angio-inhibitory therapeutics. Several agents are now under clinical investigation for their anti-angiogenic activity and most have been found to be cytostatic to the underlying tumors *(19–23)*.

WHAT ARE PHYSIOLOGIC TARGETS FOR ANGIOTHERAPY?

The development of a clinical trials paradigm for angiotherapy requires the identification and characterization of the physiologic targets involved in angio-stimulatory and angio-inhibitory activities. Understanding the physiology of angiogenesis in the context of specific disease is important in driving clinical trial design, definition, and validation of clinical endpoints, and development and validation of intermediate or surrogate markers where appropriate. For cancer, this begins with the evidence that tumor growth is angiogenesis-dependent. Numerous studies over the years have demonstrated directly or indirectly that angiogenesis is necessary relatively early in tumor development for successful progression and later for metastatic dissemination (Fig. 1) *(13,16,18,24–26)*. Further, angiogenesis is a dynamic process throughout tumor and other disease progression.

Upon activation under stimuli such as those elaborated by proliferating and invasive cancer cells, endothelial cells proliferate and the balance between apoptotic loss and proliferative gain is lost *(18)*. Tumor cells may produce angio-stimulatory cytokines such as hepatocyte growth factor (HGF/scatter factor) *(27–29)*, fibroblast growth factors (FGFs) *(30–34)*, and vascular endothelial growth factor (VEGF) *(35–39)*, among others *(40–43)*, that work in a paracrine fashion to stimulate local host endothelial cells to activate and proliferate. All angio-stimulatory factors identified to date have been found not to be restricted to endothelial cells as had been surmised originally, especially with the identification of factors such as VEGF, but also have been demonstrated in endothelial cell-free conditions to be elaborated by inflammatory cells, stromal cells, and/or tumor cells. Thus, both the growth factors and their receptors may be viable targets for angio-inhibitory treatment. These therapeutic agents may also be useful against the disease physiology as well because there is some overlap in the growth factor production and receptor location between endothelial cells and the diseased cells.

An alternative approach for angiotherapy is to target the mechanisms used by the activated endothelial cells to produce vascular tubes. Simple proliferation of endothelial cells is not adequate to produce functional vessels. In response to stimuli, endothelial cells turn on both

Table 2
A Comparison of Cytotoxic and Cytostatic Therapy for Cancer

	Cytotoxic	Cytostatic
Target	Nucleic acid and protein synthetic machinery	Selective to receptor, signal, cell type
Toxicity	Frequent normal tissue toxicity: marrow suppression, hair loss, GI mucosal damage	Less normal tissue toxicity, more constitutional symptoms
Dose	Dose escalation may increase activity	May not be as dose-dependent
Schedule	Generally intermittent administration	Maintain exposure through continuous infusion, long half-life, or frequent administration

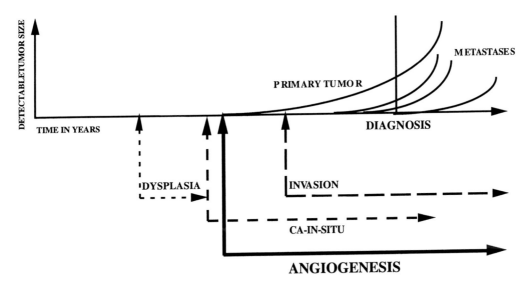

Fig. 1. Time course of development of cancer. Angiogenesis is necessary for tumor progression to a detectable size and for initiation of invasion leading to metastatic dissemination.

invasive and proliferative machinery. In order to create a capillary sprout, endothelial cells must breach their basement membrane in the direction of the stimulus. They then focus the sprout to that direction. Under differentiated and normal conditions, the basal side of an endothelial cell sits on its basement membrane. The basement membrane is an acellular complex scaffolding of extracellular matrix proteins, proteoglycans, and captured growth factors *(11,15,40)*. It is logical to consider that this barrier must be breached in tumor invasion for the process of tumor dissemination in advanced cancer *(15)*. However, this same invasive process is necessary for endothelial cells in the initiation of a vascular sprout *(11)*. The process of invasion, consisting of cellular adhesive interaction with the basement membrane, local proteolysis of the basement membrane, and migration through the site of local injury, is the same for invasive tumor cells as it is for activated and angiogenic endothelial cells. All anti-invasive therapies that have been developed for cancer treatment to date have been found to be anti-angiogenic *(19,44–49)*. Thus, the invasive behavior of activated endothelial cells may also be a therapeutic angiotherapy target.

An additional target would be to enhance mechanisms through which endothelial cell apoptosis occurs. Therefore, instead of being directly inhibitory to activated endothelial cell function, this mechanism would promote a negative physiologic event. Gene therapy approaches that introduce genes involved in the apoptotic pathway might facilitate this concept. Two endogenous proteins, angiostatin and endostatin, have been characterized that enhance endothelial cell apoptosis *(18,50–52)*. Both are effective when introduced by transfection and now there is suggestion that there may be some benefit in clinical trial and both have been successfully made into administered pharmaceuticals now in Phase I clinical trials.

WHEN SHOULD ANGIOTHERAPY BE USED?

The development of clinical trial paradigms for angiotherapy requires identification of viable targets against which the therapeutic be targeted, as well as an understanding of the pathology of the disease entity against which this treatment is used. Thus, the key question is when in the course of disease does angiogenesis begin and when in the course of disease is angiogenesis critical to its pathogenesis? Understanding disease physiology can provide the information from which to design the angiotherapy trial.

In malignancy, it is well-documented that angiogenesis is required for the tumor mass to enlarge past a defined size of 0.125 mm^2 *(53)*. It is at this size that the tumor mass has outgrown acquisition of nutrients by simple diffusion. It has been postulated that upon attainment of this stage of progression, tumors may develop or activate mechanism(s) through which to stimulate host vessels to initiate capillary sprouts in the direction of the tumor *(13,16,54,55)*. Most, if not all, defined angio-stimulatory growth factors are also tumor growth factors. For example, basic fibroblast growth factor (bFGF; FGF-2) elaborated by many cancers including breast cancer, many sarcomas, and prostate cancer is the most potent angiogenic growth factor *(31–33,56)*. Thus, in the autocrine production of FGF-2, these cancers are also elaborating paracrine angio-inducing agents. This implies that introduction of angiotherapy at the initial time frame of angio-induction, when the tumor is microscopic in size would be a critical time in the disease at which to initiate treatment that may be effective both against the neovascularization as well as directly against the tumor. Angiotherapeutics that inhibit de novo vessel production and vessel remodeling both may be effective at this time point.

A second time in the development and progression of cancer at which angiogenesis is critical is the time at which the tumor becomes invasive *(11,57)*. Without local vasculature, tumors cannot successfully shed pro-metastatic cells into the circulation. Invasive cancer cells must locally invade into the local blood vessels to initiate the process of dissemination. Although this may be a later time in general tumor development than that indicated in Fig. 1, it is still a relatively early event in tumor development, compared with the time at which patients generally come to diagnosis. At diagnosis, over half of patients will have occult or overt metastatic dissemination *(11)*. Introduction of angiotherapy agents that alter the integrity of existing blood vessels may be effective at that late time. However, simple inhibition of de novo vessel formation may not be active biologically at this point in cancer progression because the vessels have already formed. Similar paradigms can be envisioned with other pathological states in which angiogenesis plays an important role early in development and remains important as the pathology progresses. These include inflammatory diseases where there is a component of neovascularization and a component of disease where the neovessels contribute independently to the pathology.

HOW SHOULD ANGIOTHERAPY BE USED?

This leads to the next question of how to use these agents. This question is dependent on understanding of when and how angiogenesis is important to the disease, but with several additional caveats that depend on the planned endpoints of treatment. If the goal of treatment is to eradicate a disease process such as cancer, the optimal time of drug introduction, the time at which angiogenesis begins, appears to precede the time at which the disease is diagnosed. This suggests that introduction of angio-inhibitory treatment is best done in a cancer prevention mode. To test this clinical paradigm would require a very large and long clinical trial, making it prohibitive by expense in dollars and patient resources at the initiation of this important clinical treatment concept. If one were to target initiation of metastatic dissemination, a similarly early introduction of drug would be necessary and a randomized trial design most would likely be required to confirm a beneficial endpoint. If, however, the agent were administered at a time when tumor and metastases were established, this treatment might not be expected to prevent or annihilate the cancer, but may be anticipated to have a more cytostatic effect. Therefore, the physiology of disease and the physiology at the point of the intervention are important in driving the trial design.

The predominant mode of action of anti-angiogenic agents clinically tested to date in cancer trials has been cytostatic. Many but not all of the anti-angiogenesis agents under clinical investigation presently have been shown to have reversibility of their activity upon removal of the agent. This implies that the benefit of administration may be limited to that time during which a physiologically important circulating concentration of agent is available. A common theme in the administration of these agents is utilization of an approach that results in relatively constant exposure and continuous treatment until the endpoint of the trial were reached. This may require multiple daily drug doses or infrequent and intermittent dosing depending on the pharmacology and pharmacokinetic profile of the agent under investigation. This determinant is a critical point of information for anti-angiogenesis administration in clinical trial development, to optimize ease of chronic administration and patient compliance with minimal toxicity. The cytostatic and reversible nature of the action of most angio-inhibitory agents also makes them good candidates for use in nonmalignant diseases where angiogenesis plays a prominent role in the pathology. Thus, if the objective is an attenuation or prevention of neovessel growth in order to optimize the possibility of net tumor reduction, biologically the cytostatic anti-angiogenic agents must have a constant presence or constant effect. This would also be important if the angiotherapeutic was used in an adjuvant or maintenance setting to reduce or prevent tumor recurrence or progression in the period after a primary intervention. Drug and trial development would dictate logically that these agents be formulated for oral dosage or depo-dosage to provide this exposure. Intermittent treatment would have to be determined by the mechanism of action and pharmacology of the specific agent. How long to continue treatment in the context of the clinical trial may be a function of the difference expected between the treatment cohorts, size of the cohorts needed to reach adequate statistical power for analysis of the study, and long-term plans for the agent in question.

An alternative objective might be to prime a therapeutic system prior to using a more definitive intervention. For example, a period during which angiogenesis is blocked prior to a surgical extirpation of tumor might result in reduction of the potential for tumor seeding at the time of surgery. This approach might also be considered prior to and during radiotherapy done with curative intent. In this scenario, the anti-angiogenic agent would be given for a pulse period rather than continuously. Here, long-term compliance would be less important and may open up clinical opportunities for investigation.

IS THERE VALUE IN COMBINATION TREATMENT APPROACHES?

The physiology of cancer progression and similarly, that of many other chronic angiogenic but nonmalignant diseases, may require a multi-pronged therapeutic approach. Two combination treatment paradigms need be recognized, anti-angiogenic combinations and the combinations of anti-angiogenics with conventional treatments. The design of the clinical trial should reflect both the disease physiology, contribution of angiogenesis to the disease state, and finally, the expected endpoints and outcome of trial design in either combination situation. This concept is disease-independent, whether the target is cancer or nonmalignant diseases such as retinopathies, nephropathy, or inflammatory diseases wherein combination therapy is tried.

The use of a combination of anti-angiogenics with conventional chemotherapy or radiotherapy in cancer would be expected to have the benefit of nonoverlapping mechanisms and would be likely to have nonoverlapping toxicities. This takes advantage of the points raised in the Goldie-Coldman and Norton-Simon hypotheses, indicating the that intrinsic mutation rate of tumors would predict the development of a resistant clone earlier to single-agent treatment than to combination regimens, and utilization of drug scheduling in order to optimize drug exposure and reduce potential for resistance potentially also would improve outcome (58,59). One might anticipate at least an additive or perhaps a supra-additive effect of this type of combination. The anti-angiogenic agent would have the potential to maintain tumor mass reduction caused by the cytotoxic agent by removing conduits for subsequent dissemination and those vessels bringing nutrition to the tumor (60). It could be used either in conjunction with the cytotoxic chemotherapy, prior to cytotoxic treatment, between cycles of treatment in order to minimize loss of benefit for rapidly growing or resistance-developing tumors, or post-optimal treatment to maintain benefit. The literature has laboratory- and xenograft-based studies demonstrating the benefit of both concepts for the treatment of cancer. A list of in vitro and in vivo examples is found in Table 3.

The principal governing combination treatment in angiotherapy is the same as that governing combination therapy for any disease in any discipline. The combination should have benefits over single agents using defined endpoints such as response, quality of life, symptom reduction, or using newer techniques such as validated surrogate markers of outcome. Improvement can also be defined as a benefit of quality of life in which an equivalent activity against disease is demonstrated, in the setting of a net reduction in toxicity of the treatment. The development of combination therapy can use the unique properties of the cytotoxic agents, some of which have also been shown to be anti-angiogenic in their own right.

Some molecular targets have been identified that may to be synergistic targets for angiotherapy and cytotoxic chemotherapy, as targets that are shared by tumors and endothelial cells. For example, the FGFs are important tumor growth factors for a variety of cancers including prostate cancer, breast cancer, and glioblastoma multiforme (31,34,56). They are also the most potent angiogenic agents defined to date. Thus, a two-pronged approach, optimizing different mechanisms of action (Table 4), such as one that targets these active growth factors through gene therapy; chelating agents such as suramin, pentosan, or tecogalan sodium (61,62); or antibodies in combination with an anti-angiogenic that has an alternative mechanism that may or may not also have anti-cancer effects, such as TNP-470, thalidomide, or CAI (20,21,44,63–65), might have the potential to have greater anti-cancer effects than either agent alone. The toxicity profile may be sufficiently acceptable that a chemotherapeutic

Table 3
Combination Anti-Angiogenic Approaches

Author	Combination	Reference
Kohn	CAI and paclitaxel in ovarian cancer cell lines and treatment of patients with solid tumors.	(in press)
Oliver	TNP-470 and paclitaxel in treatment of arthritis	(89)
Teicher	CAI and BCNU, cyclophosphamide, cisplatin, melphalan, and radiation for cancer	(90)
Teicher	TNP-470 ± minocycline with thiotepa, cyclophosphamide, or cisplatin for cancer	(66,67)
Teicher	Multiple anti-angiogenesis agents alone or in combination with cytotoxic agents against cancer	(61)
Teicher	IL-12 ± M-CSF ± radiation therapy for cancer	(91)
Ogawa	TNP-470 with f-fluorouracil	(92)
Reed	SU5416 and carboplatin in ovarian cancer	(in preparation)

agent might also be included as has been done in xenograft models by Teicher and colleagues using minocycline, TNP-470, and either radiation or cytotoxic agents (61,66,67) or the combination of CAI and paclitaxel as we have studied (Kohn et al., in press). We found a supra-additive effect of the combination of CAI followed by paclitaxel in vitro colony-forming assays and lack of additive toxicity in animal modeling. The first phase of the clinical trial proceeded to maximum dose of CAI administered for 8 d prior to a 3 h infusion of paclitaxel. Paclitaxel dose was increased up to 250 mg/m^2 without additive toxicity. Both partial and minor responses were observed and the current protocol allows daily CAI administration with pulse 3 h paclitaxel on a 3 week basis. Preclinical work in progress has also demonstrated a more than additive effect of this combination in lung-cancer xenografts and found a reduction in VEGF expression in vitro (Kohn and Moody, manuscript in preparation). CAI treatment alone reduced circulating VEGF and IL-8 concentrations in human melanoma xenografts (Libutti and Kohn, manuscript in preparation).

Combination approaches other than concomitant combination treatment using anti-angiogenics for the treatment of cancer or other angiogenic diseases might include neo-adjuvant or adjuvant treatment with angiotherapy, maintenance therapy, or in chemoprevention when appropriate selection factors can identify patients at risk. Neo-adjuvant treatment may have an effect to reduce metastatic potential of the tumor by reducing tumor vascularity, making it more susceptible to cytotoxic chemotherapy. Adjuvant or maintenance therapy may reduce the frequency of relapse or progression, or slow the time to development of detectable or symptomatic disease by inducing dormancy of micrometastatic residual and undetectable disease (18,54). In either scenario, the patient may be afforded reduced toxicity with equivalent or greater benefit by mixing the type of treatment, toxicity profile, and therapeutic mechanisms of action.

WHAT SURROGATE MARKERS OR INTERMEDIATE ENDPOINTS SHOULD BE TESTED?

There is a general consensus within the angiogenesis developmental therapeutics field that the classical mechanism for analysis of the efficacy of anti-neoplastic activity will not be optimal nor accurate for the analysis of anti-angiogenic activity in cancer treatment

Table 4
Selected Anti-Angiogenesis Agents: Varied Mechanisms of Action

Agent	Mechanism(s) of action	Reference
CAI	Inhibition of nonvoltage-gated calcium influx, Inhibits matrix metalloproteinase-1, 2, 9 expression	(19,44,45,93–95)
Thalidomide	Undetermined, ? reactive intermediate	(21)
TNP-470	suppression cyclin D1 expression	(63,92,96,97)
IL-12	Induction of IFN-γ with induction of interferon-inducible protein 10	(98–100)
Marimastat	Inhibition of matrix metalloproteinase activity	(46,49,101)
CM-101	Polysaccharide toxin inducing inflammatory response on vasculature	(102)

(11,13,22,23,49,68,69). Similarly, it has been recognized that cytotoxic agents have not yielded cures in the large majority of cancers leading to the need for alternative mechanisms of intervention, including evaluation of cytostatic agents, such as those that inhibit angiogenesis. But if so, then how to analyze the potential benefits so as to weigh them against the possible toxicities? The fields of non-neoplastic medicine and cancer chemoprevention have used and proposed the use of intermediate endpoints and surrogate markers (19,70–72). These are biochemical activities, laboratory assays, or imaging studies that could define evolution of disease and be present in a sufficiently high frequency in the populations in question (73). Imaging modalities may allow quantification of vascularity of the tumor when compared to a control organ such as muscle (74,75). Further, they must be validated as a measure of reduction of disease activity. Demonstration that serum creatinine has improved in a diabetic with nephropathy is an example of using a biochemical activity as a marker for the renal dysfunction caused by the disease. Similarly, there are multiple serologic markers used to follow disease activity in the rheumatic diseases.

This concept is relatively new to the field of oncology and angiogenesis. However, there are several angiogenesis biomarkers for which data are available. These include microvessel counts in random tissue samples (24,76,77; A. Harris, this volume), measurement of urinary and serum FGF-2 concentrations (56), measurement of matrix metalloproteinase activity and quantity (72,78), quantitation of the presence of other angiostimulatory growth factors such as VEGF, and dynamic MRI (magnetic resonance imaging) (74,75). We have demonstrated that CAI treatment alone reduced circulating VEGF and IL-8 concentrations in human melanoma xenografts (Libutti and Kohn, manuscript in preparation) suggesting that circulating VEGF concentration measurements may be a surrogate marker in clinical trial. That hypothesis is being tested in a current Phase II trial of CAI for ovarian cancer patients. While all of these potential markers have their proponents, none have been validated as true markers of the efficacy of the antiangiogenic intervention. At best, they have been correlated retrospectively with risk of cancer or metastasis. Most of the studies are small, nonrandomized, and nonblinded. Not all of the reports are in agreement as to the validity of the potential marker. Further, these potential intermediate endpoints or surrogate markers may not truly reflect the pathophysiology in the patient as a whole.

Can a single value at a single point in time accurately reflect the isolated processes ongoing at specific disease points in the body? Matrix metalloproteinase inhibition is a very localized event in the pathology of angiogenesis of malignant and nonmalignant diseases alike and represents a dynamic balance between the varied matrix metalloproteinases, endogenous inhibitors, and administered agents. Thus, quantity or activity of matrix metalloproteinases in the serum or plasma, documented at a snippet of time during the lifetime of the cancer or serially over therapy, may or may not provide a valid assessment of the benefits of an agent.

Measurement of circulating growth factors or quantitation of growth factor expression by *in situ* hybridization or Northern-blot analysis may not give an accurate measurement of the growth factor involved in the angiogenic process. It may reflect increase in global growth-factor production overall for varied reasons, such as the host response to the presence of the cancer, and may not give an accurate measurement of the total angiogenic body burden. This is especially a problem because many angiogenic growth factors are heparin-binding proteins and are sequestered in the extracellular matrix *(40)*. A similar pitfall can be posed in the assessment of microvessel counts. This clinico-laboratory correlate, originally posed by Weidner and colleagues for breast cancer patients *(25)*, has been evaluated in numerous other malignancies (*see* adjoining chapter). This measurement has been shown generally to be a harbinger of worse prognosis with increased risk of metastatic dissemination and decreased overall survival. Given the heterogeneity of tumors and other pathologic states, it is unlikely that the single slide from a selected tissue sample assessed per patient will be either the most angiogenic area of the cancer, nor is it likely to be generally representative of the entire lesion. Recently, a report by Koukourakis and colleagues demonstrated that assessment of microvessels using an antibody that recognized the VEGF/KDR complex was selectively more accurate in predection of active microvessels *(79)*. Thus, this is where the physiology of the disease is important in deciding how to test molecular endpoints. The most important areas of neovessel formation are generally at the periphery of the tumor where the interface with normal tissue and the tumor-invasive front occurs and at the microfoci of metastatic or invasive dissemination, where in order to form a progressing metastasis, angiogenesis is necessary, otherwise tumor dormancy will ensue *(18,55)*. This needs to be considered or at least recognized in determining how to use the molecular makers.

There are a myriad of physiologic and biochemical reasons with which to find flaw with the concepts of surrogate markers or intermediate endpoints of angiotherapeutic potential. The best mechanism by which to settle these concerns is the testing and validation of putative markers in clinical trials prospectively and independently. Randomized assessments, blinded tests, and large cohorts will provide the power to determine if these alternative methods of determining drug response are valid. This issue is also pertinent to questions of molecular markers as indicators of disease, disease risk, or altered prognostic outcomes. New areas of investigation into the physiology and molecular mechanisms of angiogenesis are likely to uncover further useful surrogates for testing.

WHAT ARE THE EXPECTED TOXICITIES OF ANGIOTHERAPY?

The toxicity of a regimen must be taken into consideration in the design of clinical trials and in the development of subsequent general use dosing recommendations. The disease under treatment, underlying organ dysfunction that may already be present in to the treatment cohort, duration of treatment, clinical pharmacology of the agent, and the potential for delayed and long-term toxicities toxicity must be considered. These issues are best demonstrated looking at the history of one now promising anti-angiogenic agent, thalidomide. Preclinical development indicated that this agent was a sedative and anti-emetic and was well-tolerated. The preclinical evaluation did not uncover the teratogenic activity, although the stringency of testing required for drug approval was different during that era. Disastrous teratogenic side effects were encountered *(80,81)* that more recently have been attributed to blockade of angiogenesis necessary during limb development *(21)*. It was demonstrated that this agent required hepatic metabolism through a pathway not present in rats and mice, so rodent toxicity studies would have shown the agent to be safe. Thalidomide is now being tested in Phase I and II studies for its anti-angiogenic activity and is being administered for longer times than during its initial testing in the 1950s with a better toxicity profile in the current test cohorts. An expanded panel of side effects has been demonstrated in these cancer treatment trials, including sedation, altered mental status, fluid retention, depression, and sensory peripheral neuropathy *(82–85)* (Table 5).

The anticipated toxicities of angiotherapy, independent of the individual mechanism of action of each agent and the potential for toxicity of drug vehicles, might include some constitutional symptoms. Vessel and endothelial cell activity, while quiescent during normal adult physiology, is necessary in several normal functions, including menstrual cycles, pregnancy, and normal regeneration events such as occurs during bone remodeling, mucosal regeneration, ovulatory cyst formation, and wound healing. The importance of whether or not the anti-angiogenic agent only effects or inhibits de novo vessel production, can alter function of activated endothelial cells during vessel remodeling in response to stimuli or stresses, or can effect quiescent vessels, also will have a bearing on its potential toxicities. Agents selective to de novo vessel formation might be expected to have a more limited spectrum of toxicity directly owing to to the anti-angiogenic activity of the drug. Organs may be susceptible to toxicity from agents that may be inhibitory to activated vessels resulting in a reduction in necessary local blood flow, such as in patients with vasculopathy or atherosclerotic disease, wherein they may have reduced afferent blood flow. These include the ovary and endometrium, gastrointestinal tract, central and peripheral nervous system, bone marrow, peripheral vascular system, and the cardiopulmonary system.

Selective toxicities observed with angiotherapeutics currently in clinical trial are listed in Table 5. The broad spectrum and serious nature of some of these toxicities underscore the importance of careful analysis during early clinical trials. Careful attention to this detail is necessary in the design of clinical trials for these and upcoming agents. Until there is a body of experience with the broad variety of potential anti-angiogenic agents, their vehicles, and their schedules, the clinical investigator must be sleuthing for subtle warnings of progressive toxicity. These may be either reversible upon removal of the agent, as has been observed with the sensory peripheral neuropathy of CAI *(20,86,87)* for example, or potentially may have a lasting effect as in the fibrosis induced by matrix metalloproteinase inhibition *(48,49,69)*.

In addition to careful attention to the potential for toxicity and the pattern of toxicity development and progression, it is important to realize that there may be physiologic reasons for these toxicities that may be overcome without endangering the potential for disease benefit. For example, an unanticipated toxicity of high dose lovastatin was overcome by supplementation with coenzyme Q *(88)*. Thus, understanding both the targeted effects of the anti-angiogenic nature of these agents as well as the related biochemical targets of their mechanisms of action will lead to early recognition of specific toxicities and may further direct the investigators to mechanisms through which to overcome them.

Table 5
Toxicities of Selected Anti-Angiogenic Therapy

Agent	Common Toxicities	Rare Toxicities	Ref.
CAI	Fatigue, nausea, rare vomiting	Reversible sensory neuropathy, transient blindness	(20,86,87)
Thalidomide	Sedation, mood changes, fever, rash, constipation, nausea	Peripheral neuropathy limb swelling/erythema, limb dysgenesis	(80–85,103,104)
IL-12	Leukopenia, fever, chills, fatigue, nausea, vomiting, mucositis	Thrombocytopenia	(105)
MMPIs[a]	Peritoneal irritation with IP administration, arthralgias and stiffness, myalgias, fatigue, anorexia	Nausea and vomiting	(22,106–108)
TNP-470	Anxiety, mood changes, gait disturbance	Peripheral neuropathy urticaria	(109–111)

[a]Batimastat/Marimastat.

WHAT ARE THE TESTABLE CLINICAL HYPOTHESES, OBJECTIVES, AND ENDPOINTS FOR ANGIOTHERAPY?

The development of this important new advance to the clinical armamentarium for cancer treatment and for treatment of other diseases in which neovessel proliferation promotes or supports the disease state must be approached carefully. Clinical disciplines have defined systems for evaluation of therapeutic efficacy that may not be optimal for evaluation of angiotherapy. Hypothesis-driven clinical research with testable objectives using validated markers and endpoints is necessary so that this new intervention receives its best test. Assessment of quality of life parameters will assist in determining the utility and circumstances under which angiotherapy may be best used. It should be considered an important component of clinical trial development. Several paradigms are outlined below.

Neoadjuvant Therapy

Neoadjuvant therapy is defined as systemic treatment given prior to definitive intervention. An example is neoadjuvant chemotherapy for primary cancers of the head and neck. In this approach, systemic chemotherapy is administered to reduce net tumor burden prior to attempts at definitive surgery and/or radiotherapy. This treatment was found to improve resectability, however, it did not prolong time to recurrence or survival in patients with advanced cancers. Neoadjuvant angiotherapy might have an alternative benefit. If the anti-angiogenic agent used could target actively remodeling or newly forming vessels, then anti-angiogenic treatment for a defined time prior to intervention might reduce the viability of the local tumor, reduce local vascular access, and reduce the local metastatic spread that occurs during surgical intervention. It might also function as a radiation sensitizer. The hypothesis that neoadjuvant angiotherapy would improve primary therapy could be tested with a randomization to angiotherapy or placebo/observation prior to initiation of primary therapy. Time to recurrence, location of recurrence, and extent of recurrence would be testable endpoints. Use of angiomarkers as laboratory analyses would allow further investigation into the biologic effects of angiotherapy in this setting.

Post-Adjuvant Therapy

The ability to initiate treatment with newer drugs and in new paradigms is limited in some cases by experience to date with the agents in question. A point at which to initiate investigation is with patients for whom optimal treatments have already been exhausted as described for the Phase I clinical trials. This is a population, not just in cancer patients but in many chronic diseases, for whom benefit may be elusive independent of the agent tested. This is a population for testing safety and in whom to hope for benefit. This population of cancer patients also generally has a significant tumor burden. This places a more stringent test of benefit on agents such as anti-angiogenesis drugs. Because these agents are cytostatic and may only target those vessels that are newly forming or are remodeling, benefit in the form of tumor shrinkage may not be observed. Therefore, classical treatment objectives, such as tumor shrinkage, may not be logical endpoint. An alternative hypothesis for this population of patients is the question: Will time to disease progression be altered by use of an antiangiogenic agent at a time at which the tumor burden is minimal or nondetectable, such as after completion of treatment? This would infer that the tumor nodules exposed to the angiotherapy agent would be preangiogenic or newly angiogenic, and introduction of angiotherapy at this point in time could be proposed to maintain the smallest, nonangiogenic tumor lesions in a dormant state and through attack against the early neovessels reduce active angiogenesis. In a randomized time to progression clinical trial, the outcome measurement, a delay in the time to progression, might be expected to parallel the duration of the anti-angiogenesis treatment. Thus, design of the clinical trial would need to take into account the anticipated time to progression of the post-treatment population given no treatment, the duration of angiotherapy administration, and the potential for net loss of tumor burden from the dormant state. Additional endpoints to be incorporated into these trials are prospective tests of the utility of markers of angiogenesis in prediction of poor prognosis populations and as markers to follow response to disease.

Combination Therapy

Angiotherapy can be incorporated into clinical treatment along several approaches. A problem observed in the treatment of some aggressive cancers is the resurgence of tumor between treatment cycles. The use of angiotherapy between the cytotoxic chemotherapy cycles may provide tumor stasis without increasing toxicity at a time during which the patient may be most vulnerable. An alternative clinical hypothesis would be the inclusion of angio-inhibitory treatment into the primary treatment regimen. This may take advantage of the described additive or synergistic interactions between cytotoxic treatments and angiotherapy, utilize multiple agents with different mechanisms, or provide a more intensive regimen without increasing toxicity. Finally, inclusion of angiotherapy in a combination regimen may be used to localize and suppress the disease to improve the benefits obtained from the primary treatment. These are testable clinical hypotheses that would not require large cohort randomized trials and can be piloted with small initial patient numbers. Promising combinations can then be randomized against the regimen without anti-angiogenic therapy or the best clinical standard to define the role of combination treatments.

Prevention

The early onset of angiogenesis in the process of malignancy and other pathologic states suggests that anti-angiogenesis treatment may need to be initiated early at the time of tumor or disease development to ward off the pathologic process. Although this is an ideal situation, it may not be feasible clinically. True primary chemoprevention, either of cancer or other diseases might require initiation of treatment from childhood. It would require treatment of a large proportion of the population that might not be at actual risk in order to cover those individuals who are. This is an objective that may not be met successfully, given our present mechanisms for population risk analysis. Alternatively, identification of high-risk populations, such as those patients with family history of inflammatory diseases or malignancy, well-defined genetic risks, or in a secondary chemoprevention mode may yield populations for whom the occurrences are more common and the potential to identify a treatment benefit greater. Although early introduction of agents might still be the ideal situation, use even in adulthood or for limited duration might be able to measure benefit in a randomized time-to-onset of disease or disease progression trials.

SUMMARY

Anti-angiogenesis therapy emerges from scientific hypotheses posited over several decades. The importance of neovessel formation and vessel remodeling in many pathological states including cancer has been demonstrated by clinico-correlative studies and the early clinical trials of the first generation angio-inhibitory agents. In order to make this discipline a permanent member of the treatment armamentarium, carefully constructed clinical trials with valid endpoints need to be executed. The linkage between the laboratory and the clinic that brought this important new development to the patient must be maintained to further our understanding of the role of angiogenesis in normal physiology and disease, in order to develop and validate intermediate and surrogate markers of benefit, and to advance the discipline of angiotherapy to its optimal use. These objectives can be met through the new discoveries and continuing collaborations that have brought angiotherapy to the forefront of drug development.

REFERENCES

1. Zelen, M. (1997) Theory and practice of clinical trials, in *Cancer Medicine* (Holland, J. F., et al., eds.), Williams & Wilkins, Baltimore, MD, pp. 423–436.
2. Holland, J. F., Frei, E., Kufe, D., and Bast, R. C. (1997) Principles of medical oncology, in *Cancer Medicine* (Holland, J. F., et al., eds.), Williams & Wilkins, Baltimore, MD, pp. 755–765.
3. Labianca, R., Pancera, G., Dallavalle, G., Pessi, A., and Zamparelli, G. (1997) Response evaluation as the key-point in results interpretation. *Tumori* **83(Suppl.)**, S73–S76.
4. Frei, E. and Antman, K. (1997) Combination chemotherapy, dose and schedule, in *Cancer Medicine* (Holland, J. F., et al., eds.), Williams & Wilkins, Baltimore, MD, pp. 817–838.
5. Motzer, R. J., Reed, E., Perera, F., Tang, D., Shamkhani, H., Poirier, M. C., et al. (1994) Platinum-DNA adducts assayed in leukocytes of patients with germ cell tumors measured by atomic absorbance spectrometry and enzyme-linked immunosorbent assay. *Cancer* **73**, 2843–2852.
6. Benchekroun, M. N., Parker, R., Dabholkar, M., Reed, E., and Sinha, B. K. (1995) Effects of interleukin-1 alpha on DNA repair in human ovarian carcinoma (NIH:OVCAR–3) cells: implications in the mechanism of sensitization of cis-diamminedichloroplatinum(II). *Mol. Pharmacol* **47**, 1255–1260.
7. Sancar, A. (1995) DNA repair in humans. *Annu. Rev. Genet.* **29**, 69–105.
8. Ratain, M. and Plunkett, W. (1997) Pharmacology, in *Cancer Medicine* (Holland, J. F., et al., eds.), Williams & Wilkins, Baltimore, MD, pp. 875–890.
9. Klauber, N., Parangi, S., Flynn, E., Hamel, E., and D'Amato, R. J. (1997) Inhibition of angiogenesis and breast cancer in mice by the microtubule inhibitors 2-methoxyestradiol and taxol. *Cancer Res.* **57**, 81–86.
10. Kohn, E. C., Sandeen, M. A., and Liotta, L. A. (1992) In vivo efficacy of a novel inhibitor of selected signal transduction pathways including calcium, arachidonate, and inositol phosphates. *Cancer Res.* **52**, 3208–3212.
11. Kohn, E. C. and Liotta, L. A. (1995) Molecular insights into cancer invasion: strategies for prevention and intervention. *Cancer Res.* **55**, 1856–1862.

12. Schipper, H., Goh, C. R., and Wang, T. L. (1995) Shifting the cancer paradigm: must we kill to cure? *J. Clin. Oncol.* **13**, 801–807.
13. Folkman, J. (1971) Tumor angiogenesis: Therapeutic implications. *N. Engl. J. Med.* **285**, 1182–1186.
14. Folkman, J. and Shing, Y. (1992) Angiogenesis. *J. Biol. Chem.* **267**, 10931.
15. Liotta, L. A. and Steeg, P. S. (1991) Cancer metastasis and angiogenesis: an imbalance of positive and negative regulation. *Cell* **64**, 327.
16. Folkman, J., Hochberg, M., and Knighton, D. (1974) Self-regulation of growth in three dimensions: the role of surface area limitations, in *Control of Proliferation in Animal Cells* (Clarkson B. and Baserga, R., eds.), Cold Spring Harbor Laboratory Press, Cold Spring Harbor, NY, pp. 833–842.
17. Folkman, J., Karol, W., Ingber, D., and Hanahan, D. (1989) Induction of angiogenesis during the transition from hyperplasia to neoplasia. *Nature* **339**, 58–61.
18. Holmgren, L., O'Reilly, M. S., and Folkman, J. (1995) Dormancy of micrometastases: balanced proliferation and apoptosis in the presence of angiogenesis suppression [see comments]. *Nature Med.* **1**, 149–153.
19. Kohn, E. C., Alessandro, R., Spoonster, J., Wersto, R., and Liotta, L. A. (1995) Angiogenesis: role of calcium-mediated signal transduction. *Proc. Natl. Acad. Sci. USA* **92**, 1307–1311.
20. Kohn, E. C., Figg, W. D., Sarosy, G. A., Bauer, K. S., Davis, P. A., Soltis, M. J., et al. (1997) Phase I trial of micronized formulation CAI in patients with refractory solid tumors: pharmacokinetics, clinical outcome and comparison of formulations. *J. Clin. Oncol.* **15**, 1985–1993.
21. D'Amato, R., Loughnan, M., Flynn, E., and Folkman, J. (1994) Thalidomide is an inhibitor of angiogenesis. *Proc. Natl. Acad. Sci. USA* **91**, 4082–4085.
22. Pluda, J. M. (1997) Tumor-associated angiogenesis: mechanisms, clinical implications, and therapeutic strategies. *Semin. Oncol.* **24**, 203–218.
23. Gasparini, G. and Presta, M. (1996) Clinical studies with angiogenesis inhibitors: biologic rationale and challenges for their evaluation. *Ann. Oncol.* **7**, 441–444.
24. Liotta, L. A., Kleinerman, J., and Saidel, G. (1974) Quantitative relationships of intravascular tumor cells: tumor vessels and pulmonary metastases following tumor implantation. *Cancer Res.* **34**, 997–1003.
25. Weidner, N., Semple, J. P., Welch, W. R., and Folkman, J. (1991) Tumor angiogenesis and metastasis—correlation in invasive breast carcinoma. *N. Engl. J. Med.* **324**, 1–8.
26. Hanahan, D. and Folkman, J. (1996) Patterns and emerging mechanisms of the angiogenic switch during tumorigenesis. *Cell* **86**, 353–364.
27. Zarnegar, R. (1995) Regulation of HGF and HGFR gene expression. *EXS* **74**, 33–49.
28. Rosen, E. M. and Goldberg, I. D. (1997) Regulation of angiogenesis by scatter factor. *EXS* **79**, 193–208.
29. Polverini, P. J. and Nickoloff, B. J. (1995) The role of scatter factor and the c-met proto-oncogene in angiogenic responses. *EXS* **74**, 51–67.
30. Wang, Y. J., Shahrokh, Z., Vemuri, S., Eberlein, G., Beylin, I., and Busch, M. (1996) Characterization, stability, and formulations of basic fibroblast growth factor. *Pharm. Biotechnol.* **9**, 141–180.
31. Burgess, W. H. and Maciag, T. (1989) The heparin-binding (fibroblast) growth factor family of proteins. *Annu. Rev. Biochem.* **58**, 575–606.
32. Bikfalvi, A., Klein, S., Pintucci, G., and Rifkin, D. B. (1997) Biological roles of fibroblast growth factor-2. *Endocr. Rev.* **18**, 26–45.
33. Mignatti, P., Tsuboi, R., Robbins, E., and Rivkin, D. B. (1989) In vitro angiogenesis on the human amniotic membrane: Requirement for basic fibroblast growth factor-induced proteinases. *J. Cell Biol.* **108**, 671–682.
34. Sato, Y. and Rifkin, D. B. (1988) Autocrine activities of basic fibroblast growth factor: regulation of endothelial cell movement, plasminogen activator synthesis, and DNA synthesis. *J. Cell. Biol.* **107**, 1199–1205.
35. Plate, K. H., Breier, G., Weich, H. A., Mennel, H. D., and Risau, W. (1994) Vascular endothelial growth factor and glioma angiogenesis: coordinate induction of VEGF receptors, distribution of VEGF protein, and possible in vivo regulatory mechanisms. *Int. J. Cancer* **59**, 520–529.
36. Kim, K. J., Li, B., Winer, J., Armanini, M., Gillett, N., Phillips, H. S., and Ferrara, N. (1993) Inhibition of vascular endothelial growth factor-induced angiogenesis suppresses tumor growth in vivo. *Nature* **362**, 841–844.
37. Ferrara, N., Houck, K., Jakeman, L., and Leung, D. W. (1992) Molecular and biological properties of the vascular endothelial growth factor family of proteins. *Endocr. Rev.* **13**, 18–32.
38. Miller, J. W., Adamis, A. P., and Aiello, L. P. (1997) Vascular endothelial growth factor in ocular neovascularization and proliferative diabetic retinopathy. *Diabetes Metab. Rev.* **13**, 37–50.

39. Takahashi, Y., Kitadai, Y., Bucana, C. D., Cleary, K. R., and Ellis, L. M. (1995) Expression of vascular endothelial growth factor and its receptor, KDR, correlates with vascularity, metastasis, and proliferation of human colon cancer. *Cancer Res.* **55**, 3964–3968.

40. Furcht, L. (1986) Critical factors controlling angiogenesis: cell products, cell matrix, and growth factor. *Lab. Invest* **5**, 505–509.

41. Aaronson, S. A. (1991) Growth factors and cancer. *Science* **254**, 1146–1153.

42. Bussolino, F., Albini, A., Camussi, G., Presta, M., Viglietto, G., Ziche, M., and Persico, G. (1996) Role of soluble mediators in angiogenesis. *Eur. J. Cancer* **32A**, 2401–2412.

43. Klein, S., Roghani, M., and Rifkin, D. B. (1997) Fibroblast growth factors as angiogenesis factors: new insights into their mechanism of action. *EXS* **79**, 159–192.

44. Kohn, E. C., Felder, C. C., Jacobs, W., Holmes, K. A., Day, A. F., Freer, R., and Liotta, L. A. (1994) Stucture function analysis of signal and growth inhibition by carboxyamido-triazole, CAI. *Cancer Res.* **54**, 935–942.

45. Kohn, E. C., Jacobs, W., Kim, Y. S., Alessandro, R., Stetler-Stevenson, W. G., and Liotta, L. A. (1994) Calcium influx modulates expression of matrix metalloproteinase-2 (72 kDa type IV collagenase, gelatinase A) expression. *J. Biol. Chem.* **269**, 21,505–21,511.

46. Taraboletti, G., Garofalo, A., Belotti, D., Drudis, T., Borsotti, P., Scanziani, E., et al. (1995) Inhibition of angiogenesis and murine hemangioma growth by batimastat, a synthetic inhibitor of matrix metalloproteinases. *J. Natl. Cancer Inst.* **87**, 293–298.

47. Galardy, R., Grobelney, D., Foellmer, H. G., and Fernandez, L. A. (1994) Inhibition of angiogenesis by the matrix metalloprotease inhibitor N-{2R-2-(hydroxamidocarbonymethyl)-4 methylpentanoyl)]-L-tryptophan methylamide. *Cancer Res.* **54**, 4715–4718.

48. Eccles, S. A., Box, G. M., Court, W. J., Bone, E. A., Thomas, W., and Brown, P. D. (1996) Control of lymphatic and hematogenous metastasis of a rat mammary carcinoma by the matrix metalloproteinase inhibitor batimastat (BB-94). *Cancer Res.* **56**, 2815–2822.

49. Brown, P. D. and Giavazzi, R. (1995) Matrix metalloproteinase inhibition: a review of anti-tumour activity. *Ann. Oncol.* **6**, 967–974.

50. Folkman, J. (1995) Angiogenesis inhibitors generated by tumors. *Mol. Med.* 120–122.

51. O'Reilly, M. S., Holmgren, L., Chen, C., and Folkman, J. (1996) Angiostatin induces and sustains dormancy of human primary tumors in mice. *Nature Med.* **2**, 689–692.

52. O'Reilly, M. S., Boehm, T., Shing, Y., Fukai, N., Vasios, G., Lane, W. S., et al. (1997) Endostatin: an endogenous inhibitor of angiogenesis and tumor growth. *Cell* **88**, 277–285.

53. Fidler, I. J. and Hart, I. R. (1982) Biologic diversity in metastatic neoplasms - origins and implications. *Science* **217**, 998–1001.

54. Gimbrone, M. A. J., Leapman, S. B., Cotran, R. S., and Folkman, J. (1973) Tumor angiogenesis: iris neovascularization at a distance from experimental intraocular tumors. *J. Natl. Cancer Inst.* **50**, 219–228.

55. Gimbrone, M. A., Leapman, S. B., Cotran, R. S., and Folkman, J. (1972) Tumor dormancy in vivo by prevention of neovascularization. *J. Exp. Med.* **136**, 261–276.

56. Nguyen, M., Watanabe, H., and Budson, A. E. (1994) Elevated levels of an angiogenic peptide, basic fibroblast growth factor, in the urine of patients with a wide spectrum of cancers. *J. Natl. Cancer Inst.* **86**, 356–361.

57. Price, J. T., Bonovich, M. T., and Kohn, E. C. (1997) The biochemistry of cancer dissemination. *Crit. Rev. Biochem. Mol. Biol.* **32**, 175–253.

58. Goldie, J. H. and Coldman, A. J. (1986) Application of theoretical models to chemotherapy protocol design. *Can. Treat Rep.* **70**, 127–131.

59. Norton, L. and Simon, R. (1977) Tumor size, sensitivity to therapy, and the design of treatment schedules. *Can. Treat Rep.* **61**, 1307.

60. Folkman, J. (1996) Fighting cancer by attacking its blood supply. *Scientific American*, 150–154.

61. Teicher, B. A., Holden, S. A., Ara, G., Korbut, T., and Menon, K. (1996) Comparison of several antiangiogenic regimens alone and with cytotoxic therapies in the Lewis lung carcinoma. *Cancer Chemother. Pharmacol.* **38**, 169–177.

62. Eckardt, J., Eckardt, G., Villalona-Calero, M., Drengler, R., and Von Hoff, D. (1995) New anticancer agents in clinical development. *Oncology* **9**, 1321–1328.

63. Tanaka, Y., Kawamata, H., Fujimoto, K., and Oyasu, R. (1997) Angiogenesis inhibitor TNP-470 suppresses tumorigenesis in rat urinary bladder. *J. Urol.* **157**, 683–688.

64. Yamaoka, M., Yamamoto, T., Ikeyama, A., Sudo, K., and Fumita, T. (1993) Angiogenesis inhibitor TNP-470 (AGM-1470) potently inhibits the tumor growth of hormone-independent human breast and prostate carcinoma cell lines. *Cancer Res.* **53**, 5233–5236.

65. Fan, T.-P. D. and Brem, S. (1992) Angiosuppression, in *The Search for New Anti-Cancer Drugs* (Waring, M. J. and Ponder, B. A. J., eds.), Kluwer Academic Publishers, Lancaster, U. K., pp. 185–229.

66. Teicher, B. A., Holden, S. A., Ara, G., Sotomayor, E. A., Huang, Z. D., Chen, Y. N., and Brem, H. (1994) Potentiation of cytotoxic cancer therapies by TNP–470 alone and with other anti-angiogenic agents. *Int. J. Cancer* **57,** 920–925.

67. Teicher, B. A., Holden, S. A., Dupuis, N. P., Kakeji, Y., Ikebe, M., Emi, Y., and Goff, D. (1995) Potentiation of cytotoxic therapies by TNP-470 and minocycline in mice bearing EMT-6 mammary carcinoma. *Breast Cancer Res. Treat.* **36,** 227–236.

68. Pluda, J. M. and Parkinson, D. R. (1996) Clinical implications of tumor-associated neovascularization and current antiangiogenic strategies for the treatment of malignancies of pancreas. *Cancer* **78,** 680–687.

69. Hawkins, M. J. (1995) Clinical trials of antiangiogenic agents. *Curr. Opin. Oncol.* **7,** 90–93.

70. Kensler, T. W. and Groopman, J. D. (1996) Carcinogen-DNA and protein adducts: biomarkers for cohort selection and modifiable endpoints for chemoprevention trials. *J. Cell. Biochem.* **255,** 85–91.

71. Mark, S. D. (1996) Defining and analyzing cohorts using molecular markers of cancer risk. *J. Cell. Biochem.* **255,** 69–79.

72. Zucker, S., Lysik, R. M., DiMassimo, B. I., Zarrabi, H. M., Moll, U. M., Grimson, R., et al. (1995) Plasma assay of gelatinase B: tissue inhibitor of metalloproteinase complexes in cancer. *Cancer* **76,** 700–708.

73. Bostwick, D. G., Burke, H. B., Wheeler, T. M., Chung, L. W. K., Bookstein, R., Pretlow, T. G., et al. (1994) The most promising surrogate endpoint biomarkers for screening candidate chemopreventive compounds for prostatic adenocarcinoma in short-term phase II clinical trials. *J. Cell. Biochem.* **19(Suppl.),** 283–289.

74. Hawighorst, H., Knapstein, P. G., Knopp, M. V., Weikel , W., Brix, G., Zuna, I., et al. (1998) Uterine cervical carcinoma: comparison of standard and pharmacokinetic analysis of time-intensity curves for assessment of tumor angiogenesis and patient survival. *Cancer Res.* **58,** 3598–3602.

75. Hawighorst, H., Knapstein, P. G., Weikel, W., Knopp, M. V., Zuna, I., Knof, A., et al. (1997) Angiogenesis of uterine cervical carcinoma: characterization by pharmacokinetic magnetic resonance parameters and histological microvessel density with correlation to lymphatic involvement. *Cancer Res.* **57,** 4777–4786.

76. Weidner, N. and Folkman, J. (1996) Tumor vascularity as a prognostic factor in cancer, in *Important advances in Oncology 1996* (DeVita, V. T., Hellman, S., and Rosenberg, S. A., eds.), Lippincott-Raven, Philadelphia, PA, pp. 167–190.

77. Hollingsworth, H. C. C. K. E., Steinberg, S. M., Rothenberg, M. L., and Merino, M. J. (1995) Tumor angiogenesis in advanced stage ovarian carcinoma. *Am. J. Pathol.* **147,** 9–19.

78. Zucker, S., Lysik, R. M., Zarrabi, H. M., Moll, U., Tickle, S. P., Stetler-Stevenson, W., et al. (1994) Plasma assay of matrix metalloproteinases (MMPs) and MMP-inhibitor complexes in cancer. Potential use in predicting metastasis and monitoring treatment. *Ann. NY Acad. Sci.* **732,** 248–2062.

79. Koukourakis, M. I., Giatromanolaki, A., Thorpe, P. E., Brekken, R. A., Sivridis, E., Kakolyris, S., et al. (2000) Vascular endothelial growth factor/KDR activated microvessel density versus CD31 standard microvessel density in non-small cell lung cancer. *Cancer Res.* **60,** 3088–3095.

80. McBride, W. (1968) Thalidomide and congenital abnormalities. *Lancet* **2,** 1358.

81. Lenz, W. (1962) Thalidomide and congenital abnormalities. *Lancet* **i,** 45–46.

82. Figg, W. D., Bergan, R., Brawley, O., Tompkins, A., Linchan, M., Duray, P., et al. (1997) Randomized Phase II study of thalidomide in androgen independent prostate cancer. *Proc. ASCO* **16,** 333a.

83. Fine, H. A., Loeffler, J. S., Kyritsis, A., Wen, P., Black, P. M., Levin, V. A., et al. (1997) A phase I trial of the anti–angiogenic agent, thalidomide, in patients with recurrent high grade gliomas. *Proc. ASCO* **16,** 385a.

84. Fullerton, P. M. and O'Sullivan, D. J. (1968) Thalidomide neuropathy: a clinical, electrophysiological, and histological follow-up study. *J. Neuro. Neurosurg. Psychiatr.* **31,** 543–551.

85. Jacobson, J. M., Greenspan, J. S., Spritzler, J., Ketter, N., Fahey, J. L., Jackson, J. B., et al. (1997) Thalidomide for the treatment of oral aphthous ulcers in patients with human innumodeficiency virus infection. *N. Engl. J. Med.* **336,** 1487–1493.

86. Kohn, E. C., Reed, E., Sarosy, G., Christian, M., Link, C. J., Cole, K., et al. (1996) Clinical investigation of a cytostatic calcium influx inhibitor in patients with refractory cancers. *Cancer Res.* **56,** 569–573.

87. Berlin, J., Tutsch, K., Hutson, P., Cleary, J., Rago, R. P., Arzoomanian, R. Z., et al. (1997) Phase I clinical and pharmacokinetic study of oral carboxyamidotriazole, a signal transduction inhibitor. *J. Clin. Oncol.* **15,** 781–789.

88. Thiabault, A., Samid, D., Tompkins, A. C., Figg, W. D., Cooper, M. R., Hohl, R. J., et al. (1996) Phase I study of lovastatin, an inhibitor of the mevalonate pathway, in patients with cancer. *Clin. Cancer Res.* **2,** 483–491.

89. Oliver, S. J., Banquerigo, M. L., and Brahn, E. (1994) Suppression of collagen-induced arthritis using an angiogenesis inhibitor, AGM-1470, and a microtubule stabilizer, taxol. *Cell Immunol.* **157,** 291–299.

90. Teicher, B. A., Holden, S. A., Chen, Y. N., Ara, G., Korbut, T. T., and Northey, D. (1994) CAI: effects on cytotoxic therapies in vitro and in vivo. *Cancer Chemother. Pharmacol.* **34,** 515–521.

91. Teicher, B. A., Ara, G., Menon, K., and Schaub, R. G. (1996) In vivo studies with interleukin-12 alone and in combination with monocyte colony-stimulating factor and/or fractionated radiation treatment. *Int. J. Cancer* **65,** 80–84.

92. Zhang, Y., Griffith, E. C., Sage, J., Jacks, T., and Liu, J. O. (2000) Cell cycle inhibition by the anti–angiogenic agent TNP-470 is mediated by p53 and p21WAF1/CIP1. *Proc. Natl. Acad. Sci. USA* **97,** 6427–6432.

93. Alessandro, R., Masiero, L., Liotta, L. A., and Kohn, E. C. (1996) The role of calcium in the regulation of invasion and angiogenesis. *In vivo* **10,** 153–160.

94. Felder, C. C., Ma, A. L., Liotta, L. A., and Kohn, E. C. (1991) The antiproliferative and antimetastatic compound L651582, inhibits muscarinic acetylcholine receptor-stimulated calcium influx and arachidonic acid release. *J. Pharm. Exp. Ther.* **257,** 967–971.

95. Masiero, L., Lapidos, K. A., Ambudkar, I., and Kohn, E. C. (1999) Regulation of the RhoA pathway in human endothelial cell spreading on type IV collagen: role of calcium influx. *J. Cell Sci.* **112,** 3205–3213.

96. Taki, T., Ohnishi, T., Arita, N., Hiraga, S., Saitoh, Y., Izumoto, S., et al. (1994) Anti-proliferative effects of TNP-470 on human malignant glioma in vivo: potent inhibition of tumor angiogenesis. *J. Neuroonc.* **19,** 251–258.

97. Hori, A., Ikeyama, S., and Sudo, K. (1994) Suppression of cyclin D1 mRNA expression by the angiogenesis inhibitor TNP-470 (AGM-1470) in vascular endothelial cells. *Biochem. Biophys. Res. Comm.* **204,** 1067–1073.

98. Angiolillo, A. L., Sgadari, C., Taub, D. D., Liao, F., Farber, J. M., Maheshwari, S., et al. (1995) Human interferon–inducible protein 10 is a potent inhibitor of angiogenesis in vivo. *J. Exp. Med.* **182,** 155–162.

99. Lamers, C., Gratama, J., Ogilvie, A., Goey, H., Druit, W., Peschel, C., et al. (1997) Exogenous IL-12 induces in vivo IL-10 production, followed by downregulation of IL-12 activities. *Proc. ASCO* **16,** 435a.

100. Voest, E. E., Kenyon, B. M., O'Reilly, M. S., Truitt, G., D'Amato, R. J., and Folkman, J. (1995) Inhibition of angiogenesis in vivo by interleukin 12. *J. Natl. Cancer Inst.* **87,** 581–586.

101. Wang, X., Fu, X., Brown, P. D., Crimmin, M. J., and Hoffman, R. M. (1994) Matrix metalloproteinase inhibitor BB-94 (Batimastat) inhibits human colon tumor growth and spread in a patient-like orthotopic model in nude mice. *Cancer Res.* **54,** 4726–4728.

102. Wamil, B. D., Thurman, G. B., Sundell, H. W., DeVore, R. F., Wakefield, G., Johnson, D. H., et al. (1997) Soluble E-selectin in cancer patients as a marker of the therapeutic efficacy of CM101, a tumor-inhibiting anti-neovascularization agents, evaluated in phase 1 clinical trial. *J. Cancer Res. Clin. Oncol.* **123,** 173–179.

103. Gutierrez-Rodriguez, O., Starusta-Bacal, P., and Gutierrez-Montes, O. (1989) Treatment of refractory rheumatoid arthritis - the thalidomide experience. *J. Rheumatol.* **16,** 158–163.

104. Ochonisky, S., Verroust, J., Bastuju-Garin, S., Cherardi, R., and Revus, J. (1994) Thalidomide neuropathy incidence and clinico-electrophysiologic findings in 42 patients. *Arch. Dermatol.* **130,** 66–69.

105. Bukowski, R. M., Olencki, T., Sandstrom, K., Schwartz, L., Berg, W., Huber, M., et al. (1997) Phase I trial of subcutaneous interleukin-12 in patients with metastatic renal cell carcinoma. *Proc. ASCO* **16,** 108a.

106. Brown, P. D. (1994) Preclinical and clinical studies on the matrix metalloproteinase inhibitor, batimastat (BB94). *Clin. Exp. Metastasis* **12,** 23.

107. Bodurtha, A., Eisenhauer, E., Steward, W., Rusthoven, J., Qirt, I., Lohmann, R., et al. (1997) Phase I-II study of marimastat (BB2516) in patients with metastatic melanoma. *Proc. Am. Soc. Clin. Oncol.* **16,** 493a.

108. Rasmussen, H., Rugg, T., Brown, P., Baillet, M., and Millar, A. (1997) A 371 patient meta-analysis of studies of marimastat in patients with advanced cancer. *Proc. Am. Soc. Clin. Oncol.* **16,** 429a.

109. Dezube, B. J., Von Roenn, J. H., Holden-Wiltse, J., Remick, S., Cooley, T. P., Cheung, T. W., et al. (1997) Fumagillin analog (TNP-470) in the treatment of Kaposi's sarcoma- A phase AIDS clinical trial group study. *Proc. Natl. AIDS Malignancy Conf.* A35.

110. Pluda, J. M., Lietzau, J., and Wyvill, K. (1993) A Phase-I Trial administering TNP—470 (AGM-1470) to patients with HIV- associated Kaposi's syndrome (abstr.) *Proc. 1st Natl. Conf. Human Retroviruses Related Infect.* **1,** 61.

111. Pluda, J. M., Wyvill, K., and Figg, W. D. (1994) A Phase I study of an angiogenesis inhibitor, TNP-470 (AGM-1470), administered to patients with HIV-associated Kaposi's sarcoma (abstr.) *Proc. ASCO* **13,** 8.

29 Angiogenesis Therapies

Concepts, Clinical Trials, and Considerations for New Drug Development

William W. Li, Vincent W. Li, and Dimitris Tsakayannis

CONTENTS

BACKGROUND
CURRENT ANGIOGENESIS THERAPIES
EMERGING CONCEPTS FROM EARLY CLINICAL TRIALS OF ANGIOGENESIS
  THERAPY
UNIQUE CHALLENGES FOR THE ERA OF ANGIOTHERAPY
FUTURE ANGIOTHERAPIES
REFERENCES

BACKGROUND

Introduction

In 1971, the year that U.S. President Richard Nixon signed the National Cancer Act declaring the "war on cancer," Judah Folkman of Harvard Medical School published his seminal hypothesis in the New England Journal of Medicine speculating that "tumors are angiogenesis-dependent" (1). This hypothesis led to the development of the field of angiogenesis research, now being pursued in hundreds of academic, private, and industry laboratories worldwide. During the past three decades, scientists elucidated the fundamental mechanisms underlying angiogenesis and vascular development in a variety of human diseases ranging from cancer to ischemic cardiovascular diseases to blindness and psoriasis, among others. Beginning in the late 1980s, the biopharmaceutical industry began aggressively exploiting this field for creating new therapeutic compounds for modulating new blood-vessel growth in angiogenesis-dependent diseases.

The term "angiogenesis therapies" is used to refer to medical treatments aimed at controlling new blood-vessel growth. An increasing number of drug candidates are entering clinical trial, especially in the areas of oncology, cardiovascular medicine, and wound healing. This chapter will provide a global overview of these clinical trials, some

From: *The New Angiotherapy*
Edited by: T.-P. D. Fan and E. C. Kohn © Humana Press Inc., Totowa, NJ

new insights being gleaned from the clinical observations, and recommendations for future investigations. Portions of this work are drawn from original core education materials published on the Angiogenesis Foundation's worldwide website at http://www.angio.org.

Angiogenesis in Health

Angiogenesis is a fundamental physiological process that is required for reproduction, embryogenesis, wound healing, and tissue repair *(3)*. Heuristically, angiogenesis may be regarded as a process that involves two compartments of cells: 1) vascular endothelial cells, and 2) the surrounding cells comprising tissues and ultimately organs that depend on a blood supply. During angiogenesis, the endothelial cells comprising blood vessels undergo a sequence of coordinated events that include proliferation, migration, tube formation, branching, pruning, and remodeling to form functional vascular networks that bring oxygen and nutrients to tissues. New circulatory perfusion is one result of angiogenesis. There is also a second function of angiogenesis. Vascular endothelial cells produce and secrete more than 20 paracrine molecules that can influence the growth of adjacent cell types, as shown in Table 1 *(3)*. Therefore, a new angiogenic population of endothelial cells serves to act directly on, as well as bring perfusion to, local cells. In the healthy state, the angiogenic process may be viewed as the provision of a dual lifeline for sustaining critical tissues, such as myocardium, brain, endometrium, and the developing embryo.

The physiological control of angiogenesis involves a complex balance of endogenous molecules that stimulate or inhibit neovascularization. At least 20 angiogenic growth factors (cytokines) have now been identified that stimulate new blood-vessel growth in vitro and in vivo, shown in Table 2. Endogenous angiogenesis inhibitors have also been identified, some of which are present in the extracellular matrix or found in the circulation, shown in Table 3 *(4–7)*. The phenotype of angiogenesis in the body represents the net effect of these countervailing forces. Loss of this balance — resulting in either excessive or insufficient new blood-vessel growth—leads to disease or to disease progression. This concept is known as the "angiogenesis model for homeostasis" *(8)*.

Angiogenesis in Disease

In many pathological states, an imbalance occurs in the normal regulation of angiogenesis, resulting in either an overproduction of angiogenic growth factors or a relative deficiency of angiogenesis inhibitors. Cancer is perhaps the most striking example of a disease displaying exuberant angiogenesis. The onset of angiogenesis in a colony of cancer cells enables a tumor mass to escape growth restriction (1–$2 mm^3$ size), to become locally invasive, and to metastasize to distant organs *(9)*. Excessive angiogenesis also results in loss of vision in patients with age-related macular degeneration or diabetic retinopathy. Neovascularization invading the joint space contributes to cartilage and bone destruction in rheumatoid arthritis (RA). New blood-vessel growth beneath the epidermis drives the growth of the disfiguring lesions of psoriasis and other skin conditions *(2,10,11)*. Angiogenesis is also associated with the invasion of endometrial explants into the female peritoneum in endometriosis.

Inadequate angiogenesis can have equally devastating clinical consequences. In patients with progressive coronary artery stenosis, angiogenesis and its correlate, arteriogenesis, are required to maintain perfusion via generation of a collateral

Table 1
Bioactive Molecules from Endothelial Cells with Paracrine Effects

Platelet-derived growth factor (PDGF)
Connective-tissue growth factor
Basic fibroblast growth factor (bFGF or FGF-2))
Endothelial-derived growth factor (EGF)
Heparin-like inhibitor
Hepatocyte growth factor
Transforming growth factor-β (TGF-β)
Insulin-like growth factor-1
Insulin-like growth factor-2
Heparin-binding epidermal growth factor
Burst promoting factor
Interleukin-1 (IL-1)
Interleukin-6 (IL-6)
Interleukin-7 (IL-7)
Interleukin-8 (IL-8)
Interleukin-9 (IL-9)
Leukemia inhibitory factor (LIF)
Granulocyte-colony stimulating factor (G-CSF)
Macrophage-colony stimulating factor (M-CSF)
Granulocyte-macrophage colony stimulating factor
Steel factor
Melanoma-growth stimulatory activity
Macrophage chemotactic peptide
Transferrin
Endothelin-1
C3b complement fragment
Survivin
Soluble Fas Ligand

Table 2
Angiogenic Growth Factors

Angiogenin
Angiopoietin-1
Del-1
Fibroblast growth factors: acidic (aFGF or FGF-1) and basic (bFGF or FGF-2)
Follistatin
Granulocyte colony-stimulating factor (G-CSF)
Hepatocyte growth factor (HGF)/scatter factor (SF)
Interleukin-8 (IL-8)
Interleukin-8 (IL-8)
Leptin
Midkine
Placental growth factor
Platelet-derived endothelial- cell growth factor/thymidine phosphorylase (PD-ECGF/TP)
Platelet-derived growth factor-BB (PDGF-BB)
Pleiotrophin (PTN)
Proliferin
Transforming growth factor-α (TGF-α)
Transforming growth factor-β (TGF-β)
Tumor necrosis factor-α (TNF-α)
Vascular endothelial growth factor (VEGF)/vascular permeability factor (VPF)

Table 3
Endogenous Angiogenesis Inhibitors

Angiostatin (plasminogen fragment)
Antiangiogenic antithrombin III
Canstatin
Cartilage-derived inhibitor (CDI)
CD59 complement fragment
Endostatin (collagen XVIII fragment)
Fibronectin fragment
Gro-β
Heparinases
Heparin hexasaccharide fragment
Human chorionic gonadotropin
Interferon (IFN)- α/β/γ
Interferon-inducible protein (IP-10)
Interleukin-4 (IL-4)
Interleukin-10 (IL-10
Interleukin-12 (IL-12)
Kringle 5 (plasminogen fragment)
Maspin
Met-1
Met-2
Metalloproteinase inhibitors (TIMPs)
2-Methoxyestradiol
Pigment epithelium derived factor (PEDF)
Placental ribonuclease inhibitor
Plasminogen activator inhibitor
Platelet factor-4
Prolactin 16kD fragment
Proliferin-related protein
Retinoids
Tetrahydrocortisol-S
Thrombospondin-1
Transforming growth factor-β (IGF-β)
Troponin-I
Tumstatin
Vasculostatin
Vasostatin (calreticulin fragment)

circulation to the myocardium beyond atherosclerotic blockages. Insufficient collateral formation can lead to angina, myocardial infarction, and death *(12–14)*. In stroke, angiogenesis occurs in response to brain hypoxia. Increased brain angiogenesis after ischemic stroke is correlated with improved survival in patients *(15)*. Insufficient neovascularization in the extremities causes poor wound healing, leading to gangrene and subsequent limb amputation in patients with severe peripheral vascular disease and diabetes.

New angiogenesis-based therapies address these excesses or deficiencies through pharmacological manipulation of endothelial cells, using therapeutic angiogenic growth factors or antiangiogenic compounds. The following sections will review the important issues under study in our institution and discuss how new insights gleaned from current clinical trials are being used to guide development of angiogenesis therapy.

CURRENT ANGIOGENESIS THERAPIES

Three primary forms of angiogenesis therapy are currently under development by the biopharmaceutical industry. One class of therapies is designed to "turn on" new blood-vessel growth. This is known, in various circles, as pro-angiogenic therapy, angiogenesis stimulation, or therapeutic angiogenesis. We collectively term this "molecular revascularization." Another class of therapies "turns off" new blood-vessel growth, called antiangiogenesis, antiangiogenic therapy, or angiogenesis inhibition. Both forms are in human clinical trials, outlined in Tables 4, 5, and 6. A third class of therapy, vascular stabilization, still at the preclinical stage, aims to stabilize the architecture of newly formed blood vessels when angiogenesis is absolutely required but where fragile vessels have undesirable clinical consequences, such as excessive permeability, edema, or hemorrhage.

Angiogenesis Stimulation (Molecular Revascularization)

Clinicians are now testing angiogenic growth factors for their ability to stimulate therapeutic angiogenesis in patients suffering from ischemic tissues. Six of the 20 known angiogenic cytokines have been produced in recombinant form for clinical use: acidic fibroblast growth factor (aFGF or FGF-1), basic fibroblast growth factor (bFGF or FGF-2), vascular endothelial growth factor (VEGF), transforming growth factor-β (TGF-β), granulocyte macrophage colony-stimulating factor (GM-CSF), and platelet-derived growth factor (PDGF-BB). The latter (sold under the tradename Regranex) is the first commercially available growth-factor therapy Food and Drug Administration (FDA)-approved for promoting granulation and healing of diabetic neuropathic foot ulcers. PDGF-BB is both a direct and indirect modulator of endothelial-cell growth *(16–21)*.

Five major diseases are now being treated using therapeutic angiogenesis:

ISCHEMIC HEART DISEASE

Cardiac specialists are now studying the effects of therapeutically-administered recombinant peptides (FGF-1, FGF-2, and VEGF), their genes (FGF, VEGF), or mediators (HIF-1α) in the myocardium of patients with advanced coronary-artery disease (*see* Table 4). The clinical goal is to stimulate local neovascularization, promote collateral channel formation, decrease myocardial ischemia, ameliorate ischemic symptoms (angina pectoris), and increase the functional exercise capacity of patients *(22–24)*.

PERIPHERAL ARTERIAL DISEASE

Vascular surgeons and cardiologists are administering VEGF and FGF-2 to patients with severe peripheral vascular disease (*see* Table 4). The clinical goal is to increase regional limb perfusion, reduce ischemic symptoms (claudication and rest pain), heal chronic wounds, and avert the need for limb amputation *(25,26)*.

CHRONIC WOUNDS

Surgeons are applying topical growth factors (rhPDGF-BB, FGF-2, GM-CSF, TGF-β and growth factor modulating compounds (e.g., sucralfate) to stimulate wound neovascularization and granulation in patients with diabetic, venous, and pressure ulcers (*see* Table 4). Living skin equivalents (Apligraf and Dermagraft) are bioengineered tissue constructs that express angiogenic cytokines such as FGF-2, VEGF, PDGF, TNF-α, TGF-β, IL-8, and angiopoietin. Environmental modulators such as hyperbaric oxygen (HBO) therapy are also used to accelerate wound healing angiogenesis. The clinical goal of all these agents and devices is to accelerate wound closure *(27,28)*.

Table 4
Major Angiogenesis Drugs in Clinical Trials (as of 3/01)

Therapeutic Angiogenic Drugs

Ischemic Heart Disease
    Peptide therapies
        FGF1
        FGF2
        VEGF
    Gene therapies
        FGF4
        gtVEGF2
        $Ad_{GV}VEGF121.1$
        $VEGF_{121}$
        HIF1-α
Critical Limb Ischemia
    Peptide therapies
        FGF2
        VEGF
    Gene therapies
        gtVEGF2
Chronic Wounds
    Peptide therapies
        FGF-2
        rbFGF
        rhPDGR-BB
        TGF-β2
    Gene Therapies
        VEGF

Adapted with permission from The Angiogenesis Foundation, Drug Database.

Angiogenesis Inhibition (Antiangiogenesis)

Antiangiogenic drugs are being aggressively developed by the biopharmaceutical industry, with cancer as a primary target. Ophthalmic, dermatologic, rheumatologic, gynecologic, and AIDS applications are also under development.

CANCER

Oncologists throughout North America, Europe, Asia, and Australia are testing more than 50 antiangiogenic drugs in patients with a wide variety of solid tumors, including breast, brain, prostate, cervical, colon, ovarian and pancreatic carcinomas, as well as hematologic malignancies such as acute myelogenous leukemia, lymphoma, and multiple myeloma *(29,30)* *(see* Table 5).

Because of the growing number of agents that possess antiangiogenic properties, the U.S. National Cancer Institute (NCI) uses a classification system, published on their website (http://cancertrials.nci.nih.gov) to identify compounds based on their action on particular components of the angiogenic pathway. This proposed classification system categorizes antiangiogenic drugs into five subgroups: (i) agents that inhibit endothelial cells directly; (ii) agents that block activators of angiogenesis; (iii) agents that block

Table 5
Major Angiogenesis Drugs in Clinical Trials (as of 3/01

Antiangiogenic Drugs

Cancer
  Angiozyme
  Angiostatin
  Avicine
  BMS275291
  Carboxyamidotriazole
  Cilengitide
  CGP 41251
  CM101
  Col-3 (Metastat)
  Combretastatin A4 Prodrug
  CT-2584
  D-Penicillamine
  EMD 121974
  Endostatin
  Flavopiridal
  Genistein Concentrated Polysaccharide (GCP)
  IM862
  Interferon-α (IFN-α)
  Interleukin-12 (IL-12)
  Marimastat
  Neovastat
  Octreotide
  OSI-774
  PI-88
  Prinomastat
  PTK787
  RhuMab-VEGF
  Solimastat
  Squalamine
  SU5416
  SU6668
  Tetrathiomolybdate
  Thalidomide
  TNP-470
  Vitaxin

Adapted with permission from The Angiogenesis Foundation, Clinical Trials Database.

extracellular matrix breakdown; (iv) agents that inhibit endothelial-specific integrin signaling; and (v) agents with nonspecific mechanisms of action. Table 7 contains a list of some antiangiogenic agents as classified by the NCI scheme. This classification system does not easily accommodate antiangiogenic drugs that have multiple mechanisms of action, or those that act indirectly via regulation of host gene-expression activities (e.g., upregulation of IP-10). Importantly, the mechanism of action of many antiangiogenic drugs remains poorly understood.

Table 6
Major Angiogenesis Drugs in Clinical Trials (as of 3/01)

Antiangiogenic Drugs
Neovascular Eye Disease
AG3340
Anecortave acetate
EYE001
ISV-120
LY333531
Neoretna
Thalidomide
Psoriasis
Paclitaxel
Neovastat
ABX-IL8
Verteporfin

Adapted with permission from The Angiogenesis Foundation, Clinical Trials Database.

The clinical goal of antiangiogenic therapy in cancer is to improve patient survival and quality of life through tumor regression, disease stabilization, and suppression of metastasis. Currently, most clinical trials enroll patients with advanced metastatic cancer who have failed standard cytotoxic chemotherapy or radiation therapy *(31)*.

OCULAR NEOVASCULARIZATION

Ophthalmologists are administering anecortave acetate, AG3340, IFN-α-2a, ISV-120, thalidomide, Neovastat, EYE001, and somatostatin to patients suffering from neovascular eye diseases, including: age-related macular degeneration, diabetic retinopathy, and recurrent pterygium (*see* Table 6). The photodynamic agent verteporfin (Visudyne) accumulates selectively in neovascular lesions and destroys abrerrant vessels. This agent was FDA-approved in 1999. The clinical goal of these agents is to improve vision or to prevent progressive visual loss *(8,32)*.

HEMANGIOMAS OF CHILDHOOD

Pediatricians are administering intravenous steroids or IFN-α-2a to children suffering from hemangiomas of infancy *(38,39)*. Both represent antiangiogenic strategies to suppress hemangioma growth. Although hemangiomas in children usually regress spontaneously by 8 years of age, aggressive treatment of massive or precariously situated lesions may be life- or vision-saving *(33,34)*.

AIDS-KAPOSI'S SARCOMA

AIDS specialists are administering hCG (human choriogonadotropin), captopril, TNP-470, thalidomide, IM862, IFN-α-2a, and paclitaxel to patients with Kaposi's sarcoma *(35–37)* (*see* Table 5). Paclitaxel is a well-established cytotoxic agent with antiproliferative activity on endothelial cells. The clinical goal is regression of these vascular lesions, which are disfiguring when located on the skin and potentially life-threatening when present in the viscera or lungs.

PSORIASIS

Dermatologists are testing formulations of paclitaxel, Neovastat, and antibody to IL-8 (ABX-IL8) in patients with moderate to severe psoriasis (*see* Table 6). The clinical goal is to alleviate cutaneous symptoms of itching, and to suppress recurrent flares of the disease *(38)*.

EMERGING CONCEPTS FROM EARLY CLINICAL TRIALS OF ANGIOGENESIS THERAPY

The Challenge of Disease Selection

A major challenge for developers of molecular-targeting angiogenesis-based agents is the appropriate matching of a drug with a specific disease. Two approaches to drug development are 1) the "top-down" approach (first selecting a prevalent disease representing an attractive market, and then developing a drug to treat that condition); or 2) the "bottom-up" approach (first identifying a molecular or cellular drug target, and then selecting a disease to treat). Rational drug design combines both strategies, whereby a disease-related cellular event, such as receptor tyrosine kinase signaling, is targeted, followed by the systematic high-throughput screening of large chemical libraries to identify candidate drug molecules for further in vitro, in vivo, and human testing.

Identifying the disease most likely to respond to a given antiangiogenic drug, however, is not obvious, and this problem poses a formidable challenge in the angiogenesis field. For example, the fundamental mechanisms governing the angiogenic switch in specific solid tumor types are still not well-understood. It remains unclear whether antagonism of one angiogenic factor or its receptor pathway is sufficient to ablate the tumor's ability to induce angiogenesis. Furthermore, although many antiangiogenic agents have defined mechanisms of action, it is not yet known which molecular steps are the most critical lynch pins in the angiogenic process. A detailed understanding of the molecular pathways in angiogenesis and their relevance in different disease conditions will be required to optimize rational drug design. The limitations of the current knowledge are illustrated in the following case studies drawn from early clinical trials in the angiogenesis field.

CASE STUDY: IFN-α-2A

The drug IFN-α-2a was first reported to inhibit endothelial cell locomotion in 1980 *(33)*. In 1989, pediatricians seized on its antiangiogenic properties in a last-ditch effort to regress a life-threatening vascular tumor in a child dying from pulmonary hemangiomatosis. The effort was successful *(34)*. Subsequently, other pediatric specialists have successfully employed IFN-α-2a as an antiangiogenic agent to treat a variety of hemangiomas in children *(33)*.

It was assumed, incorrectly, that interferon's antiangiogenic effect in hemangioma patients would translate directly into efficacy as an antiangiogenic treatment for choroidal neovascularization in patients with age-related macular degeneration (AMD). A single case report of success fueled early optimism among ophthalmologists *(40)*, but those results were not reproduced in a randomized, prospective double-masked clinical trial *(41,42)*. Elderly patients experienced adverse reactions (flu-like symptoms) from interferon use and damage to the retina was even observed, leading to discouragement of its use for the treatment of ocular neovascularization.

Table 7
Antiangiogenic Agent Classification System Utilized by the U.S. National
Cancer Institute and Some Examples of Drugs in Development

1. Agents that inhibit endothelial cells directly
    Angiostatin
    Endostatin
    Squalamine
    Thalidomide
2. Agents that block activators of angiogenesis
    Anti-VEGF Antibody
    IFN-α
    SU-5416
    SU-6668
3. Agents that block extracellular matrix breakdown
    BMS275291
    COL-3
    Marimastat
    Neovastat
4. Agents that inhibit endothelial-specific integrin signaling
    EMD 121974
5. Agents with nonspecific mechanisms of action
    CAI
    IL-12
    IM862

Adapted with permission from NCI website: http://nci.nih.gov.

Why should this disparity of effectiveness exist for a single antiangiogenic agent in two angiogenic diseases? One explanation is that interferon is only a weak angiogenesis inhibitor. In mouse studies using the Lewis lung carcinoma, for example, IFN-α produces only 25% inhibition of tumor growth by antiangiogenesis, compared with other more potent agents, such as TNP-470 (>50% inhibition), and angiostatin or endostatin (>90% inhibition) *(43)*. The treatment of neovascularization in AMD may require a more potent antiangiogenic drug than IFN-α.

Alternatively, choroidal neovascularization may involve a different angiogenic mechanism, such as mediation by VEGF, compared to hemangiomas, which appear to be primarily FGF-2 mediated, and this mechanistic difference may account for different therapeutic results *(44)*. Indeed, interferon therapy was reported as ineffective in regressing a testicular hemangioma found to express VEGF but not FGF-2, in contrast to liver and skin hemangiomas in the same patient that did express FGF-2 and that did respond to interferon therapy *(45)*. Furthermore, drug delivery to target tissues plays a significant role in clinical-trial design. For example, in the multicenter study of interferon for AMD, the drug was administered systemically. When endocrinologists at the University of Florida administered long-term IFN-α subcutaneously, they reported that the drug stabilized the progression of diabetic retinopathy, another disease of ocular neovascularization *(46)*. Other significant factors include drug dosing, schedule of administration, and selection of clinical endpoints used to determine drug efficacy.

The impact of such complex factors for the development of angiogenesis therapies can be significant. When the multicenter study's negative results on interferon and AMD were published in a leading ophthalmology journal, many ophthalmologists lost interest in investigating interferon as a potential treatment for neovascular eye disease. The lesson is that a drug that is effective in treating angiogenesis in one disease may not be successful for treating another angiogenic condition. Ultimately a more sophisticated knowledge of the molecular basis of new blood vessel growth in a given disease combined with well thought-out clinical trials will be required for success.

CASE STUDY: BATIMASTAT

The drug Batimastat, a nonselective metalloproteinase inhibitor, was initially developed to treat malignant effusions and ascites in lung and ovarian cancer, respectively. Batimastat's antiangiogenic activity results from its disruption of extracellular matrix remodeling during tumor-induced neovascularization. In early clinical trials enrolling cancer patients, Batimastat did not show any significant therapeutic benefit; moreover, its route of administration (intracavitary injection into pleural space or the peritoneum) caused patients intense pain. The sponsoring company later discontinued the Batimastat program when a better-tolerated oral analog, Marimastat, became available *(47)*. Batimastat therefore is an angiogenesis inhibitor that did not succeed in the initially selected therapeutic area, oncology.

Nevertheless, prior to its discontinuation in cancer studies, Batimastat was licensed to a company developing ocular therapeutics. Under a new name (ISV-120) and with a topical ophthalmic formulation, Batimastat was tested in patients with recurrent pterygium, a disfiguring, benign fibrovascular membrane growing over the conjunctiva that afflicts over three million people in the United States alone. In these studies, ISV-120 exhibited no significant toxicity in Phase I trials, and Phase II trials showed signs of efficacy. ISV-120 thus showed "proof of concept" in an angiogenesis-dependent disease in an entirely different therapeutic area (ophthalmology) from the one for which it was initially developed (oncology).

An angiogenesis-modulating drug that fails in its initial application may therefore possess therapeutic value for an alternate disease indication, and may require different drug formulations. Had Batimastat not been licensed for ophthalmic use, its effects in pterygium may have never been found. Significantly, the programs of other antiangiogenic drugs, including thalidomide, AG-3340, SU 5416, and Neovastat, initially aimed at cancer have been diversified to include ophthalmic conditions as concurrent disease targets.

Challenges Posed by Multiple Angiogenic Factors in Human Disease

A diverse array of angiogenic cytokines is known to be present in pathological tissues and in patient body fluids. Large investments have been made to treat disease by targeting a single angiogenic factor, such as FGF-2, VEGF, or TNF-α or their receptors, for the therapeutic control of angiogenesis. In the field of ophthalmology, considerable emphasis has been placed on targeting VEGF as the "culprit" molecule underlying ocular neovascularization, even though other angiogenic factors (TGF-β, FGF-1, FGF-2, and HGF) have been identified in both normal and pathological eye tissues *(48–52)*.

Within the oncology field, there is similar enthusiasm to target VEGF, despite mounting evidence that multiple angiogenic growth factors participate in tumor angiogenesis

(53,54). Relf and colleagues showed that human primary breast cancers express as many as six angiogenic factors (VEGF, FGF-1, FGF-2, TNF-β, platelet-derived endothelial cell growth factor/thymidine phosphorylase [PD-ECGF/TP], placenta growth factor, and pleiotrophin) simultaneously *(55)*. In another study, Barton and colleagues found that in 39 patients with advanced epithelial ovarian cancer, they could detect three angiogenic factors (angiogenin, FGF-2, and VEGF) in their serum and ascites fluid *(56)*. In the study of Wakabayshi and colleagues, human glioma cells were found to produce FGF-2, VEGF, and interleukin-8 (IL-8) as mediators of angiogenesis *(57)*.

Solid tumors and other angiogenic pathologies exploit redundant mechanisms to induce angiogenesis, and neutralization of multiple factors may be required to suppress tumor growth. Moreover, the downregulation of endogenous angiogenesis inhibitors (such as thrombospondin-1, angiostatin, endostatin, interferons, and vasostatin) may play an equally important role. Therefore, repleting the local supply of angiogenesis inhibitors may be as important as antagonizing a particular angiogenic growth factor for antiangiogenic therapy. A number of growth factor-specific drugs (rhuMAb-VEGF, SU-5416, Angiozyme) are now in clinical trial for solid tumors, and their results will shed light on the advantages and limitations of growth factor-specific antiangiogenic strategies.

Angiogenesis Modulation: Physiological and Adverse Effects

EARLY CLINICAL FINDINGS

Angiogenesis Inhibitors. Since the 1980s, antiangiogenic compounds have been described in the scientific literature as "nontoxic" in animal studies. Indeed, oncology Phase 2 clinical trials have demonstrated that, as a class, these agents are much safer and better tolerated than conventional cytotoxic cancer chemotherapy. Like all pharmaceuticals however, most angiogenesis inhibitors do have dose-related adverse effects that have been documented in human testing. Examples of such adverse effects described for individual agents include fatigue, cerebellar ataxia, peripheral neuropathy, sedation, anorexia, fever, vomiting, hypertension, leukopenia, thrombocytopenia, and liver-function abnormalities. Severe, unexpected events such as pulmonary hemorrhage and thrombosis have been noted in some trials, but no clear causative association with antiangiogenic drug exposure has been determined.

Interestingly, neurotoxicities are sometimes observed in clinical trials of anti-angiogenic agents, and we believe it is worthy of special discussion. Neuropathic pain is a well-known adverse reaction with thalidomide treatment. Reversible ataxia and peripheral neuropathies have been observed with TNP-470 administration. Approximately 10% of children treated with IFN-α for infantile hemangioma experience spastic diplegia or other neurotoxicities, which are generally reversible when the medication is discontinued *(58,59)*.

We propose that angiogenesis may play a more important role than is currently appreciated in maintaining the homeostasis of the peripheral and central nervous system. Recent molecular findings support our hypothesis. Exogenously-administered FGF-2 has been shown to enhance functional recovery and increased expression of neuronal sprouting markers (GAP-43) after focal cerebral infarction *(60)*. The angiogenic factor VEGF is known to be expressed in cortical neurons and pial cells *(61)*.

VEGF binds to human neuropilin-1, a receptor for the collapsin/semaphorin family that guides neuronal outgrowth, which is also expressed on vascular endothelial cells (62). The expression of this receptor is upregulated in vascular endothelium by another angiogenic cytokine, TNF-α (63). Furthermore, two neurokines, midkine and pleiotrophin, are also considered angiogenic factors (64). Clearly, the role of angiogenesis, its growth factors, and their receptors in neuronal growth and function merits future investigation.

Angiogenesis Stimulators. Recombinant human platelet-derived growth factor-BB (rhPDGF-BB) is the first FDA-approved angiogenic growth-factor therapy, indicated for healing diabetic lower extremity ulcers. This topical agent is virtually devoid of toxicities. Pharmacokinetic studies using rats showed < 3% systemic bioavailability of rhPDGF-BB following topical applications of the drug. Human clinical trials showed no increased incidence in rhPDGF-BB-treated patients of ulcer-related adverse events such as skin, bone, or systemic infection compared to placebo control (65). There was a 2% incidence of erythematous rash in rhPDGF-BB users, which may be a hypersensitivity to the paraben preservative present in the methylcellulose vehicle gel. Topical rhPDGF-BB has not been studied in carcinogenesis or teratogenicity assays (66).

FGF-2 has been well-studied in animals for its systemic and local effects and it is being clinically tested for its ability to induce molecular revascularization in ischemic hearts and limbs. Systemically-administered FGF-2 has been observed to cause reversible, dose-dependent hematological abnormalities and glomerulopathy (67), as well as hypotension (68). Although FGF-2 has been reported to produce a negative ionotropic effect on the rat cardiac myocyte (69), this has not been observed in clinical trials employing the drug as an intracoronary or an epicardial sustained-release agent.

The VEGF peptide, its gene, and regulatory inducers (HIF-1α) are being studied in humans as a therapeutic angiogenic strategy. Administration of VEGF peptide causes systemic hypotension in experimental animals, and this reversible, dose-dependent effect is also observed in human clinical trials. In contrast, systemic blood pressure does not appear to be altered after the *VEGF* gene is introduced into directly into the myocardium or ischemic limb, and VEGF peptide is locally expressed (25,70).

The plasmid for the *VEGF* gene, when injected into the rat myocardium, causes local angiomas at the injection site as well as regional angiogenesis (71). Distal angioma formation on the foot of a human patient was reported following arterial *VEGF* gene transfer to an ischemic limb (25). Such observations raised concern about possible exacerbation of neovascular eye disease during VEGF therapy. A longitudinal ophthalmologic follow-up of eight diabetic patients with documented baseline retinopathy participating in clinical trials administering intramuscular, arterial, or intramyocardial *VEGF* gene therapy, however, showed no progression of retinopathy or change in visual acuity up to 18 mo following *VEGF* gene transfer (72). Similarly, there has been no increase in cancer incidence noted in cardiac patients receiving VEGF therapy.

OPTIMAL BIOLOGICAL DOSE VS MAXIMAL TOLERATED DOSE IN PHASE I TRIALS OF ANTIANGIOGENIC AGENTS FOR CANCER

Antiangiogenic therapy for cancer represents a new paradigm for oncology drug development. The target is the vascular endothelial cell rather than the tumor cell. Antiangiogenic agents are generally cytostatic rather than cytotoxic.

Phase I oncology clinical trials, however, have traditionally aimed to identify a drug's "Maximal Tolerated Dose" (MTD). Therefore, many of the antiangiogenic drugs used in cancer patients to date have been intentionally dosed at near-toxic levels.

We believe a therapeutic antiangiogenic response is likely to be found at doses much lower than those causing toxicity. We have proposed that an alternative Phase I clinical trial strategy should be exploited: clinical investigators should seek the "Optimal Biologic Dose" (OBD), instead of the MTD, and employ the OBD as the starting dose in Phase II studies *(73)*. For oncologic drug development, this strategy represents a significant shift from conventional Phase I clinical-trial design and requires clear markers to determine biological effects of angiogenesis inhibition in patients. To date, reliable and definitive markers remain elusive, although many candidates (serum/urine VEGF or FGF-2 levels, TUNEL analysis of serial tumor biopsies, functional imaging parameters) have been proposed. This issue is discussed in a later section of this chapter. Clearly, biopharmaceutical companies, clinical investigators, and regulatory agencies must carefully consider the new paradigms introduced by antiangiogenic therapy.

The Host Response to Angiogenesis Modulation

DELAYED RESPONSE TIME TO ANTIANGIOGENIC THERAPY

The clinical experience to date with IFN-α-2a, Marimastat, IM862, Neovastat, thalidomide, and TNP-470 suggests that the disease response to antiangiogenic therapy may require prolonged treatment to become clinically evident. After antiangiogenic treatment begins, disease progression (tumor or hemangioma growth) may continue to progress for weeks or even months, albeit at a slower rate, prior to disease regression *(74)*. The first cancer patient showing a complete response to TNP-470 therapy did not show evidence of a partial response until 12 wk of therapy, for example, and tumor regression did not occur until after 18 wk of treatment *(75)*. For infantile hemangiomas, complete regression of a lesion refractory to standard intervention may take up to 1 yr of treatment with IFN-α *(33)*. This observation is consistent with the concept that antiangiogenic therapy does not directly attack tumor cells but rather causes tumor attrition indirectly, via depletion of vascular endothelial cells.

This insight impacts on clinical trial design, length of therapy, evaluation of endpoints, and requires the education of both clinical investigators and their patients. Early discontinuation of an antiangiogenesis drug may lead to treatment failure owing to an insufficient treatment duration.

RESPONSE TIME TO THERAPEUTIC ANGIOGENESIS

rhPDGF-BB in Chronic Wounds. Topical administration of rhPDGF-BB to nonhealing diabetic foot ulcers leads to wound granulation within days to weeks. In the pivotal Phase II clinical trials of rhPDGF-BB, significant acceleration of complete wound closure compared to controls was noted beginning at 6 wk after treatment initiation *(72)*. This growth-factor therapy was FDA-approved in 1997 for the treatment of diabetic ulcers, and widespread off-label prescribing of rhPDGF-BB has demonstrated its utility for venous stasis and pressure ulcers. There is significant patient-to-patient variation in terms of time to complete wound healing using this agent, attributed to factors such as patient drug compliance, suboptimal wound care (e.g., lack of sharp debridement, lack of off-loading, poor nutritional status), and wound infection *(65)*. Successful angiogenic therapy for wounds requires diligent management of the host condition, a principle that will certainly translate to angiogenesis therapy of other diseases as well.

***VEGF Gene* Transfer in Ischemic Myocardium.** Direct myocardial injection of plasmid DNA for VEGF into ischemic myocardium has been successfully undertaken in human patients *(77)*. In a study of 5 patients, there was evidence of increased collateral blood flow at 30 d post-gene transfer by coronary angiography, and increased myocardial perfusion in ischemic regions documented by SPECT-sestamibi imaging at 60 d. Functional improvement, assessed by decrease in angina (ischemic chest pain) was noted as early as 10 d after *VEGF* gene transfer, with symptoms completely abolished in two patients. Notably, several clinical trials (VIVA and FIRST) showed that anginal symptoms also improve in control patients, suggesting a strong placebo effect that may limit the utility of this endpoint in drug testing. Other clinical trials employing protein and gene VEGF and FGF-2 are ongoing, and their results will yield additional information on patient response to delivery of an angiogenic therapy to ischemic tissues.

LACK OF DRUG RESISTANCE TO ANTIANGIOGENIC THERAPY

The development of drug resistance to conventional cancer chemotherapy is a formidable problem in cancer patients. The multi-drug resistance (*MDR*) gene is upregulated in tumor cells exposed to exposure to conventional cytotoxic agents. Clonal expansion of increasingly resistant cancer-cell populations leads to eventual ineffectiveness of the chemotherapeutic drugs. Antiangiogenic therapies, in contrast, are aimed at normal proliferating endothelial cells, and are therefore thought to be at low risk for developing drug resistance. Experimental studies employing long-term (> 1 yr) cycled administration of angiostatic therapy (angiostatin and endostatin) to treat mice bearing Lewis lung carcinomas showed no evidence of drug resistance *(78)*. In a patient who received long-term (greater than 2 yr) TNP-470 therapy, prolonged tumor regression was noted without the emergence of drug resistance *(79)*. Anecdotal clinical observations do not, however, adequately address the issue of drug resistance, and carefully designed basic laboratory investigations are underway to explore this hypothesis further. For example, endothelial cells chronically suppressed with a VEGF inhibitor may upregulate FGF-2 or other growth factors to achieve an angiogenic "escape."

Interactions Between Angiogenesis Therapies and Common Medications

COMMON DRUGS AFFECT ENDOTHELIAL-CELL GROWTH CONTROL

Many formulary medications available to physicians possess angiogenesis-modulatory activity. For example, several commonly prescribed diuretic agents inhibit endothelial-cell proliferation in vitro, including spironolactone *(80)*, furosemide, and bumetanide *(81)*. Antihypertensive medications, such as captopril, also inhibit angiogenesis *(82)*. Bruno Vogt and colleagues deliberately prescribed captopril (at a oral dose of 50 mg/d) and successfully regressed Kaposi's sarcoma lesions in a renal transplant patient *(36)*. Other formulary medications with endothelial anti-proliferative activities include: minocycline *(83)*, vitamin D3 *(84)*, retinoic acid *(85)*, octreotide *(86)*, amiloride *(87)*, isosorbide *(88)*, irsogladine *(89)*, cimetidine *(90)*, gold thiomalate *(91)*, and nonsteroidal anti-inflammatory agents *(92)*. The selective Cox-2 inhibitors celecoxib and rofecoxib are potent inhibitors of angiogenesis with direct endothelial effects and indirect effects through suppression of inflammation.

The recognition by clinicians of the angiogenesis-modulatory properties of common drugs is important in the development and future application of both inhibitory and stimulating angiogenesis therapies. Patients receiving pro-angiogenic drugs may need to avoid medications that could exhibit antiangiogenic effects, and vice versa *(93)*. The Angiogenesis Foundation maintains a comprehensive database of all prescription medications reported to stimulate or inhibit endothelial-cell proliferation.

Case Study: *rhVEGF* Gene Therapy. Recombinant human VEGF (rhVEGF) was introduced into a patient's ischemic leg via a percutaneous balloon angiocatheter and this resulted in new collateral formation by 4 wk, as documented by serial angiography, as well as development of lower extremity peripheral edema *(25)*. VEGF is a potent vascular permeability factor *(94)*. Twelve weeks later, clinical investigators noted that the newly generated vessels regressed. Although the precise factors governing durability of the therapeutic angiogenic response remains poorly understood, it is noteworthy that cardiovascular patients often receive formulary medications that may inhibit angiogenesis, including the aforementioned diuretic, afterload reduction, and vasodilator medications *(81)*. Clinical trials of pro-angiogenic agents may need to be designed to control for the concomitant prescription of standard cardiac drugs that possess anti-endothelial-cell activity *(95)*.

UNIQUE CHALLENGES FOR THE ERA OF ANGIOGENESIS THERAPIES

Surrogate Markers for Cancer Therapy

Surrogate markers of disease and its response to treatment are useful when direct measurement of the pathologic condition is limited. Such markers should correlate with disease biology, and should reflect the progression, stabilization, or regression of the disease process.

The search for new surrogate markers for cancer in antiangiogenic drug development is driven by the need for tools to evaluate pharmacologic effects on the neovasculature per se. Conventional imaging modalities —computed tomography (CT), magnetic resonance imaging (MRI)— are capable of assessing the tumor vasculature but are generally used only to assess tumor size. Anatomical and functional imaging of tumor angiogenesis is now a major research priority and this topic has served as the focus of a U.S. National Cancer Institute sponsored Expert Consensus Panel named AIM (Angiogenesis Imaging Methodologies in Clinical Trials).

The clinical utility of some conventional tumor markers, such as prostate-specific antigen (PSA), in clinical trials of antiangiogenic agents is also being challenged. Thalidomide, for example, appears to increase expression of PSA in LNCaP cell lines in tissue culture *(96)*. In contrast, clinical observations suggest that PSA levels may decline in some prostate-cancer patients after thalidomide treatment. This paradoxical behavior of thalidomide on PSA expression in vitro and in vivo remains unexplained. TNP-470 also causes upregulation in the expression and secretion of PSA in vitro. TNP-470 treatment of prostate cancer patients has been associated with a rise in serum PSA, a finding that has led to discontinuation of the drug in those cases *(97)*. It is unknown, however, whether the TNP-470-associated increase in PSA levels actually correlated with disease progression in those patients.

The direct measurement of angiogenic factors circulating in the serum, cerebrospinal fluid, and urine of patients is under investigation. A growing body of scientific literature suggests that the serum of cancer patients contains elevated levels of angiogenic factors *(98–100)*. In a prospective study of cerebrospinal fluid from children with brain tumors, the presence of FGF-2 was correlated with biological activity, increased intratumoral angiogenesis, and poor prognosis *(101)*. In children with acute lymphoblastic leukemia, urinary FGF-2 levels were also found to be increased compared to healthy controls *(102)*. Nyugen and colleagues showed in a study of 950 patients seen at Boston's Dana-Farber Cancer Institute that 38% of patients with multiple solid tumor types had elevated FGF-2 excreted in their urine *(103)*. Moreover, elevated levels of FGF-2 detected in the urine of bladder-cancer patients were associated with extent and status of disease. Furthermore, a reduction of urinary FGF-2 in response to antiangiogenic therapy has been reported in bladder-cancer patients receiving the antiangiogenic drug pentosan polysulfate *(104)*. The urine of patients with hemangiomas contains up to 100 times the normal levels of FGF-2 and these levels have been found to decline with regression of vascular lesions treated with IFN-α-2a *(74,105)*. Similar studies are underway to measure the levels of VEGF and other angiogenic factors in the body fluids of cancer patients *(106)*. Serial tumor biopsies have been conducted in Phase I studies of endostatin, employing immunohistochemical techniques to examine drug-induced tumor cell and endothelial cell apoptosis and to quantify changes in microvessel density. This novel approach extracted useful data, but may be impractical for large-scale clinical studies, e.g. Phase II and III trials.

Drug Delivery

ANTIANGIOGENIC DRUGS

Antiangiogenic drugs will require efficient delivery systems to optimize effects in target organs and tissues. Having a diverse armamentarium of drug-delivery systems is important because each target — whether tumor, retina, skin, or joint — possesses unique barriers that limit drug penetration to the desired site *(107,108)*. These tissue barriers include the blood-brain barrier, the blood-retina barrier (BBB), gastric mucosa, and the keratinized epithelium. Diverse drug-delivery routes are being explored in ongoing human clinical trials of antiangiogenic drugs: intravenous, subcutaneous, topical, oral, and nasal inhalation. Although endothelial proliferation is localized to the pathological site, systemic, rather than local, drug delivery remains the most common route under development.

Antiangiogenic therapy for cancer is envisioned to become a chronic intervention, perhaps requiring lifelong treatment. Drug candidates that are orally bioavailable are considered highly attractive, although drug reimbursement may become a formidable issue for self-administered outpatient medicines. Currently, Neovastat and thalidomide are oral antiangiogenic agents in advanced clinical development for cancer. One potential adverse effect of an oral antiangiogenic agent may be interference with ulcer healing in the stomach *(109)*. Therefore, close monitoring should be conducted of patients receiving oral antiangiogenic drugs for gastric or duodenal ulcers.

THERAPEUTIC ANGIOGENESIS

Angiogenic growth factor peptide and gene therapies are under development for therapeutic angiogenesis. Both are novel biotechnologies requiring special considerations for effective drug delivery. Large molecular size, electrical charge, and proteolytic susceptibility are major challenges posed by angiogenic peptide drugs. The first commercially available angiogenic peptide is a topical growth factor (rhPDGF-BB) applied to cutaneous wounds *(65)*. Growth-factor delivery through intact skin for deep tissue or systemic delivery would require special technologies to enhance transdermal peptide penetration. In clinical trials of angiogenic peptides for ischemic heart disease, agents have been delivered by: 1) direct injection into the myocardium at the time of thoracotomy; 2) intracoronary infusion; 3) intravenous infusion; or 4) epicardial implantation of growth factor impregnated heparin-alginate, sustained-release microspheres *(110–113)*. The results of these clinical studies will help reveal which, if any, of these routes is effective or superior.

Gene-transfer therapy, employing the delivery of bioengineered adenoviral vectors, naked plasmid DNA, or gene-plasmid/liposomes of angiogenic factors has led to successful therapeutic angiogenesis in animal studies, and these are now under study in human clinical trials *(70,114)*. Remarkably, the intramuscular delivery of VEGF naked plasmid DNA (into ischemic limbs and heart) has been reported to result in clinically significant collateral formation localized only to ischemic regions in several nonplacebo controlled clinical trials *(77,115)*. This site-specific gene expression remains poorly understood.

Clinical Endpoints

A major challenge facing both pro- and anti-angiogenic drug development is the selection of appropriate clinical trial endpoints. Functional endpoints being used in therapeutic angiogenesis studies in the heart include improvement in exercise capacity, decreased angina, and improved nuclear perfusion in ischemic territories. Clinical trials of ocular and skin agents incorporate endpoint measurements that can be directly visualized (e.g., retinal and choroidal angiography, skin examination). Ongoing studies will reveal whether any of these measurements correlate with clinical improvement.

Special consideration of endpoint selection is warranted in the field of oncology. Conventional oncological drug development aims for disease "cure," i.e. tumor regression. For antiangiogenic therapy of cancer, other endpoints may be appropriate, such as disease stabilization, delayed time to progression, or diminution of systemic toxicity related to treatment. All ongoing clinical trials should include increased survival and quality of life endpoints. Both endpoints may be attainable if tumor growth is stabilized; thus stable disease (SD) may be viewed as a true "response" for antiangiogenic therapy. With the exception of a few isolated cases, none of the human studies have to date shown the consistent tumor regressions found in the basic angiogenesis research literature, i.e. mice studies. Efforts to evaluate and standardize endpoint measurements will help facilitate regulatory evaluation of angiogenesis-based drugs in oncology and other clinical disciplines.

Adverse Reactions

Because of the differential role of angiogenesis in various organ pathologies, suppression of angiogenesis in one tissue may theoretically lead to compromise of necessary neovascularization in another tissue. It is not yet known whether the prolonged administration of antiangiogenic therapy in cancer patients will inhibit coronary collateral formation, delay wound healing, or diminish brain angiogenesis caused by carotid artery stenosis. Under what clinical situations might pharmacologically induced antiangiogenesis itself be considered an adverse reaction? Are there any absolute contraindications to either anti-angiogenic or pro-angiogenic therapy? Although clinical trial protocols are initially designed to exclude patients that might be harmed by these agents owing to co-morbidities, only the eventual widespread use of angiogenesis therapies for label and off-label indications will reveal the answer to these questions. Therefore, Phase IV monitoring of angiogenesis-based drugs will be important for long-term evaluation of safety. Furthermore, early signs of adverse reactions are more likely to be detected during the clinical development stage if the trial protocol requires enrolled patients to be evaluated by multidisciplinary teams of medical specialists (e.g., oncologists, cardiologists, dermatologists, neurologists, ophthalmologists, and rheumatologists). Although these additional evaluations add complexity and cost to clinical trials, there will be long-term benefits to an earlier grasp of both the beneficial and adverse events in different end-organ systems, regardless of the primary indication being investigated.

Durability of Therapeutic Effects and Long-Term Consequences

The durability of response to angiogenesis therapies is an important issue to clinicians and to patients. For pro-angiogenic therapies, the induction of a permanent, stable, vascular network capable of perfusion is desirable. Whether attainment of this goal can be achieved with a single course of treatment, or whether chronic therapy will be necessary remains unknown. The current clinical trials of growth factor peptides in ischemic hearts and limbs mostly involve single, or just a few, doses of drug. The durability of response has not yet been adequately studied in either animal system or in man.

In most diseases where antiangiogenic therapy is required, pathological tissues such as tumors continuously produce and release angiogenesis growth. Exogenous angiogenesis inhibitors are aimed at overcoming the effects of these stimuli. The current opinion among experts is that antiangiogenic treatment of cancer will necessitate chronic, life-long, angiosuppressive therapy to maintain disease control. Could gene therapy delivery of antiangiogenic drugs provide continuous drug delivery to metastatic tumors? Will durable antiangiogenic responses have long-term untoward effects in maturing adolescents, in females of reproductive age, or in elderly patients? The answers to these questions will require difficult, long-term clinical studies and years of longitudinal tracking of large cohorts of patients. Properly coordinated preclinical animal studies may provide early insights and guide clinical development.

FUTURE ANGIOTHERAPIES

The potential of angiogenesis therapies reaches far beyond the current disease targets of cancer, macular degeneration, arthritis, hemangioma, psoriasis, coronary-artery disease, stroke, and wound healing. Controlled vascular development is a central component to normal organ development and maintenance, reproductive health, and many diseases. The discovery of angiopoietins, a family of peptides involved in the regulation of endothelial-cell, perivascular smooth-muscle cell and pericyte behavior during angiogenesis through the Tie2 endothelial-cell receptor, suggests that "vascular stabilization" may be another angiogenesis therapy *(116,117)*. Vascular stabilization therapy might be used to treat conditions characterized by a fragile, unstable vascular architecture, where there is a risk of hemorrhage and loss of tissue function. Such conditions include Moya-Moya *(118)*, berry aneurysms *(119)*, proliferative diabetic retinopathy *(120)*, and stroke.

Reproductive medicine may be another proving ground for certain angiogenesis therapies. Certain types of infertility may be associated with insufficient or abnormal angiogenesis in the corpus luteum or in the placenta. A pro-angiogenic drug may promote conditions required for successful conception, implantation, and fetal development. In the condition known as pre-eclampsia, malformed spiral arteries in the placenta pose a life-threatening risk for both the mother and fetus. Vascular growth strategies for normalizing spiral-artery development may benefit patients at high risk for pre-eclampsia. Other potential problems of female reproduction are associated with excessive angiogenesis, include ectopic pregnancy, teratoma, cervical dysplasia, menorrhagia, and endometriosis *(121)*. Additionally, the angiogenesis inhibitor TNP-470 has been shown to interfere with decidualization, placental and yolk-sac formation, and embryonic vascular development *(122)*, raising the possibility that antiangiogenic drugs may find a role as female contraceptive agents.

As attention increases on primary disease prevention through strategies such as chemoprevention, angiogenesis inhibitors may play a role in suppressing neovascularization in patients at high risk for certain conditions. While pharmacologic chemoprevention is already under development, a future strategy may also include dietary chemoprevention. Various food compounds have been found to possess angiogenesis inhibitory activity, including soy beans (genistein), licorice (isoliquitrin), cumin, tumeric, garlic, ginseng (ginsenoside), and green tea (epigallo-catechin-3 gallate) *(123,124)*. The oral bioavailability of these antiangiogenic compounds through routine food consumption is not yet known, nor has the stability of bioactivity been characterized when the parent food substance has been prepared through cooking. Nonetheless, an angiogenesis-based dietary chemoprevention strategy is an appealing concept worthy of scientific exploration.

An enormous momentum is now propelling the translation of the scientific principles of angiogenesis research into a new class of therapeutic agents. Although many challenges and problems remain unsolved, it seems certain that angiogenesis-based drugs and devices will form the basis for a new frontier in 21st century healthcare. Observers and participants in angiogenesis research are thus witnessing a new era emerging in clinical medicine.

REFERENCES

1. Folkman, J. (1971) Tumor angiogenesis: therapeutic implications. *N. Engl. J. Med.* **285,** 1182–1186.
2. Folkman, J. (1995) Angiogenesis in cancer, vascular, rheumatoid and other disease. *Nature Med.* **1,** 27–31.
3. Rak, J., Filmus, J., and Kerbel, R. S. (1996) Reciprocal paracrine interactions between tumour cells and endothelial cells: the 'angiogenesis progression' hypothesis. *Eur. J. Cancer* **32A,** 2438–2450.
4. O'Reilly, M. S., Boehm, T., Shing, Y., Fukai ,N., Vasios, G., Lane, W. S., et al. (1997) Endostatin: an endogenous inhibitor of angiogenesis and tumor growth. *Cell* **88,** 277–285.
5. Holmgren, L., O'Reilly, M. S., Folkman, J. (1995) Dormancy of micrometastases: balanced proliferation and apoptosis in the presence of angiogenesis suppression. *Nature Med.* **1,** 149–153.
6. Holmgren, L. (1996) Antiangiogenesis restricted tumor dormancy. *Cancer Metastasis Rev.* **15,** 241–245.
7. Pike, S. E., Yao, L., Jones, K. D., Cherney, B., Appella, E., Sakaguchi, K., et al. (1998) Vasostatin, a calreticulin fragment, inhibits angiogenesis and suppresses tumor growth. *J. Exp. Med.* **188,** 2349–2356.
8. Casey, R. and Li, W. (1997) Factors controlling ocular angiogenesis. *Am. J. Ophthalmol.* **124(4),** 521–529.
9. Fidler, I. J. and Ellis, L. M. (1994) The implications of angiogenesis for the biology and therapy of cancer metastasis. *Cell* **79,** 185–188.

10. Li, V. W. and Li, W. W. (1996) Cyclosporine and angiogenesis in psoriasis. *J. Am. Acad. Dermatol.* **35**, 1019–1020.

11. Li, V. W. and Barnhill, R. L. (1995) Angiogenesis in dermatology: pathophysiology and clinical implications. *Prog. Dermatol.* **29**, 1–12.

12. Simons, M. and Ware, J. A. (1996) Food for starving hearts. *Nature Med.* **2**, 519–520.

13. Ware, J. A. and Simons, M. (1997) Angiogenesis in ischemic heart disease. *Nature Med.* **3**, 158–164.

14. Sasayama, S. and Fijita, M. (1992) Recent insights into coronary collateral circulation. *Circulation* **85**, 1197–1204.

15. Krupinski, J., Kaluza, J., Kumar, P., Kumar, S., and Wang, J. M. (1994) The role of angiogenesis in patients with cerebral ischemic stroke. *Stroke* **25**, 1794–1798.

16. Lindner, V. and Reidy, M. A. (1995) Platelet-derived growth factor ligand and receptor expression by large vessel endothelium in vivo. *Am. J. Pathol.* **146**, 1488–1497.

17. Nicosia, R. F., Nicosia, S. V., and Smith, M. (1994) Vascular endothelial growth factor, platelet-derived growth factor, and insulin-like growth factor-1 promote rat angiogenesis in vitro. *Am. J. Pathol.* **145**, 1023–1029.

18. Bar, R. S., Boes, M., Booth, B. A., Dake, B. L., Henley, S., and Hart, M. N. (1989) The effects of platelet-derived growth factor in cultured microvessel endothelial cells. *Endocrinology* **124**, 1841–1848.

19. Beitz, J. G., Kim, I. S., Calabresi, P., and Frackelton, A. R., Jr. (1991) Human microvascular endothelial cells express receptors for platelet-derived growth factor. *Proc. Natl. Acad. Sci.* **88**, 2021–2025.

20. Lindahl, P., Johansson, B. R., Leveen, P., and Betsholtz, C. (1997) Pericyte loss and microaneurysm formation in PDGF-B-deficient mice. *Science* **277**, 242–245.

21. Kimura, I., Tsuneki, H., Okabe, M., and Ogasawara, M. (1997) Platelet-derived growth factor blocks the cell-cycle transition from the G0 to G1 phase in subcultured angiogenic endothelial cells in rat thoracic aorta. (1997) *Japn. J. Pharmacol.* 74, 303–311.

22. Yanagisawa-Miwa, A., Uchida, Y., Nakamura, F., Tomaru, T., Kido, H., Kamijo, T., et al. (1992) Salvage of infarcted myocardium by angiogenic action of basic fibroblast growth factor. *Science* **257**, 1401–1403.

23. Harada, K., Grossman, W., Friedman, M., Edelman, E. R., Prasad, P. V., Keighley, C. S., et al. (1994) Basic fibroblast growth factor improves myocardial function in chronically ischemic porcine hearts. *J. Clin. Investig.* **94**, 623–630.

24. Lopez, J. J. and Simons, M. (1996) Local extravascular growth factor delivery in myocardial ischemia. *Drug Delivery* **3**, 143–147.

25. Isner, J. M., Pieczek, A., Schainfeld, R,. Blair, R., Haley, L., Asahara, T., et al. (1996) Clinical evidence of angiogenesis after arterial gene transfer of phVEGF(165) in patient with ischaemic limb. *Lancet* **348(9024)**, 370–374.

26. Isner, J. M., Baumgartner, I., Rauh, G., Schainfeld, R., Blair, R., Manor, O., et al. (1998) Treatment of thromboangiitis obliterans (Beurger's Disease) by intramuscular gene transfer of vascular endothelial growth factor: preliminary clinical results. *J. Vasc. Surg.* **28**, 964–975.

27. Robson, M. C. (1996) Exogenous growth factor application effect on human wound healing. *Prog. Dermatol.* **30**, 1–7.

28. Steed, D. L. and the Diabetic Ulcer Study Group. (1995) Clinical evaluation of recombinant human platelet-derived growth factor for the treatment of lower extremity diabetic ulcers. *J. Vasc. Surg.* **21**, 71–81.

29. Rak, J. and Kerbel, R. S. (1996) Treating cancer by inhibiting angiogenesis: new hopes and potential pitfalls. *Cancer Metastasis Rev.* **15**, 231–236.

30. Pluda, J. M. (1997) Tumor-associated angiogenesis: mechanisms, clinical implications and therapeutic strategies. *Semin. Oncol.* **24**, 203–218.

31. Nelson, N. J. (1998) Inhibitors of angiogenesis enter Phase III testing. *J. Natl. Cancer Instit.* **90**, 960–963.

32. Mollet, B., Vialettes, B., Haroche, S., Escoffer, P., Gastaut, P., Tanbert, J. P., and Vague, P. (1992) Stabilization of severe proliferative diabetic retinopathy by long-term treatment with SMS 201-995. *Diabetes Metab.* **18**, 438–444.

33. Ezekowitz, R. B. A., Mulliken, J. B., and Folkman, J. (1992) Interferon alpha-2a therapy for life-threatening hemangiomas of infancy. *N. Engl. J. Med.* **326**, 1456–1463.

34. White, C. W., Sondheimer, H. M., Crouch, E. C., Wilson, H., and Fan, L.L. (1989) Treatment of pulmonary hemangiomatosis with recombinant interferon alfa-2a. *N. Engl. J. Med.* **320**, 1197–1200.

35. Gill, P. S., Lunardi-Iskandar, Y., Louie, S., Tulpule, A., Zheng, T,. Espina, B. M., et al. (1996) The effects of preparation of human chorionic gonadotropin on AIDS-related Kaposi's sarcoma. *N. Engl. J. Med.* **335,** 1261–1269.

36. Vogt, B. and Frey, F. J. (1997) Inhibition of angiogenesis in Kaposi's sarcoma by captopril. *Lancet* **349,** 1149.

37. Pluda, J. M., Feigal, E., and Yarchoan, R. (1993) Noncytotoxic approaches to the treatment of HIV-associated Kaposi's sarcoma. *Oncology* **7,** 25–33.

38. Dupont, E., Savard, P. E., Jourdain, C., Juneau, C., Thibodeau, A., Ross, N., et al. (1998) Antiangiogenic properties of a novel shark cartilage extract: potential role in the treatment of psoriasis. *J. Cutaneous Med. Surg.* **2,** 146–152.

39. Brouty-Boye, D. and Zetter, B. R. (1980) Inhibition of cell motility by interferon. *Science* **208,** 516–518.

40. Fung, W. E. (1991) Interferon alfa-2a for treatment of age-related macular degeneration. *Am. J. Ophthalmol.* **112,** 349–350.

41. Guyer, D. R., Tiedeman, J., Yannuzzi, L. A., Slakter, J. J., Parker, D., Kelley, J., et al. (1993) Interferon-associated retinopathy. *Arch. Ophthalmol.* **111,** 350–356.

42. Guyer, D. R., Adamis, A. P., Gragoudas, E. S., Folkman, J., Slakter, J. S., and Yanuzzi, L. A. (1992) Systemic antiangiogenic therapy for choroidal neovascularization. What is the role of interferon alpha? *Arch. Ophthalmol.* **110,** 1383–1384.

43. Holaday, J. (1997) Conference proceedings. Angiogenesis antagonists: current clinical trials, drug development and regulatory issues (Bermuda). Cambridge Healthtech Institute, Cambridge, Massachusetts.

44. Bielenberg, D. R., Bucana, C. P., Sanchez, R., Donawho, C. K., Kripke, M. L., and Fidler, I. J. (1998) Molecular regulation of UVB-induced cutaneous angiogenesis. *J. Investig. Dermatol.* **111,** 864–872.

45. Uchida, K., Takahashi, A., Miyao, N., Takeda, K., Tsutsumi, H., Satoh, M., and Tsukomoto, T. (1997) Juvenile hemangioma of the testis: analysis of expression of angiogenic factors. *Urology* **49,** 285–286.

46. Skowsky, W. R., Siddiqui, T., Hodgetts, D., Lambrou, F. H., Stewart, M. Y., and Foster, M. T. (1996) A pilot study of chronic recombinant interferon-alpha 2a for diabetic proliferative retinopathy: metabolic effects and ophthalmologic effects. *J. Diabetes Complic.* **10,** 94–99.

47. Rassmussen, H. S. and McCann, P. (1997) Matrix metalloproteinase inhibition as a novel anticancer strategy: a review with special focus on batimastat and marimastat. *Pharmacol. Therapeut.* **75,** 69–75.

48. Miller, J. W. (1997) Vascular endothelial growth factor and ocular neovascularization. *Am. J. Pathol.* **151,** 13–23.

49. Aiello, L., Avery, R., Arrigg, P., Keyt, B., Jampoel, H., Shah, S., et al. (1994) Vascular endothelial growth factor in ocular fluid of patients with diabetic retinopathy and other retinal disorders. *N. Engl. J. Med.* **331,** 1480–1487.

50. Adamis, A. P., Miller, J. W., Bernal, M.-T, D'Amico, D. J., Folkman, J., Yeo, T.-K., and Yeo, K.-T. (1994) Increased vascular endothelial growth factor levels in the vitreous of eyes with proliferative diabetic retinopathy. *Am. J. Ophthalmol.* **118,** 445–450.

51. Tolentino, M. J., Miller, J. W., Gragoudas, E. S., Chatzistefanou, K., Ferrara, N., and Adamis, A. P. (1996) Vascular endothelial growth factor is sufficient to produce iris neovascularization and neovascular glaucoma in a non-human primate. *Arch. Ophthalmol.* **114,** 964–970.

52. Adamis, A., Shima, D., Tolentino, M., Gragoudas, E., Ferrara, N., Folkman, J., et al. (1996) Inhibition of VEGF prevents ocular neovascularization in a non-human primate. *Arch. Ophthalmol.* **114,** 66–71.

53. Kumar, R., Kuniyasu, H., Bucana, C. P., Wilson, M. R., and Fidler, I. J. (1998) Spatial and temporal expression of angiogenic molecules during tumor growth and progression. *Oncol. Res.* **10,** 301–311.

54. Kumar, R., Yoneda, J., Bucana, C. P., and Fidler, I. J. (1998) Regulation of distinct steps of angiogenesis by different angiogenic molecules. *Intl. J. Oncol.* **12,** 749–757.

55. Relf, M., Lejeune, S., Scott, P. A. E., Fox, S., Smith, K., Leek, R., et al. (1997) Expression of the angiogenic factors vascular endothelial cell growth factor, acidic and basic fibroblast growth factor, tumor growth factor b-1, platelet-derived endothelial cell growth factor, placenta growth factor, and pleiotrophin in human primary breast cancer and its relation to angiogenesis. *Cancer Res.* **57,** 963–969.

56. Barton, D. P. J., Cai, A., Wendt, K., Young, M., Gamero, A., and De Cesare, S. (1997). Angiogenic protein expression in advanced epithelial ovarian cancer. *Clin. Cancer Res.* **3,** 1579–1586.

57. Wakabayashi, Y., Shomo, T., Isono, M., Hori, S., Matsuchima, K., Ono, M., and Kuwano, M. (1995) Dual pathways to tubular morphogenesis of vascular endothelial cells by human glioma cells: vascular endothelial growth factor/basic fibroblast growth factor and interleukin-8. *Japn. J. Cancer Res.* **86,** 1189–1197.

58. Barlow, C. F., Priebe, C. J., Mulliken, J. B., Barnes, P. D., MacDonald, D., Folkman, J., and Ezekowitz, R. A. (1998) Spastic diplegia as a complication of interferon alpha-2a treatment of hemangiomas of infancy. *J. Pediatr.* **132,** 527–530.

59. Enjolras, O. (1998) Neurotoxicity of interferon alfa in children treated for hemangiomas. *J. Am. Acad. Dermatol.* **39,** 1037–1038.

60. Kawamata, T., Dietrich, W. D., Schaller, T., Gotts, J. E., Cocke, R. R., Benowitz, L. I., and Finkelstein, S. P. (1997) Intracisternal basic fibroblast growth factor enhances functional recovery and up-regulates the expression of a molecular marker of neuronal sprouting following focal cerebral infarction. *Proc. Natl. Acad. Sci. USA* **94,** 8179–8184.

61. Hayashi, T., Abe, K., Suzuki, H., and Itoyama, Y. (1997) Rapid induction of vascular endothelial growth factor gene expression after transient middle cerebral artery occlusion in rats. *Stroke* **28,** 2039–2044.

62. Soker, S., Takushima, S., Mino, H. P., Neufeld, G., and Klagsbrun, M. (1998) Neuropilin-1 is expressed by endothelial and tumor cells as an isoform-specific receptor for vascular endothelial growth factor. *Cell* **92,** 735–745.

63. Gipaudo, E., Primo, L., Audero, E., Gerber, H. P., Koolwijk, P., Soker, S., et al. (1998) Tumor necrosis factor-alpha regulates expression of vascular endothelial growth factor receptor-2 and of its co-receptor neuropilin-1 in human vascular endothelial cells. *J. Biol. Chem.* **273,** 22,128–22,135.

64. Choudhuri, R., Zhang, D. T., Donnini, S., Ziche, M., and Bicknell, R. (1997) An angiogenic role for the neurokines midkine and pleiotrophin in tumorigenesis. *Cancer Res.* **57,** 1814–1819.

65. Wieman, T. J., Smiell, J. M., and Su, Y. (1998) Efficacy and safety of a topical gel formulation of recombinant human platelet-derived growth factor-BB (becaplermin) in patients with chronic neuropathic diabetic ulcers. A phase III randomized placebo-controlled double blind study. *Diabetes Care* **21,** 822–827.

66. REGRANEX package insert, Ortho-McNeil Pharmaceuticals, February 1998.

67. Mazue, G., Bertolero, F., Garofano, L., Brughera, M., and Carminati, P. (1992) Experience with the preclinical assessment of basic fibroblast growth factor (bFGF). *Toxicol. Lett.* **64/65,** 329–338.

68. Cuevas, P., Carceller, F., Ortega, S., Zazo, M., Nieto, I., and Giminez-Gallego, G. (1991) Hypotensive activity of fibroblast growth factor. *Science* **250,** 1208–1210.

69. Ishibashi, Y., Urabe, Y., Tsutsui, H., Kinugawa, S., Sugimachi, M., Takahashi, M., et al. (1997) Negative ionotropic effect of basic fibroblast growth factor on adult cardiac myocyte. *Circulation* **96,** 2501–2504.

70. Vale, P. R., Losordo, D. W., Symes, J. F., and Isner, J. M. (1998) Gene therapy for myocardial angiogenesis. *Circulation* **98(Suppl.),** 322.

71. Schwarz, E. R., Speakman, M. T., Patternson, M., Kedes, L., and Kloner, R. A. (1998) Effect of intramyocardial injection of DNA expressing vascular endothelial growth factor in myocardial infarct tissue in the rat heart: angiogenesis and angioma formation. *Circulation* **98(Suppl.),** 456.

72. Vale, P. R., Rauh, G. F., Wuensch, D. I., Pieczek, A. M., and Schainfeld, R. M. (1998) Influence of vascular endothelial growth factor on diabetic retinopathy. *Circulation* **98(Suppl.),** 353.

73. Li, W. W., Li, V. W., Casey, R., Tsakayannis, D., Kruger, E. A., Lee, A., et al. (1998) Clinical trials of angiogenesis-based therapies: overview and new guiding principles, in *Angiogenesis: Models, Modulators and Clinical Applications* (Maragoudakis, M., ed.), Plenum, New York, NY, pp. 475–492.

74. Folkman J. (1997) Antiangiogenic therapy, in *Cancer: Principles & Practice of Oncology, 5th ed.* (DeVita, Jr., V. T., Hellman, S., Rosenberg, S. A., ed.), Lippincott-Raven, Philadelphia, PA, pp. 3075–3085.

75. Kudelka, A. P., Levy, T., Verschraegen, C. F., Edwards, C. L., Piamsomboon, A., Termrungruanglert, W., et al. (1997) A phase I study of TNP-470 administered to patients with advanced squamous cell cancer of the cervix. *Clin. Cancer Res.* **3,** 1501–1505.

76. Li, V. Unpublished data.

77. Losordo, D. W., Vale, P. R., Symes, J. F., Dunnington, C. H., Esakof, D. D., et al. (1998) Gene therapy for myocardial angiogenesis. Initial clinical results with direct myocardial injection of phVEGF165 as sole therapy for myocardial ischemia. *Circulation* **98,** 2800–2804.

78. Boehm, T., Folkman, J., Browder, T., and O'Reilly, M. S. (1997) Antiangiogenic therapy of experi-
     mental cancer does not induce acquired drug resistance. *Nature* **390,** 404–407.

79. Kudelka, A. P., Verschraegen, C. F., and Loyer, E. (1998) Complete remission of metastatic cervical
     cancer with the angiogenesis inhibitor TNP-470. *N. Engl. J. Med.* **338,** 991–992.

80. Klaubner, N., Browne, F., Anand-Apte, B., and D'Amato, R. J. (1996) New activity of spironolactone.
     Inhibition of angiogenesis in vitro and in vivo. *Circulation* **94,** 2566–2571.

81. Panet, R., Marks, M., and Atlas, H. (1994) Bumetanide and furosemide inhibited vascular endothelial
     cell proliferation. (1994) *J. Cell Physiol.* **158,** 121–127.

82. Bouck, N. and Campbell, S. (1998) Anti-cancer dividends from captopril and other inhibitors of
     angiogenesis. *J. Nephrol.* **11,** 3–4.

83. Tamargo, R. J., Bok, R. A., and Brem, H. (1991) Angiogenesis inhibition by minocycline. *Cancer
     Res.* **51,** 672–675.

84. Fujioka, T., Hasagawa, M., Ishikura, K., Matsushita, Y., Sato, T. M., and Tanji, S. (1998) Inhibition
     of tumor growth and angiogenesis by vitamin D3 agents in murine renal cell carcinoma. *J. Urol.* **160,**
     247–251.

85. Liaudat-Coopman, E. D. E., Berchem, G. J., and Wellstein, A. (1997) In vivo inhibition of angiogenesis
     and induction of apoptosis by retinoic acid in squamous cell carcinoma. *Clin. Cancer Res.* **3,** 179–184.

86. Danesi, R., Agen, C., Benelli, U., Paolo, A. D., Nardini, D., Bocci, G., et al. (1997) Inhibition of
     experimental angiogenesis by the somatostatin analogue octreotide acetate (SMS 701-995). *Clin.
     Cancer Res.* **3,** 265–272.

87. Alliegro, M. C., Alliegro, M. A., Crague, E. J., Jr., and Glaser, B. M. (1993) Amiloride inhibition of
     angiogenesis in vivo. *J. Exp. Zool.* **267,** 245–252.

88. Pipili-Synetos, E., Papageorgiou, A., Sakkoula, E., Sotiropoulou, G., Fotsis, T., Karakinlakis, G., and
     Maragoudakis, M. E. (1995) Inhibition of angiogenesis, tumor growth and metastases by the
     NO-releasing vasodilators, isosorbide mononitrate and dinitrate. *Br. J. Pharmacol.* **116,** 1829–1834.

89. Ono, M., Kawahara, N., Goto, D., Wakabayashi, Y., Ushiro, S., and Sato, Y. (1996) Inhibition of tumor
     growth and neovascularization by an antigastric ulcer agent, irsogladine. *Cancer Res.* **56,**
     1512–1516.

90. Tsuchida, T., Tsukamoto, Y., Sagawa, K., Goto, H., and Hase, S. (1990) Effects of cimetidine and
     omeprazole on angiogenesis in granulation tissue of acetic acid-induced gastric ulcers in rats. *Diges-
     tion* **47,** 8–14.

91. Koch, A. E., Burrows, J. C., Polverini, P. J., Cho, M., and Leibovich, S. J. (1991) Thiol-containing
     compounds inhibit the production of monocyte and macrophage-derived angiogenesis activity. *Agents
     Actions* **34,** 350–357.

92. Sakamoto, T., Soriano, D., Nassaralla, J., Murphy, T. L., Oganesian, A., Spee, C., et al. (1995) Effects
     of intravitreal administration of indomethicin on experimental subretinal neovascularization in the
     subhuman primate. *Arch. Ophthalmol.* **113,** 222–226.

93. Li, V. W., Jaffe, M. P., Li, W. W., and Haynes, H. A. (1998) Off-label dermatologic therapies. Usage,
     risks, and mechanisms. *Arch. Dermatol.* **134,** 1449–1454.

94. Keck, P. J., Hauser, S. D., Krivi, G., Sanzo, K., Warren, T., Feder, J., and Connolly, D. T. (1989)
     Vascular permeability factor, an endothelial cell mitogen related to PDGF. *Science* **246,** 1309–1312.

95. Li, W. W., Li, V. W., Casey, R., and Tsakayannis, D. (1996) Arterial gene therapy [letter]. *Lancet*
     348(9038), 1381.

96. Dixon, S. C., Kruger, E. A., Bauer, K. S., and Figg, W. D. (1999) Thalidomide up-regulates prostate-
     specific antigen secretion from LNCaP cells. *Cancer Chemother. Pharmacol.* **43(Suppl.),**
     S78–S84.

97. Horti, J., Dixon, S. C., Logothetis, C. J., Guo, Y., Reed, E., and Figg, W. D. (1999) Increased transcrip-
     tional activity of prostate-specific antigen in the presence of TNP-470, an angiogenesis inhibitor.
     Br. J. Cancer **79(9–10),** 1588–1593.

98. Meyer, G. E., Yu, E., Siegal, J. A., Petteway, J. C., Blumenstein, B. A., and Brawer, M. K. (1995)
     Serum basic fibroblast growth factor in men with and without prostate carcinoma. *Cancer* **76,**
     2304–2311.

99. Sliutz, G., Tempfer, C., Obermair, A., Reinthaller, A., Gitsch, G., and Kainz, C. H. (1995) Serum
     evaluation of basic fibroblast growth factor in cervical cancer patients. *Cancer Lett.* **94,** 227–231.

100. Watanabe, H., Nguyen, M., Schizer, M., Li, V., Hayes, D. F., Sallan, S., and Folkman, J. (1992) Basic
     fibroblast growth factor in human serum: a prognostic test for breast cancer. *Mol. Biol. Cell* **3,** 234a.

101. Li, V. W., Folkerth, R. D., Watanabe, H., Yu, C., Rupnick, M., Barcus, P., et al. (1994) Basic fibroblast growth factor in the cerebrospinal fluid of children with brain tumours: correlation with microvessel count in the tumour. *Lancet* **344,** 82–86.

102. Perez-Atayde, A. R., Sallan, S. E., Tedrow, U., Conners, S., Allred, E., and Folkman, J. (1997) Spectrum of tumor angiogenesis in the bone marrow of children with acute lymphoblastic leukemia. *Am. J. Pathol.* **150,** 815–821.

103. Nyugen, M., Watanabe, H., Budson, A. E., Richie, J. P., Hayes, D. F., and Folkman, J. (1994) Elevated levels of an angiogenic peptide, basic fibroblast growth factor, in the urine of patients with a wide spectrum of cancers. *J. Natl. Cancer Inst.* **86,** 356–361.

104. Barrington, J. W., Fulford, S., Fraylin, L., Fish, R., Shelley, M., and Stephenson, T. P. (1996) Reduction of urinary basic fibroblast growth factor using pentosan polysulphate sodium. *Br. J. Urol.* **78,** 54–56.

105. Folkman, J. (1993) Diagnostic and therapeutic applications of angiogenesis research. *Life Sci.* **316,** 914–918.

106. Obermair, A., Tempfer, C., Hefler, L., Preyer, O., Zeillinger, R., Leodolter, S., and Kainz, C. (1998) Concentration of vascular endothelial growth factor (VEGF) in the serum of patients with suspected ovarian cancer. *Br. J. Cancer* **77,** 1870–1874.

107. Jain, R. K. (1996) Delivery of molecular medicine to solid tumors. *Science* **271,** 1079–1080.

108. Langer, R. (1996) Controlled release of a therapeutic protein. *Nature Med.* **2,** 7443.

109. Folkman, J., Szabo, S., Stovroff, M., McNeil, P., Li, W., and Shing, Y. (1991) Duodenal ulcer: discovery of a new mechanism and development of angiogenic therapy that accelerates healing. *Ann. Surg.* **214,** 414–427.

110. Edelman, E. R., Nugent, M. A., and Karnovsky, M. J. (1993) Perivascular and intravenous administration of basic fibroblast growth factor: vascular and solid organ deposition. *Proc. Natl. Acad. Sci. USA* **90,** 1513–1517.

111. Edelman, E. R., Mathiowitz, E., Langer, R., and Klagsbrun, M. (1991) Controlled and modulated release of basic fibroblast growth factor. *Biomaterials* **12,** 619–626.

112. Lai, P., Sahota, H., Nokilaychik, V., Chekanov, V., Keelan, M. H., and Kipshidze, N. N. (1998) Therapeutic angiogenesis in patients with advanced coronary artery disease. *Circulation* **98(Suppl.),** 352–353.

113. Henry, T. D., Rocha-Singh, K., and Isner, J. M. (1998) Results of intracoronary recombinant human vascular endothelial growth factor (rhVEGF) administration trial. *J. Am. College Cardiol.* **31,** 65A.

114. Laitinen, M., Hartikainen, J., Eranen, J., Kiviniemi, M., Hiltunen, M. O., Laakso, M., and Yla-Herttuala, S. (1998) Catheter-mediated VEGF gene transfer to human coronary arteries after angioplasty. Safety results from phase I Kuopio angioplasty gene transfer trial (KAT trial). *Circulation* **98(Suppl.),** 322.

115. Baumgartner, I., Pieczek, A., Manor, O., Blair, R., Kearney, M., Walsh, K., and Isner, J. M. (1998) Constitutive expression of phVEGF165 after intramuscular gene transfer promotes collateral vessel development in patients with critical limb ischemia. *Circulation* **97,** 1114–1123.

116. Davis, S., Aldrich, T. H., Jones, P. F., Acheson, A., Compton, D. L., Jain, V., et al. (1996) Isolation of angiopoietin-1, a ligand for the TIE2 receptor, by secretion-trap expression cloning. *Cell* **87,** 1161–1169.

117. Risau, W. (1997) Mechanisms of angiogenesis. *Nature* **386,** 671–674.

118. Hasuo, K., Tamura, S., Kudo, S., Uchino, A., Carlos, R., Matsushima, T., et al. (1985) Moya moya disease: use of digital subtraction angiography in its diagnosis. *Radiology* **157,** 107–111.

119. Pollock, B. E., Flickinger, J. C., Lunsford, L. D., Bissonette, D. J., and Kondziolka, D. (1996) Factors that predict bleeding risk of cerebral arteriovenous malformations. *Stroke* **27,** 1–6.

120. Neely, K. A., Quillen, D. A., Schachat, A. P., Gardner, T. W., and Blankenship, G. W. (1998) Diabetic retinopathy. *Med. Clin. N. Am.* **82,** 847–876.

121. Reynolds, L. P., Killilea, S. D., and Redner, D. A. (1992) Angiogenesis in the female reproductive system. *FASEB J.* **6,** 886–892.

122. Klauber, N., Rohan, R. M., Flynn, E., and D'Amato, R. J. (1997) Critical components of the female reproductive pathway are suppressed by the angiogenesis inhibitor AGM-1470. *Nature Med.* **3,** 443–446.

123. The Angiogenesis Foundation. Natural Compounds Database, 2001.

124. Cao, Y. and Cao R. (1999) Angiogenesis inhibited by drinking tea. *Nature* **398,** 381.

30 Angiostatin and Endostatin

Recent Advances in Their Biology, Pharmacokinetics, and Potential Clinical Applications

Jesus V. Soriano and B. Kim Lee Sim

CONTENTS

INTRODUCTION

A Novel Class of Proteins: Fragments of Precursor Proteins that Inhibit Endothelial Cell Activities

The generation of endogenous inhibitors of angiogenesis that are specific for endothelial cells from larger precursor molecules with entirely different functions, appears to be a recurrent theme. Early reports on such a novel class of inhibitors came from the study of the 16 kDa fragment of prolactin *(1,2)*, and the 29 kDa heparin-binding fragment of fibronectin *(3)*. Subsequently, a cleavage fragment of the chemokine platelet factor-4 *(4)*, Angiostatin, a fragment of plasminogen *(5)*, Endostatin, the carboxy-terminal fragment of collagen XVIII *(6)* and ATIII *(7)* have shown potent endothelial specific inhibitory activities. Both plasminogen and collagens are substrates of plasminogen activators (tissue-type and urokinase-type) and interstitial collagenase, respectively. These substrates can be co-induced by VEGF to generate a pro-degradative environment that facilitates migration and sprouting of endothelial cells *(8,9)*. Pepper and Montesano (1990) had proposed that plasminogen activator inhibitor-1 can provide a negative regulatory step that serves to balance the proteolytic process (Reviewed in ref. *10*). Cleavage of the substrate plasminogen by macrophage metalloelastase or tumor derived serine proteases generate Angiostatin™ protein *(11,12)*. Elastase cleavage of plasminogen also results in other fragments of plasminogen such as kringle 4, which has been reported as having slight angiogenic activity on bovine endothelial cells in culture *(5)*. It is possible that cleavage of the substrates plasminogen and collagen XVIII results in fragments of

From: *The New Angiotherapy*
Edited by: T.-P. D. Fan and E. C. Kohn © Humana Press Inc., Totowa, NJ

proteins that, together with the parent molecule, provide both the positive and negative balance that control physiologic angiogenesis.

ANGIOSTATIN

Biology and Mechanism of Action

Plasminogen is the proenzyme form of the serine protease plasmin which represents the major fibrinolytic enzyme in humans *(13)*. The complex structure of plasminogen consists of 5 highly disulfide bonded triple looped domains termed kringles at the N-terminal half. Cleavage of the Arg561-Val562 bond of plasminogen with urokinase or tissue-type plasminogen activator forms the active 2 chain plasmin linked by two disulfide bonds (14). Angiostatin is described as comprising kringles 1–4 (for reviews, *see* refs. *5, 15–20*).

There may be multiple pathways of Angiostatin generation. It seems that more than one enzyme can cleave plasminogen to generate Angiostatin in vivo *(20)*. The enzymes that have been identified appear to be generated by circulating macrophages as well as by various tumor types. Matrix metalloproteinases (MMPs) as well as serine proteases in conjunction with a free sulfhydryl donor can also catalyze the proteolysis of plasmin to generate Angiostatin *(20–22)*. Another possible mechanism of endogenous generation of Angiostatin by tumors is alternative transcription. We analyzed several tumor lines including T241 and LLC-LM, the tumor line that first reported the identification of Angiostatin for transcripts by method of RT-PCR. Transcripts of Angiostatin have not been detected and thus we believed that Angiostatin in circulation, is a product of the proteolysis of plasminogen (Sim, unpublished). Plasminogen is bound to endothelial surface receptors *(23)*. Annexin II and enolase are known cellular receptors of plasminogen. Whether Angiostatin is generated from cleavage of receptor-bound plasminogen or plasminogen in circulation or both is unknown. The role of the kringles of plasminogen in activities other than angiogenesis remains unclear, but the kringle domains have been shown to bind to several proteins such as fibrin *(24)* or thrombospondin, and to endothelial cells, platelets, neutrophils, and lymphocytes.

As with the multiple pathways that can generate Angiostatin, recent studies show that there may also be multiple mechanisms that lead to its potent antiangiogenic effects. Early reports had shown that tumor inhibition caused by systemic treatment with Angiostatin was found to be a result of an increased tumor cell apoptotic index even though tumor cell proliferative rates remained constant *(25)*. Subsequently, it was shown that Angiostatin directly induced apoptosis of endothelial cells in a dose dependent manner without a compensatory increase in proliferation, resulting in a net reduction of viable endothelial cells *(26,27)*. Endothelial cell apoptosis resulting from Angiostatin therapy was associated with increased tyrosine kinase activity of focal adhesion kinase that results in disruption of the normal turn over of focal adhesion contacts *(26)*. Angiostatin has been shown to induce an upregulation of E-selectin protein expression in proliferating endothelial cells with a corresponding increase in cell adhesion suggesting a role in cell migration *(28)*. It has also been proposed that the inhibition of tumor growth upon systemic treatment with Angiostatin is a result of endothelial cell mitosis arrest at the G_2/M phase *(27,29)*. In addition, Angiostatin also inhibits the bFGF and VEGF activation of extracellular signal-regulated kinase (ERK)-1, ERK-2, and other phosphoproteins by transient dephosphorylation specifically in human microvascular endothelial cells *(30)*.

But is Angiostatin's ability to inhibit angiogenesis the result of a receptor-ligand interaction? Are there proteins that interact with Angiostatin as transport molecules or substrates through which Angiostatin exerts its effect? Using ligand blot analysis, Angiostatin was found to bind to the a/b subunits of ATP synthase that was localized to the surface of human umbilical vein endothelial (HUVE) cells *(31)*. The binding of Angiostatin was distinct and did not compete with that of plasminogen's binding to annexin II on the surface of HUVE cells. These studies speculate that ATP synthase activity on the endothelial cell surface provides for an extracellular source of ATP that diffuses into and contributes to the intracellular ATP pool. Maintenance of high intracellular ATP levels render endothelial cells resistant to hypoxic stress that in itself can induce the generation of angiogenic growth factors at tumor sites. Thus Angiostatin binding to ATP synthase could disrupt the production of ATP and thus deprive endothelial cells of this alternative source of ATP upon which their survival within the tumor microenvironment is dependent *(31)*. Even though the experiments described in this study show the association of Angiostatin generated from elastase cleavage of human plasminogen to ATP synthase, the proposed mechanism does not justify the potent antiangiogenic effects and tumor growth inhibition that have been described upon systemic rhAngiostatin treatment (*see* review in ref. *19)*. Furthermore, while this hypothesis for the first time attempts to correlate an activity of Angiostatin to a biochemical mechanism, it over looks a couple facts. First, the binding of Angiostatin to HUVE cells inhibits the proliferation of endothelial cells in vitro when oxygen is not deficient. If endothelial cells use surface ATP synthase to supplement ATP generation in low oxygen environments, Angiostatin treatment would not be expected to inhibit the proliferation of endothelial cells in vitro where oxygen is not a limiting factor. Furthermore, the transport of protons and the synthesis of ATP by ATP synthase are mechanically coupled such that the generation of ATP is driven by a gradient of protons across the membrane that requires the flow of protons from interior of the membrane to the exterior. Because of the acidic extracellular environment of tumors and the relatively alkaline intracellular pH of tumor cells, the H^+ concentration gradient favors proton entry and consequently would not support the generation of ATP *(32)*.

Angiostatin has also been known to bind to a novel protein termed Angiomotin that has been shown to be expressed in endothelial cells of capillaries and of human placenta *(33)*. Angiomotin is localized to the ruffled edges of migrating endothelial cells implicating its role in the angiogenesis cascade. Most interesting is the fact that in a limited study, angiomotin was found expressed in endothelial cells of vessels infiltrating a Kaposi's sarcoma lesion but not the surrounding normal dermal vessels. This finding argues for a mechanism that results in the specificity of Angiostatin, and its ability to target endothelial cells of tumor origin. There are some obvious unanswered questions. The interaction of Angiostatin with angiomotin that lacks a typical signal peptide and transmembrane domain argues against the fact that angiomotin is a membrane receptor. Thus this leaves the possibility of another as yet undefined "first-step" in the mechanistic pathway of angiogenesis inhibition conferred by Angiostatin. Furthermore, the downstream process(s) subsequent to the interaction of Angiostatin to angiomotin that leads to angiogenesis blockade and tumor growth inhibition is undefined.

Safety and Pharmacokinetic Profile of Recombinant Human Angiostatin

Recombinant human (rh) Angiostatin produced in the yeast Pichia pastoris inhibits B16BL6 experimental metastases in a dose-dependent fashion, with greater than 90% inhibition obtained after daily systemic administration of 4.5 mg/kg in mice (34).

In correlative pharmacokinetic studies, there was a similar increase in circulating levels of Angiostatin that was dose dependent. Effects of Angiostatin on tumor neovascularization and tumor growth in late stage disease involving established lung metastases (11 d after tumor cell seeding) was further studied by delaying rhAngiostatin therapy until tumors had established a vascular bed. RhAngiostatin inhibited the growth of macrometastases and essentially arrested their development to fulminant disease as scored by lung weights (>65%). Immunohistological staining with antibodies against Von Willebrand factor showed an inhibition of angiogenesis in lung metastases of mice treated with Angiostatin indicating that inhibition of tumor growth was a direct result of angiogenesis inhibition (34).

Clinical grade rhAngiostatin has been produced in quantities that currently support on-going phase I trials (see below). In range finding toxicity studies of this rhAngiostatin in Cynomolgus monkeys, a formulation at 11.2 mg/mL in isotonic saline was administered intravenously (iv) to four monkeys in a range-finding toxicity study prior to the design of IND-directed toxicology studies (35). Two monkeys were dosed with Angiostatin™ protein at 112 or 56 mg/kg (1344 or 672 mg/m^2) by iv push (5 min) in a total volume of 10 mL/kg. Two additional monkeys were dosed with Angiostatin™ protein at 280 or 140 mg/kg (3360 or 1680 mg/m^2) by continuous iv infusion (1 h) in a total volume of 25 kg/kg. Blood samples were collected for hematology, coagulation, chemistry, and serum drug determinations prior to study, 4 h, 1 d, and 3 d post-dosing. Cardiovascular telemetry in these animals did not reveal any acute or long-term changes in HR, BP, or EKG measurements. No rhAngiostatin™ related effects were noted on any of the standard hematology, coagulation, or blood chemistry parameters. Ancillary studies indicated a transient increase in circulating tissue plasminogen activator concentration. In addition, Angiostatin™ protein increased plasma tissue factor pathway inhibitor concentration in a dose-dependent manner.

RhAngiostatin was also shown to be safe in a separate 60-d chronic daily dosing study performed in Cynomolgus monkeys. In this study, study groups that included both male and female monkeys were dosed with either 4.5, 150, or 300 mg/m^2/d of rhAngiostatin (Fortier et al, unpublished). There were no mortalities or unscheduled sacrifices during the course of the study. In addition, there were no adverse clinical observations that were related to the administration of rhAngiostatin protein. No rhAngiostatin protein-related effects were noted on any of hematology or blood chemistry parameters. The results of these studies indicated that rhAngiostatin can be administered safely in high doses to monkeys and that clinical Phase I studies could be designed that would incorporate effective levels as determined in preclinical tumor models.

In a separate study using radiolabeled Angiostatin derived from elastase cleavage of human plasminogen, the short-term pharmacokinetics and distribution in rats with far lower doses of 10–50 mg showed conflicting information, with "instant blood coagulation" at the tip of a permanent cannula used for easy access to pharmacokinetic measurements (36). In this same study, immunohistochemical analysis showed a fraction of larger pulmonary vessels contained undefined fibrous material that was also found in lungs of control animals. It should be pointed out that the source of human Angiostatin used in this study was a reagent grade commercial lysine-binding site I fraction of elastase cleaved plasminogen, that consists of a high proportion of a nonprotein fraction *(36,37)*.

Angiostatin in New Anti-Neoplasic Strategies: Single Anti-Angiogenesis vs Neoadjuvant Therapy

Human cancers with poor prognosis often fail to respond to radiotherapy, chemotherapy or hormone therapy due to the development of tumor resistance. In many cases poor prognosis is associated with high microvascular density *(36,38–40)*. Like Endostatin, Angiostatin is a potent inhibitor of tumor angiogenesis highly effective at shrinking tumors and resilient to the development of resistance *(41,42)*. Recent studies suggest that the administration of Angiostatin in combination with cytotoxic therapies may prove advantageous in resistant tumors. When Lewis lung carcinoma and the human-tumor xenografts D54, SQ-20B, or PC3 are treated with Angiostatin in combination with doses of radiation similar to those used in radiotherapy, the result is a synergistic reduction in tumor volume *(43–45)*. Remarkably, the combination of treatments entails no increase in toxicity for normal tissues *(43)*.

How does radiation enhance the anti-tumor activity of Angiostatin? To be effective, Angiostatin must be already acting on the tumor vasculature at the time of irradiation. Combinatorial studies have shown that Angiostatin delivered concomitantly with radiation for 2 d is as effective at suppressing primary tumor growth as a 14-d course of Angiostatin combined with an identical course of radiation. In contrast, Angiostatin is less effective if delivered after radiation. Interestingly, no difference is observed when radiation is associated with either a high or a low dose of Angiostatin *(44)*. In vitro studies of their mechanism of action have shown that the combination of radiation and Angiostatin had additive cytotoxic effects on primary endothelial cells, and that these effects are more predominant on dividing endothelial cells. In contrast, the same doses of both agents, applied either in combination or individually, did not induce any cytotoxicity in tumor cells. In related in vivo studies, the inhibition of tumor growth induced by this combined treatment was correlated with a marked decrease of tumoral microvascular density *(43–46)*. It follows that the combination of radiation and Angiostatin primarily affects tumor vasculature.

Because it targets tumor vessels, which are genetically stable and unlikely to develop resistance *(47,48)*, the combination of radiotherapy and Angiostatin may represent a new strategy against refractory cancer, especially at late stages of tumor development *(49)*. This hypothesis is supported by the finding that the combination of radiotherapy with intratumoral Angiostatin gene therapy dramatically inhibits tumor growth in well-established C6 gliomas, which are relatively resistant to irradiation *(45,50)*. Currently, we are assessing the benefits of this combination for oncological patients in Phase I clinical trials.

Finally, Angiostatin is also an adjuvant candidate in the treatment of nononcological conditions, as in photodynamic therapy (PDT) of choroidal neovascularization, a condition responsible for vision loss during macular degeneration *(51)*. PDT involves the systemic administration of a photosensitizer dye that accumulates in proliferating tissues such as tumors or newly formed vessels. The target tissue is subsequently irradiated with low-intensity, nonthermal light at a wavelength corresponding to the absorption peak of the dye. Excitation of the dye leads to the formation of reactive oxygen species causing photochemical damage of the target tissue *(52)*. When tested in vitro, Angiostatin and PDT had combined cytotoxic effects on retinal capillary endothelial cells, but not on pigment epithelial cells. In addition, as in the combination of Angiostatin and radiotherapy, no synergism between Angiostatin and PDT was observed when Angiostatin was administered after PDT *(51)*. Finally, it has been suggested that local release of Angiostatin and down-regulation of vascular endothelial growth factor in human vitreous mediate the therapeutic effects of retinal photocoagulation in proliferative diabetic retinopathy *(53)*.

In conclusion, the use of Angiostatin as an adjuvant of other cytotoxic modalities may be a strategy for increasing the damage done to pathological neovascularization, and reducing the deleterious effects on normal tissues.

Clinical Evaluation of (rh)Angiostatin

Phase I clinical trials assessing the safety, pharmacokinetics and pharmacodynamics of rhAngiostatin in patients with solid, refractory malignancies have been initiated. The following section reports results presented at a recent meeting. In one of these trials, the dose levels under evaluation ranged from 15 mg/m^2 to 240 mg/m^2 administered daily as a 10 min infusion in groups of 3–6 patients *(54)*. The patients were assessed for effects on urine and plasma VEGF/βFGF, tumor size, blood flow and vascularity determined by tumor biopsies and other noninvasive techniques that included contrast ultrasound and MRI. Extensive coagulation parameters were monitored and no clinically significant thrombotic or bleeding events have been noted to date. No dose limiting toxicities have been observed to date. Further, six patients had surgical wounds that healed while on continued therapy with rhAngiostatin. Pharmacokinetics of rhAngiostatin was found to be linear as demonstrated by dose-proportionate increases in both the area under the serum concentration-time profile, and the peak serum concentration. In this study, 7/10 patients had 15–92% decrease in urine bFGF levels and 5/10 patients had 30–64% decrease in urine VEGF levels *(54)*.

Other Phase I trials include investigating the use of rhAngiostatin protein in combination with radiation therapy for the treatment of patients with solid tumors, as well as studies of lower doses (7.5 mg/m^2, 15 mg/m^2, 30 mg/m^2) administered subcutaneously have been initiated. Promising preclinical data indicates that in addition to being an inhibitor of angiogenesis, and tumor growth, rhAngiostatin may potentiate radiotherapy *(43–45)*. Phase I studies of an Angiostatin generating "cocktail" that induces the direct in vivo conversion of plasminogen to Angiostatin by administration of a sulfhydryl donor in concert with a plasminogen activator has been recently reviewed *(20)*.

ENDOSTATIN PROTEIN

How is Endostatin Generated?

Endostatin is generated from its precursor, collagen XVIII, by a mechanism of limited proteolytic processing comparable to that of Angiostatin *(6,15)*. Collagen XVIII is the core protein of a heparan sulfate proteoglycan. It is widely distributed in different tissues and localizes in vessel walls, and in endothelial and epithelial basement membranes. Together with collagen XV, it forms the multiplexin subfamily of collagens, characterized by a central triple-helicoidal region interrupted by multiple noncollagenous domains and a unique C-terminal noncollagenous (NC1) domain *(55–62)*. The NC1 domain of collagen XVIII comprises an N-terminal domain that is implicated in the homotrimerization of collagen XVIII, a central protease-sensitive hinge region, and the active C-terminal endostatin domain *(60)*.

The mechanism whereby Endostatin is released from collagen XVIII is starting to be understood. Several in vitro studies have suggested that different proteases participate in this process. The cysteine-type protease cathepsin L is secreted by EOMA cells, and generates a 22 kDa Endostatin from collagen XVIII in an acidic extracellular milieu similar to that existing in the tumor microenvironment. This process occurs parallel to a metalloproteinase activity, but is independent of it *(63)*. Endostatin can also be generated by means of a two-step cleavage: an initial matrix metalloproteinase (MMP)-mediated release of NC1 and other intermediate Endostatin-containing fragments, followed by a second elastase–mediated *(64)* or cathepsin-mediated *(63)* release of Endostatin. Finally, human Endostatin-related fragments can be obtained in vitro by incubating recombinant human NC1 with a wide range of proteinases, such as cathepsins B, K, and D, MMP-2, MMP-3, MMP-9, MMP-12, MMP-13, MMP-14, and MMP-20 *(65)*. The following in vivo observations suggest that several proteolytic pathways may participate in this process: the presence of 11 different protease-sensitive sites in the N-terminal hinge region of recombinant and endogenous circulating Endostatins and Endostatin-containing fragments; the cleavage, by an unknown protease, of one or two C-terminal basic residues in Endostatins that are released from collagens XVIII and XV; and the existence in tissues, plasma, and urine of different endostatin proteins with a heterogineous distribution in molecular weight (19.5 kDa to 38 kDa), N- and C-terminal sequences, and glycosylation patterns *(6,60,61,66,67)*.

Is Endostatin's generation regulated? Different reports indicate that Endostatin is not incidently released during the proteolytic breakdown of basement membranes, but that it is instead the product of a coordinated process. First, Endostatin has lower binding affinity fo fibulin-2, nidogen-1, nidogen-2, laminin-1, sulfatides, and the heparan sulfate perlecan than its 38 kDa NC1 precursor *(60,62)*, which indicates that the proteolytic release serves to modify the ability of Endostatin to bind with the extracellular matrix. Upon release from collagen, XV retains almost the same binding properties as its precursor, the NC1-XV domain *(62)*. Hence, the proteolytic release of endostatins may modulate their respective binding affinities, a process which may determine their bioavailability. Third, it was unclear until now whether released NC1 had intrinsic biological activity *(6,71)*. The recent observation that Endostatin is more active than its precursor NC1 in a FGF-2-stimulated chick chorioallantoic membrane assay *(62)* suggests that this proteolytic processing is also Endostatin's mechanism of activation. Finally, given that serum concentrations of Endostatin (100–300 ng/mL) are similar to the concentrations inhibiting endothelial cell proliferation in vitro *(60)*, this process may serve to control blood levels of Endostatin.

Together these findings indicate that Endostatin and its related fragments are generated by a tightly regulated mechanism that participates in the homeostatic control of angiogenesis.

Leads into the Mechanism of Action of a Potent Angiogenesis Inhibitor

The various proposed mechanistic activities ascribed to Endostatin has been recently reviewed *(19)*. Endostatin, a potent inhibitor of angiogenesis and tumor growth, has been shown to inhibit endothelial cell migration in vitro *(6,42,72)*. In a recent study, a potential modulator of this anti-angiogenic activity of Endostatin has been identified *(73)*. In that

Table 1A
Pharmacokinetics of rhEndostatin in Mice

Dose and Route (mg/kg)	1.5–iv	1.5–sc	1.5–iv	1.5–sc
Dose (mg/m^2)	4.5	4.5	150	150
C_{max} (ng/mL)	5512	161	59,434	4582
$t_{1/2\,ka}$ (h)	–	5.45	–	4.19
$t_{1/2\,\alpha}$ (h)	0.85	–	4.18	–
$t_{1/2\,\beta}$ (h)	41.1	53.1	77.0	75.2
$t_{1/2\,z}$ (h)	–	–	919	760
$AUC_{0->inf.}$	16.6	16.0	660	700
F (%)	–	96.4	–	106
CI_{TB} (mL/h/kg)	90.4	–	75.8	–
V_B (mL/kg)	5365	–	8422	–

study, a phage-display library was screened to identify polypeptides that mimic the binding domains of proteins with which Endostatin interacts. A conformed peptide (E37) was identified that shared an epitope with human tropomyosin implicating tropomyosin as an Endostatin binding protein. Also, rhEndostatin was shown to bind to tropomyosin and to tropomyosin-associated microfilaments in a variety of endothelial cell types in vitro (74). Tropomyosin is expressed by multiple cell types and functions in association with actin to regulate cell morphology and migration, and has been localized at the ruffled edge of migrating cells. The most compelling evidence that tropomyosin modulates Endostatin's activity was demonstrated when E37 blocked greater than 84% of Endostatin's tumor-growth inhibitory activity in a dose-dependent fashion, in a B16BL6 murine tumor model. It was proposed that the E37 peptide mimicked the Endostatin-binding epitope of tropomyosin and blocked Endostatin's anti-tumor activity by competing for Endostatin binding. It was postulated that Endostatin's interaction with tropomyosin resulted in disruption of microfilament integrity leading to inhibition of cell motility, induction of apoptosis, and ultimately inhibition of tumor growth.

This study leaves open the possibility for an initial step at the endothelial cell surface prior to Endostatin's interaction with intracellular tropomyosin. Further, the mechanism by which Endostatin is internalized is also undefined. It is also possible that processing may occur and only a fragment of Endostatin is internalized. However, it is of interest to note that there have been reports that tropomyosin is expressed on the surface of endothelial cells. Alternatively, integrins (a_5 and a_v) have been implicated in the interaction of Endostatin with the surface of endothelial cells, allowing Endostatin to function as an integrin antagonist (75). The fact that Endostatin binds heparin as well as zinc and speculations and controversies as to the role of these binding in the activities attributed to Endostatin have been described (71,72,75–79).

The Pharmacokinetic Profile of Recombinant Human Endostatin

We have determined the pharmacokinetics of rhEndostatin™ protein in mice and male Cynomolgus monkeys (Table 1) (72). Male mice were dosed either via the iv or subcu-

Table 1B
Pharmacokinetics of rhEndostatin in Cynomolgus Monkeys

Dose and Route (mg/kg)	0.375–iv	3.75–sc	12.5–iv	12.5–sc
Dose (mg/m^2)	4.5	4.5	150	150
C_{max} (ng/mL)	1226	254	55,137	605
$t_{1/2\,ka}$ (h)	–	145	–	197
$t_{1/2\,\alpha}$ (h)	1.78	–	5.55	–
$t_{1/2\,\beta}$ (h)	15.6	–	23.8	–
$t_{1/2\,z}$ (h)	–	228	291	231
$AUC_{0->inf.}$ (ug min/mL)	13.5	184	896	507
F (%)	–	68.4	–	56.6
CI_{TB} (mL/h/kg)	27.8	–	13.9	–
V_B (mL/kg)	625	–	5836	–

taneous (sc) route with 1.5 and 50 mg/kg, two doses that inhibit primary xenograft tumors and experimental metastasis (72). Peak serum levels of rhEndostatin for both sc doses occurred 30 min following injection into mice. C_{max} values were 161 and 4582 ng/mL after doses of 1.5 and 50 mg/mL/kg, respectively (Table 1A). Following iv injection, peak serum drug levels occurred within 2 min. C_{max} values were 5512 and 59.434 ng/mL after doses of 1.5 and 50 mg/kg, respectively. The elimination of rhEndostatin was triexponential following the 50 mg/kg iv doses with a terminal life of 919 min. Not all phases of elimination were evident at lower doses and/or sc administration. The calculated values for total body clearance and apparent volume of distribution for the two iv doses were reasonably consistent, varying by 1.2-fold and 1.56-fold, respectively. rhEndostatin was rapidly and extensively absorbed following sc administration to mice, with an apparent absorption half-life of 4.19–5.45 min. The bioavailability was essentially 100%. AUC was 16.6 and 16.0 mg × mL/min for the 1.5 mg/kg dose given iv and sc, respectively, and 660 and 700 mg × mL/min for the 50 mg/kg dose given i.v. and sc, respectively (Table 1A). We subsequently studied the pharmacokinetics of rhEndostatin in Cynomolgus monkeys, following iv administration of rhEndostatin at 0.375 and 12.5 mg/kg (Table 1B). These doses represent an equivalent mg/m^2 dose given to mice. C_{max} occurred within 2 min of iv bolus injection and 4 h or more after sc administration. The calculated C_{max} for both iv and sc administration were reasonably proportional to the 0.375 and 12.5 mg/m^2 dose levels (Table 1B). The elimination of rhEndostatin was triexponential following the 12.5 mg/m^2 iv dose, with a terminal half-life of 291 min. However, with the lower doses and/or sc administration, not all phases of elimination could be discerned. The calculated values for total body clearance and apparent volume of distribution varied substantially between the two iv doses. rhEndostatin was well absorbed following sc administration, with an apparent absorption half-life of 145–197 min. The calculated bioavailability was 56.6–68.4% (relative to the 12.5 mg/m^2 iv dose). The terminal half-life was nearly identical at the two sc dose levels and was comparable to that observed following the 12.5 mg/m^2 iv dose. AUC was 896 and 507 mg × mL/min for the 12.5 mg/kg dose given iv and sc, respectively (72).

Antitumor Activity Devoid of Drug-Related Adverse Effect
in Animal Models

Preclinical studies in animal models have shown a unique feature of Endostatin, namely, the rare combination of high anti-tumor efficacy with the absence of drug-related adverse effects such as acquired drug resistance and toxicity.

Early studies by Boehm et al., demonstrated that systemic administration of Endostatin to xenografts-bearing mice was able to inhibit the growth, and reduce the volume, of established tumors. Noteworthy, neither toxic effects nor the development of drug resistance was observed at doses sufficient to eradicate the tumors (42). Endostatin was administered subcutaneously to mice bearing Lewis lung carcinoma (LLC), T241 fibrosarcoma, or B16F10 melanoma, until tumors regressed to a microscopic size. Treatment was discontinued and the tumors were allowed to grow. Then, a new cycle of Endostatin was administered. Cyclic administration of Endostatin repeatedly reduced tumors to barely visible subcutaneous nodules, did not induce drug resistance, and resulted in tumor dormancy after 6 (LLC), 4 (T241), or 2 (B16F10) cycles of treatment. Tumor dormancy persisted indefinitely after therapy. In contrast, mice treated with cyclophosphamide developed drug resistance after one or two cycles of chemotherapy and died of rapidly progressing tumors (42). In primary tumor xenografts, orthotopic tumor implantation and experimental metastasis murine models, subcutaneous treatment with Endostatin™ protein elicited its anti-tumor and anti-angiogenic activities over a broad concentration range (1.5–300 mg/m^2) that was devoid of any drug-related adverse effects (19,72). Moreover, systemic treatment with Endostatin (20 mg/m^2/d) did not alter serum cholesterol levels and body weight in ApoE lipoprotein-deficient mice (80).

The anti-tumor efficacy of rhEndostatin™ protein depends on the route and schedule of administration. Planar scanning of breast tumor bearing rats after iv injection of 99Tc-EC-labelled rhEndostatin showed that, after 30 min, tumor uptakes significant amounts of rhEndostatin, which remain detectable for more than 4 h (81). Using the B16BL6 experimental metastasis model, we have studied the relationship between therapeutic activity and pharmacokinetics of rhEndostatin™ protein. Intravenous administration of 1.5 mg/kg/d of rhEndostatin™ protein resulted in C_{max} and AUC_{last} of 1219 ng/mL and 204.31 h × ng/mL, respectively, while subcutaneous administration resulted in C_{max} 188 ng/mL and AUC_{last} 289.71 h × ng/mL. Interestingly, the anti-tumor efficacies (T/C) were 0.31 and 0.33, respectively, which demonstrates that both ways of administration result in similar inhibition of metastasis. Using the BxPc3 human pancreatic carcinoma xenograft mouse model, Kisker et al., compared the anti-tumor efficacy of rhEndostatin™ protein (2, 6, and 20 mg/kg/d) administered either as an intra-peritoneal bolus or in intraperitoneal continuous infusion. For the three doses tested, the anti-tumor efficacy (T/C) of rhEndostatin™ protein was significantly higher when administered as continuous infusion (82). These findings demonstrate that the extent of rhEndostatin™ protein is a determining factor for anti-tumor activity. Finally, we have found that low doses of rhEndostatin™ protein given by continuous infusion can generate equivalent anti-tumor activities at lower AUCs. Whereas a 20 mg/kg/d of rhEndostatin™ protein administered via intraperitoneal bolus yielded a T/C of 0.34, a 2 mg/kg/d dose administered in intraperitoneal continuous infusion yielded a T/C of 0.32. However, C_{max} and AUC_{7d}, were 51-fold and 3-fold smaller, respectively, at the 2 mg/kg/d dose (Table 2).

Table 2
Low Dose rhEndostatin Protein Given by Continuous Infusion
Can Generate Equivalent Antitumor Activities at Lower AUCs

Dose (Mg/kg/d)	Route	Mode	T/C	C ng/mL	AUC_{7d} (hr.ng/mL)
20	ip	bolus	0.34	980.63	7011.69
20	ip	ci	0.03	366.54	38,555.36
2	ip	ci	0.32	19.03	2,371.73

We have assessed the absence of drug related adverse effects of rhEndostatin™ protein in non-human primates. In an initial dose range finding study (72) Cynomolgus monkeys were given a single iv bolus of rhEndostatin™ protein at 5, 25, and 100 mg/kg, and observed for five days (Table 3). Monkeys dosed at 5 and 25 mg/kg were normal throughout the study. At the 100 mg/kg dose level, the monkey appeared agitated but returned to normal within 10 min after injection. A subsequent monkey fitted for cardiac telemetry was administered an iv infusion of either formulation vehicle alone or 300 mg/kg rhEndostatin™ protein. There were no adverse effects attributed to rhEndostatin™ protein. Serum drug levels for the monkeys receiving bolus injections of rhEndostatin ranged from 52 to 604 ng/mL on day 2 to 20 to 83 ng/mL on day 4. Serum drug levels in the monkey that received an iv infusion of rhEndostatin at 300 mg/kg ranged from 7180 ng/mL 4 h postinfusion to 62 ng/mL on day 4. There were no significant alterations in hematology or serum chemistry parameters in any monkey treated with rhEndostatin™ protein (72).

We subsequently assessed the safety of a 28-d subchronic iv administration of Endostatin™ protein to Cynomolgus monkeys (83). Doses were derived from the pharmacodynamic assessments in preclinical murine tumor models and the dose range finding studies in primates described above. Male and female monkeys were assigned to 4 treatment groups, comprised of control, formulation vehicle or Endostatin™ protein at 4.5, 150, or 300 mg/m²/d. All doses were administered in an equivalent volume (3.12kg/kg) at an infusion rate of 2 min/min. Physical examinations were performed once weekly and blood samples were collected for hematology, coagulation, chemistry, and serum drug and antibody determination prior to study initiation and on study days 2, 15, and 28. There were no mortalities or unscheduled sacrifices during the course of the study. In addition, there were no adverse clinical observations that were related to the administration of Endostatin™ protein. No Endostatin™ protein-related effects were observed on any of hematology, coagulation or blood chemistry parameters. A slight reversible decrease in total and ionized serum Ca^{2+} 'vas seen in both control and treated monkeys without corresponding alterations in electrocardiogram recording. Anatomic pathology was unremarkable in all monkeys treated with Endostatin™ protein. Circulating levels of Endostatin™ protein were dose-dependent with mean values on day 28 of 226; 8225; and 20,745 ng/mL 20-min postinjection of 4.5, 150 and 300 mg/m²/d, respectively. Serum through level determination of circulating Endostatin™ protein during the course of the study revealed drug accumulation (Fig. 1). Low-titer anti-Endostatin™ protein IgM and IgG antibodies (<1:800) were elicited in 4/20 and 16/20 monkeys respectively (83).

Table 3
Dose Range Finding Study of rhEndostatin in Cynomolgus Monkeys

Dose (mg/kg)	Dose (mg/m2)	Route	Drug-Related Clinical Pathology	Serum Levels (ng/mL)			
				Pre-Dose	4th	2d	4d
5	60	iv bolus	None	12	–	52	20
25	300	iv bolus	None	12	–	169	65
100	1200	iv bolus	None	11	–	604	83
300	3600	1 h infusion	None	–	7180	244	62

A

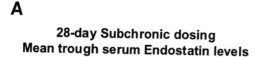

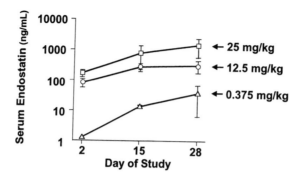

B

28-day Subchronic dosing
Mean post-dose serum Endostatin levels

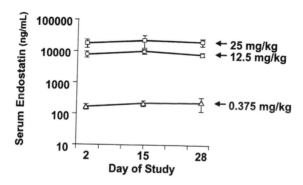

Fig. 1. Drug serum levels in Cynomolgus monkeys treated with Endostatin™ protein for 28 consecutive days. (**A**) Through serum drug levels indicate drug accumulation to levels as high as 1 mg/mL in the 25 mg/kg dose cohort. (**B**) Peak serum levels of Endostatin™ protein, measured at 20 min post dose, reached 20 mg/mL.

The 28-d subchronic administration study was subsequently extended to assess the safety of 90-d chronic iv administration of Endostatin™ protein (*84*). Blood samples were collected for hematology, coagulation, chemistry and serum drug, and antibody determination prior to the study and on study days 1, 15, 29, 57, and 85. There were no mortalities or unscheduled sacrifices during the course of the study. In addition, there were neither adverse clinical observations nor alterations in hematology, coagulation, blood chemistry parameters, or anatomical pathology related to Endostatin™ protein. Circulating levels of Endostatin™ protein were dose-dependent: mean values on day 85 were 462; 15,378; and 19,527 ng/mL 20-min post-injection of 4.5, 150, and 300 mg/m²/d,

A

90-day chronic i.v.
Mean trough serum Endostatin level

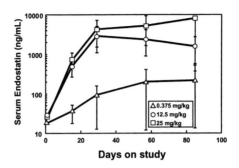

B

90-day chronic i.v.
Mean post-dose serum Endostatin level

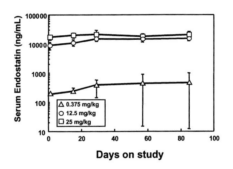

Fig. 2. Drug serum levels in Cynomolgus monkeys treated with Endostatin™ protein for 90 consecutive days. (**A**) Through serum drug levels indicated drug accumulation during the initial 28 d of dosing then reaching and maintaining a dose-dependent plateau. (**B**) Peak serum levels of Endostatin™ protein, measured at 20 min post dose, were dose-dependent.

respectively. Serum through level determination of circulating Endostatin™ protein during the course of the study revealed drug accumulation during the first 28 d of dosing followed by sustained plateau concentrations on days 57 and 85 (Fig. 2). At study day 85, anti-Endostatin™ protein IgM and IgG antibodies were detected in 20/20 and 8/20 monkeys treated with Endostatin™ protein, respectively *(84)*. These data demonstrated that subchronic and chronic daily intravenous administration of Endostatin™ protein to Cynomolgus monkeys is without significant toxicological effects and supported the initiation of Phase I clinical trials.

In conclusion, no toxicity has been observed in any anti-angiogenic or anti-tumor efficacy preclinical study performed to date with Endostatin™ protein. In fact, in our pharmacokinetic studies in monkeys, the peak serum levels achieved were up to 340-fold greater and AUCs about 56-fold higher than the levels that caused inhibition of metastases in mice, with no observed drug related effects seen in the monkeys *(72)*.

Combination Studies with Other Chemotherapeutics

It has been previously shown in vitro that recombinant human Endostatin specifically inhibits endothelial cell proliferation, migration and cord formation and, in vivo, that it exhibits a potent inhibitory effect on angiogenesis and tumor development *(6,19,72)*. More recently, we assessed whether two conventional chemotherapeutics, Adriamycin and Taxol,, modulate the antiangiogenic activity of Endostatin™ protein *(85)*.

When added to cultures of HUVE cells incubated on a reconstituted extracellular (Matrigel) matrix, both compounds potently inhibited the formation of capillary-like cords in a dose-dependent manner. A significant ($P < 0.05$) inhibition of cord formation was observed with concentrations as low as 100 ng/mL of Adriamycin and 10 ng/mL of Taxol (Fig. 3A). The antiangiogenic effects of Adriamycin and Taxol, are not cytotoxicity-dependent, given the high viability of HUVECs upon treatment (at least 90% viable cells at 10 mg/mL, and at least 80% at 100 mg/mL). Thus, when used at low doses, Adriamycin and Taxol are potent, noncytotoxic inhibitors of endothelial cell function *(85)*.

Next we assessed the effect of suboptimal doses (1 and 10 mg/mL) of Endostatin™ protein used in combination with either Adriamycin or Taxol,. HUVECs were incubated with rhEndostatin and increasing doses (0.01, 0.1, and 1 mg/mL) of each chemotherapeutic. Cord formation was subsequently analyzed using the method of Chou and Talalay to determine the synergistic, additive, or antagonistic effects of the two drugs in combination. A synergistic interaction was observed when rhEndostatin was combined with Adriamycin or Taxol® (Fig. 3B,C) *(85)*.

The benefits of combining Endostatin and cytotoxic therapies have been demonstrated in a model of human, high-grade non-Hodgkin lymphoma (NHL). In this model, the sequential administration of rhEndostatin induces tumor stabilization after therapy with cyclophosphamide or with anti-CD20 (rituximab) chimerical antibody. Most importantly, tumor growth was blocked so long as Endostatin was administered *(86)*. B-cell NHL is an angiogenesis-dependent malignancy that is responsive to both cyclophosphamide and rituximab. However, because patients who have achieved remission have a 50% risk of relapse, Endostatin represents a sequential and/or long-term treatment devoid of toxicity *(83,84; see above)* and drug resistance *(42)*. One can hypothesize that sequential administration of chemotherapy and Endostatin would be indicated in patients with bulky disease, whereas the less toxic sequential administration of rituximab and Endostatin would be indicated in patients with limited disease *(86)*. Finally, the observation that cyclophosphamide can be scheduled to provide more sustained apoptosis of vascular endothelial cells within the tumor bed *(87)* indicates that cytotoxic strategies can be designed to potentiate the anti-tumor activity of Endostatin.

Anti-Angiogenic Therapy with rhEndostatin
Does Not Impair Wound Healing

Because oncological patients often undergo extensive surgery, it is critical to determine whether anti-angiogenic therapy could hinder the wound-healing process. Murine preclinical studies, have assessed the effect of subcutaneous administration of endostatin during wound healing by primary intention *(88,89)*. We evaluated the effects of administering Endostatin protein at either 20 mg/kg/dose (once a day for 16 d) or 50 mg/kg/dose (twice a day for 14 d) using a cutaneous tensile strength model. We observed that Endostatin™ proein does not affect either the wound-breaking strength or the vascular

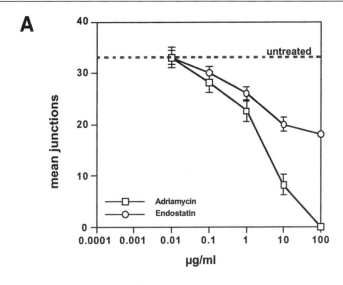

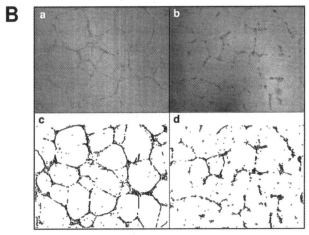

C

Combination	Endo Alone (T/C)	Drug Alone (T/C)	Expected (T/C)	Actual (T/C)	C.I.
Endo 1ug/mL + Adriamycin 0.01ug/mL	0.99	0.73	0.72	0.29	0.05
Endo 1ug/mL + Taxol 0.01ug/mL	0.91	0.67	0.61	0.41	0.12
Endo 1ug/mL + Cyclophosphamide 0.01ug/mL	0.82	0.72	0.59	0.4	0.04

Combination indecies (CI) for combinations of Endostatin with the chemotherapeutics used in this study. Each CI (CI=1-, additive effect; CI>1-, antagonist effect; CI<1, synergistic effect) was determined by the method of Chou and Talalay using JMP statistical software (SAS Institute, Cary, NC).

Fig. 3. Synergistic effects of Endostatin™ protein and conventional chemotherapeutics. (**A**) Adriamycin and Taxol block formation of capillary-like cords by HUVE cells on Matrigel. Endothelial cell viability was never less than 80%. (**B**) Morphological effects of Endostatin™ protein and Taxol on in vitro Angiogenesis. (a) HUVE cells incubated on Matrigel for 16 hr at 370°C under control conditions form a continuous network of cords. (b) Effect of Endostatin (1 mg/mL) and Taxol® (0.01 mg/mL). (a,b) Phase contrast microscopy; (c,d) images (a) and (b), respectively, after image analysis. (**C**) Combination indices (CI) for combinations of Endostatin™ protein with the chemotherapeutics used in this study.

density of PVA sponges implanted at the wound site *(88,89)*, it altered blood vessel morphology in the granulation tissue *(89)*. As to the mechanism involved, Endostatin did not affect the expression of either VEGF, angiopoietin-1, or angiopoietin-2 during the angiogenic phase of wound repair. This indicates that other factors are implicated in the capillary abnormalities seen by Bloch et al. In addition, Endostatin down-regulated the expression of fibronectin and collagen types I and III at the wound site, which resulted in improved scar quality *(89)*.

We can conclude that wound healing is not impaired during endostatin treatment. On the contrary, endogenous Endostatin may play a homeostatic role in wound healing, probably by controlling excessive angiogenesis, thus preventing unnecessary growth of granulation tissue and excessive deposition of connective scar tissue.

Potential Endostatin Indications in Nononcological Angiogenic Diseases

The involvement of Endostatin in relevant non-neoplasic conditions is not limited to the regulation of wound healing. On the contrary, Endostatin plays an important role as a physiological inhibitor of angiogenesis during tissue development and homeostasis. In addition, several angiogenesis-dependent, nononcological diseases have emerged as potential therapeutic indications for Endostatin.

Atherosclerosis

In healthy humans, vassa vasorum in large vessels are restricted to the outer media and to the adventitia. During atherosclerosis, this microvascular network develops, branching out mainly from the adventitia, and invading the intima in at least 40% of atherosclerotic lesions. When apolipoprotein E-deficient hypercholesterolemic mice are treated subcutaneously with recombinant mouse endostatin (20 mg/kg/d for 16 wk), this prevents intimal neovascularization and growth of atherosclerotic plaques, resulting in a plaque growth inhibition of 85%. Endostatin did not alter either serum cholesterol levels or body weight, two risk factors in atherosclerosis *(80)*. This observation corroborates our preclinical safety studies *(72)* and shows that Endostatin prevents atherosclerosis by directly inhibiting angiogenesis. Studies on endothelial cell proliferation have shown that vessels within the atherosclerotic plaque are at different stages of development *(90)*, which indicates that neovascularization is an active process in established atherosclerosis lesions. In addition, the inhibitory effect of endostatin was less pronounced when early lesions devoid of intimal neovascularization (rather than older, already vascularized lesions) were treated *(80)*. Thus, endostatin is a safe candidate for the prevention and treatment of atherosclerosis as well as for the prevention of its main complications, myocardial infarction and ischemic stroke.

Rheumatoid Arthritis

Angiogenesis is an essential process in rheumatoid arthritis *(91)*. Pathologically, RA is characterized by chronic inflammatory changes such as pilling up and villous proliferation of synovial lining cells and neovascularization of the synovial stromal tissue *(91)*. In the serum and joint fluid of patients with rheumatoid arthritis, the ratio of VEGF to endostatin levels is significantly increased, while serum levels of endostatin correlate with the rate of C-reactive protein and erythrocyte sedimentation, both of which are markers of inflammation and clinical activity in Rheumatoid Arthritis. Interestingly, treatment with prednisolone and either bucillamine or salazosulfapyridine, two disease modifying antirheumatic drugs, decreased VEGF levels and increased endostatin levels in peripheral blood *(92)*. This important observation indicates that endostatin is a protective factor against chronic arthritis and a potential therapeutic approach to rheumatoid arthritis.

New Hope for Macular Degeneration?

As discussed previously, choroidal neovascularization of the retina is a condition responsible for vision loss in macular degeneration. Recent studies have shown both that collagen XVIII-null mice have little or no circulating levels of endostatin-like fragments, and that they suffer from developmental eye defects. Because of a lack of endothelial cell apoptosis, hyaloid vessels in the vitreous fail to regress shortly after birth, leading to the postnatal persistence of some blood vessels in the vitreous, and to incomplete development of the retinal vessel plexus (N. Fukai and B. Olsen, personal communication). This phenotype closely resembles some features of Knobloch syndrome, an autosomal recessive human condition caused by a splice site mutation affecting the short form of collagen XVIII that involves, among other defects, high myopia, macular abnormalities, and vitroretinal degeneration *(93)*. These findings demonstrate that endostatin plays a physiological role during retinal vascular remodeling, and that it may be a new treatment of macular degeneration and other angiogenesis-dependent ophthalmologic diseases.

Clinical Evaluation of rhEndostatin

Toxicology studies in monkeys evaluating the pharmacokinetic profile, as well as acute and chronic effects of a continuous administration of recombinant rhEndostatin for 90 d demonstrate a total absence of toxicity *(72,84)*. Multi centered Phase I trials in patients with refractory solid malignancies have been initiated. The primary goal of these Phase I studies was to determine safety, toxicity and the pharmacokinetics of rhEndostatin. Dose levels evaluated ranged from 15 mg/m^2 to 600 mg/m^2 administered daily as an IV bolus, as well as studies of lower doses (3.75 mg/m^2 to 15 mg/m^2) administered subcutaneously or as a continuous infusion. Other correlative investigations performed in these Phase I studies include noninvasive imaging techniques such as perfusion magnetic resonance imaging as a noninvasive measure of tumor blood flow, Doppler Ultrasound, dynamic CT, also evaluation of surrogate serum markers, tumor biopsies for vessel densities and endothelial cell activities, and sequential skin biopsies for effects on wound healing. To date, there are no surrogate markers that predict efficacy in any anti-angiogenesis clinical trials, it was important to ask if these extensive correlative studies could perhaps yield correlates that could be used to guide other anti-angiogenesis trials in general. In the following paragraphs, the results of these on-going Phase I studies are discussed together as a summary of results reported at recent meetings *(94–101)*.

It is clear that the Phase studies show the unequivocal safety of rhEndostatin in the treatment of clinical patients. Pharmacokinetics (AUC and C_{max}) was shown to be linear at all doses studied, and were comparable to the equivalent levels obtained in preclinical models of tumor inhibition. T1/2 of elimination is approximately 11 hr, mean values ($\pm$ SEM) of volume of distribution and total body clearance were 336.9 ± 48.7 l/m^2 and 22.9 ± 3.9 $l/h/m^2$ respectively *(101)*. Urine levels of βFGF and VEGF showed a dose dependent decline from baseline values for doses greater than 60 mg/m^2 generating a decrease in 8 of 9 patients analyzed *(98)*. O15 PET and dynamic CT measuring blood flow at 56 d showed a statistically significant decrease in blood flow versus dose ($p = 0.009$

and $p = 0.03$ respectively). Analysis of biopsy specimens for CD31 and TUNEL demonstrate an increase in endothelial cell apoptosis in 3 of 6 patients examined at dose levels from 120 –300 mg/m^2 *(99).*

Prolonged stable disease and even radiographic regression of advanced, refractory, metastatic disease has been demonstrated in patients receiving rhEndostatin. Of interest is the fact that in sequential skin biopsies performed on patients treated with rhEndostatin, skin wounds did not show a decrease in vascularity (Ki67 positive/CD31 positive), endothelial cell proliferative index nor apoptotic index at dose levels up to 300 mg/m^2 *(100).* These studies pave the way for Phase II trials and will allow delineation of our Phase II trial designs.

ACKNOWLEDGEMENTS

We thank Drs. Edward R. Gubish, Anne Fortier, William Fogler and Barbara Nelson, Mr. Art Hanson, Ms. Sauda Ayub and all the team of Entremed for their outstanding work.

REFERENCES

1. Ferrara, N., Clapp, C., and Weiner, R. (1991) The 16K fragment of prolactin specifically inhibits basal or fibroblast growth factor stimulated growth of capillary endothelial cells. *Endocrinology* **129,** 896–900.
2. Clapp, C., Martial, J. A., Guzman, R. C., Rentier-Delure, F., and Weiner, R. I. (1993). The 16-kilodalton N-terminal fragment of human prolactin is a potent inhibitor of angiogenesis. *Endocrinology* **133,** 1292–1299.
3. Homandberg, G. A, Williams, J. E., Grant, D., Schumacher, B., and Eisenstein, R. (1985) Heparin-binding fragments of fibronectin are potent inhibitors of endothelial cell growth. *Am J Pathol.* **120,** 327–332.
4. Gupta, S. K, Hassel, T., and Singh, J. P. (1995) A potent inhibitor of endothelial cell proliferation is generated by proteolytic cleavage of the chemokine platelet factor 4. *Proc. Natl. Acad. Sci. USA* **92,** 7799–7803.
5. O'Reilly, M. S, Holmgren, L., Shing, Y., Chen, C., Rosenthal, R. A., Moses, M., Lane, W. S., Cao, Y., Sage, E. H., and Folkman, J. (1994) Angiostatin: a novel angiogenesis inhibitor that mediates the suppression of metastases by a Lewis lung carcinoma. *Cell* **79,** 315–328.
6. O'Reilly, M. S., Boehm, T., Shing, Y., Fukai, N., Vasios, G., Lane, W. S., Flynn, E., Birkhead, J. R., Olsen, B. R., Folkman, J. (1997) Endostatin: an endogenous inhibitor of angiogenesis and tumor growth. *Cell* **88,** 277–285.
7. O'Reilly, M. S., Pirie-Shepherd, S., Lane, W. S., and Folkman, J. (1999) Antiangiogenic activity of the cleaved conformation of the serpin antithrombin. *Science* **285,** 1926–1928.
8. Pepper, M. S., Ferrara, N., Orci, L., and Montesano, R. (1991) Vascular endothelial growth factor (VEGF) induces plasminogen activators and plasminogen activator inhibitor-1 in microvascular endothelial cells. *Biochem. Biophys. Res. Commun.* **181,** 902–906.
9. Unemori, E. N., Ferrara, N., Bauer, E. A., Amento, E. P. (1992) Vascular endothelial growth factor induces interstitial collagenase expression in human endothelial cells. *J. Cell. Physiol.* **153,** 557–562.
10. Ferrara, N., and Davis-Smyth, T. (1997) The biology of vascular endothelial growth factor. *Endocr. Rev.* **18,** 4–25.
11. Dong, Z., Kumar, R., Yang, X., and Fidler, I. J. (1997) Macrophage-derived metalloelastase is responsible for the generation of angiostatin in Lewis lung carcinoma. *Cell* **88,** 801–810.
12. Gately, S., Twardowski, P., Stack, M. S., Patrick, M., Boggio, L., Cundiff, D. L., Schnaper, H. W., Madison, L., Volpert, O., Bouck, N., Enghild, J., Kwaan, H. C., and Soff, G. A. (1996) Human prostate carcinoma cells express enzymatic activity that converts human plasminogen to the angiogenesis inhibitor, angiostatin. *Cancer Res.* **56,** 4887–4890.
13. Saksela, O. (1985) Plasminogen activation and regulation of pericellular proteolysis. *Biochim. Biophys Acta.* **823,** 35–65.
14. Ponting, C. P., Marshall, J. M., and Cederholm-Williams, S. A. (1992) Plasminogen: a structural review. *Blood Coagul. Fibrinolysis.* **5,** 605–614.

15. Sim, B. K., O'Reilly, M. S., Liang, H., Fortier, A. H., He, W., Madsen, J. W., Lapcevich, R., Nacy, C. A. (1997) A recombinant human angiostatin protein inhibits experimental primary and metastatic cancer. *Cancer Res*. **57,** 1329–1334.

16. Cao, Y. (1998) Endogenous angiogenesis inhibitors: angiostatin, endostatin, and other proteolytic fragments. *Prog. Mol. Subcell. Biol*. 20, 161–1761. O'Reilly, M. S., Pirie-Shepherd, S., Lane, W. S., and Folkman, J. (1999) Antiangiogenic activity of the cleaved conformation of the serpin antithrombin. *Science*. **285,** 1926–1928.

17. Sim, B. K. L. (1998a) Angiostatin protein and other plasminogen fragments. In: B. A. Teicher (ed.) Antiangiogenic Agents in Cancer Theraphy, vol. 14 pp. 225–236. Humana, Totowa, NJ.

18. Sim, B. K. L. (1998b) Angiostatin and Endostatin : endothelial cell-specific endogenous inhibitors of angiogenesis and tumor growth. *Angiogenesis* **2,** 37–48.

19. Sim, B. K. L., MacDonald, N. J., and Gubish, E. R. (2000) Angiostatin and Endostatin: Endogenous inhibitors of tumor growth. *Cancer and Metastasis Reviews* **19,** 181–190.

20. Soff, G. A. (2000) Angiostatin and angiostatin-related proteins. *Cancer Metastasis Rev*. **19,** 97–107.

21. Stathakis, P., Fitzgerald, M., Matthias, L. J., Chesterman, C. N., and Hogg, P. J. (1997) Generation of angiostatin by reduction and proteolysis of plasmin. Catalysis by a plasmin reductase secreted by cultured cells. *J. Biol. Chem*. **272,** 20,641–20,645.

22. Stathakis, P., Lay, A. J., Fitzgerald, M., Schlieker, C., Matthias, L. J., and Hogg, P. J. (1999) Angiostatin formation involves disulfide bond reduction and proteolysis in kringle 5 of plasmin. *J. Biol. Chem*. **274,** 8910–8016.

23. Hajjar, K. A. (1991) The endothelial cell tissue plasminogen activator receptor. Specific interaction with plasminogen. *J. Biol. Chem*. **266,** 21,962–21,970.

24. Cesarman, G. M., Guevara, C. A, and Hajjar, K. A. (1994) An endothelial cell receptor for plasminogen/tissue plasminogen activator (t-PA). II. Annexin II-mediated enhancement of t-PA-dependent plasminogen activation. *J. Biol. Chem*. **269,** 21,198–21,203.

25. Holmgren, L., O'Reilly, M. S., and Folkman, J. (1995) Dormancy of micrometastases: balanced proliferation and apoptosis in the presence of angiogenesis suppression. *Nat. Med*. **2,** 149–153.

26. Claesson-Welsh, L., Welsh, M., Ito, N., Anand-Apte, B., Soker, S., Zetter, B., O'Reilly, M., and Folkman, J. (1998) Angiostatin induces endothelial cell apoptosis and activation of focal adhesion kinase independently of the integrin-binding motif RGD. *Proc. Natl. Acad. Sci. USA* 95, 5579–5583.

27. Lucas, R., Holmgren, L., Garcia, I., Jimenez, B., Mandriota, S. J., Borlat, F., Sim, B. K., Wu, Z., Grau, G. E., Shing, Y., Soff, G. A., Bouck, N., and Pepper, M. S. (1998) Multiple forms of angiostatin induce apoptosis in endothelial cells. *Blood* **92,** 4730–4741.

28. Luo, J., Lin, J., Paranya, G., and Bischoff, J. (1998) Angiostatin upregulates E-selectin in proliferating endothelial cells. *Biochem. Biophys. Res. Commun*. **245,** 906–911.

29. Griscelli, F., Li, H., Bennaceur-Griscelli, A., Soria, J., Opolon, P., Soria, C., Perricaudet, M., Yeh, P., and Lu, H. (1998) Angiostatin gene transfer: inhibition of tumor growth in vivo by blockage of endothelial cell proliferation associated with a mitosis arrest. *Proc. Natl. Acad. Sci. USA* **95,** 6367–6372.

30. Redlitz, A., Daum, G., Sage, E. H. (1999) Angiostatin diminishes activation of the mitogen-activated protein kinases ERK-1 and ERK-2 in human dermal microvascular endothelial cells. *J. Vasc. Res* **36,** 28–34.

31. Moser, T. L., Stack, M. S., Asplin, I., Enghild, J. J., Hojrup, P., Everitt, L., Hubchak, S., Schnaper, H. W., and Pizzo, S. V. (1999) Angiostatin binds ATP synthase on the surface of human endothelial cells. *Proc. Natl. Acad. Sci. USA* 96, 2811–2816.

32. Gillies, R. J. (1999). Angiostatin's partners. *Science*. **284,** 434.1.

33. Troyanovsky, B., Levchenko, T., Mansson, G., Matvijenko, O., and Holmgren, L. (2001) Angiomotin. An angiostatin binding protein that regulates endothelial cell migration and tube formation. *J. Cell Biol*. **152,** 1247–1254.

34. Fogler, W. E., Grella, D., Liang, H., Plum, S., Chang, A., Lu, M., Fortier, A., Trail, P., Lewin, A., and Sim, B. K. L. (1999). Recombinant human Angiostatin™: Dose-dependent inhibition of early and late stage established metastasis in mice. *Proc. Am. Assoc. Cancer Res*. **40,** .

35. Fogler, W. H., Fortier, A. H., Hassler, C. R., Tuner, N., and Sim, B. K. L. (2000) Range finding toxicity studies of recombinant human Angiostatin™ in Cynomolgus monkeys. *Proc. Am. Assoc. Cancer Res*. **41,** #2083.

36. Molema, G., van Veen-Hof, I., van Loenen-Weemaes, A. M., Proost, J. H., de Leij, L. F., and Meijer, D. K.(2001) Pharmacokinetics and whole body distribution of elastase derived angiostatin (K1-3) in rats. *Int. J. Cancer*. **91,** 1–7.

37. Sigma Catalog of Biochemicals and reagents for life science research (2001) Cat. No.: P1667, p. 808.

38. Harris, A. L. (1998) Anti-angiogenesis therapy and strategies for integrating it with adjuvant therapy. *Recent Results Cancer Res.* **152**, 341–352.

39. Gasparini, G. (1999) The rationale and future potential of angiogenesis inhibitors in neoplasia. *Drugs* **58**, 17–38.

40. Griffioen, A. W., and Molema, G. (2000) Angiogenesis: potentials for pharmacologic intervention in the treatment of cancer, cardiovascular diseases, and chronic inflammation. *Pharmacol Rev.* **52**, 237–268.

41. O'Reilly, M. S., Holmgren, L., Chen, C., and Folkman, J. (1996) Angiostatin induces and sustains dormancy of human primary tumors in mice. *Nat Med.* **2**, 689–692.

42. Boehm, T., Folkman, J., Browder, T., and O'Reilly, M. S. (1997) Antiangiogenic therapy of experimental cancer does not induce acquired drug resistance. *Nature* **390**, 404–407.

43. Mauceri, H. J., Hanna, N. N., Beckett, M. A., et al. (1998) Combined effects of angiostatin and ionizing radiation in anti-tumor therapy. *Nature* 394, 287–291.

44. Gorski, D. H., Mauceri, H. J., Salloum, R. M., Gately, S., Hellman, S., Beckett, M. A., Sukhatme, V. P., Soff, G. A., Kufe, D. W., and Weichselbaum, R. R. (1998) Potentiation of the anti-tumor effect of ionizing radiation by brief concomitant exposures to angiostatin. *Cancer Res.* **58**, 5686–5689.

45. Griscelli, F., Li, H., Cheong, C., Opolon, P., Bennaceur-Griscelli, A., Vassal, G., Soria, J., Soria, C., Lu, H., Perricaudet, M., and Yeh, P. (2000) Combined effects of radiotherapy and angiostatin gene therapy in glioma tumor model. *Proc Natl. Acad. Sci USA* **97**, 6698–6703.

46. Hari, D., Beckett, M. A., Sukhatme, V. P., Dhanabal, M., Nodzenski, E., Lu, H., Mauceri, H. J., Kufe, D. W., and Weichselbaum, R. R. (2000) Angiostatin induces mitotic cell death of proliferating endothelial cells. *Mol. Cell. Biol. Res. Commun.* **3**, 277–282.

47. Denekamp, J. (1982) Endothelial cell proliferation as a novel approach to targeting tumour therapy. *Br. J. Cancer* **45**, 136–139.

48. Kerbel, R. S. (1991) Inhibition of tumor angiogenesis as a strategy to circumvent acquired resistance to anticancer therapeutic agents. *Bioessays* **13**, 31–36.

49. Bergers, G., Javaherian, K., Lo, K.-M., Folkman, J., and Hanahan, D. (1999) Effects of angiogenesis inhibitors on multistage carcinogenesis in mice. *Science* **284**, 808–812.

50. Black, P. M. Brain tumor. Part 2. (1991) *N. Engl. J. Med.* **324**, 1555–1564.

51. Renno, R. Z., Delori, F. C., Holzer, R. A., Gragoudas, E. S., and Miller, J. W. (2000) Photodynamic therapy using Lu-Tex induces apoptosis In vitro, and its effect is potentiated by angiostatin in retinal capillary endothelial cells. *Invest. Ophthalmol. Vis. Sci.* **41**, 3963–3971.

52. Oleinick, N. and Evans, H. (1998) The photobiology of photodynamic therapy: Cellular targets and mechanisms. *Radiat. Res.* **150**, S146– S156.

53. Spranger, J., Hammes, H. P., Preissner, K. T., Schatz, H., and Pfeiffer, A. F. (2000) Release of the angiogenesis inhibitor angiostatin in patients with proliferative diabetic retinopathy: association with retinal photocoagulation. *Diabetologia* **43**, 1404–1407.

54. De Moraes, E. D., Fogler, W. E., Grant, D., et al. (2001). Recombinant human angiostatin (rhA): A phase I clinical trial assessing safety, pharmacokinetics (PK) and pharmacodynamics (PD). *Proc. Am. Soc. Clin. Oncol.* 20, (In press).

55. Oh, S. P., Warman, M. L., Seldin, M. F., Cheng, S. D., Knoll, J. H., Timmons, S., and Olsen, B. R. (1994) Cloning of cDNA and genomic DNA encoding human type XVIII collagen and localization of the alpha (XVIII) collagen gene to mouse chromosome 10 and human chromosome 21. *Genomics* **19**, 494–499.

56. Rehn, M., Hintikka, E., and Pihlajaniemi, T. (1994) Primary structure of the alpha 1 chain of mouse type XVIII collagen, partial structure of the corresponding gene, and comparison of the alpha 1(XVIII) chain with its homologue, the alpha 1(XV) collagen chain. *J. Biol. Chem.* **269**, 13,929–13,935.

57. Muragaki, Y., Timmons, S., Griffith, C. M., Oh, S. P., Fadel, B., Quertermous, T., and Olsen, B. R. (1995) Mouse Col18a1 is expressed in a tissue-specific manner as three alternative variants and is localized in basement membrane zones. *Proc. Natl. Acad. Sci. USA* **92**, 8763–8767.

58. Halfter, W., Dong, S., Schurer, B., and Cole, G. J. (1998) Collagen XVIII is a basement membrane heparan sulfate proteoglycan. *J. Biol. Chem.* **273**, 25,404–25,412.

59. Saarela, J., Ylikarppa, R., Rehn, M., Purmonen, S., and Pihlajaniemi, T.(1998) Complete primary structure of two variant forms of human type XVIII collagen and tissue-specific differences in the expression of the corresponding transcripts. *Matrix Biol.* **16**, 319–328.

60. Sasaki, T., Fukai, N., Mann, K, Gohring, W., Olsen, B. R., and Timpl, R. (1998) Structure, function and tissue forms of the C-terminal globular domain of collagen XVIII containing the angiogenesis inhibitor endostatin. *EMBO J.* **17**, 4249–4256.

61. Miosge, N., Sasaki, T., and Timpl, R. (1999) Angiogenesis inhibitor endostatin is a distinct component of elastic fibers in vessel walls. *FASEB J.* **13**, 1743–1750.

62. Sasaki, T., Larsson, H., Tisi, D., Claesson-Welsh, L., Hohenester, E., and Timpl, R. (2000) Endostatins derived from collagens XV and XVIII differ in structural and binding properties, tissue distribution and anti-angiogenic activity. *J. Mol. Biol.* **301,** 1179–1190.

63. Felbor, U., Dreier, L., Bryant, R. A., Ploegh, H. L., Olsen, B. R., Mothes, W. (2000) Secreted cathepsin L generates endostatin from collagen IVIII. *EMBO J.* **301,** 1179–1190.

64. Wen, W., Moses, M. A., Wiederschain, D., Arbiser, J. L., and Folkman, J. (1999) The generatin of endostatin is mediated by elastase. *Cancer Res.* **59,** 6052–6056.

65. Ferreras, M., Felbor, U., Lenhard, T., Olsen, B. R., and Delaisse, J.-M. (2000) Generation and degradation of human endostatin protein by various proteinases. *FEBS Lett.* **486,** 247–251.

66. Standker, L., Schrader, M., Kanse, S. M., Jurgens, M., Forssmann, W. G., and Preissner, K. T. (1997) Isolation and characterization of the circulating form of human endostatin. *FEBS Lett.* **420,** 129–133.

67. John, H., Preissner, K. T., Forssmann, W. G., and Standker, L. (1999) Novel glycosylated forms of human plasma endostatin and circulating endostatin-related fragments of collagen XV. *Biochemistry* **38,** 10,217–10,224.

68. Ding, Y. H., Javaherian, K., Lo, K. M., Chopra, R., Boehm, T., Lanciotti, J., et al. (1998) Zinc-dependent dimers observed in crystals of human endostatin. *Proc. Natl. Acad. Sci. USA* **95,** 10,443–10,448.

69. Hohenester, E., Sasaki, T., Olsen, B. R., and Timpl, R. (1998) Crystal structure of the angiogenesis inhibitor endostatin at 1.5 A resolution. *EMBO J.* **17,** 1656–1664.

70. Hohensester, E., Sasaki, T., Mann, K., and Templ. T., (2000) Variable zinc coordination inendostatin. *J. Mol. Biol.* **297,** 1–6.

71. Yamaguchi, N., Anand-Anand-Apte, B., Lee, M., Sasaki, T., Fukai, N., Shapiro, R., et al. (1999) Endostatin inhibits VEGF-induced endothelial cell migration and tumor growth independently of zinc binding *EMBO J.* **18,** 4414–4423.

72. Sim, B. K. L., Fogler, W. E., Zhou, X., Liang, H., Madsen, J. W., Luu, K. (1999) Zinc ligand-disrupted recombinant human endostatin: Potent inhibition of tumor growth, safety and pharmacokinetic profile. *Angiogenesis* **3,** 41–51.

73. MacDonald, N. J., Shivers, W. Y., Narum, D. L. Plum, S. M., Wingard, J. N., Fuhrmann, S. R., et al. (2001) Endostatin binds tropomyosin: A potential modulator of the anti-tumor activity of Endostatin. (Submitted).

74. French, F., Pryor, K. C., and Penny, R. (1990) Antibodies to the cytoskeleton proteins tubulin, actin and tropomyosin bind to the surface of human capillary endothelial cells and human lung fibroblasts. *J. Cell Biochem. Suppl.* 14, part A, #B311.

75. Rehn, M., Veikkola, T., Kukk-Valdre, E., Nakamura, H., Ilmonen, M., Lombardo, C. R., et al. (2001) Interaction of endostatin with integrins implicated in angiogenesis. *Pro. Natl. Acad. Sci. USA* **98,** 1024–1029.

76. Boehm, T., O'Reilly, M. S., Koeugh, K., Shiloach, J., Sharpiro, R., and Folkman, J. (1998) Zinc-binding of endostatin is essential for its antiangiogenic activity. *Biochem. Biophys. Res. Commu.* **252,** 190–194.

77. Sasaki, T., Larsson, H., Kreuger, J., et al. (1999) Structural basis and potential role of heparin/heparan sulfate binding to the angiogenesis ihnibitor endostatin. *EMBO J.* **18,** 6240–6248.

78. Chang, Z., Choon, A., and Friedl, A. (1999) Endostatin binds to blood vessels in situ independent of heparan sulfate and does not compete for fibroblast growth factor-2 binding. *Am. J. Pathol.* **155,** 71–76.

79. Dixelius, J., Larsson, H., Sasaki, T., Holmqvist, K., Lu, L., Engstrom, A., Timpl, R., Welsh, M., and Claesson-Welsh, L. (2000) Endostatin-induced tyrosine kinase signaling through the Shb adaptor protein regulates endothelial cell apoptosis. *Blood* **95,** 3403–3411.

80. Moulton, K. S, Heller, E., Konerding, M. A., Flynn, E., Palinski, W., and Folkman, J. (1999) Angiogenesis inhibitors endostatin or TNP-470 reduce intimal neovascularization and plaque growth in apolipoprotein E-deficient mice. *Circulation* **99,** 1726–1732.

81. Yang, D. J., Herbst, R., Fogler, W. E., Abbruzzese, J., Azhadarinia, A., Mullani, N. A., Kalimi, S. K., Kim, E. E., and Podoloff, D. A. (2001) Targeted angiogenesis tumor vascular imaging with radiolabeled Endostatin. *J. Nucl. Med.* **41,** (In press).

82. Kisker, O., Becker, C. M., Fannon, M., D'Amato, R., Fogler, W. E., Pirie-Shepherd, S. R., and Folkman, J. (2000) continuous administration improves efficacy of Endostatin therapy in mice. 11th NCI-EORTC-AACR symposium on new drugs in cancer therapy, #577.

83. Fortier, A. H., Fogler, W. H., Tomaszewski, J. E., et al. (1999) Recombinant human Endostatin™ protein in Cynomolgus monkeys produces no toxicological effects following i.v. administration for 28 consecutive days. *Clin. Cancer Res.* **5,** 3813s.

84. Fortier, A. H., Fogler, W. E., Ruiz, A., Kough, E., and Sim, B. K. L. (2000) Recombinant human Endostatin™ in Cynomolgus monkeys produces no toxicological effects following i.v. administration for 90 consecutive days. *Proc. 25th Congress Eur. Soc. Med. Oncol.* **75P**.

85. Hanson, A. D., Plum, S. M., Vu, H. A., Nelson, B. J., and Fortier, A. H. (2000) Synergistic effects of rhEndostatin and conventional Chemotherapeutics *In vitro*. *Proc. Am. Assoc. Cancer Res.* #3928.

86. Bertolini, F., Fusetti, L., Mancuso, P., Gobbi, A., Corsini, C., Ferrucci, P. F., Martinelli, G., and Pruneri, G. (2000) Endostatin, an antiangiogenic drug, induces tumor stabilization after chemotherapy or anti-CD20 therapy in a NOD/SCID mouse model of human high-grade non-Hodgkin lymphoma. *Blood* **96**, 282–287.

87. Browder, T., Butterfield, C. E, Kraling, B. M., Shi, B., Marshall, B., O'Reilly, M. S., and Folkman, J. (2000) Antiangiogenic scheduling of chemotherapy improves efficacy against experimental drug-resistant cancer. *Cancer Res.* **60**, 1878–1886.

88. Berger, A. C., Feldman, A. L., Gnant, M. F., et al. (2000) The angiogenesis inhibitor, endostatin, does not affect murine cutaneous wound healing. *J. Surg. Res.* **91**, 26–31.

89. Bloch, W., Huggel, K., Sasaki, T., Grose, R., Bugnon, P., Addicks, K., Timpl, R., and Werner, S. (2000) The angiogenesis inhibitor endostatin impairs blood vessel maturation during wound healing. *FASEB J.* **14**, 2373–2376.

90. O'Brien, E. R., Garvin, M. R., Dev, R., Stewart, D. K., Hinohara, T., Simpson, J. B., and Schwartz, S. M. (1994) Angiogenesis in human coronary atherosclerotic plaques. *Am. J. Pathol.* **145**, 883–894.

91. Koch, A. E. (1998) Review: angiogenesis: implications for rheumatoid arthritis. *Arthritis Rheum.* **41**, 951–962.

92. Nagashima, M., Asano, G., and, Yoshino, S. (2000) Imbalance in production between vascular endothelial growth factor and endostatin in patients with rheumatoid arthritis. *J. Rheumatol.* **27**, 2339–2342.

93. Sertie, A. L., Sossi, V., Camargo, A. A., Zatz, M., Brahe, C., Passos-Bueno, M. R. (2000) Collagen XVIII, containing an endogenous inhibitor of angiogenesis and tumor growth, plays a critical role in the maintenance of retinal structure and in neural tube closure (Knobloch syndrome). *Hum. Mol. Genet.* **9**, 2051–2058.

94. Eder, J. P., Clark, J. W. Supko, J. G., et al.(2000) Recombinant human Endostatin demonstrates safety, linear pharmacokinetics and biological effects on tumor growth factors : Results of a phase I clinical trial. 11th NCI-EORTC-AACR symposium on new drugs in cancer therapy, #258.

95. Herbst, R., Tran, H., Hess, K., et al. (2000). A phase I clinical trial of recombinant human Endostatin (rHE) in patients (PTS) with solid tumors: Pharmacokinetic (PK), safety and efficacy analysis. 11th NCI-EORTC-AACR symposium on new drugs in cancer therapy, #259.

96. Herbst, R., Hess, K., Mullani, N. A, et al. (2000). A phase I clinical trial of recombinant human Endostatin (rHE) in patients (PTS) with solid tumors: Surrogate analysis to determine a biologically effective dose (BED). 11th NCI-EORTC-AACR symposium on new drugs in cancer therapy, #578.

97. Thomas, J. P., Schiller, J., Lee, F., Perlman, S., Friedl, A., Winter, T., et al. (2000). A phase I pharmacokinetic and pharmacodynamic study of recombinant human Endostatin. 11th NCI-EORTC-AACR symposium on new drugs in cancer therapy, #260.

98. Eder, J. P., Clark, J. W. Supko, J. G., Shulman, L. N., Garcia-Carbonero, R., Roper, K., Proper, J., Keogan, M., Kinchla, N. M., Schnipper, L. S. Connors, S., Butterfield, C., Fogler, W., Xu, G., Puchalski, T. A., Janicek, M. J., Gubish, E., Soker, S., Folkman, J., and Kufe, D. W. (2001) Phase I pharmacokinetic and pharmacodynamic trial of recombinant human Endostatin. *Proc. Am. Soc. Clin. Oncol.* **20**, (In press).

99. Herbst, R., Tran, H., Mullani, N. A, Chamsangavej, Hess, K., Davis, D., et al. (2001) A phase I clinical trial of recombinant human Endostatin (rHE) in patients (PTS) with solid tumors: Pharmacokinetic (PK), Safety and efficacy analysis using surrogate endpoints of tissue and radiologic response. *Proc. Am. Soc. Clin. Oncol.* **20**, (In press).

100. Mundhenke, C., Thomas, J. P., Neider, R., Sebree, L. A., Wilding, G., and Friedl, A. (2001) Endothelial cell kinetics in skin wounds and tumors of patients receiving Endostatin. *Proc. Am. Soc. Clin. Oncol.* **20**, (In press).

101. Fogler, W. E., Song, M., Supko, J. G., Eder, J. P., Kufe, D. W., Tran, H. T., Madden, T., Herbst, R., Abbruzzese, J. L., Tutsch, K., Thomas, J. P., Wilding, G. Pluda, J., and Gubish, E. (2001) recombinant human Endostatin demonstrates consistent and predictable pharmacokinetics following intravenous bolus administration to cancer patients. *Proc. Am. Soc. Clin. Oncol.* **20**, (In press).

Index